Atlas of Adult Autopsy

S. Kim Suvarna (represented by Grace Horne)
Abigail K. Sharp
Editors

Atlas of Adult Autopsy

A Guide to Modern Practice

Second Edition 2024

Springer

Editors
S. Kim Suvarna (*deceased*) (represented by Grace Horne)
Department of Histopathology
Royal Hallamshire Hospital, Sheffield Teaching Hospitals
Sheffield, South Yorkshire, UK

Abigail K. Sharp
Department of Histopathology
Royal Hallamshire Hospital, Sheffield Teaching Hospitals
Sheffield, South Yorkshire, UK

ISBN 978-3-031-72209-7 ISBN 978-3-031-72207-3 (eBook)
https://doi.org/10.1007/978-3-031-72207-3

This Springer imprint is published by the registered company Springer Nature Switzerland AG
The registered company address is: Gewerbestrasse 11, 6330 Cham, Switzerland

Dr. Abigail K. Sharp—To Tom, Dad, Jo, and Chrissy, my biggest cheerleaders.
Prof. S. Kim Suvarna—To Seonaid, Maxine, and Grace, for all their support.

In Memoriam

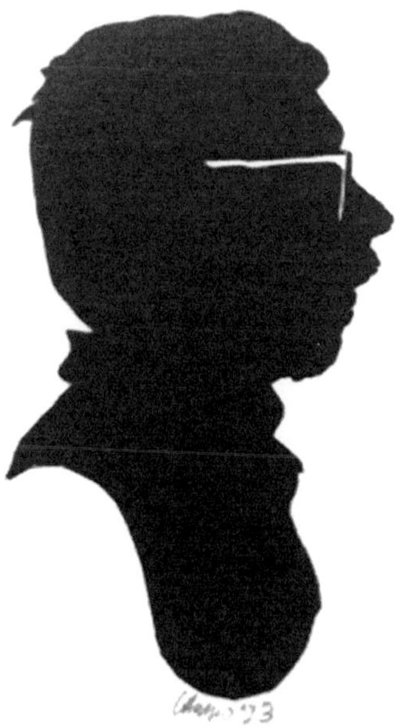

Lauren Muney—silhouette artist

Professor S. Kim Suvarna
1960–2024
Professor Suvarna was diagnosed with an incurable malignancy whilst in the early stages of working on this second edition. He continued to work on this book until a few weeks before his death in January 2024 because he believed it to be a valuable contribution to the literature on autopsy, particularly as a guide for those learning evisceration and dissection techniques.

Preface

The autopsy, and indeed the training in this area of medical practice, for me has always been a particular area of interest. This aspect of pathology straddles consent and medicolegal autopsy practice and has been a bedrock of understanding disease for the past few centuries. Unlike virtually every other aspect of medical practice, it remains like that performed historically (certainly over the last 100 or more years).

Despite this, it is clear that the classic dissection-style autopsy is in decline. This decline reflects advances in antemortem special tests (blood work, surgical biopsies, radiological techniques, etc.) that provide an improved insight into internal pathology than previously existed. Another factor has been the objections from some religious groups and the public disquiet about the practice of a few pathologists who have created a scandal at some centres, with the result that a number of 'consented' autopsies, relying on permission from relatives, have fallen. Contrastingly, and certainly in the UK, the medicolegal autopsy has continued to be used widely.

It is still considered to have a vital place in terms of the evaluation of disease and can highlight undeclared pathologies. The autopsy also has a role in teaching pathologists and students of medicine, providing access to tissues for research, helping with medicolegal queries and in validating antemortem tests.

What has changed in the past century is that the macroscopic autopsy is now assisted by a variety of special tests. Furthermore, the autopsy can be augmented not only by the standard of microscopy but also by immunohistochemistry, microbiology (for bacteria, fungi, viruses, and other organisms), serological studies, genetic studies, and mass spectroscopy to name but a few of the available tests, and all can be recorded by photography.

However, it could be argued that the autopsy is at a crossroads currently. Alongside the better understanding of disease, driven by molecular antemortem tests and modern imaging, there is a view that the 'gold standard' invasive autopsy may be less relevant. Certainly, digital autopsy techniques, especially CT radiology, are now coming into play, and diminishing the need for invasive studies.

If the autopsy is in decline, then the opportunity to learn by seeing and doing will diminish and pathologists are coming to active practice with far less experience than previous trainees enjoyed. In an arena where competence is recognized to be experience-driven, this could be a problem. The aim of this book is therefore to provide a training standard of the protocol for an autopsy in the form of a manual of current practice. The atlas layout hopes to provide insight into the pathological lesions that may be found at autopsy to aid in case examination. It attempts to deal with the various aspects of the autopsy in terms of grouped areas for dissection and special investigations. It also endeavours to cover the basics of forensic pathology, the radiological autopsy, histology, and toxicology. It is hoped that it will support students and provide trained practitioners with a ready reference. It is primarily aimed at practising pathologists, particularly in training grades. It may have value to those working as anatomical technicians in autopsy suites, as well as parties with a legal interest in autopsy practice. I would hope this atlas will be a helpful resource for those approaching the practical examination of autopsy practice assessment in the UK and the equivalent further afield.

The images and data in a book of this size cannot be all-encompassing, but the majority of common lesions are displayed, along with some rarities. Most of the images are derived from autopsy cases, with a few images from surgical cases. Most images are largely left to speak for themselves, but, where provided, the red reference bar is 10 mm.

Suggestions for further reading and references are also provided. One is mindful that autopsy pathology is often the same pathology as seen in the living, but simply demonstrated in the deceased. It follows that a good grounding in general surgical pathology is required to be a competent autopsy practitioner. There are so many books one could recommend in this arena, but only a few are cited, and it is left to the readers to select their favourites to add to their understanding of autopsy cases.

It is important, given occasional scandals (Alder-Hey, Bristol) and conflicts with social and religious custom, that each autopsy is appropriate and respectful. It is vital to remember that the deceased was someone's mother, father, daughter, or son. This author believes that the deceased should be afforded the same status as any other patient. Due respect must always be given, and one must have an open attitude about discussing cases with the bereaved and with medicolegal agencies, other relevant medical authorities, family practitioners, and society in general. That does not mean open access, and it is important that the autopsy is not abused for inappropriate commentary or gratuitous display.

Knowledge of the method by which one undertakes a high-quality autopsy will undoubtedly remain part of twenty-first-century medical practice, but this expensive and time-consuming technique needs to find its place in the ever-increasing range of medical investigations that can be performed. Ultimately, it is hoped that this atlas will be of use as a reference for the next generation of pathologists and anatomical pathology technicians, as well as for medicolegal practitioners and others.

Sheffield, UK S. Kim Suvarna

Acknowledgements

A book such as this, especially in the circumstances it was prepared, is an example of team effort and the culmination of many people's hard work.

Weeks after learning of Kim's devastating cancer diagnosis, he asked if I would join him as a co-editor for this second edition. Kim believed passionately that this book was a valuable addition to the autopsy literature, and he worked on his chapters tirelessly in his final months of life. He showed me the ropes of editing and built my competence and confidence to continue after he died. I am grateful to him for this mammoth opportunity. His pathology legacy continues in this book and in the minds of many of us who were trained by him.

To the chapter authors of this edition, my appreciative thanks for sharing your expertise, contributing images and your attention to detail. I could not have completed this without you all. Your efforts have been instrumental in compiling this work and I have appreciated every encouraging email you have sent, of which there have been many. This enthusiastic group of colleagues, near and far, has risen to the challenges of their chapters, sometimes in the face of significant personal grief around the time of Kim's death. The chapters have received updates with inclusion of new images to complement and upgrade the previous edition's content. Kim was especially excited for the addition of a post-mortem histology chapter and I am particularly grateful to Esther for providing a whole chapter's worth of high-quality images and commentary.

My grateful thanks go to the staff at Springer (especially Anand Shanmugam, Dhanushya Vijayakandeepan, Robert Donkersteeg, Melissa Morton, and Emily Wong), for your patience as you have guided me in this role and worked to bring this project to completion.

The entire medicolegal autopsy team in Sheffield has been pivotal in seeing this book to completion. A giant thank you to my supportive autopsy pathologist colleagues and the autopsy-interested trainees in Sheffield, UK. Special thanks go to those working in the dissection room in the mortuary in Sheffield: Maxine Coe, Joanne Dawn, Nigel Prestidge, Sally Smith, Tim Wild, and Paul Wood. I know Seonaid Ashby provided her usual outstanding secretarial support in preparation for this second edition and I am indebted to you for typing Kim's dictations, making the process significantly smoother. Additional thanks are expressed to the various coroners across the UK, but in particular, Mrs. Rawden (HM Coroner for South Yorkshire, West). The coroners have provided us with the opportunity to work and train with very interesting cases. I expect there are people who contributed to this project even before I became involved; to those who assisted in any way, I give my thanks.

One must not lose sight of the fact that the images from this book are almost all derived from the deceased. Immense gratitude is expressed to the relatives who have given consent for images to be retained and used to teach the pathologists of the future. This generosity cannot be understated.

Thanks also go to Grace, Miranda, and Elara Horne for welcoming me into your home at the most difficult of times and supporting Kim in working on this book in his final months. He often spoke of the three of you, whilst at the dissection bench or in the histopathology department, recounting your current goings on and celebrating your achievements in the workshop, university, school, and work. He was so proud of each of you. I am indebted to Elara Horne for her photo editing skills, ensuring that confidentiality has been afforded to the deceased and giving uniformity to the figures in this book.

And finally, to my family and friends, who treated me with understanding and supported me to choose my laptop over quality time for the sake of completing this book, a chunk of which was written with baby Henry in one arm, I am so grateful. Thank you for your gentleness in the face of a difficult time.

Sheffield, UK Abigail K. Sharp

Contents

Contributors

Julian L. Burton Medical Education, Division of Clinical Medicine, School of Medicine and Population Health, The University of Sheffield, Sheffield, UK

Maxine S. Coe Public Mortuary, Medicolegal Centre, Sheffield, UK

Kirsty L. Lloyd Department of Histopathology, Sheffield Teaching Hospitals NHS Foundation Trust, Sheffield, UK

Philip D. Lumb Department of Forensic Pathology, Medicolegal Centre, Sheffield, UK

Stephen R. Morley Forensic Toxicology Unit, Leicester Royal Infirmary, Leicester, UK

Ian S. D. Roberts Department of Cellular Pathology, Oxford University Hospitals Foundation Trust, John Radcliffe Hospital, Oxford, UK

Abigail K. Sharp Department of Histopathology, Sheffield Teaching Hospitals NHS Foundation Trust, Sheffield, UK

S. Kim Suvarna Department of Histopathology, Sheffield Teaching Hospitals NHS Foundation Trust, Sheffield, UK

Eu-Wing Toh Department of Histopathology, Sheffield Teaching Hospitals NHS Foundation Trust, Sheffield, UK

Zoë C. Traill Department of Radiology, Oxford University Hospitals Foundation Trust, Churchill Hospital, Oxford, UK

Stephen B. Wharton Division of Neuroscience, School of Medicine and Population Health, University of Sheffield, Sheffield, UK

Department of Histopathology, Sheffield Teaching Hospitals NHS Foundation Trust, Sheffield, UK

Esther Youd Forensic Medicine and Science, University of Glasgow, Glasgow, UK

General Considerations and Safety

1

Maxine S. Coe and S. Kim Suvarna

Introduction

Preparation for the autopsy and consideration of the case, before entering the autopsy room or putting knife to skin, are key in getting the best results from the examination. This chapter commences with the components of an instruction to perform an autopsy. The relevant paperwork (usually legal and/or consent permissions) is discussed.

The practical realities of completing an autopsy require a modern, well-lit, ventilated and dedicated room or facility for this examination; views of some facilities are shown. Other requirements are appropriate clothing, protective face masks, gloves, and other body-wear. The standard tools and the workstation are presented. This process permits a safe working environment for the autopsy practitioner and will enable the pathologist or technician to efficiently examine the case.

All these efforts will maximize macroscopic information, but additional tests are often required to realize the full potential of the autopsy. The role of specialist investigations (histology, toxicology, microbiology) is described, and macroscopic photography is also considered. Finally, the methods for recording the data derived are described.

S. Kim Suvarna was deceased at the time of publication.

M. S. Coe (✉)
Public Mortuary, Medicolegal Centre, Sheffield, UK
e-mail: maxine.coe@sheffield.gov.uk

S. K. Suvarna (Deceased)
Department of Histopathology, Sheffield Teaching Hospitals NHS Foundation Trust, Sheffield, UK

Paperwork: Permissions and Instructions

Before starting the autopsy, it is vital to confirm that there is a clear instruction to perform the examination from the relevant authorities. This data may come from legal sources (e.g. for the United Kingdom; HM Coroner or Procurator Fiscal), the police, or another state body. Alternatively, it may be driven by a request from the medical staff or relatives; in the form of a "consent" autopsy.

Identification

As with all medical procedures, identification of the body in question is required, using a variety of different case identifier data. The name, date of birth and relevant hospital number may be important. However, other identifying information may come from third parties (confirming the identity of the deceased). Specific body features, including piercings, tattoos, dentures, and other identification elements, may be relevant in allowing certification of identity. Correlation with a previous photographic record (e.g. passport, identity cards, or other resources) is sometimes of use.

Ideally, bodies are retrieved soon after death, and little decomposition will have occurred. However, some bodies will have been significantly degraded with autolysis and maggot infestation. In such circumstances, other data such as dental record comparison, registry numbers of implants or evidence of prior disease events or correlates may be needed.

Once confirmation of identity has been established, the body is 'booked-in'. This necessitates the assignment of the body to a unique case identification number (e.g., 679H/24, reflecting the case number given, with a check letter and the year).

The body, usually identified by a name label or bracelet, is then stored to await examination. Bodies are normally stored in refrigerators, generally at 4 °C (40 °F). Alternatively, if storage is needed for a prolonged period, then freezing at −20 °C (−4 °F) is appropriate.

S. K. Suvarna (represented by Grace Horne), A. K. Sharp (eds.), *Atlas of Adult Autopsy*,
https://doi.org/10.1007/978-3-031-72207-3_1

The Background Story

The examination generally follows review of information from those requesting the examination, and/or consideration of the clinical record and medical history data. This may yield not only information to guide the examination in terms of likely pathology, but also information that may be pertinent to various infection risks for those working in the autopsy suite. Consideration of potential risks in the form of various viral infections (drug users, those brought back from abroad, etc.) may be of importance. Nevertheless, *in all cases* the various risks of infection must be assessed before examining a body.

Cases with category 1 and 2 infections can proceed without special measures. Category 3 risk cases need additional clothing and protection. Ideally, such cases should be performed by those with appropriate experience. Category 4 risk cases should be examined only by experienced practitioners in specialist facilities with the appropriate techniques and safety measures. It cannot be over-emphasized that caution with all cases must be the standard for working in the mortuary, and relevant immunizations are mandatory for all personnel.

Getting Ready

One cannot perform autopsies wearing one's own clothing. The mortuary must provide clothing designed to be comfortable and yet protective for the staff. At this point, it is worth stressing that there should always be at least two people in the autopsy room when it is active, for safety reasons.

Fresh clothing (usually theatre scrubs, stored in dedicated changing rooms with wash and shower facilities) should be worn, with an outer gown. Layers of flexible waterproof and stab-resistant (Kevlar/chainmail) gloves must be worn. Additional waterproof lower arm covers are recommended. Face covers (generally masks and visors) are required, and one may also select hair/beard nets or caps. Specialist masks may be required for various infection risks. It should be noted that facial hair (including beards and stubble) can cause difficulties with some respiratory protective equipment requiring a good seal to the face which may necessitate alternative equipment such as a battery-operated full facial unit. A waterproof apron must be worn, covering the torso and legs, down to below the top of waterproof wellington boots (with toe protection).

The Autopsy Room, Workbench, and Autopsy Table

The autopsy room, along with adjoining dedicated transitional rooms, must be available. The layout of an autopsy room needs good lighting, down-draft ventilation, running water, work surfaces capable of being chemically cleaned and sterilized, nonslip flooring, and space to work.

The workstation should be equipped with a range of scalpel blades and other long knives. There should be scissors (various sizes) and 'toothed' forceps. A ruler, measuring jug and accurate electronic scales are vital. A range of bowls, ladles, string, wire-cutters, saws, shears, and other instruments must be available.

A digital camera is particularly valuable in the autopsy room to record the stages of dissection, as well as specific lesions or gross morphology. Imaging is of vital importance in some cases that have a legal bearing, such as in cases of surgical procedures with complications, retained foreign bodies, and to demonstrate absence of such occurrences.

Additional Testing Materials

Within easy reach should be containers for swabs, culture bottles, toxicology kits, formalin pots and tissue cassettes.

Histological examination is a common adjunct to the autopsy. This test requires the availability of formalin and appropriately numbered cassettes for securing the samples taken. The cassettes should be identified in terms of the case number and the cassette number (e.g., case 679H/24 A1, where the designator A1 is the cassette number that can be specified with regard to the contents). The tissue type and number of tissue fragments should be recorded for the content of each cassette. Standard paraffin-based tissue processing is commonplace. However, glutaraldehyde for electron microscopy may also be relevant. Handling tissues for frozen section must also be possible.

Microbiology samples may be taken in possible cases of bacterial, fungal, or viral disease. Those with a significant infection risk (e.g., Category 3 risk) must be labeled accordingly.

Toxicology tests may also be needed, with samples of various body fluids (vitreous, blood, cerebrospinal fluid, urine) and tissues being reserved for analysis.

Rarely, other specialist techniques find their way into the autopsy room. For example, samples may be taken for mass spectroscopy (e.g., metal analysis) or serology (e.g., hormone assay, serum tryptase).

The Results

Examining a body will generate a lot of information, such as organ weights, pathology descriptions and measurement. These must be annotated, by tape or digital recording or by writing onto a standard proforma (see Appendix).

The paperwork or recording must itemize whether samples have been taken. If so, the type and number of samples should be stated. At this point, one may be able to provide a cause of death, which should be in the standard format (i.e., 1a, 1b, 1c, 1d and 2).

Figures 1.1, 1.2, 1.3, 1.4, 1.5, 1.6, 1.7, 1.8, 1.9, 1.10, 1.11, 1.12, 1.13, 1.14, 1.15, 1.16, 1.17, 1.18, 1.19, 1.20, 1.21, 1.22, 1.23, 1.24, 1.25, 1.26, 1.27, 1.28, 1.29, 1.30, 1.31, 1.32, 1.33, 1.34, and 1.35 illustrate the points made in this chapter.

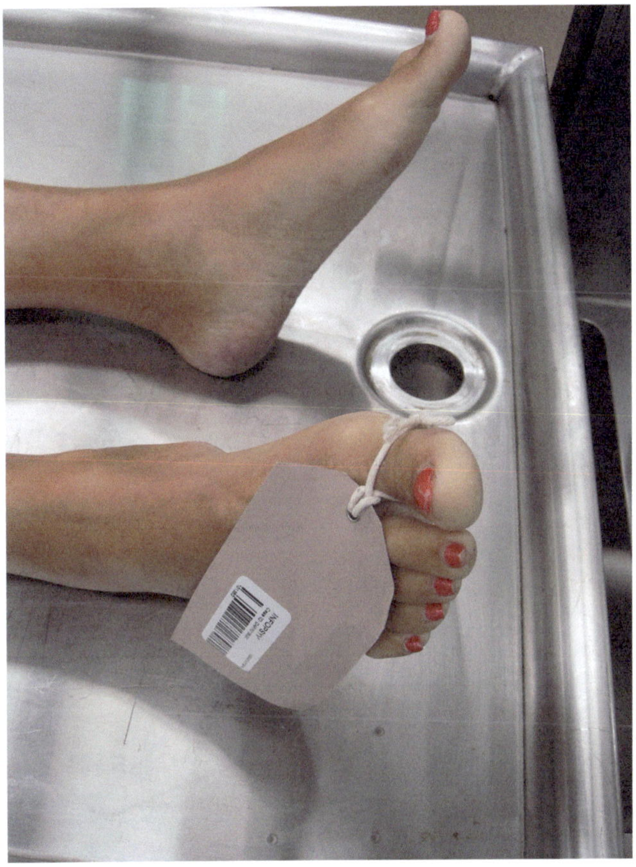

Fig. 1.1 A toe tag attached to the body is seen with some of the numerical patient data of the deceased. The patient's name is on the reverse of this form

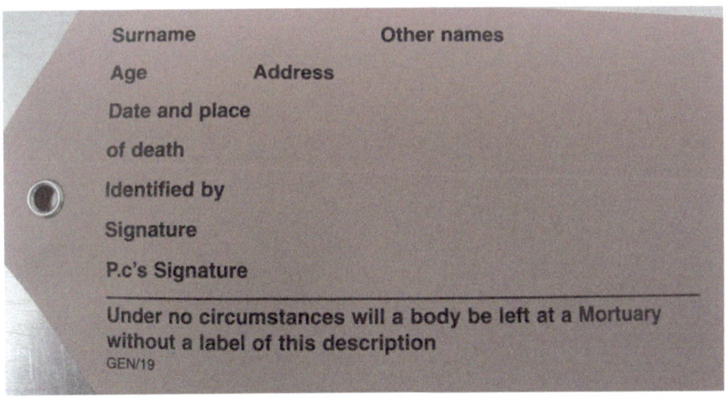

Surname Other names
Age Address
Date and place
of death
Identified by
Signature
P.c's Signature

Under no circumstances will a body be left at a Mortuary without a label of this description
GEN/19

Fig. 1.2 The tag should show relevant identifier data: full name, place and date of death, address and confirmation as to how the identification was verified

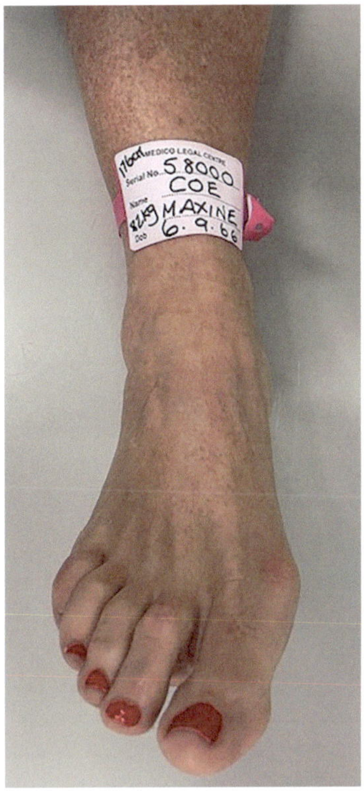

Fig. 1.3 Additional data may be added to the body, such as this coloured band added to the wrist or ankle containing relevant details of the deceased, including the case number, height, and weight

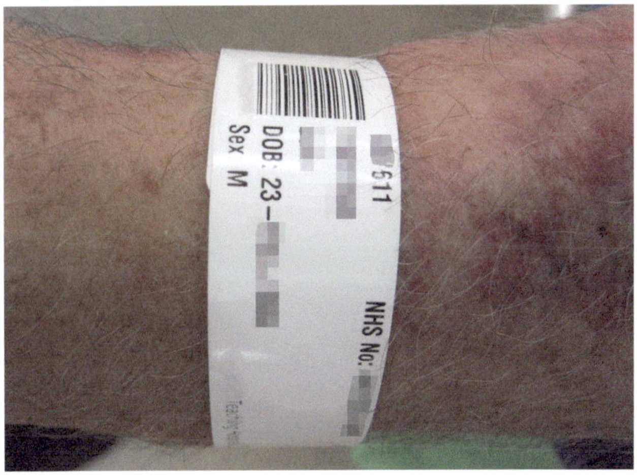

Fig. 1.4 The arrival of a body from a medical unit often comes with bar-coded identifier wrist bands and other information. The name in this case has been obscured intentionally

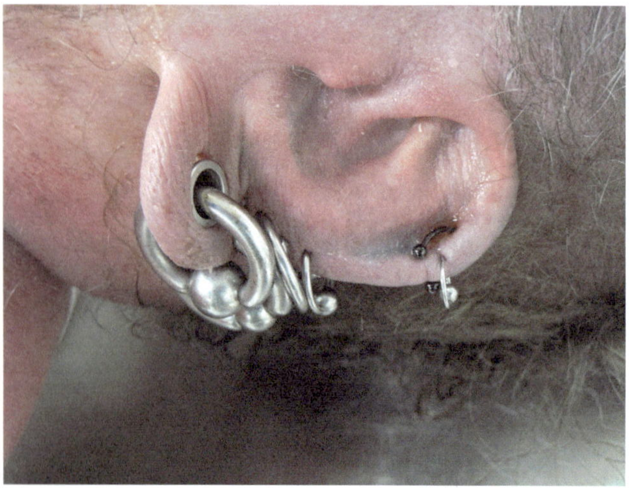

Fig. 1.5 Additional information confirming the person's identity may be seen in the form of external jewellery (e.g. metal ear rings or piercings)

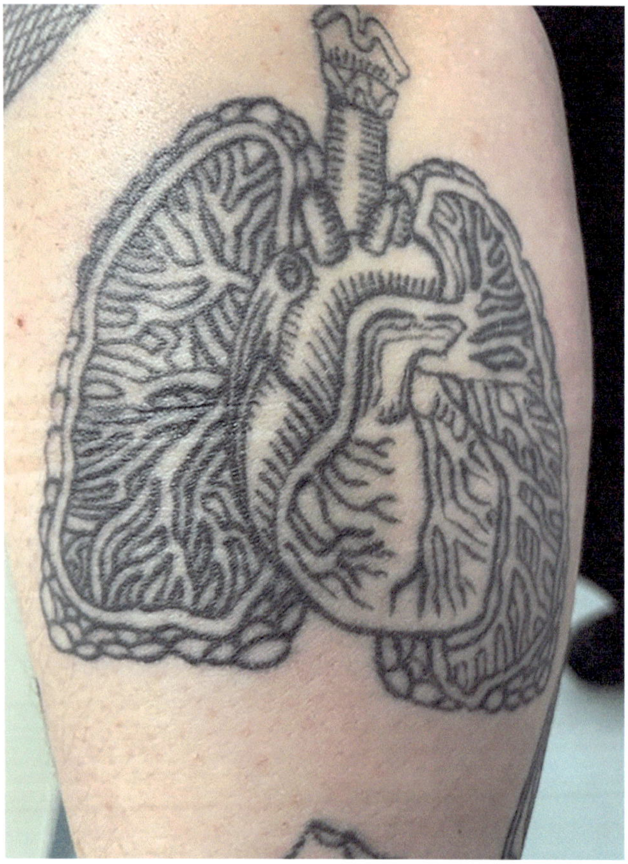

Fig. 1.6 Tattoos are also a good identifier, particularly if unique or unusual. This arm tattoo of the heart and lungs is not a common design and may be helpful when correlating to other information about the deceased or photographs taken in life

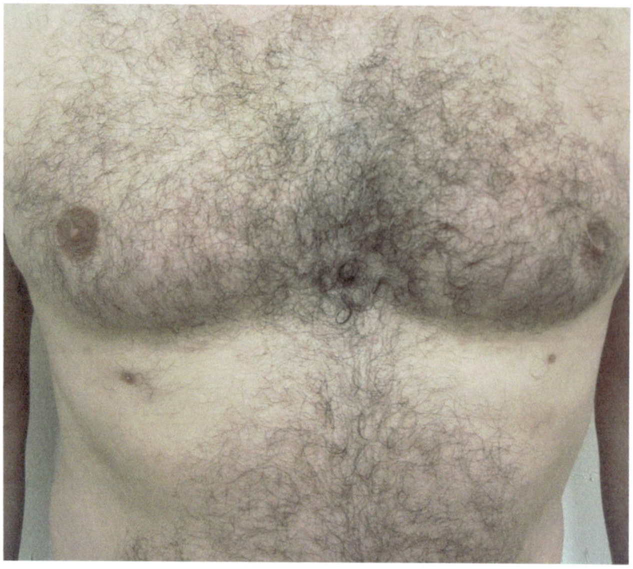

Fig. 1.7 The body may have a variety of distinguishing marks that aid identification. This image shows the front of the chest with multiple nipples

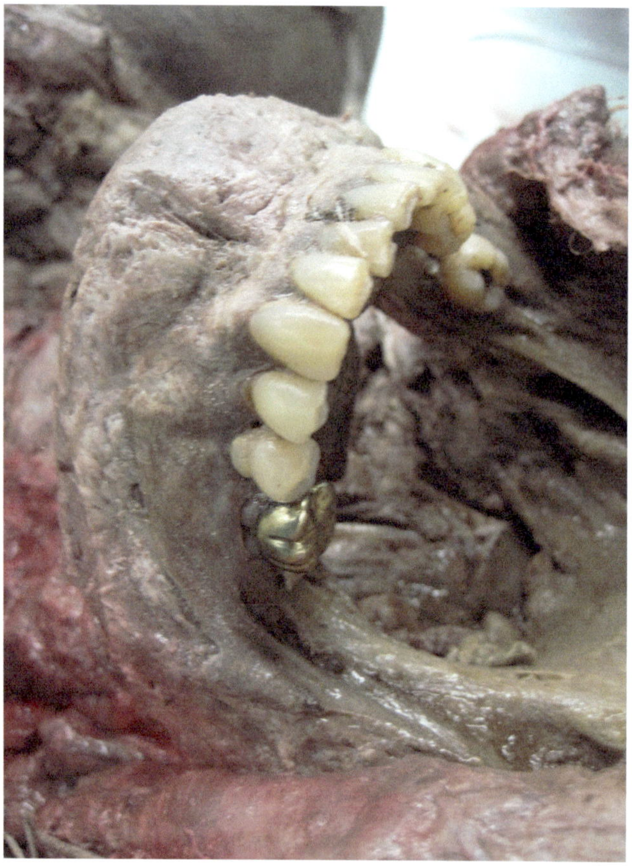

Fig. 1.8 Even badly decomposed bodies may contain useful clues for identification, including dental work. Here the mouth is seen to have dental amalgam filling and a gold tooth

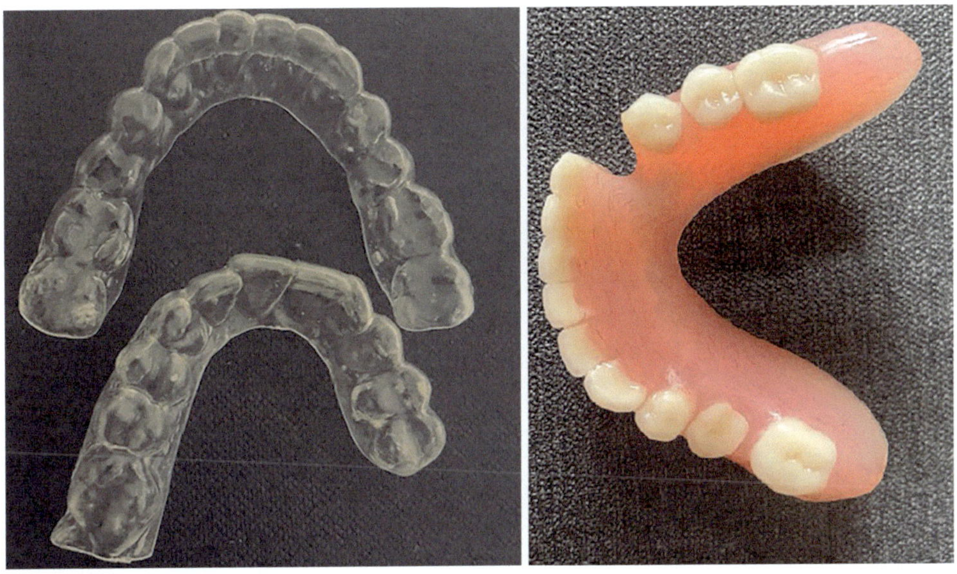

Fig. 1.9 Teeth-straightening retainers and dentures, as seen here, are common at autopsy and can be used for identification purpose

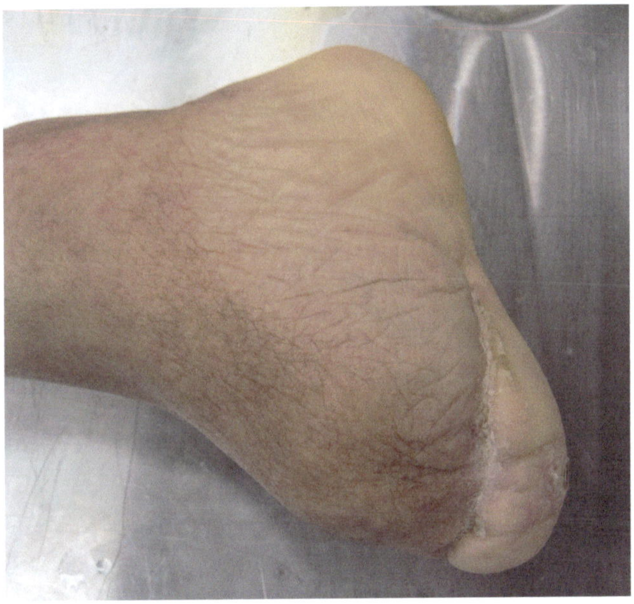

Fig. 1.10 Amputations and other scars may serve to confirm identity, particularly when matched to hospital records

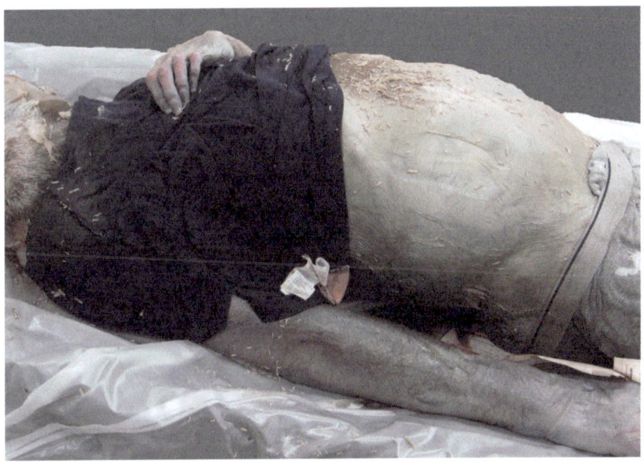

Fig. 1.11 Often the body may be fully or partly dressed. This can be mapped against witness information as to the clothes the deceased was last seen wearing. Precautions must be taken when removing clothing from a body. The pockets may contain sharp objects or may be covering jagged, protruding bone. One should use forceps to expose pocket contents

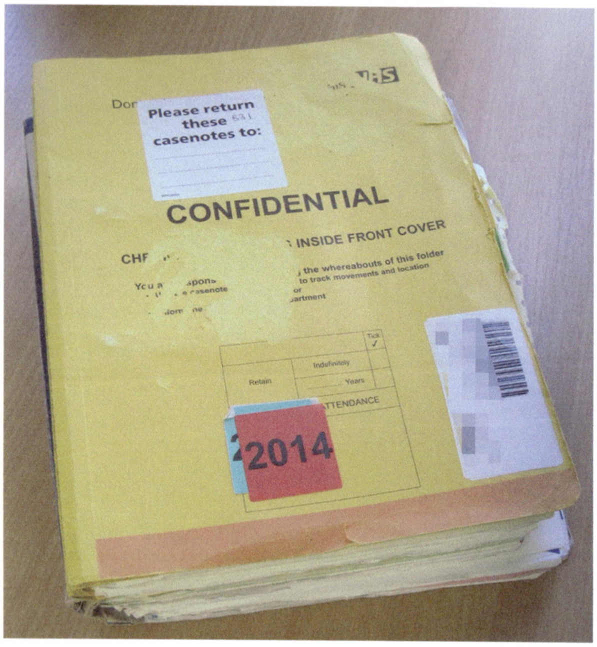

Fig. 1.12 The notes of the deceased often contain the abundant medical, nursing, and other data that help to identify the deceased. The clinical record may also point to hazards to be considered before the autopsy (e.g., infection risks)

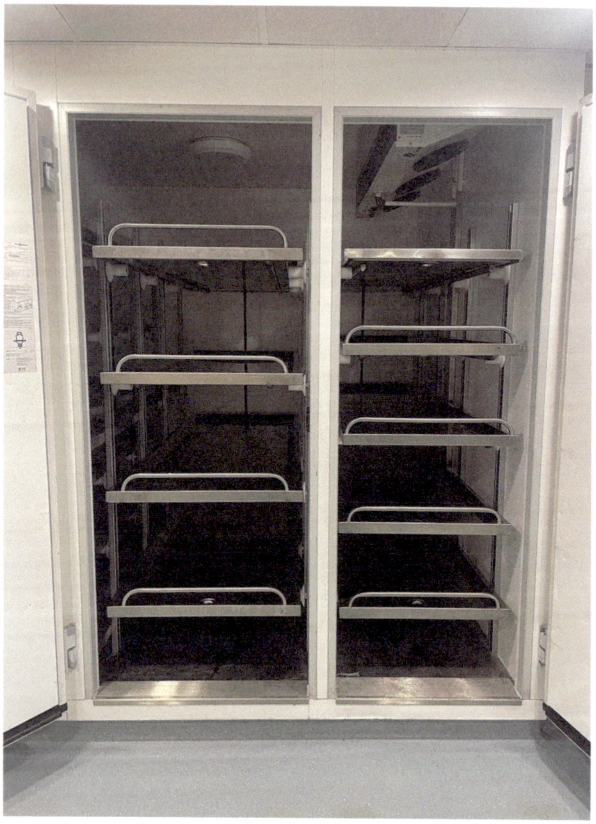

Fig. 1.13 An example of body storage is shown here, with a refrigerated compartment containing horizontal tiers of roll in/roll out trays. The tray travels with the body during the stay in the mortuary. The trays and bodies are usually arranged in tiers of three to five and vary in size to accommodate bariatric bodies. The units have doors at the head and feet ends. They are run at a temperature of 4 °C (40 °F) or freezer temperature of −20 °C (−4 °F)

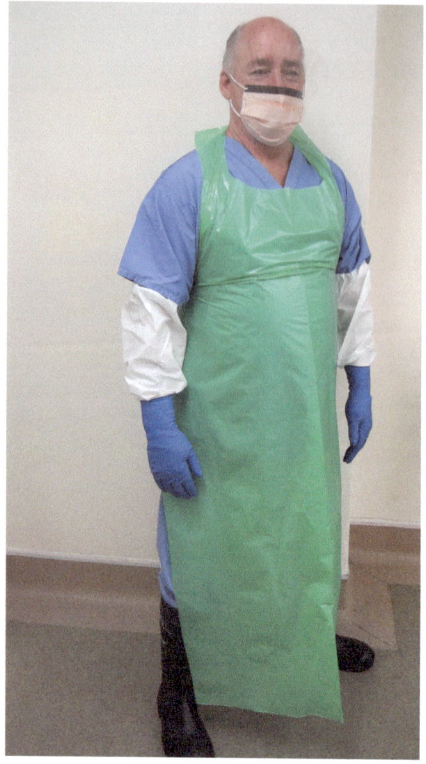

Fig. 1.14 The acceptable minimum protective clothing to perform a post mortem: scrub (tunic and trousers); trousers tucked inside reinforced (toe-cap) wellingtons and plastic apron close to the floor; gloves and oversleeves. There should be a mask with an attached or integral clear plastic visor to cover the face

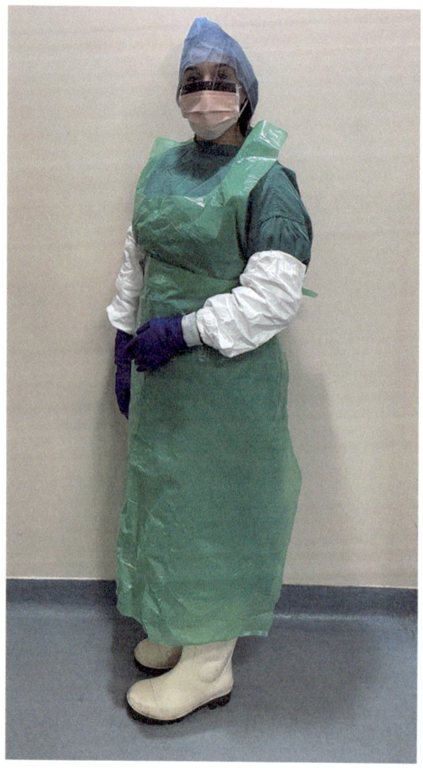

Fig. 1.15 Pathologists wear an additional gown that helps to differentiate them from the technicians

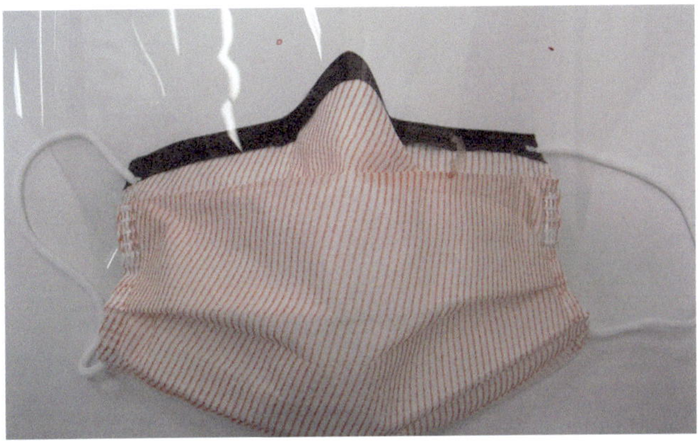

Fig. 1.16 This photograph of a mask and inbuilt visor shows the importance of protecting the eyes and the mouth. The visor has prevented small blood splashes from striking the face

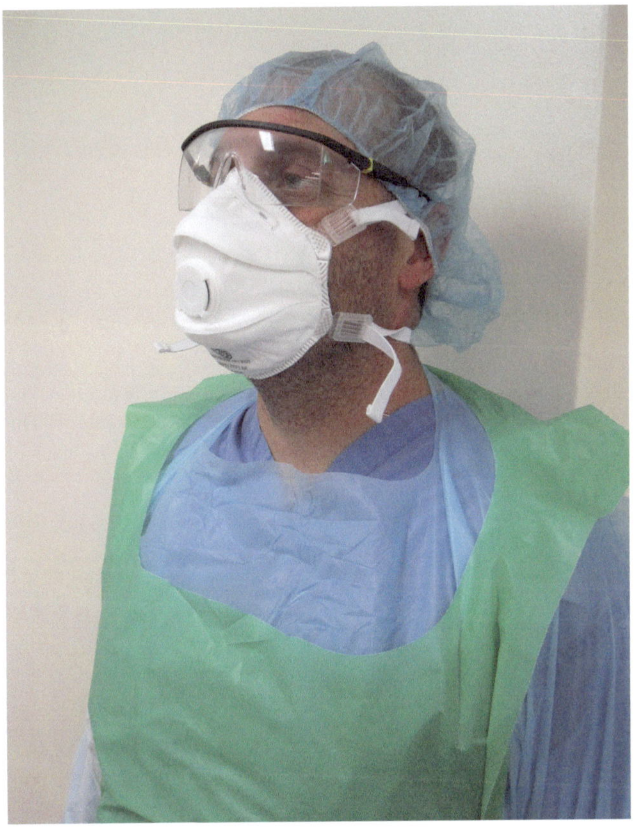

Fig. 1.17 This image shows a specialised mask being used in Category 3 risk cases, with separate clear goggles, and a hair net. Covering the hair provides additional protection

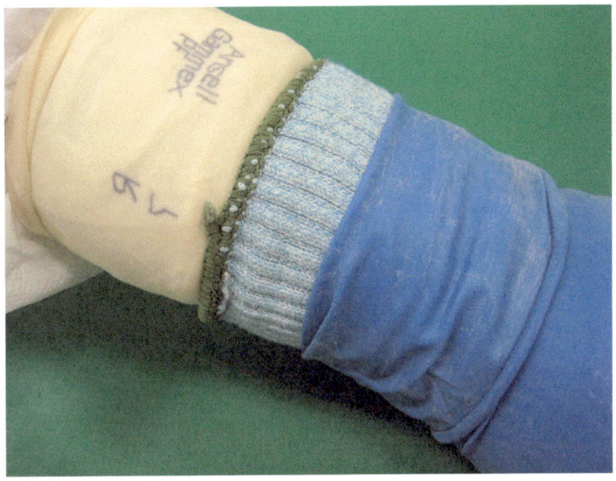

Fig. 1.18 Layering of the gloves limits the risk of cutting and of tissue fluid penetration to the operator's skin. Here, the inner beige surgical glove sits next to the skin. Then there is a Kevlar (or chainmail as an alternative) glove. Finally, there is a heavy duty waterproof blue glove. This ensemble will interlock with the oversleeves and afford good protection for those working with body dissection

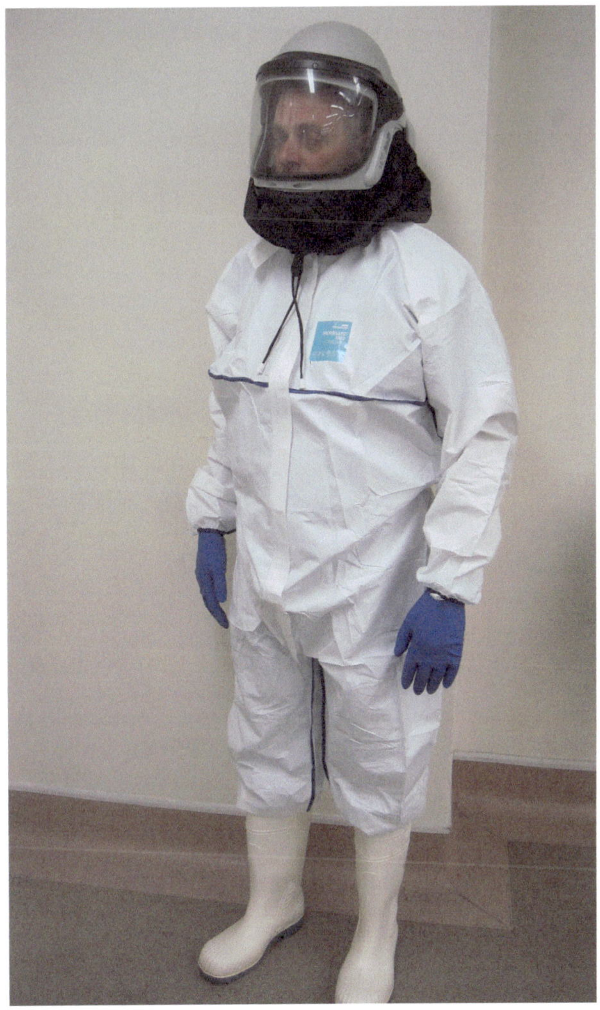

Fig. 1.19 Dealing with high-risk cases may require additional measures for protection. Here, a disposable suit is worn over the standard mortuary wear. In cases with high risk of infection, if one wishes to use a battery-operated full facial unit, it should be put in place before entering the autopsy room

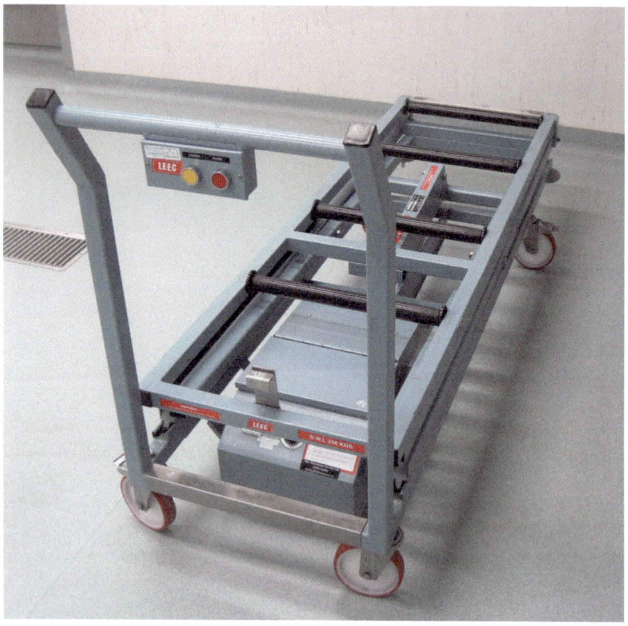

Fig. 1.20 Moving bodies around in the mortuary requires safe working practices to avoid mortuary staff injury. A hydraulic unit, as shown here, is employed to allow the fridge tray and body to be moved safely to the operating station

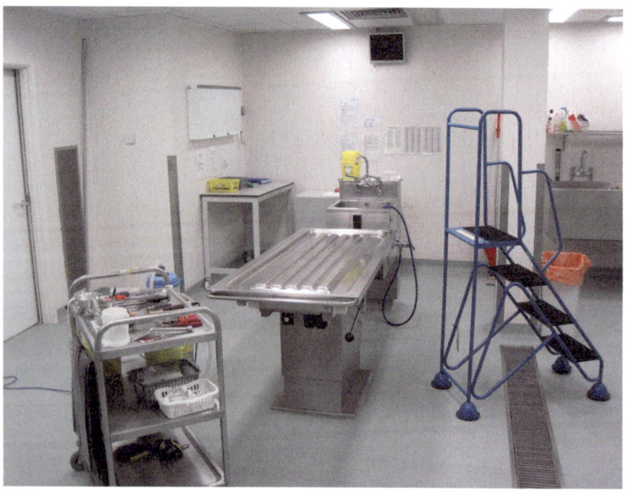

Fig. 1.21 The general layout of a post mortem facility is seen, with a central dissecting station. There is good lighting, drainage and access to fridges and other equipment. For illustration purposes in this view, there is a ladder for an assistant to take photographs during dissection. Dissection tools and other equipment are on a mobile trolley

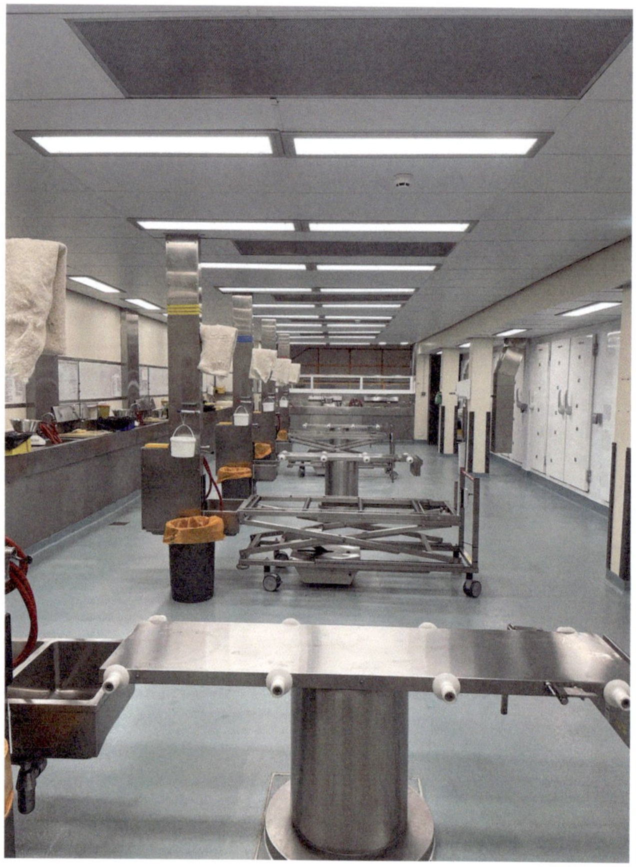

Fig. 1.22 Shown here is an example of a 3-fixed station and 2-trolley station post mortem suite, allowing for multiple autopsy examinations to occur simultaneously, sometimes with multiple pathologists. This type of set up is particularly important with consideration for major incidents, allowing for the disaster victim identification team to work collaboratively

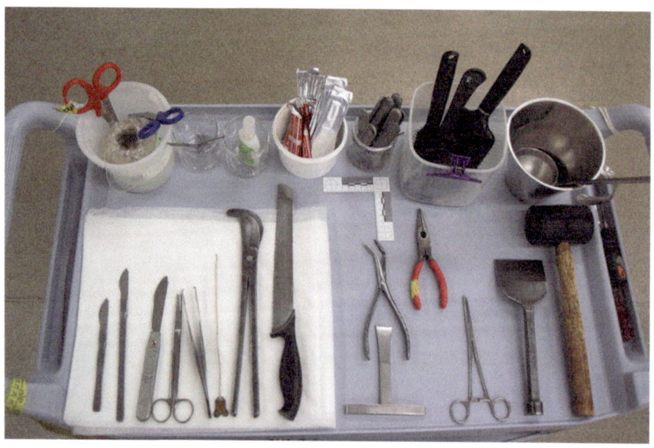

Fig. 1.23 The dissection trolley layout shows the instruments that can be used during the autopsy

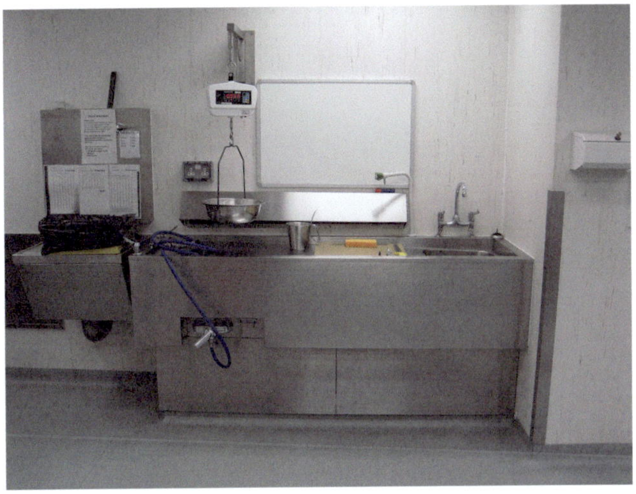

Fig. 1.24 After evisceration, the organs are often carried to a separate work area, allowing the autopsy assistant to start reconstructing the body. The work area should be well lit, with down-draft ventilation and good access to running water and drainage. All surfaces (as with other areas in the mortuary) are capable of chemical cleaning and sterilisation later

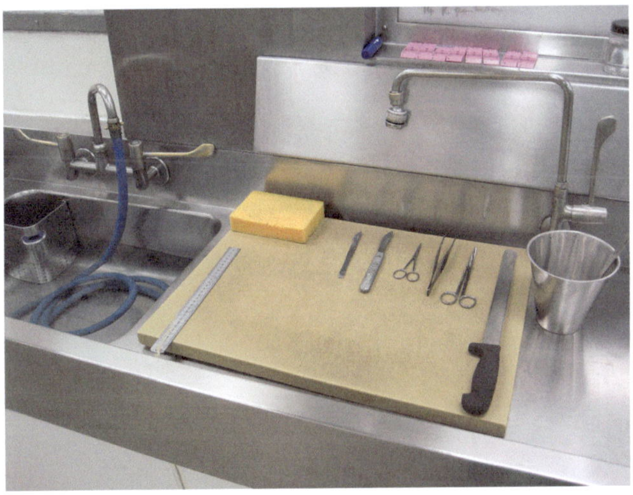

Fig. 1.25 The pathologist dissection bench is shown with the essential instruments for examination. These include a large or long knife, scissors, small and large scalpels, forceps, sponge, and ruler. Also needed are local access to running water, a measuring jug and histology cassettes

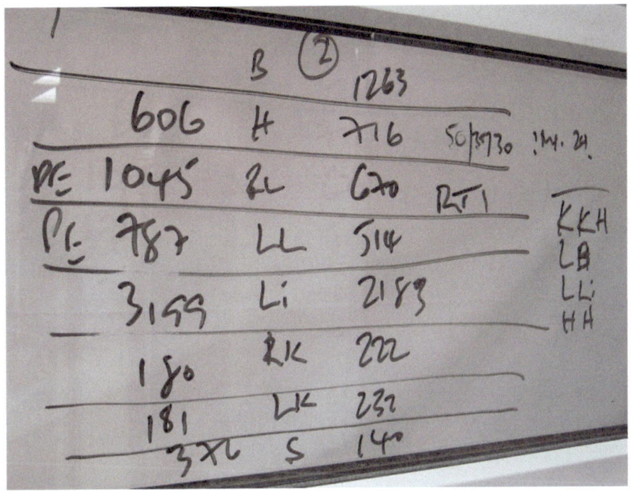

Fig. 1.26 Recording of weights and other notes during the examination can be made on wipe-clean surfaces using nonpermanent markers

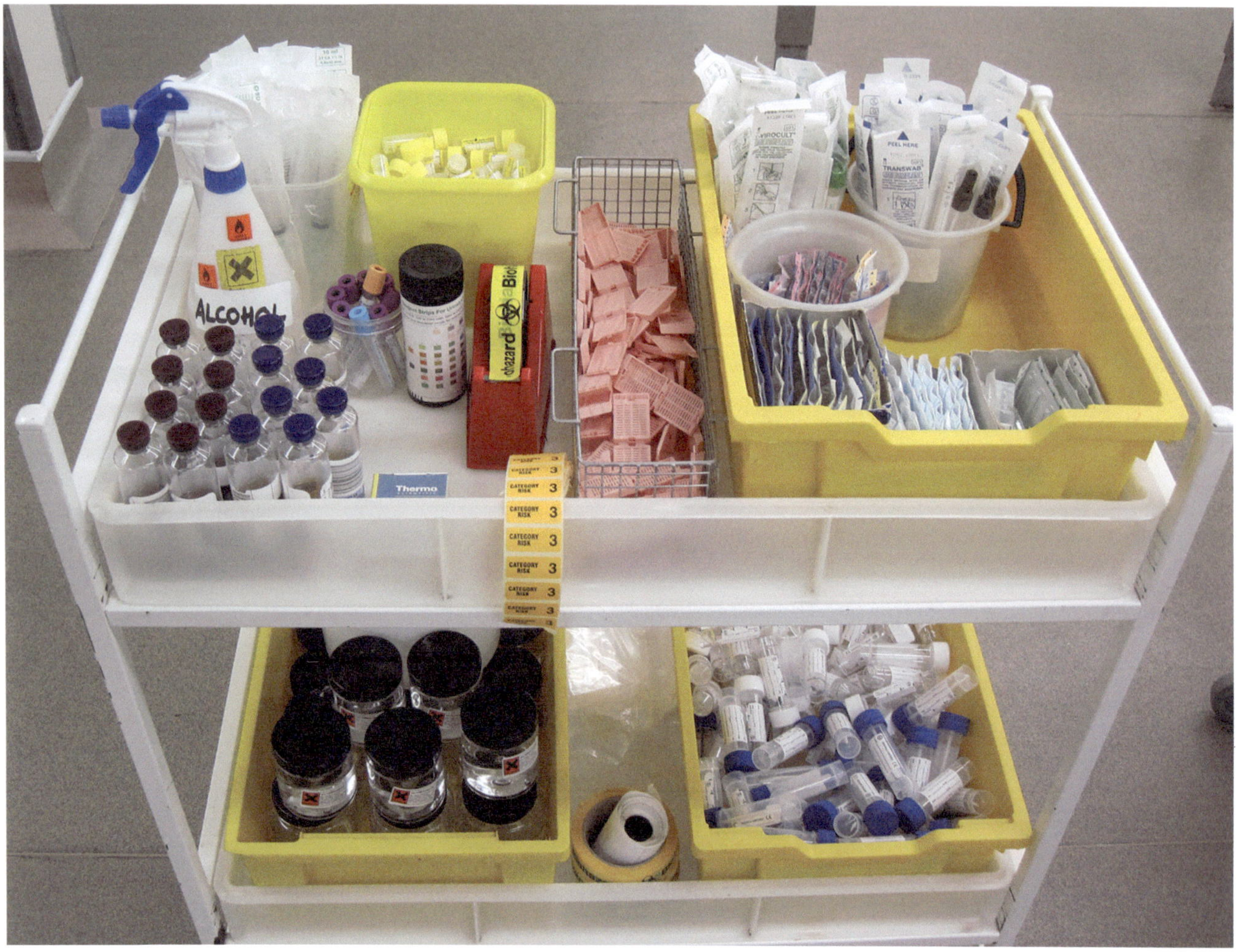

Fig. 1.27 This two-tiered sample trolley contains materials for additional tests. The upper shelf has syringes, needles, blood culture bottles, cassettes for histology, and swabs for bacteriology and virology. The lower tier holds specimen pots for histology samples, together with containers or tubes for blood, urine, tissue, and faeces

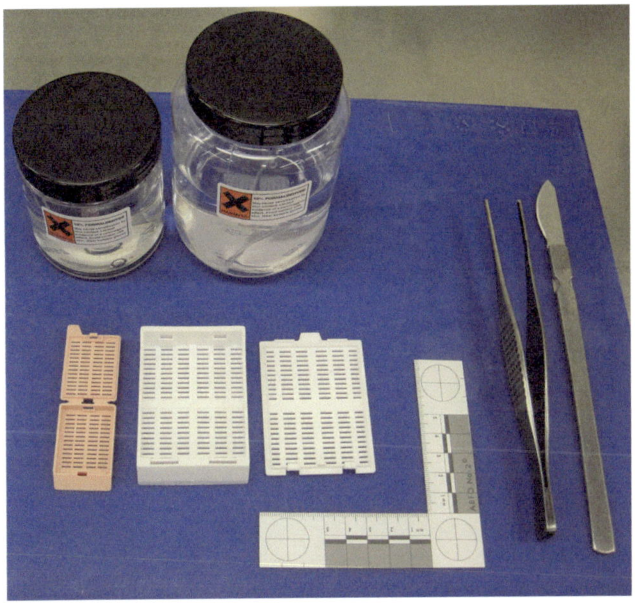

Fig. 1.28 Histology cassettes of different sizes are used to ensure that the amount of tissue taken can be processed appropriately. The smaller (standard) pink cassettes are generally used for thumbnail or smaller tissue fragments. The larger white cassettes are useful for larger samples that merit large area architecture analysis (e.g., samples of brain, lung, and heart). Sharp scalpel blades and forceps should be used when samples are taken for histology

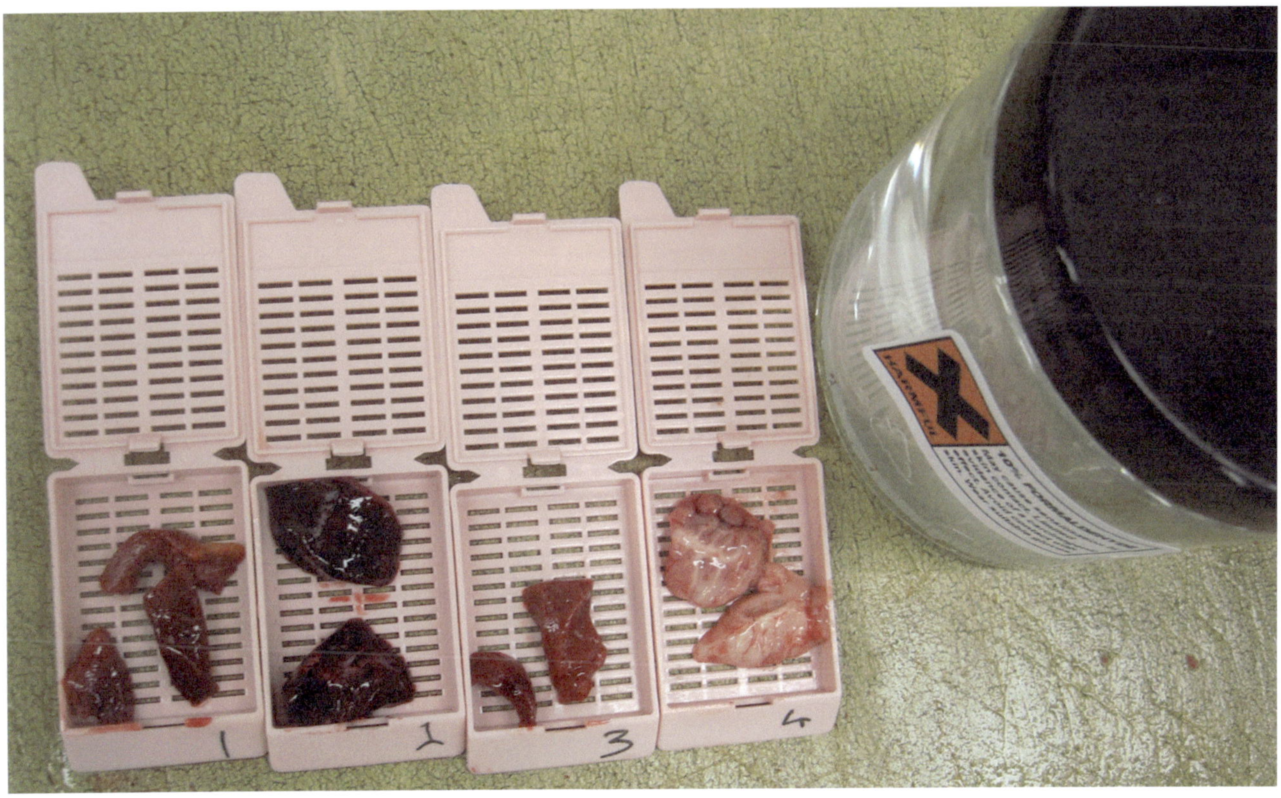

Fig. 1.29 The samples of tissue for histology may be placed in cassettes in single pieces, or, as in this case, as multiple fragments. The tissue samples should be recorded ideally. This multiple sample technique means that special stains may be used on multiple bits of tissue with only one additional slide per stain being needed

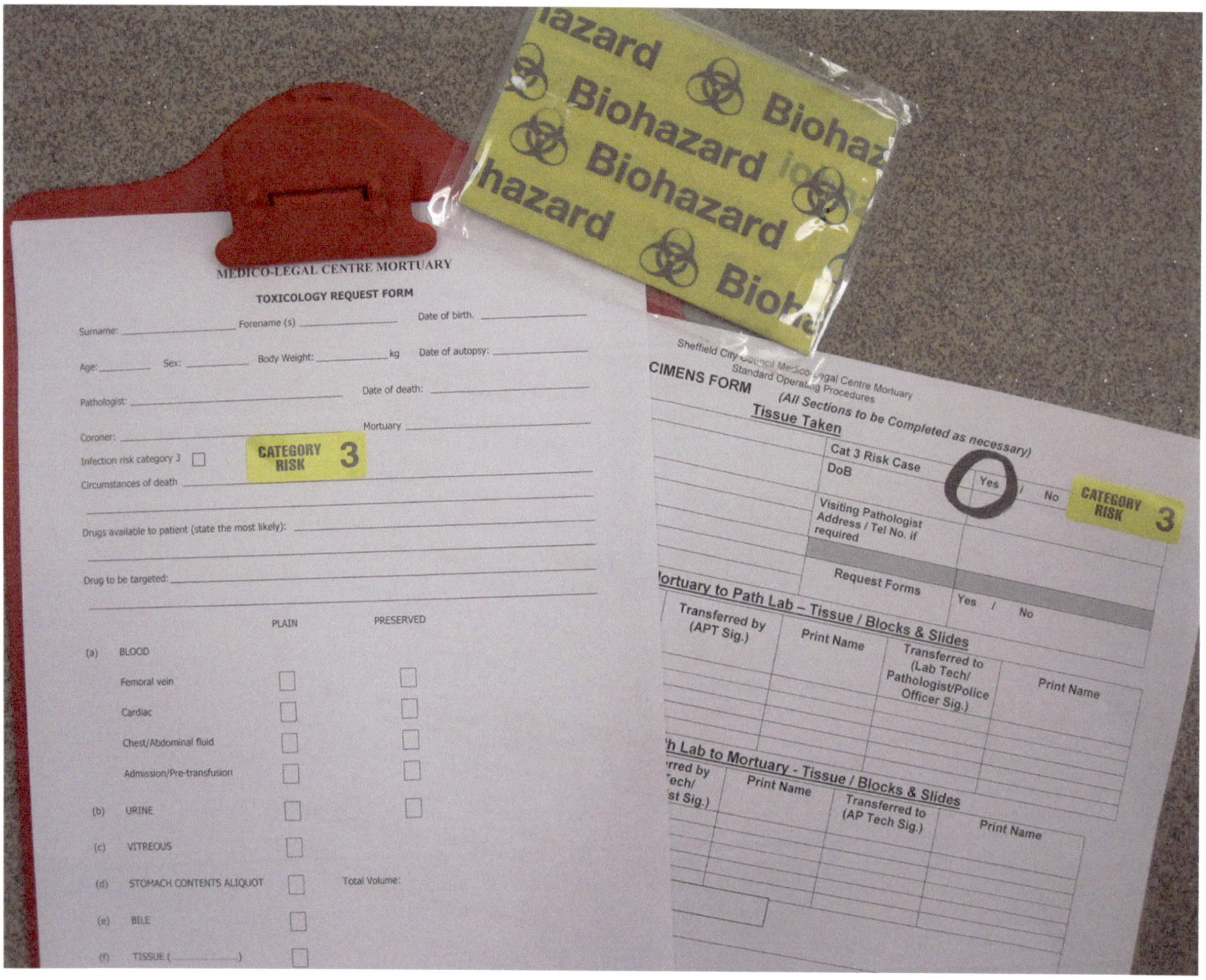

Fig. 1.30 Any samples that are taken must have the correct corresponding paperwork to accompany the specimen to the laboratory. High risk cases must be labelled with high risk (yellow) stickers to alert laboratory staff to risks and dangers

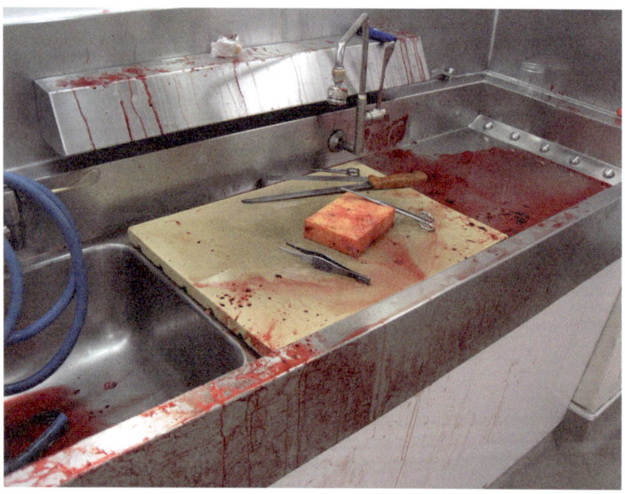

Fig. 1.31 A messy workstation (here mocked-up for illustration purposes) poses a risk to others. Aside from the widespread contamination of the work area, the discarded and contaminated blades pose a significant hazard. This is not good practice

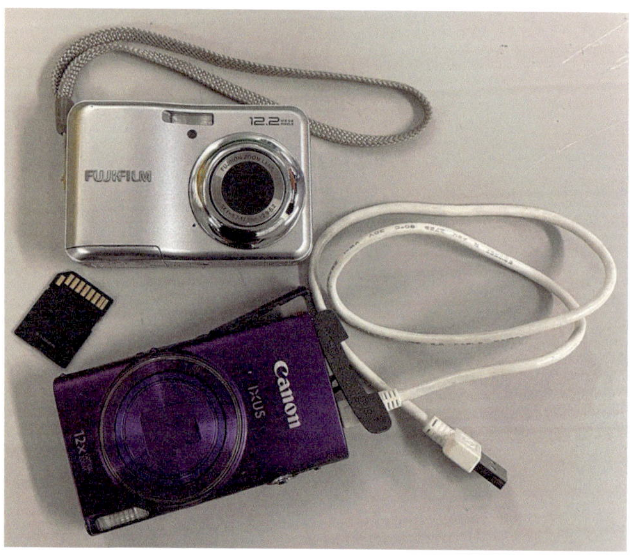

Fig. 1.32 Different types of camera can be used in the autopsy room. In recent years, compact digital cameras have good resolution and autofocus, comparing favourably with single lens reflex type cameras. For health and safety reasons, cameras ideally should not be removed from the autopsy room. Data should be remotely downloaded and stored onto a secure (often encrypted) computer

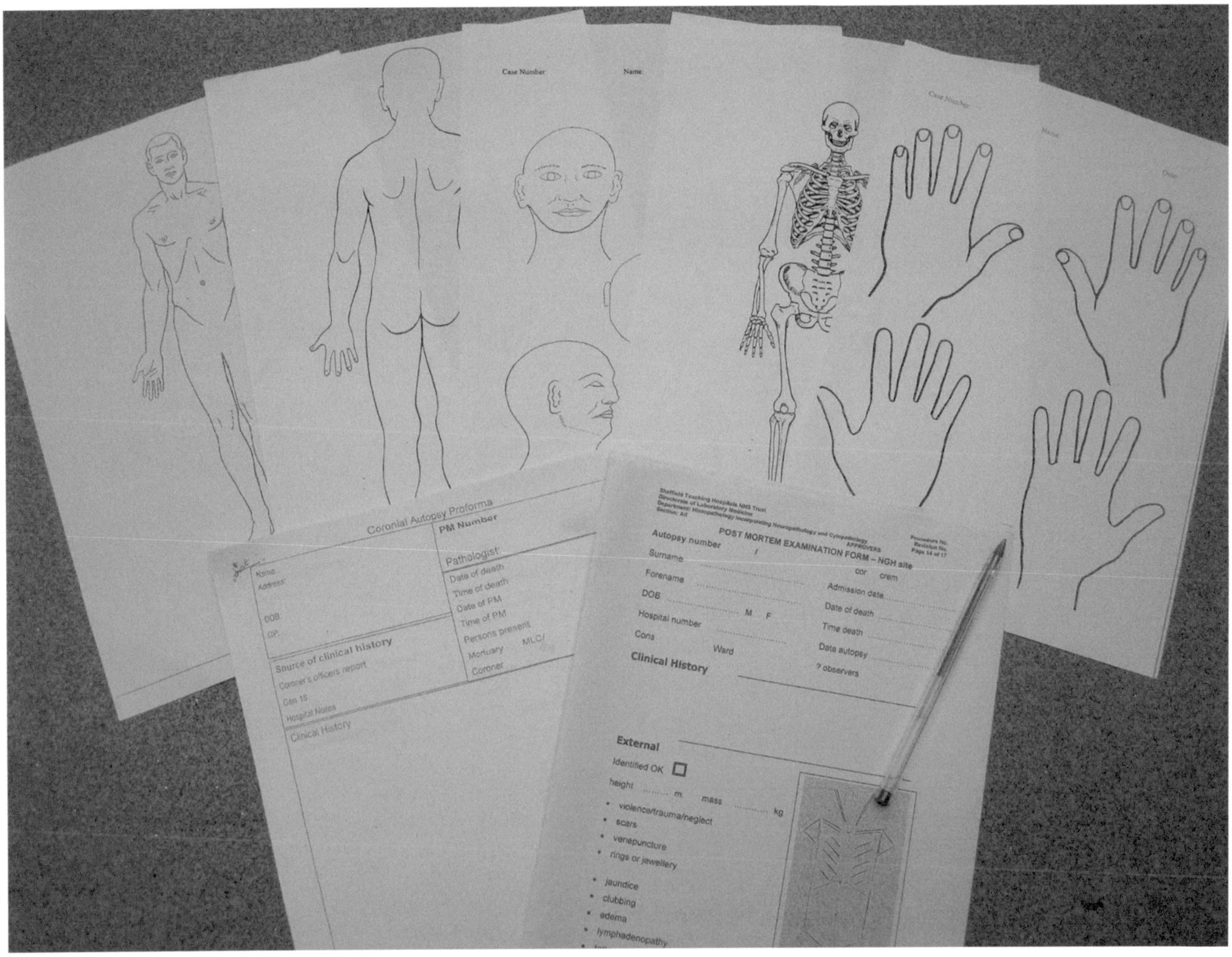

Fig. 1.33 Paperwork at the completion of the examination will vary depending on the standard operating procedures of the department. The basic paperwork includes sheets for data and results, and anatomical diagram proformas

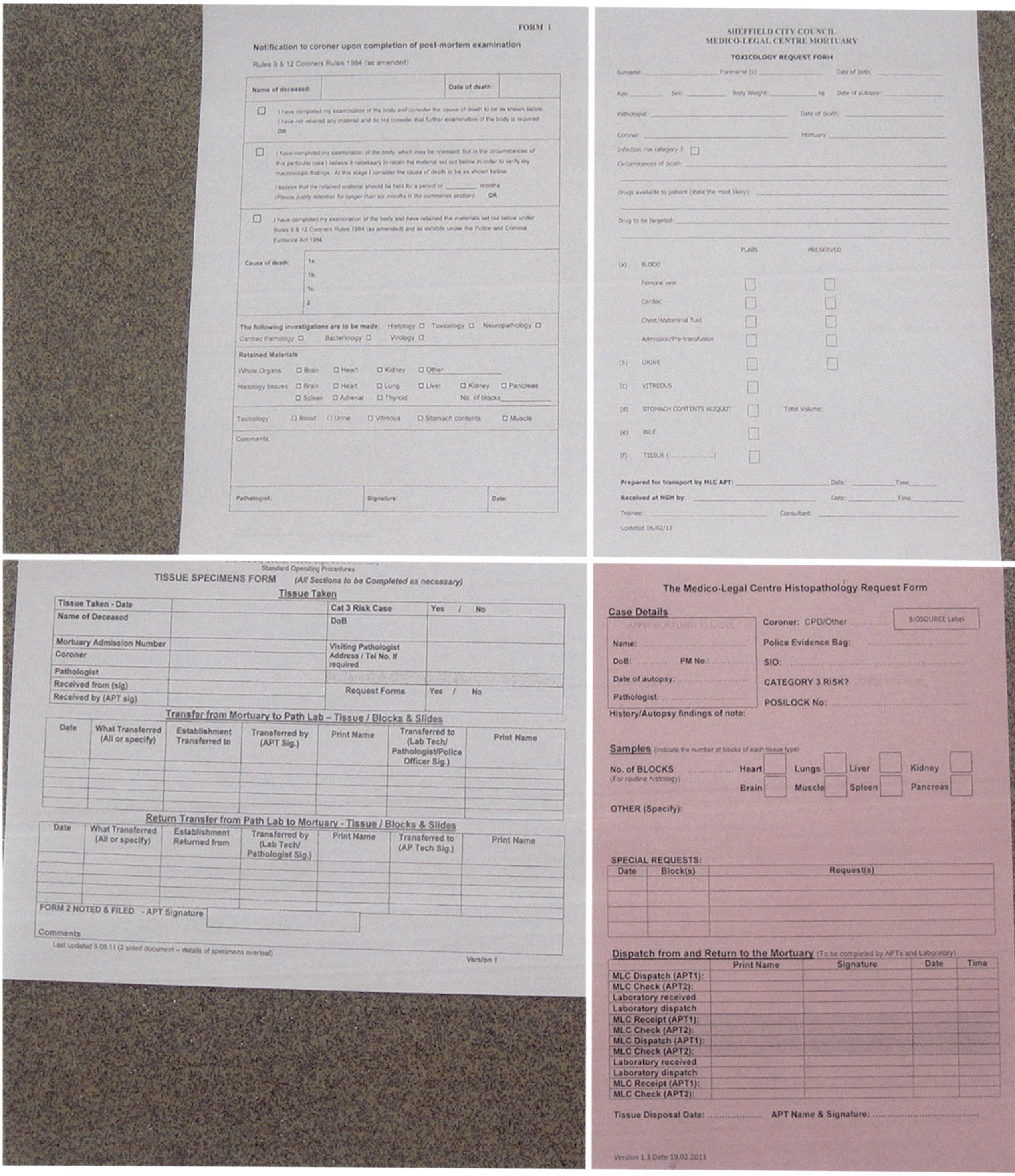

Fig. 1.34 The paperwork also includes 'cause of death' documents, histology tissue sheets (i.e., the record of tissues sampled), microbiology specimen forms, toxicology sample documents, and other items

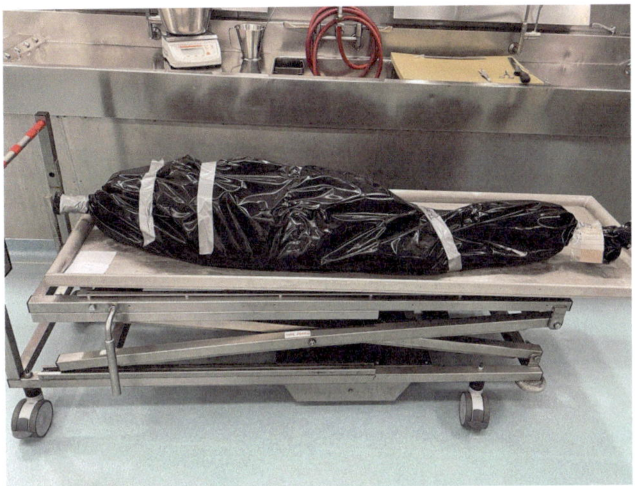

Fig. 1.35 After the examination, bodies are reconstituted and returned to the shelving in the fridges. Those with significant tissue degradation and decomposition may require heavy bagging ('cracker-wrapping') to avoid tissue leakage. Contaminated waste materials should be placed into clearly marked bags for incineration

Suggested Reading

Connolly AJ, Finkbeiner WE, Ursell PC, Davis RL, editors. Autopsy pathology: a manual and atlas. 3rd ed. Philadelphia, PA: Elsevier; 2016.

Health and Safety Executive. Managing infection risks when handling the deceased (HSG 283). Jul 2018.

Hoffman PN, Healing TD. Guide to infection control in the healthcare setting. The infection hazards of human cadavers. International Society for Infectious Diseases; 2022.

Knight B. The post-mortem technician's handbook: a manual of mortuary practice. Oxford: Blackwell Scientific Publications; 1984.

Leadbeatter S, Lucas S, Lowe J. Standards for Coroners' pathologists in post-mortem examinations of deaths that appear not to be suspicious. The Royal College of Pathologists; 2014.

Ludwig J. Handbook of autopsy practice. 3rd ed. Ottawa: Humana Press; 2002.

Royal Institute of Public Health & Hygiene. A handbook of mortuary practice and safety for anatomical pathology technicians. 1991.

Saukko P, Knight B, editors. Knight's forensic pathology. 4th ed. Boca Raton: CRC Press; 2015.

The Royal College of Pathologists. Autopsy guidelines series by multiple authors. A rolling 5-year programme. https://www.rcpath.org/profession/guidelines/autopsy-guidelines-series.html.

External Examination

2

Kirsty L. Lloyd and S. Kim Suvarna

Introduction

The aim of the external examination is to identify the deceased, and to formally document relevant positive and negative findings related to natural disease or injury. The examination of the outer surfaces of a body provides supporting information for later clinicopathological correlation, and it may (in its own right) help to determine the cause of death.

The 2006 report from the National Confidential Enquiry into Patient Outcome and Death (a national review of the UK autopsy system) [1] states 'Before evisceration of a body, the pathologist must inspect the body first. This is to confirm identity, to observe any external features that might modify the process of examination and to consider the possible need for a forensic examination.' Guidance from The Royal College of Pathologists [2] also emphasises that this is a vital part of the autopsy.

The images in this chapter are organised in the manner of one starting with initial impressions and then going around the body at the start of an autopsy examination, finishing with changes seen with decomposition:

- Initial impression (Figs. 2.1, 2.2, 2.3, 2.4, 2.5, 2.6, 2.7, 2.8, 2.9, 2.10, 2.11, and 2.12)

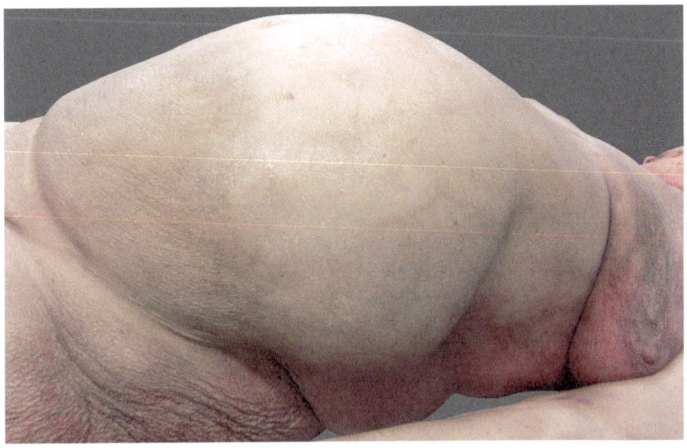

Fig. 2.1 It is important to take a moment for an 'end of the bed assessment' at the beginning of the external examination. In this case, obese body habitus was linked to poor mobility and the finding of deep vein thrombosis and pulmonary embolism

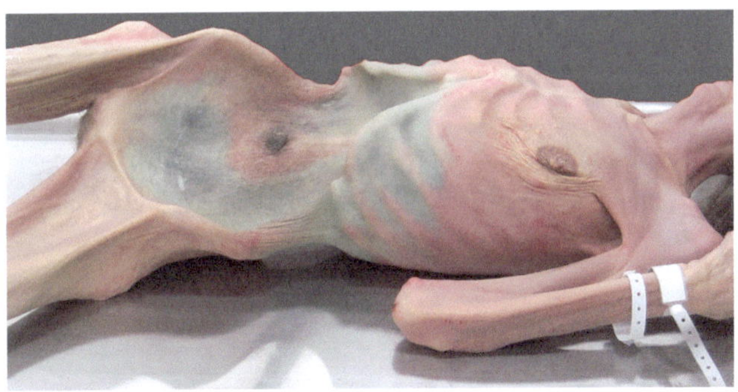

Fig. 2.2 The general state of nutrition can be assessed by looking at the abdomen. This patient is emaciated (cachectic). Note the green skin discoloration, which is an early sign of decomposition

S. Kim Suvarna was deceased at the time of publication.

K. L. Lloyd (✉) · S. K. Suvarna (Deceased)
Department of Histopathology, Sheffield Teaching Hospitals NHS Foundation Trust, Sheffield, UK
e-mail: kirsty.lloyd@nhs.net

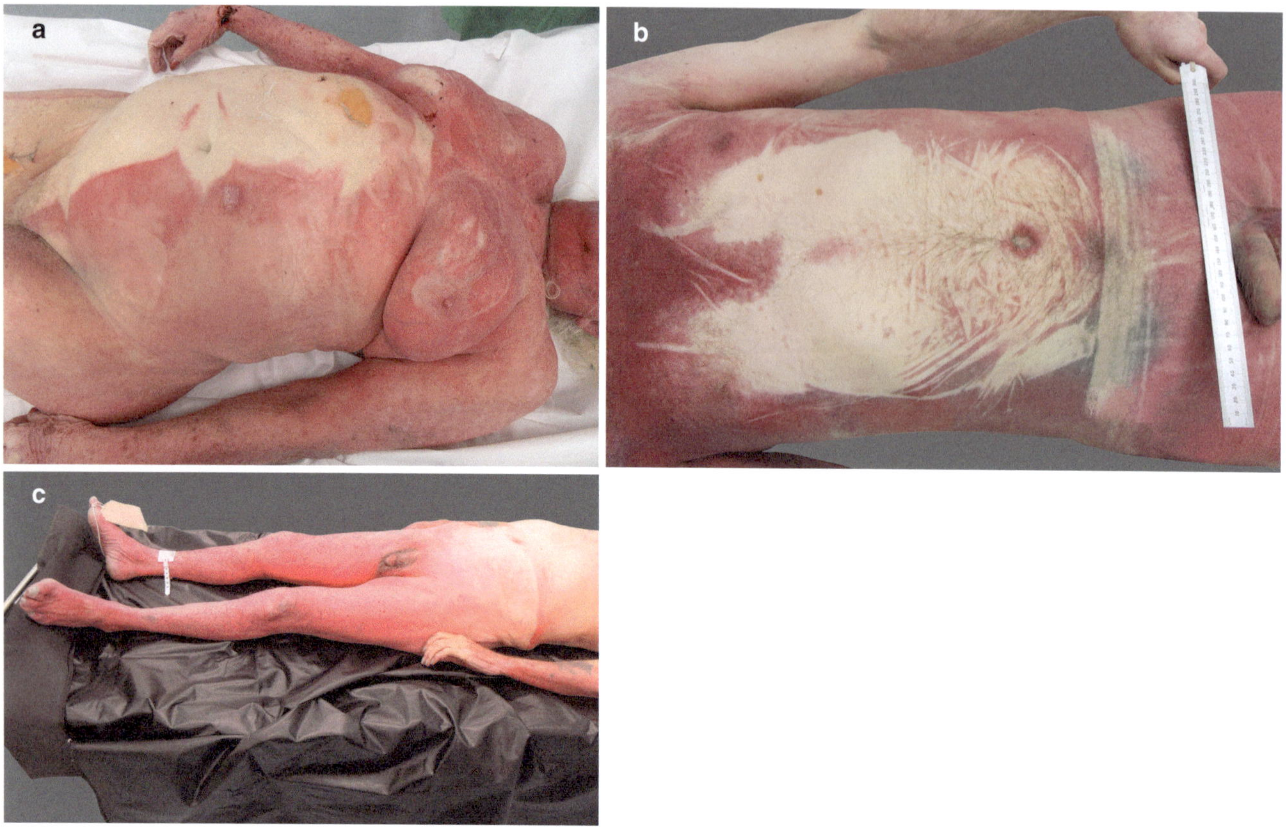

Fig. 2.3 The distribution of hypostasis and lividity can provide information as to the position a person was in when they died. (**a**) In the first image, the spared, pale, area reflects this woman lying on something on her lateral side leaving a 'negative' imprint. Note also the parchment-like area of skin on the upper abdomen which represents a postmortem abrasion, with absence of vital reaction in the tissues. (**b**) The second image shows irregular imprints from clothing/fabric. The waistband of his trousers is readily identifiable. (**c**) The third photograph illustrated pronounced inferiorly distributed lividity over the abdomen and legs in a hanging case where the body was suspended above the ground

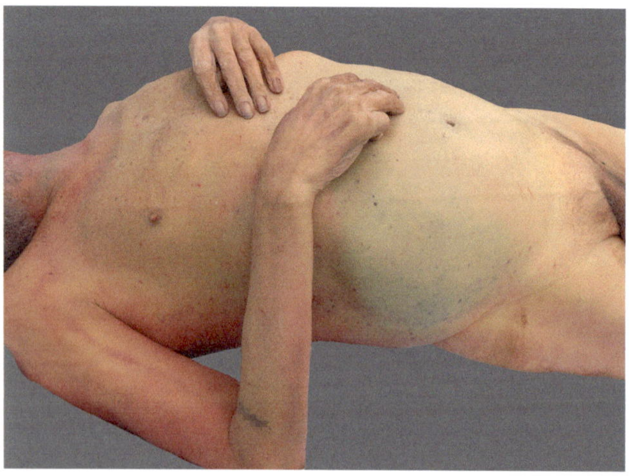

Fig. 2.4 Jaundice is an indicator of hepatobiliary and pancreatic disease. It may be seen in people with decompensated alcoholic liver disease. Jaundice can be challenging to notice in the skin, unless very pronounced, as in this case. Yellow discolouration of the sclera would also be present

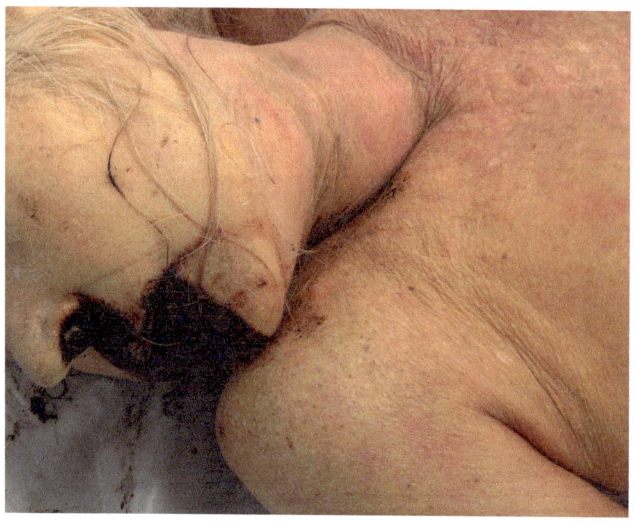

Fig. 2.5 Fluids and material noted around or in the body's natural orifices are useful indicators of internal disease. The dark red/brown material from the mouth represents upper gastrointestinal haemorrhage. Note the accompanying jaundice in the skin. The cause of death was decompensated liver disease with acute upper gastrointestinal haemorrhage

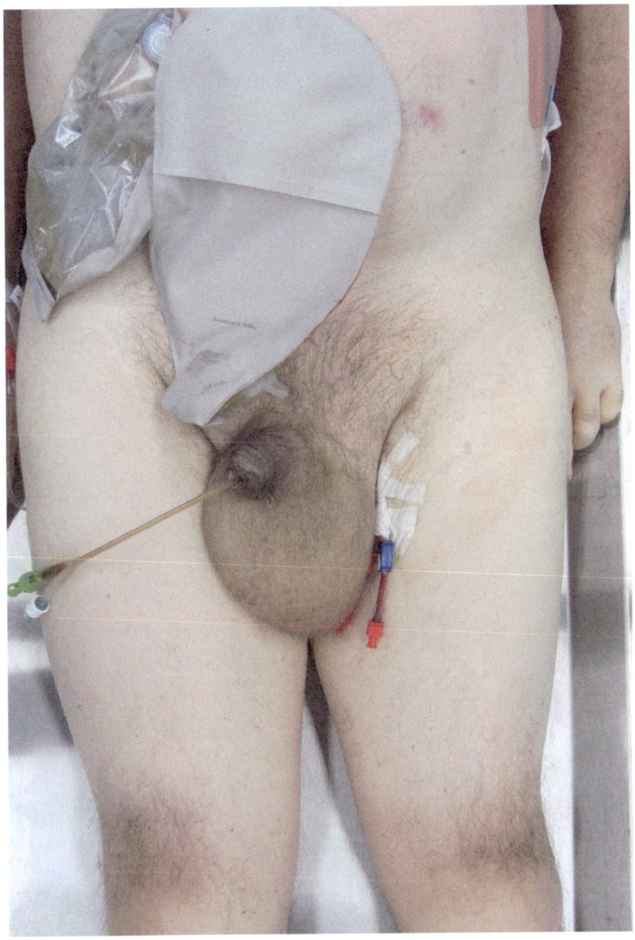

Fig. 2.6 The presence of multiple medical devices points to recent hospital admission and death possibly in a post-operative period. Each device is documented and the approach to internal examination may be modified to suit the circumstances and check device placement. In this case, the grey stoma bag is covering an open surgical wound, rather than stoma. The clear bag in the right upper quadrant is collecting yellow fluid from a drain site and a further drain site is just visible at the left flank. Also seen are a urinary catheter and left femoral arterial line

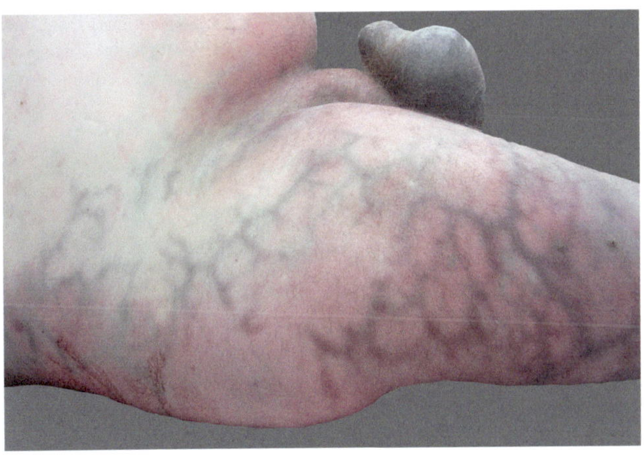

Fig. 2.7 This is pronounced skin marbling from bacterial load in the circulatory system ante-mortem, with subsequent intravascular erythrocyte haemolysis. It can be an indicator of pre-mortem sepsis

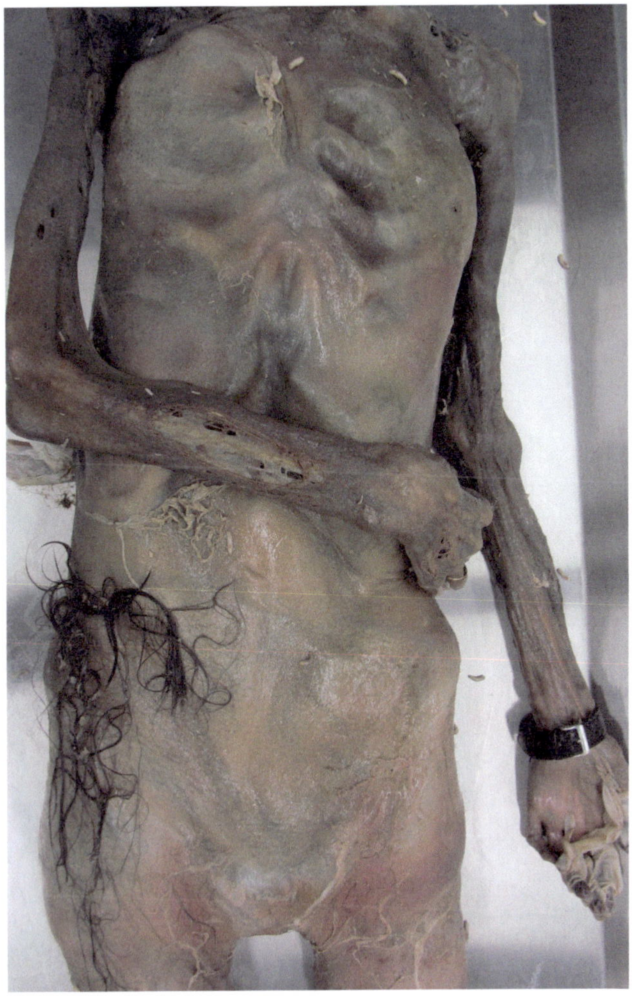

Fig. 2.8 This decomposed body shows generalised putrefaction and skin discolouration. Note the degloving skin slippage of the left hand, and loss of body hair. The hair over the right hip has detached from the scalp. Breakdown of the tissues and maggot infestation leaves small holes in the skin and underlying tissues. The organs can be surprisingly well preserved in this situation. In this case there was evidence of a recent myocardial infarction, myocardial rupture and haemopericardium

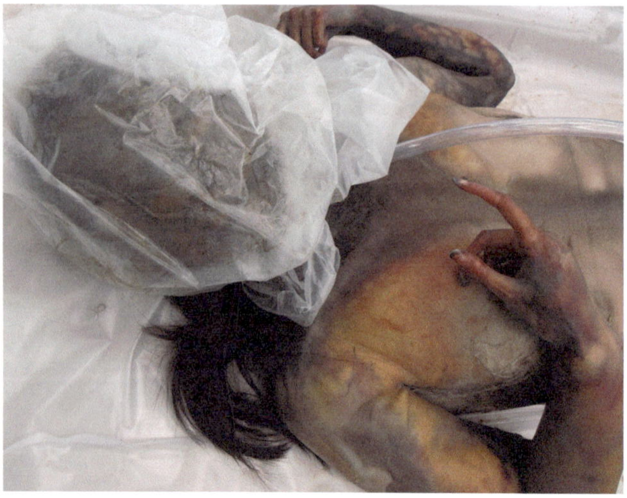

Fig. 2.9 This is an uncommon method of self harm where the plastic bag has enabled suffocation by a noxious gas delivered through the plastic tubing. A risk assessment is necessary, and appropriate hazard protective personal equipment might be needed

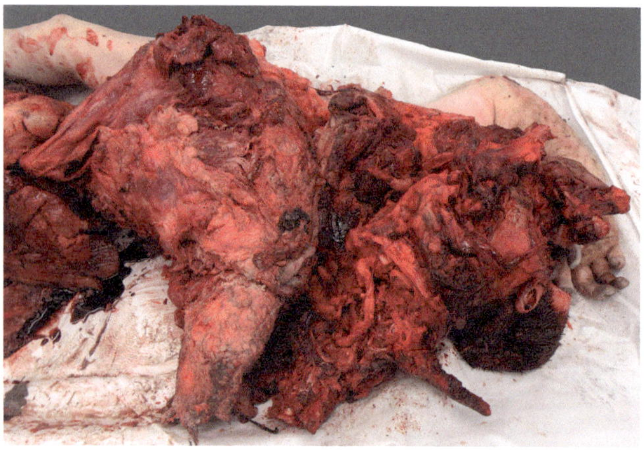

Fig. 2.10 High impact trauma deaths, such as those seen in road traffic or train collisions, are usually reported as due to multiple trauma or multiple injuries. It is still important to document external findings and identify internal organs for tissue sampling. There is unlikely to be blood available for toxicological sampling, necessitating alternative samples, for example using liver tissue or psoas muscle (see Chap. 15)

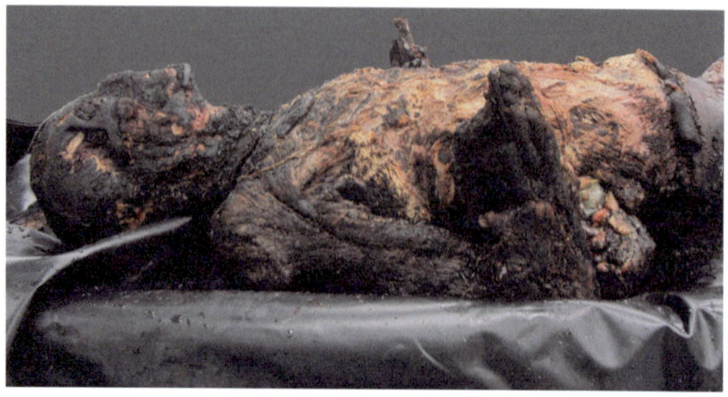

Fig. 2.11 In a fire death, the aim is to establish whether there is evidence that a person died prior to the fire or as a result of the fire. This elderly man died in a shed fire. The complete loss of skin and subcutaneous tissues over the chest is consistent with him falling onto a stove. Note the pugilistic arm posture and loss of the forearm and hand structures. The bowel can be seen protruding from the right flank. Autopsy confirmed acute coronary artery thrombus as the most probable reason for his collapse

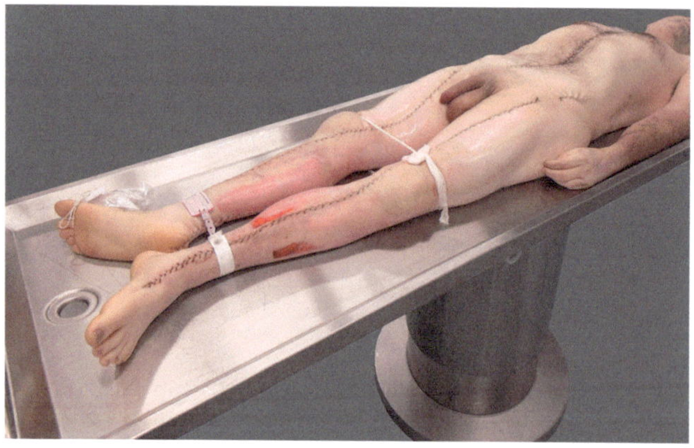

Fig. 2.12 In the UK, the Coroner must give permission for organ donation prior to autopsy examination. Following discussion with the autopsy pathologist (general or forensic) a decision will be made about which, if any, organs can be donated without disrupting the death investigation. The long central incision is used to retrieve the major intrathoracic and intraabdominal organs (heart, lungs, liver, kidneys, pancreas, small bowel). The long incisions over the limbs are for blood vessel and bone retrieval. The pale pink rectangular areas over the calves represent areas of skin retrieval. After corneal retrieval the eyes will contain small plastic shields under the eyelids (not seen)

- Head (Figs. 2.13, 2.14, 2.15, 2.16, 2.17, 2.18, and 2.19)

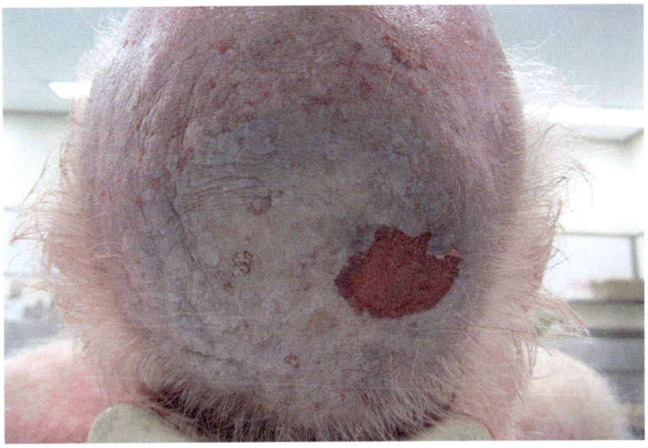

Fig. 2.13 When there is not much hair, scalp injuries are easily visible. Note the lack of vital reaction in the tissues around this injury which was sustained after death when the deceased was moved from the bed where he died onto the floor for attempted CPR. It is important to be aware of the circumstances at the scene, so as not to misinterpret injuries

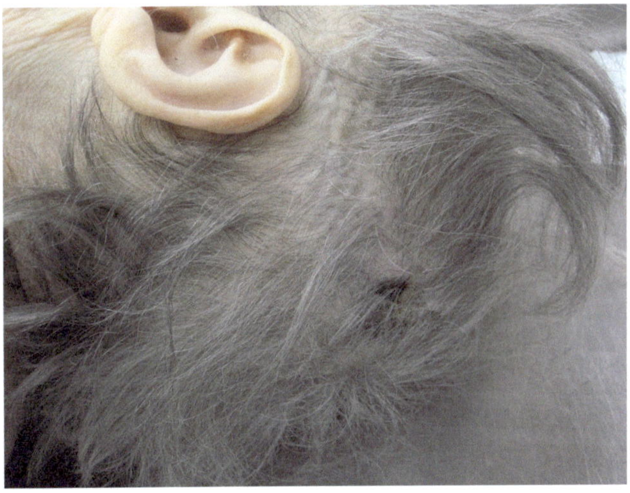

Fig. 2.14 Careful examination of the head can reveal features of prior neurosurgery. Here, palpable and visible in the scalp, is a metal mesh support used to maintain skull integrity after significant injury. The old craniotomy scar was hidden under the hair. This case illustrates the importance of palpating the skull to identify features such as surgical implants or fractures, which may be hidden by hair

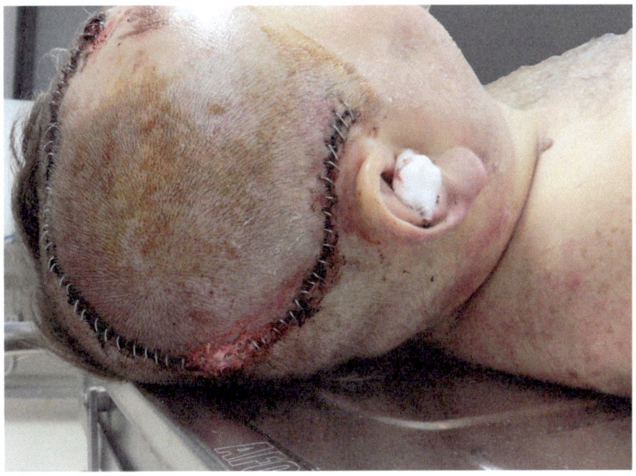

Fig. 2.15 Staple closure over a surgical incision following neurosurgery is shown. This wound is fresh and congealed blood is seen around the staple line

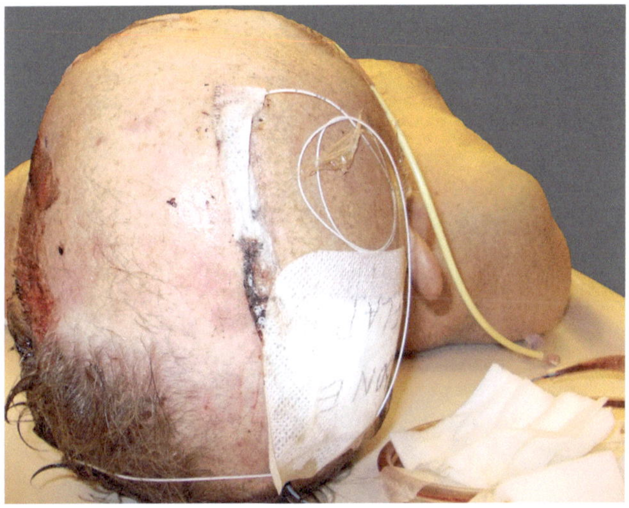

Fig. 2.16 This is an intracranial pressure monitor and ventricular catheter. Part of the wound is visible and healing. The dressings are removed but the catheter remains in place

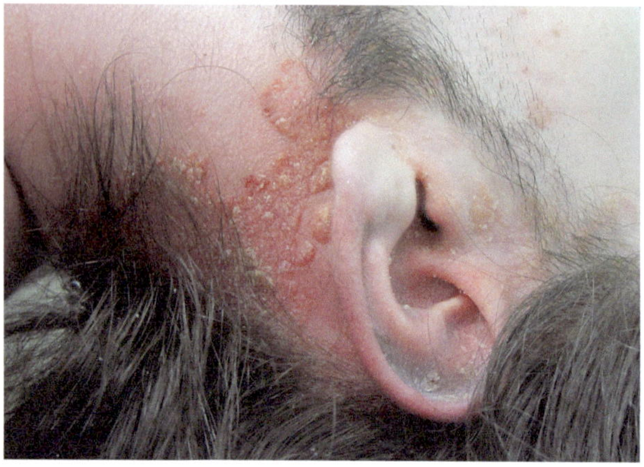

Fig. 2.17 Skin conditions may manifest on the head. Psoriasis usually presents with symmetrically distributed, red, scaly plaques with well-defined edges. The scale is typically silvery white, except in skin folds where the plaques often appear shiny with a moist peeling surface. The most common sites are the scalp, elbows, and knees, but any part of the skin can be involved. Whilst unlikely to be the cause of death, skin changes can be linked to systemic disorders and drug treatments (*e.g.*, biological therapies) that may be relevant

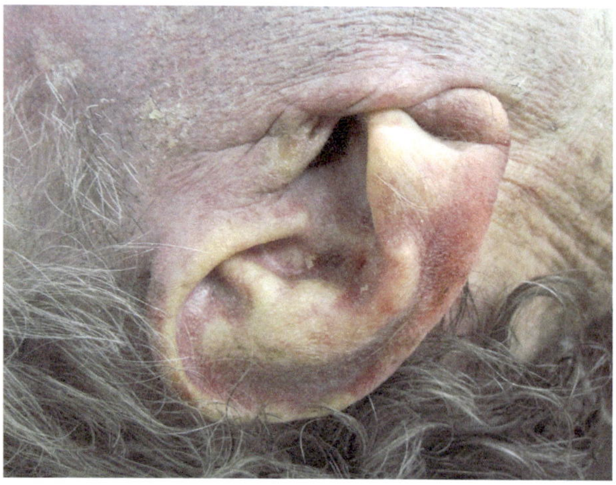

Fig. 2.18 Diagonal earlobe creases are considered a potential indicator of coronary artery disease and cardiovascular causes of death [13–15]

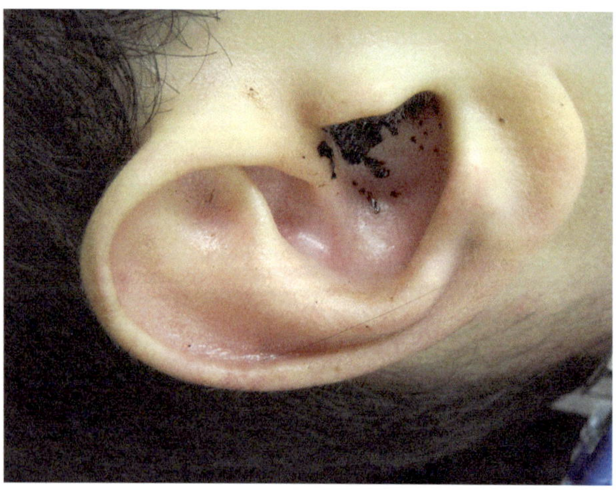

Fig. 2.19 Cerebrospinal fluid and/or blood in the external auditory meatus often indicates a basal skull fracture. However, one must check that the blood has not come from a facial or scalp wound

- Face (Figs. 2.20, 2.21, 2.22, 2.23, 2.24, 2.25, 2.26, 2.27, 2.28, 2.29, 2.30, 2.31, 2.32, 2.33, 2.34, 2.35, 2.36, and 2.37)

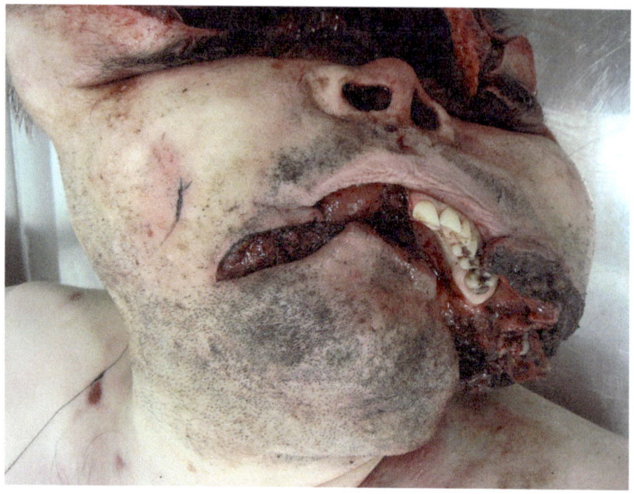

Fig. 2.20 Face trauma is shown here. Injury resulting from high-velocity accidents leads to loss of skin, soft tissue, and skeletal integrity

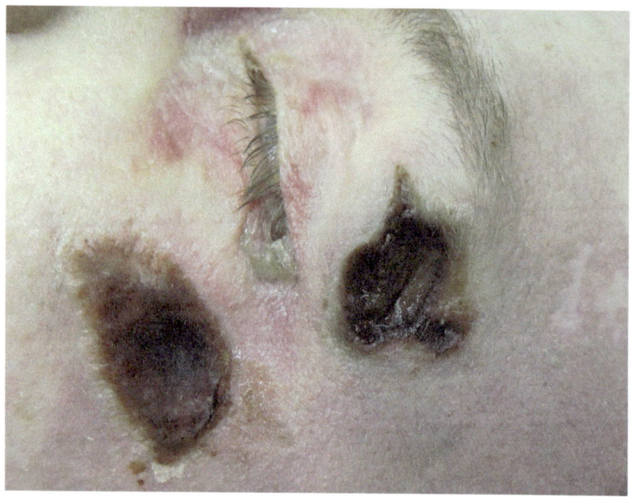

Fig. 2.21 The face may show signs of injury. These pressure areas over bony prominences occurred after death. One notes that the edges of the lesions lack vital skin reaction, confirming post-mortem injury

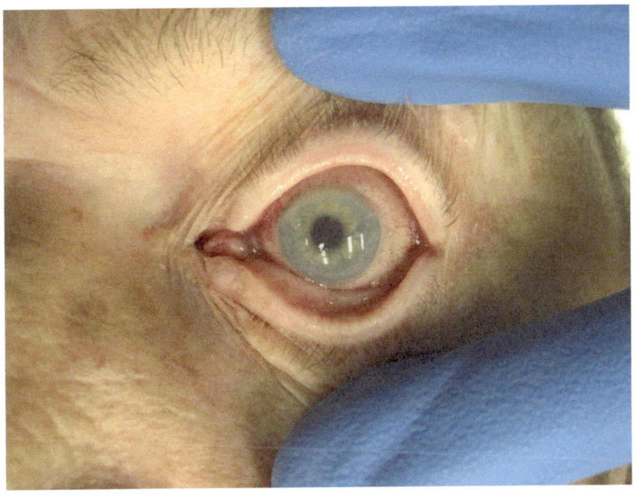

Fig. 2.22 The skin around the eye, the iris, conjunctiva and sclera are examined for haemorrhages or jaundice. The eyelids need to be partly retracted

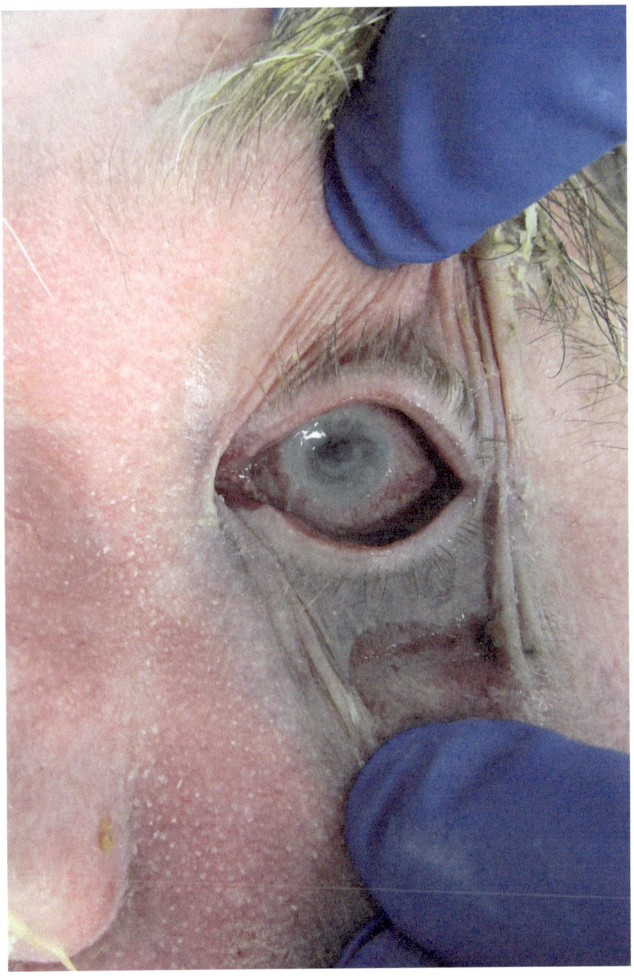

Fig. 2.23 The eyelids are retracted to examine the conjunctiva, which in this case reveals prominent capillaries, usually described as 'suffused'. This finding is commonly noted in cases of respiratory and cardiac arrest

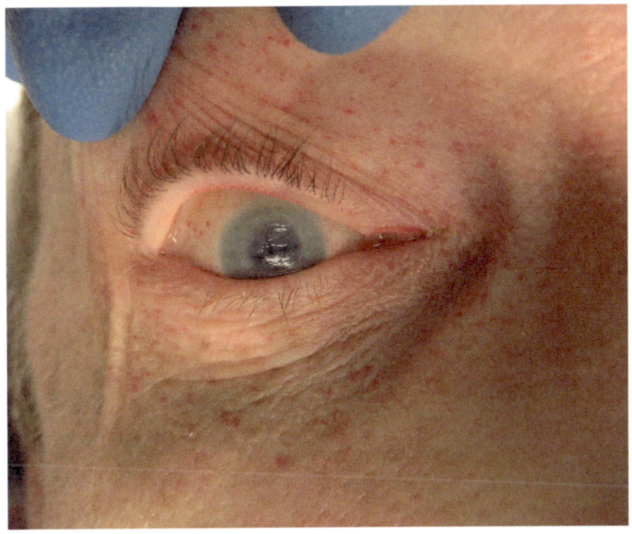

Fig. 2.24 The rupture of small capillaries may cause petechial haemorrhages, seen here in the sclera and periocular skin. They are associated with venous overpressure and may reflect severe coughing or asphyxia due to respiratory disease or cardiac arrest

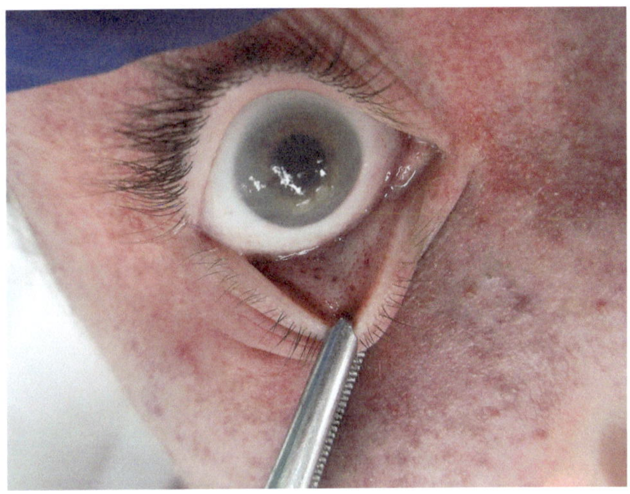

Fig. 2.25 The eyelids are retracted to examine the conjunctiva, which in this case reveals petechial haemorrhages noted in a hanging case

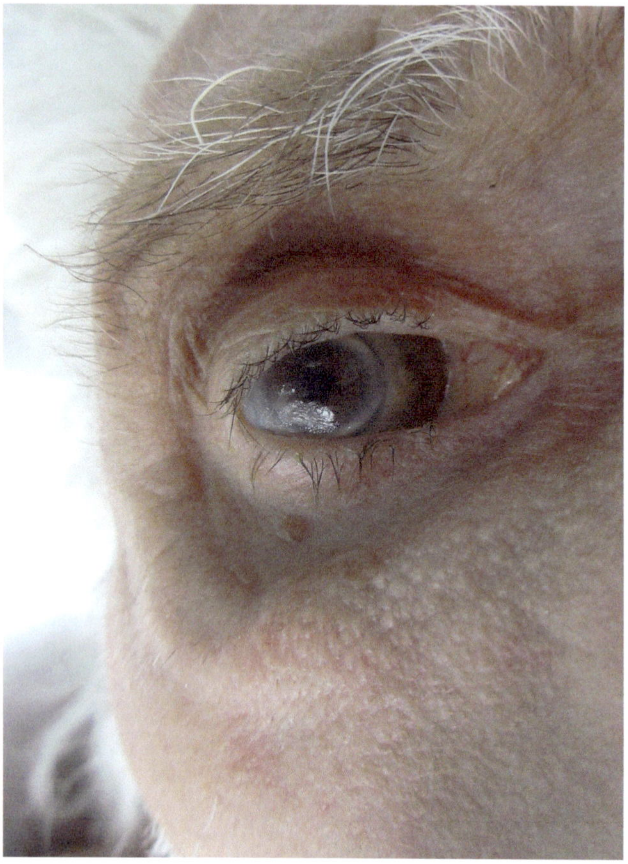

Fig. 2.26 Systemic diseases can manifest in the eye. Corneal arcus (arcus senilis) is deposition of lipid in the peripheral cornea. It is generally considered a feature of the normal ageing process and is to be expected in the elderly patient. In a person under the age of 50, this finding may have more significance

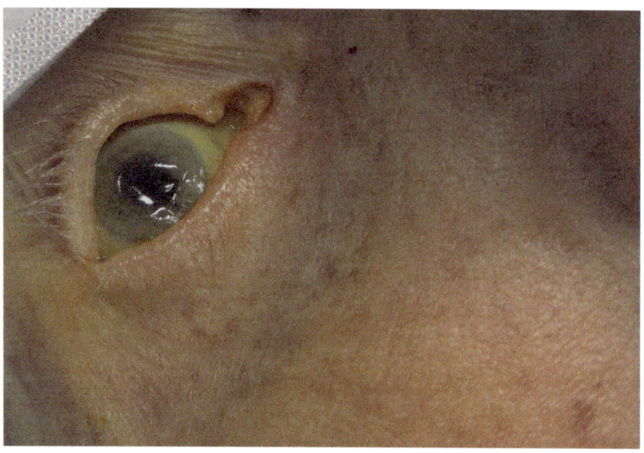

Fig. 2.27 Yellow discolouration of the sclera due to jaundice

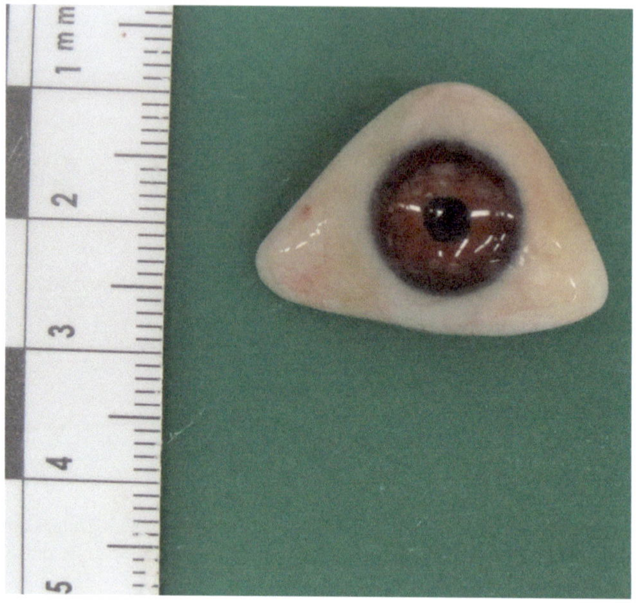

Fig. 2.28 False eye. It is not necessary to remove prostheses, but it is important to identify this, if present

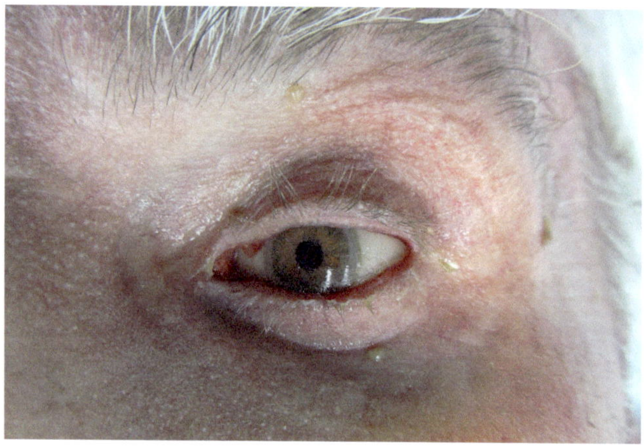

Fig. 2.29 Here is another example of a false eye. Modern prosthetic eyes are excellently matched to the natural eye, and careful comparison is recommended

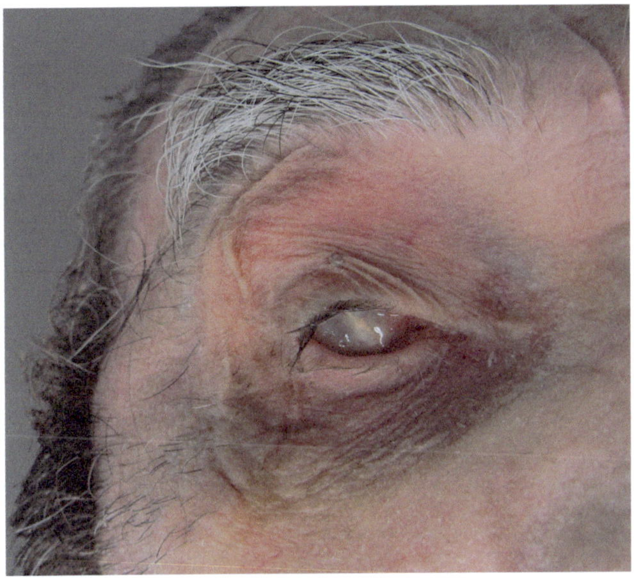

Fig. 2.30 This is a non-functioning, or phthisical, eye. The background history to account for this finding was not available in the medical records

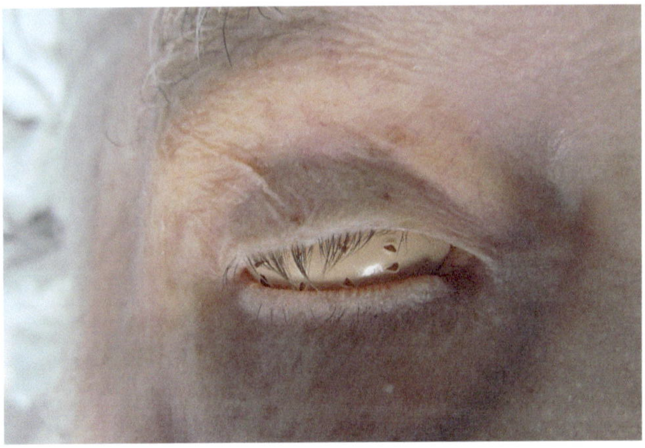

Fig. 2.31 An eye cap has been inserted underneath the eyelids to maintain the rounded contour of a normal eye and to keep the eyelids from opening. Such caps might be placed following corneal donation or by funeral directors

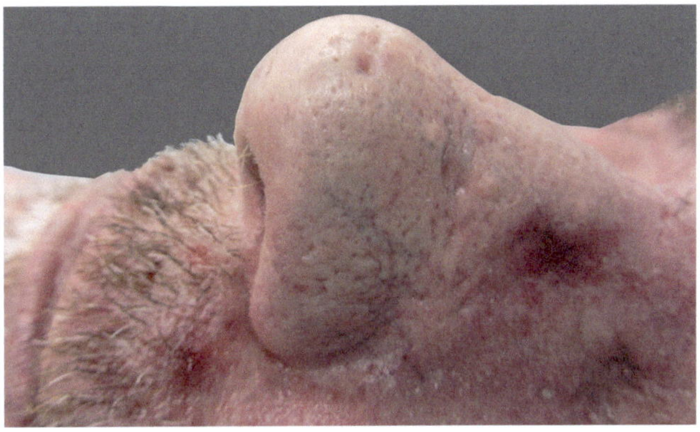

Fig. 2.32 False clues: This man has features of rhinophyma, a disfiguring nasal deformity due to the proliferation of sebaceous glands and underlying connective tissue. There is a commonly presumed link to excessive alcohol use. However, the direct causal relationship between rhinophyma and alcohol has not been substantiated and it is a result of rosacea

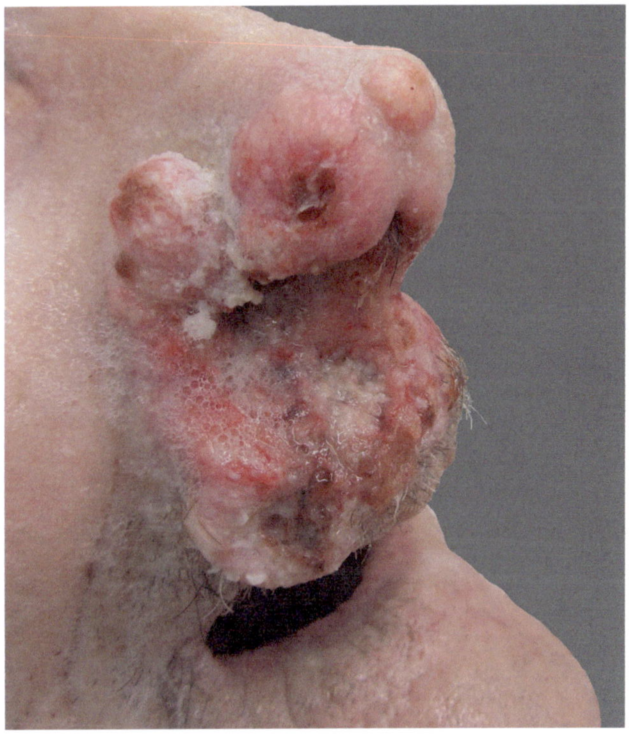

Fig. 2.33 The skin is examined for tumours: the site, size and appearance are recorded. This is a recurrent nasal squamous carcinoma showing local recurrence affecting the tissues of the nose

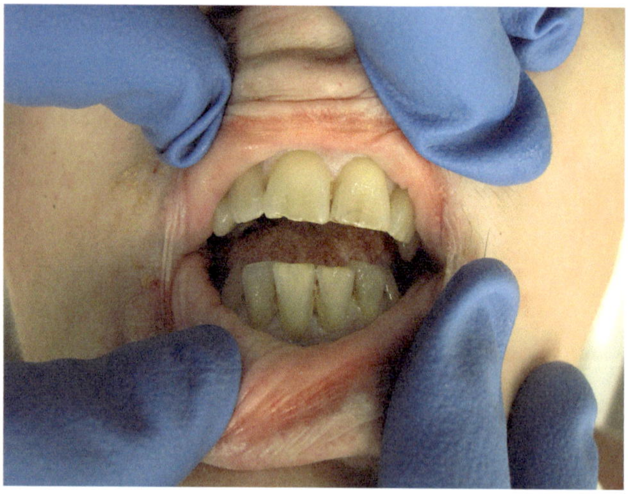

Fig. 2.34 The presence and condition of teeth or dentures is recorded. Loose-fitting dentures may be a feature of weight loss

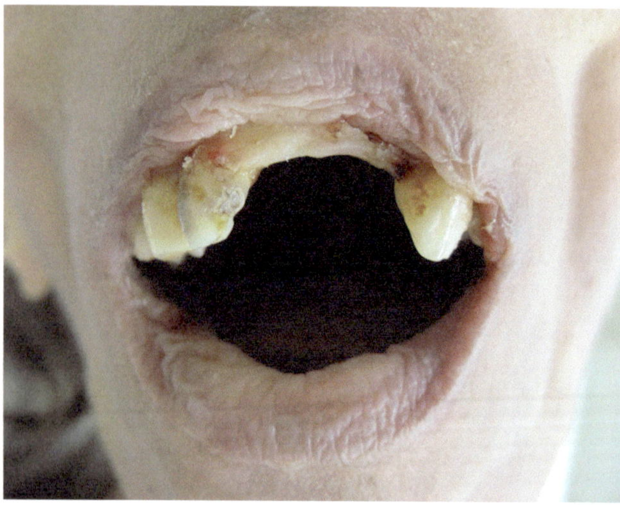

Fig. 2.35 Severe dental caries is a source of bacteremia and can cause generalised sepsis and endocarditis

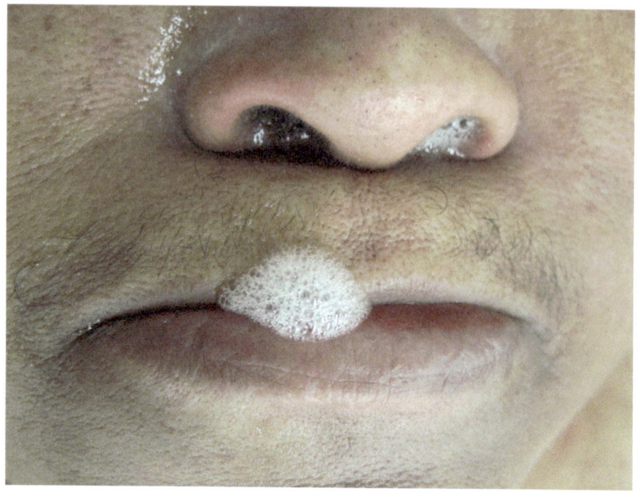

Fig. 2.36 There is frothy fluid in the nose and mouth of this patient who died of acute left ventricular failure. With drowning, a frothy 'plume' is also often seen in the oropharynx. There may be some blood staining

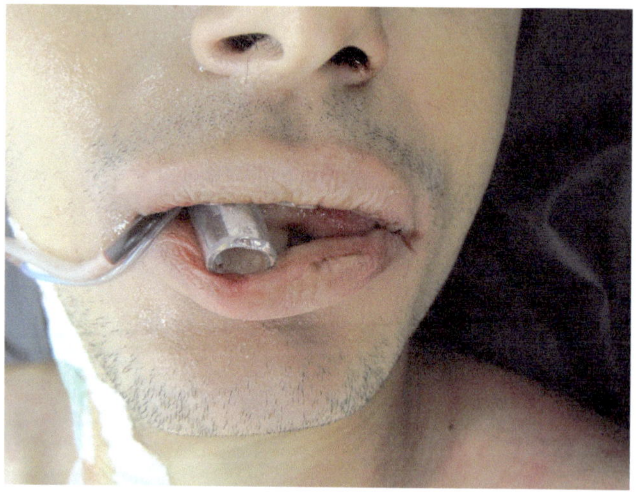

Fig. 2.37 The end of an endotracheal tube has been trimmed to aid evisceration. Note that the narrow, clear inflating tube remains intact to help prevent the tube from becoming dislodged

- Neck (Figs. 2.38, 2.39, 2.40, 2.41, 2.42, 2.43, 2.44, 2.45, 2.46, 2.47, and 2.48)

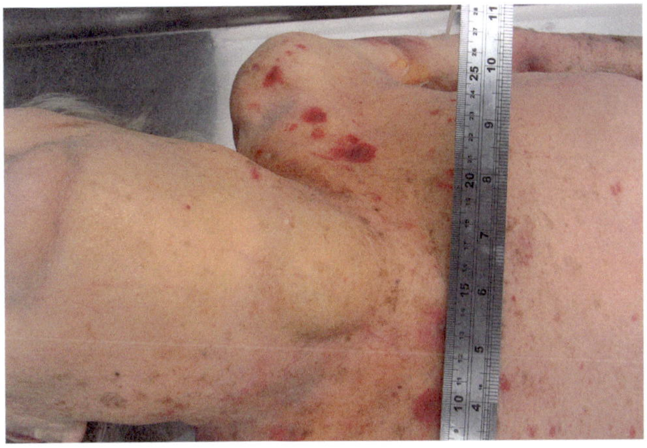

Fig. 2.38 The neck is visually inspected and palpated for masses (thyroid gland, cysts, lymph nodes). A large goitre, seen here, usually represents benign disease but may have implications on the patient's swallowing and/or respiratory function. Unilateral enlargement of the cervical glands prompts careful examination of the throat, and hard immobile nodes may indicate underlying metastatic malignancy

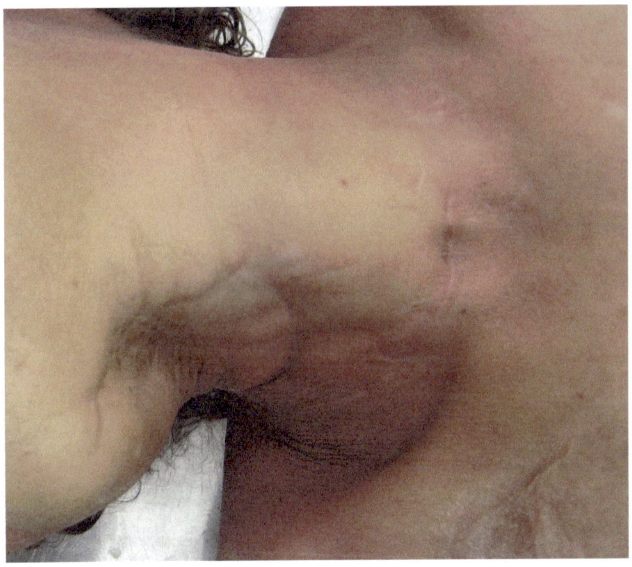

Fig. 2.39 The large area of surgical scarring with underlying loss of tissue is due to a radical neck dissection for head and neck cancer. Note the healed tracheostomy scar in the midline

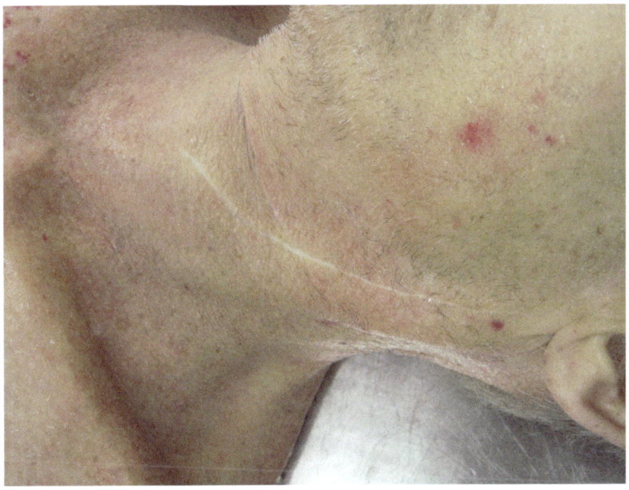

Fig. 2.40 Carotid surgery. Shown here is a surgical scar in the anterior triangle of the neck, due to carotid atheromatous disease surgery

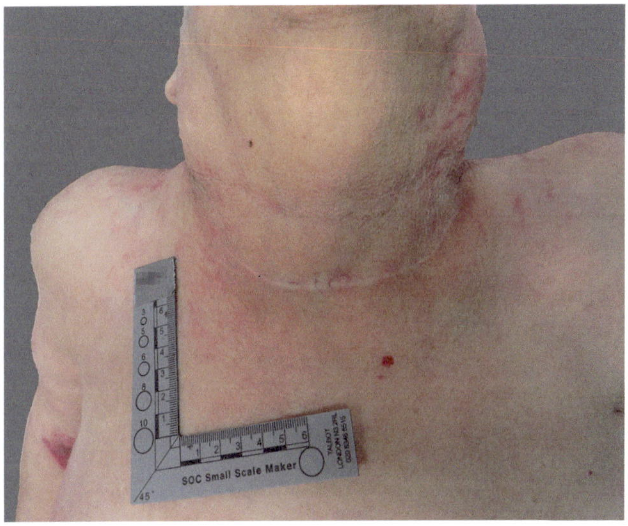

Fig. 2.41 A transverse scar at the base of the neck is often due to thyroid surgery

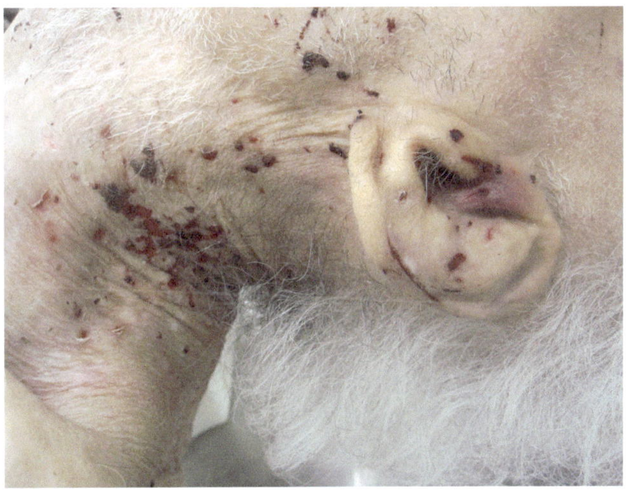

Fig. 2.42 Scratch marks may reflect a confused state of delirium or dementia, pruritus, or skin infestation

Fig. 2.43 Carbon monoxide poisoning without burn injury is shown. The cherry red discolouration of carbon monoxide poisoning is most pronounced in the neck and upper chest of this person, indicating that he was alive during the time when the fire was active nearby

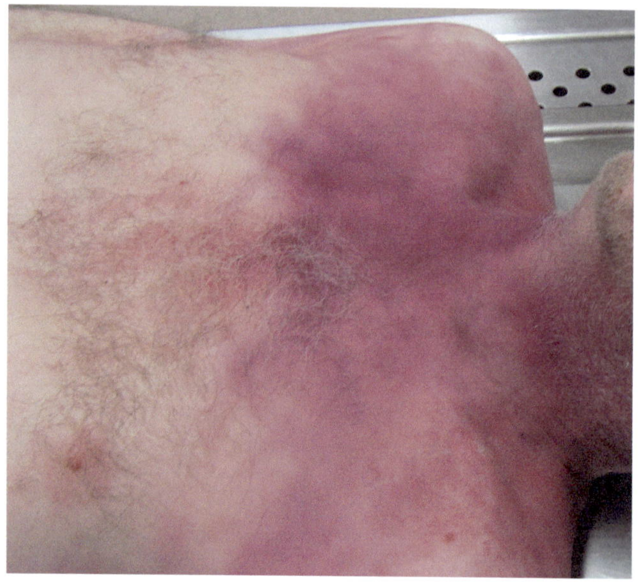

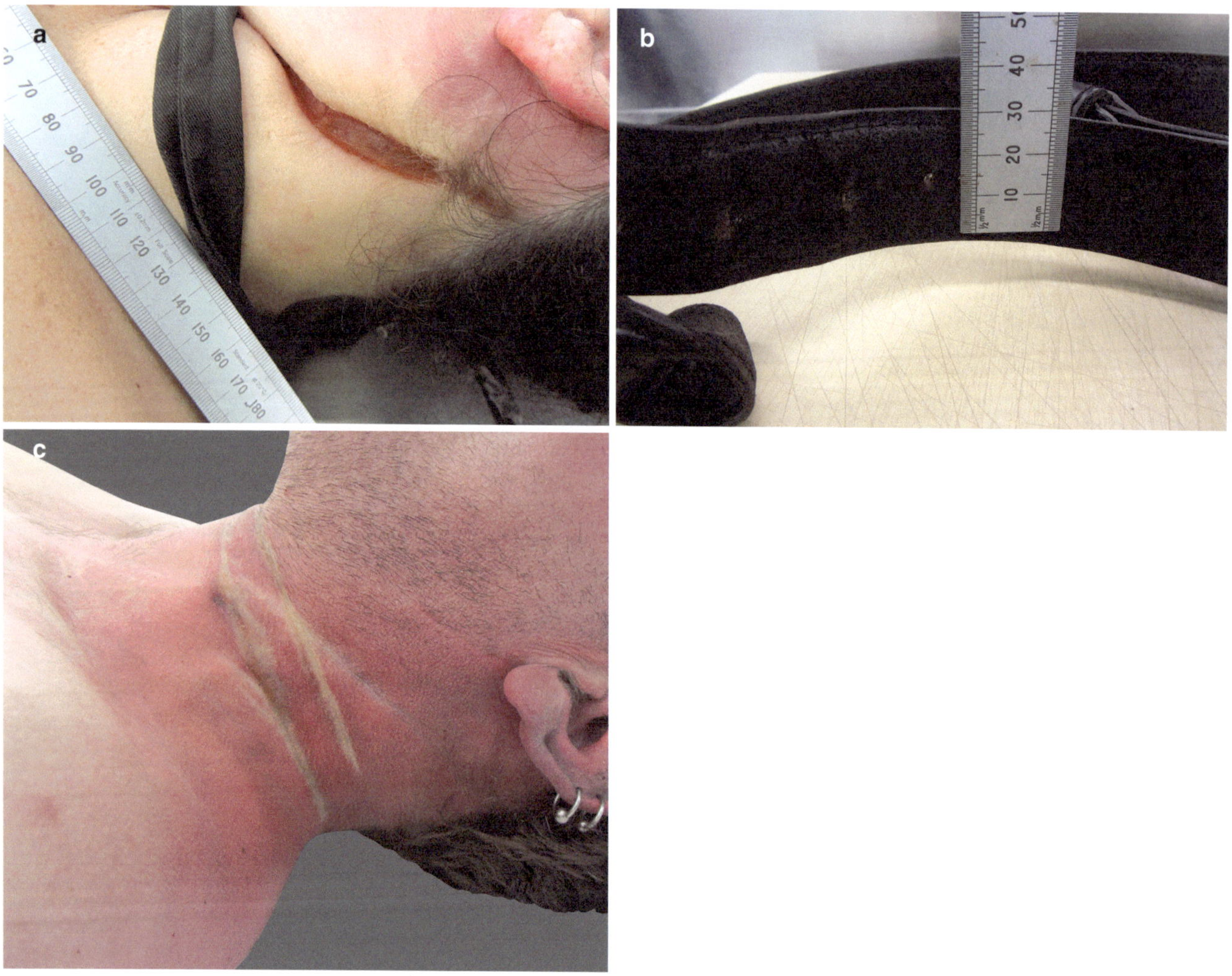

Fig. 2.44 (**a**–**c**) Noose-type ligatures around the neck must be documented before removal, with subsequent examination of the ligature mark after the noose is removed (see also Chap. 12)

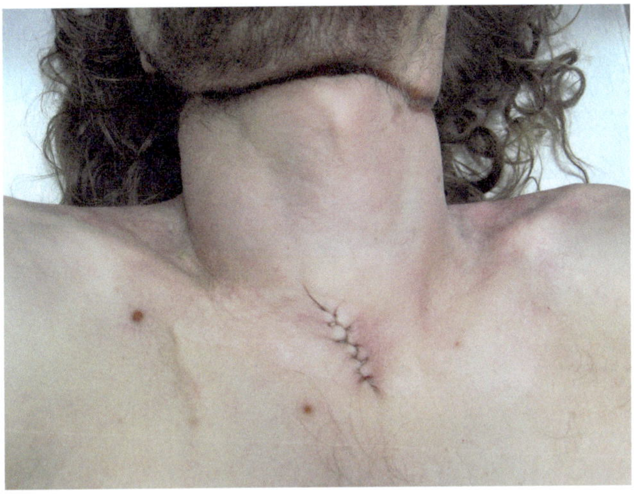

Fig. 2.45 Ligature mark and embalming incision. Following removal, the marks made in the high neck by the ligature in a case of hanging can be examined. This case also shows a sutured low neck incision from embalming

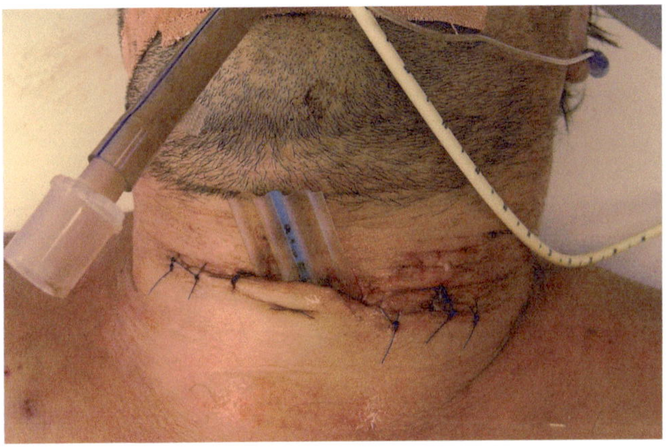

Fig. 2.46 Self-inflicted neck wounds. Several initial incised wounds and a deeper cut are seen here on the neck, alongside evidence of surgical intervention. A corrugated drain is present, as well as sutures. Endotracheal and nasogastric tubes are also present

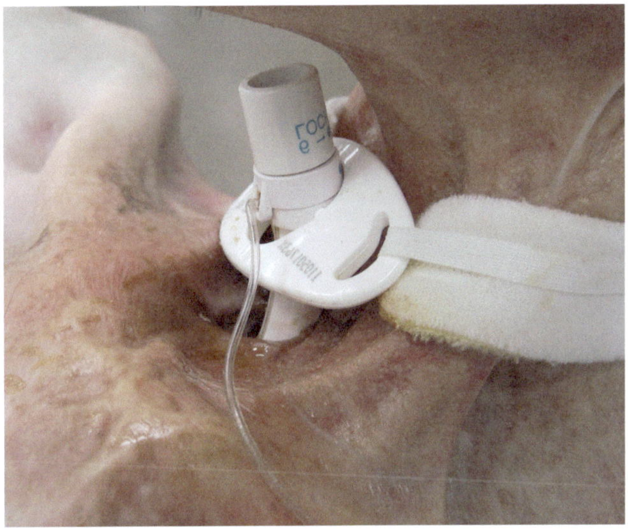

Fig. 2.47 Tracheostomy tube. These tubes have an outer cannula with an inflatable cuff and inner cannula that can be removed for cleaning. The device is often removed prior to evisceration, making sure to examine the tube and distal end for obstruction (mucus, inflammatory matter, tumour, etc.)

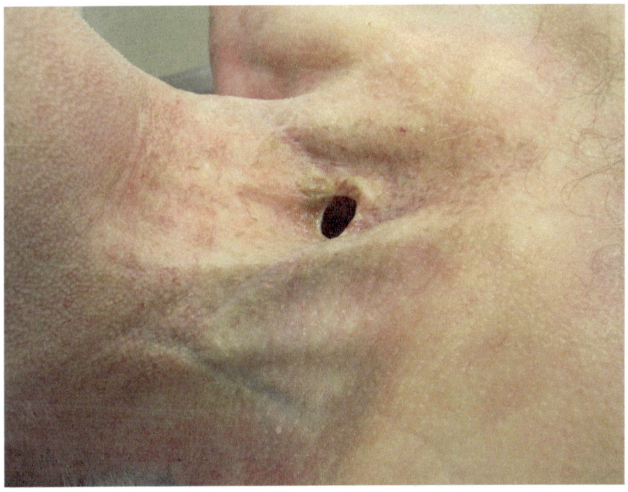

Fig. 2.48 A surgical airway (tracheostomy) may be seen in patients for a wide number of underlying conditions, both acute and chronic. Fistula formation between the posterior tracheal wall and the oesophagus can occur in long-standing tracheostomies

- Upper limbs (Figs. 2.49, 2.50, 2.51, 2.52, 2.53, 2.54, 2.55, 2.56, 2.57, 2.58, 2.59, 2.60, and 2.61)

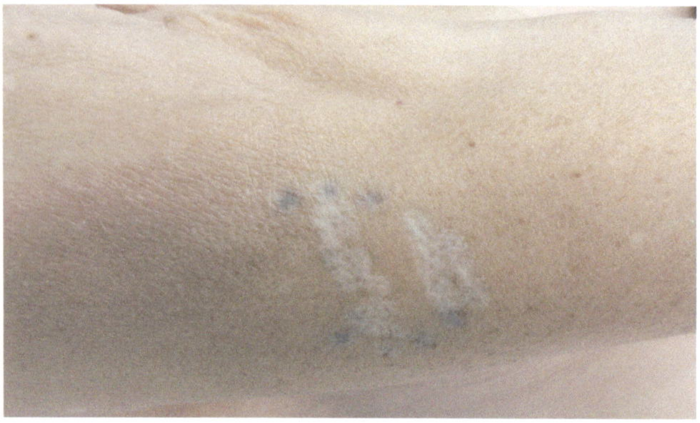

Fig. 2.49 Tattoo removal. Laser removal of tattoos is noted as pallor and scarring of the skin; some residual pigment is seen

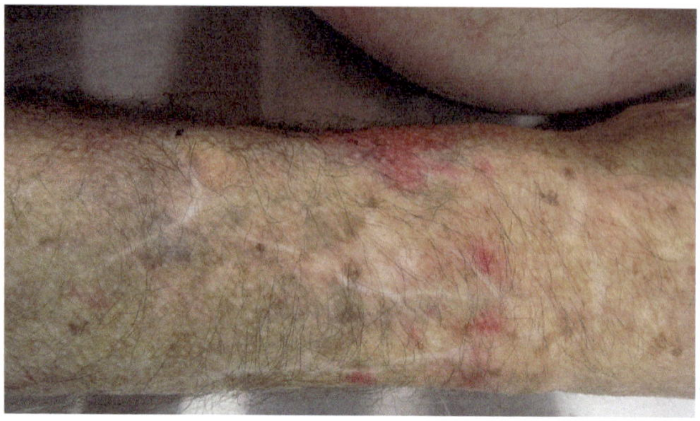

Fig. 2.50 Old injuries, with irregularly distributed scars of previous traumatic injury, which may include healed skin tears

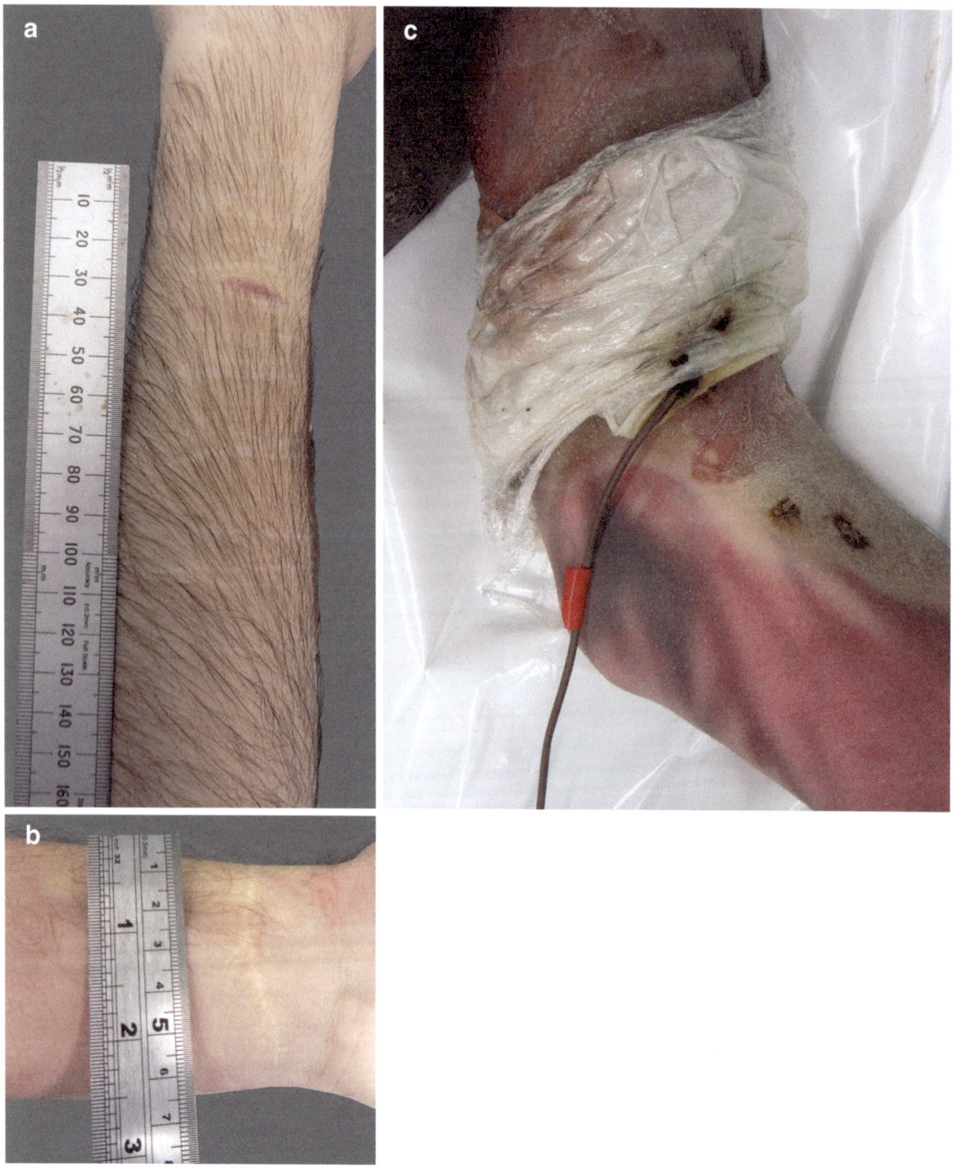

Fig. 2.51 Self-harm injury. Multiple, superficial, parallel incisions are indicative of self-harming. They can be found anywhere, but the upper limbs, thighs, abdomen and breasts are more common. The limbs need to be examined carefully as body fluids, hair and tattoos can mask old injuries (Image **a**). The injury in image (**b**) has features of surgical scarring suggestive of surgical repair. Other types of injury may be self-inflicted, such as burns or insertion of foreign objects such as broken glass. In the case shown in image (**c**), this man connected wires to his body to take his life via electrocution

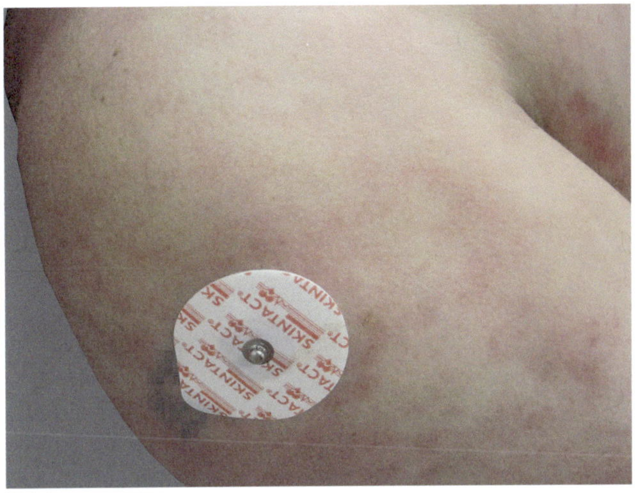

Fig. 2.52 ECG stickers are often placed on all four limbs and around the chest. They should be removed and discarded at the start of the autopsy. This sticker is overlying a tattoo which has been blurred

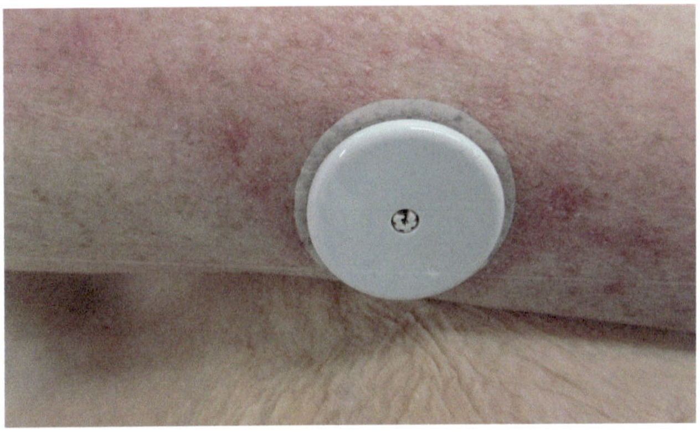

Fig. 2.53 This is a continuous glucose monitor used by people with insulin dependent diabetes mellitus

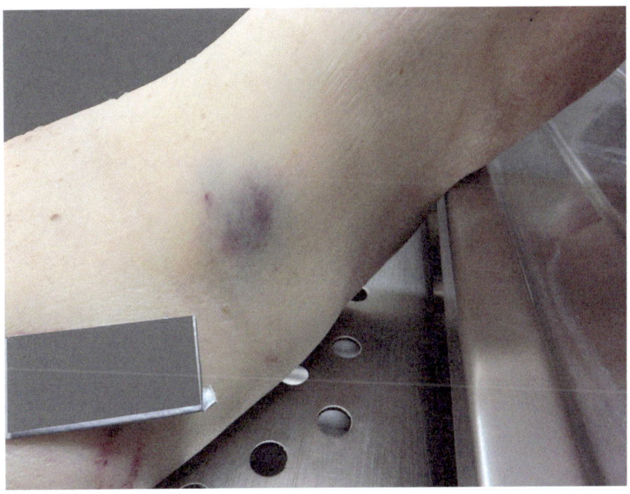

Fig. 2.54 Venepuncture marks are often associated with localised bruising

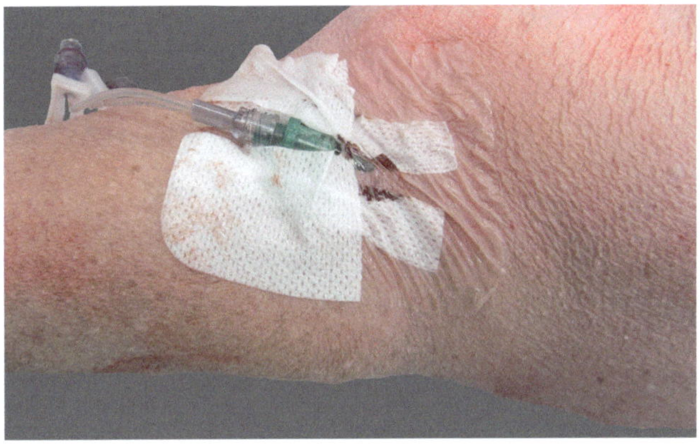

Fig. 2.55 Intravenous cannulas are often found in the upper limb. If the patient has spent some time in hospital, there may be previous sites showing bruising and or swelling

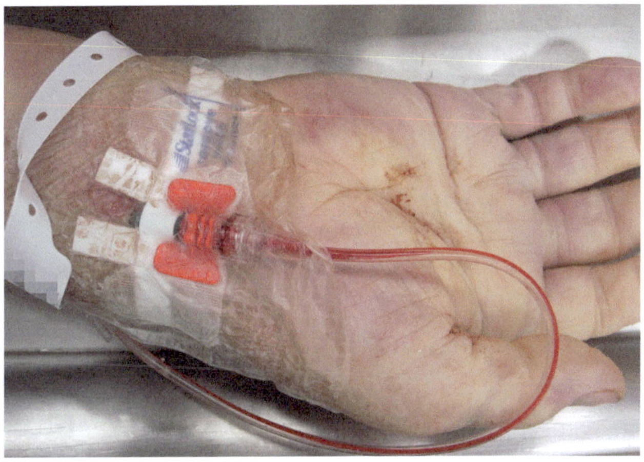

Fig. 2.56 Arterial lines can be placed in any accessible artery. The catheter tube has a red stripe along the surface to indicate to clinical staff that it is an arterial line. Superficial lines are removed and discarded prior to evisceration, if the pathologist is satisfied the placement was correct

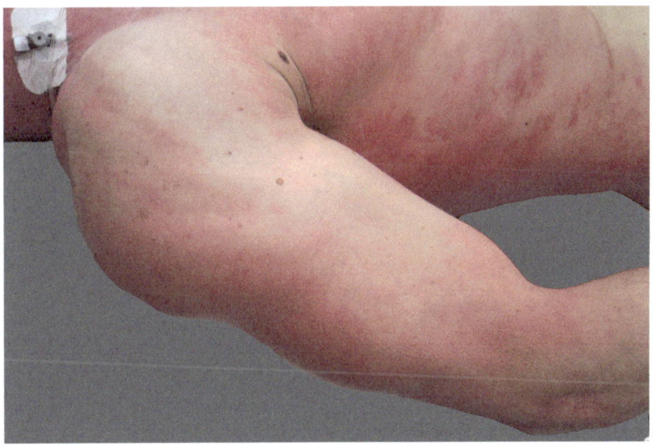

Fig. 2.57 The limbs are good for assessing physical build. Increased muscle bulk may be due to general athleticism, or potentially to anabolic steroid use. A venous line is noted in the neck, used during the attempted resuscitation

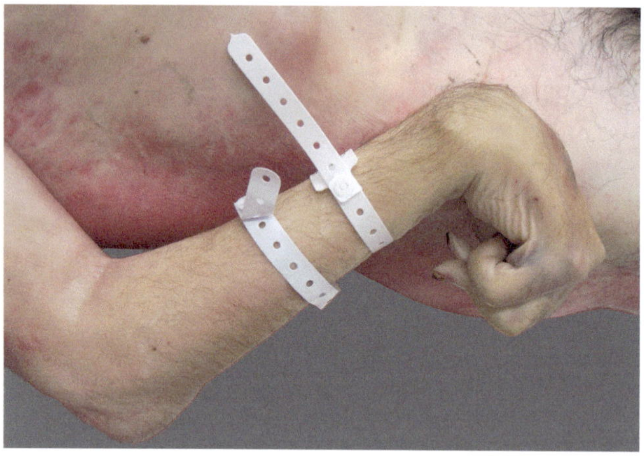

Fig. 2.58 Neurological disease may be assessed externally, with this abnormal limb posture often seen following a cerebrovascular event, resulting in an upper motor neuron lesion

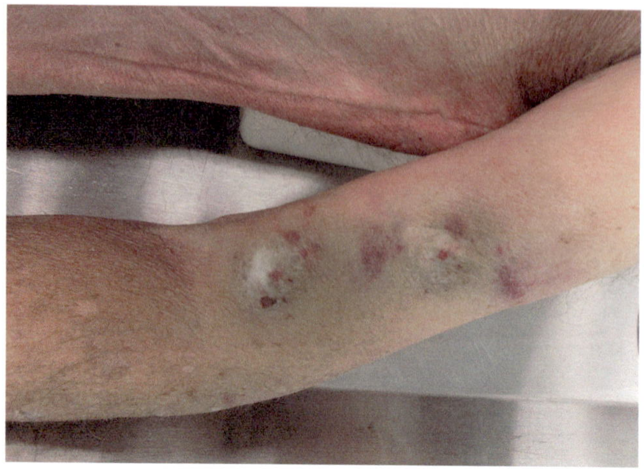

Fig. 2.60 A renal dialysis fistula and associated scarring from repeated use

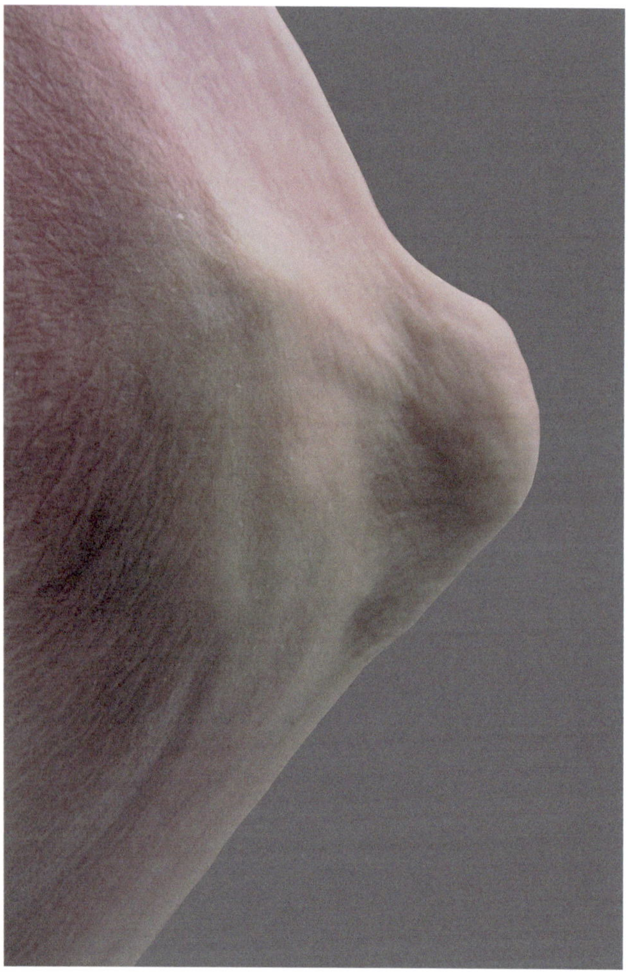

Fig. 2.59 Olecranon bursitis has possible associations with acute trauma, repetitive injury, systemic inflammatory processes, or crystal deposition. This was noted along with multiple other joint deformities in a patient with gout

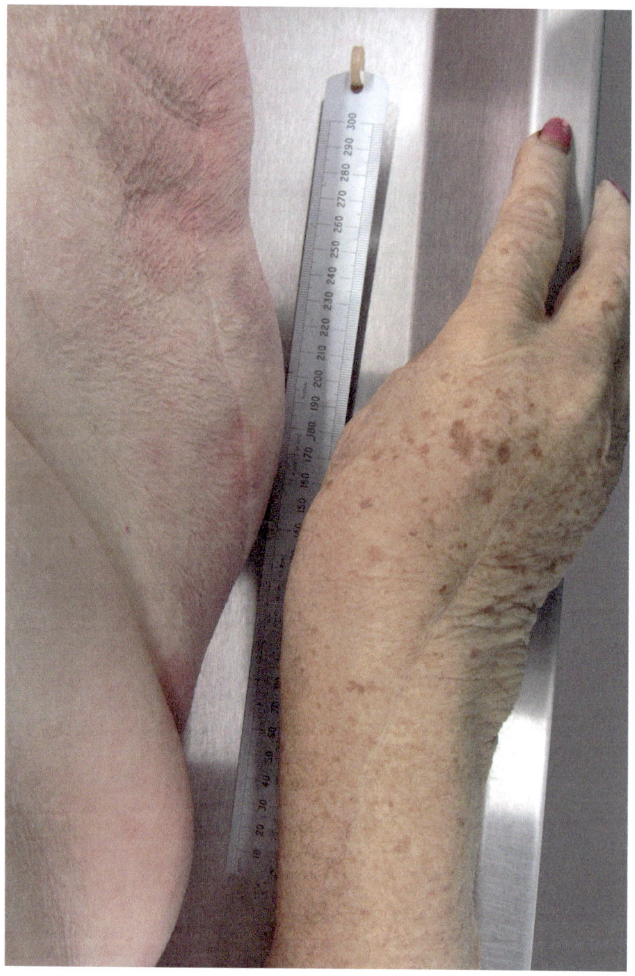

Fig. 2.61 Joint scars. Hip and wrist scars are present, indicating previous surgery related to inflammatory arthropathy and prompting a review of the drug treatment history. In such cases, consideration of external and internal manifestations of the disease and side effects of steroids, biological treatments and disease-modifying anti-rheumatic drugs is important

- Hands (Figs. 2.62, 2.63, 2.64, 2.65, 2.66, 2.67, 2.68, 2.69, 2.70, and 2.71)

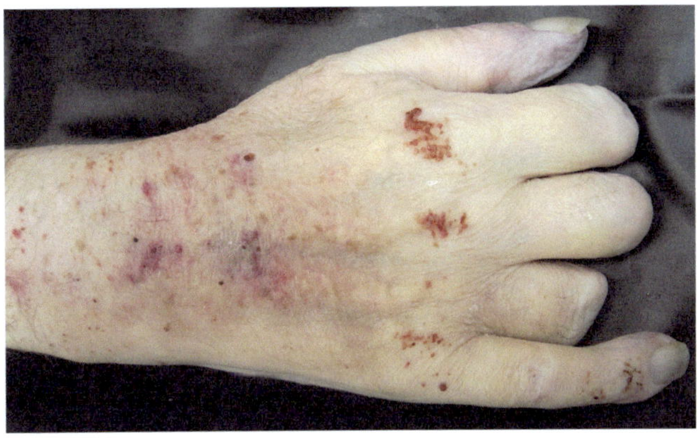

Fig. 2.62 The hands are common sites for injury, which may be incidental or due to the circumstances surrounding death. This degree of damage reflected a workplace accident many years previously

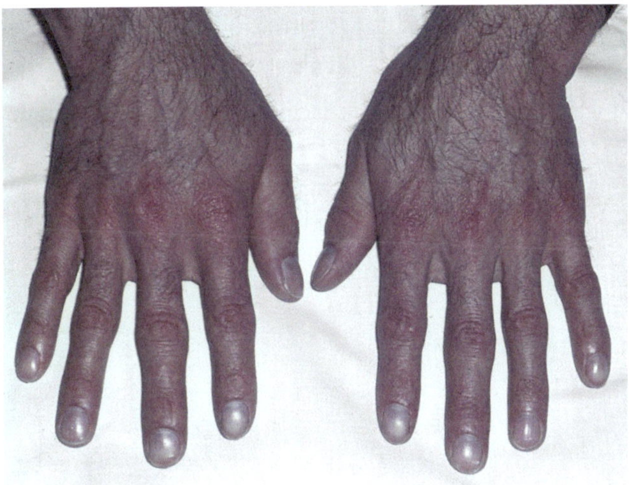

Fig. 2.63 This ante-mortem image depicts argyria. This unusual blue/grey discolouration of the skin is due to exposure to silver-containing preparations

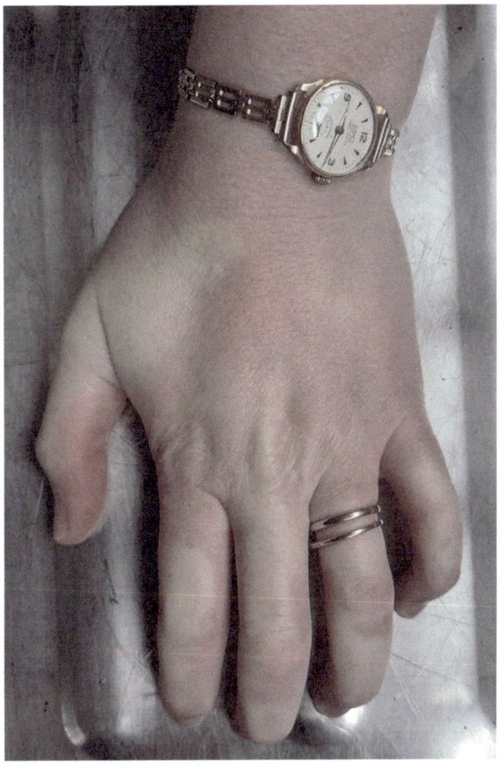

Fig. 2.64 Assumptions regarding the nature of jewellery should be avoided. It is best to describe watches and jewellery as "yellow metal" rather than gold

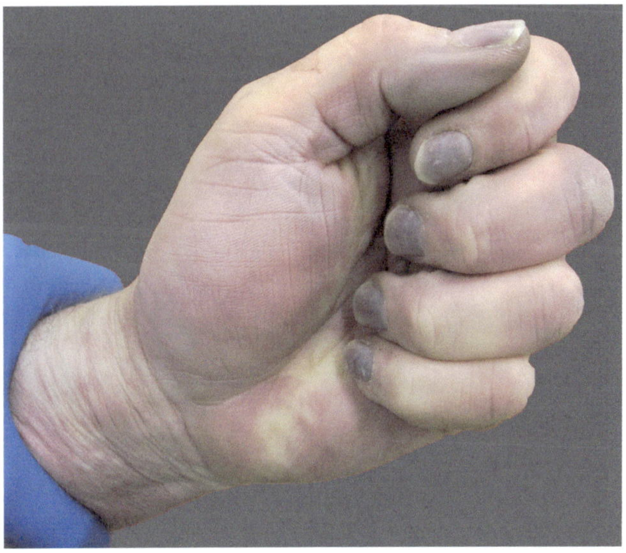

Fig. 2.65 The nails often have a dusky appearance after death, which should not be over-interpreted as peripheral cyanosis

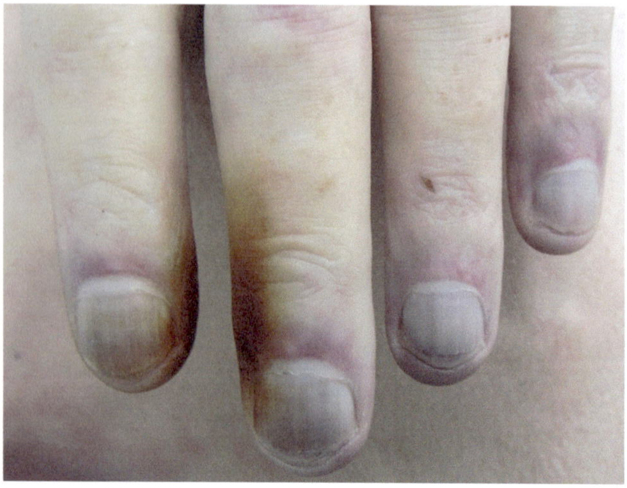

Fig. 2.66 Not all cigarette smokers get tar-stained fingers. However, when present, it is usually an indication of heavy smoking

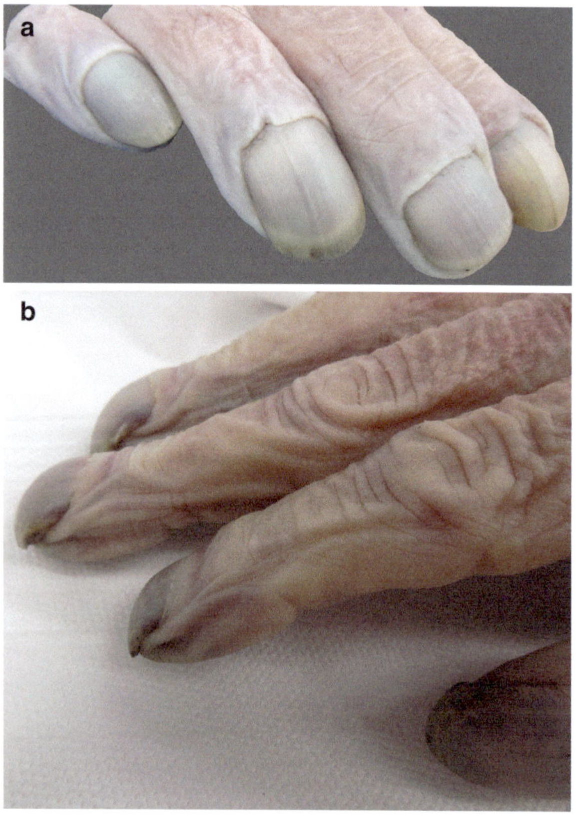

Fig. 2.67 (**a**, **b**) Digital clubbing may be idiopathic or associated with a variety of clinical conditions including bronchiectasis, lung cancer, liver cirrhosis, congenital heart disease, inflammatory bowel disease and others

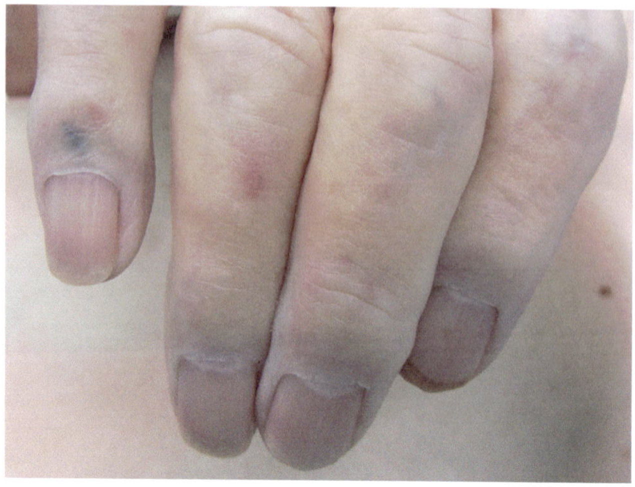

Fig. 2.68 Irregular pigmentation may be occupation-related such as in this example of coal tattooing on the hands of a retired miner. This should raise the possibility of occupational lung disease

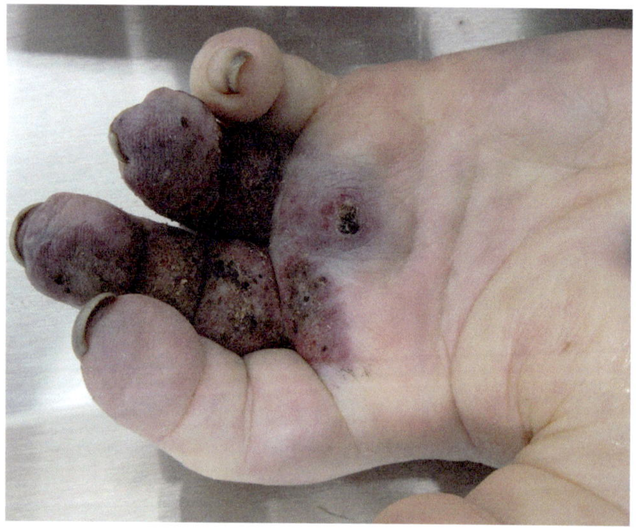

Fig. 2.69 Digital ischaemia. Non-healing injury at the base of these ischaemic fingers suggests underlying vasculopathy, thrombosis or diabetes mellitus

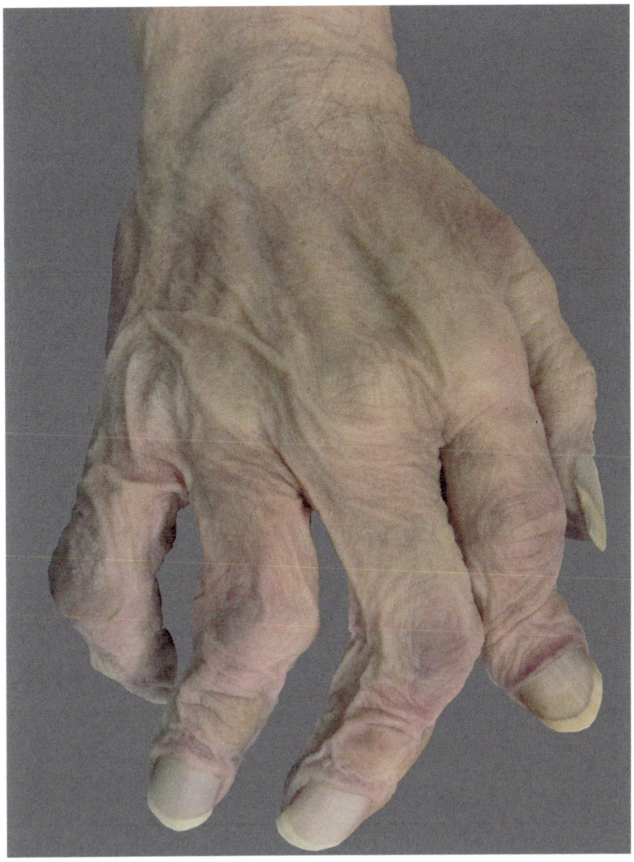

Fig. 2.70 Rheumatoid arthritis causes bone and joint destruction, which in turn leads to specific joint deformity. In this case there is deviation of the metacarpophalangeal joints and swan-neck deformities at the proximal interphalangeal joints. There is also wasting of the small muscles of the hand

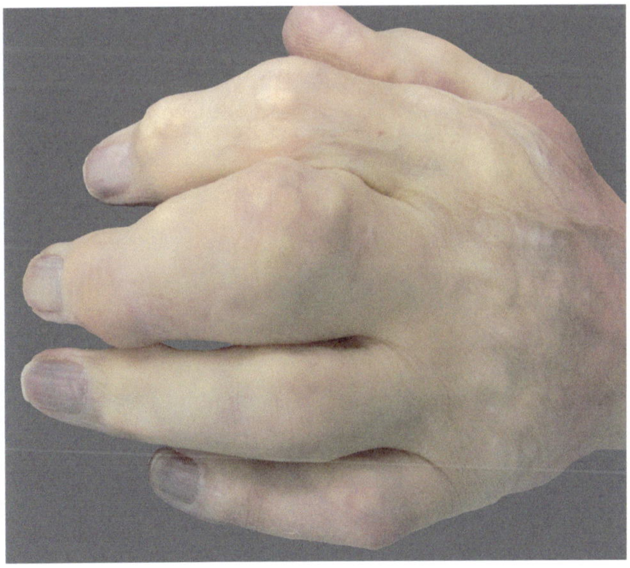

Fig. 2.71 Gouty tophi are nodular masses of monosodium urate crystals deposited in the soft tissues of the body. They contain a white pasty material which can work its way towards the skin surface to drain. Small sinus tracts can be noted

- Chest (Figs. 2.72, 2.73, 2.74, 2.75, 2.76, 2.77, 2.78, 2.79, 2.80, 2.81, and 2.82)

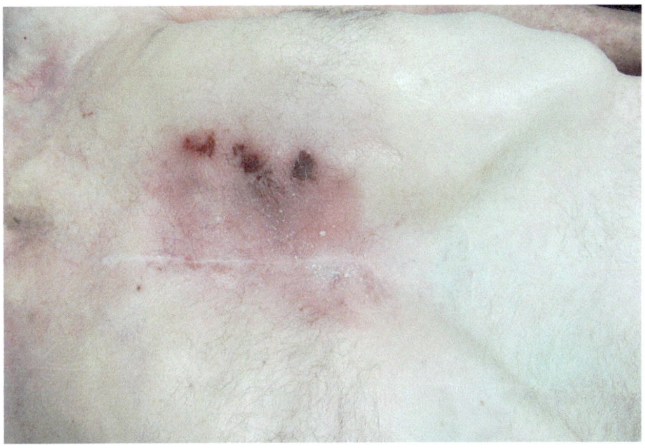

Fig. 2.72 Marks left by cardiopulmonary resuscitation (CPR) are not unusual. The chest hair is shaved to improve electrode conduction. The defibrillator pads are extremely sticky and can cause superficial skin loss when removed. By the time of autopsy, these areas of skin loss will have the appearance of an abrasion with parchment texture

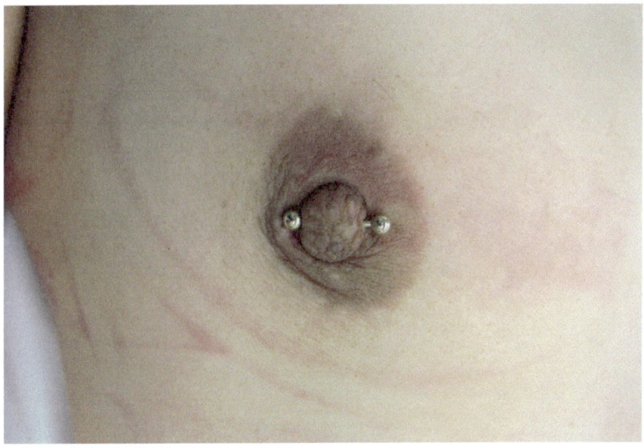

Fig. 2.73 Various rings, studs and implantable jewellery may be noted as part of the external examination, such as this metal bar nipple piercing. These findings should be documented and left in situ (unless otherwise requested by the relatives). They can be useful for identification purposes

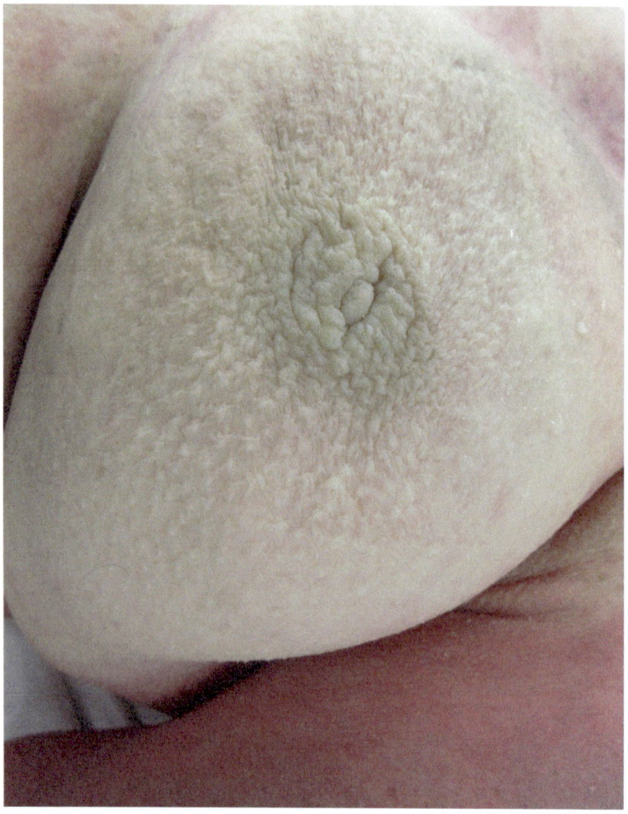

Fig. 2.74 Shown here is peau d'orange skin change and a tethered nipple indicating underlying breast malignancy

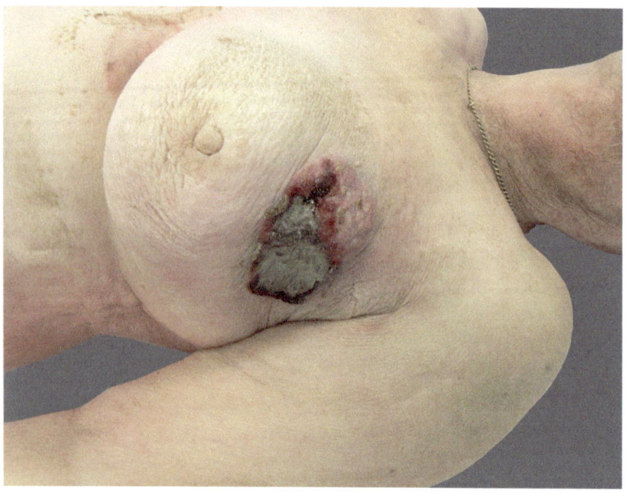

Fig. 2.75 Untreated breast cancer is seen with a fungating wound over the breast

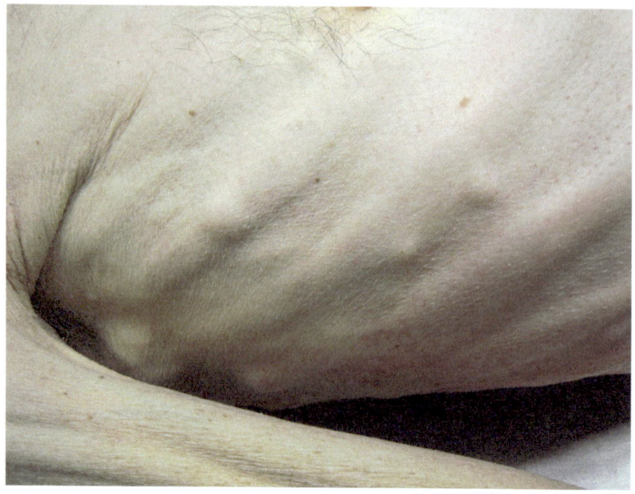

Fig. 2.76 Many malignancies metastasise to the skin and subcutaneous tissues. These are deposits of malignant mesothelioma

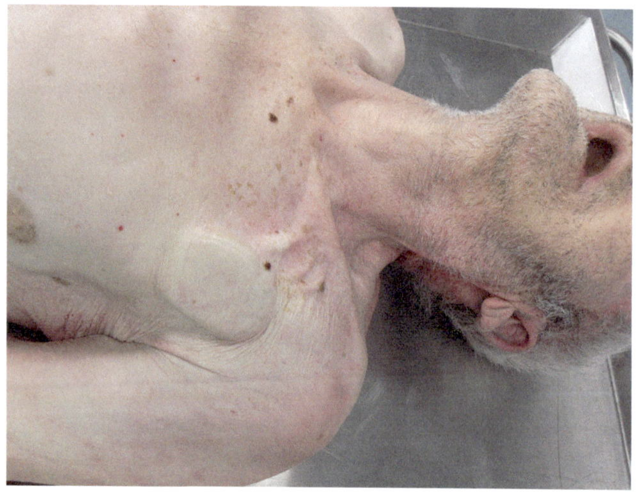

Fig. 2.77 A check needs to be made for pacemaker devices. In this case, the device is clearly visible on the left chest. In patients with larger habitus they are not as obvious

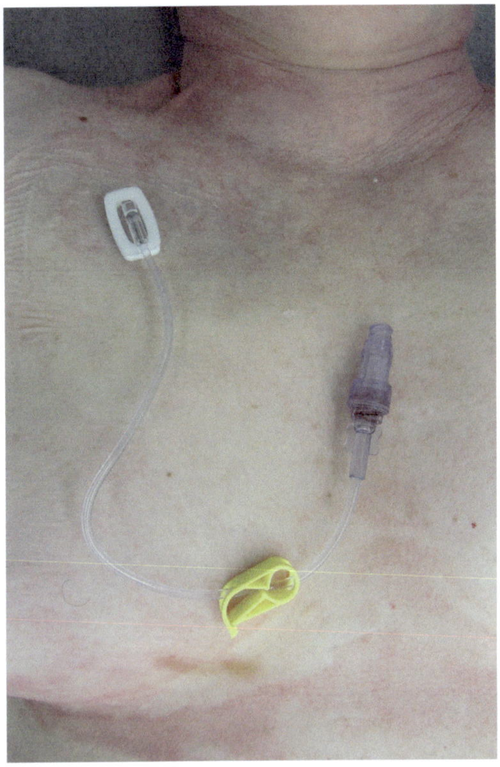

Fig. 2.78 This is a Hickman line used to administer drugs, blood products and other fluids intravenously. The tip of the line can be sent for microbiology if line sepsis is a consideration in the cause of death

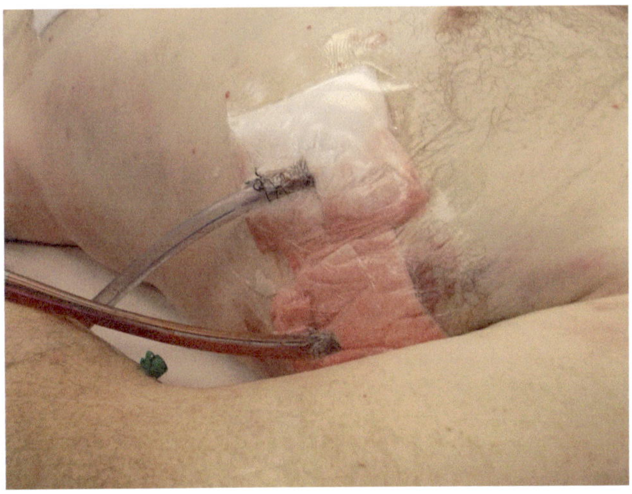

Fig. 2.79 Large intrathoracic chest drains (with protective dressings) should remain in situ until the internal placement has been confirmed. The volume and nature of fluid in any drain bag should be documented. The dressings are removed to examine the skin surrounding the incisions. Surgical drains are often sutured in place and care must be taken not to tear the skin during removal

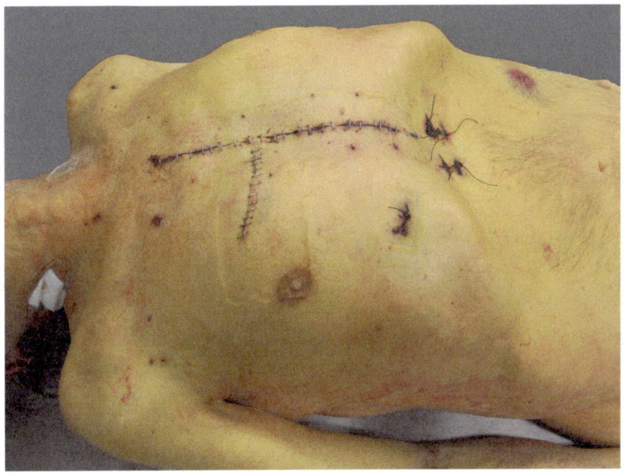

Fig. 2.80 Elective thoracotomy. These are fresh surgical incisions of cardiothoracic surgery. The lateral horizontal incision is used for a minimally invasive approach, which appears in this case to have been converted into a central sternotomy approach. The sutured incisions are port or catheter sites. Note also the severe jaundice of the skin

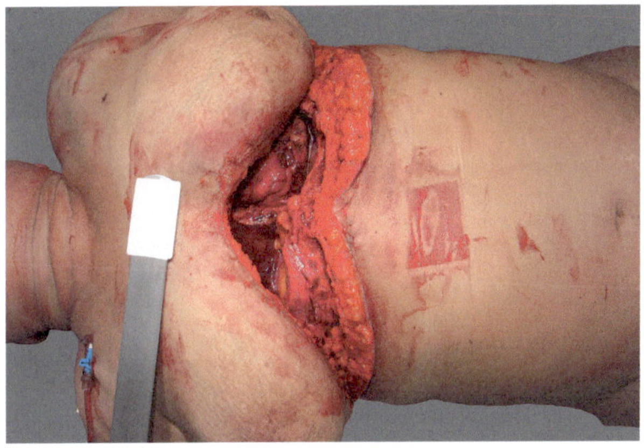

Fig. 2.81 Emergency thoracotomy. Performed only in an emergency trauma setting, usually for penetrating (and rarely blunt force) chest trauma, an emergency thoracotomy gives access to the chest to enable control of reversible causes of cardiac arrest (haemorrhage, cardiac tamponade). The sutures should be removed and the incision examined. This is a 'clam-shell' incision. Subsequent examination of internal organs will need to differentiate iatrogenic versus traumatic wounds

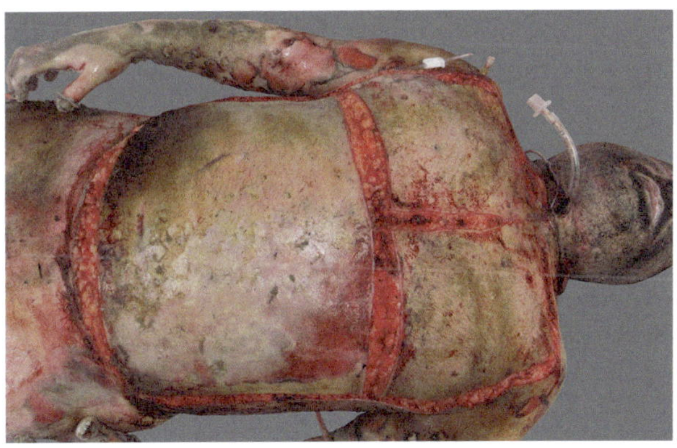

Fig. 2.82 Escharotomy is an emergency surgical procedure involving incising through areas of burnt skin to release the eschar and its constrictive effects, restore distal circulation, and allow adequate ventilation. Note the emergency tracheostomy airway, and partial full thickness loss of the epidermis over the limbs

- Abdomen (Figs. 2.83, 2.84, 2.85, 2.86, 2.87, 2.88, 2.89, 2.90, 2.91, 2.92, 2.93, 2.94, and 2.95)

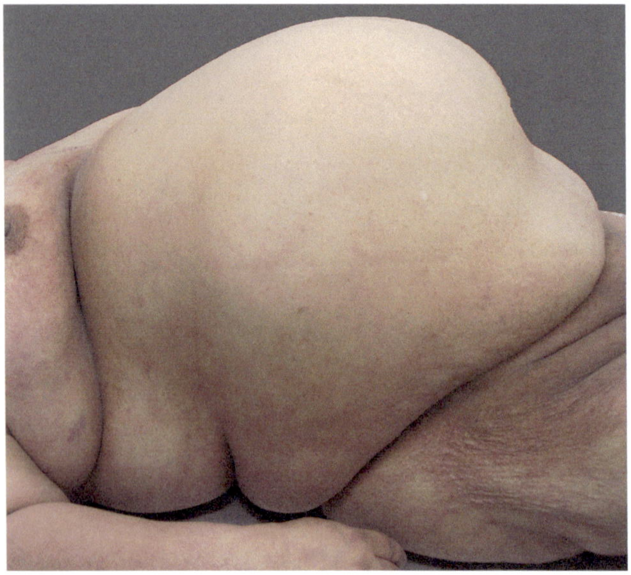

Fig. 2.83 Abdominal distention may be due to fat, fluid, faeces, fetus, or gas. In this case it was clearly shown to be fat

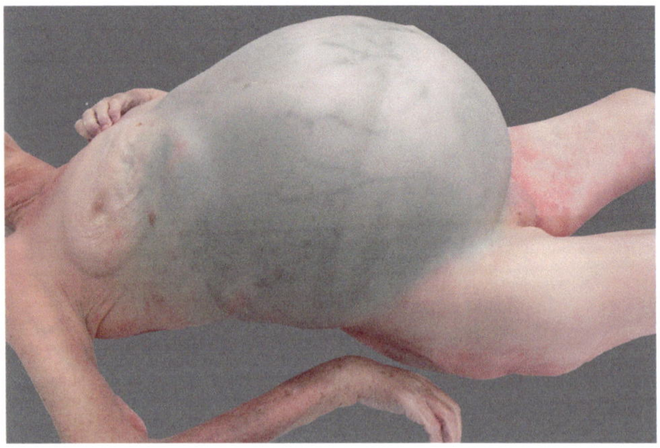

Fig. 2.84 Mass ascites may be seen, in this case due to ovarian malignancy

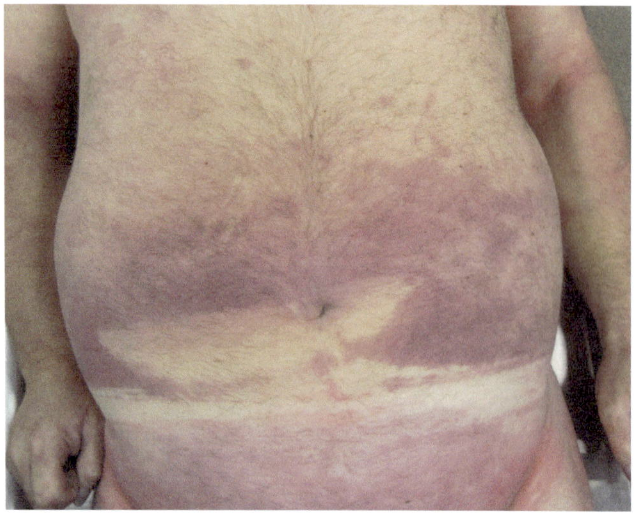

Fig. 2.85 In this case of hanging, the post-mortem lividity/blood collection is inferiorly distributed over the abdomen and legs. Note also the negative imprint from some clothing

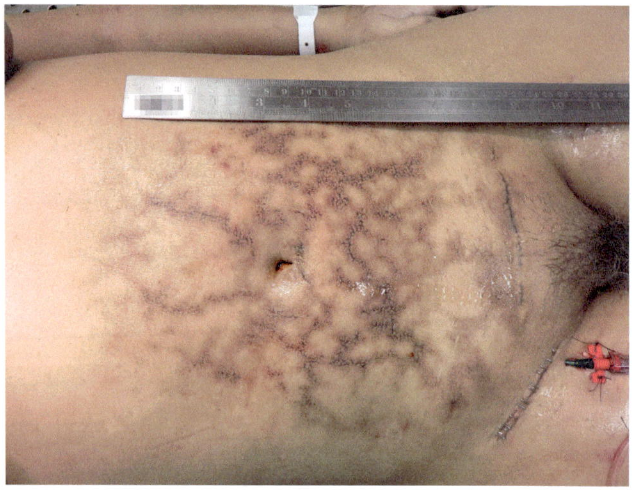

Fig. 2.86 Erythema ab igne. Prolonged exposure of the skin to heat (hot water bottle, electric fires, laptop, etc.) can lead to the development of reticulated erythema, hyperpigmentation, scaling and telangiectasia in the affected area. This patient had chronic abdominal pain due to endometriosis, relieved using a hot water bottle. Note also the recently healed suprapubic Pfannenstiel scar and the fresh right groin incision closed by staples

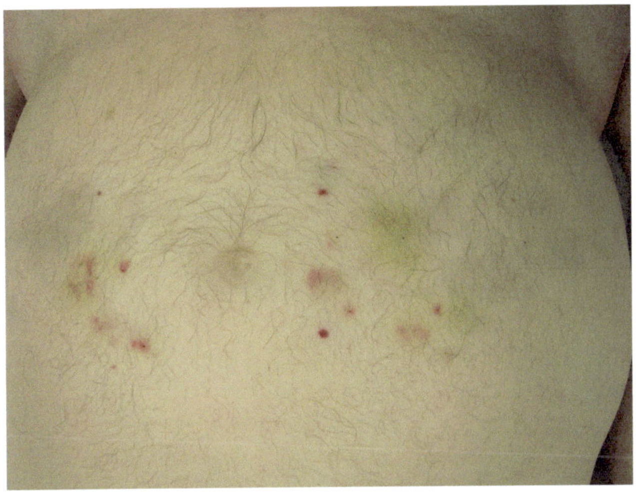

Fig. 2.87 These bruises represent subcutaneous injection sites. Low molecular weight heparin (LMWH) is delivered as a subcutaneous injection into the abdominal tissues. Hospital patients are at increased risk of deep vein thrombosis and receive daily LMWH as a risk-reducing measure, albeit with some minor bruising at the sites of drug delivery

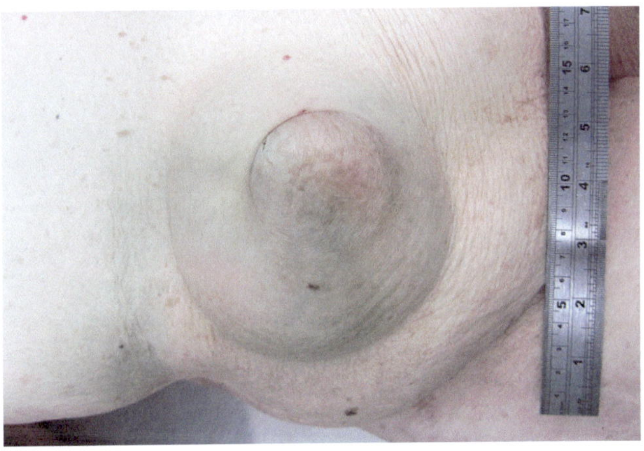

Fig. 2.88 This is a paraumbilical hernia in a case of previous laparoscopic surgery with an incisional hernia at the umbilicus. There is distention and subtle discolouration of the skin, suggesting incarceration

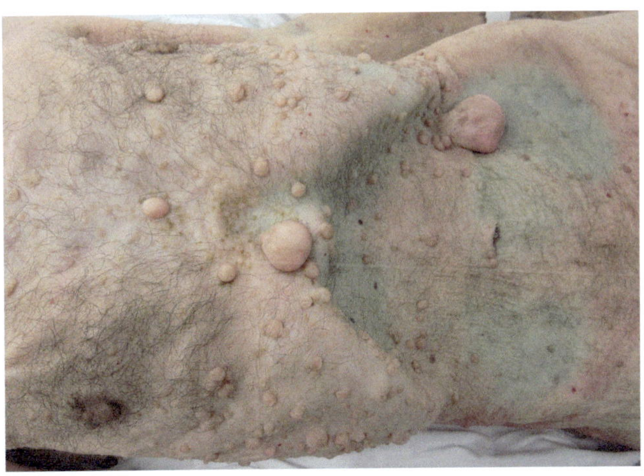

Fig. 2.89 A spot diagnosis in many clinical medical exams, this multisystem genetic disorder of neurofibromatosis can be associated with an increased risk for several malignancies, including gastrointestinal stromal tumours and malignant peripheral nerve sheath tumours

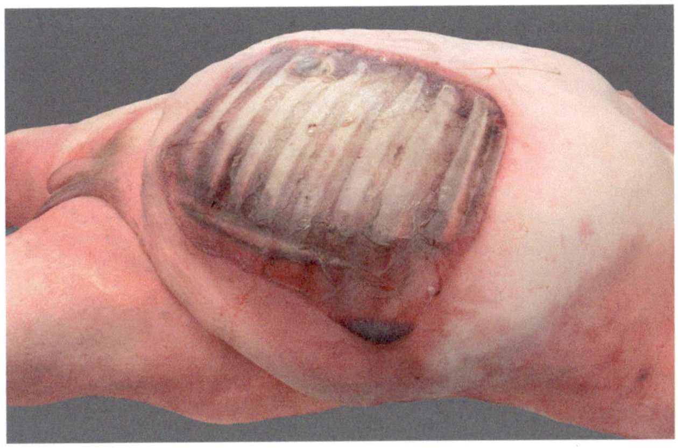

Fig. 2.90 Burn injury. If there is any doubt about unusual injuries noted during the external examination, it is important to seek additional information before proceeding with evisceration or internal examination. The imprint, size and associated burns suggest this injury was caused by a portable heater

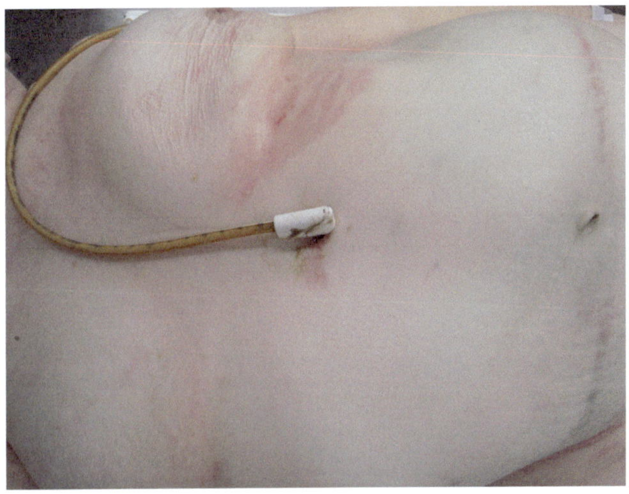

Fig. 2.91 Percutaneous endoscopic gastrostomy (PEG) devices enable enteral nutrition. There is a balloon cuff on the internal side of the device, which prevents the tube from falling out

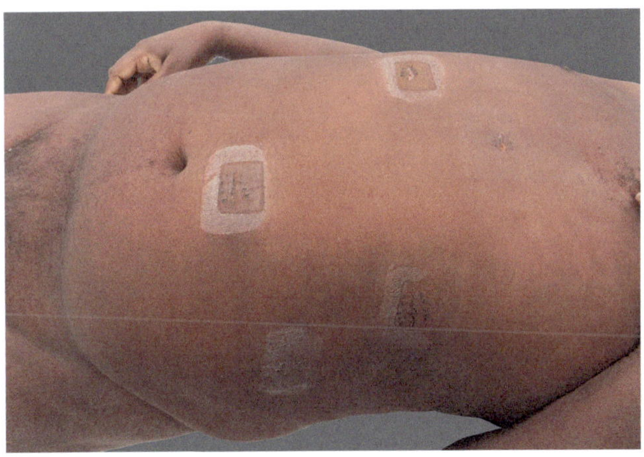

Fig. 2.92 Laparoscopic surgery port scars are seen. The wounds are healing and show no signs of infection. They were covered with postoperative dressings, indicating recent surgery. Close examination of the abdomen is needed to identify older port scars as they can be almost invisible and single port surgery techniques are practised in some centres. Sometimes the lack of an appendix or gallbladder prompts a 'relook' of the skin

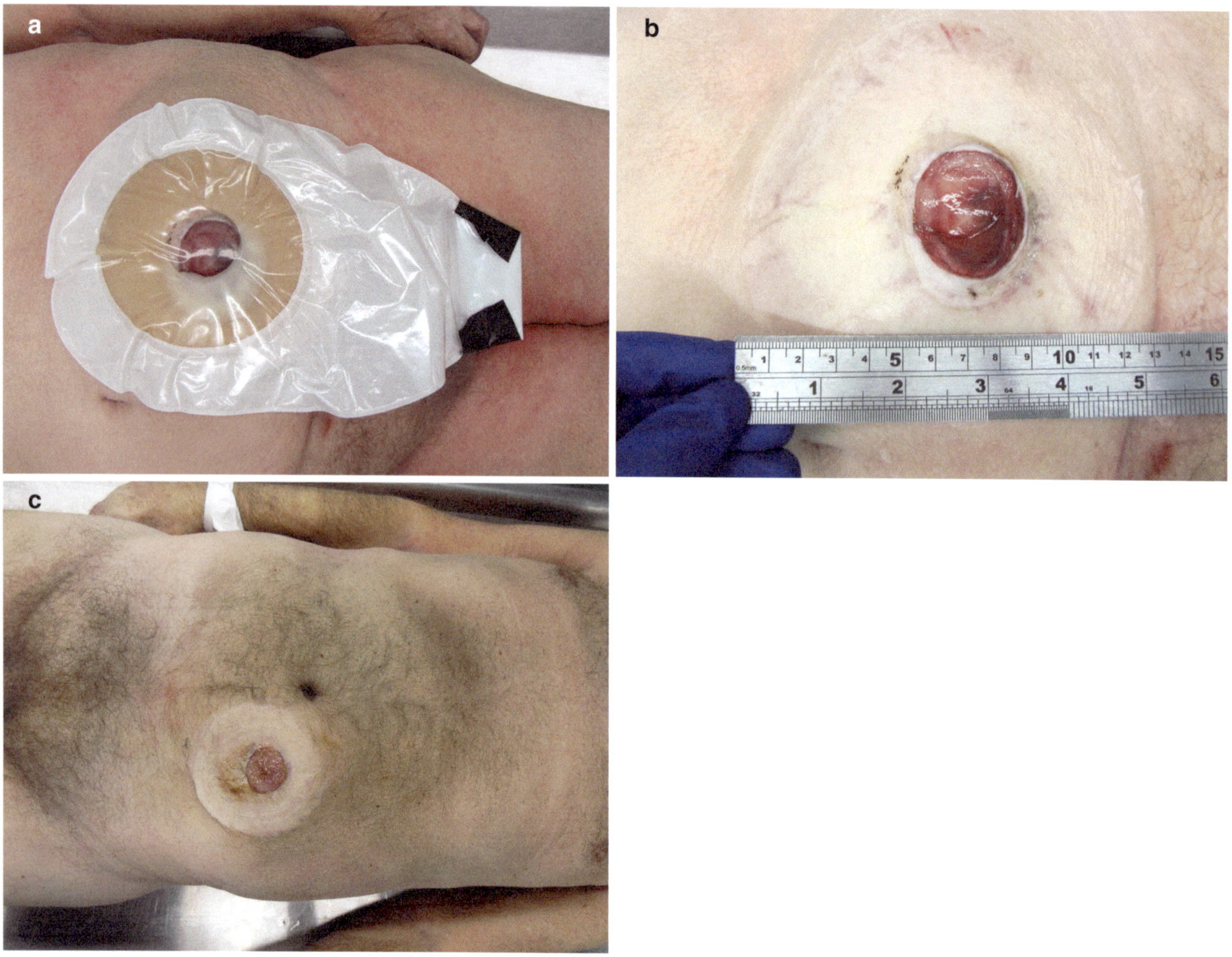

Fig. 2.93 Stomas. Bags covering stomas (Image **a**) are removed to examine the stoma. It should be noted whether the mucosal tissues are healthy, if there are signs of inflammation in the surrounding skin, wound dehiscence, or subtle hernia formation. In standard surgical procedures the site can be indicative of the type of stoma, for example in image (**b**) there is a sigmoid colostomy in the left lower quadrant following an emergency bowel resection due to obstruction. Image (**c**) shows a urostomy diverting urine from the kidney following bladder removal. The right lower abdomen is the more conventional location for urostomy

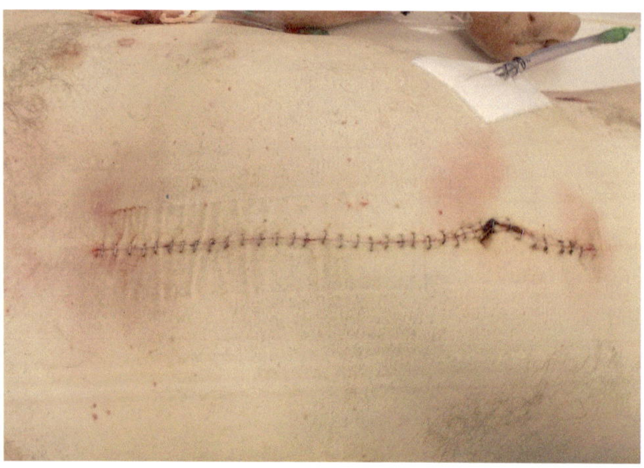

Fig. 2.94 Dressings over wounds should be removed and the condition of the skin (healthy or inflamed or healing, etc.) should be considered. The length of the scar should be documented. The type of closure (here stapled) merits comment. A surgical drain is seen in the left lower quadrant

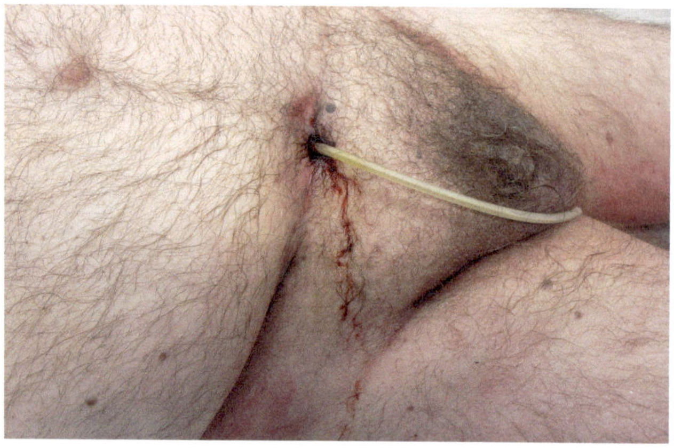

Fig. 2.95 There is some reddening of the skin at the site of this suprapubic catheter. Urine spillage and local bacterial sepsis causes skin irritation, similar to 'nappy rash' seen in infants

- Groin and external genitalia (Figs. 2.96, 2.97, 2.98, 2.99, 2.100, 2.101, 2.102, 2.103, 2.104, 2.105 and 2.106)

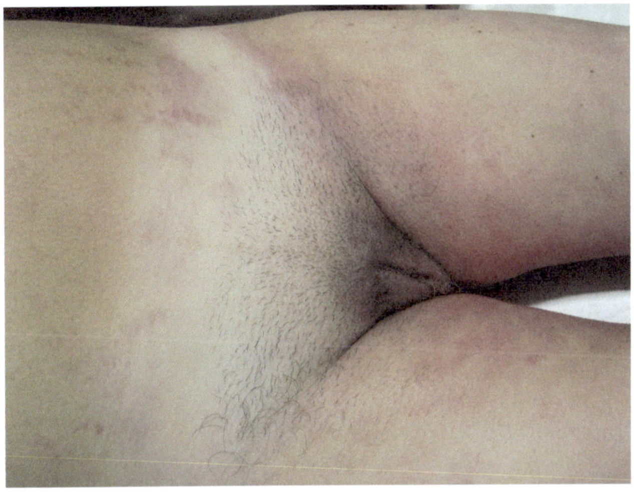

Fig. 2.96 Female genitalia. Examine the vulva for gross pathology, piercings and tattoos. In this case, the pubic hair has been shaved. Some pathologists comment on the distribution and nature of body hair of both sexes

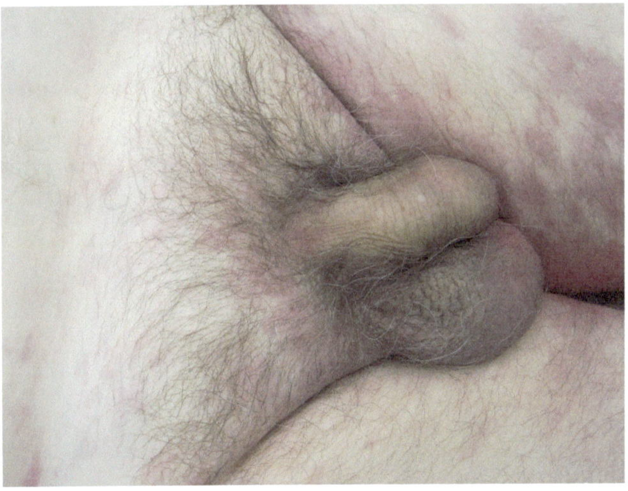

Fig. 2.97 Male genitalia. The penis is lifted to examine the scrotum and testes. Scrotal oedema is seen in heart failure and fluid overload. One should also check for genital tattoos or piercings

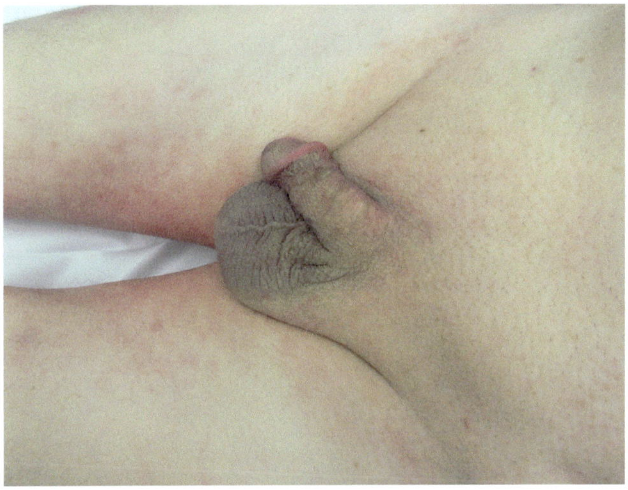

Fig. 2.98 In this case with a lack of pubic hair, the hair loss is secondary to radiotherapy treatment for prostate cancer

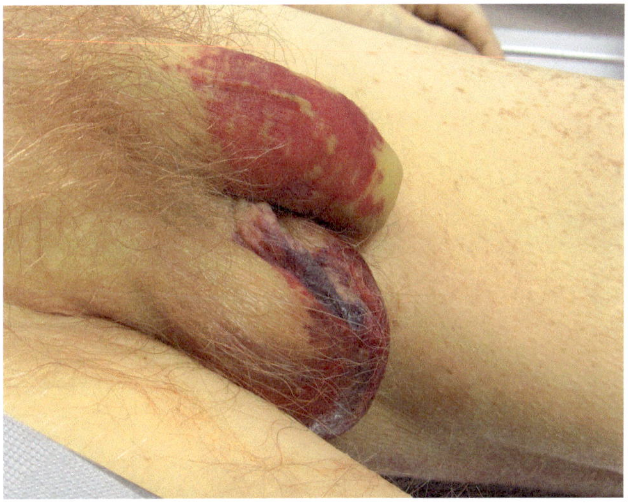

Fig. 2.99 Genital ecchymosis. Consideration must be given to genital bruising. Generalised and diffuse bruising may be due to trauma, intraperitoneal haemorrhage or surgery. In this case, the bruising is irregular yet localised, reflecting thrombocytopenia due to a haematological malignancy. Note also the severe jaundice in the skin, which makes the red colour stand out

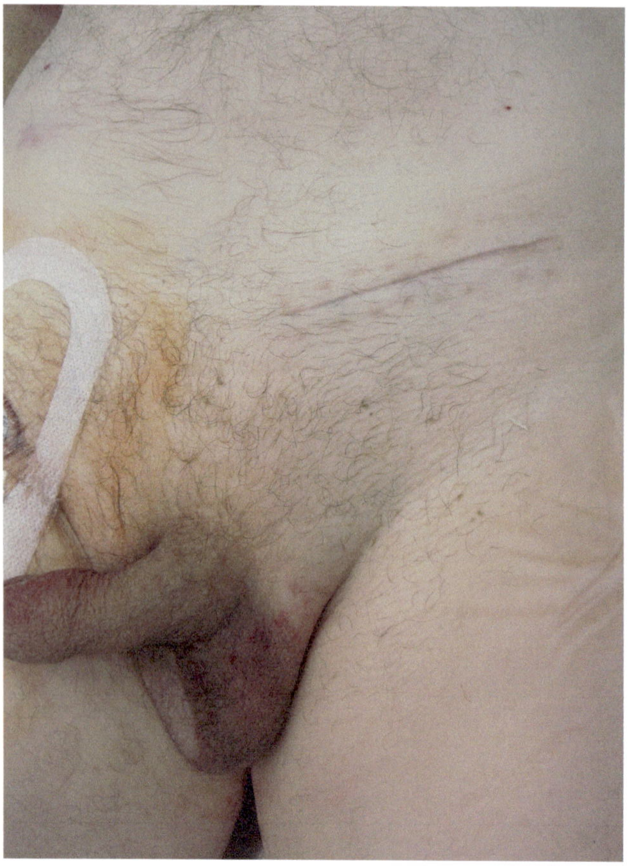

Fig. 2.100 An inguinal scar provides a clue to previous orchidectomy. In this case, the loss of volume in the scrotum is visible, but palpation of the scrotum will confirm whether the testes are present and normal. One should remember that prosthetic testicles can be implanted. One should also be looking for hydrocele and tumours

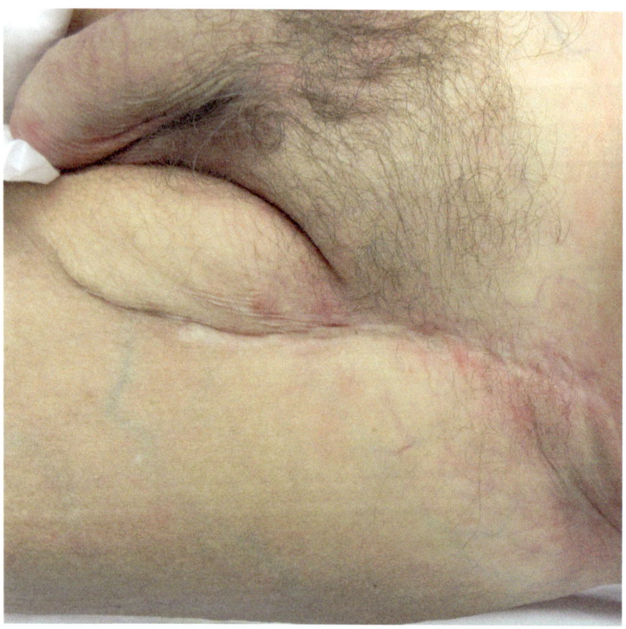

Fig. 2.101 Groin scar. There was a history of femoral artery surgery. Deformity of the tissue is palpated to assess whether this is a mass, or hernia

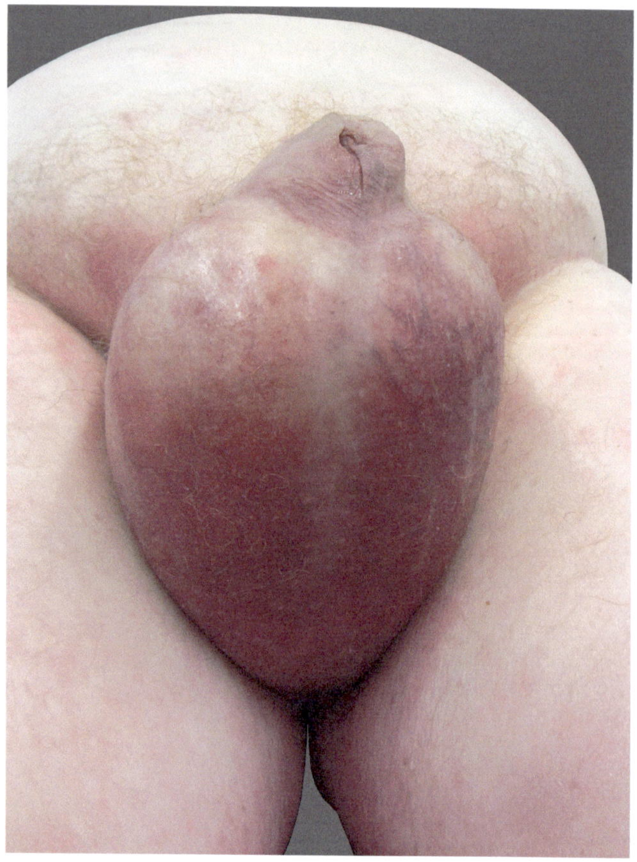

Fig. 2.102 In this case there is marked scrotal swelling due to a hydrocele. Fluid can be drained for investigations such as cytology and microbiology, if relevant to the history and examination

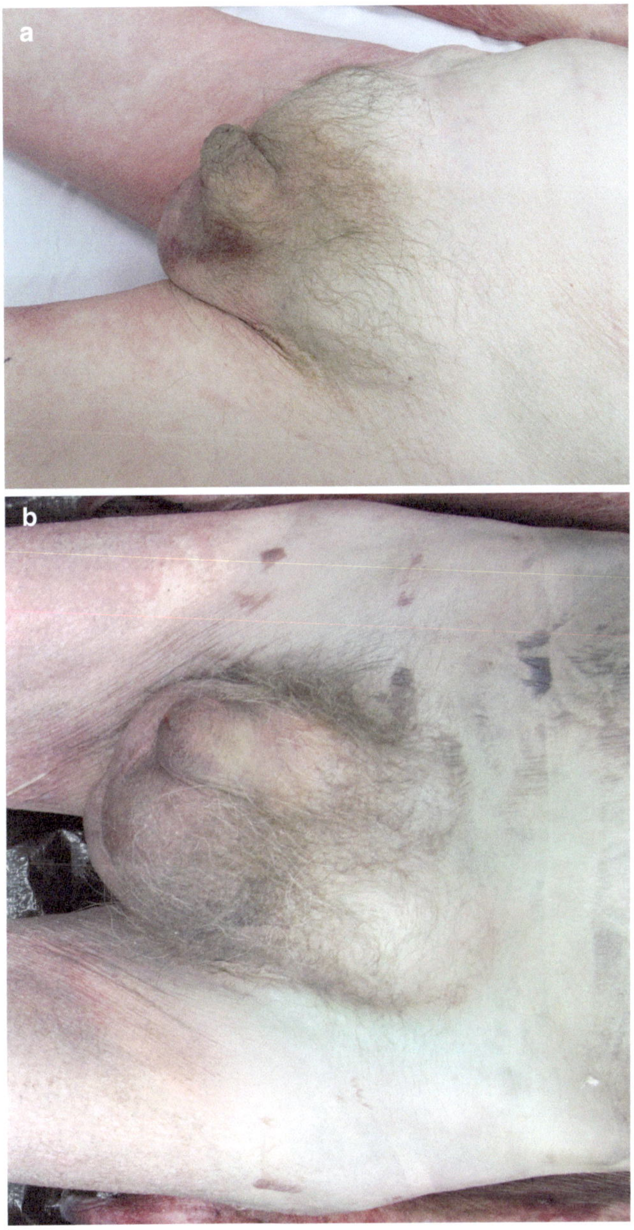

Fig. 2.103 A fullness of the inguinal area or scrotum consistent with a hernia. Hernias can be subtle (Image **a**) or obvious (Image **b**). The evisceration technique can be modified in order to examine the contents of the hernial sac and identify bowel infarction or incarceration

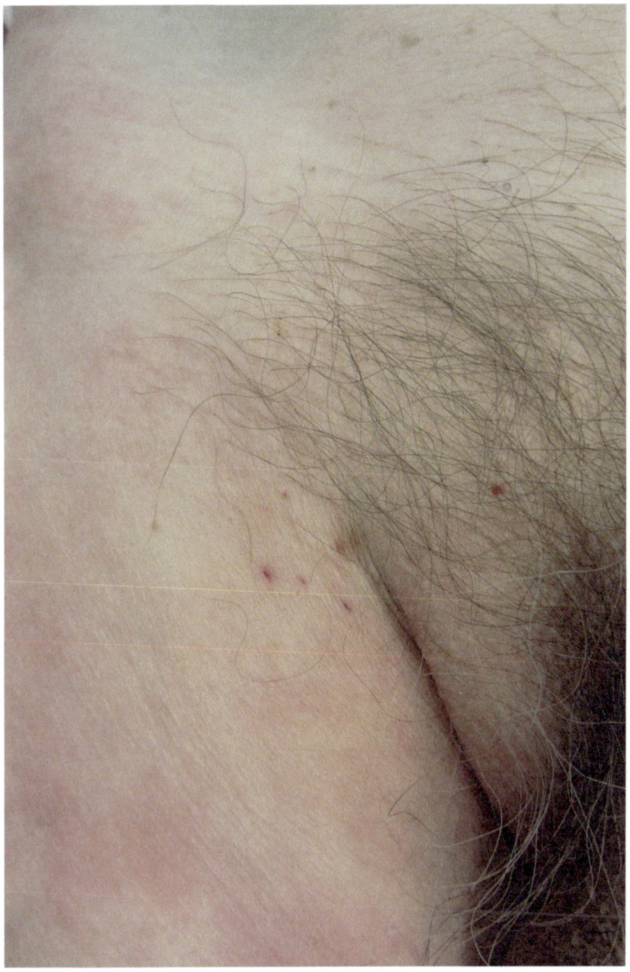

Fig. 2.104 Medical puncture wounds. 'Femoral stab' sites noted in the groin following emergency resuscitation, in an attempt to sample blood when peripheral vessels are shut down

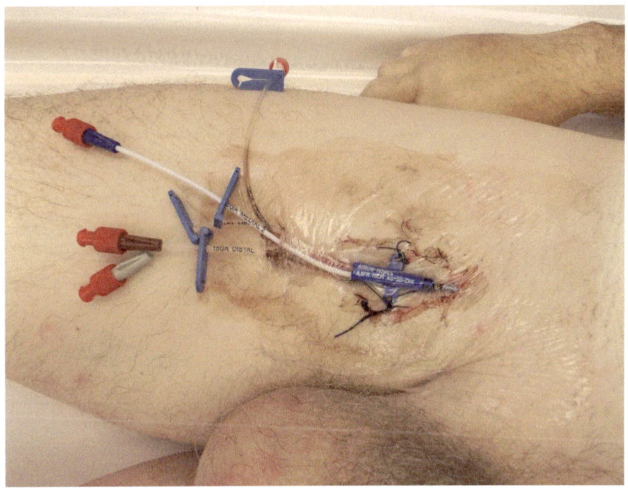

Fig. 2.105 This is a groin-sited intravenous central line used for fluid delivery. It should be remembered that needle puncture marks may be from emergency care (as in this case) or from intravenous drug use. One should also check the groin for hernias, but unless large, these are unlikely to be palpable in a prone dead body. One should always palpate for enlarged inguinal lymph nodes

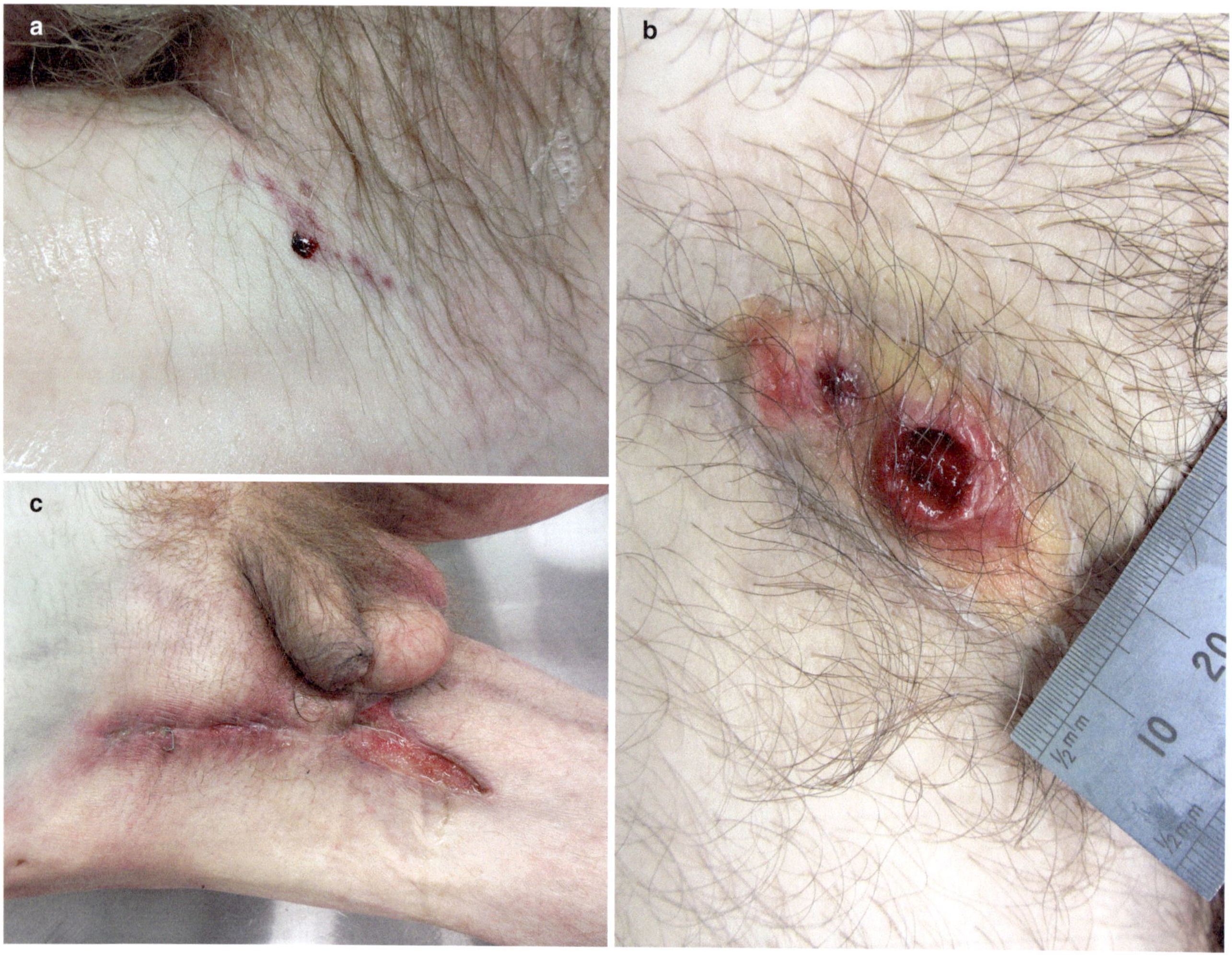

Fig. 2.106 The groin in an intravenous drug user often shows evidence of repeated injections in the same site (Image **a**) with inflammation and bruising. Late changes will involve sinus formation (Image **b**), which can risk developing sepsis necessitating surgical intervention (Image **c**). This wound is healing by secondary intention and the base shows healthy granulation tissue

- Lower limbs (Figs. 2.107, 2.108, 2.109, 2.110, 2.111, 2.112, 2.113, 2.114, 2.115, 2.116, 2.117, 2.118, 2.119, 2.120, 2.121, 2.122, 2.123, 2.124, 2.125, 2.126, 2.127, 2.128, 2.129, 2.130, 2.131, 2.132, 2.133, and 2.134)

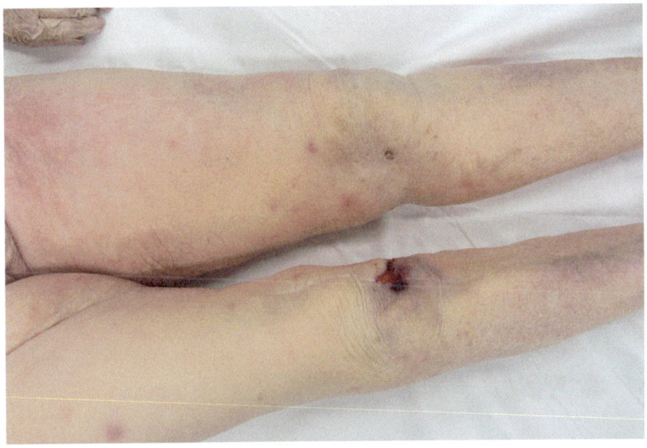

Fig. 2.107 There is leg asymmetry with the left side appearing bigger than the right. If legs are asymmetrical, one should ideally measure mid-thigh or calf circumference (10 cm below the tibial tuberosity). A difference of 3 cm or more raises the possibility of deep vein thrombosis and potentially pulmonary thromboembolism. A scar from previous knee replacement surgery is noted on the right side

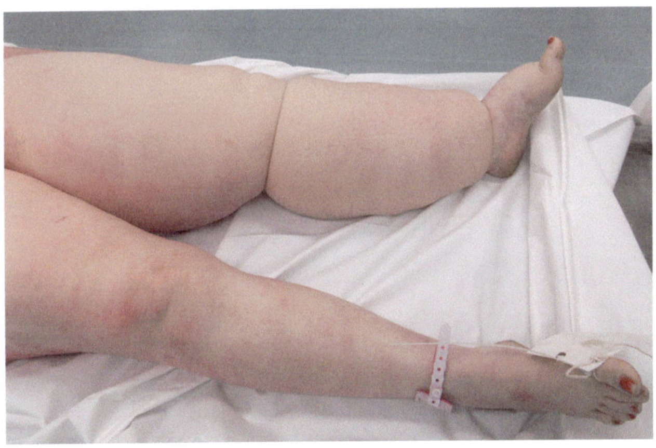

Fig. 2.108 Chronic venous obstruction and lymphoedema. This may reflect obstruction to the venous and/or lymphatic outflow from the leg. It may be associated with previous lymphadenectomy during cancer surgeries. Ulceration may also be seen

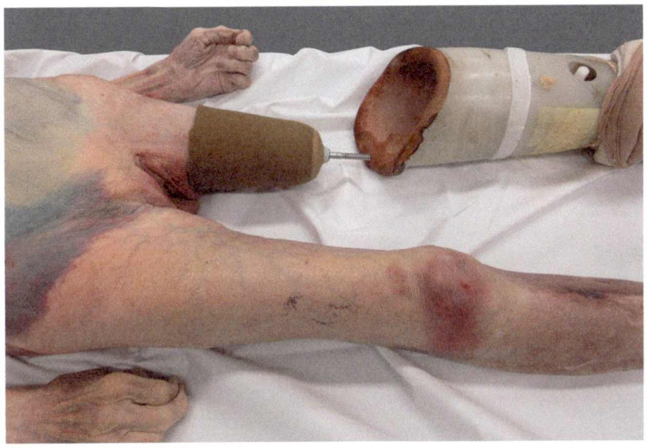

Fig. 2.109 Limb amputation can be associated with complications of diabetes mellitus, infection, peripheral arterial disease and trauma. Note the right groin scarring, subcutaneous haematoma and lower left abdominal scar. The deceased had severe arterial disease, underwent previous arterial surgeries, and was on anti-coagulant medications

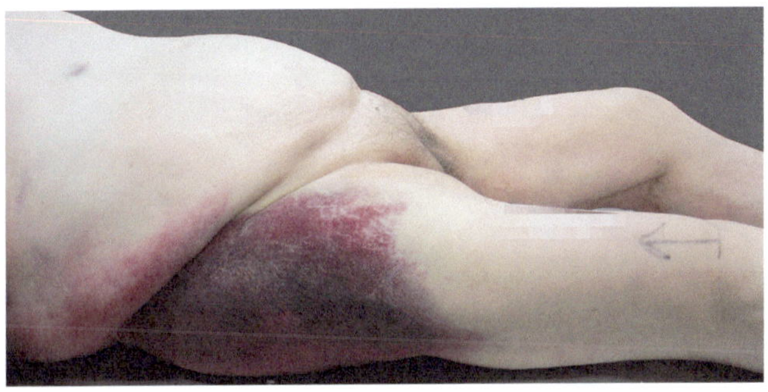

Fig. 2.110 In the post-mortem room, as in life, a shortened and externally rotated lower limb provides a clue to a fractured neck of femur. In this case, there is massive haemorrhage around the hip, which has leaked into the subcutaneous tissues. Internal haemorrhages can progress after death as the blood pools in the dependent areas. Note the arrow drawn on the right leg by the surgical team to identify the correct site for planned surgery. Care must be taken when examining fracture sites internally as there may be sharp bony edges

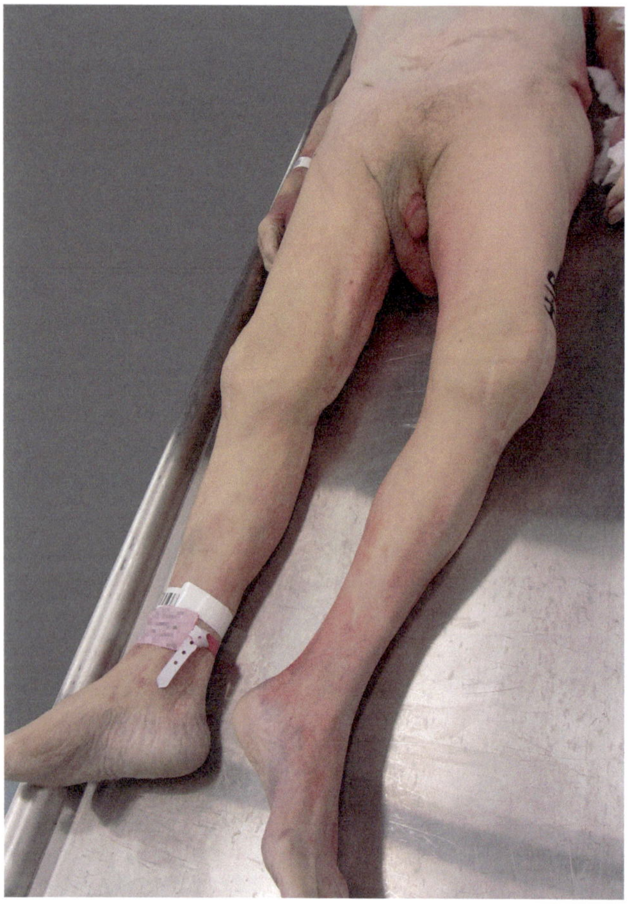

Fig. 2.111 Hip fracture. The left leg is shortened and externally rotated. Correct-site surgical marking of the affected limb will provide a clue if the positioning was not immediately obvious. There is also previous knee replacement scarring over the left knee

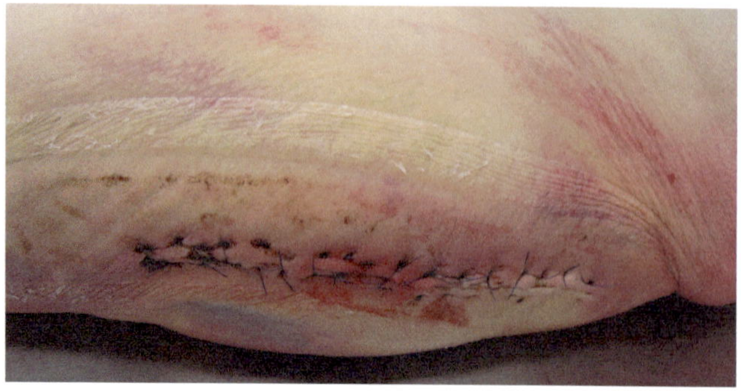

Fig. 2.113 This surgical wound overlying the hip shows features of erythema and oedema. Releasing the sutures revealed purulent fluid, which should be collected in a sterile container and sent to microbiology. A wound swab is acceptable, but a volume of pus is preferred

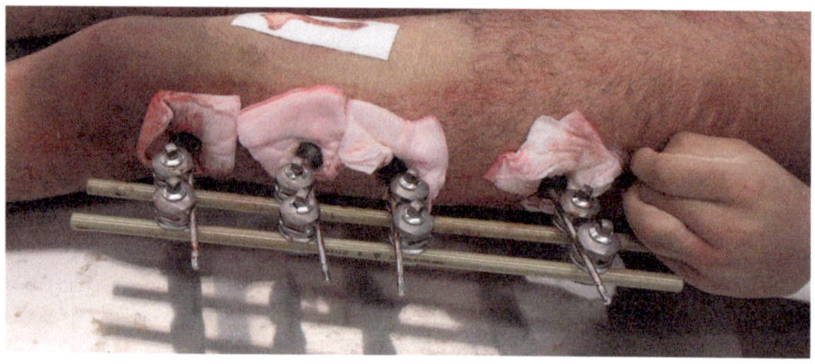

Fig. 2.114 External orthopaedic fixation devices need to be removed by the appropriate technical department in the hospital prior to the body being released for burial or cremation

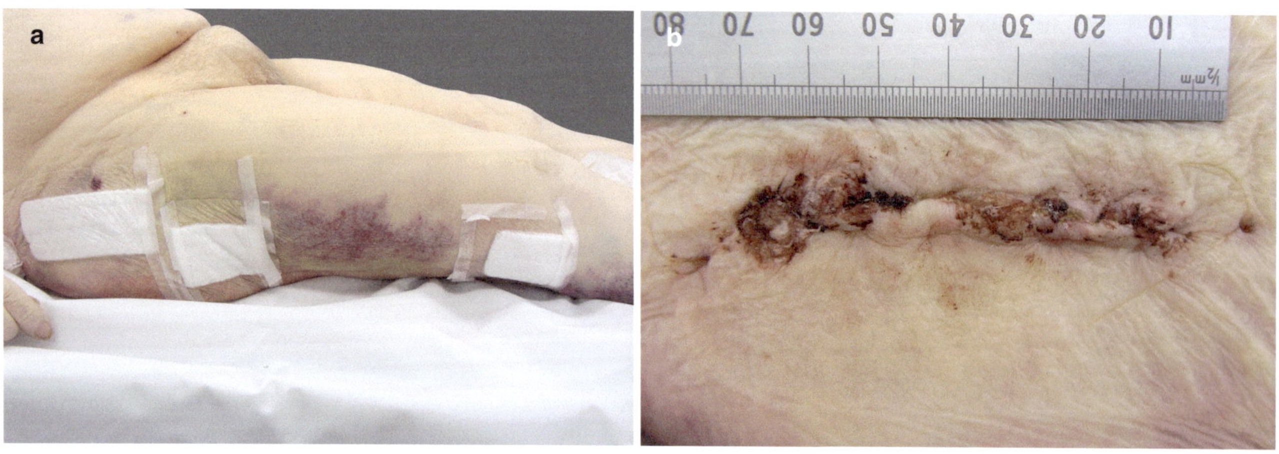

Fig. 2.112 Hip surgery. Recent hip surgery with dressings in place (Image **a**). All dressings are removed to examine surgical incisions checking for wound integrity, healing and signs of infection. In this case the wound looks healthy (Image **b**). Swabs or fluid can be collected for microbiology testing if there are signs of infection

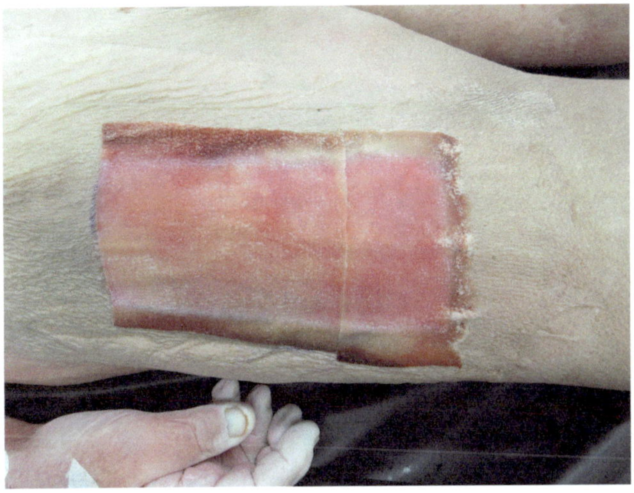

Fig. 2.115 A split thickness skin graft donor site is shown. These grafts are utilised in wound closures for burns, trauma, and reconstruction

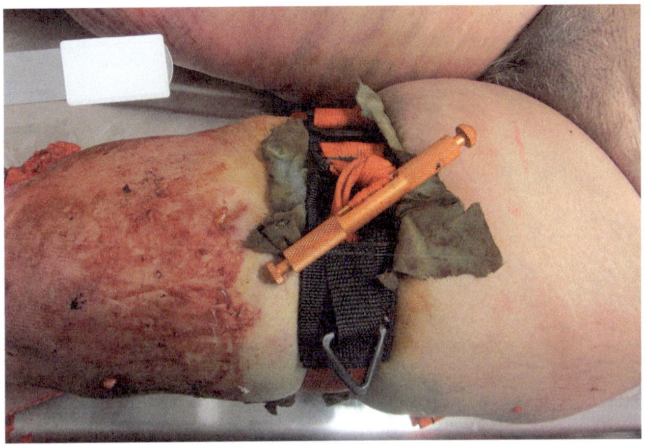

Fig. 2.116 This limb tourniquet was applied at the scene of a road traffic collision following a traumatic below-knee amputation

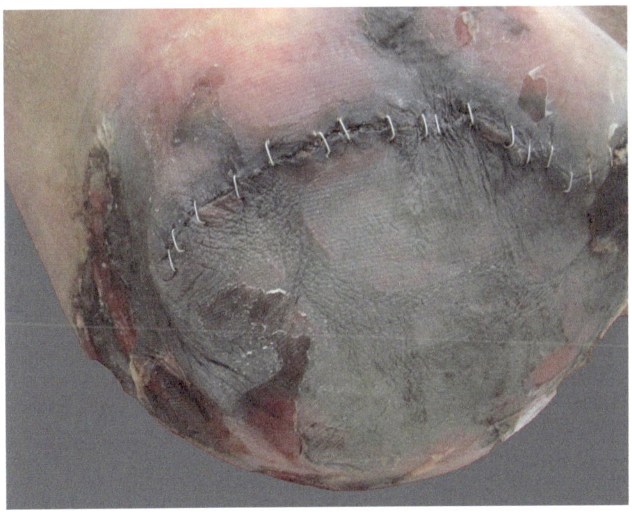

Fig. 2.117 It is advisable to note the level of any amputation and comment on the condition of the stump. This is a fresh surgical wound (staples are still in place) showing signs of local tissue necrosis, suggesting sepsis (possibly necrotising fasciitis) and/or critical ischaemia

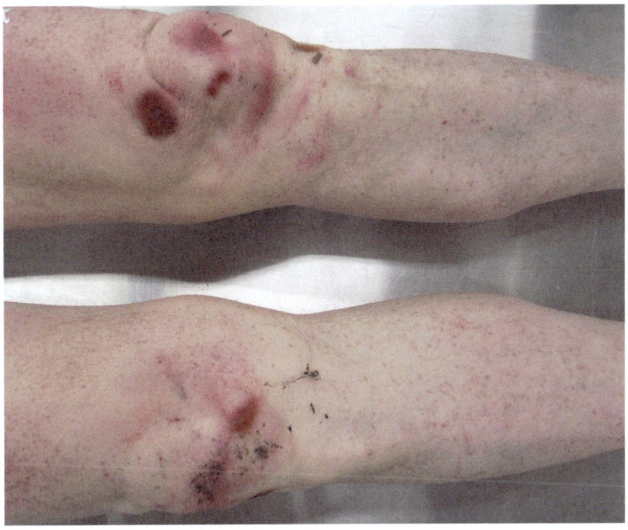

Fig. 2.118 Multiple injuries over the knees at varying stages of healing may suggest chronic or repeated bouts of intoxication (*e.g.*, alcohol) and frequent falls

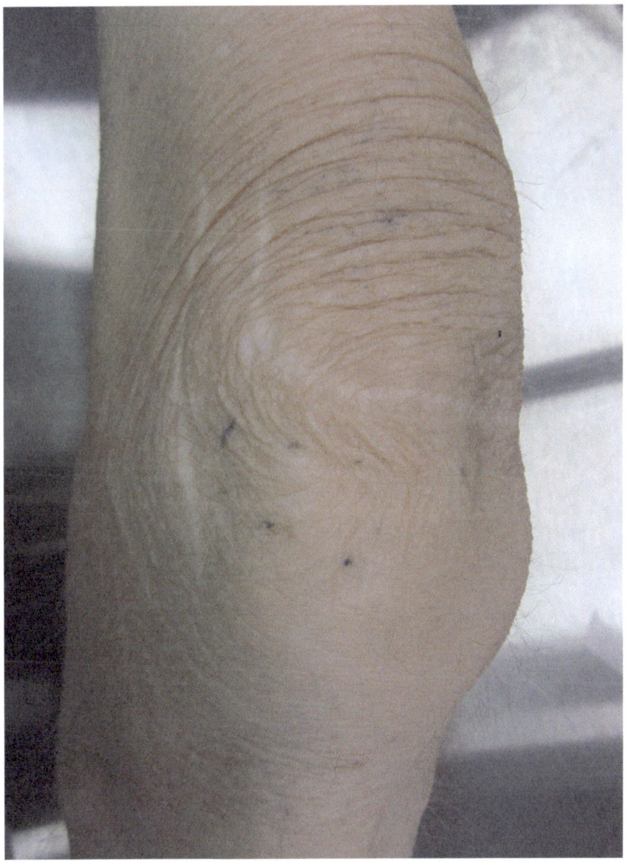

Fig. 2.119 These irregular scars are in keeping with previous trauma. Noting the coal pigment tattooing on the knee of a retired underground coal miner

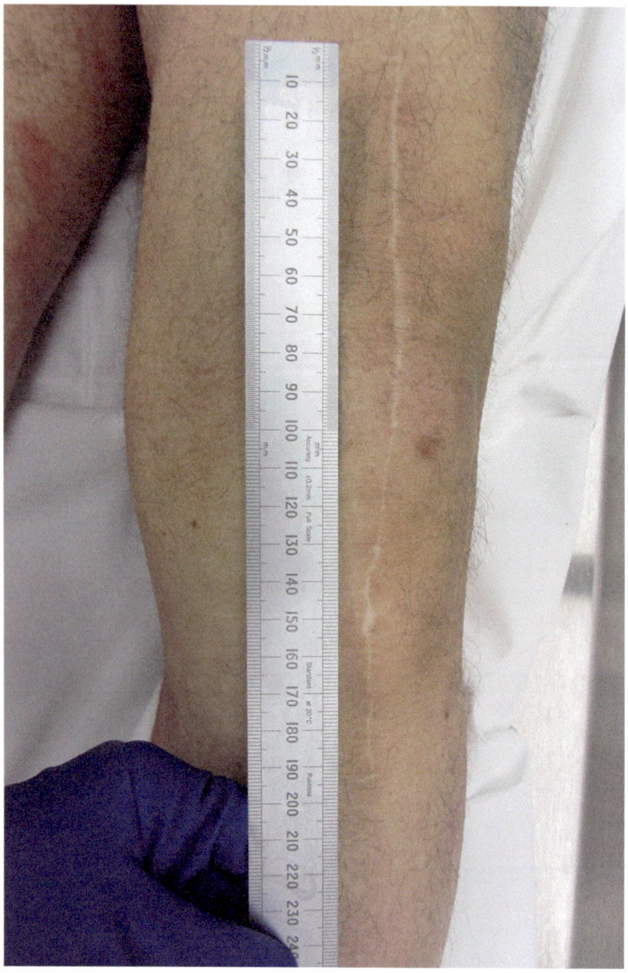

Fig. 2.120 Joint replacement surgery of the knee. Hip and knee joint replacement is often bilateral

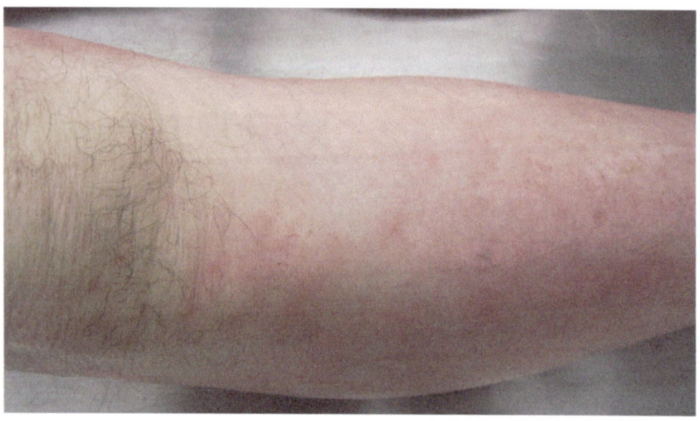

Fig. 2.121 Peripheral vascular disease can lead to natural hair loss in the lower leg, often with diminished soft tissue and muscle bulk

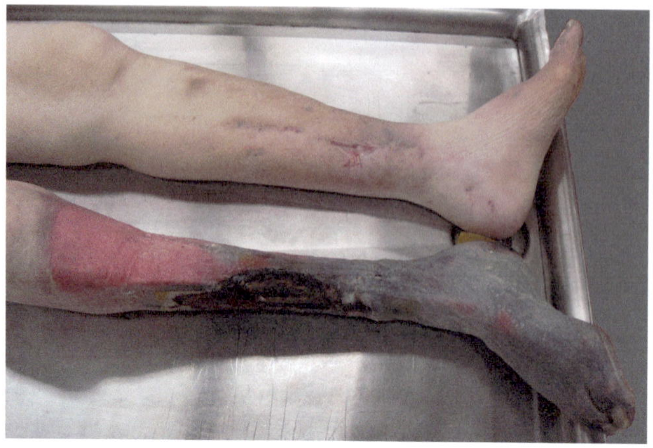

Fig. 2.122 Severe peripheral vascular disease in a patient with poorly controlled diabetes. Note that the left leg is hairless and there is ulceration present. The right leg shows extensive gangrene with ulceration through to the tibia. The back of the right heel is discoloured at the site of a pressure ulcer

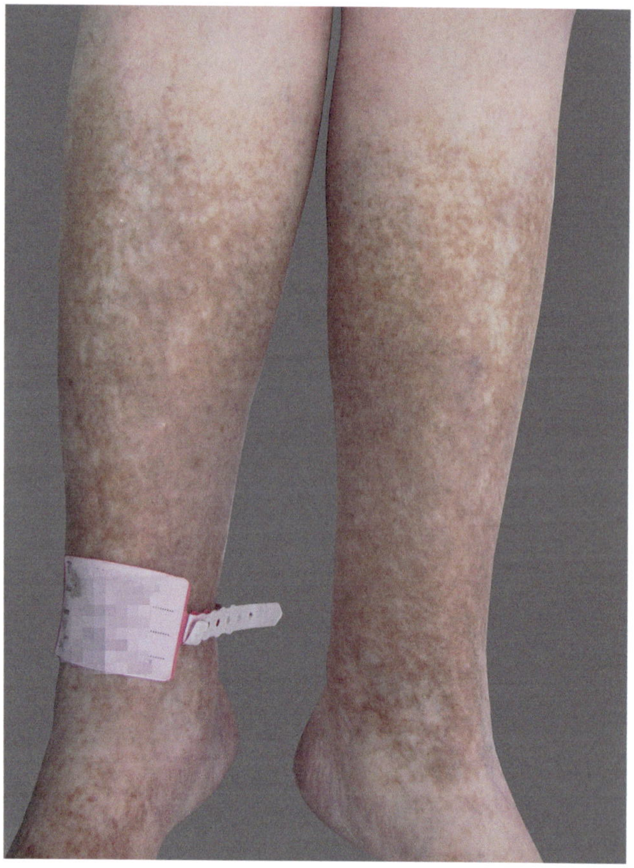

Fig. 2.123 Chronic venous eczema is a sign of chronic venous insufficiency. It can have a variable appearance: orange-brown macular pigmentation due to haemosiderin deposition (seen here); red, blistered and crusted plaques; or dry fissured and scaly plaques on one or both lower legs. The classic 'Champagne bottle' shape of the lower leg due to narrowing at the ankles and induration (lipodermatosclerosis) may also be identified. Secondary infection and cellulitis can complicate the disorder

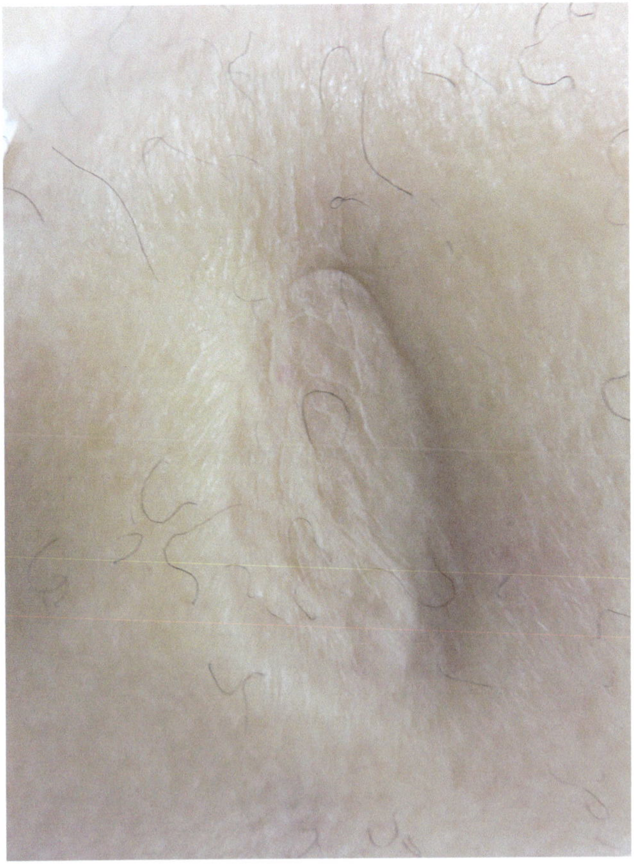

Fig. 2.124 Pitting pedal oedema. Apply firm digital pressure (for at least 10 s) over a distal bony prominence to assess for pitting oedema

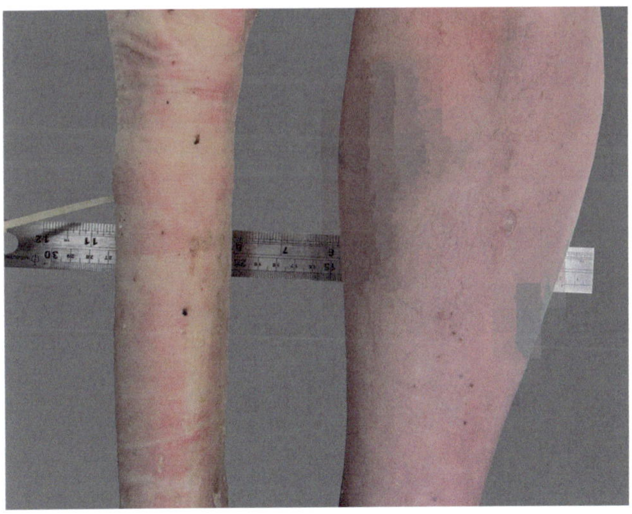

Fig. 2.125 The cause of this unilateral limb atrophy was not clear in the medical records examined and had been present from childhood

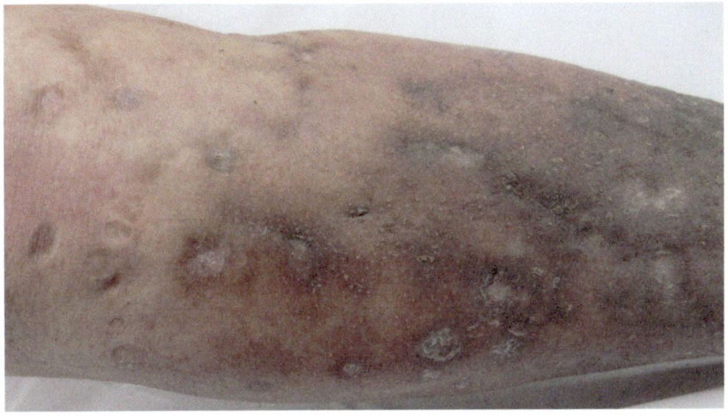

Fig. 2.126 Skin popping. These marks are due to the injection of 'street drugs' into intradermal or subcutaneous tissues, causing hyperpigmented, fibrotic, depressed, round plaques on the extremities. Drug absorption is slower via this method and reduces the risk of overdose. These lesions are an important clue to illicit drug use and contribute information to the autopsy risk assessment

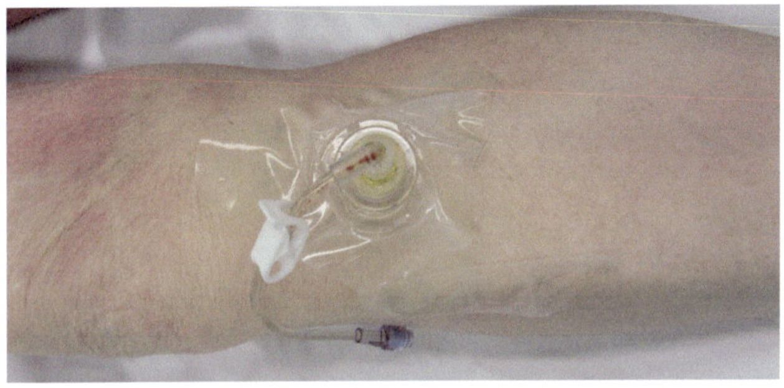

Fig. 2.127 This is an intraosseous needle in the tibial site. The intraosseous infusion route is commonly used in paediatric patients but is also seen in acute/trauma adult settings [16]

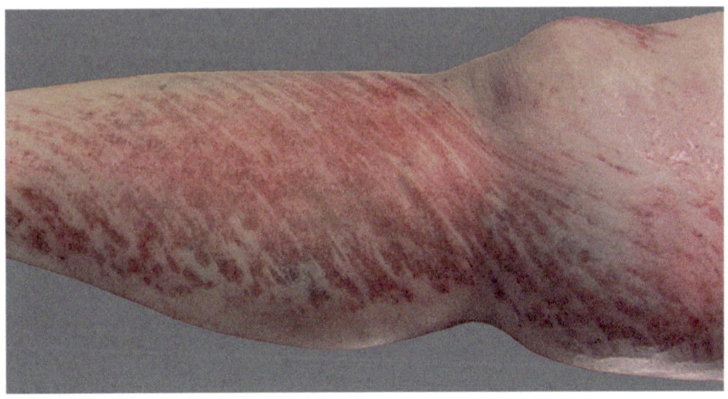

Fig. 2.128 Superficial skin abrasions sustained in a road traffic collision. The direction of force can be established by looking this injury. Skin abrasions may occur during the accident but also might occur afterwards, when the body is moved

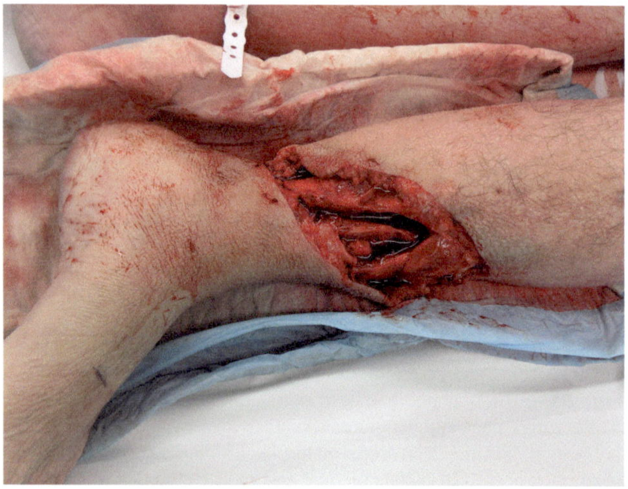

Fig. 2.129 Limb deformity may be due to congenital or acquired musculoskeletal or neurological diseases. However, this is an open compound fracture causing deformity

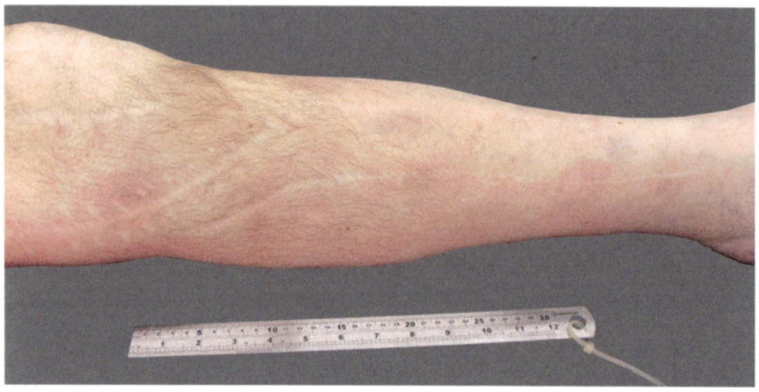

Fig. 2.130 Finding a sternotomy scar should prompt you to look at the legs to identify vein graft harvest sites for coronary bypass surgery

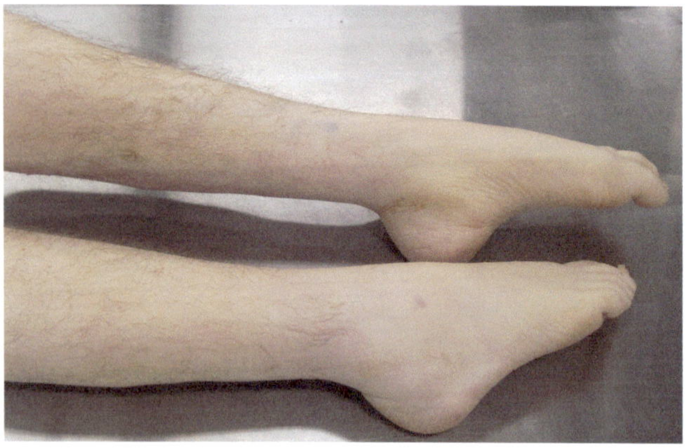

Fig. 2.131 A spinal cord injury has led to bilateral (spastic-style) extension of the feet and muscle wasting

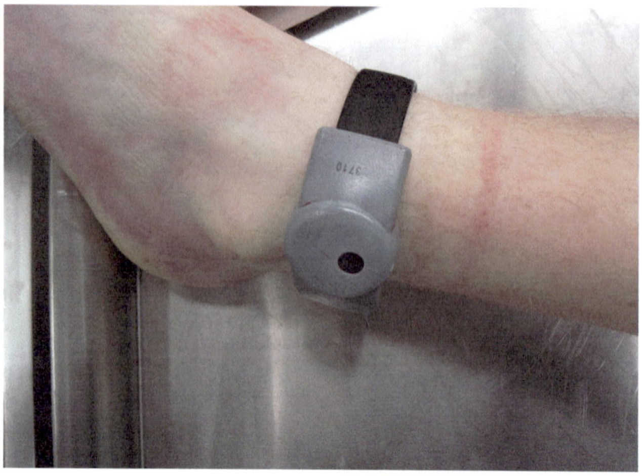

Fig. 2.132 Monitoring (offender) tag. This is an electronic tag used to provide information on the geographic position of convicted persons present in the community and subject to control orders

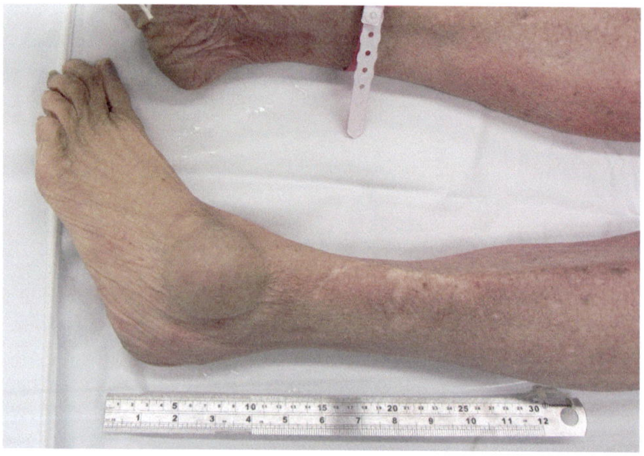

Fig. 2.133 Inspection and palpation of 'lumps', noting the characteristics as one would do in a clinic setting, will provide a good indication of the nature of the mass. This was a firm mobile mass on the ankle with smooth circumscribed edges, in keeping with a benign mesenchymal tumour, of no relevance to the cause of death

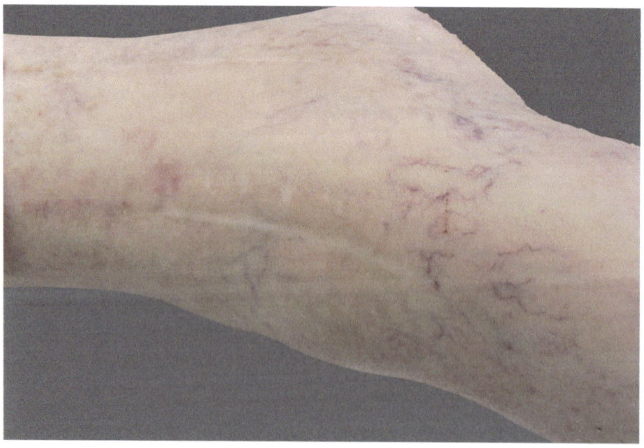

Fig. 2.134 A scar following ankle surgery

- Feet and toes (Figs. 2.135, 2.136, 2.137, 2.138, 2.139, 2.140, 2.141, and 2.142)

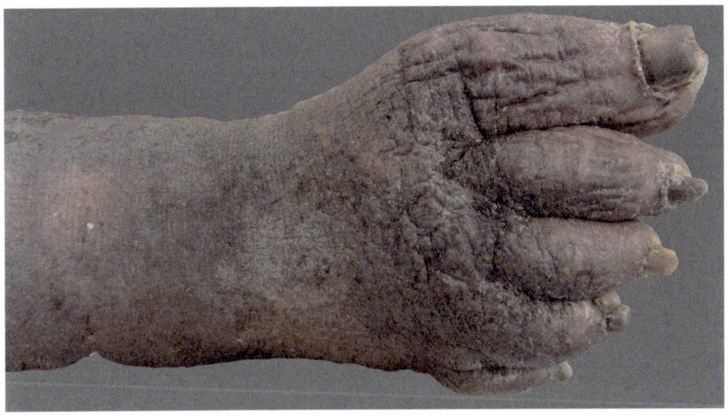

Fig. 2.135 Although feet may appear unremarkable, one should always look for missing toes, positional deformity (neurological, musculoskeletal), arthritis effects (rheumatoid or osteoarthritis, etc.), scabies, and needle puncture marks (*e.g.*, intravenous drug use). If there is a known history of diabetes, then one should check the feet carefully for signs of injury, ulceration and/or infection. The condition of the feet can also reflect social circumstances and physical mobility

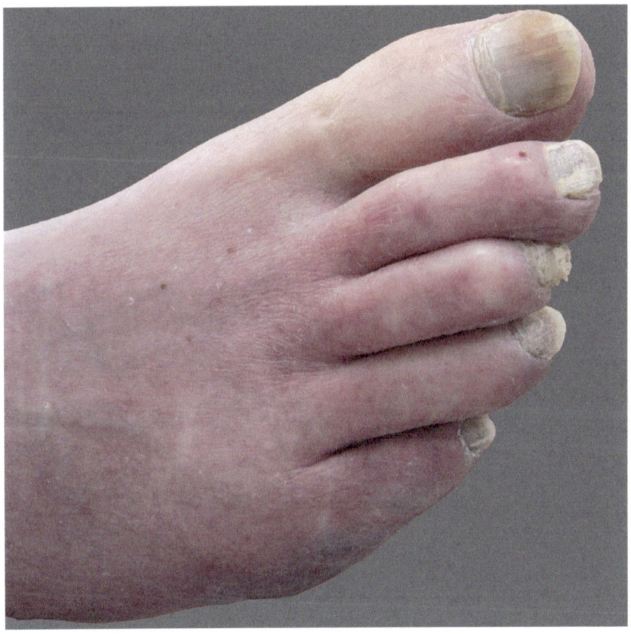

Fig. 2.136 Fungal infection of the toenails is not uncommon in the adult population, but it can be associated with diabetes mellitus and with arterial and venous insufficiency

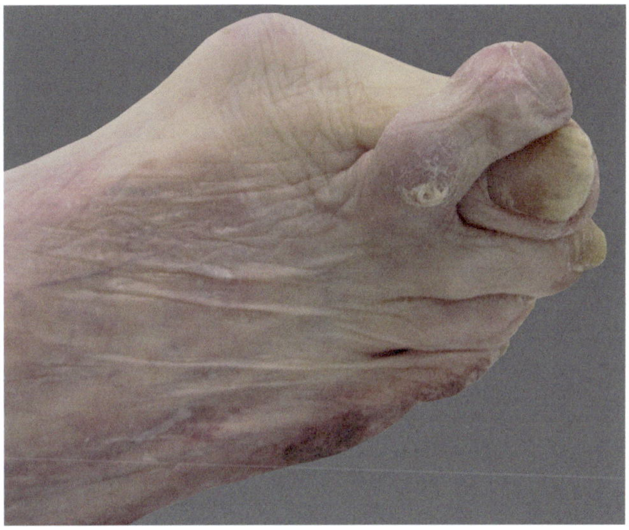

Fig. 2.137 Malalignment of toes. Positional deformity of the toes can be a cause of trips and falls in the elderly

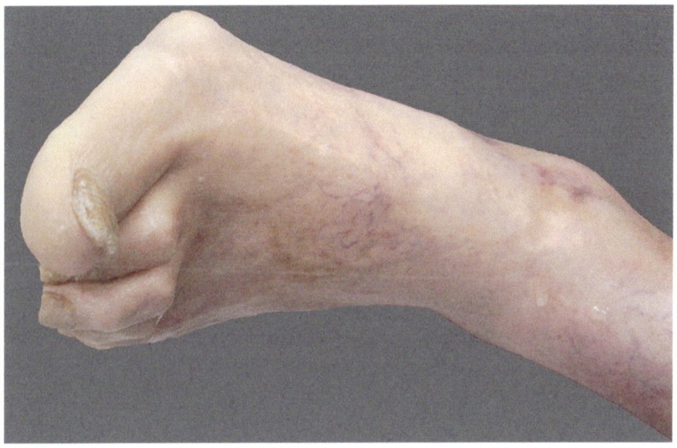

Fig. 2.138 The small joints in the feet may show deformities of arthritis

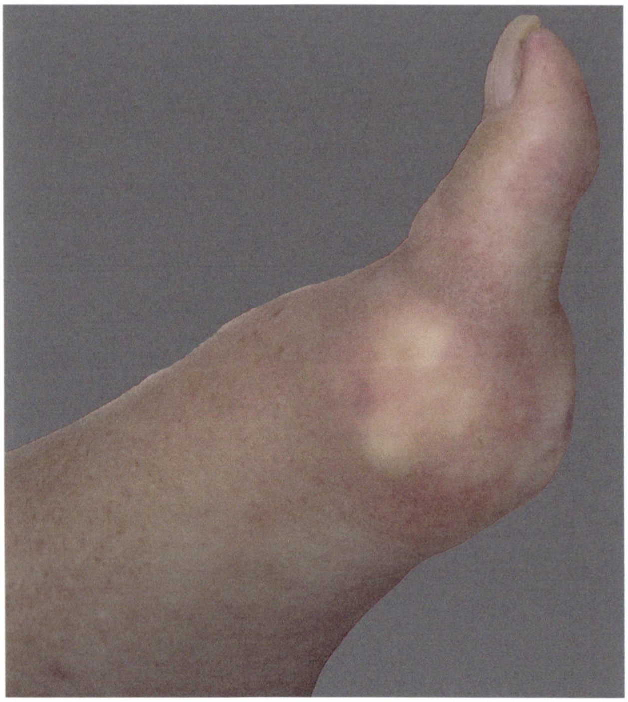

Fig. 2.139 Gout. These subcutaneous nodules are gouty tophi in the classic disease site

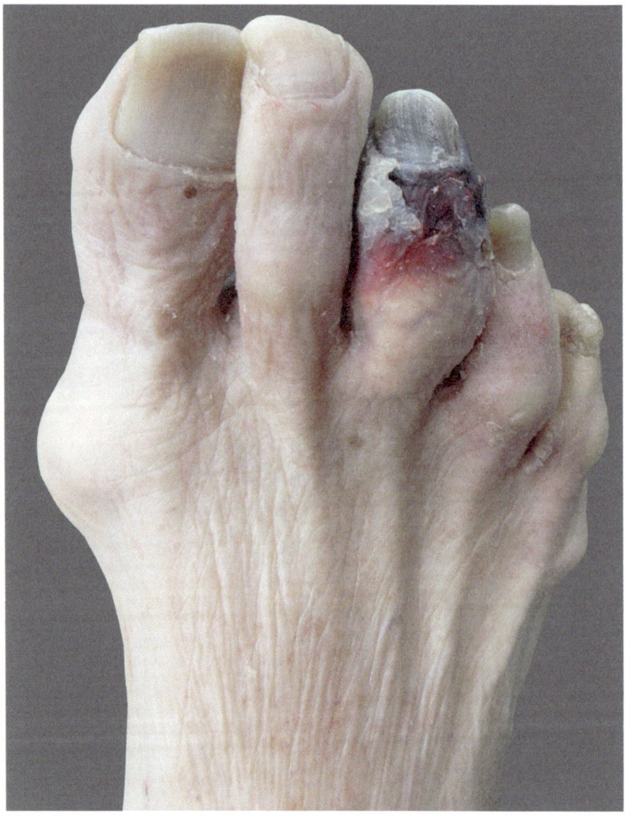

Fig. 2.140 Ischaemic toe. Blue toe syndrome is a sign of lower extremity emboli. In this case it followed aortic surgery

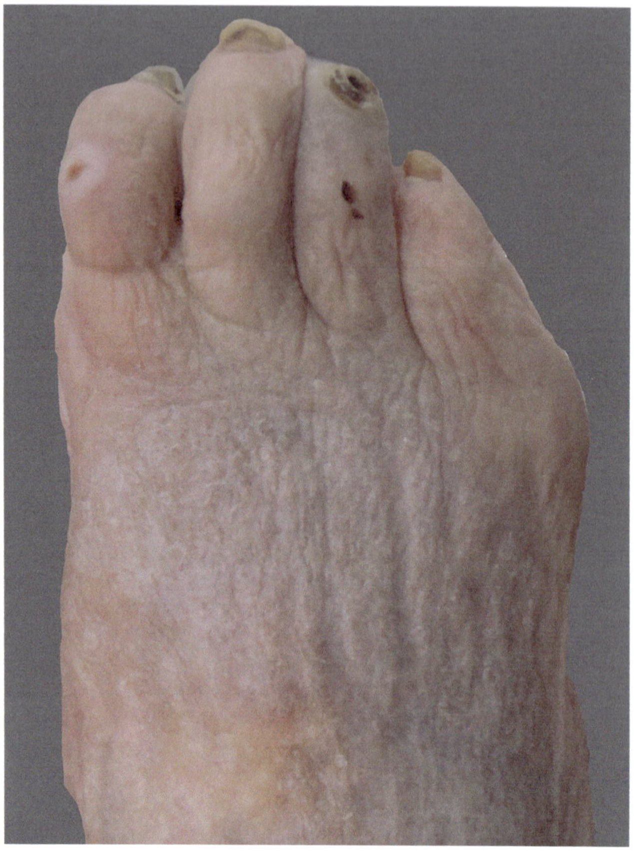

Fig. 2.141 In this diabetic foot, the big toe has been previously amputated, perhaps because of trauma or infection. There is toenail disease due to fungal infection. Ulceration is noted over the second toe, in keeping with diabetic neuropathy

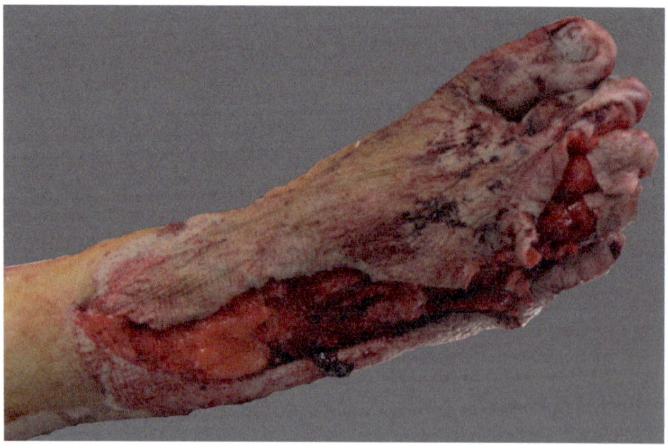

Fig. 2.142 In this traumatic foot injury, there is partial de-gloving of the skin overlying the foot and ankle, several of the toes are broken and one is partially amputated

- Lateral aspect (Figs. 2.143, 2.144, 2.145, 2.146, and 2.147)

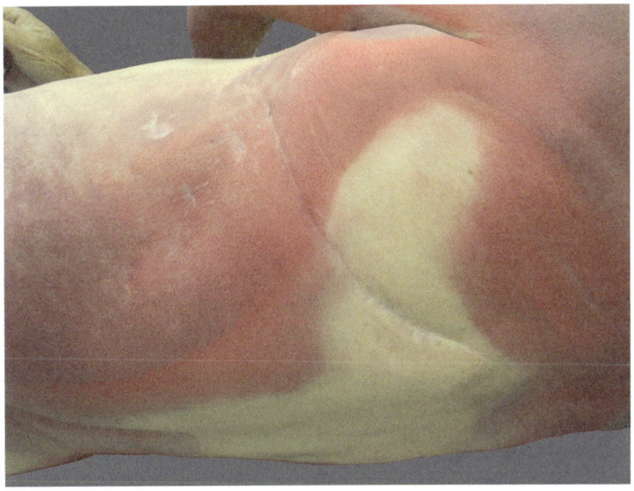

Fig. 2.143 It is all too easy to look at the body only from the front or back. Old lateral-aspect thoracotomy scars can be overlooked. Note the separate smaller scars from previous chest drains

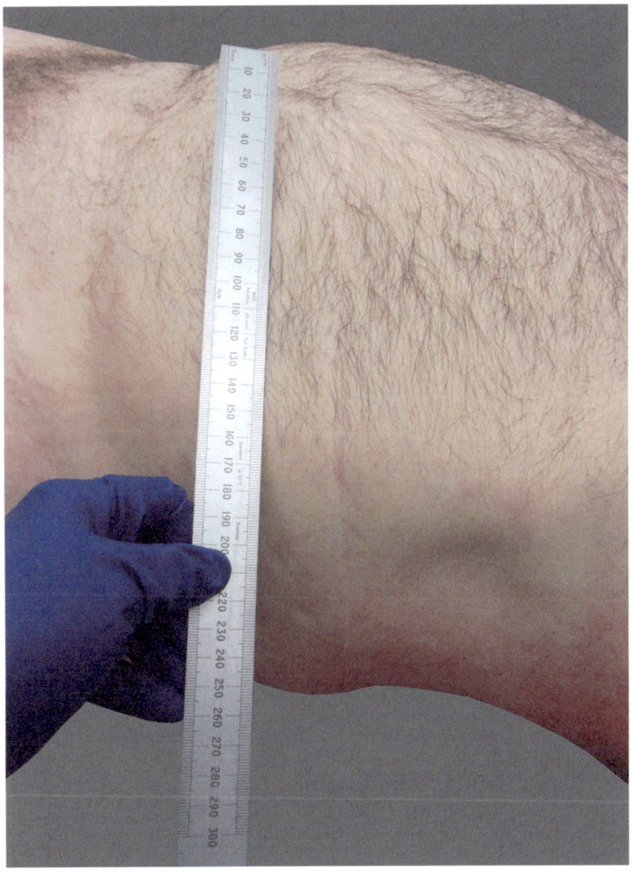

Fig. 2.144 Renal surgery. The flanks are easily overlooked and faded scars may be missed. There was a history of nephrectomy for a benign renal tumour

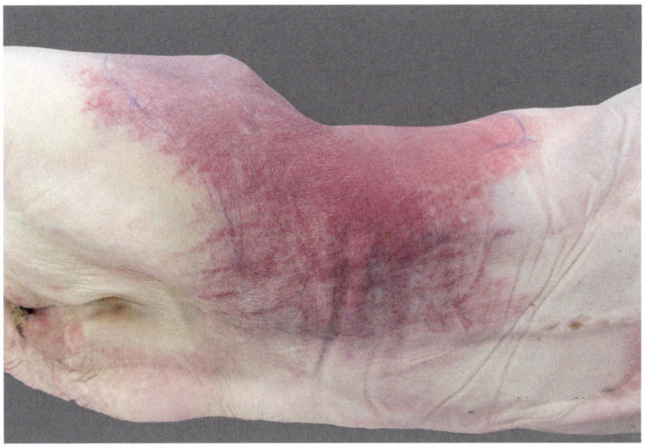

Fig. 2.145 Grey Turner's sign is shown here. There was a massive retroperitoneal haemorrhage due to dissection of the internal iliac artery

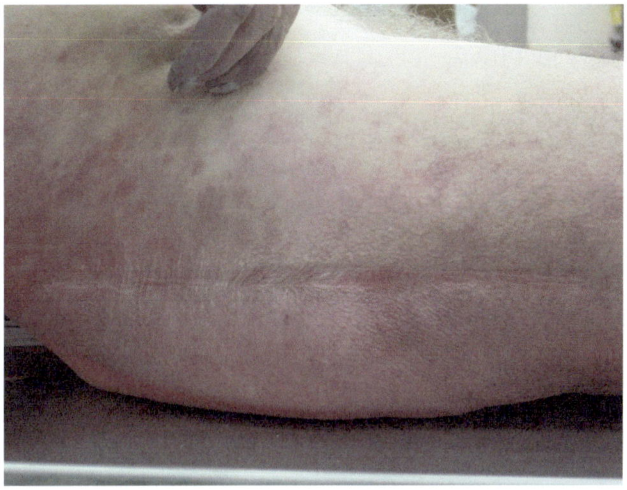

Fig. 2.146 Hip replacement scar may be missed unless one looks at the sides of the body. Old hip replacement scars can be faded and difficult to appreciate

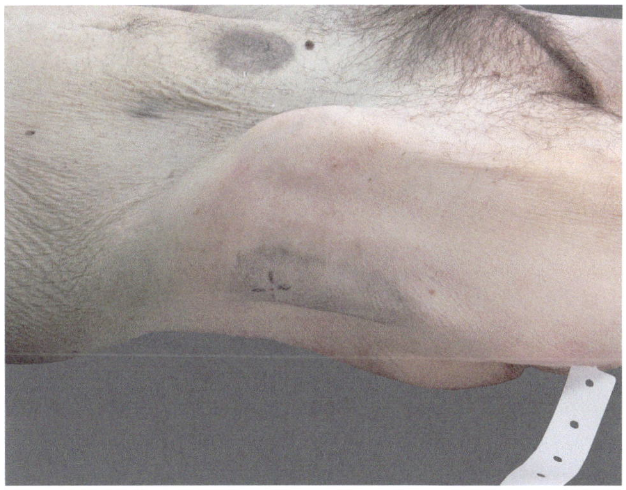

Fig. 2.147 A radiotherapy tattoo marking for pelvic radiotherapy treatment

- Back (Figs. 2.148, 2.149, 2.150, 2.151, and 2.152)

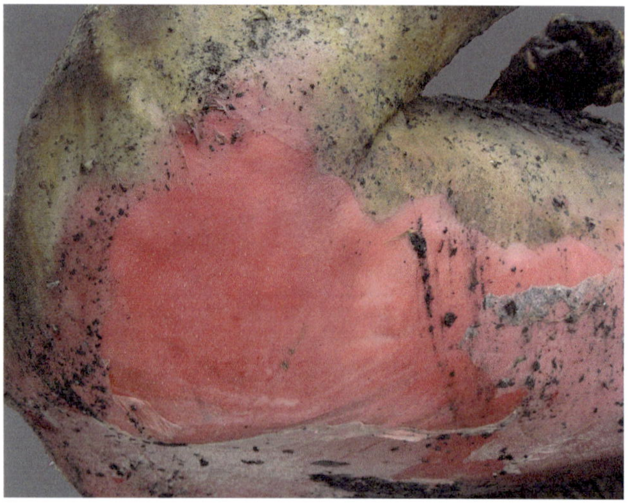

Fig. 2.148 Turning the body to the side. This body has been rotated onto the left side. It shows extensive burn injury affecting the hand (top right corner). This injury is seen in association with the cherry red discolouration of carbon monoxide poisoning on the back (in the area where the skin surface has been lost). There is widespread soot deposition on the attached skin surfaces

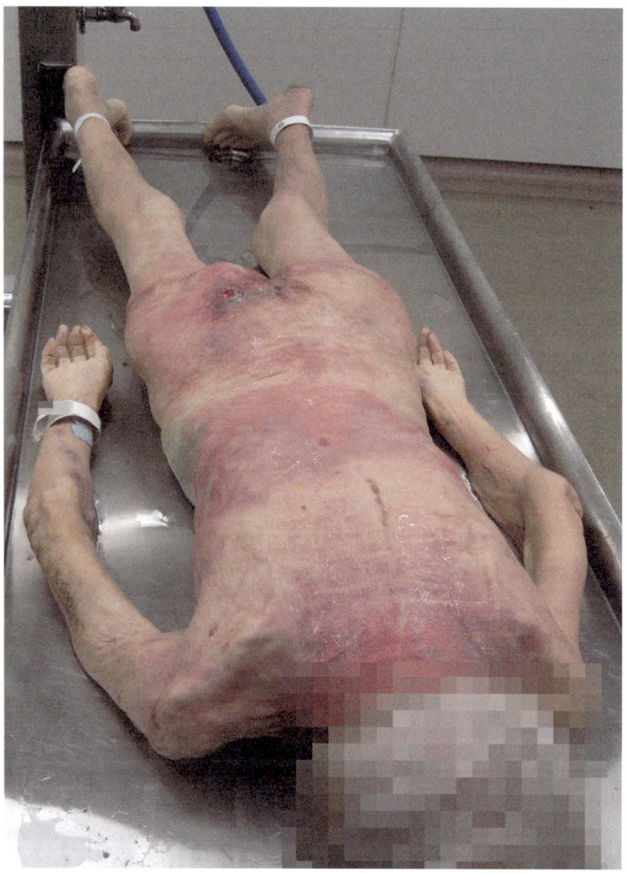

Fig. 2.149 Prone examination. The body can be turned onto the front (prone) to get a good view of all the posterior tissues, especially if photography is needed. Note the pressure areas over the buttock and sacrum, which were photographed. However, as above, turning the body by 90° (right or left side) often suffices and is simpler

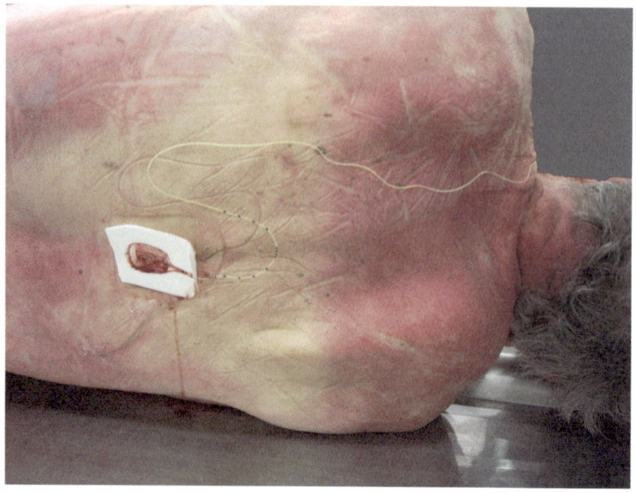

Fig. 2.150 The dressing over this epidural catheter will be removed to examine the insertion point

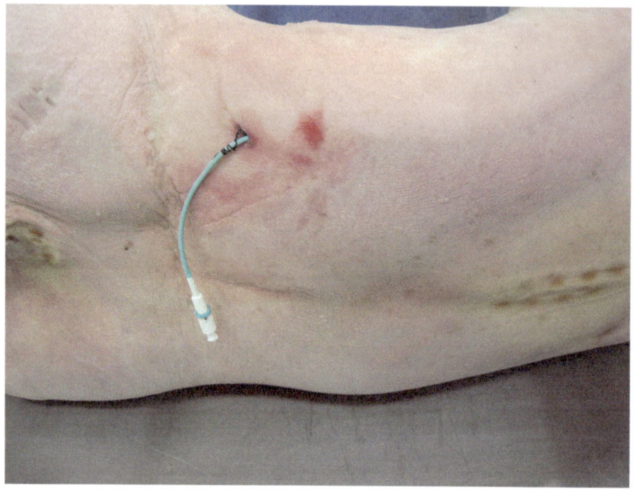

Fig. 2.151 Direct drainage from the kidney pelvis via a nephrostomy catheter is seen. The tube is left in situ until the internal placement is confirmed. Note the early pressure changes to the skin over the spine and sacrum in this patient reflecting a period of inactivity

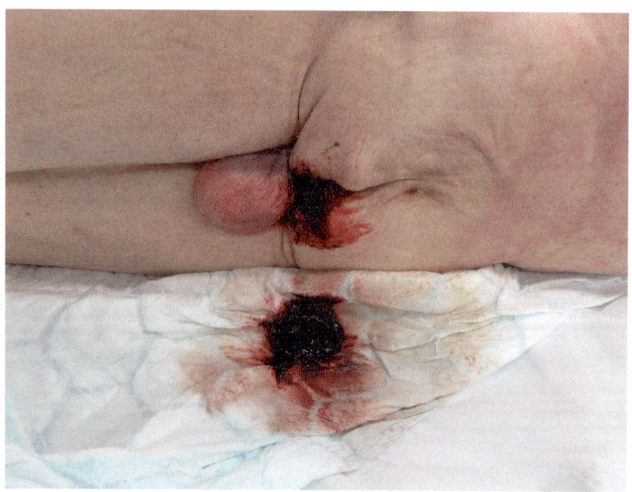

Fig. 2.152 Acute gastrointestinal haemorrhage. Examination of the tissues around the anus and any associated fluid/matter are noted in this case to be a result of acute gastrointestinal haemorrhage which caused hypovolaemic shock

- Decomposition (Figs. 2.153, 2.154, 2.155, 2.156, 2.157, 2.158, and 2.159)

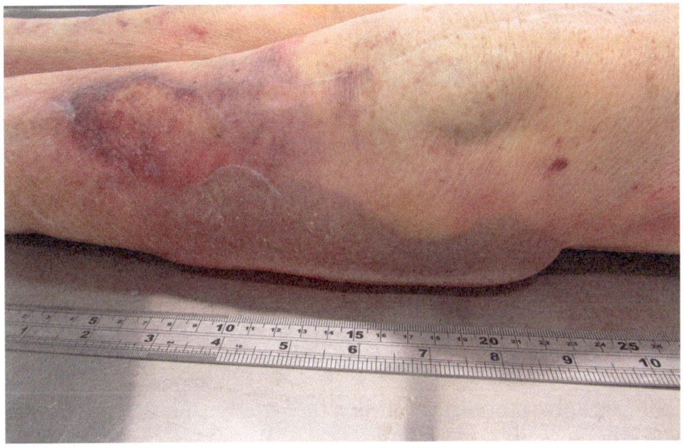

Fig. 2.153 Skin slippage occurs as a result of autolytic release of hydrolytic enzymes at the junction of the epidermis and dermis. This results in loosening and sloughing of the epidermis. This may be seen initially as the formation of vesicles or blisters

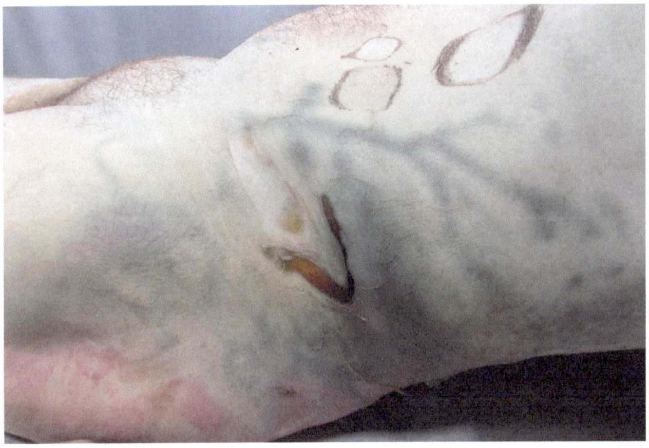

Fig. 2.154 Skin marbling is shown. In this situation the skin changes reflect the progression of decomposition

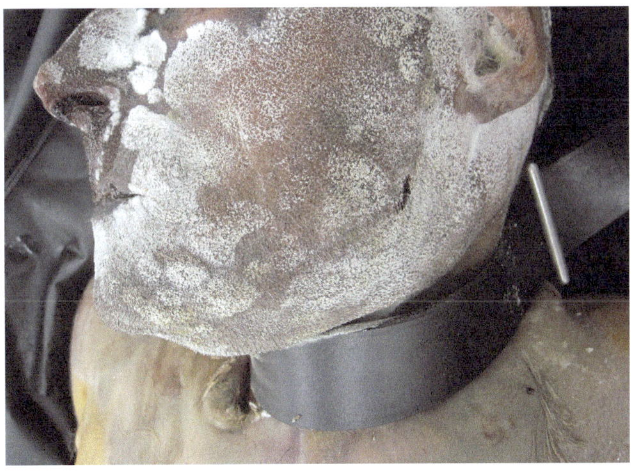

Fig. 2.155 Decomposition is affected by environmental factors such as temperature, but also microbes, organisms and insects. This is fungal bloom over the head and neck of a man found hanged

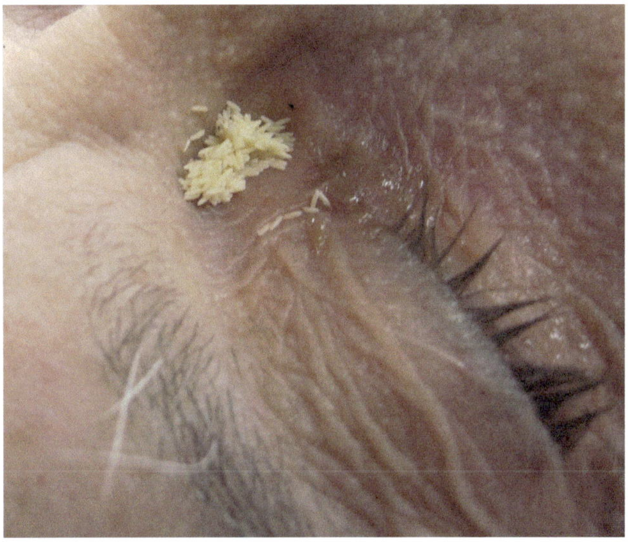

Fig. 2.156 Early decomposition. The presence of a body in the open often leads to flies laying eggs at mucocutaneous junctions early—in this case, at the eye. These eggs will hatch after a short period and the maggots will degrade the decomposing flesh

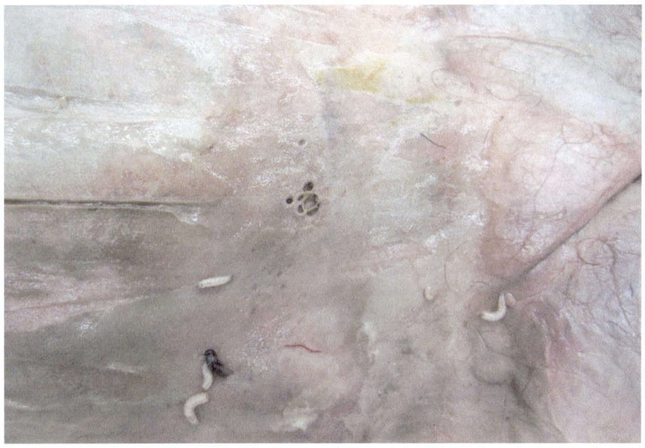

Fig. 2.157 Maggot infestation is seen initially in natural orifices but this will spread throughout the body. The small holes on the skin surface here represent sites of maggot burrowing into deeper tissues

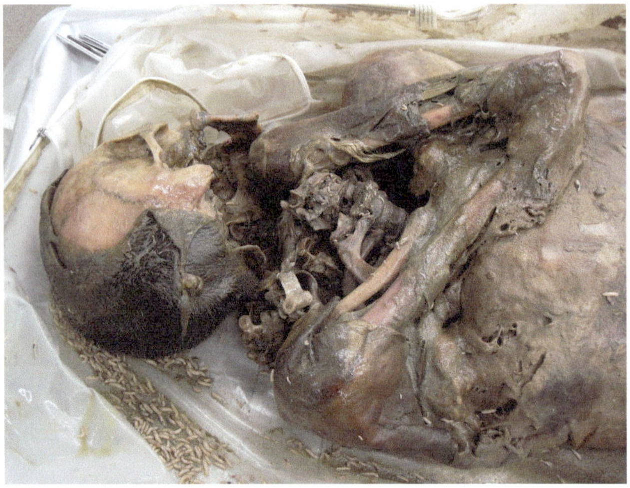

Fig. 2.158 Infestation and decomposition. The external tissues soften and become brown-black as they putrefy. Maggots flee from light and are best assessed when the body bag is first opened. There are holes seen on the skin surface where the maggots have burrowed into deeper tissues

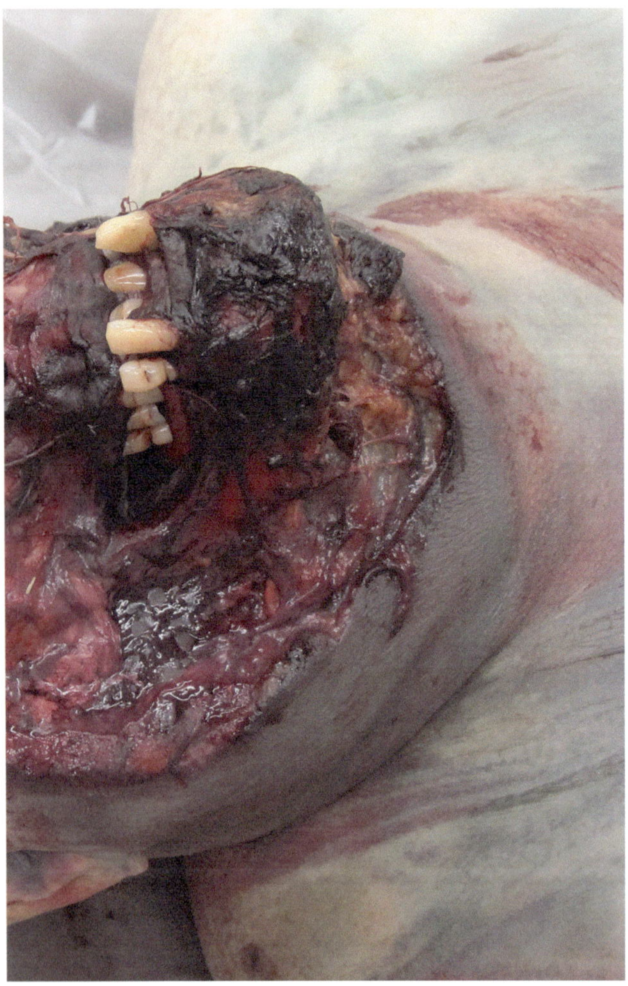

Fig. 2.159 Animal marks. Domestic, wild and marine animals may scavenge tissue from the dead. In this case, a domestic pet was responsible for the loss of tissue over the face

Practical Realities of the External Examination

Any relevant external features are usually documented on a body diagram, using a combination of text, drawing, and shorthand symbols. The site and appearance of each feature is noted, along with relevant measurements. The diagram and descriptive information serve as an aide-mémoire for the final report and act as contemporaneous evidence of findings at the time of examination. Some may find it preferable to contemporaneously dictate the external examination using a voice recorder.

Photography is important as it provides a permanent record for future reference. Photographing every detail with a scale rule is not necessary in a general autopsy case. All photographs should include the case reference number (either in the image or as coding digitally) and should be taken in accordance with good medical practise guidelines and local legal/consent realities. Taking photographs on personal smartphones is not advisable.

The Examination in Stages

The external examination is akin to how one approaches external examination of a patient in a clinical setting, starting with an 'end of the bed assessment', each organ system is then given consideration. External stigmata of many diseases may remain after death, but some do not. Some features (*e.g.*, cyanosis) no longer hold relevance in the post-mortem setting. Palpation and articulation of the body is also necessary, akin to the clinical examination.

It does not matter in which order the examination is completed, but it is recommended that the approach is logical and done in a standard fashion so that nothing is missed. The anterior, posterior and lateral aspects are examined from head to toe.

Findings fall under broad headings: demographics (apparent age, ethnicity, sex, height, weight), descriptors (eye colour, hair colour, nutritional state, signs of neglect of personal hygiene), items attached to the body (clothing, jewellery, medical and surgical devices, ligatures, etc.), surgical and nonsurgical modifications (hair extensions, breast implants, etc.), body adornments (tattoos, piercings, etc.), signs of natural disease, signs of injury (new and old), signs of decomposition.

The documents written at the time of the external examination should be kept as part of the autopsy record according to local and national guidelines. In the UK, they are ideally kept for a period of up to 30 years [3, 4]. All medicolegal autopsy reports in the UK belong to the HM Coroner (or Procurator Fiscal), and permission is required to share them with any interested person, including family or medical staff.

General Observations in All Reports

Identification of the body (see Chap. 1) is confirmed by using identification bands and case paperwork. A note is made of the height, weight, apparent age (some diseases cause premature aging), habitus (*i.e.*, general nutritional state), sex, and ethnicity.

The sex is recorded according to the external genitalia, with appropriate adjustment made in the final report to account for transgender status. Ethnicity is recorded either according to skin tone and bone structure (white, brown, black) or ethnicity (Caucasian, African, African-Caribbean, Indian subcontinent, Oriental, South American Indian, Polynesian, Inuit, etc.). If one is uncertain, describe the skin and hair, and be prepared to ask the family about the family tree.

In a mortuary setting, most of the deceased are already naked. If clothing is present, each item should be recorded prior to removal. Pockets should be examined using forceps, so as to avoid inadvertent sharps injury. Assumptions regarding the nature of jewellery should be avoided. For example, refer to a yellow metal ring with a clear stone, rather than a gold ring containing a diamond.

The position of the patient may be relevant and the distribution of post-mortem hypostasis should be noted. Comment on mild, moderate, or pronounced rigor mortis. Fluids around the body are documented.

For repatriated bodies, there may have been an autopsy in the country of death and the external examination will reflect previous embalming and evisceration.

Medical and Surgical Intervention Devices

The purpose of recording medical and surgical devices is to confirm the interventions, exclude iatrogenic injury, and seek information about disease treatment and management. See also Chap. 11.

Medical devices are documented by site and name. If the device has a specific registration code, this too is noted. Advances in medical technology may mean that the pathologist is faced with an unfamiliar device. Photography for future reference and review of the clinical/medical record should be considered.

Devices are commonly related to medical emergencies (ECG stickers), surgical treatment (drains) and organ monitoring (urinary catheters). However, there are also devices for chronic disease management, treatment, and drug delivery (Table 2.1). One is advised to record the drug name, dose, and location of drug delivery devices such as transdermal patches. Remember that some medical devices, such as haemodialysis fistulas, Hickman line, cardiac pacemakers, and intrathecal shunts, may be visible below the skin or palpable. If a cardiac pacemaker is known to be present, then it is important to clarify whether it is a defibrillator (ICD) device, as these devices must be deactivated prior to evisceration because there is a finite risk of electrical shock to the prosector [5]. Orthopedic external fixation devices may require specialist removal.

Table 2.1 Examples of medical and surgical devices found during the external examination

Type of device	Examples
Implantable devices	Pacemaker ICD Contraceptive Insulin pump Intrathecal shunt AV haemodialysis shunt
Drug/nutrition delivery devices	Transdermal patch Intravenous line Hickman line NG tube PEG tube
Organ monitoring/ support devices	Arterial line Urinary catheter (indwelling/suprapubic) ET tube Tracheostomy Intracranial pressure inducer
Surgical devices	Chest drains Surgical drains Colostomy, urostomy, ileostomy bags Nephrostomy line
Emergency treatment	ECG stickers Defibrillator pads Limb tourniquets

AV arteriovenous, *ET* endotracheal, *ICD* implantable cardioverter defibrillator, *NG* nasogastric, *PEG* percutaneous endoscopic gastrostomy

Bandages, dressings, and plaster casts must be removed to enable examination of any underlying wound. Interventional devices (*e.g.*, endotracheal tube, nasogastric tube, chest drain, peritoneal drain, surgical drains, etc.) remain in situ until the internal location is confirmed, but they may be cut flush with the skin to facilitate examination. Intravascular lines can also be cut flush to the skin if necessary, to aid assessment after evisceration. Superficial devices are removed and may be safely discarded if they are not required as evidence.

The volume and colour of fluid in drain bags should be recorded before it is discarded. The skin adjacent to devices or wounds is examined for signs of infection, haemorrhage, surgical emphysema, and damage. If there are features of infection, one may consider whether a microbiology swab is appropriate (although handling of the body post-mortem and skin commensals often provide a mixed flora result).

The common sites of venous access are the dorsum of the hand, anterior wrist, antecubital fossa, anterior neck, and groin, but any vessel may have been cannulated in patients with limited venous access. Intraosseous needles are usually left in situ and are more common in patients from an emergency setting. One should always look for needle puncture marks (which might suggest illicit drugs), bruising, thrombophlebitis, and localized accumulation of fluid in subcutaneous tissues.

Medical devices may have been removed recently, and marks on the skin provide clues or indeed may cause concern; for example, deep bruising over the anterior triangle of the neck (from a central line) should not be misinterpreted as a sign of assault.

Cardiopulmonary Resuscitation

Marks left by cardiopulmonary resuscitation (CPR) are not unusual. In order to be effective, CPR is a physically forceful procedure. It may leave marks externally and internally. Chest hair is shaved to improve electrical conduction. The defibrillator pads are extremely sticky and can cause superficial skin loss when removed. By the time of autopsy, the areas of skin loss will have the appearance of an abrasion with parchment texture. The ribs fracture during chest compressions. Palpation of the anterior chest wall may demonstrate loss of ribcage integrity, leaving the internal examination to clarify which ribs are fractured. There may be numerous needle puncture marks due to attempted venous and arterial sampling. The location and dimensions of skin abrasions and the location of ECG stickers and so forth are recorded, but in the report are often summarised as 'features consistent with CPR'.

Scars

Scars are identifying marks, they may be a result of surgery, minor trauma, tribal marking, or self-harm. The site, size and state of the skin affected (fresh, healing, healed) is documented for each mark, and the surrounding skin is examined for signs of infection or surgical emphysema. Scarring that does not fit with the history provided or that is unusual in type or distribution should raise the possibility of injury that is not accidental or self-inflicted. Further information should be obtained before proceeding.

Scars have particular characteristics that allow presumption of origin. Incised surgical wounds heal by primary intention and leave a narrow, linear scar. Those that heal by secondary intention have a wider profile. The pathologist should be aware of the common surgical approaches in major surgery and therefore be able to predict which internal organs may be missing or repaired. One should pay close attention to the lateral aspects of the body so as not to miss nephrectomy, hip surgery, and/or thoracotomy scars. The type of wound closure and the state of healing is documented, with or without photography.

Autopsy practitioners should be aware that surgical techniques and approaches have changed over time and continue to do so. Thus, large laparotomy scars have been replaced by laparoscopic processes, so one must therefore diligently hunt out faint 10–20 mm port scars across the abdomen.

Stretch marks and skin creases can be problematic; palpation of the mark and finding fibrous subcutaneous tissue should help determine a true scar. Old, healed scars may show hypertrophic or keloid changes.

Scars from old minor trauma are usually less regular in outline and can be found almost anywhere on the body. Self-inflicted injury, such as repeated cutting of the skin, leads to multiple linear scars that are usually located on the arms and legs, but the breast and abdomen are not unusual sites. The scars are likely to be clustered together and arranged in parallel lines. It may be difficult to determine the exact number. One approach is to record the location of the scars, the longest and shortest measurement, and the nature of the arrangement.

Identifying Marks

The main purpose of recording identifying marks is for identification, but they also serve as clues to previous operations or procedures (*e.g.*, radiotherapy marking) or health risks (*e.g.*, street-art cosmetic tattoos, with a potential risk of blood borne viruses). One should document the type of identifying mark (Table 2.2), its location, description, size, and state of healing (fresh, healing, healed), remembering to look for signs of infection.

One should always consider identifiers with cultural or society realities. There are some good texts on this material [6] dealing with body modifications and piercings and cultural body modifications. One advises caution about commenting on specific details of artistic adornments or nonsurgical modifications. Stating there is a tattoo on the left

Table 2.2 Examples of identifying marks

Type of marks	Examples
Adornments	Tattoos (artistic, related to radiation therapy, related to occupation; record text, style, position of tattoo) Piercings Scarification Branding
Nonsurgical modifications	Cosmetics Hair treatments/extensions Nail extensions
Surgical modifications	Implants Prostheses Gender reassignment surgery
Scars	Surgical Old injury Self-harm

forearm measuring up to 30 mm is unlikely to cause problems, but incorrectly interpreting text or figurative drawings may lead to confusion, irritation, anger or distress for the family.

Indicators of Internal Disease and General Health

The skin provides information about the age, general health, nutrition status, and mobility of the deceased, primary dermatological diseases, and systemic illness. As the largest provider of information during the external examination, it is considered separately in this section.

In older individuals, the skin is thinner, more fragile, and more likely to be damaged, even during handling after death. Signs of aging include an increase in seborrheic keratosis, loss of elasticity and Campbell de Morgan spots (cherry haemangiomas).

General and nutritional health, care, and neglect may be reflected in the general appearance, condition, and cleanliness of the skin. Pressure ulcers over bony prominences and the sacrum (due to immobility and occasionally to limited nursing care) are described by site and degree of skin breakdown (ideally take a photograph with a scale rule). Poorly controlled diabetes mellitus may cause nonhealing arterial or neuropathic ulcers in the lower limbs, which have a characteristic punched-out appearance. Both diabetes and severe peripheral vascular disease may result in hair loss over the lower limb, gangrene, or distal surgical amputations.

Features that might indicate potential neglect of the deceased should be considered carefully before any further examination takes place, particularly if the individual has been in social, nursing, or hospital care facilities. In such cases, forensic/specialist practitioners may need to be involved.

The site, size, location, and description of primary skin pathology, such as individual skin tumours (whether benign or malignant), should be recorded. Multiple skin tumours may be associated with underlying genetic disease (*e.g.*, neurofibromatosis) or immunosuppression (*e.g.*, renal transplant patients). In some cases, the changes clearly indicate a potential cause of death (*e.g.*, malignant melanoma). Chronic inflammatory diseases of the skin such as psoriasis and eczema are usually not life-threatening but should prompt one to look for the effects of chronic steroid use. These conditions may point towards an 'Addisonian-type' crisis as a mode of death. Clearly, any generalised skin inflammatory process will debilitate an individual, and in cases of infection a rash may suggest fatal bacteraemia (*e.g.*, the rash of meningococcal sepsis which remains after death).

A variety of color changes are useful clues as to internal disease. As in life, bright yellow discolouration of jaundice is an indicator of raised bilirubin, consistent with red cell lysis, biliary obstruction and/or liver failure. It should be noted that the classical skin stigmata of chronic liver disease, such as palmar erythema and spider naevi, fade when the circulation ceases, but abdominal varices and clubbing will persist.

Pallor is a good indicator of anaemia in the living, but it is a less specific sign after death. Gross pallor may nevertheless be due to massive internal haemorrhage.

In situations of carbon monoxide poisoning, the skin takes on a cherry-red colour due to carboxyhaemoglobin formation.

The blue discolouration of cyanosis, seen ante-mortem in chronic respiratory illnesses, is less specific after death [7]. Indeed, the peripheries are often noted to have a dusky hue in those both with and without chronic lung disease. Other colour clues include focal skin discolouration, such as tar staining on fingers in those who are heavy tobacco smokers, or coal tattoos affecting miners and a few other occupations.

The distribution and quality of petechial haemorrhages in the skin should always be assessed. Those resulting from asphyxia are likely to be distributed in the face and neck, whereas those from disorders causing thrombocytopenia have an irregular distribution across the body and are likely to be accompanied by larger purpura changes. In addition, the petechial haemorrhages seen within areas of dependent lividity have a coarse appearance. Disorders of coagulation (liver failure, haematological malignancy) may lead to widespread purpuric bruising.

Autoimmune diseases may cause scarring and skin deformity (*e.g.*, scleroderma).

If the external examination raises the possibility of an infectious disease, it is important to notify other people working with you so that appropriate safety measures can be taken.

Schematic Examination Guides the Assessment of Internal Pathology

Each part of the body is carefully examined for external features of disease (Table 2.3). Pathologists ideally should be familiar with many of the external stigmata of systemic diseases. This book cannot cover all possibilities; other texts [8] and a clinical examination textbook should be consulted where necessary [9]. Site-specific or device-specific medical or surgical intervention related to underlying disease processes should be simultaneously considered.

Positive findings immediately guide the internal examination, and relevant supporting internal pathology should be sought to corroborate external findings. For example, an abdominal surgical scar should make one consider not only visceral gastrointestinal surgery but also hernia repair. In the

Table 2.3 Considerations at specific body sites during the external examination[a]

Body site	Considerations during examination
Skin	Assess age, general health, nutrition, and cleanliness Look for signs of immobility or neglect. Describe the site and size of primary skin pathology (tumours, rashes, etc.) Look for signs of systemic diseases: autoimmune, infectious, haematological, etc. Identify signs pointing to specific illnesses: *e.g.*, chronic liver disease, peripheral vascular disease, diabetes mellitus
Hair	Colour, length, hair loss
Scalp	Look and feel for injury
Face	Note characteristics of congenital syndromes. Feel integrity of the facial skeleton. Look for xanthelasma
Ears	Look for fluid in the external auditory canal, earlobe creases (associated with cardiovascular disease), postauricular bruising
Eyes	Surrounding tissues: periorbital oedema, panda eye bruising Iris: colour (if difficult to decide, use pale *vs* dark) Sclera: colour, petechial haemorrhages Conjunctiva: colour, congestion (commonly seen in cardiac arrests), petechial haemorrhages (invert the lower lids) Cornea: cataract, corneal arcus (significant if <40 years), eyeliner/tache noire (discolouration occurring when eyelids are left open after death) Pupils: symmetry no longer relevant after death
Nose	Integrity of the nasal septum (can disintegrate with heavy cocaine use)
Lips	Angular stomatitis (vitamin deficiency)
Tongue	Injury (epilepsy), glossitis (vitamin deficiency), candida infection (immunosuppression, steroid use)
Teeth	The presence and condition of teeth/dentures
Gums	Gingivitis, hypertrophy (phenytoin treatment)
Mouth	Note fluid around or in the mouth. Look for foreign body, enlarged tonsils, and aphthous ulcers (inflammatory bowel disease). Check for a high arched palate (Marfan's)
Neck	Feel for masses: lymph nodes, thyroid gland, cysts, tumours Check trachea: central (deviated in pneumothorax), tracheostomy
Shoulders, clavicles	Articulate to reveal closed fracture/dislocations
Upper and lower arms	Compare sides, assessing symmetry and colour (upper limb DVT, limb ischaemia). Palpate axillary lymph nodes. Examine elbow for rheumatoid nodules. This is common site for intravenous access; check for thrombophlebitis and localised fluid accumulation from 'tissued' cannulas. Palpate scars to reveal AV fistulas of renal dialysis
Hands, fingers	Check for missing digits, muscle wasting (may be neurological or musculoskeletal). Assess bony deformities of rheumatoid and osteoarthritis. Examine interdigital web spaces for scabies and needle puncture marks in IVDU cases. Feel for Dupuytren's contracture (liver disease)
Nails	Nail signs remain after death: leukonychia (hypoalbuminemia), koilonychia (iron deficiency), splinter haemorrhages (infective endocarditis, manual work), pitting (psoriasis), paronychia, onychomycosis, digital clubbing
Chest	Assess shape: barrel chest (chronic lung disease), pigeon chest (congenital). Palpate left upper chest for pacemaker. Compress ribs to elicit fractures. Check lateral chest for old chest drain scars
Breast	Palpation may reveal breast masses, implants, or gynecomastia. Look for skin changes associated with breast disease. Lift breast to check for scars or skin infection
Abdomen	Distention may be due to fat, fluid, faeces, fetus, or gas. Lift the abdominal apron to examine skin creases for infection, obscured medical paraphernalia, and injury. Look for bruising caused by common subcutaneous injections (insulin, low molecular weight heparin). Examine each quadrant carefully, looking for scars and hernias (epigastric, umbilical, inguinal, incisional). Note surgical drains, recording volume and appearance of fluid in drain bags. Removal of stoma bags is necessary; check that a replacement bag is available for reconstruction post autopsy. Cullen's sign (umbilical/periumbilical bruising) is a rare sign of retroperitoneal haemorrhage (ectopic pregnancy, acute pancreatitis, etc.)
Groin	Needle puncture marks may be from emergency care or IVDU; deep sinus formation is due to chronic drug misuse. Check for hernias (unlikely to be palpable in a prone dead body unless very large). Palpate for inguinal lymph nodes. This is a common site for interventional radiological access, so be alert for iatrogenic injury
External genitalia	Lift the penis to examine the scrotum and testes Scrotal oedema is seen in heart failure and fluid overload. Palpate the scrotum to identify both testes (prosthetic testicles can be implanted after orchiectomy), swellings (hydrocele), and tumours. Examine penis and vulva for gross pathology, piercings, and tattoos
Upper and lower legs	Limb deformity may be due to congenital or acquired musculoskeletal or neurological diseases. Note the level of any amputation and comment on the condition of the stump Examine over joints for surgical scars. If legs are asymmetrical, measure calf circumference (10 cm below tibial tuberosity); a difference of $\geq$3 cm raises possibility of DVT. Comment on surface changes: unilateral skin mottling due to critical limb ischaemia remains after death; venous insufficiency leads to hair loss, venous eczema/stasis dermatitis, hyperpigmentation, oedema, varicose veins, and/or cellulitis. Distinguish between arterial, venous, and pressure ulcers. Apply firm pressure over a distal bony prominence to assess for pitting oedema. Moving proximally, repeat to find most proximal level (remembering that there will be dependent pooling of plasma on the posterior surface)

(continued)

Table 2.3 (continued)

Body site	Considerations during examination
Feet, toes	Check for missing toes, positional deformity (neurological, musculoskeletal). Look for changes related to rheumatoid and osteoarthritis. Examine interdigital web spaces for scabies and needle puncture marks in IVDU cases. In diabetics, check the feet carefully for signs of injury and infection
Toenails	Note if the toenails are extremely long; this can lead to falls in the elderly. Long nails can also damage the skin and have been implicated in variable haemorrhage and/or local skin sepsis
Lateral surfaces	Grey-Turner's sign (bruising over the flank) is due to retroperitoneal blood (*e.g.*, acute pancreatitis). Bruising in this area also can be due to trauma (fight or accident) and may not have been noticed by the police. Scars from nephrectomy or thoracotomy are found at this location
Posterior surfaces	A visual assessment of the back will reveal spinal deformity, surgical scars, and intrathecal devices. Attention should be paid to the sacral pressure areas, particularly in bedbound and elderly people. Pressure areas are measured, and the depth of epidermal damage is noted. The posterior surfaces of the limbs should be examined for injury and tattoos
Anus	Haemorrhoids and skin tags are not uncommon. There may be faecal matter or melena around the anus. Remember to be alert for injury

AV arteriovenous, *DVT* deep vein thrombosis, *IVDU* intravenous drug use
[a] Injuries, identifying marks, and devices are noted for all locations

same way, information from the clinical history should be corroborated with the external examination; a clinical diagnosis of pulmonary embolism, for instance, should direct one to carefully examine the symmetry of the lower limbs. Documenting important negative findings is also prudent, based on what is expected when one reviews the clinical ante-mortem data.

Generalised features such as muscle wasting may indicate malnutrition or musculoskeletal or neurological disease. There are many causes of pitting peripheral oedema. The lymph nodes in the neck, axilla and groin are palpated to identify widespread or focal lymphadenopathy.

A constellation of findings may provide good supporting evidence for a specific internal or systemic pathological process, such as a distended abdomen with incarcerated and discoloured incisional hernia, which is in keeping with bowel obstruction and fatal toxaemia. Similarly, a constellation of findings may point to a narrow differential, as when shiny, hairless skin on the lower leg with distal ulceration, gangrene and previous toe amputation point to chronic peripheral vascular disease and diabetes mellitus.

Trauma and Injury

Traumatic injury can result in direct, indirect, or delayed death. The pathologist may be examining injuries from a recent accident or one that happened in the past. It is important to record findings accurately (Table 2.4), and photography is extremely useful in this instance. The types of injuries and their relevance to the cause of death is discussed in Chap. 12.

Table 2.4 Terminology of wounds and fractures

Injury	Definition
Abrasion	Superficial graze or scratch
Bruise	Result of blunt trauma without skin breakage, causing discolouration through various stages: red → blue → green → yellow → brown
Laceration	Result of blunt trauma causing the skin to tear
Incision	A wound caused by a sharp edge
Closed fracture	Bone does not protrude through skin
Open fracture	Bone protrudes through skin
Amputation	Limb or digit missing; may be traumatic or surgical

Bony injury may be visible or may be revealed by palpation or articulation of the limbs, thoracic cage, pelvis, and scalp. The identification of any closed fractures should be communicated to the person eviscerating the body so as to guard against injury from sharp-edged bony fragments. Injury sustained once blood flow has ceased will lack a surrounding skin reaction, helping to differentiate between pre-mortem and post-mortem injuries.

Recognising that the general autopsy may take place with an incomplete or limited history of the events leading up to death, it is vital to be alert for findings that do not quite fit the story given. Very careful consideration is paid to the mechanism of any traumatic injury and how it relates to the clinical history provided.

Specifically, the external examination is to ensure the correct post-mortem examination is carried out. Unexpected or unusual findings should be discussed with police or legal representatives or relevant medical staff. It is better to pause an examination in order to gather more information than to go ahead with the evisceration and potentially destroy evidence.

External Examination as Part of the Radiological Autopsy

Post-mortem imaging is being increasing used as an adjunct to autopsy examination (see Chap. 13). This evolving specialist technique has demonstrated good results in assessing traumatic injury [10]. Accessing hospital pre-mortem emergency scans may also be feasible in some settings. A forensic text should be consulted for in-depth descriptions of traumatic injuries and their common mechanisms [7].

Post-mortem Changes and Decomposition

Post-mortem changes and decomposition will be the least familiar external features to the uninitiated pathologist. Importantly, the pathologist must guard against over-interpreting decomposition and post-mortem damage as injury related to the death. Therefore, an understanding of the basic physiological changes in anatomical tissues after death and an overview of the macroscopic appearances is required.

The features may be documented in some detail at the time of external examination but are often summarised carefully in the final report so as to give accurate information to the reader whilst minimising unnecessary distress to the bereaved, should they read the report.

The complexity of organic matter decomposition is beyond the scope of this brief text, as it is affected by a multitude of environmental and endogenous conditions. The literature refers to various sequential stages of decomposition, but there is usually a degree of heterogeneity in external decomposition [11].

Once circulation ceases, the blood and plasma fall to the dependant areas of the body (hypostasis). Haemoglobin breakdown gives a red-blue hue to the skin (lividity), and plasma pooling leads to dependent oedema. Small, pinpoint, coarse haemorrhages may be seen within the post-mortem hypostasis, and these should not be over-interpreted as petechial haemorrhages of asphyxiation, which are finer and more discrete. Any item exerting pressure on the skin at the time of death will leave a negative imprint in the area of lividity.

Large, superficial, fragile skin blisters are due to the pooled plasma moving into subcutaneous and epidermal tissues. These blisters may break or coalesce, leading to small or large areas of skin slippage. Areas of superficial epidermal loss become dry and attain a parchment-like quality. These areas may resemble superficial burns, but confusion is unlikely when the clinical history and circumstances of death are considered.

The actions of endogenous cellular mechanisms (autolysis) and microbial proliferation (putrefaction) gradually break down cellular tissue components. Liquefaction of mucosal linings happens rapidly, and brown fluid seen in or around the mouth and nasopharynx should not be over-interpreted as evidence of upper gastrointestinal haemorrhage. Haematemesis is not usually a subtle finding and there will be internal findings to support the diagnosis.

Green discolouration of the skin is usually an early sign of internal decomposition. Red blood cells leak into the subcutaneous tissues and bacteria convert haemoglobin into sulphaemoglobin. Because the caecum contains a high concentration of gut flora and is located relatively near to the skin surface, this process commonly begins in the right lower quadrant of the abdomen and spreads across the abdomen and flanks. Venous marbling is due to decomposition of haemoglobin within blood vessels and gas assisting the travel of sulphaemoglobin through vessels and lymphatics [12]. The result is a striking appearance of superficial vessels against the usual skin tone of the deceased, giving a marbled appearance, which can be very pronounced in a very short time in those who die in circumstances of overwhelming sepsis. Gas formation also leads to abdominal bloating, and the internal soft tissues appear 'bubbly' (similar to surgical emphysema see in vivo).

Sometimes bodies are remarkably well-preserved, even if they have come to the attention of the authorities some time after death. This state may be due to mummification, as occurs in dry or cold environments, or the formation of apodicere (a waxlike organic substance formed by the anaerobic bacterial hydrolysis of fat), more common in wet environments.

In general, external tissues soften and become black as they putrefy. Maggot infestation begins in natural orifices but spreads throughout the body. Maggots flee from light and are best assessed when the body bag is first opened. Care is taken to ensure all maggots that escape from the post-mortem table are cleared up, so as to prevent fly infestations within the mortuary. Whilst entomology is a central topic of interest in forensic dramas, it is very rarely relevant to the general autopsy. One only needs to comment on the presence of eggs, maggots or flies; it is not necessary to document the stages of pupation or number of adult insects.

After putrefaction, all that remains of the deceased is musculoskeletal or skeletal tissue. If the body is not yet identified, a specialist odontologic examination is required. Even with very little human remains, a careful external examination with appropriate sampling is required.

In most cases, as a general rule, the pathologist needs only to comment on early or late decomposition changes and to document specific findings such as maggot infestation or bite marks left by domestic, wild, or marine animals. It is unlikely that the pathologist would be asked to provide a time of death based on decomposition; such cases should be handled by those with experience in decomposition changes.

References

1. Lucas SB, Cooper H, Emmett S, Hargraves C, Mason M. The coroner's autopsy: do we deserve better? National Confidential Enquiry into Patient Outcome and Death; 2006. http://www.ncepod.org.uk.
2. Leadbeatter S, Lucas SB, Lowe J. Standards for Coroners' pathologists in post-mortem examinations of deaths that appear not to be suspicious. The Royal College of Pathologists; 2014. https://www.rcpath.org/static/1b02cfb9-000a-4b2f-b6b80256b719a5ee/Standards-for-Coroners-pathologists-in-post-mortem-examinations-of-deaths-that-appear-not-to-be-suspicious.pdf.
3. Wilkins B. The retention and storage of pathological records and specimens. 5th ed. Guidance from The Royal College of Pathologists and The Institute of Biomedical Science; 2015. https://www.rcpath.org/static/049ea966-df5c-4a9f-9353ba24a69bb808/The-retention-and-storage-of-pathological-records-and-specimens-5th-edition.pdf.
4. The Transformation Directorate of NHS England. Records management code of practice. 2023. https://transform.england.nhs.uk/information-governance/guidance/records-management-code/.
5. Suvarna SK, Lloyd KL, Toh EW. Guidance for pathologists conducting post-mortem examinations on individuals with implanted electronic medical devices. The Royal College of Pathologists; 2022. https://www.rcpath.org/static/4f04f871-257e-446b-b94f38095defaf0d/guidance-for-pathologists-conducting-post-mortem-examinations-on-individuals-with-implanted-medical-devices.pdf.
6. Rutty GN. The external examination. In: Burton JL, Rutty GN, editors. The hospital autopsy. 3rd ed. London: Hodder Arnold; 2010. p. 99–101.
7. Saukko P, Knight B, editors. Knight's forensic pathology. 4th ed. Boca Raton: CRC Press; 2015.
8. Connolly AJ, Finkbeiner WE, Ursell PC, Davis RL, editors. Autopsy pathology: a manual and atlas. 3rd ed. Philadelphia, PA: Elsevier; 2016.
9. Thomas J, Monaghan T, editors. Oxford handbook of clinical examination and practical skills. 2nd ed. Oxford: Oxford University Press; 2014.
10. Scholing M, Saltzherr TP, Fung Kon Jin PH, Ponsen KJ, Reitsma JB, Lameris JS, et al. The value of post-mortem computed tomography as an alternative for autopsy in trauma victims: a systematic review. Eur Radiol. 2009;19(10):2333–41.
11. Burton JL. The decomposed body and the unascertained autopsy. In: Burton JL, Rutty GN, editors. The hospital autopsy. 3rd ed. London: Hodder Arnold; 2010. p. 292–307.
12. Pinheiro J. Decay process of a cadaver. In: Schmidt A, Cumha E, Pinheiro J, editors. Forensic anthropology and medicine. Ottawa: Humana Press; 2006. p. 85–116.
13. Frank ST. Aural sign of coronary-artery disease. N Engl J Med. 1973;289(6):327–8.
14. Kirkham N, Murrells T, Melcher DH, Morrison EA. Diagonal earlobe creases and fatal cardiovascular disease: a necropsy study. Br Heart J. 1989;61(4):361–4.
15. Edston E. The earlobe crease, coronary artery disease, and sudden cardiac death: an autopsy study of 520 individuals. Am J Forensic Med Pathol. 2006;27(2):129–33.
16. Day MW. Intraosseous devices for intravascular access in adult trauma patients. Crit Care Nurse. 2011;31(2):76–89.

Evisceration

3

Maxine S. Coe and S. Kim Suvarna

The Process of Opening the Torso and Removing the Tissues

The process of evisceration involves the removal of the organs from the mouth down to the anus with preservation of anatomical organ and tissue relationships. The process is performed in stages, allowing the consideration of various pathological constructs, such as the presence of pneumothorax, examination of the cavities for fluid collections, and direct inspection of the tissues for hemorrhage or other focal lesions.

The process also allows staged reduction of the tissue volume, as the majority of the bowel tissues are removed prior to the thoracic, upper gastrointestinal tract, retroperitoneal, and pelvic contents. The images in this chapter detail the stages in the recommended dissection pathway, although it is accepted that many practitioners have their own variations and/or protocols. The technique presented is recommended as suitable for most autopsies.

Following inspection of the cavities, the body may be prepared for reconstruction whilst dissection of the main organs continues.

There are many different permutations for organ removal, some advising removal of tissues in single block format and others suggesting smaller blocks. Although it is possible to extract the mouth/neck and thoracic tissues in one piece, extract the abdominal bowel tissues, resect the retroperitoneal content down to the pelvic rim, and remove the pelvic organs in sequential and separate parts, doing so will necessarily alter anatomical relationships and is not advocated for standard autopsy purposes. One should always dissect tissues in a manner likely to maximize the data to be collected and to assist sampling.

Finally, it should be remembered that high-risk infection cases may merit limited tissue handling or minimal dissection and direct tissue sampling once the torso has been opened.

Samples and Investigations to Be Taken During Evisceration

The advised dissection protocol provides the opportunity to consider pathology as it becomes visible and permits the operator to adapt the dissection according to the needs of the case and/or the pathology under consideration.

The role of digital photography cannot be overemphasized in this regard, as initial views and then dissected images of pathology processes are a vital adjunct to both standard pathology and medico-legal cases. They also serve as a valuable resource for teaching.

It is possible to gather microbiology, toxicology, and other tissue samples at various stages during the dissection. Benefits include direct vision collection of the sample and a minimal manipulation field as the samples are retrieved.

This illustrated dissection protocol with some pathologies encountered during evisceration (Figs. 3.1, 3.2, 3.3, 3.4, 3.5, 3.6, 3.7, 3.8, 3.9, 3.10, 3.11, 3.12, 3.13, 3.14, 3.15, 3.16, 3.17, 3.18, 3.19, 3.20, 3.21, 3.22, 3.23, 3.24, 3.25, 3.26, 3.27, 3.28, 3.29, 3.30, 3.31, 3.32, 3.33, 3.34, 3.35, 3.36, 3.37, 3.38, 3.39, 3.40, 3.41, 3.42, 3.43, 3.44, 3.45, 3.46, 3.47, 3.48, 3.49, 3.50, 3.51, 3.52, 3.53, and 3.54) also allows direct inspection of the inner aspect of the torso and thoracic walls. Later access to the vertebral column (for bone/marrow samples) is also possible. It is relatively easy to progress onwards to the spinal cord following removal of the vertebral column, psoas musculature, and liver tissues if toxicology samples are required (*e.g.*, decomposed cases). The process also allows one to see the undersurface of the palate and tissues of the postnasal space.

S. Kim Suvarna was deceased at the time of publication.

M. S. Coe (✉)
Public Mortuary, Medicolegal Centre, Sheffield, UK
e-mail: maxine.coe@sheffield.gov.uk

S. K. Suvarna (Deceased)
Department of Histopathology, Sheffield Teaching Hospitals NHS Foundation Trust, Sheffield, UK

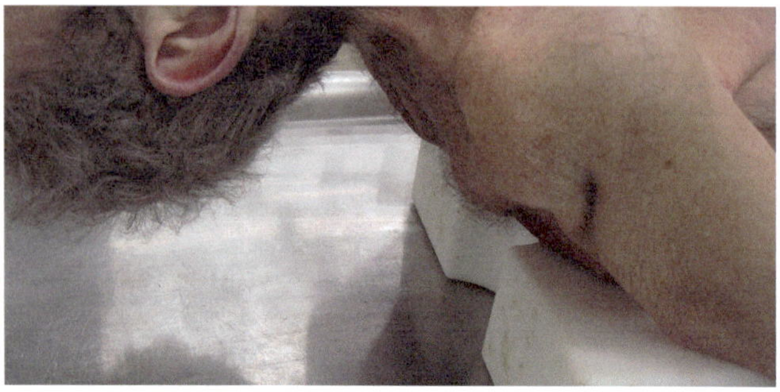

Fig. 3.1 The evisceration process starts with a block being placed under the shoulders of the individual so that the head is pulled backwards by gravity into a hyperextended posture. This allows direct inspection of the anterior neck tissues and identification of any scars, which are often hidden within skin creases at this site

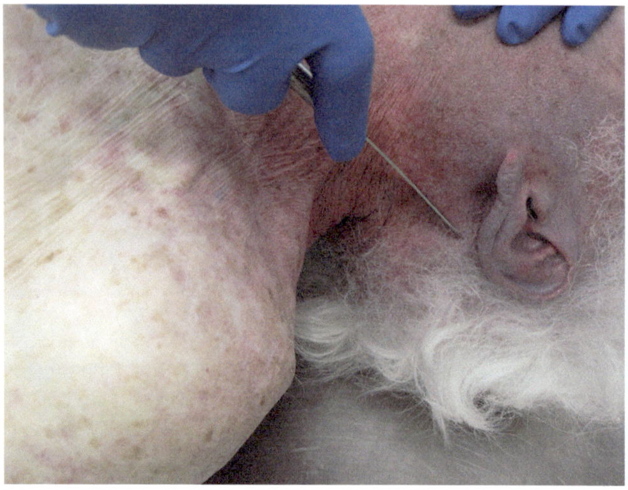

Fig. 3.2 An incision is passed from the mastoid process downwards and forwards, along the edge of the sternomastoid muscle and down across the neck. The cut should be made as perpendicular to the skin as possible, although it is recognized that the neck is a complicated three-dimensional structure

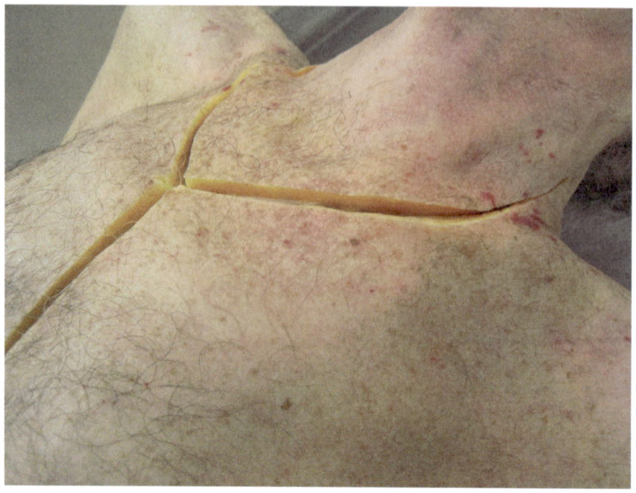

Fig. 3.3 The cuts from either side can join in a V-shaped interface at the manubrium level and then pass as a single cut along the front of the chest and downwards towards the pubis/low abdomen centrally

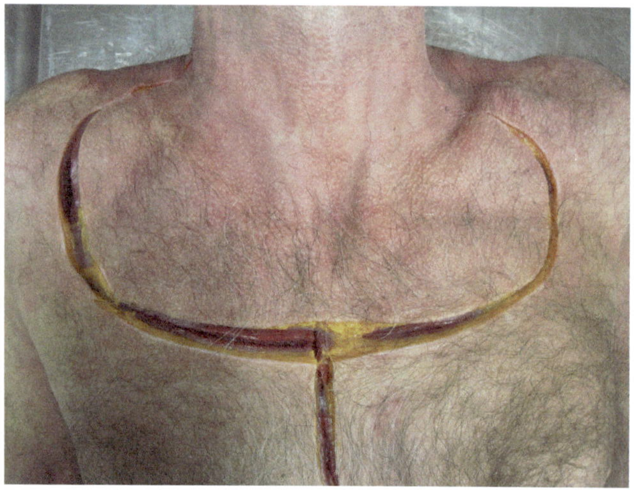

Fig. 3.4 An alternative method for dissection involves the cuts from the mastoid processes running behind the sternomastoid musculature and then swinging in a U-shaped fashion across the front of the chest. These cuts then continue down the midline of the central chest and abdomen

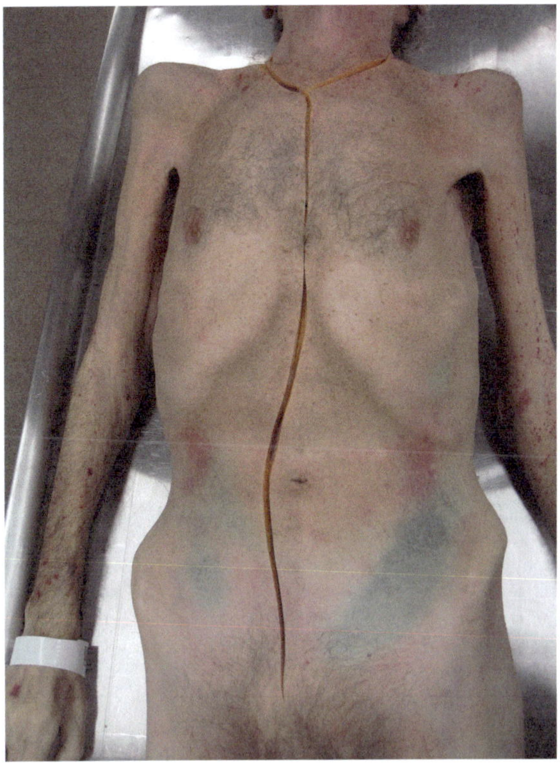

Fig. 3.5 The midline dissection, usually by knife, passes down to the suprapubic region, avoiding the umbilicus

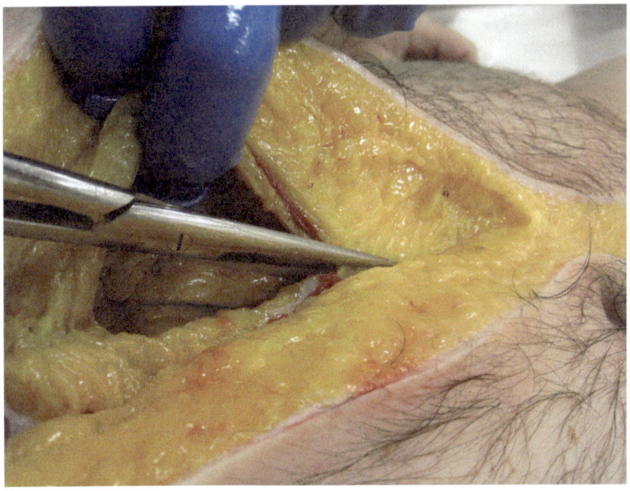

Fig. 3.6 One can open directly into the abdominal cavity at this point, with scissors, allowing direct inspection of the abdominal cavity

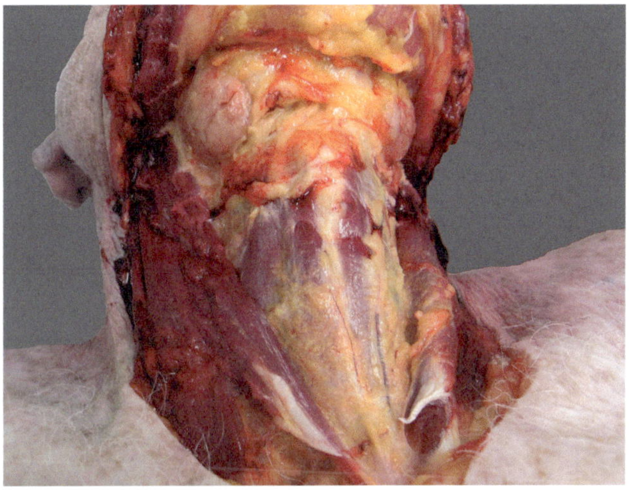

Fig. 3.7 In this case, the V-shaped dissection has allowed the soft tissues of the skin and fatty subcutis to be dissected free of the local neck structures. These are lifted upwards towards the jaw. The dissection in this plane of tissue should continue up to the edge of the mandible, thereby exposing the strap muscles around the hyoid bone as well as the submandibular salivary gland tissues superiorly. At this point, one can consider whether to dissect the strap musculature sequentially, in order to consider damage to the hyoid bone/larynx (*e.g.*, in medico-legal or assault cases). It is also possible to approach the thyroid from the front, although dissection of the thyroid and related tissues often is left until later (see Chap. 8)

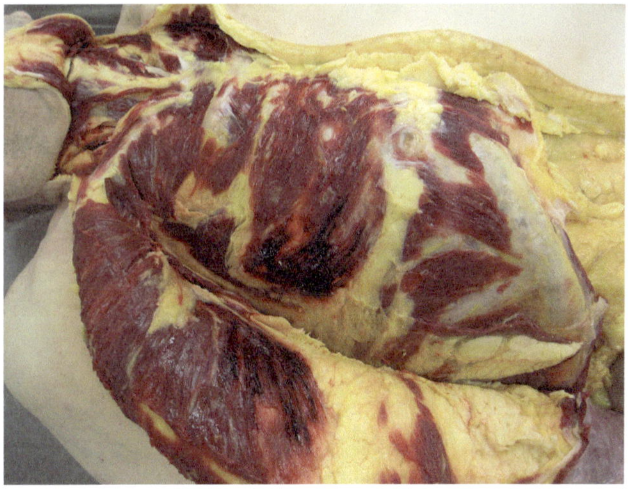

Fig. 3.8 The tissues of the thorax are incised directly onto the sternum, with lateral undermining of the muscles and other soft tissues of the chest. These are reflected further laterally to expose the intercostal musculature and ribs. This dissection plane also allows identification of any pacemaker or other devices that penetrate into the vasculature or soft tissues around the chest. In this case, haemorrhage and fracturing of the ribs is evident focally

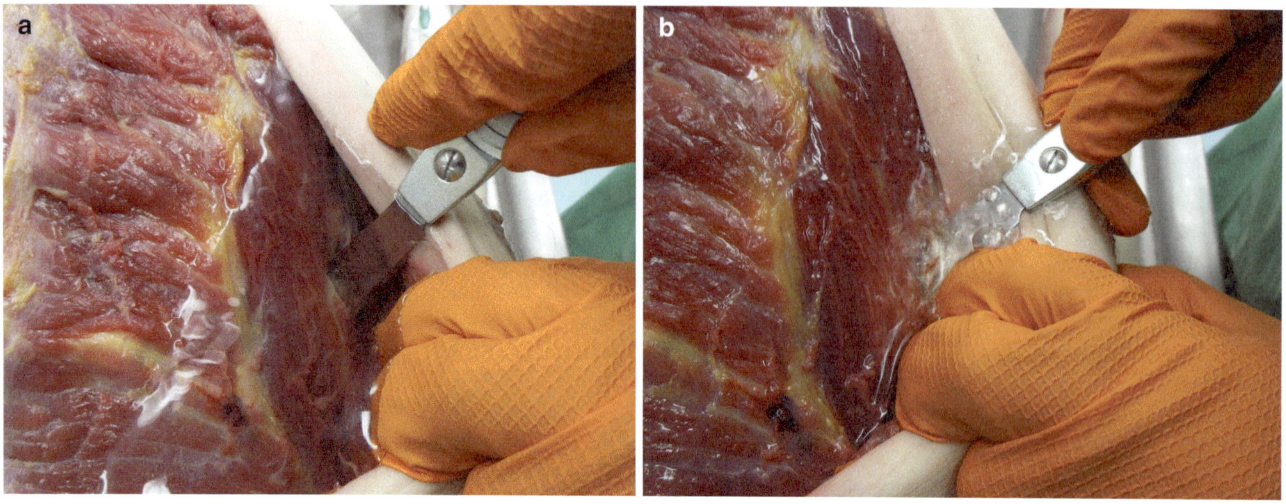

Fig. 3.9 (**a**, **b**) To test for pneumothorax, before the body is further opened, one dissects around the chest wall and reflects the soft tissue, thereby creating a pocket, which may be filled with water. The next step is to insert a blunt instrument, such as scissors or a bullnose PM40, into the intercostal musculature between the ribs, below the water level, penetrating into the pleural space. It is possible to facilitate the examination by turning the knife or scissors through one quarter turn and gently pressing on the front of the chest to check for air. Tension pneumothorax will be evident as a rush of gas being released at this point. Small, nonsignificant pneumothoraces may not be identified by this technique, but a normal pleural cavity will characteristically suck inwards some of the fluid without bubbles. One should also be aware that pushing a knife or scissors deeply into the chest will inevitably damage any underlying lung tissue or pathology

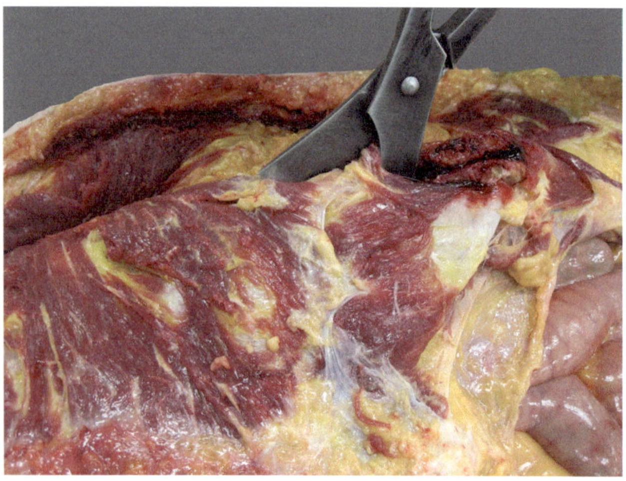

Fig. 3.10 The chest wall is removed by inserting bone shears into the chest at the lower edge of the rib cage and then cutting across the musculature and bone tissues along the lateral aspect of the chest and towards the manubrioclavicular junction

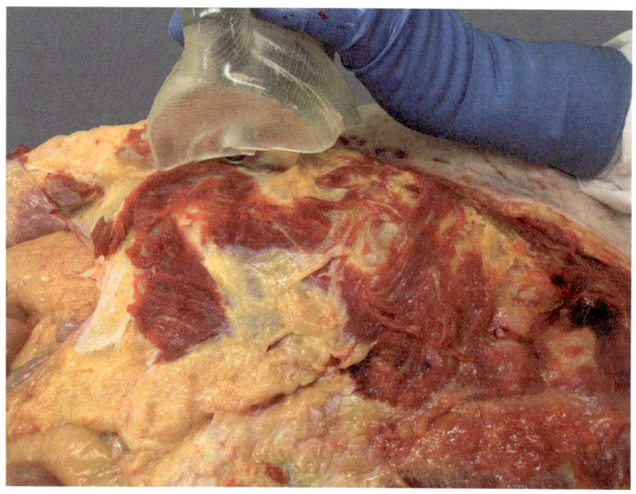

Fig. 3.11 It is also possible to use a mechanical or hand saw to cut through rib tissues, although rib shears are quick and efficient. Note that the saw is fitted with an extractor hood to reduce bone dust aerosolisation

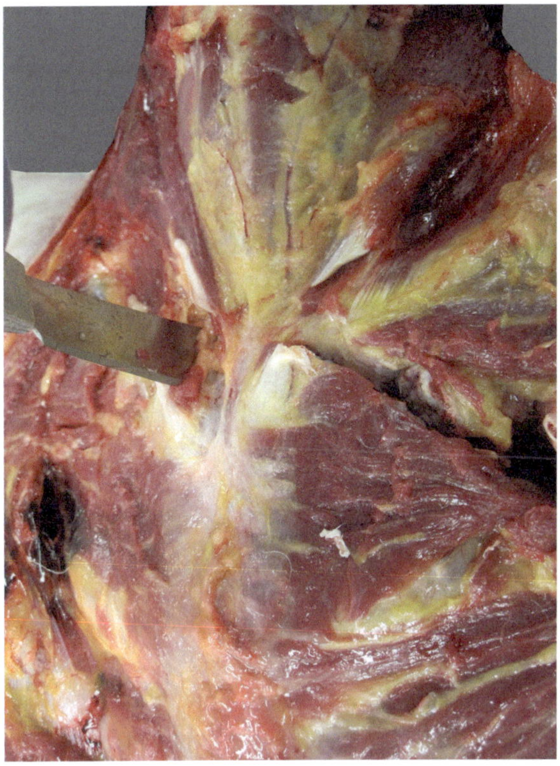

Fig. 3.12 The removal of the chest bony tissues and front of the rib cage initially requires the manubrioclavicular joint to be freed from its attachments. This joint can be identified by moving the ipsilateral shoulder slightly and feeling for the joint space at the manubrioclavicular junction. In this process, a knife blade is inserted vertically downwards and moved around the joint, allowing this tissue to be freed. In this image, the cutting of the ribs and that at the manubrioclavicular junction join up

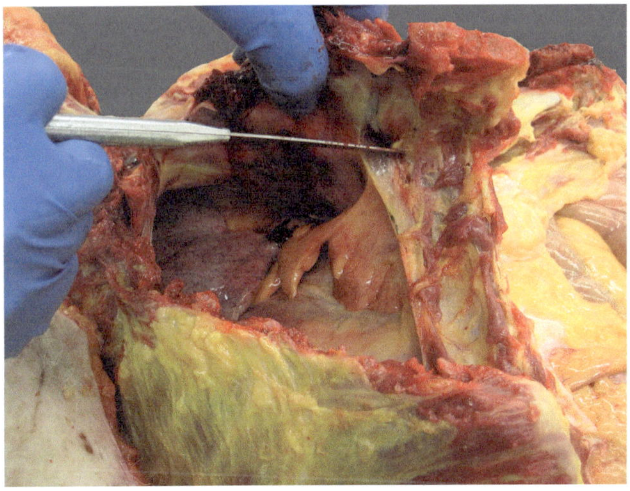

Fig. 3.13 The lateral aspect of the rib cage is now lifted upwards, allowing a knife to be used to free up the mediastinal content tissues from the inner aspect of the chest contents. If the individual has undergone coronary bypass surgery, attention should be paid to the origin of the left internal mammary artery (LIMA), which is often used as part of the revascularisation technique. If relevant, a suture placed around the end of the artery may be useful in the subsequent examination of cardiac tissue (see Chap. 4)

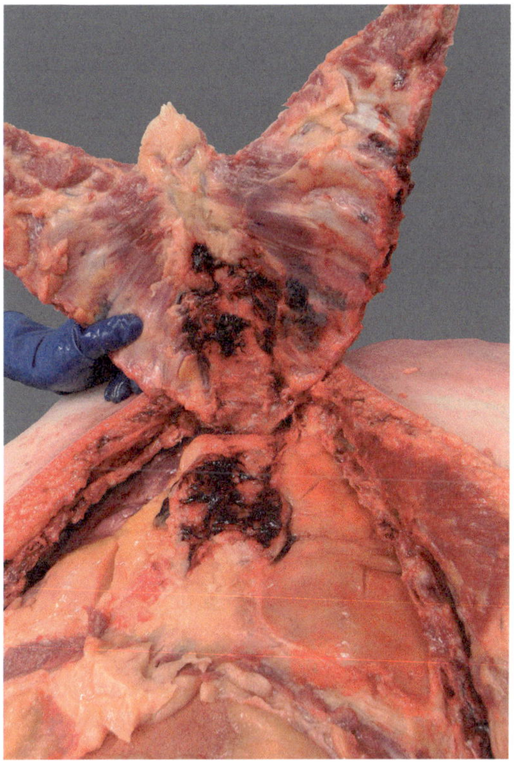

Fig. 3.14 Bruising from chest compressions during cardiopulmonary resuscitation may be seen at this point in the evisceration

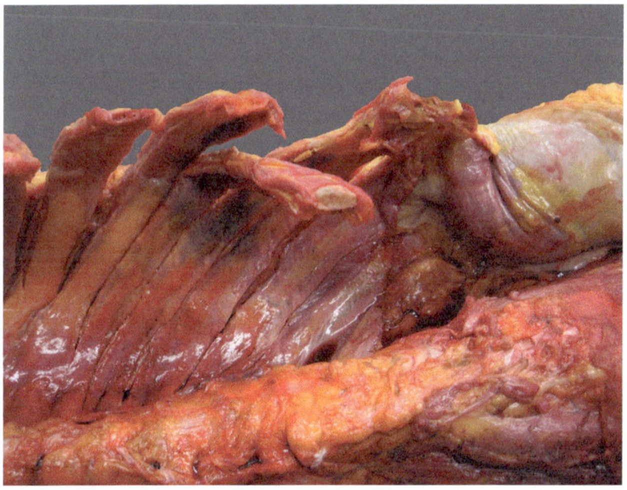

Fig. 3.15 During the evisceration, fractures of the ribs may become obvious. There is bruising locally, in keeping with these fractures occurring ante-mortem. They are best demonstrated by incision through the intercostal muscles

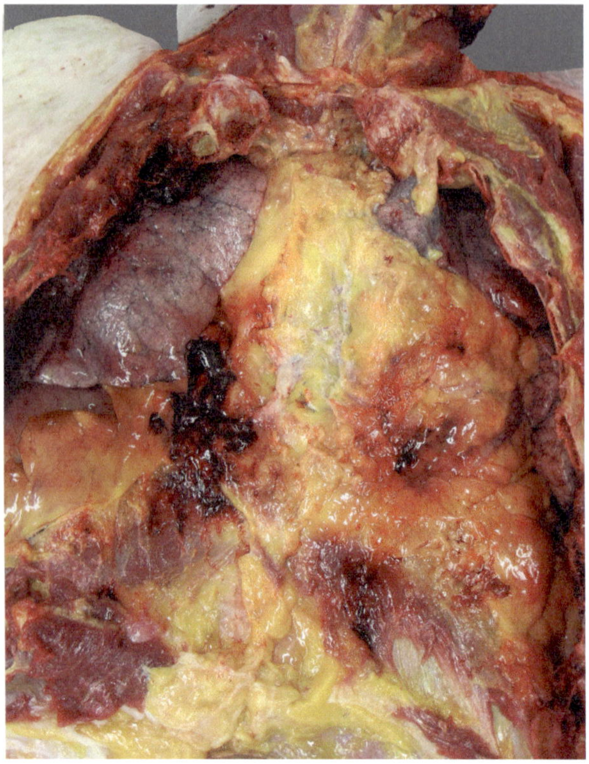

Fig. 3.16 The rib cage has now been removed from the front of the body, exposing the lungs, heart, and upper abdominal vasculature. The pleural cavities should be inspected for fluid collections and sepsis. The pericardial tissue should be looked at from the external/outer aspect and may be opened at this point. If there is a fluid collection, then it may be appropriate to aspirate the content. This image also shows some blood related to rib fractures incurred during attempted resuscitation

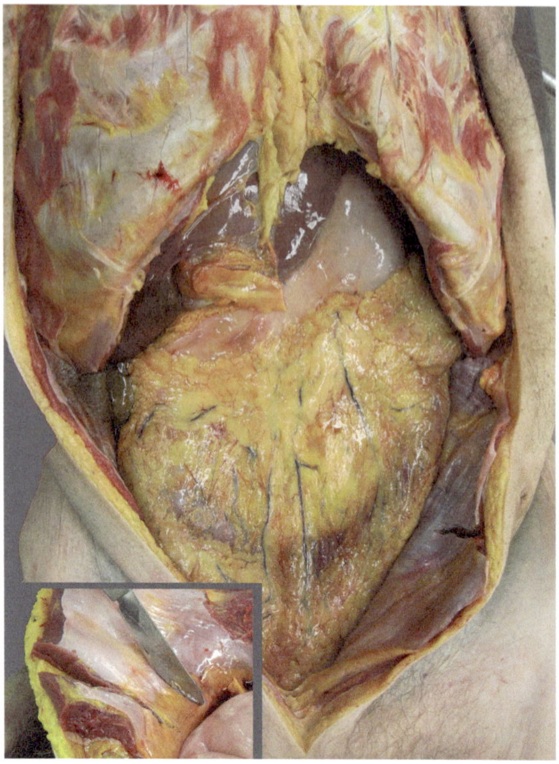

Fig. 3.17 The abdominal tissues have been opened using the cut running along the front of the abdomen, which has been extended into the peritoneal cavity. The abdominal incision edges have been pulled to the sides, exposing the liver and small bowel. The small bowel is often seen to have a moderate amount of fatty tissue. The lower left inset image shows transverse cuts into the lower abdominal wall, which facilitate laying the abdominal wall outwards

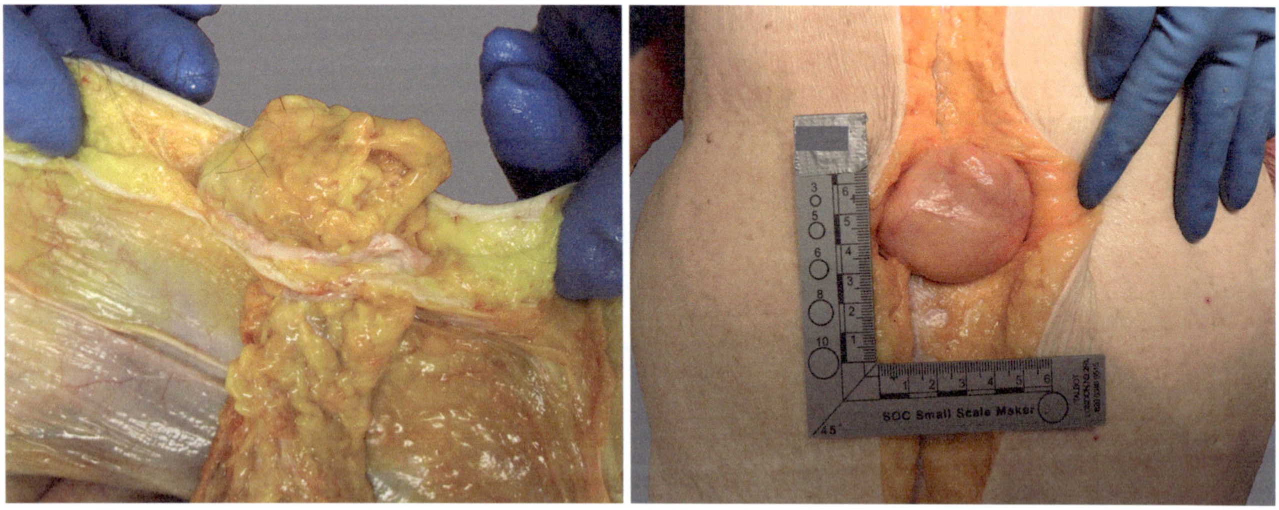

Fig. 3.18 At the time of opening the abdomen, one may identify hernias at various points. They are common around the groin, where the abdominal wall is weak, but following surgery, soft tissues of a mesenteric nature (*left*) or potentially bowel (*right*) can protrude into defects in the abdominal wall lining in some cases despite surgical closure by sutures

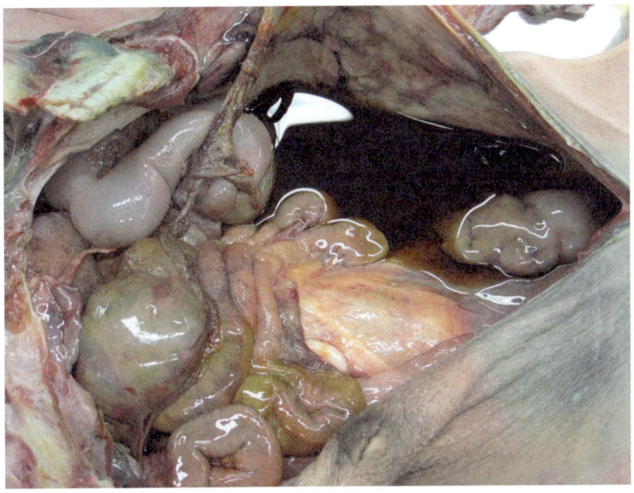

Fig. 3.19 The examination of the abdominal content may often identify variable fluid collections. These may be serous (*i.e.*, clear yellow), turbid/purulent or haemorrhagic. This case shows some altered blood on a serous background. Fluid for cytological or microbiological tests can be sampled at this point, before any contamination by further dissection. The color and consistency of the fluid may give an indication as to likely intra-abdominal pathology. In all cases, the total volume of fluid should be assessed

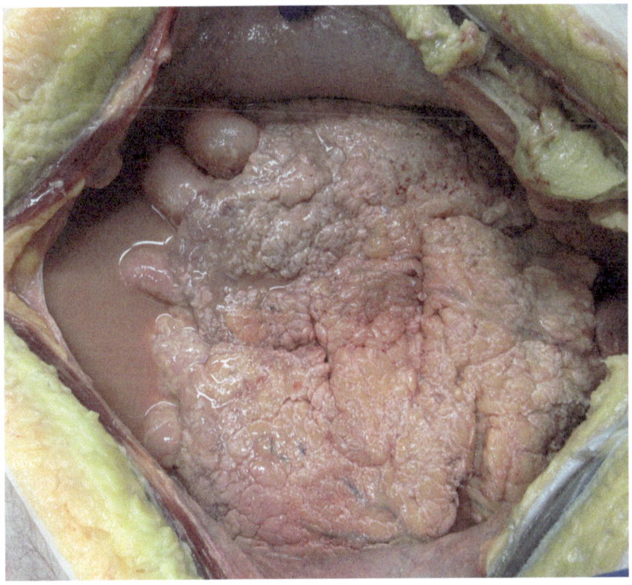

Fig. 3.20 This image shows an abnormal appearance upon the opening of the abdomen of turbid fluid with peritonitis, indicative of viscus rupture. Further exploration will identify the cause for this pathology. Consideration of fluid collection at this point may be prudent for bacteriology

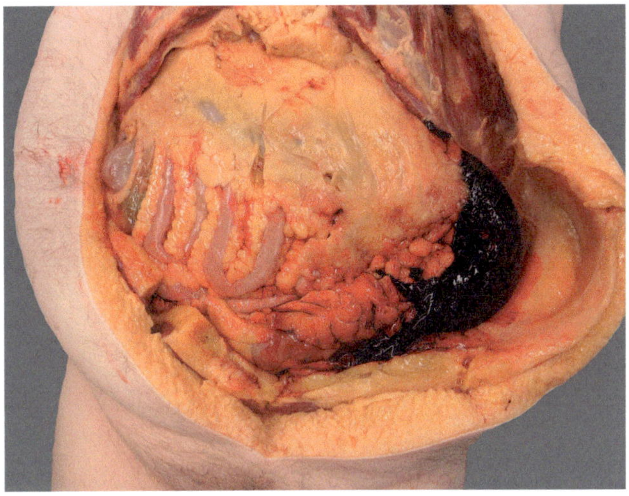

Fig. 3.21 Intraabdominal haemorrhage is easily detected at this stage of evisceration, prompting examination of the tissues in situ with a view to identifying the source of the blood. The clot can be collected with a jug and ladle for estimation of volume of extra-circulatory blood loss

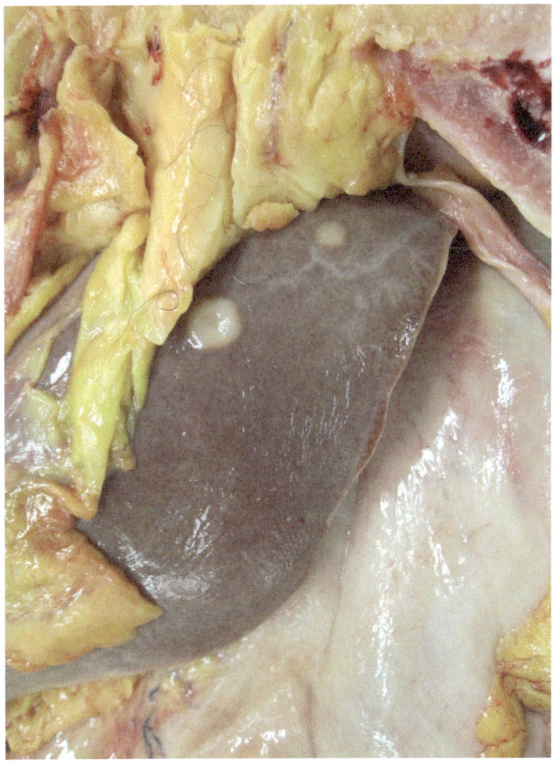

Fig. 3.22 Another apparent cause of death seen early in the examination is seen here. The liver appears slightly enlarged and has several foci of cream tumor on the surface. This points towards carcinomatosis, subsequently determined to be disseminated lung cancer

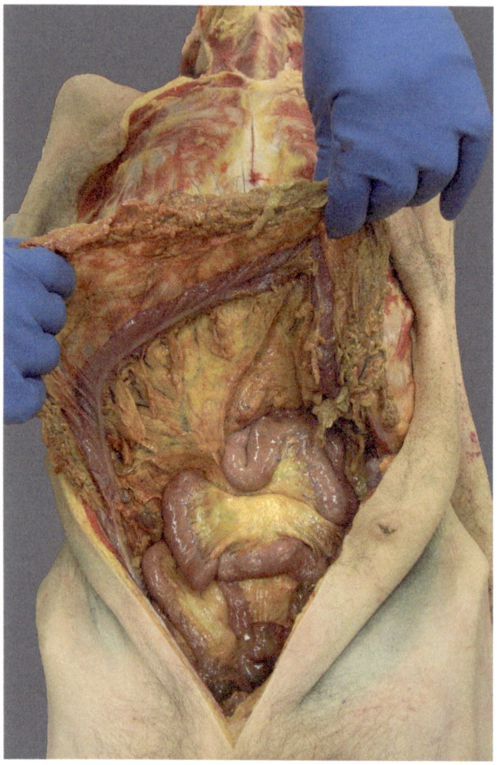

Fig. 3.23 In most cases, the abdominal tissue content appears broadly normal with regard to the contents and architecture. To continue the examination, the proximal jejunal and distal duodenal tissues are identified by pulling the transverse colon upwards towards the head. After this manipulation, most of the small bowel is moved gently towards the right side, exposing the root of the mesentery

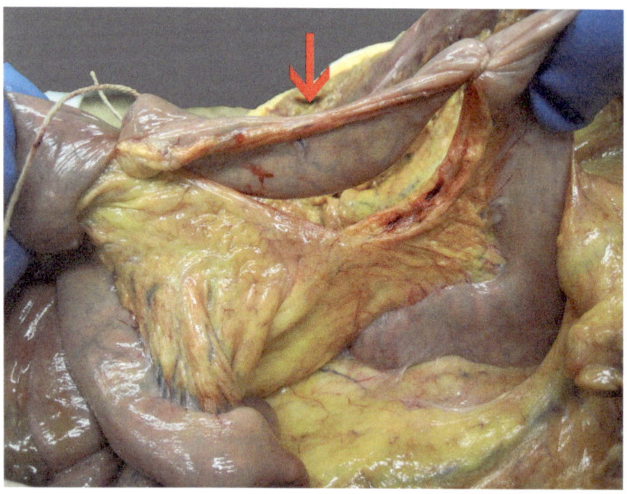

Fig. 3.24 By making a single cut into the proximal jejunal mesentery, one can insert ties that will prevent bowel content leakage. One then cuts across the centre of this small bowel zone (*red arrow*)

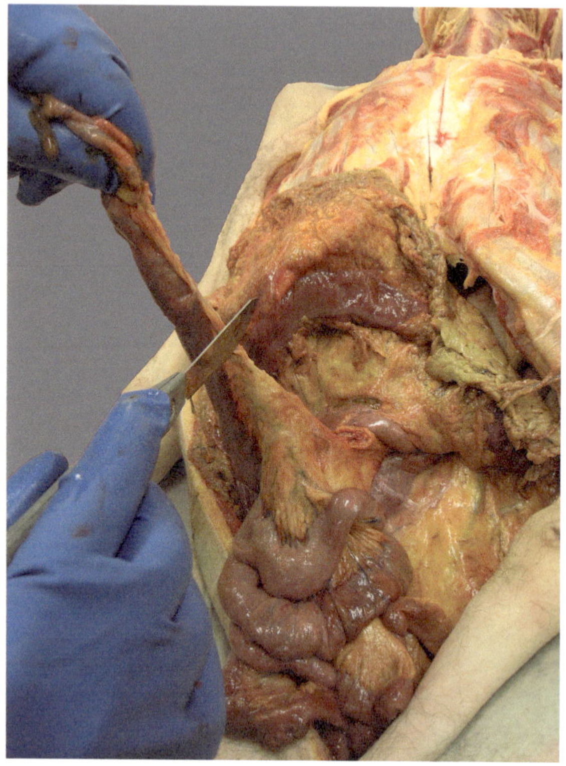

Fig. 3.25 The small bowel (from jejunum to distal ileum) is dissected free by cutting through the mesentery adjacent to the edge of the small bowel. The cut allows the bowel to be removed proximal to distal. The bowel is lifted outwards and out of the body cavity

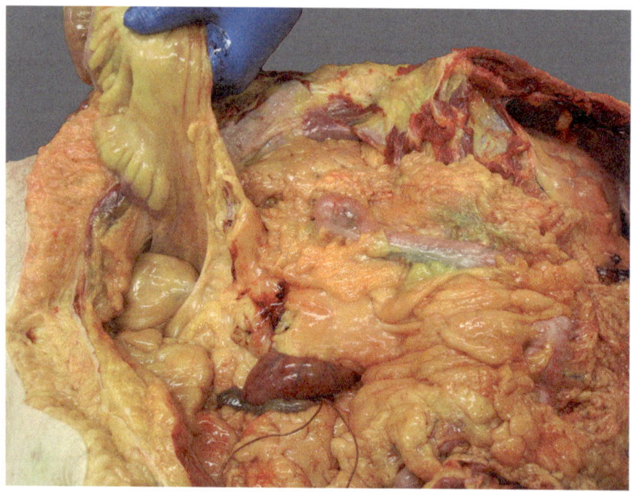

Fig. 3.26 Alternatively, one can dissect the small bowel tissues by cutting close to the vascular origin. This process allows review of the vasculature in relation to the bowel tissues

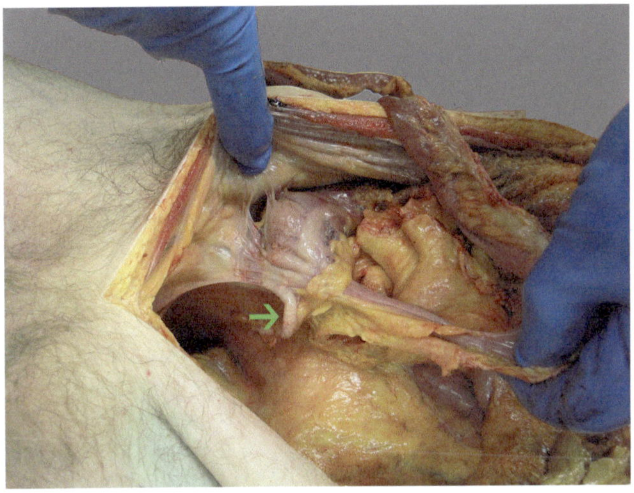

Fig. 3.27 It is to be remembered that the cecum and ascending colon are retroperitoneal. When one has dissected down to the level of the terminal ileum, it is necessary to pull gently and bluntly dissect (with fingers/scissors) into the retroperitoneal compartment around the cecum, freeing the proximal colon tissues. At this point, the appendix (*arrow*) should be directly inspected to confirm normality and absence of inflammation

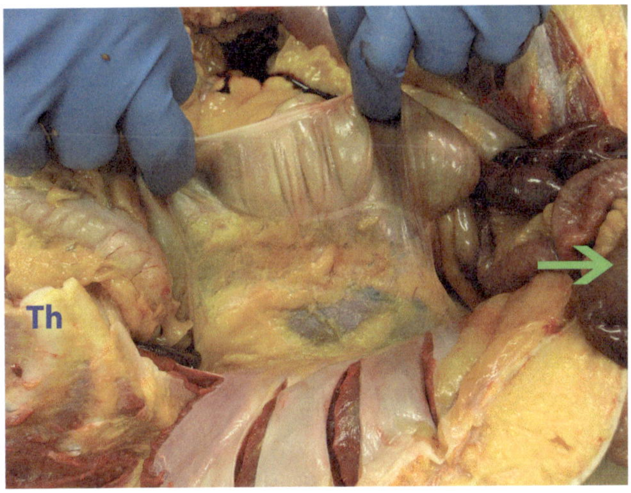

Fig. 3.28 Looking from the right side of the opened abdomen, with the small bowel pulled downwards towards the feet (in the line of the *green arrow*), and with the part of the already opened thoracic rib cage (Th) in this view; one pulls the right side colon tissues medially and frees the bowel gently. This blunt dissection progresses up to the hepatic flexure

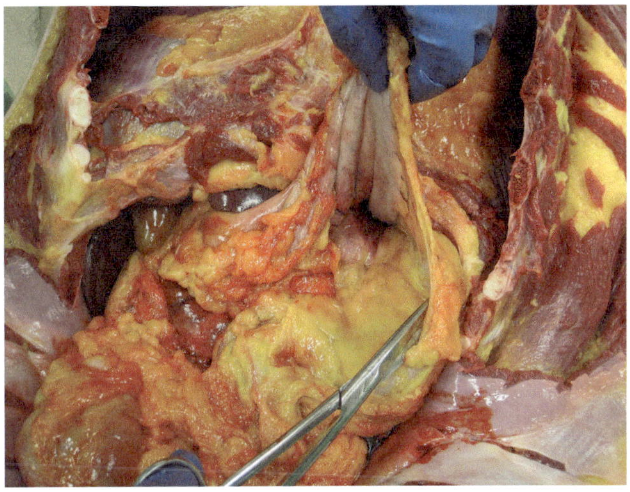

Fig. 3.29 The cut passes across the top of the lesser sac using scissors, separating the stomach and transverse colon tissues. One can then look onto the anterior surface of the pancreas, to check for inflammation. The colonic tissues are then mobilized onwards, around the splenic flexure and down the descending colon in a similar manner to that on the right side, with the retroperitoneal descending colon tissues being mobilized downwards towards the sigmoid

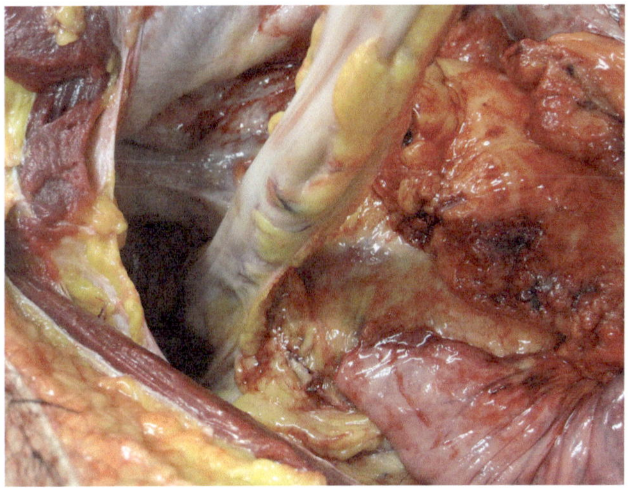

Fig. 3.30 The pelvic tissues and sigmoid colon are freed and pulled upwards, freeing the sigmoid colon at the mesenteric root. One may then cut off the colon tissues down to the upper rectum level, with or without tying the bowel at this point. All the bowel tissues are now removed and put to one side. Some may require further dissection (see Chap. 5)

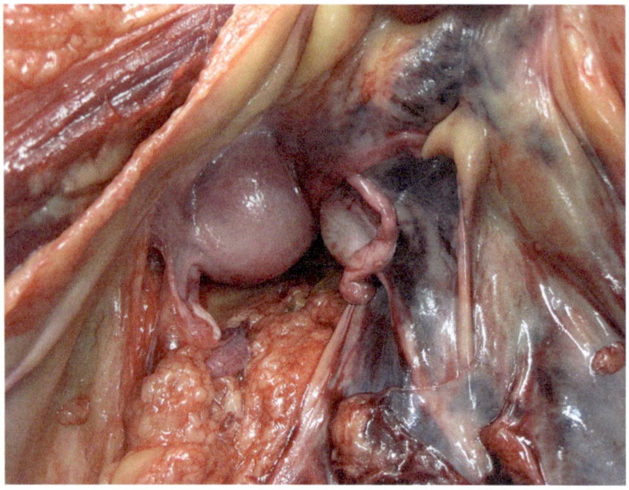

Fig. 3.31 Once the colon and proximal tissues are removed, one can inspect the internal genital organs in females. In this case, the superior aspect of the uterus, the tubes and ovaries can be seen

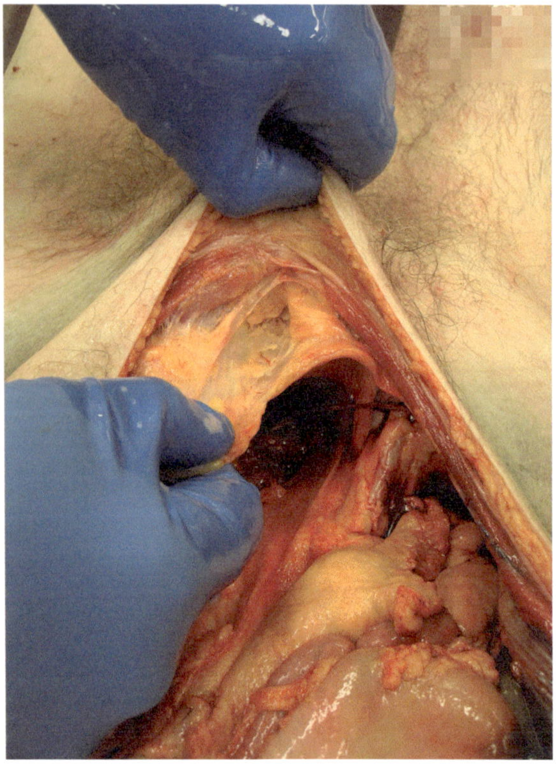

Fig. 3.32 The pelvic tissues are removed with the bladder and rectal parenchyma intact. In starting this maneuver, the soft tissue plane in front of the bladder is identified at the distal end of the original abdominal incision

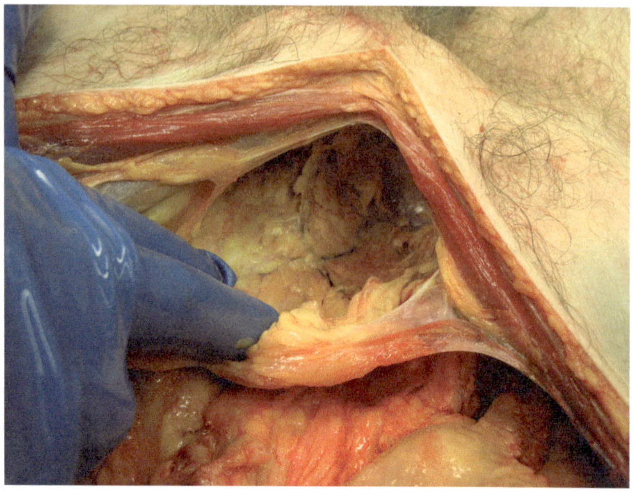

Fig. 3.33 Using finger dissection down around the bladder neck, one creates a plane between the inner aspect of the pelvis anteriorly and the bladder

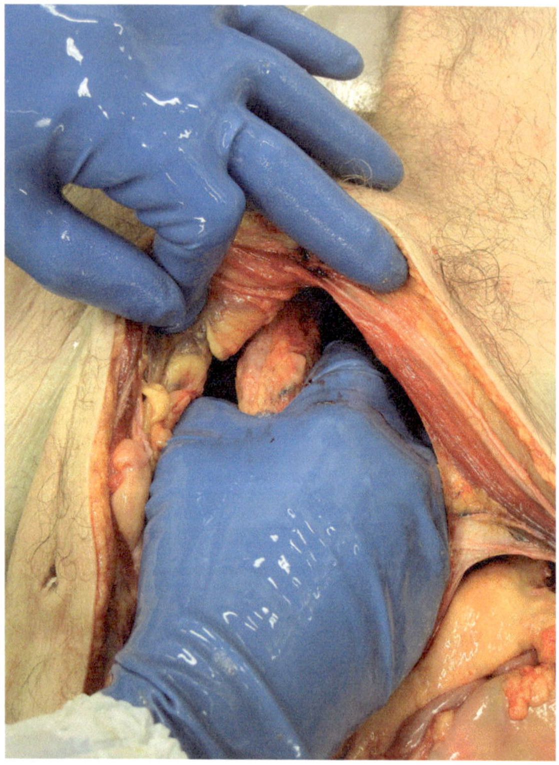

Fig. 3.34 The finger dissection passes downwards and around the bladder neck/prostate (in men) or around the bladder/cervix (in women). The fingers from both hands continue to bluntly dissect the soft tissues around the pelvic floor until one reaches behind the rectum. The fingers (from both hands) should now be able to be in direct contact with each other, in front of the sacral bony tissues. The next manoeuvre is to pull this entire group of tissues upwards, thereby increasing the separation of the rectum/bladder from the pelvis. Performing this technique means that one should be able to mobilize the bladder, rectum, and internal genital tissues (prostate and seminal vesicles in males; uterus/cervix, tubes, and ovaries in females) without having disturbed the relationship between the tissues

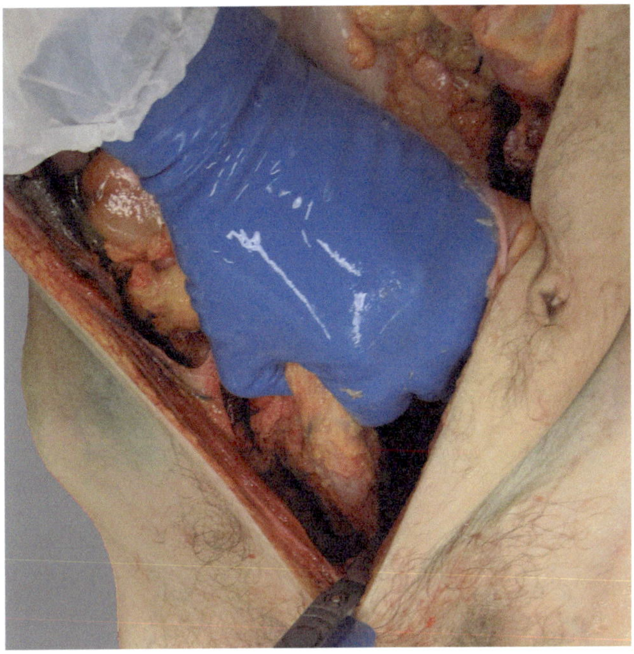

Fig. 3.35 Although it is difficult to look into the pelvis directly, one now must run a knife behind the pubic bone, making a cut transversely across the pelvic floor tissues to free the bladder (with prostate in men) and internal genital organs (in women), and transversely across the rectum—ideally in one motion

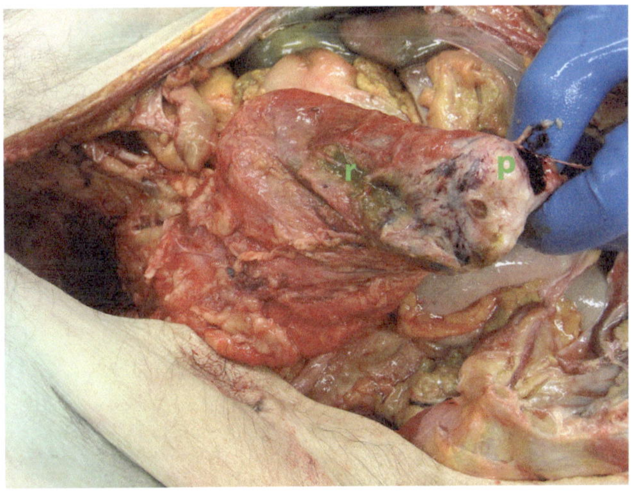

Fig. 3.36 The anteriorly freed tissues are then pulled upwards and cranially with blunt dissection across the pelvic bony tissues towards the posterior pelvic brim. The cut end of the prostate (p) and the rectum (r) are seen in this view

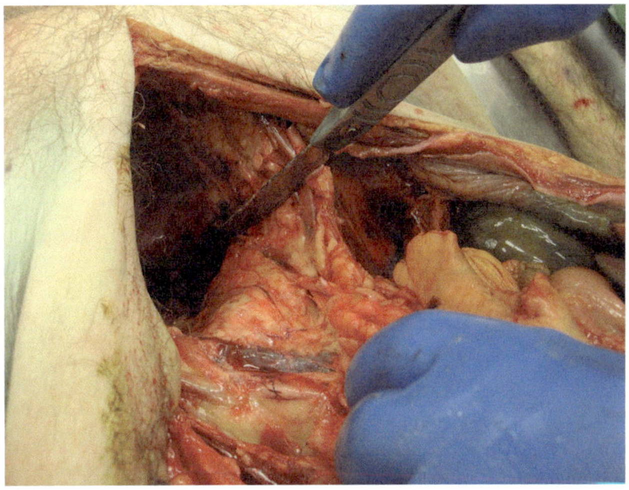

Fig. 3.37 Having applied tension to the pelvic tissues upwards in a cranial direction, an oblique cut is made through the soft tissues at 45° at the pelvic brim, keeping the knife close to the bone. This cut transects the common iliac artery and vein but leaves the medially placed ureter intact

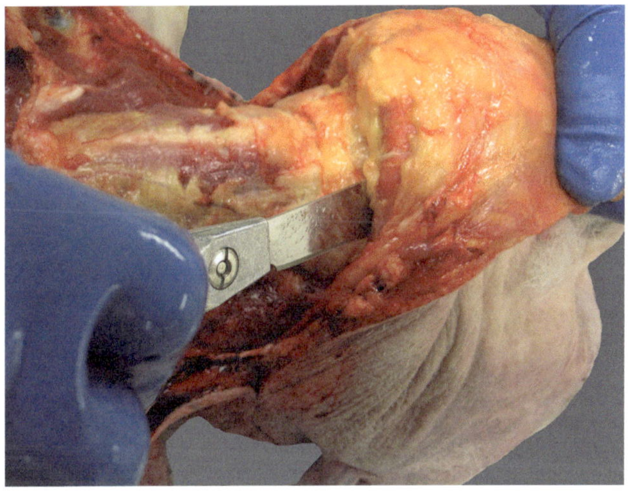

Fig. 3.38 The mouth tissues are dissected by passing a knife around the inner aspect of the mandible, thereby freeing up the tongue and related salivary glands. Cutting the soft tissues and vasculature around this site may cause some degree of blood loss into the operating field, but this blood often can be mopped up to allow clear inspection of the next set of cuts

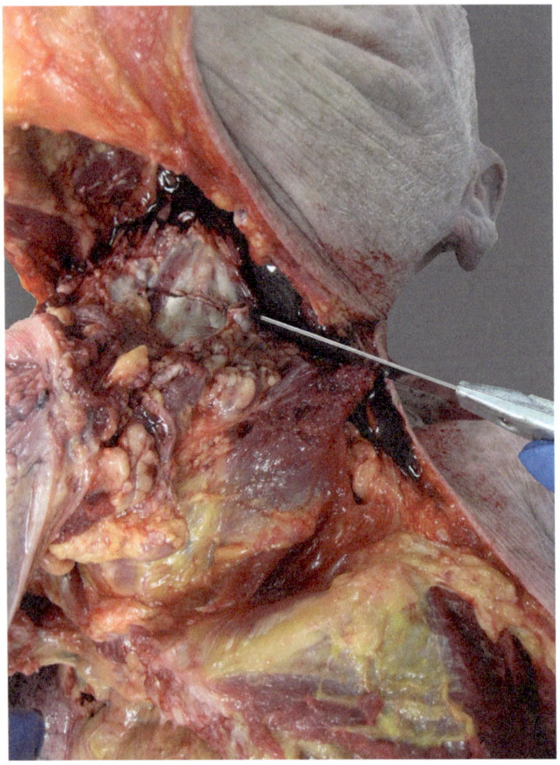

Fig. 3.39 The next step is a transverse cut made across the back of the pharynx, which will then divide/transect the carotid vasculature above the carotid bulb. It will also cut across the internal jugular vein and around onto the soft tissues adjacent to the cervical spine

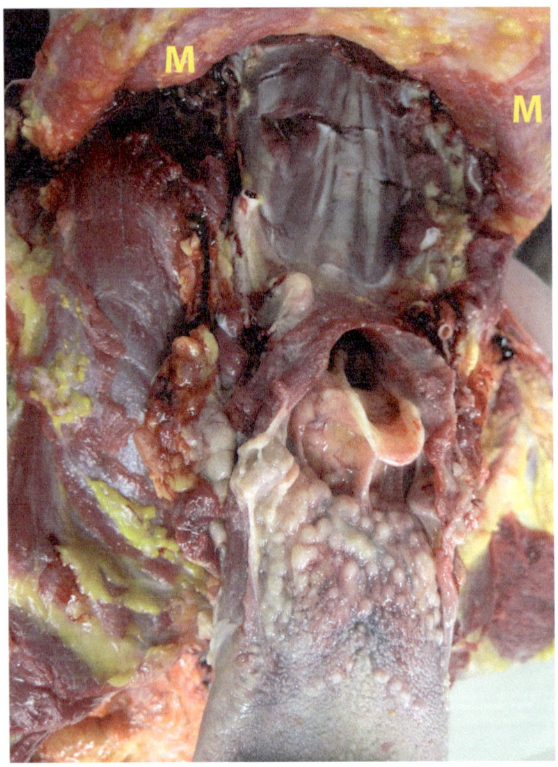

Fig. 3.40 The mouth tissues are pulled downwards and away from the inner jaw tissues. (The mandible is marked *M*.) The epiglottis and larynx can be inspected for obstructive pathology

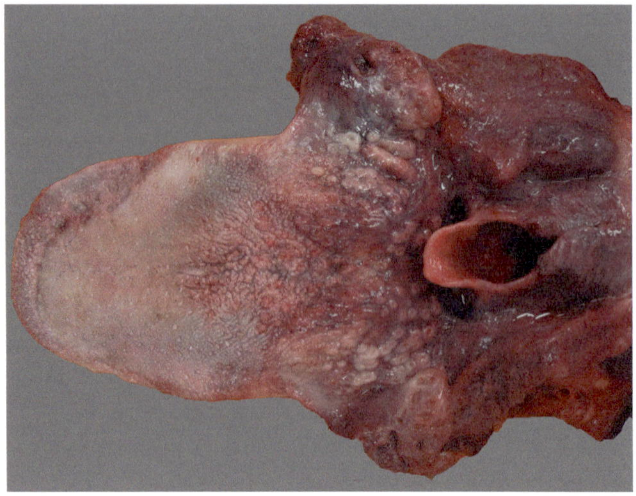

Fig. 3.41 The cause of death may also be demonstrated early during evisceration by simple observation of the tissues. This case clearly showed a tooth pattern on the tongue, in keeping with tongue-biting. This individual was known to have epilepsy, and this evidence points toward an epilepsy-related death

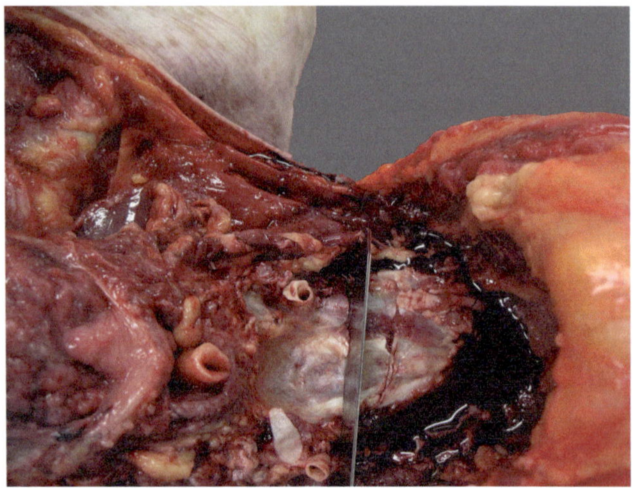

Fig. 3.42 The cut on both sides should be made down onto the bony tissues, to guarantee preservation of these structures, which will be considered later. The process should be undertaken on both sides equally. One should look for atheromatous disease at the cut ends of the carotid vasculature

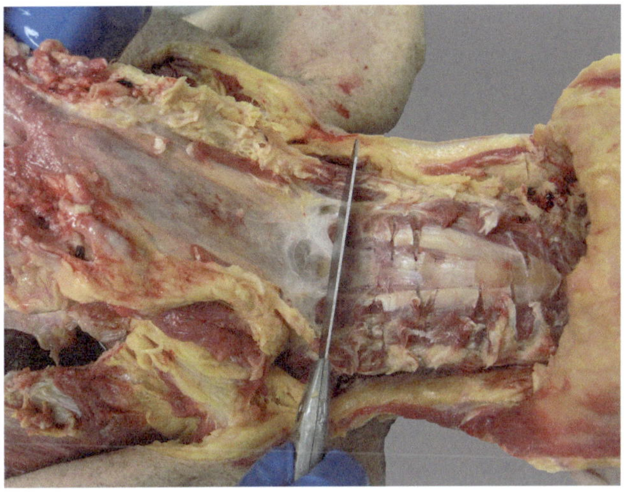

Fig. 3.43 To free the neck tissues requires the transverse oropharyngeal cut to be extended downwards on both sides and laterally at the side of the vertebral column. Cutting directly onto the lateral aspect bony tissues of the vertebral bodies means that all relevant medially placed and important neck structures will be kept intact

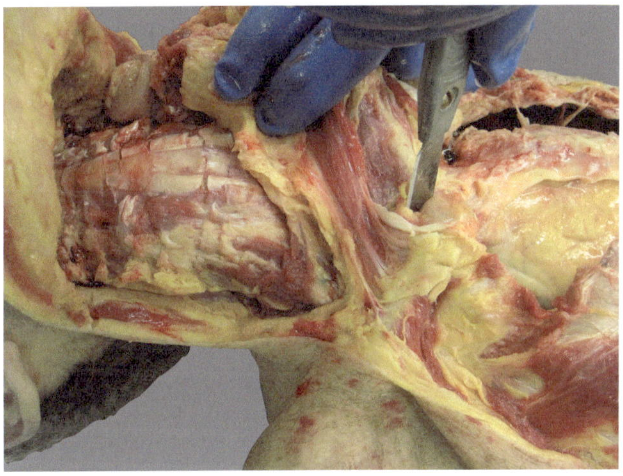

Fig. 3.44 The soft tissues at the thoracic inlet are now cut by running the knife around the inner aspect of the first rib. All the neck structures now will be freely mobile

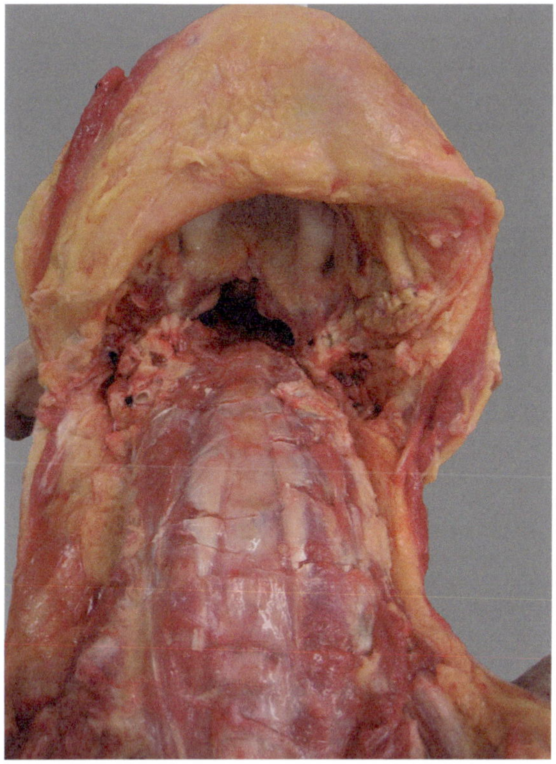

Fig. 3.45 The neck structures have been removed and one can look upwards into the mouth, up to the hard/soft palate

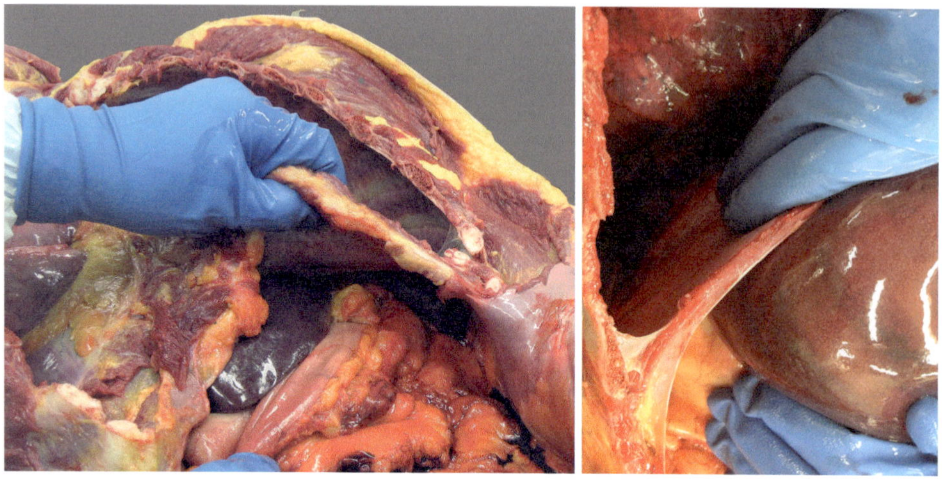

Fig. 3.46 The diaphragm tissues are freed by running a knife around the inner aspect of the lower rib cage, and around towards the lateral aspect of the vertebral bodies on both sides. In these two images, the diaphragm is being identified and pulled taut before the cut is made. On the left side (*left*), one protects the spleen and kidney by pulling this tissue upwards and away from the knife. The same approach applies on the right (*right*) for the liver and kidney

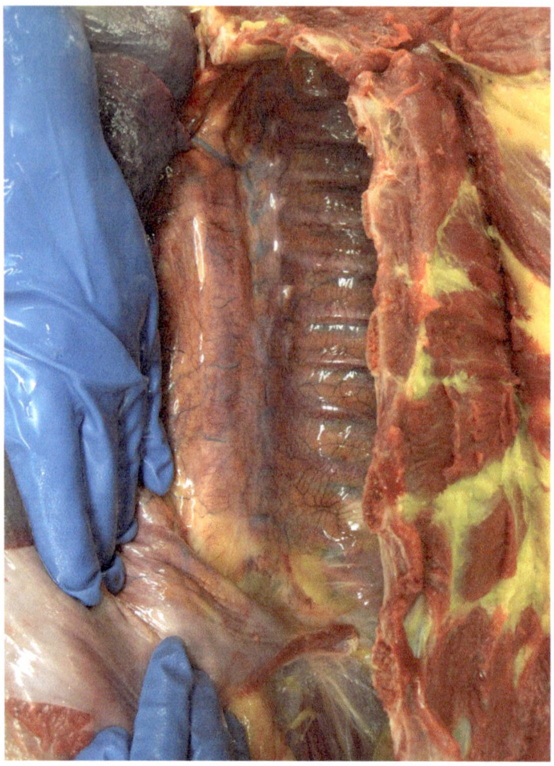

Fig. 3.47 To avoid any tearing of inflexible thoracic content (*e.g.*, atheromatous aorta) during the next phase, one reflects the thoracic content to one side and cuts along the lateral aspect of the vertebral bodies. Note how the diaphragm has been cut around the edge and onto the vertebral column

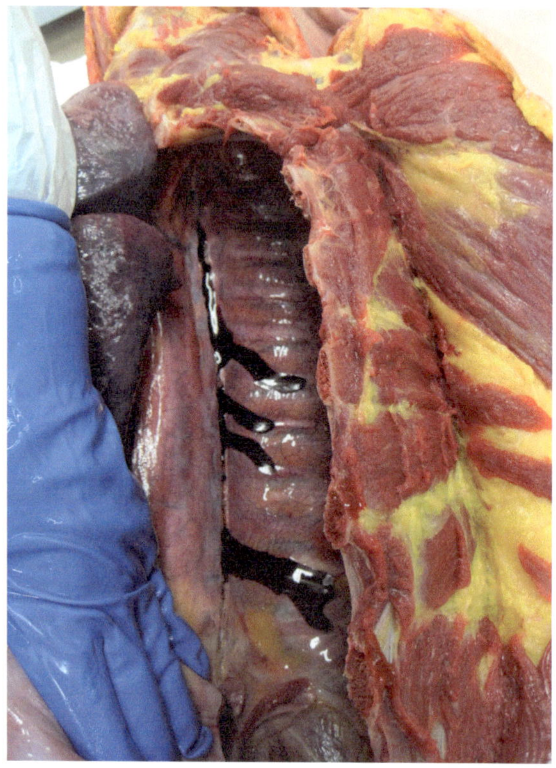

Fig. 3.48 This image shows the long cut made onto the vertebral tissues

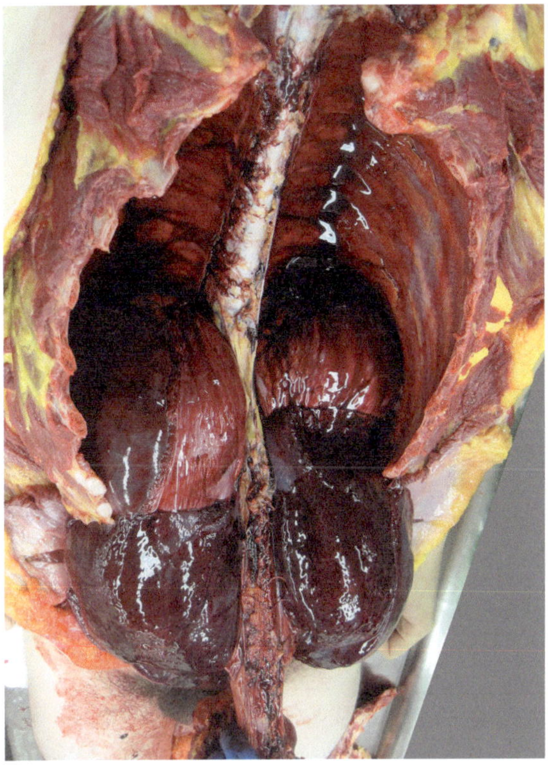

Fig. 3.49 Grasping the neck content firmly, one now pulls the thoracic tissues downwards towards the pelvis. There should be minimal resistance, as the tissues are free at the thoracic inlet and around the vertebral column, but some additional cuts may be needed to ease the tissues out

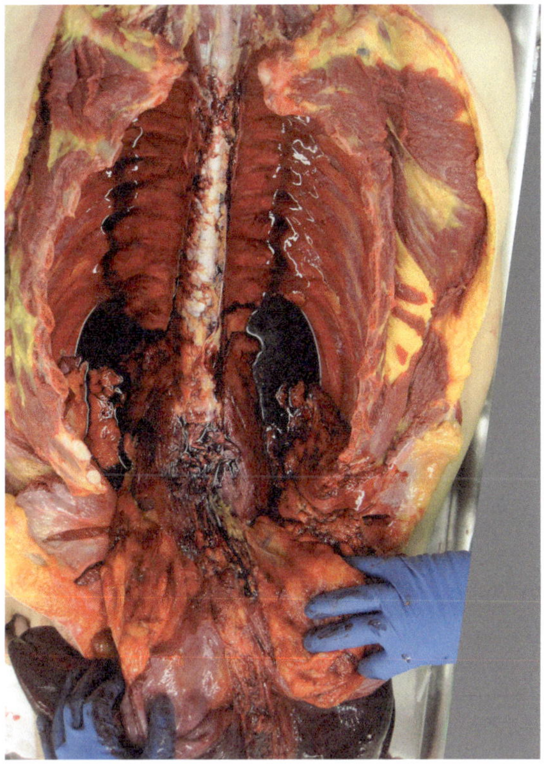

Fig. 3.50 The tissues can be pulled further downwards, towards the pelvis. This is often facilitated by an earlier light incision into the psoas muscle on both sides. This cut continues down towards the pelvic brim, where it will intersect with the prior dissection of the pelvic tissues and iliac vessels. Again, in some cases, some cuts around the vertebral column are required to assist the tissue extraction. Now all the thoracic, abdominal, and retroperitoneal tissues can be removed in one piece

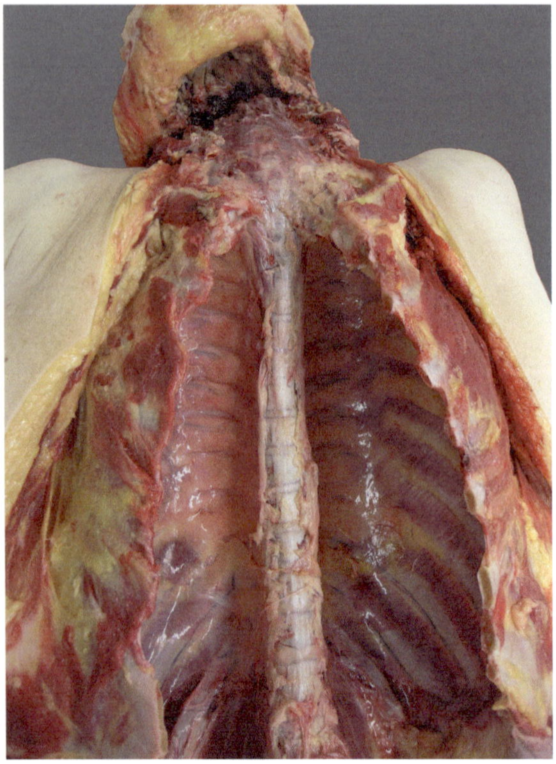

Fig. 3.51 Once the viscera from the thorax, abdomen, and retroperitoneum have been removed, it is possible to inspect the back of the torso. This view allows one to confirm the normality of the pleura and the integrity of the vertebral column and to assess the state of the musculature and fat. The same examination should follow for the lower vertebral column and pelvis. Note how the examination is enhanced by having cleaned the inner tissues of body fluids

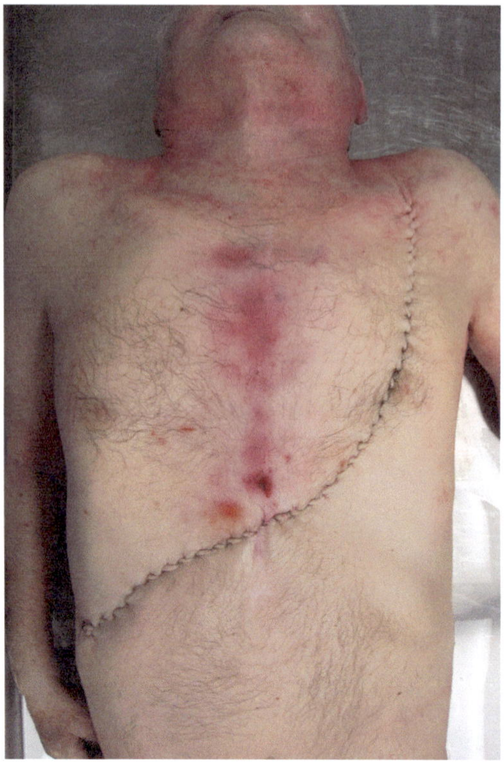

Fig. 3.52 Limited autopsy examination is increasingly common, given the range and abilities of ante-mortem investigations. This case was chest-limited but permitted access to the abdomen. By running the incision downwards and obliquely across the chest, the incision was hidden but good access to the chest was still available to remove the heart, lungs, and mediastinal content. Opening directly through the diaphragms also allowed sampling of the liver and kidneys

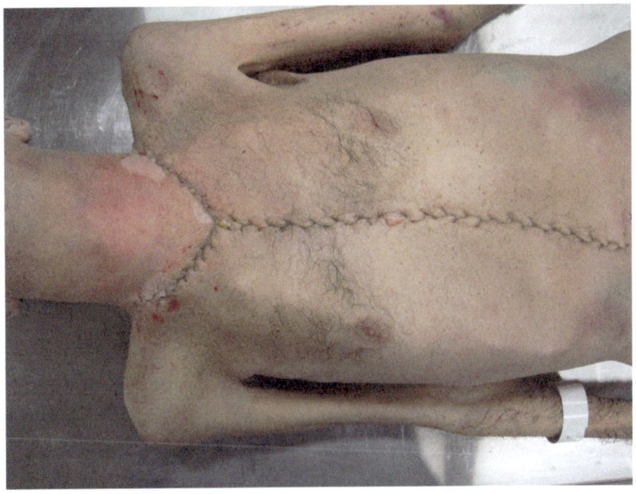

Fig. 3.53 Following evisceration, tissue examination, and the taking of samples, the body is reconstituted with all the tissue contents placed into bags within the thorax/abdomen cavity. This includes the central nervous system, as leakage from cranial reconstitution would not be acceptable. The tissues can be split into bowel and other tissues to limit the rate of tissue degradation if a second autopsy is likely. The evisceration incisions should be closed by twine in a secure manner so that skin integrity is complete. Thereafter, the body should be washed, dried and shrouded. It is then returned to the refrigerator

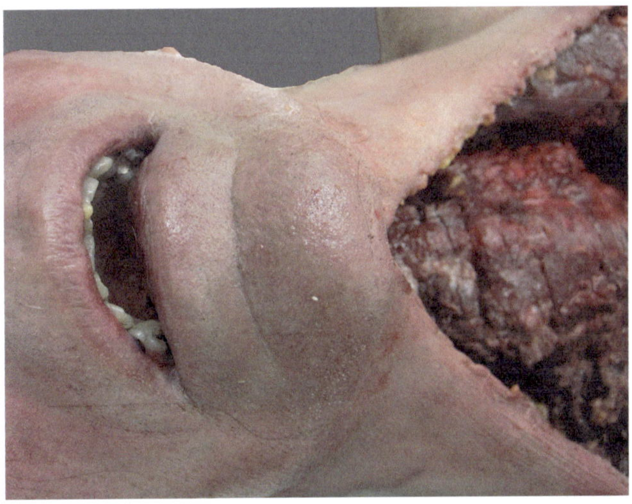

Fig. 3.54 This second autopsy case shows a particularly poor evisceration incision that ran up to the mandibular tissues and chin in the midline. This should be avoided if possible, as it is very difficult to achieve a good cosmetic reconstruction result after the autopsy

Suggested Reading

Burton JL, Rutty G. The hospital autopsy. 3rd ed. London: Hodder Arnold; 2010. p. 115–35.

Knight B. The post-mortem technician's handbook. Oxford: Blackwell Scientific Publications; 1984.

Ludwig J. Autopsy practice. 3rd ed. Ottawa: Humana Press; 2002.

Royal Institute of Public Health and Hygiene. A handbook of mortuary practice and safety: for anatomical pathology technicians. London: Royal Institute of Public Health and Hygiene; 1991.

Thorax: Heart, Lungs, Mediastinum, and Pleura

4

S. Kim Suvarna and Kirsty L. Lloyd

General Principles of Examining the Thorax

At the start, it is important to emphasize that a thorough knowledge of normal anatomy, physiology, and general pathology is required if one is to understand any thoracic autopsy findings. This background allows the examination to progress with understanding of any pathology, mapped against the patient's clinical data and history.

To fully appreciate cardiac and lung disease, it is important to separate the tissues carefully and sequentially, looking for disease as one proceeds. It is fair to say that the heart and lungs can best be regarded as a single unit, in that the heart has two halves with the lungs operating between the right and left side cardiac chambers.

The first part of this chapter (Figs. 4.1, 4.2, 4.3, 4.4, 4.5, 4.6, 4.7, 4.8, 4.9, 4.10, 4.11, 4.12, 4.13, 4.14, 4.15, 4.16, 4.17, 4.18, and 4.19) allows one to inspect the thoracic parenchymal units and to then start to break them down into smaller components. In this way, certain disorders (pulmonary embolism, congenital variations, and upper respiratory infections) can be spotted early in the case examination. Thereafter, the chapter looks specifically at the lung and heart tissues.

Photography is paramount in thoracic cases, and ideally should be used during the entirety of the dissection process, recording different aspects of the tissues. Histological sampling is also important, alongside microbiology assessment.

S. Kim Suvarna was deceased at the time of publication.

S. K. Suvarna (Deceased) · K. L. Lloyd (✉)
Department of Histopathology, Sheffield Teaching Hospitals NHS Foundation Trust, Sheffield, UK
e-mail: Kirsty.lloyd@nhs.net

S. K. Suvarna (represented by Grace Horne), A. K. Sharp (eds.), *Atlas of Adult Autopsy*,
https://doi.org/10.1007/978-3-031-72207-3_4

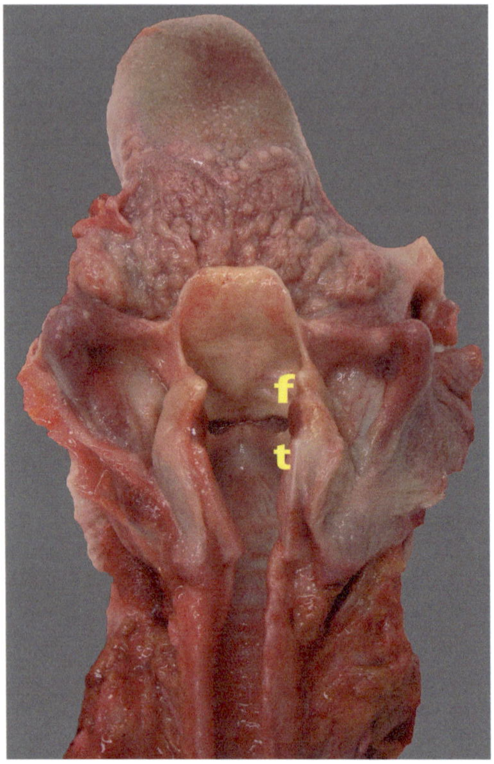

Fig. 4.1 Examination of the thoracic block of tissues should ideally start with the upper airway tissues. Placing tissues in a posterior-anterior position (*i.e.*, inspecting from the back), one can see the posterior wall of the trachea and laryngeal tissues. The epiglottis is noted proximally, and the tongue also may be inspected at this point. The airway should be checked for oedema, secretions, foreign matter or food debris, and tumours. The laryngeal cartilages are opened, using scissors, along the midline and the vocal cords (*t*, true; *f*, false) are seen in their correct position. The proximal tracheal tissues are now available for inspection

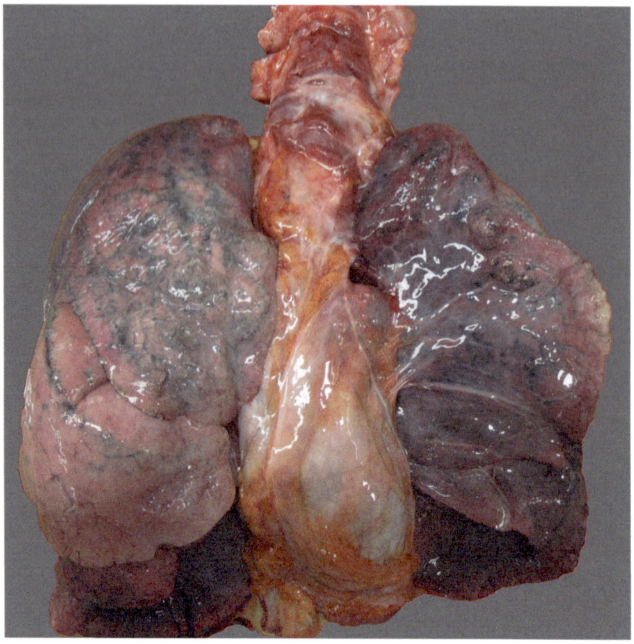

Fig. 4.2 The thoracic contents are seen from the front, having been removed from the body. The heart, within the pericardial sac, is centrally placed, with the lungs either side. The general architecture should be checked, with attention to congenital variations and external pathology

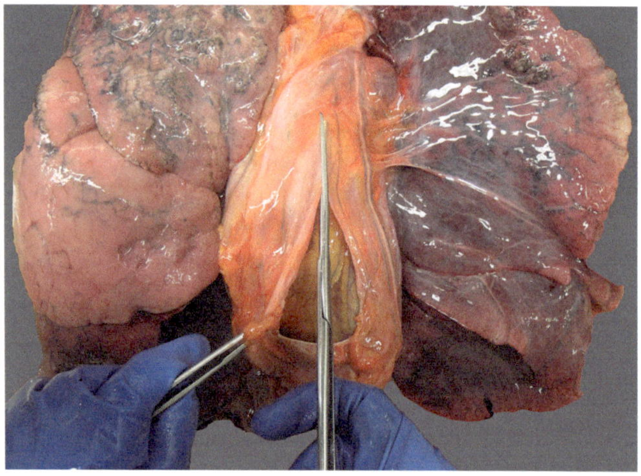

Fig. 4.3 The pericardium is opened, making sure that any fluid content is assessed (volume/type). If there is fluid of significance, then samples may be taken for microbiology and cytology

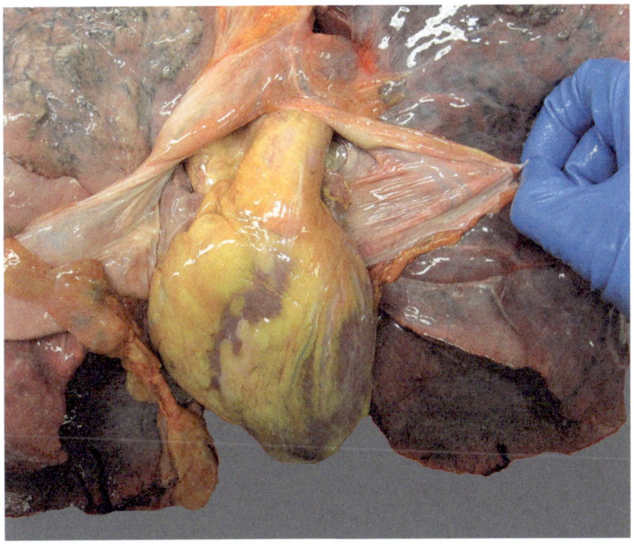

Fig. 4.4 The internal aspect of the pericardium should be inspected for possible tumour foci and fibrinous deposits. This inspection also allows a view of the heart, again allowing one to assess isomerism and other congenital cardiac variants

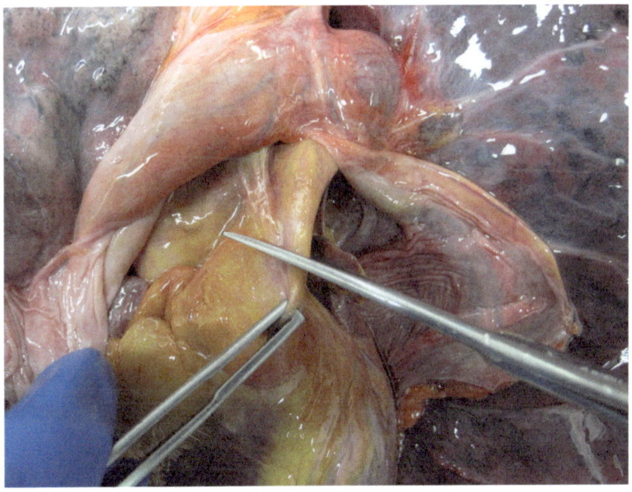

Fig. 4.5 The pulmonary artery is put under slight tension and the vessel is opened anteriorly using scissors to permit examination of the vessel for large pulmonary emboli

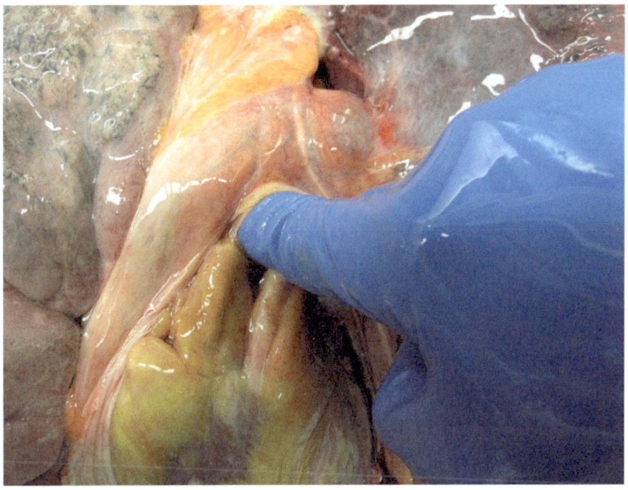

Fig. 4.6 A single finger may be introduced into the pulmonary artery to palpate into the branches on either side. Pulmonary emboli often can be felt before being visualized in this technique, and they may be pushed slightly into the artery to avoid their loss when the lungs are separated from the mediastinal content

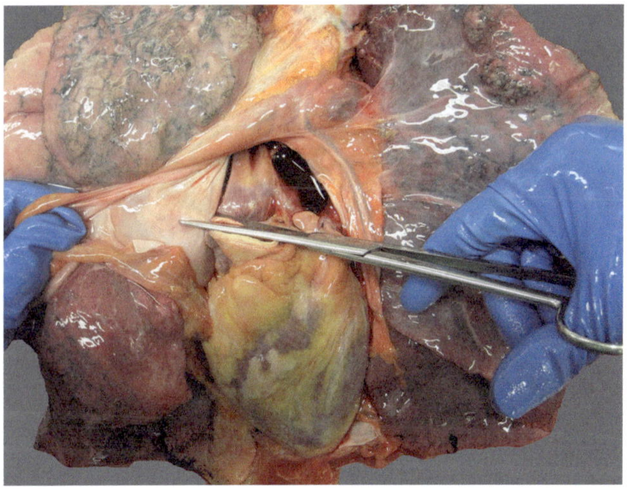

Fig. 4.7 After the examination of the pulmonary artery, the heart may be removed from the block of tissue by completing the cut across the pulmonary artery trunk and aorta, in sequence

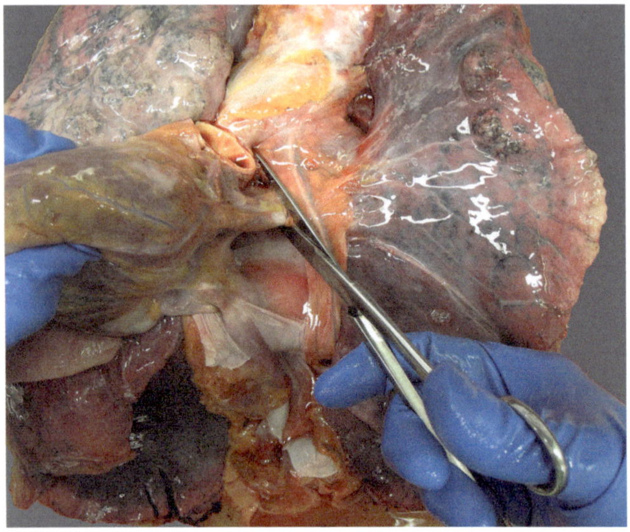

Fig. 4.8 Next, the heart is lifted upwards and towards the right side. The dissection proceeds with cutting across the pulmonary veins. These are transected, ideally with scissors, above the left atrial roof and posterior wall

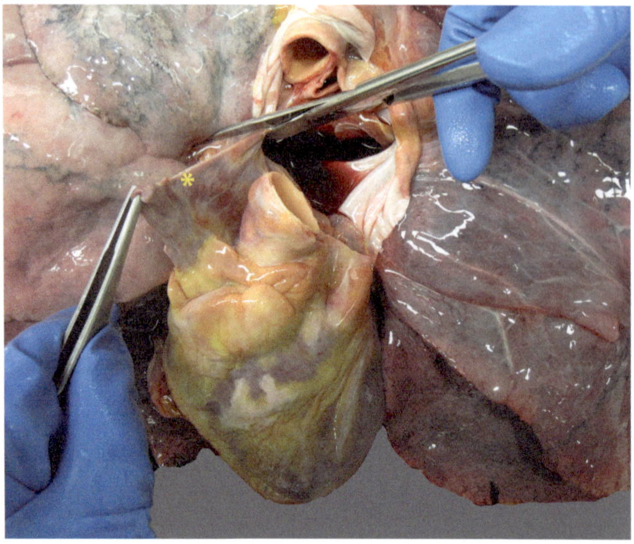

Fig. 4.10 The superior vena cava (SVC) must be cut above the sinoatrial node (SAN). The SAN is at the interface of the SVC and the right atrium anteriorly (*asterisk*). By gently putting the SVC under tension, one can ensure that the cut across the SVC is at least 10 mm above the SAN

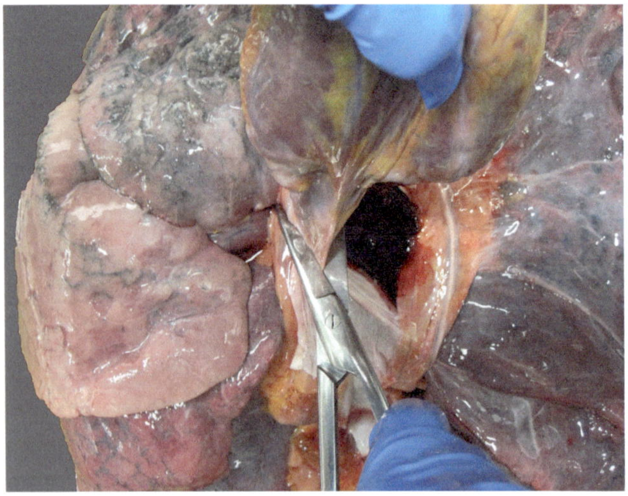

Fig. 4.9 Lifting the heart upwards (towards the head) allows the inferior vena cava to be cut where it enters the right atrium

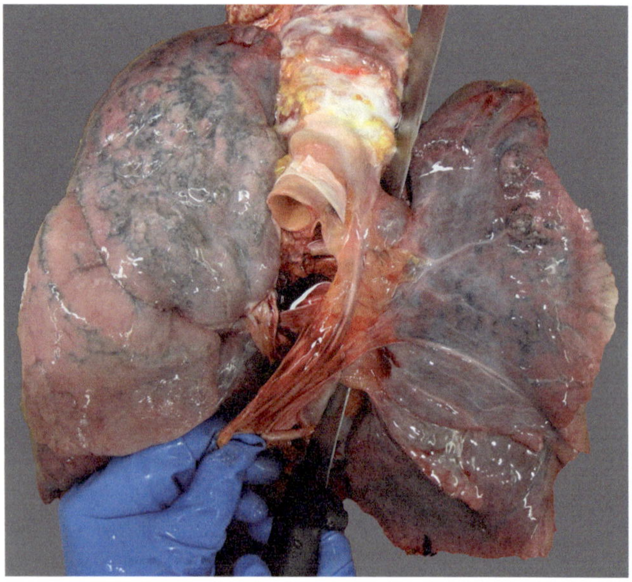

Fig. 4.11 The next step is to separate the lungs. In this case, the left lung is resected first, by placing a long knife under the left lung hilum. It is safest to put the knife in position with the blunt side upmost and then rotate the blade so the cutting edge is upward when the knife is in position. The lung should be removed with one slice, rather than a sawing motion

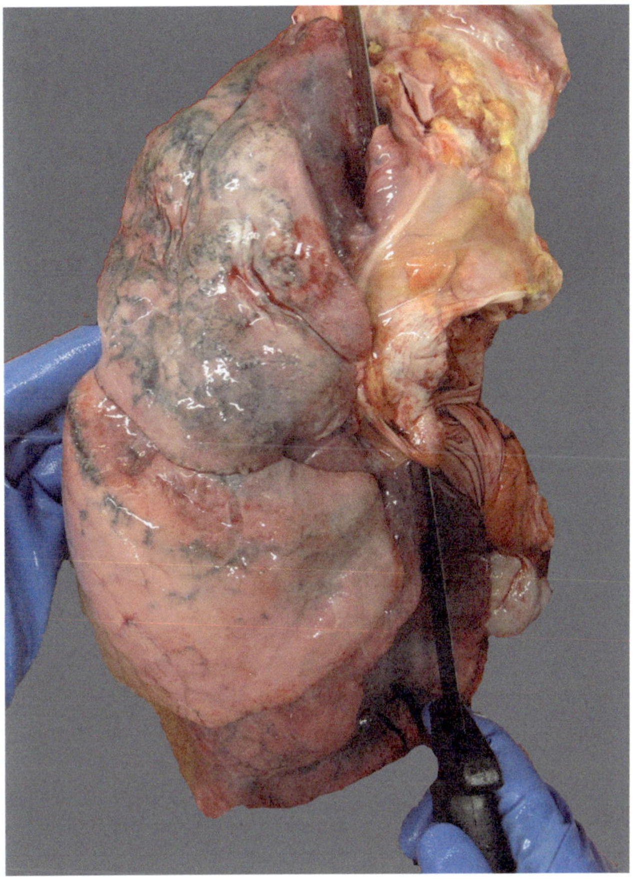

Fig. 4.12 The right lung is now removed by repeating the process at the right lung hilum

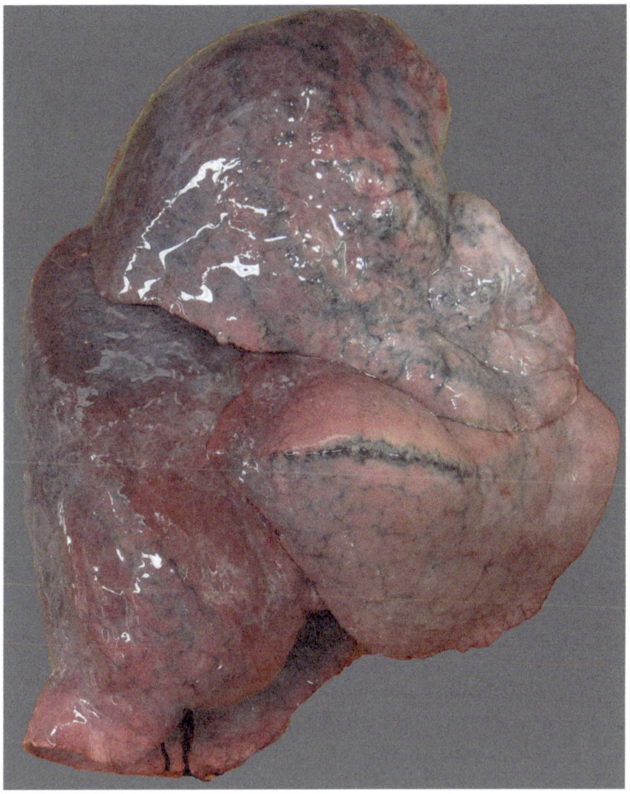

Fig. 4.13 The right lung is seen from the lateral aspect, with an unremarkable pleural surface. Note the three lobes

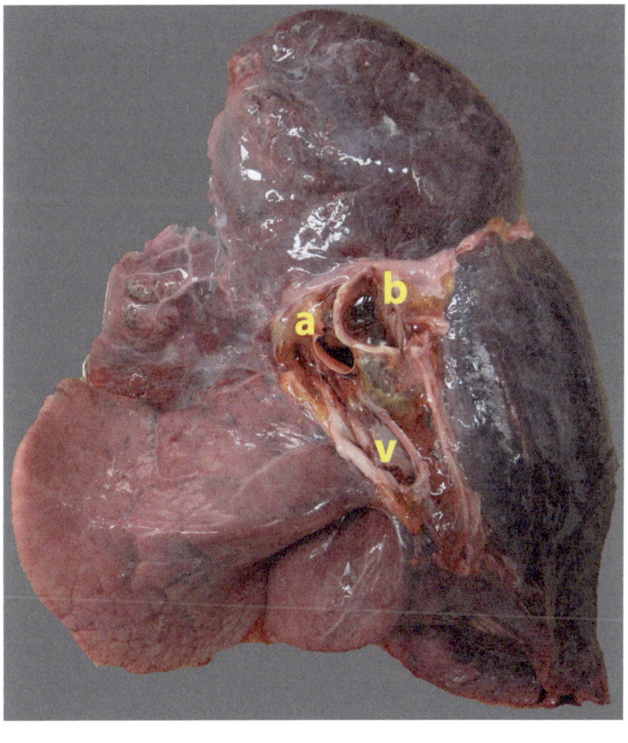

Fig. 4.14 The mediastinal view of the right lung shows the normal bronchus (*b*) and vasculature (*a*, artery; *v*, vein)

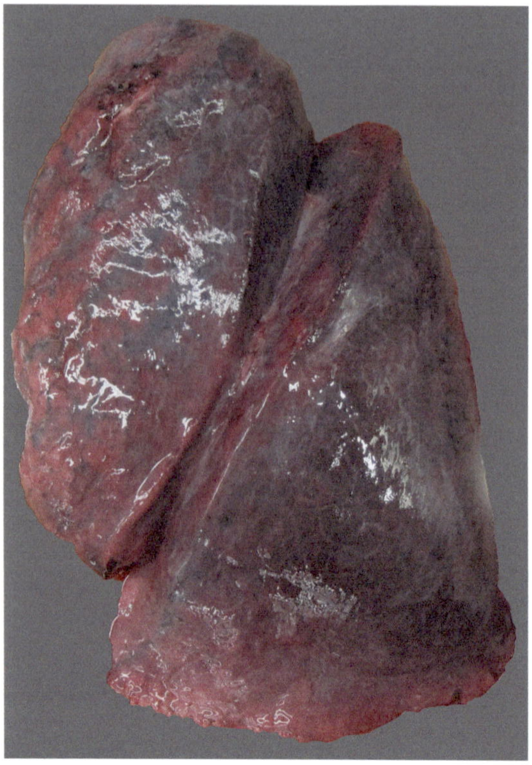

Fig. 4.15 The external surface of the left lung lateral aspect is seen; the two lobes show a normal pleural surface

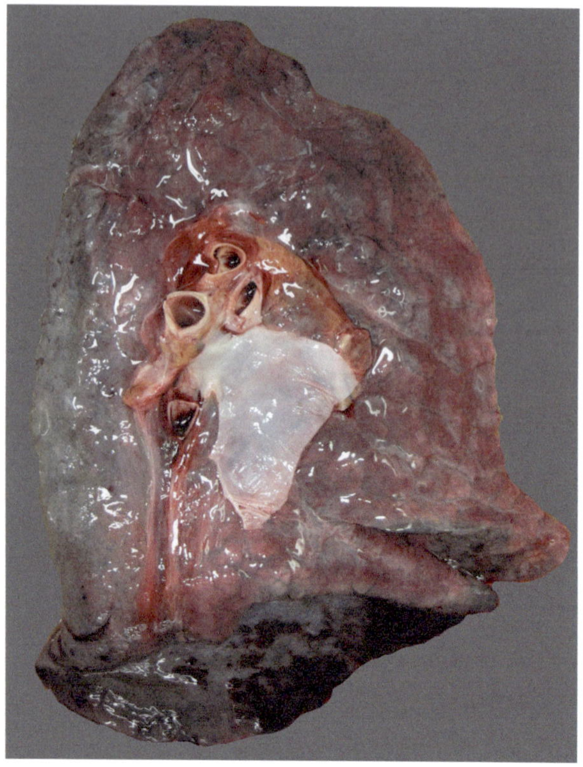

Fig. 4.17 This mediastinal view of the left lung shows part of the pericardium attached, highlighting the proximity of the lung to the heart tissues

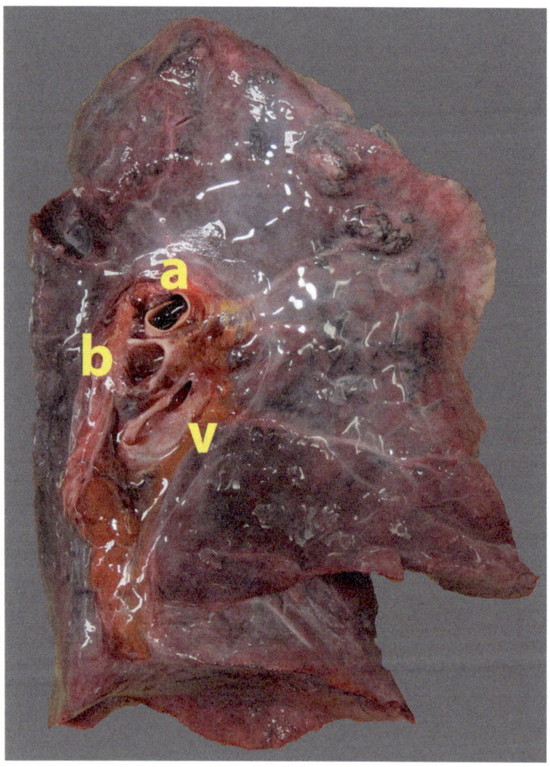

Fig. 4.16 The mediastinal view shows the normal bronchus (*b*) and vasculature (*a*, artery; *v*, vein)

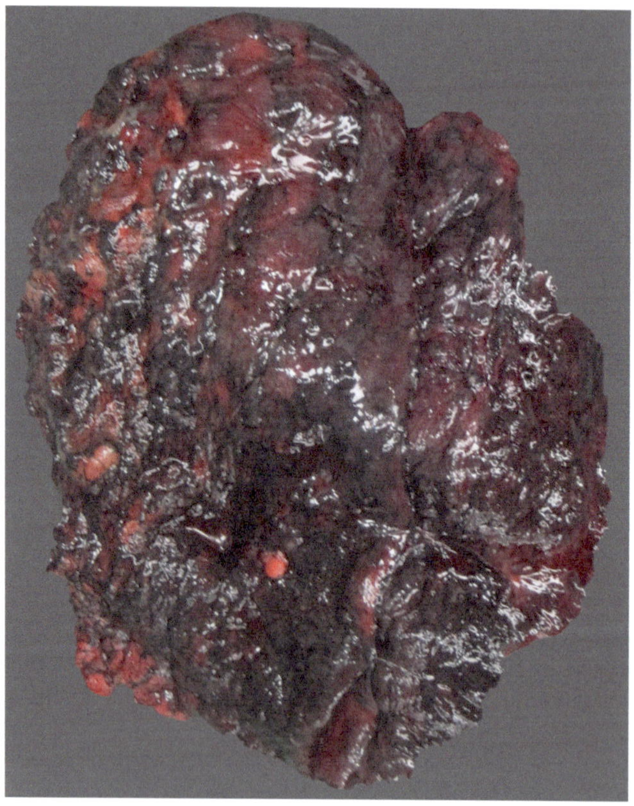

Fig. 4.18 Modern urban life rarely leaves individuals in a low-pollution environment. Consequently, many lungs show some anthracotic (black) dust accumulation, generally reflecting pollution from fossil fuels and general dusts

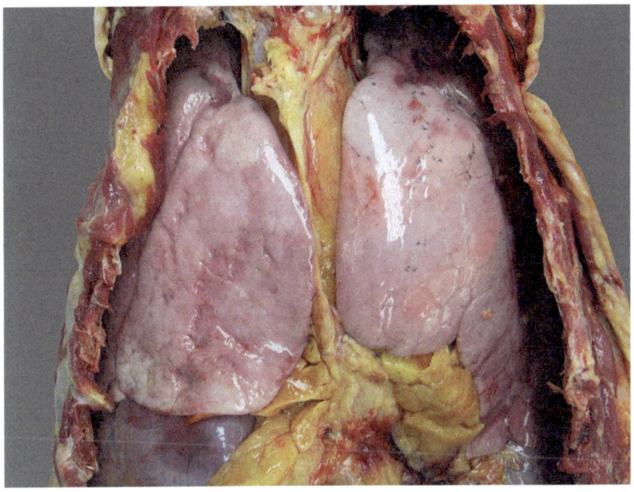

Fig. 4.19 These lungs are relatively clear of dust; they are from an individual who lived in a very rural setting without significant soot staining

The Lung Tissues: Acute and Infective Processes

Examination of the lung tissues (Figs. 4.20, 4.21, 4.22, 4.23, 4.24, 4.25, 4.26, 4.27, 4.28, 4.29, 4.30, and 4.31) is primarily concerned with initially confirming normality and then by seeking out any pathology issues. The lung tissues must be considered carefully, with attention to the vasculature as well as the airways. Consideration of the pleural membranes and chest wall may also be necessary if one is to fully appreciate pulmonary function.

Common culprits in terms of pathology include embolic disorders (Figs. 4.32, 4.33, 4.34, 4.35, 4.36, 4.37, 4.38, 4.39, 4.40, 4.41, 4.42, 4.43, 4.44, 4.45, 4.46, and 4.47), with large emboli being common lesions in the autopsy room. If large, they are almost instantly fatal.

Lung infections (standard community-acquired pneumonic conditions as well as atypical bacterial, fungal, and viral diseases) are common lesions in the autopsy room (Figs. 4.48, 4.49, 4.50, 4.51, 4.52, 4.53, 4.54, 4.55, 4.56, 4.57, 4.58, 4.59, 4.60, 4.61, 4.62, 4.63, 4.64, and 4.65). With any infective process, samples should be taken for microbiological assessment and histology.

The placement of chest drains, septic and haemorrhagic complications from surgical intervention, and the impact of fractures are important aspects of assessing the thoracic tissues. The role of photography is highlighted.

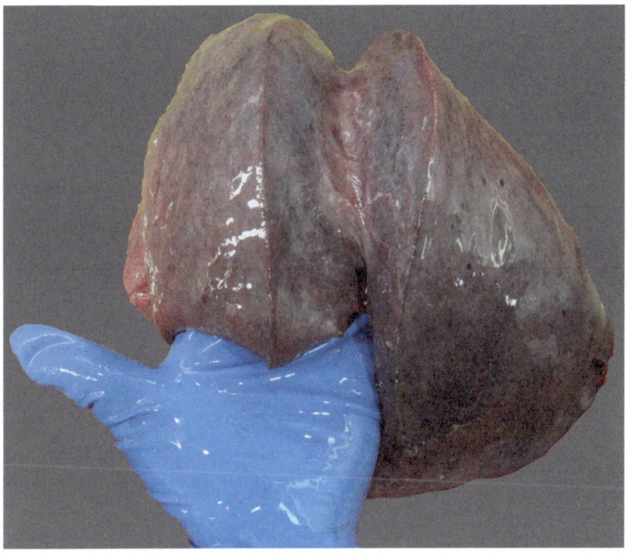

Fig. 4.20 Dissection of the internal aspect of the lung tissues is commenced with the vasculature. The examination of the pulmonary vasculature is best appreciated by exposing the interlobar fissure, accomplished by holding the lung at the hilum and letting the lobes fall on either side of the hand

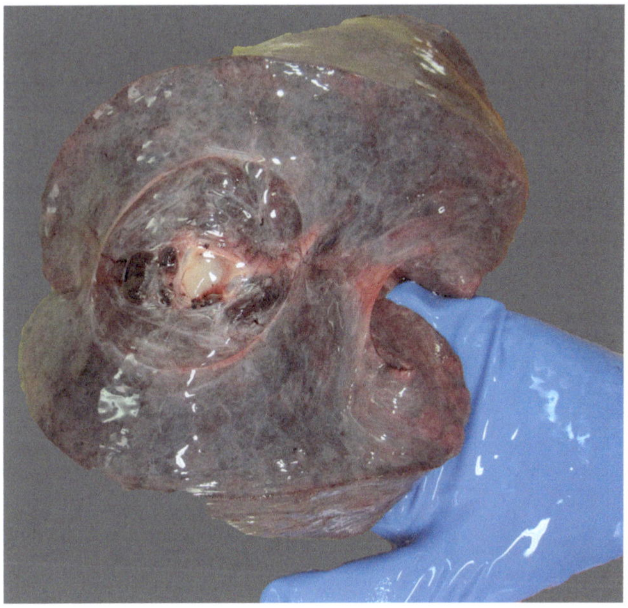

Fig. 4.21 An incision is made into the interlobar fissure over the pulmonary artery, opening the bifurcation point of the pulmonary artery. The lung tissues fall either side of the cut, if one holds the lung centrally from below at the hilum

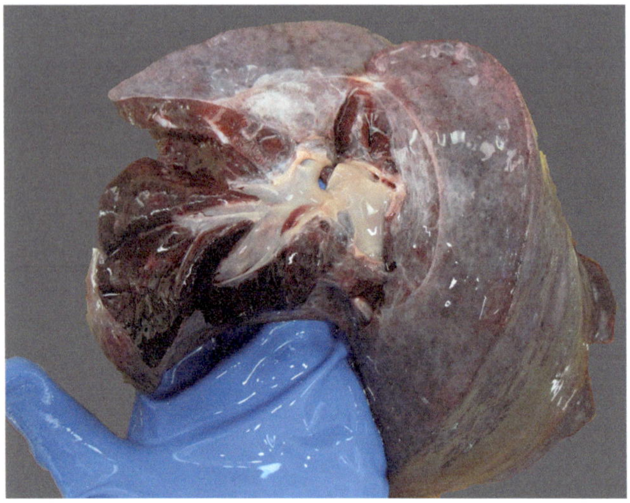

Fig. 4.22 By gently inserting scissors into the vessels and only then cutting, the pulmonary arteries can be carefully exposed along the lengths of the vessels towards the lung edge. One should consider the extent of any atheromatous change and the presence of thromboemboli or other focal lesions

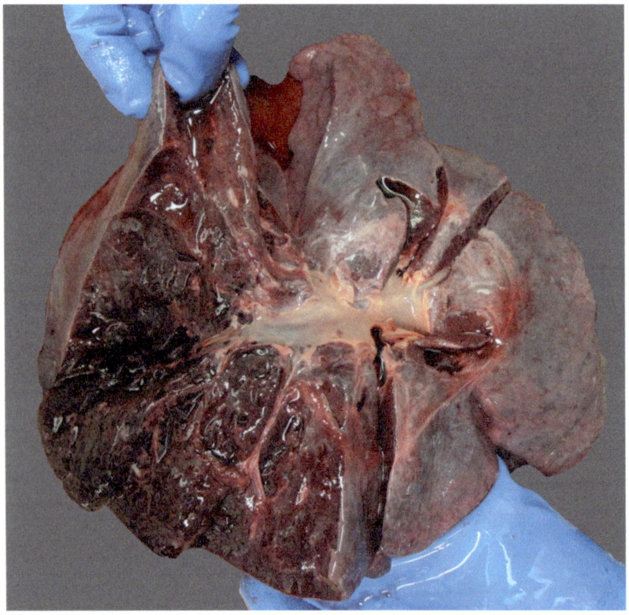

Fig. 4.23 The arteries should be explored outwards towards the periphery of the lung tissue, not simply 10–20 mm from the centre of the lung. This allows examination of a significant amount of lung parenchyma

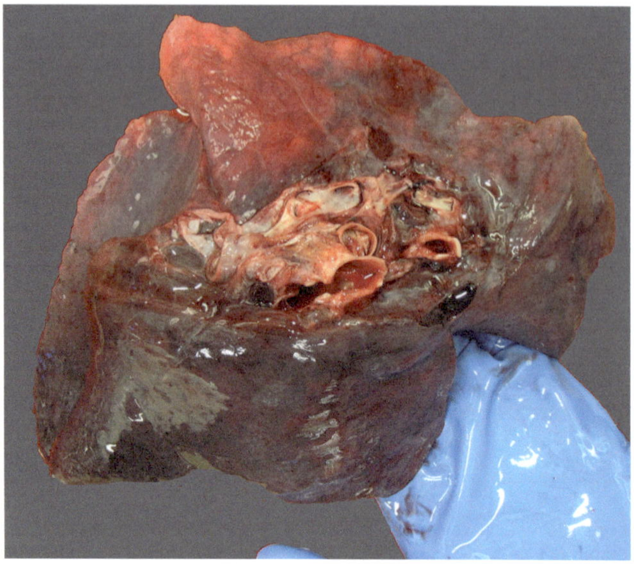

Fig. 4.24 The lung tissues are now turned over to show the mediastinal aspect uppermost. The bronchi are inspected initially, looking for obstructing tumours or foreign material

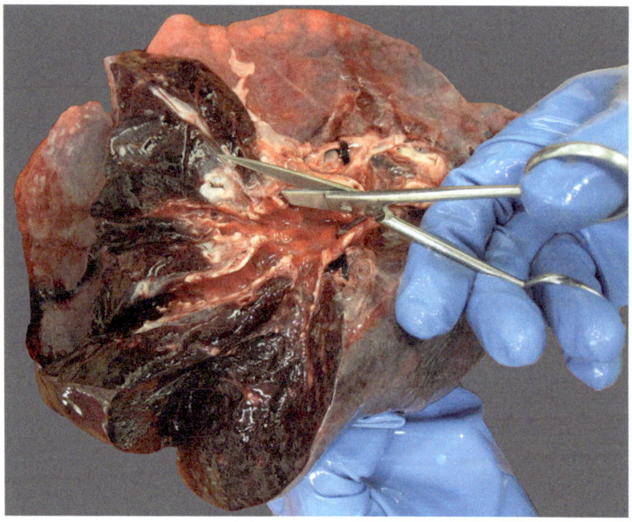

Fig. 4.25 In a similar manner, the next step involves the scissors being gently inserted into the bronchi, with cuts being made onwards and outwards towards the periphery of the lung tissue

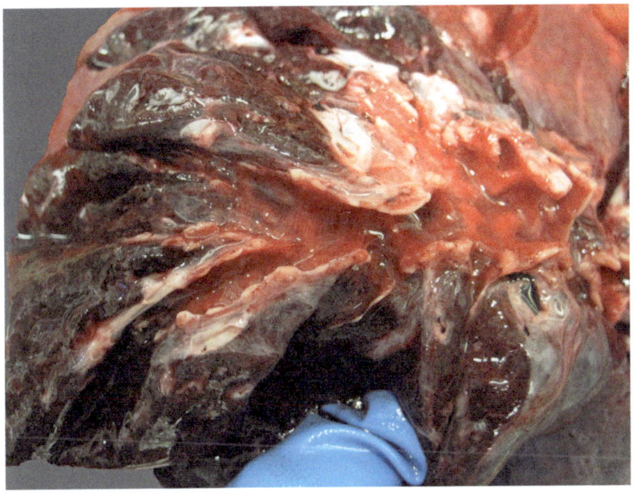

Fig. 4.26 The surfaces of the bronchial tree should be inspected with regard to sepsis, tumour, or obstructive lesion. The airways shown are clear of tumour and inflammatory exudate, but there is a degree of bronchial congestion, raising the possibility of some bronchitis

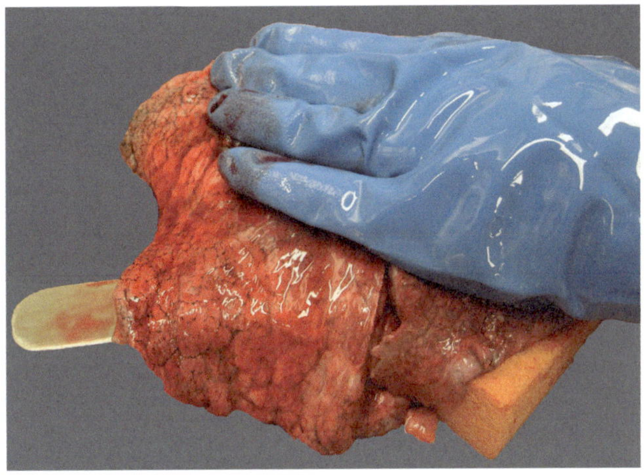

Fig. 4.28 One can slice lung along its long (parasagittal) axis in order to display the tissues. This method is quicker, but it clearly cannot fully assess the bronchi and vasculature. It is particularly useful, however, when considering interstitial and diffuse lung disease

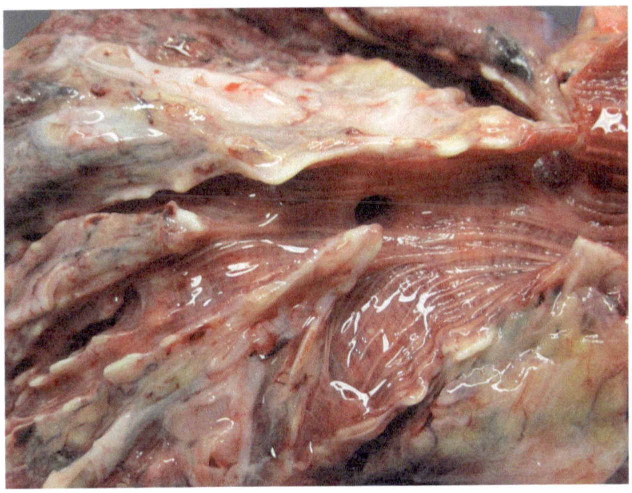

Fig. 4.27 The airways (in health) generally are seen to have a ridged or corrugated surface quality, which assists drainage of secretions

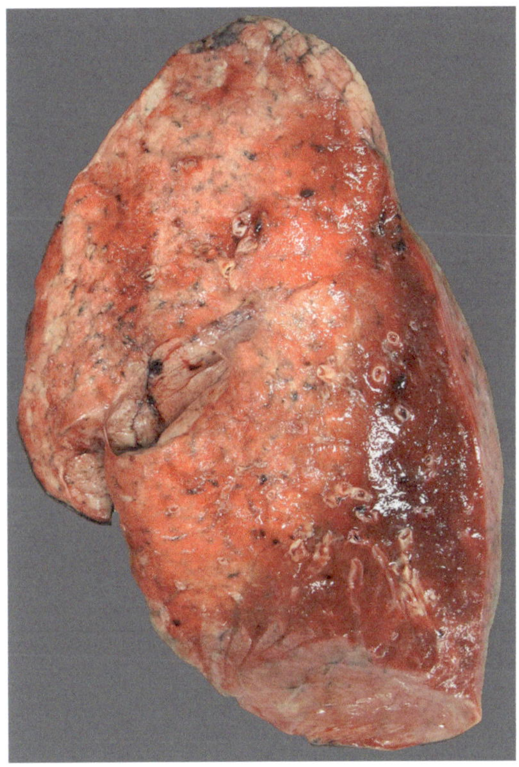

Fig. 4.29 The cut surface of the lung seen in parasagittal section is shown here. The lung tissues appear largely normal, but hypostasis affects the lungs in the same way as it does the rest of the body. Blood has accumulated in the posterior and dependent part of the lung following death. This technique, apart from being quicker, does allow a more global view of the parenchyma

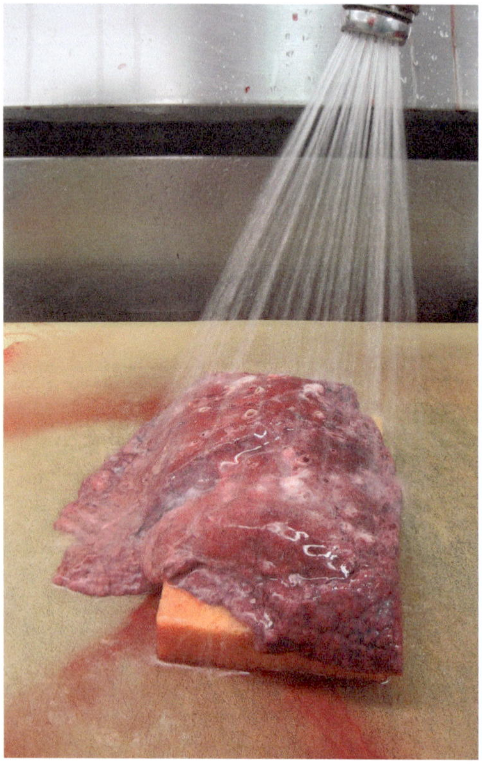

Fig. 4.30 Lung tissues contain a lot of blood and often are rich in secretions, so lung detail may be obscured macroscopically. One solution is to gently spray water onto the cut surface for about 3–5 min

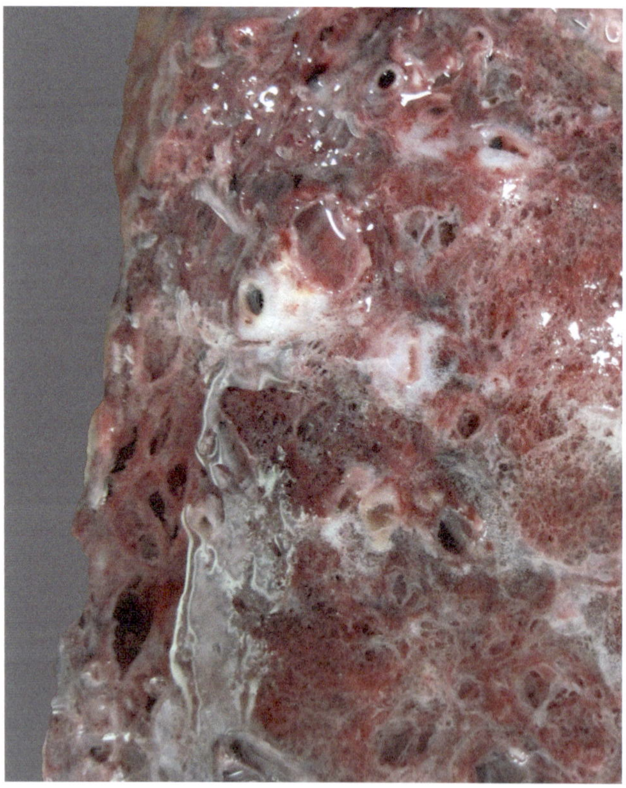

Fig. 4.31 After gentle washing, more detail is apparent in the washed lung

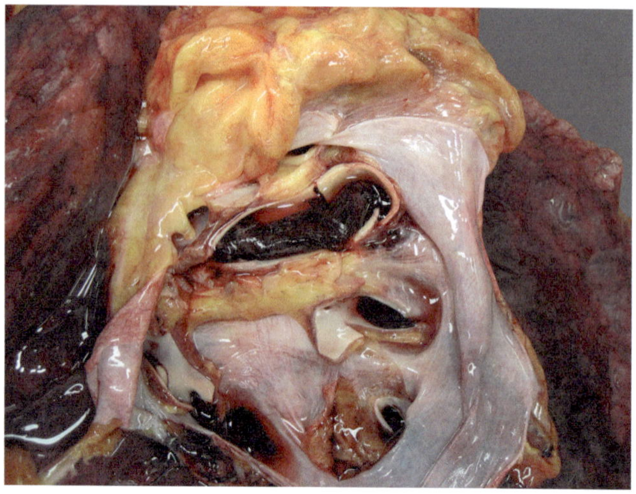

Fig. 4.32 Shown is a saddle embolus, clearly occluding the branch of the pulmonary artery and causing sudden death. This is evident before the lungs are removed, but after the heart has been separated from the mediastinal content

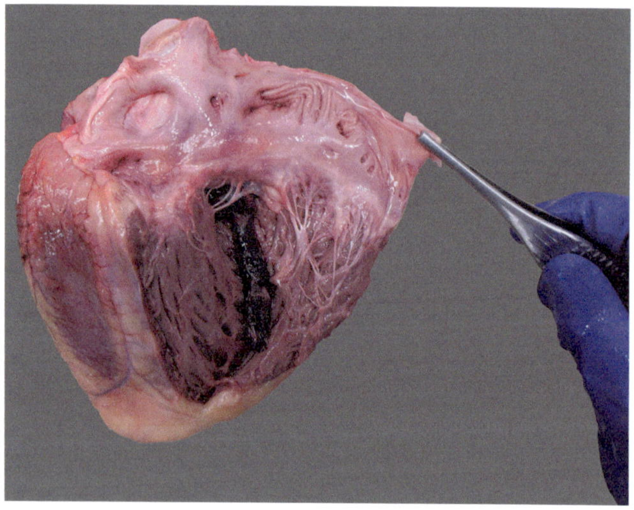

Fig. 4.33 This shows a case of pulmonary embolism with part of the thromboembolus caught within the right ventricle, largely blocking the outflow tract

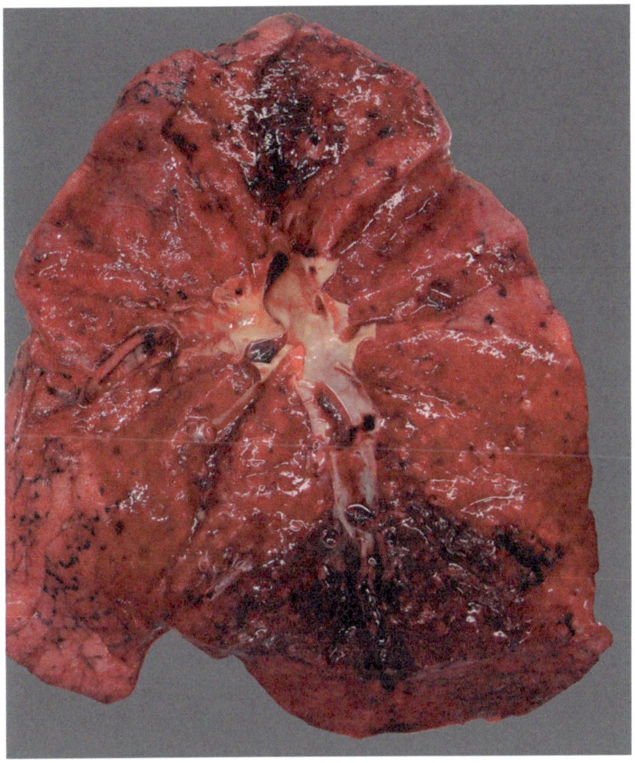

Fig. 4.34 The lung tissues have been opened from the blood vessel aspect. There are two zones of haemorrhagic infarction towards the top and bottom of the lung fields. Some adherent thrombus is also seen attached to one of the segmental pulmonary arteries

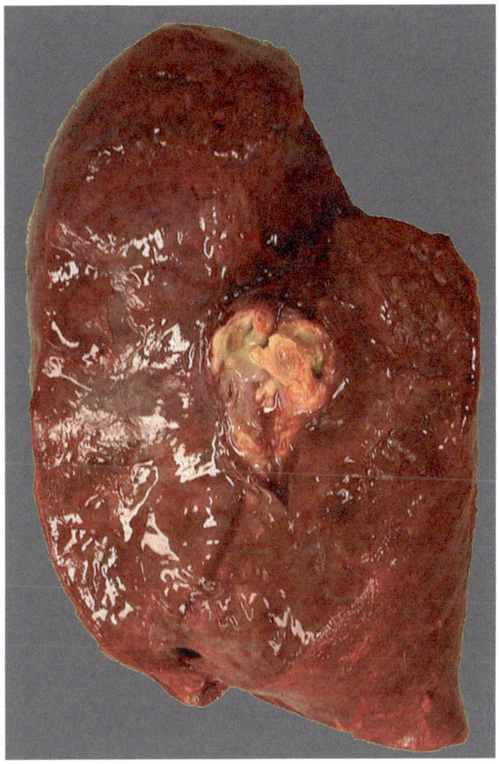

Fig. 4.36 Thrombotic material can be complicated by septic findings. Bacterial infection can localize within dead tissue or thrombus at the root of the lung

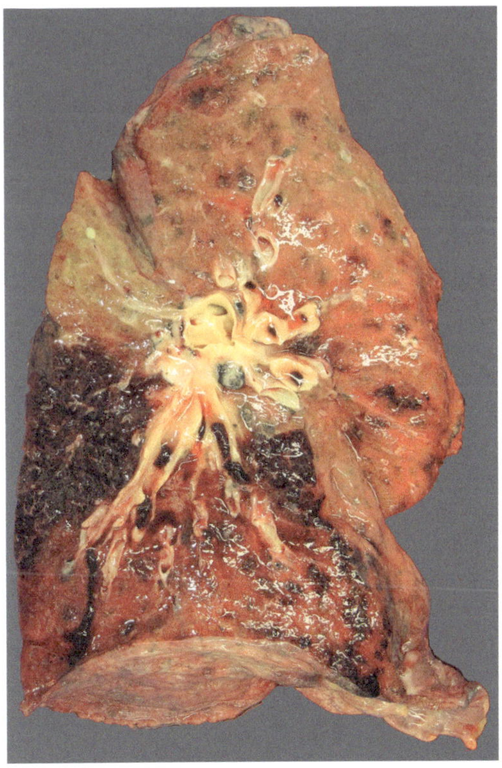

Fig. 4.35 The classic wedge-shaped pulmonary infarct is seen after a few days in a case of pulmonary embolism. Note the partially adherent thrombotic material in the proximal artery. The local viable lung showed consolidation and septic changes histologically

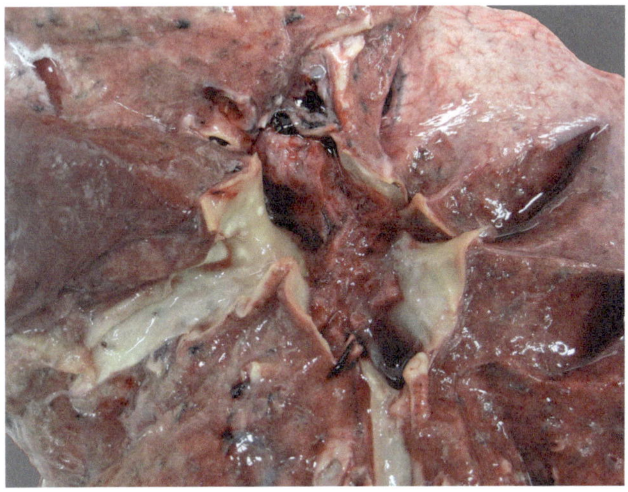

Fig. 4.37 Thromboembolic matter may reflect longstanding thrombotic events within the venous circulation. This very firm and pale thrombus was found in a patient who collapsed suddenly and who had a chronic history of recurrent deep vein thrombotic change. This thrombus had likely formed in the large veins many weeks beforehand

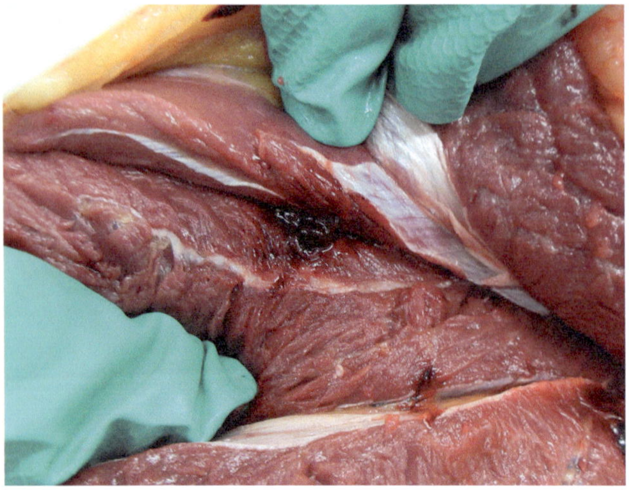

Fig. 4.38 A deep vein thrombus is seen within one of the calf muscles of the leg in a case of pulmonary embolism

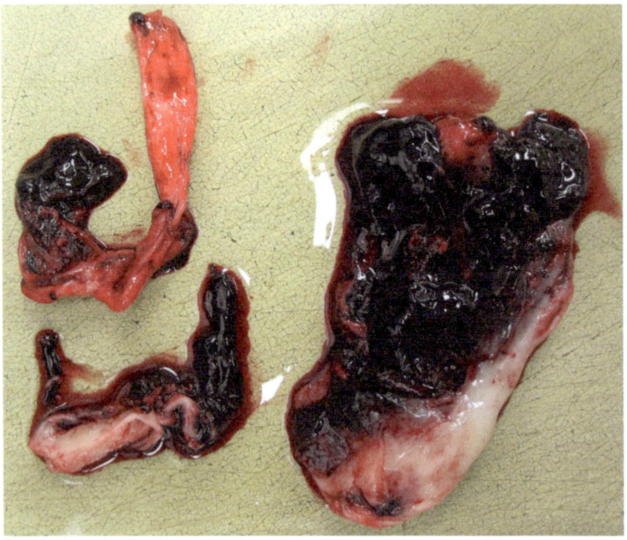

Fig. 4.39 Post-mortem coagulum, in the form of semisolid protein and blood cells, is often seen at autopsy. The coagulum is layered (owing to post-mortem settling out of erythrocytes and other cells) and generally quite soft; it should not be confused with thrombus

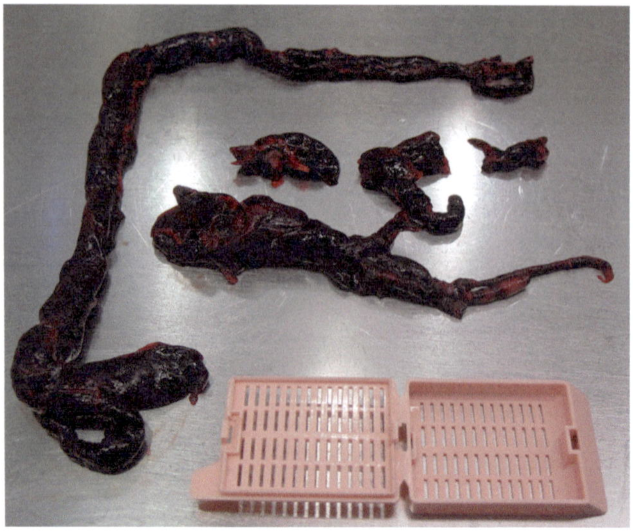

Fig. 4.40 Thromboembolic matter is seen with the venous radicle configuration, which allows one to map the thrombi (by virtue of their size) to the likely source within the venous circulation

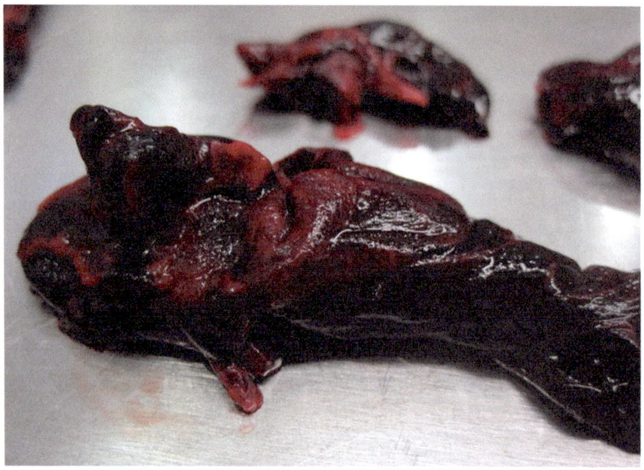

Fig. 4.41 Close up of venous thromboembolic material shows irregularities in keeping with valve projections in the venous circulation at the sites where the thrombus is formed

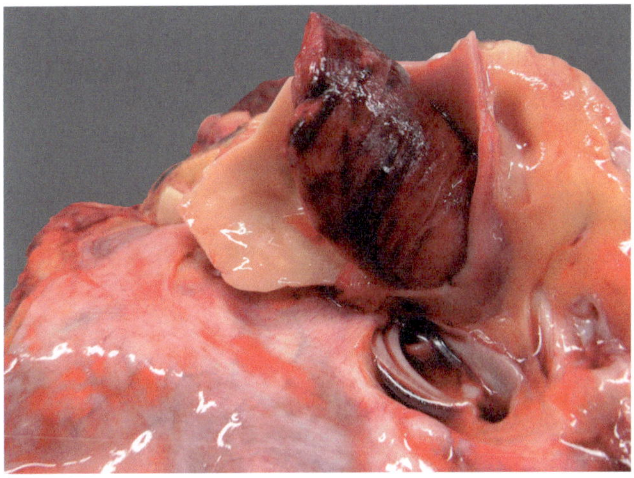

Fig. 4.42 Laminated thrombus is seen in this pulmonary artery, in keeping with chronic pulmonary embolism which has lodged and partially occluded this pulmonary artery

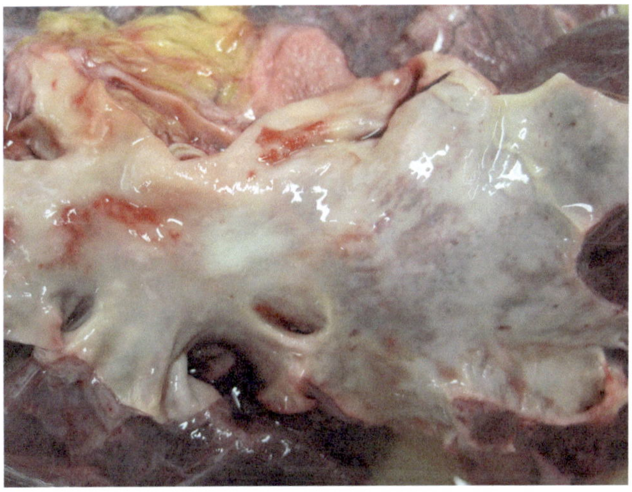

Fig. 4.43 This is a view of the opened pulmonary artery. The intimal surface appears irregular and variably thickened and fibrotic. This patient had surgery for recurrent and significant pulmonary embolism approximately 6 months before death. The surgery had involved opening the pulmonary artery and extracting partially adherent clot material directly, thereby causing intimal scarring

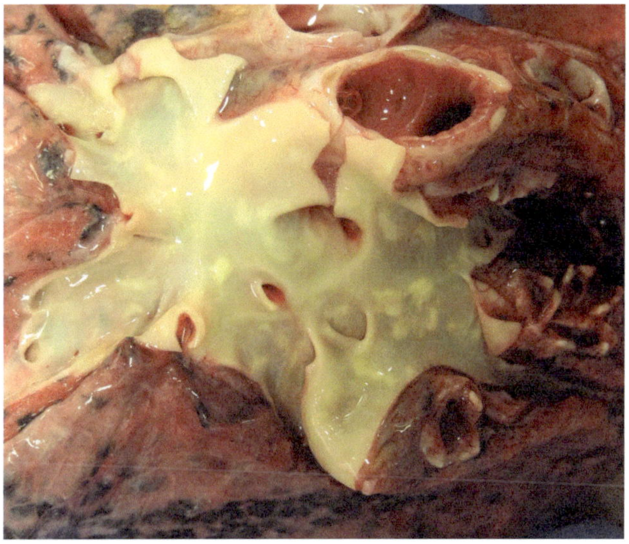

Fig. 4.44 The pulmonary artery in this case shows some atheroma deposits. This may be commonly noted in the pulmonary artery root but if these are present through into the deeper segmental arteries then the atheroma may indicate pulmonary hypertension. Additional evidence of pulmonary hypertension will require histological examination of the alveolated lung vasculature

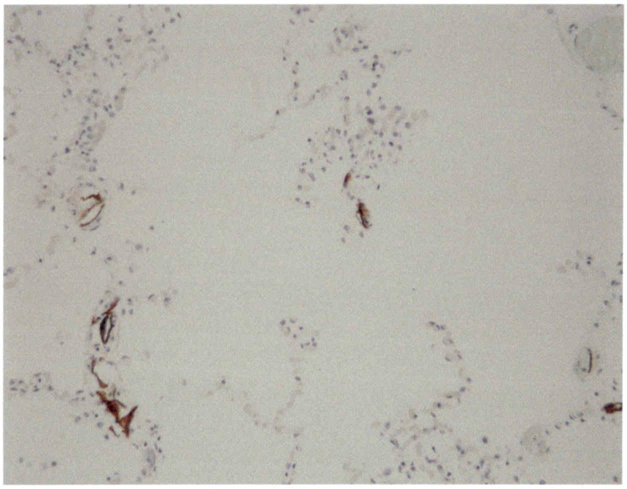

Fig. 4.45 Histology of lung tissues, using high molecular weight cytokeratin immunohistology, clearly defines fetal epithelial cells (*stained brown*) from amniotic fluid embolism. These cells are present within the capillary vasculature of the lung tissues

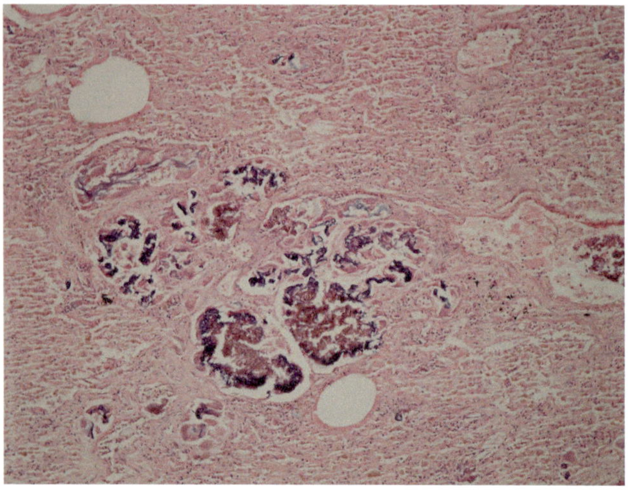

Fig. 4.46 In cases of intravenous drug use, irregular foreign material concretions are often seen in and around the pulmonary vasculature. The somewhat corrugated and partially calcified debris seen in this view reflects fragments of gelatin-type matrix from partially dissolved drug capsule matrix, which was directly injected into the venous circulation some time previously

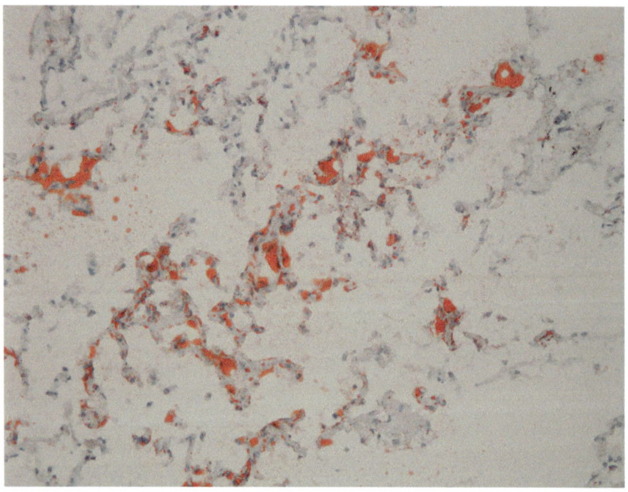

Fig. 4.47 Frozen section of fresh tissues from the autopsy, followed by Oil Red O staining, serves to highlight fat fragments in a case of fat embolism. It is not possible to use this technique after formalin fixation and paraffin processing, as the fat droplets are removed during tissue processing

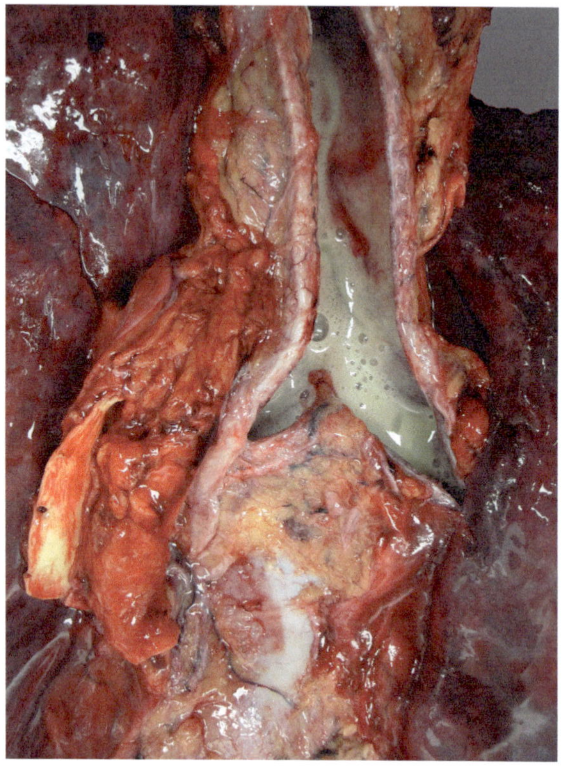

Fig. 4.48 Bronchopneumonia is seen in the distal trachea at the bifurcation into the lobar bronchi. The mucopurulent secretions are clearly thick and tenacious; they largely obstruct both major airways. This obstruction is a potent cause of death, particularly in the elderly and debilitated

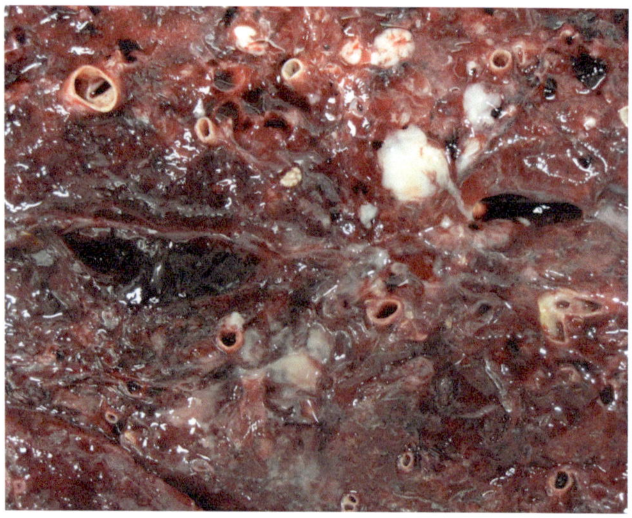

Fig. 4.49 The cut surface of lobar and bronchopneumonia often shows consolidation, with mucopurulent secretions involving the airways

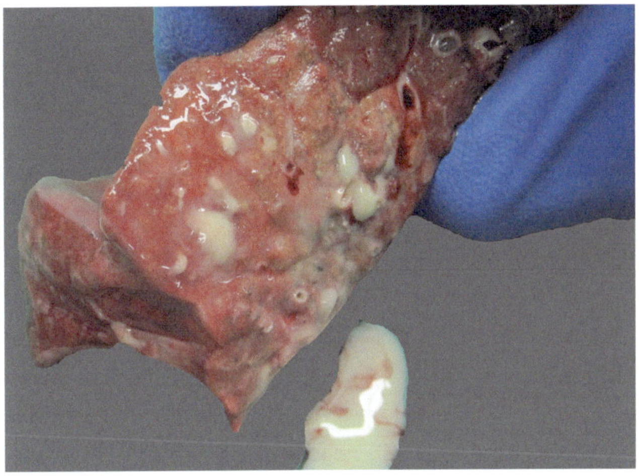

Fig. 4.50 With gentle pressure, the lung tissues will exude pus from the cut surface, confirming the macroscopic interpretation and allowing sampling of the infected material

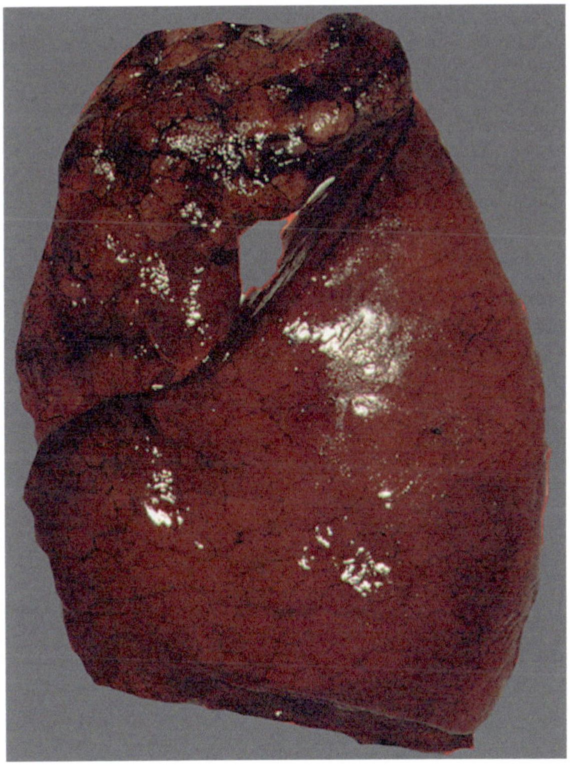

Fig. 4.51 Lobar pneumonia, with a classic engorged and consolidated lobe of lung, is seen; compare the adjacent upper lobe

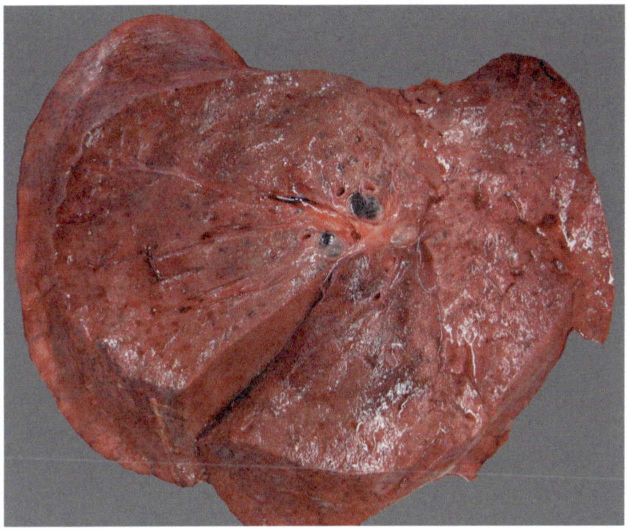

Fig. 4.52 Consolidation of the lung tissue is often appreciated as solid-appearing lung, but it also can be appreciated as palpably firm tissues

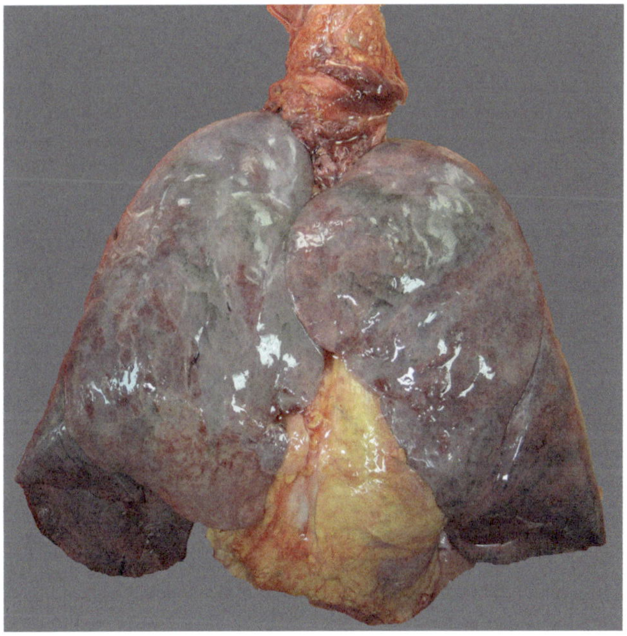

Fig. 4.53 In this case of influenza pneumonia with bilateral lung consolidation, the distended lungs project across the front of the mediastinum

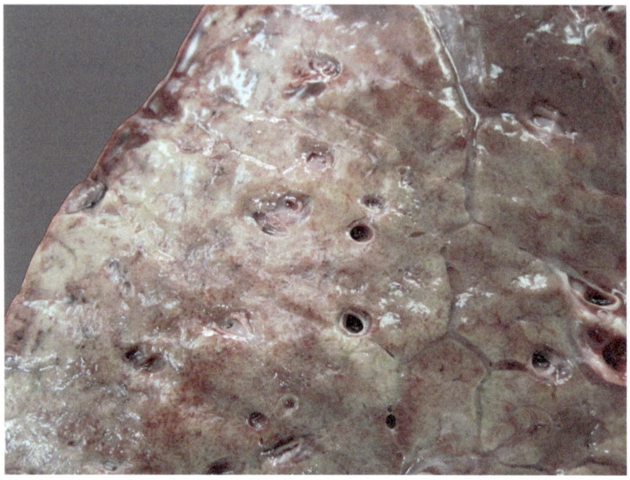

Fig. 4.54 Influenza may produce diffuse lung consolidation. This H1N1 influenza case shows extreme consolidation of the lung tissues, with grey hepatisation. Histologically, a range of inflammatory cells are often present, together with fibrin and spilled erythrocytes

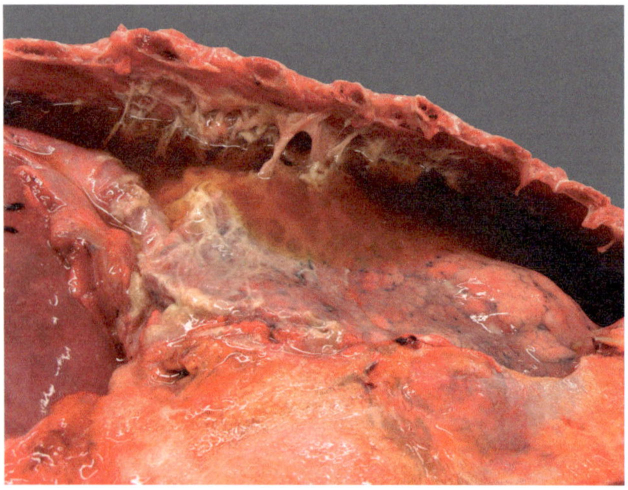

Fig. 4.55 Acute on chronic pleuritis is seen with fibrinous strands tying the visceral and lateral pleural surfaces together. The fluid is brown and slightly turbid in keeping with ongoing infection

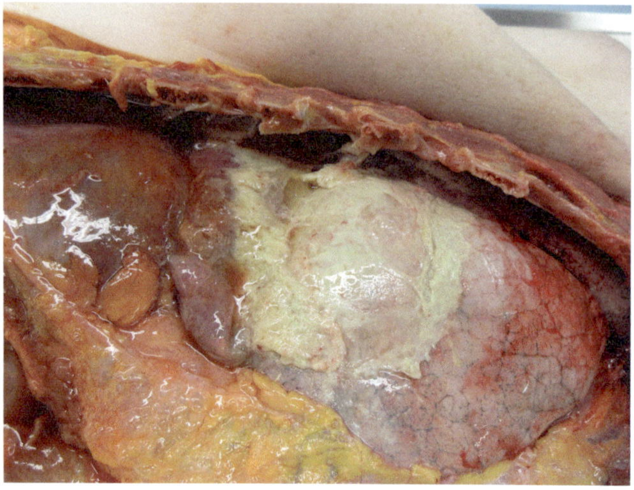

Fig. 4.56 On removing the sternum, it is apparent that there is an infective process, prompting a pause in the dissection to consider risk factors for tuberculosis and review the personal protective equipment for all staff in the dissection room. In this case, the deceased was found in the community with no known medical history so pulmonary infection was not suspected. There is a right lower zone fibrinous exudate with loculations and associated purulent fluid, subsequently shown to be related to tuberculosis

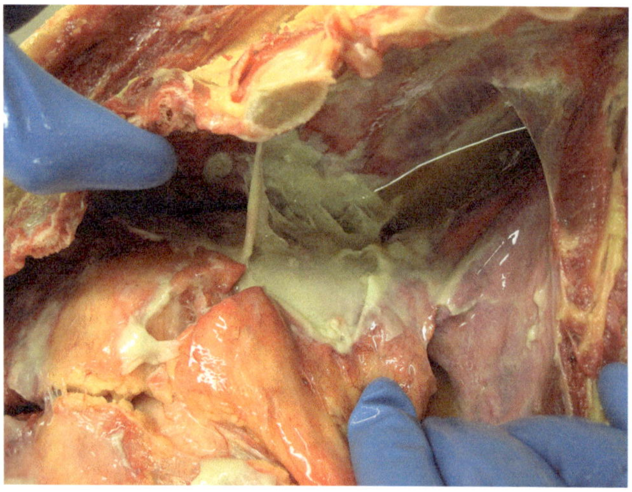

Fig. 4.57 Septic collections are common in the pleural cavity and are often best examined immediately after the chest has been opened. A septic collection is present at the base of this hemithorax, which contains both turbid fluid and clearly purulent material at the costophrenic angle

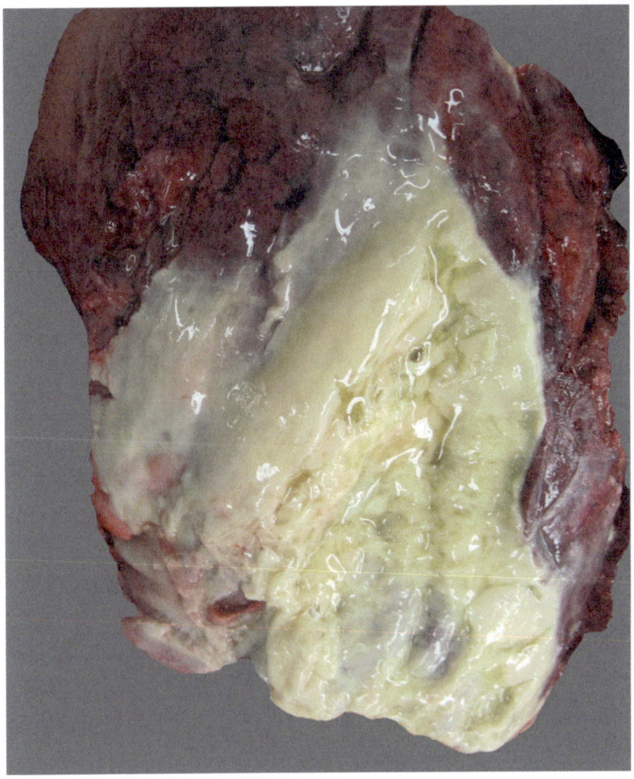

Fig. 4.58 Empyema can be tenacious and can encase lung tissues. This area of subacute empyema was in the process of organising, with semi-solid and gelatinous/mucoid components being evident. Swab samples should be taken to consider the nature of the infective agent. In addition, histology of the underlying lung and infected substrate may prove useful

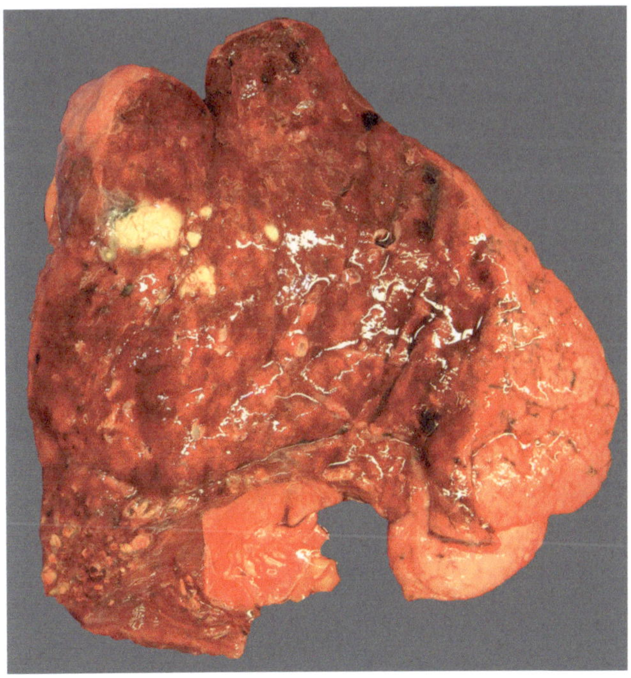

Fig. 4.59 Peripheral lung tissue is seen in a case of old tuberculosis. There is a focus of fibrosis and old granulomatous change in the lung parenchyma, with smaller nodules of similar inflammation adjacent. No active parenchymal sepsis is present, and the appearances are in keeping with previous tuberculosis

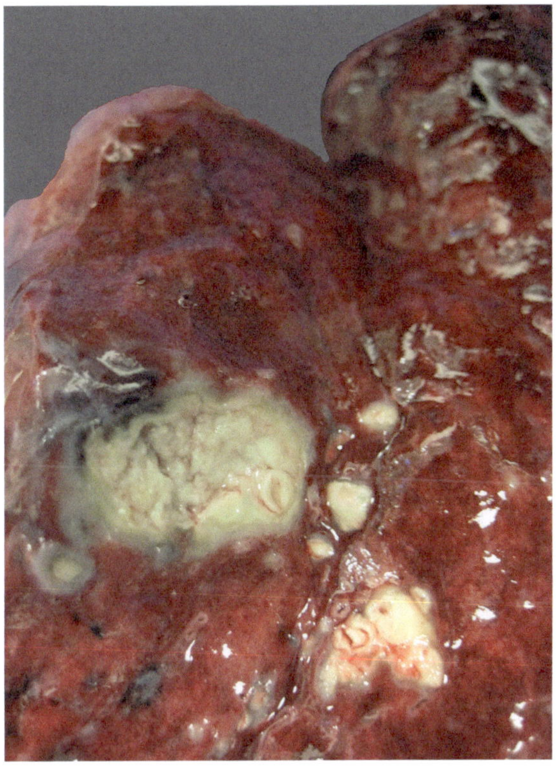

Fig. 4.60 Higher magnification of the Ghon focus, highlighting old caseous necrosis and local fibrosis

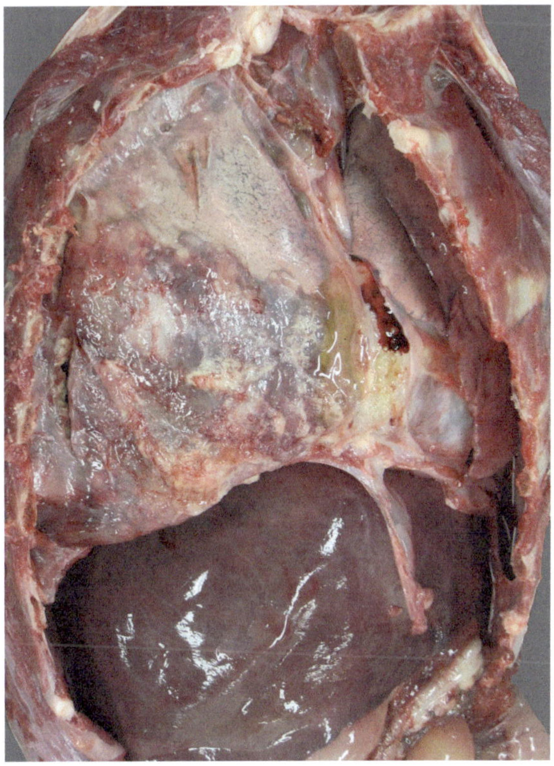

Fig. 4.61 The chest has been opened in another tuberculosis case, revealing largely consolidated lung tissue that was tightly bound to the chest wall

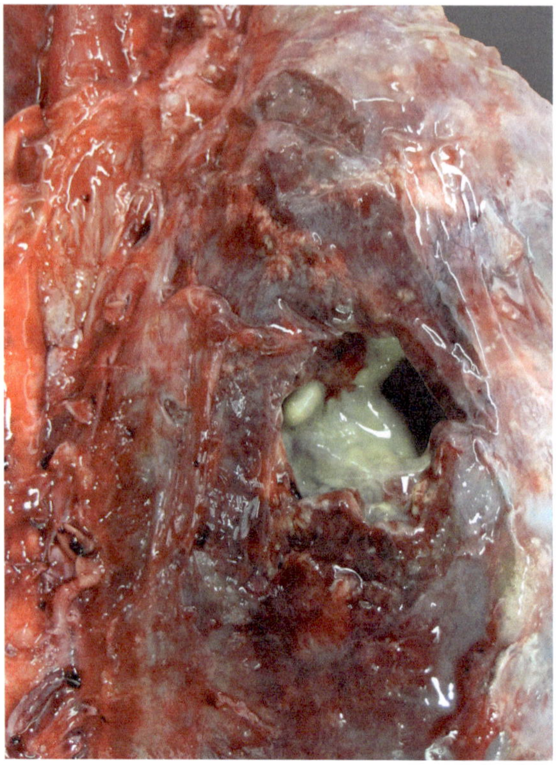

Fig. 4.62 Further dissection of this case has revealed a cavitated area, which should be regarded as tuberculosis until proven otherwise. Standard cultures as well as specialist culture for mycobacteria and fungi should follow

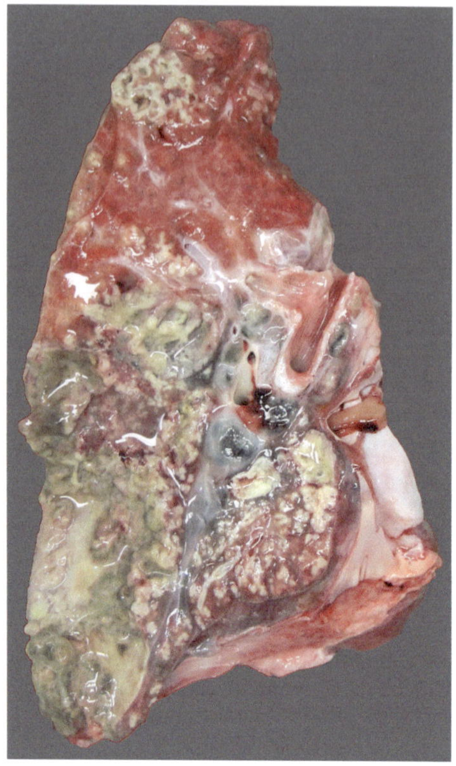

Fig. 4.63 This case of tuberculosis with overwhelming lung sepsis shows necrotising pneumonia, consolidation, and destruction of the pulmonary parenchyma

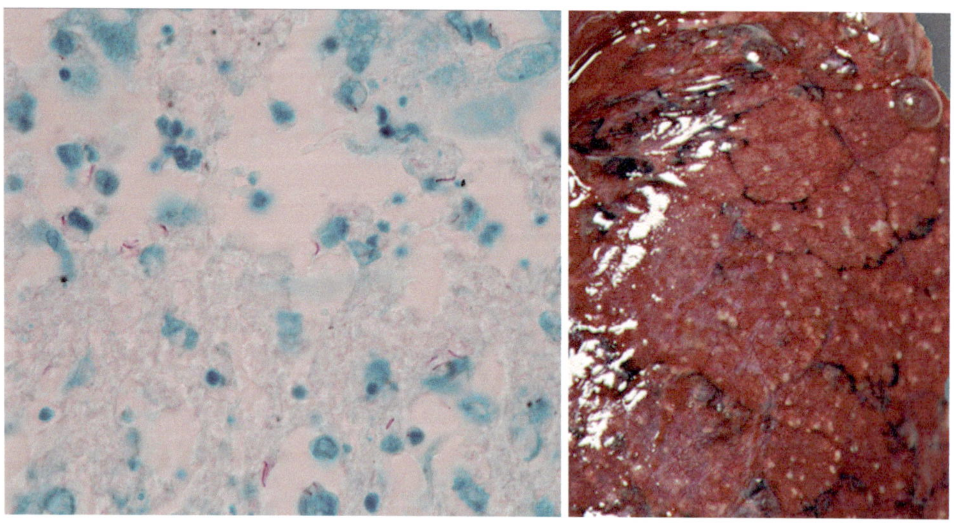

Fig. 4.64 Miliary (millet seed–like) tuberculosis is seen, with fine, small flecks of yellow discolouration diffusely distributed across the lung parenchyma. Acid-fast bacilli are seen with characteristic elongated, red-stained forms in a Ziehl-Neelsen stain

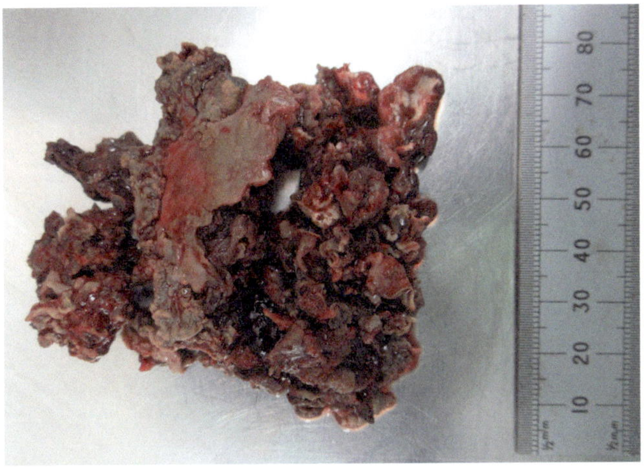

Fig. 4.65 Granular grey/brown contents are seen from this cystic lesion in the lung, subsequently confirmed to be aspergillus

Degenerative Lung Conditions

The chapter gives examples of degenerative lung conditions (Figs. 4.66, 4.67, 4.68, 4.69, 4.70, 4.71, 4.72, 4.73, 4.74, 4.75, and 4.76). It deals first with obstructive pulmonary disease, a group that includes asthma, bronchiectasis, chronic bronchitis, and emphysema in variable format. Both macroscopic and histological assessment may be pertinent in fully appreciating the relevance to the cause of death.

The lung can be also involved by diffuse fibrosing processes of primary or secondary type (Figs. 4.77, 4.78, 4.79, 4.80, 4.81, 4.82, 4.83, 4.84, and 4.85). Many of these conditions have an autoimmune background, although dust-related diseases (pneumoconiosis) also are important, particularly with exposure to coal dust, silica, or asbestos (Figs. 4.86, 4.87, 4.88, 4.89, 4.90, 4.91, 4.92, 4.93, 4.94, 4.95, 4.96, 4.97, 4.98, 4.99, 4.100, 4.101, 4.102, 4.103, 4.104, 4.105, 4.106, 4.107, and 4.108).

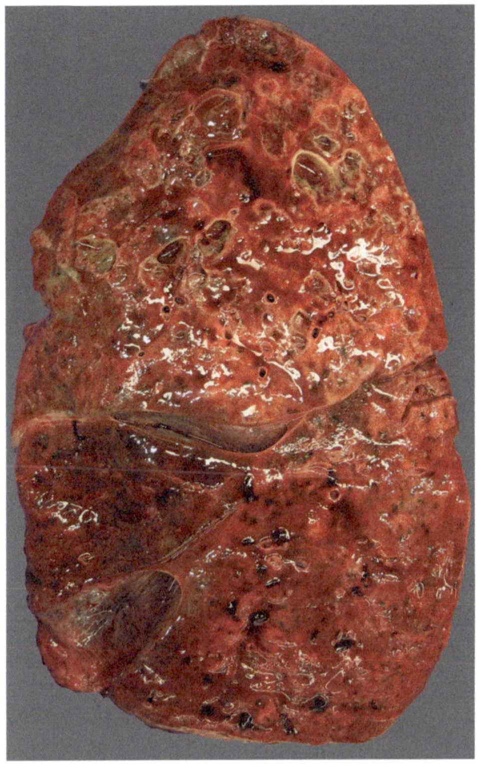

Fig. 4.66 Bronchiectasis can be lobe-limited or diffuse. Dilatation of many of the airways is seen, often with some collapse of the parenchymal tissues and persistent sepsis. In this case, the lung is markedly infected, and swabs or lung tissue should be taken to assess microbiological content

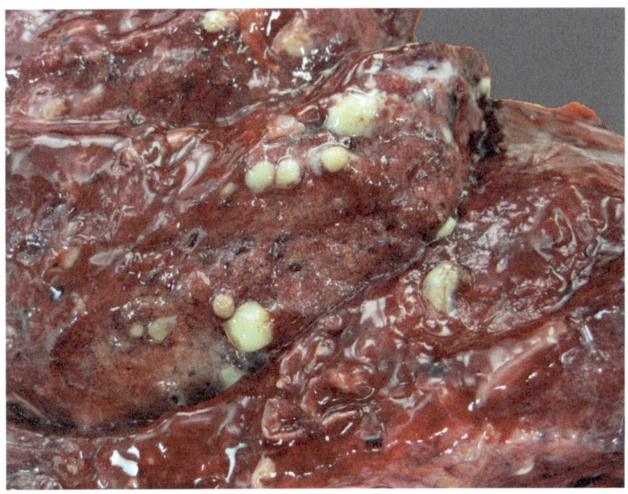

Fig. 4.67 Bronchiectasis is often complicated by persistent sepsis with significantly pathogenic bacteria. The lung tissue in this young individual, suffering with cystic fibrosis, shows marked bronchopneumonia associated with bronchiectasis. The degree of bronchiectasis is masked by the pronounced infected secretions

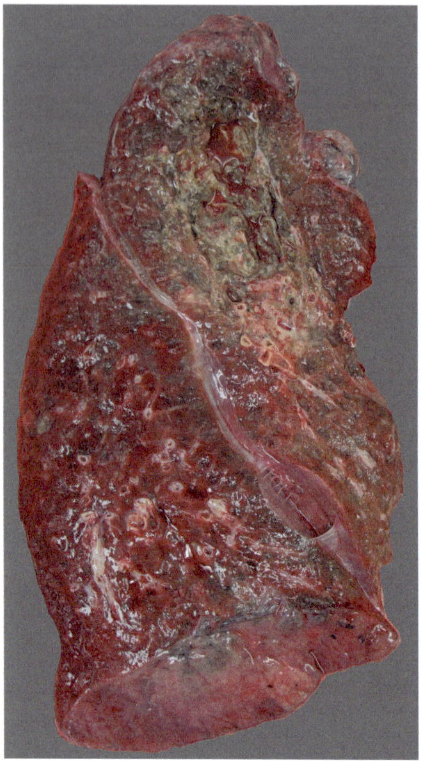

Fig. 4.68 This lobe-limited zone of bronchiectasis had developed into a persistent zone of sepsis with necrotizing pneumonia and finally abscess formation

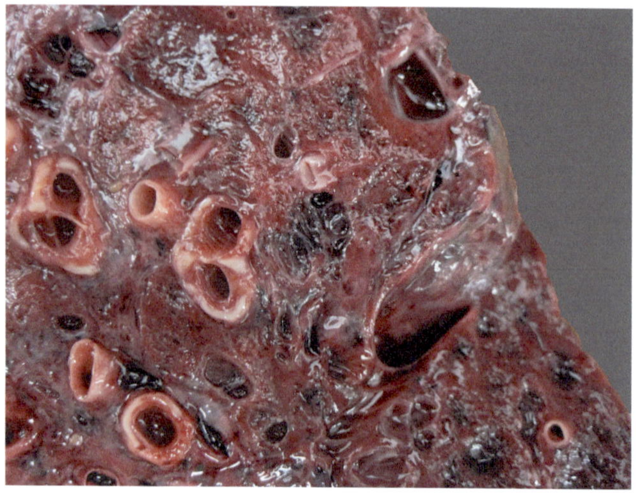

Fig. 4.69 Close inspection of the cut surface of this lung in a case of mild bronchiectasis shows somewhat fibrotic-walled airways, which are dilated and congested. In addition, there is local, patchy emphysema with some cystic change and interstitial scarring. Many cases of lung disease do not show a single, pure format

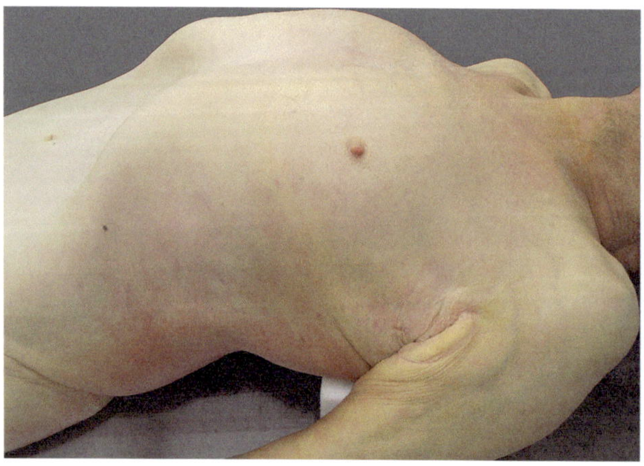

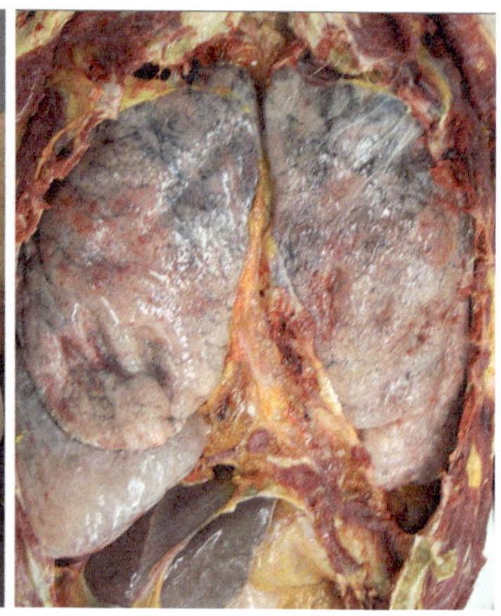

Fig. 4.70 The external examination of the chest of a patient with emphysema (*left image*) often starts with the appreciation of a 'barrel chest' reflecting pulmonary hyperinflation. The *right image* shows a case of emphysema with lung hyperinflation filling the chest cavities and extending across the anterior mediastinal soft tissues. Bullous change is noted peripherally at the base of the right lung

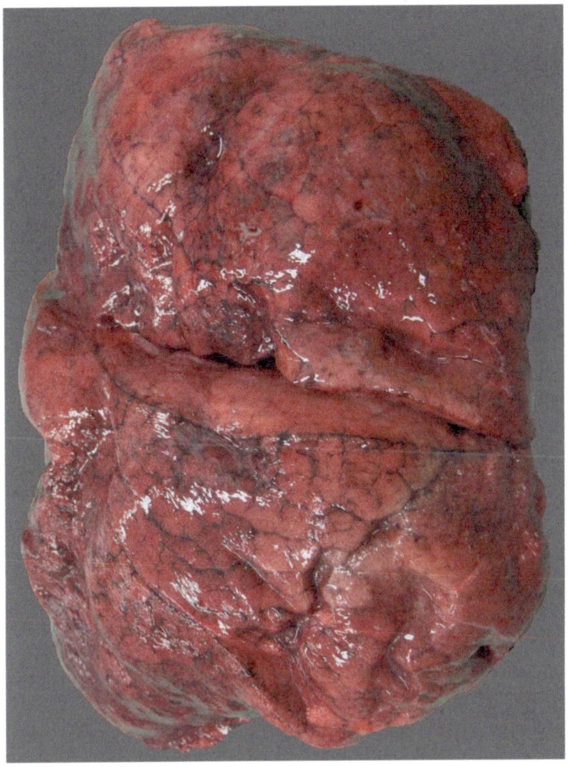

Fig. 4.71 Emphysematous lungs often remain inflated despite dissection from the mediastinal content

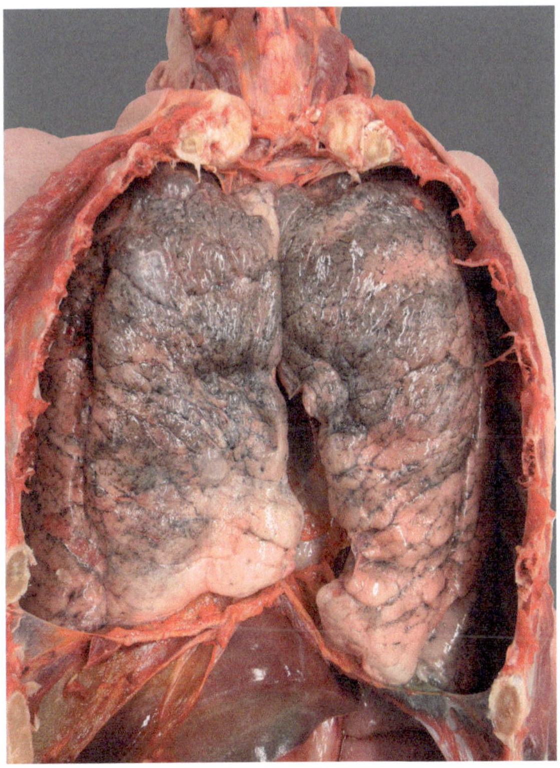

Fig. 4.72 Marked emphysema is seen in these lung tissues. The presence of moderate brown/black soot staining raises the possibility of industrial exposure, although some degree of anthracosis is not uncommon in those living in an urban environment

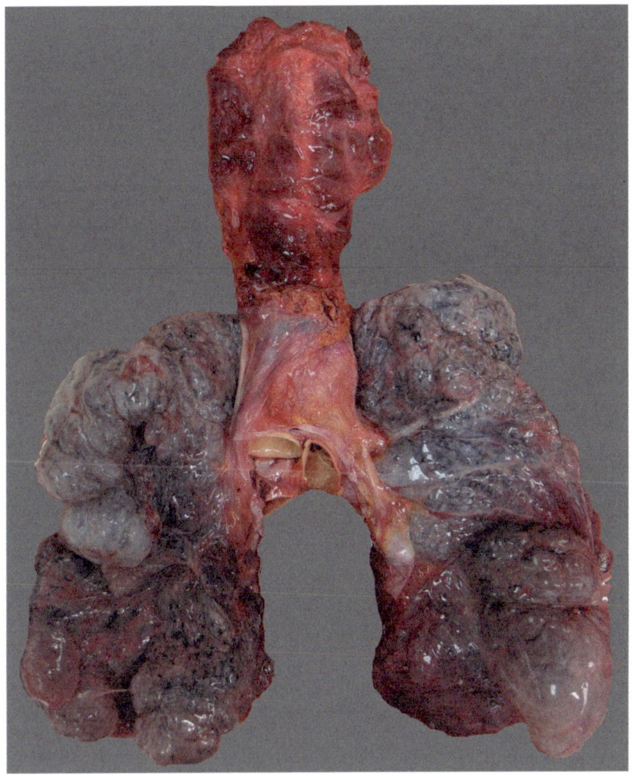

Fig. 4.73 End-stage pulmonary emphysema is seen with widespread bullous change affecting the tissues of both the upper and lower lobes

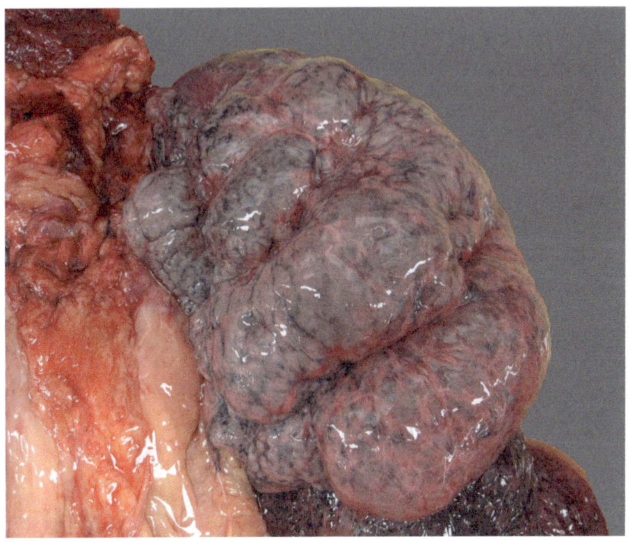

Fig. 4.74 Large bullae are often evident when lungs are examined; an assessment of the overall size is useful in the report

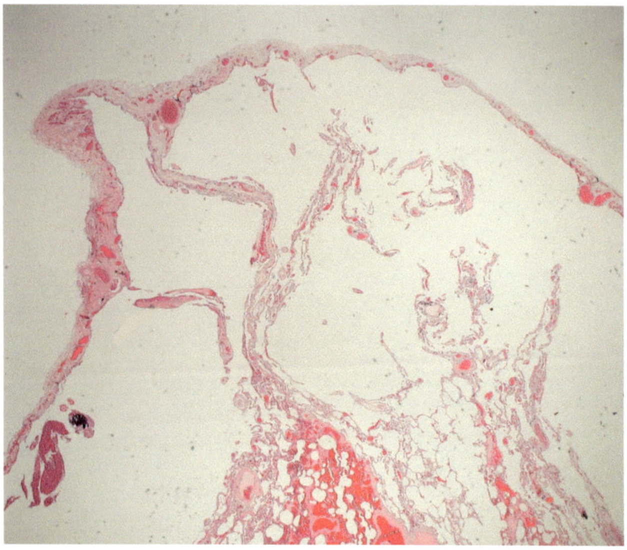

Fig. 4.75 Histological examination of emphysematous tissue reveals the characteristic alveolar wall loss and airspace dilatation

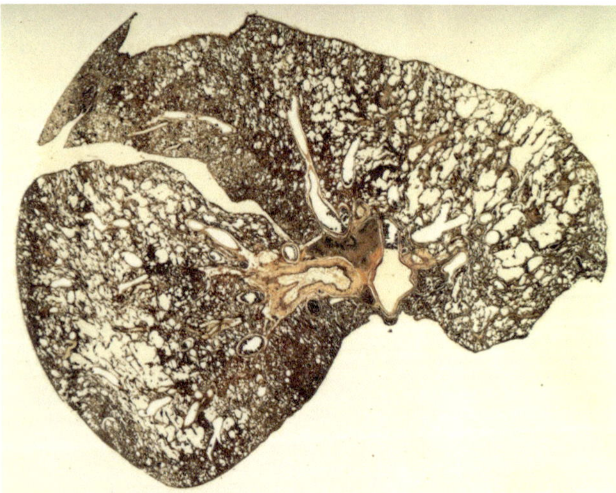

Fig. 4.76 This Gough and Wentworth section shows evidence of widespread emphysematous change. This historical technique is rarely used now, given the significant advances of radiology, including high-resolution CT scanning (HRCT)

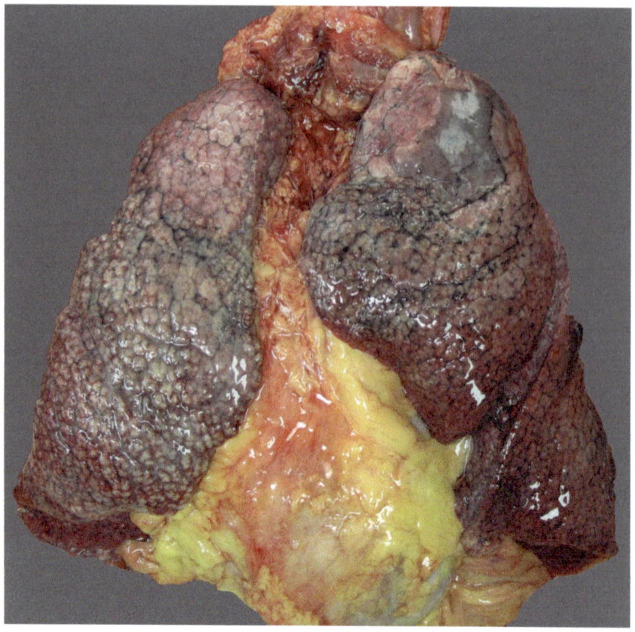

Fig. 4.77 The lung parenchyma shows firm lungs with a somewhat bosselated pleural surface quality, akin to morocco leather (or cobble-stoning). The tissues are palpably firm and will stand without support on the bench. This is typical for diffuse pulmonary fibrosis

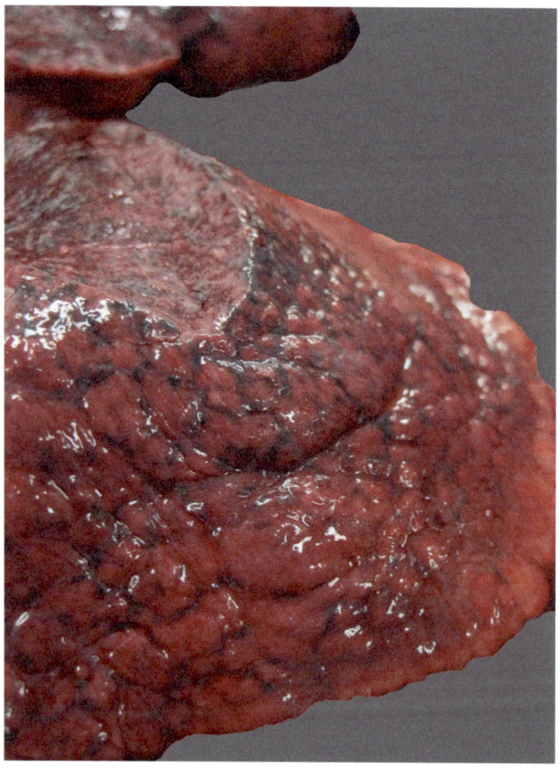

Fig. 4.78 Lung tissues with interstitial fibrosis often maintain their architecture even after slicing into the lung tissue at the periphery

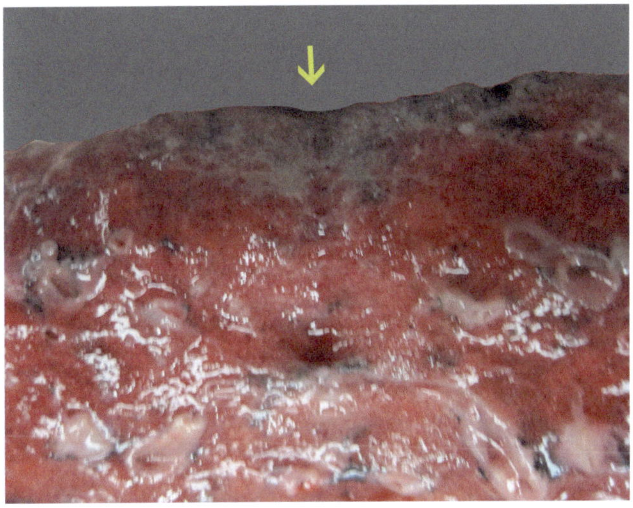

Fig. 4.79 Usual interstitial pneumonia (UIP) is a term used to describe histological and radiological patterns in the assessment of interstitial lung diseases (as opposed to being a clinical diagnosis). Idiopathic pulmonary fibrosis is a clinical diagnosis with a UIP pattern. Interstitial lung disease MDT meetings bring together all the data for a diagnosis. The post mortem may be the first opportunity to examine the lung parenchyma, as in day to day practice these fibrosing diseases are not often biopsied. The peripheral fibrosis is markedly grey (*arrow*). This area has been highlighted by washing the lung tissue under running water

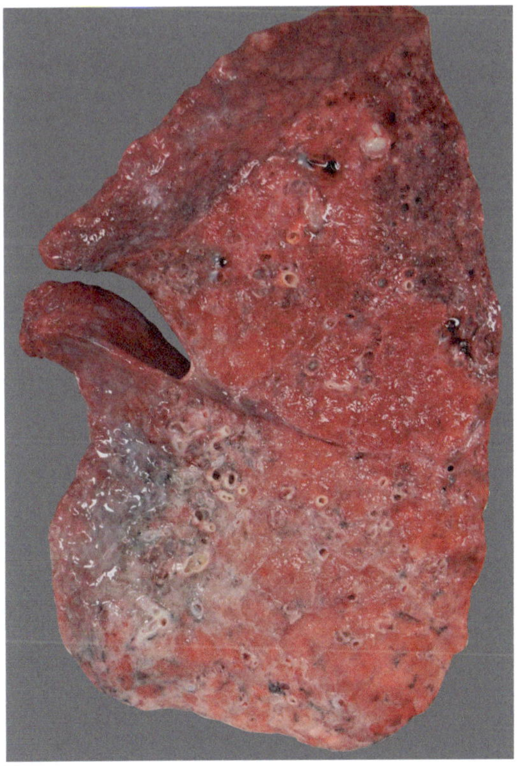

Fig. 4.80 The lung shows peripheral fibrosis, some cystic change and a somewhat grey discolouration, in keeping with idiopathic pulmonary fibrosis. There also appears to be some chest infection changes in the upper lobe anterior aspect

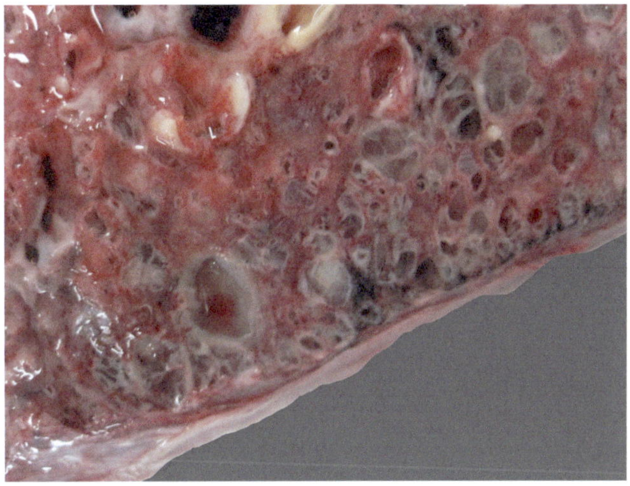

Fig. 4.81 This lung tissue has been washed carefully. It shows pronounced loss of the normal tissues, fibrosis, and airspace dilatation/retraction artefact, manifest as peripheral cystic changes. This appearance is seen in end stage fibrosing lung diseases. Note that the consistency of the lung parenchyma is stiff

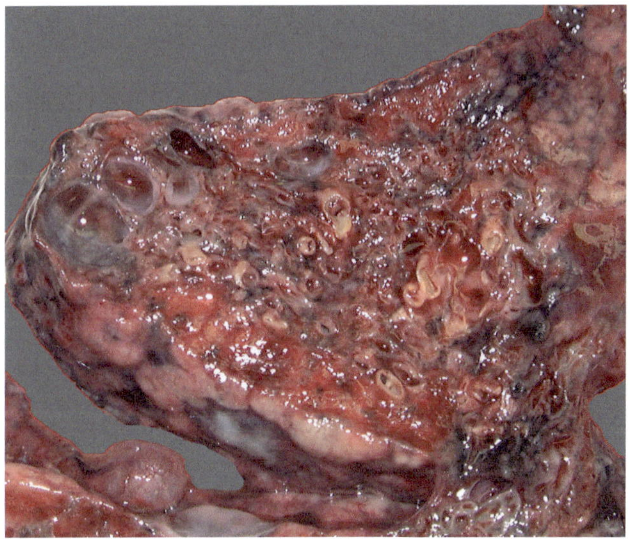

Fig. 4.82 Lung tissues with extensive or end-stage fibrosis generally all look similar, with honeycomb change, fluid collections in cystic spaces, and some sepsis. This case of lung disease had a background of exposure to metal dust and fumes. From the macroscopic perspective, it looks no different from naturally occurring lung fibrosis

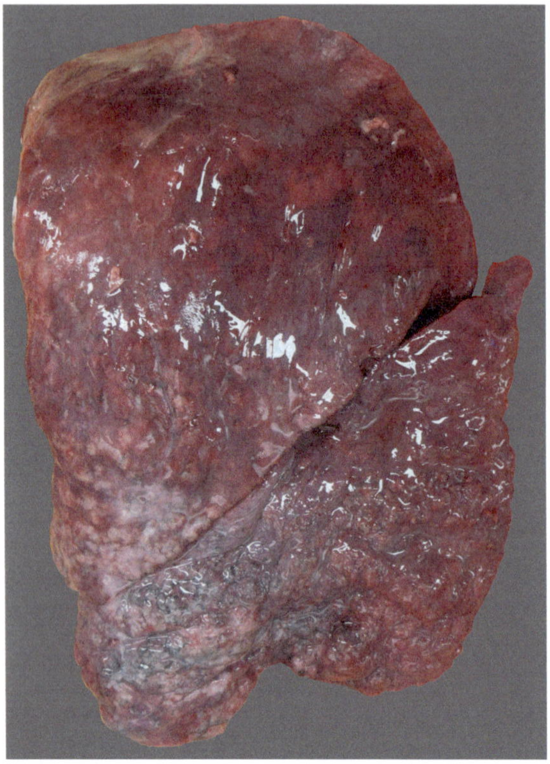

Fig. 4.83 This is a case of lung fibrosis and some cystic change, complicated by a lower lobe pneumonia. External examination of this lung gives the impression of a solid texture with nodularity below the pleural surface, giving an appearance of cobblestoning (due to underlying fibrosis). Pale discoloration in the lower lobe corresponded to a focus of pneumonia. The case was subsequently confirmed as that of Langerhans' cell histiocytosis which had progressed to pulmonary fibrosis

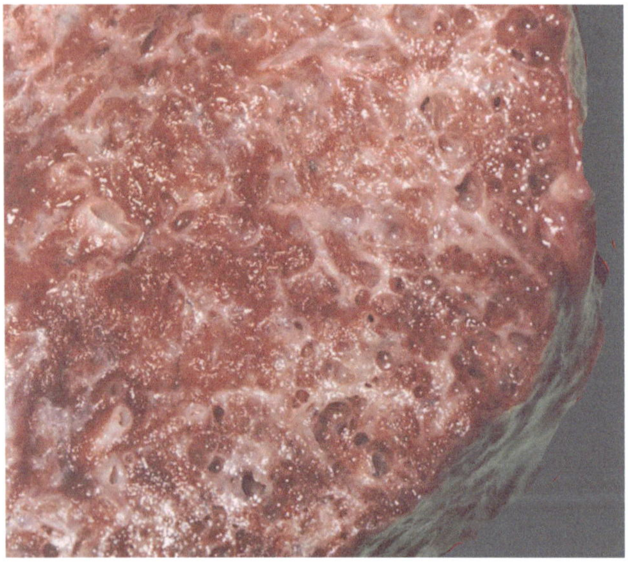

Fig. 4.84 A surgical sample is seen in a case of Langerhans cell histiocytosis (LCH). The cut surface of the lung has widespread cystic and fibrotic change characteristic of this condition. LCH is often similar morphologically to lymphangioleiomyomatosis (LAM)

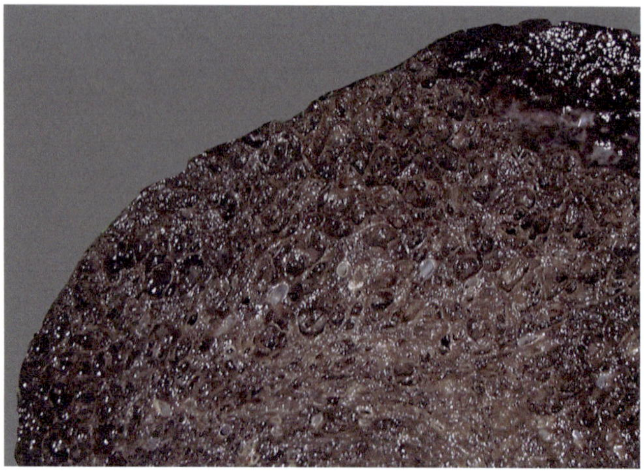

Fig. 4.85 The fibrotic and cystic disease features of lymphangioleiomyomatosis (LAM) are seen in this lung tissue, which has been fixed and then sectioned. In some ways, the appearance is akin to Langerhans cell histiocytosis (LCH). LAM is rarely seen in men

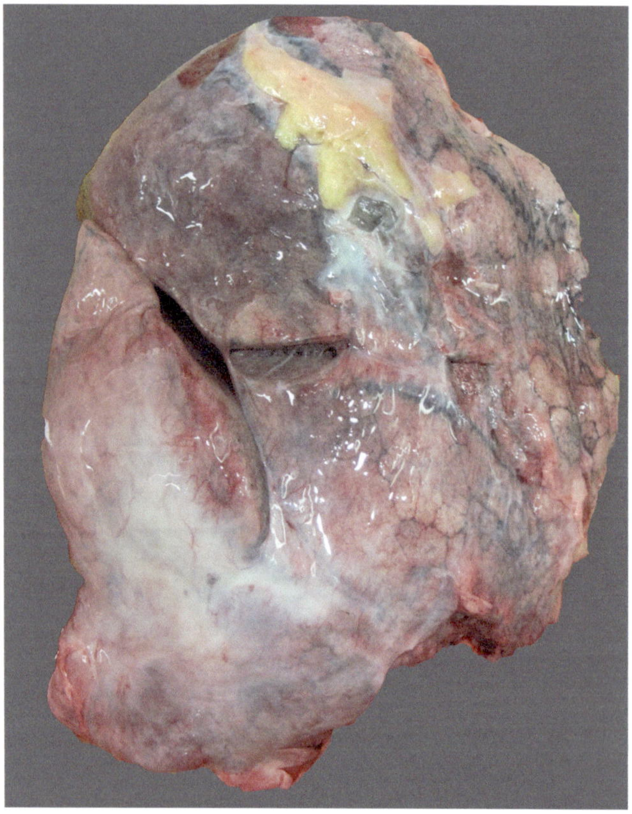

Fig. 4.86 In some cases of asbestos exposure, persistent pleural effusions can cause protein deposition, which produces a slow accumulation of fibrous matrix around the dependent parts of the visceral pleural surface. This sometimes manifests as diffuse pleural fibrosis, one of the components of asbestos-related disease

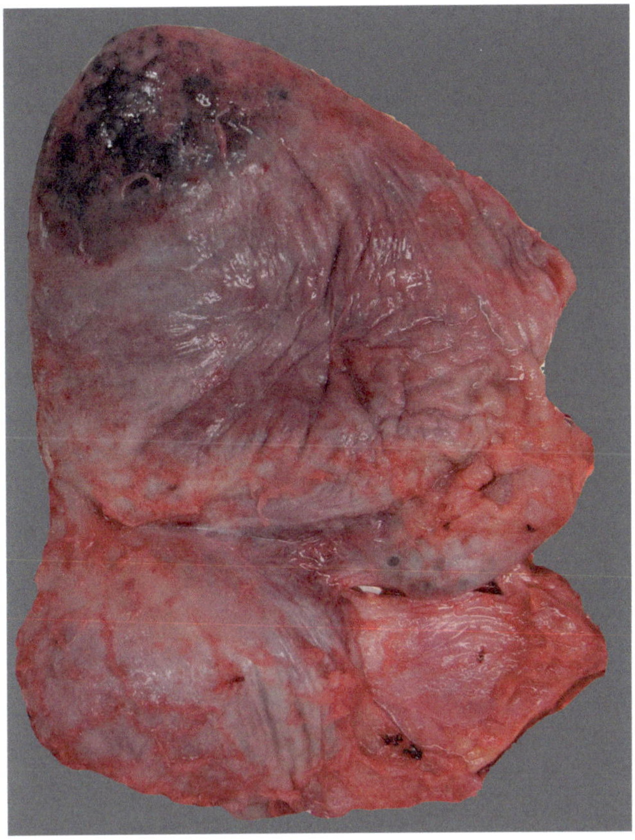

Fig. 4.87 Diffuse pleural fibrosis in a case of asbestos disease. This should not be confused with mesothelioma or other pleural neoplasia

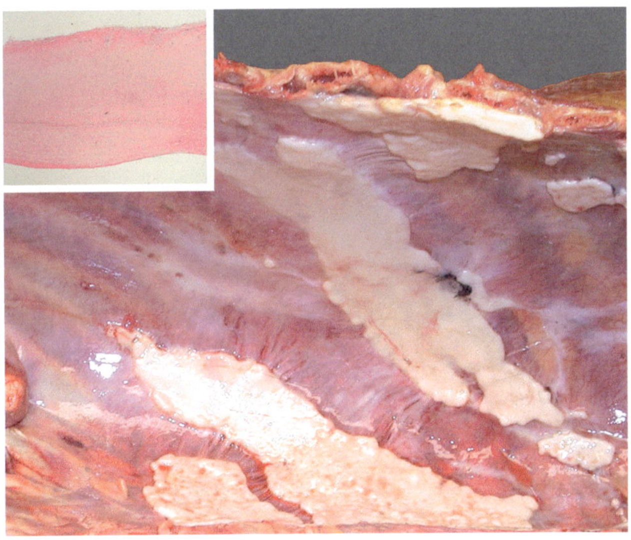

Fig. 4.88 Benign pleural plaques are dense zones of fibrous tissue fixed onto the pleural surface. They are often parietal tissue biased but may be widespread on the visceral pleural surfaces. The plaques may be calcified. The *inset* shows the histological appearance of dense hyaline collagen, with a somewhat 'basketweave' quality. Asbestos is linked with formation of pleural plaques, but they can occur with mild or trivial exposures. The presence of plaques does not automatically imply significant exposure to asbestos fibres

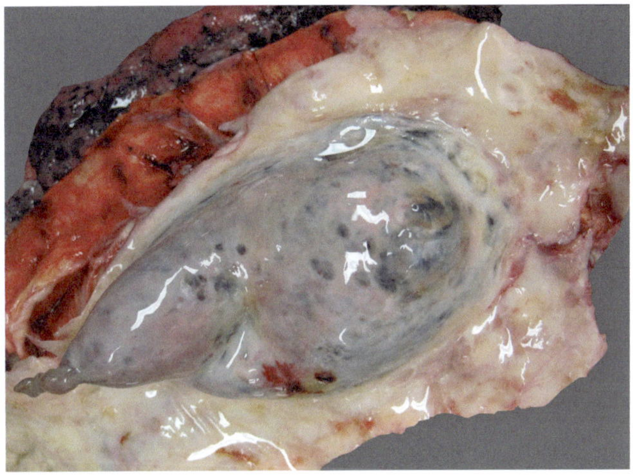

Fig. 4.89 Pleural mesothelioma commonly surrounds and compresses lung tissue. This case had a persistent effusion, with tumour widely infiltrating the chest wall. This lung was firmly encased within a dense, fibrous tumour capsule. The tumour has compressed the lung to roughly one third of its original volume

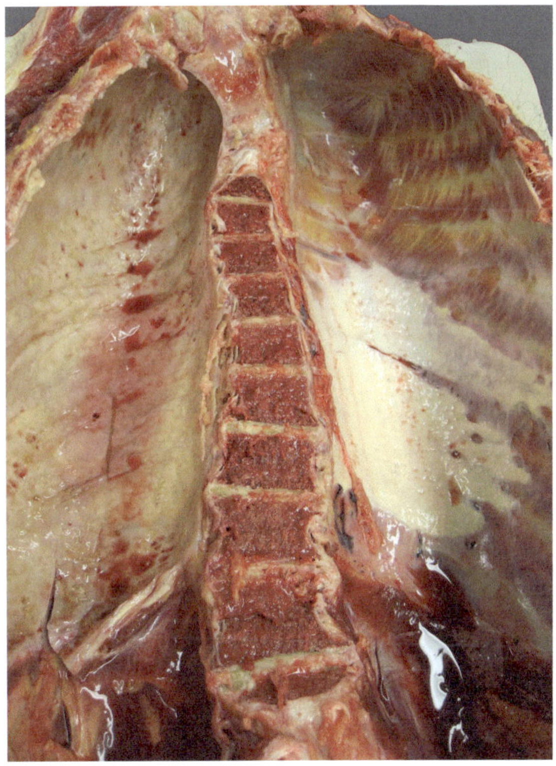

Fig. 4.90 The opened chest in a case of mesothelioma (right hemithorax) is seen with the left hemithorax containing pleural plaques. Confirmation of plaques is important in cases of asbestos disease, and can be usefully described as a percentage (%) of pleural involvement, as opposed to measuring each plaque. In this image a strip of vertebral tissue has been removed to assess for vertebral metastasis

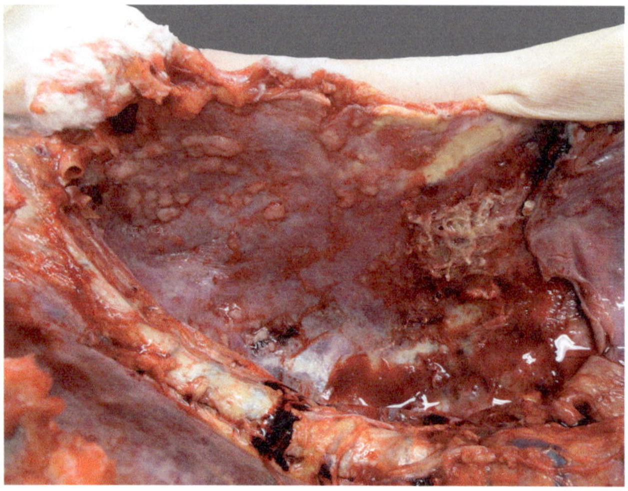

Fig. 4.91 Mesotheliomatous infiltration of the pleural tissues is seen in this view

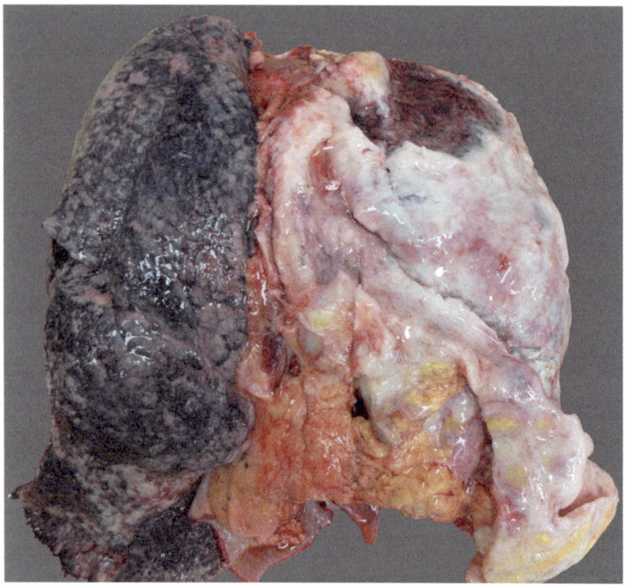

Fig. 4.92 Extensive pleural mesothelioma is seen involving the posterior right chest tissues

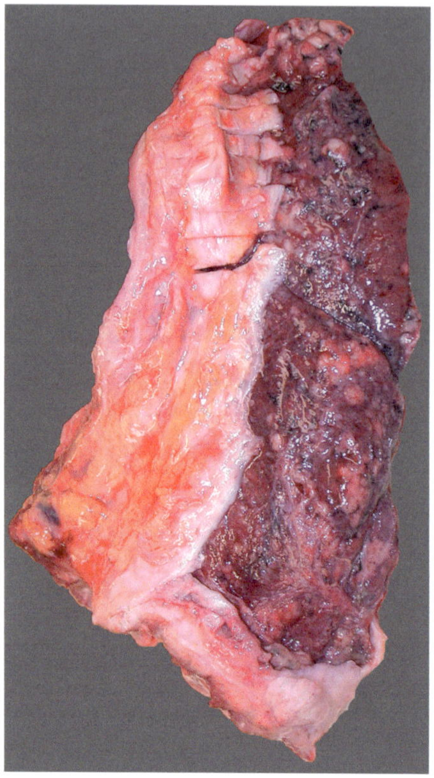

Fig. 4.93 Mesothelioma tissue is seen running around the lung parenchyma, tightly binding together the tumour, chest wall, and lung tissue. The lung itself is compressed and atelectatic, with nodularity representing tumour infiltrating in a lymphangitis-like fashion throughout the tissues

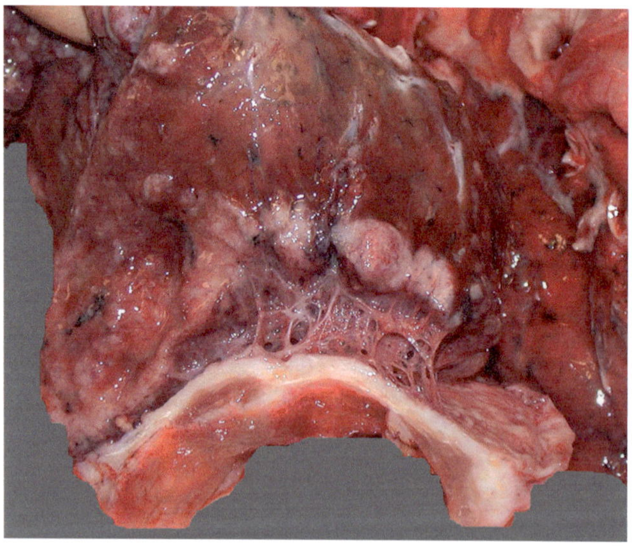

Fig. 4.94 Mesothelioma characteristically produces a rind of tumour on the outer aspect of the lung, involving the visceral pleura. Tumour foci are also seen here eroding into the lung tissue, with bands of tumour linking the visceral and parietal pleural tissue

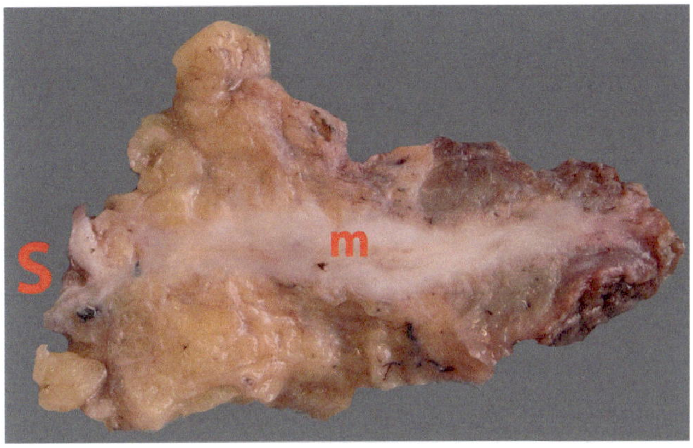

Fig. 4.95 Mesothelioma (grey tissue, *m*) may often extend out along thoracotomy tracts to involve chest wall tissues and skin surface. This is a perpendicular section of chest wall tissues highlighting the path of the mesothelioma towards the skin surface (*S*). For this reason, radiotherapy is often given to the port site of thoracoscopic intervention

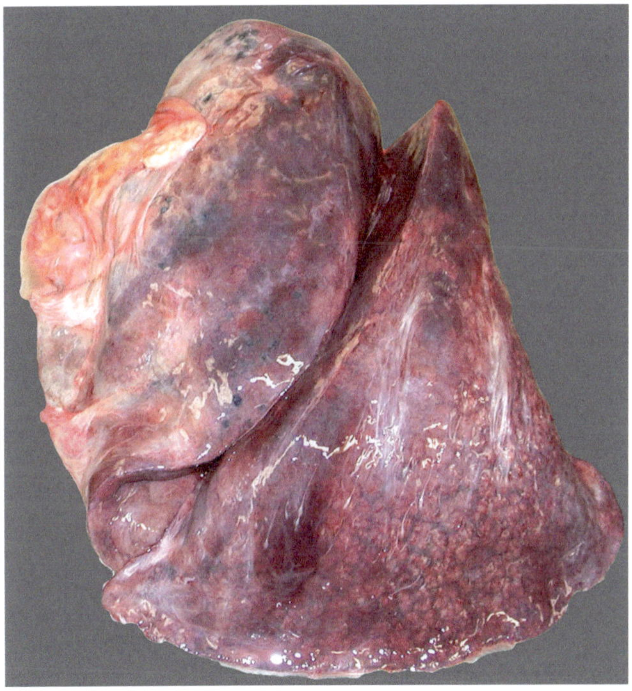

Fig. 4.96 Pulmonary fibrosis due to asbestos appears morphologically similar to pulmonary fibrosis or interstitial lung disease from other causes. The occupational history, clinical history of the disease, histology and special tests such as lung fibre analysis may be required to evaluate asbestos related diseases further

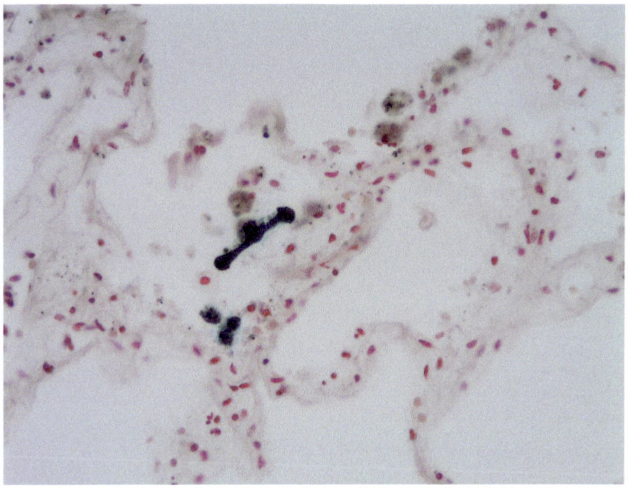

Fig. 4.97 A coated fibre is seen in a case of asbestosis. There are published and designated levels of fibre that are required to be seen in the plane of section or within lung digests/analyses in order to determine whether the case merits consideration as industrial lung disease

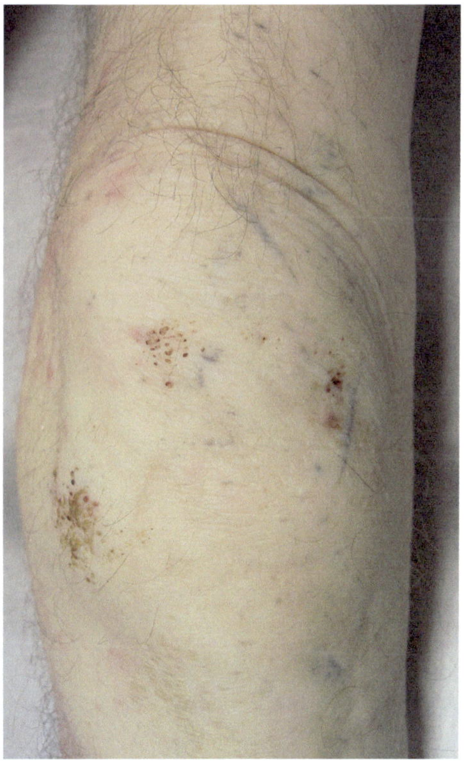

Fig. 4.98 Aside from considering the lung tissue in cases of coal workers' disease, it is important to look for coal-dust tattoos, which are usually present on the shoulders, elbows, hands, and knees. This view of the knee shows irregular, black discolouration of the dermal tissues in keeping with coal dust 'inoculation' into the dermal tissues during underground coal mining

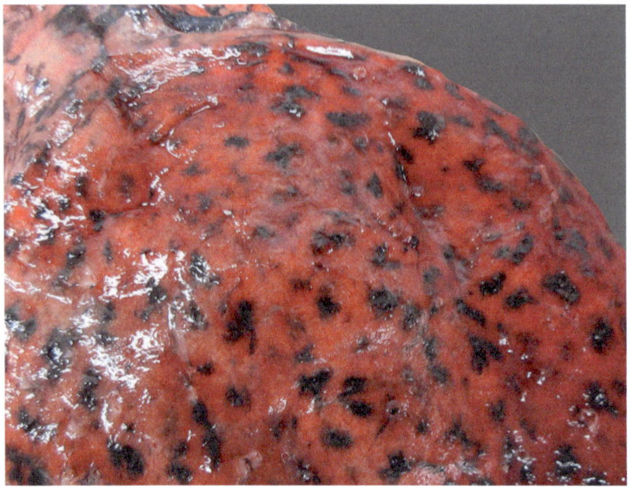

Fig. 4.99 The cut surface of this lung shows patchy macular anthracosis. This man had a brief history of underground coal working with some soot deposition but not to the level as to cause functional deficit within his lung parenchyma or indeed alteration to his lung function tests

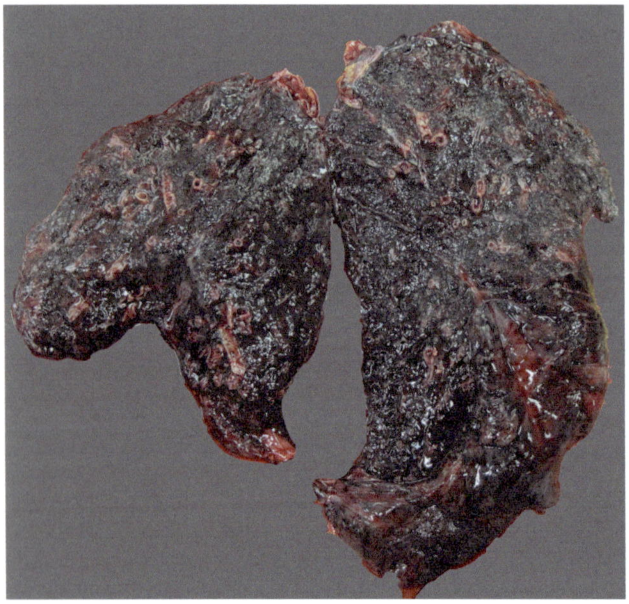

Fig. 4.100 Coal workers' lungs can be variably affected by the dust (coal workers' pneumoconiosis). Extreme forms have heavy anthracosis and distortion of the lung tissue and formation of conglomerate masses (progressive massive fibrosis)

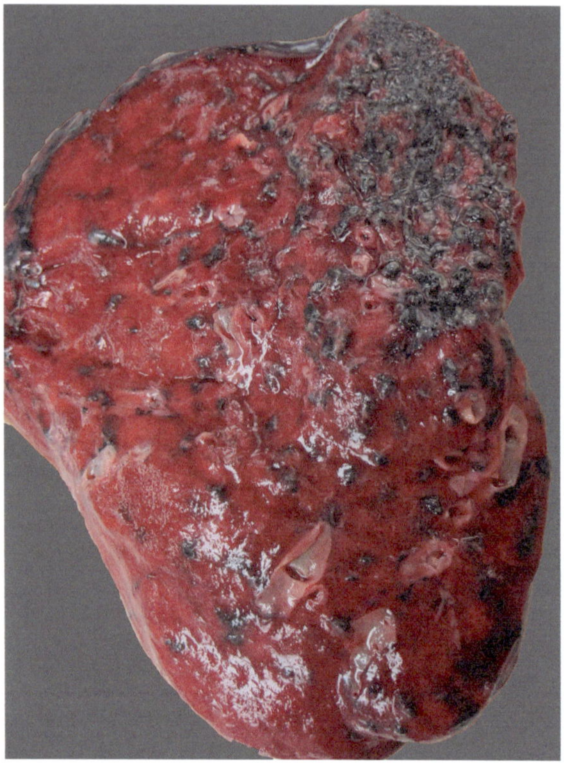

Fig. 4.101 The lung parenchyma in a coal worker shows gradation of nodularity, with a zone of complex nodularity bordering on progressive massive fibrosis in the upper part of the lung. Small nodularity with anthracosis is present in the lower part of the lung tissues

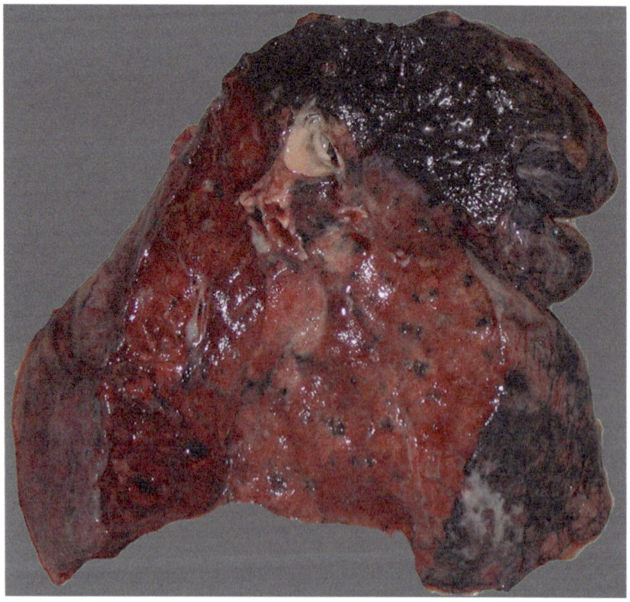

Fig. 4.102 This is a case of progressive massive fibrosis within the upper lobe tissues

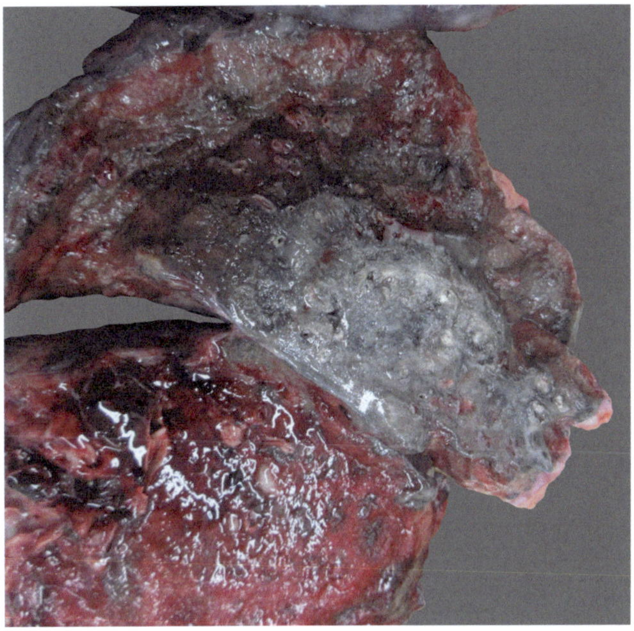

Fig. 4.103 Progressive massive fibrosis is seen in this lung upper lobe with collapse and fibrosis of the parenchyma. There is no overt sepsis or neoplasia

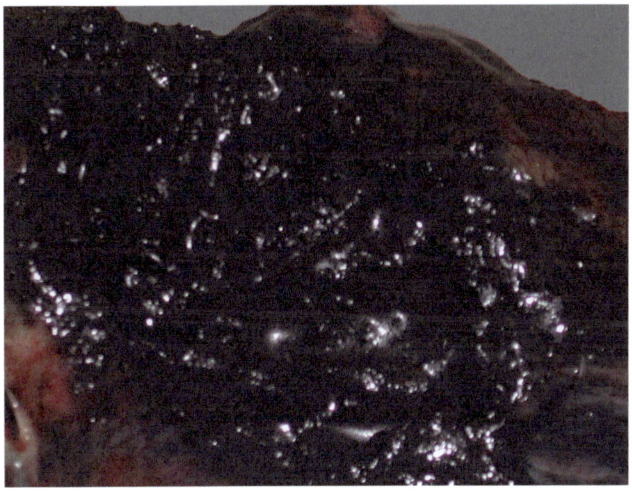

Fig. 4.104 Progressive massive fibrosis, seen close up, reveals the solid and rather gritty mass replacing lung parenchyma. The cut surface often has no substructure; after being sectioned, it may ooze black fluid

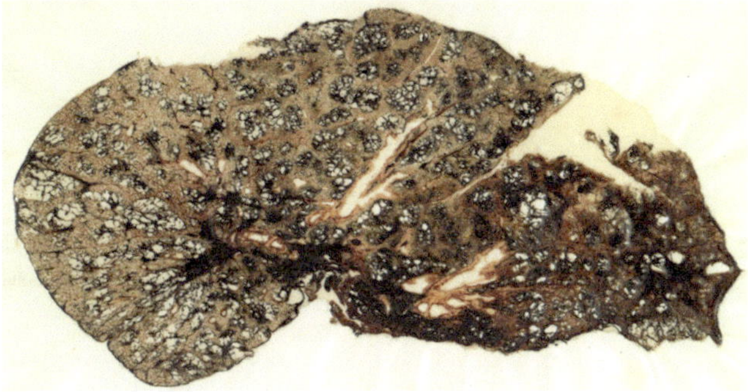

Fig. 4.105 Classically, Gough-Wentworth lung slides were used to assess the broad detail of lung parenchyma, but this technique is no longer commonly used. The heavy dust accumulation in this case is mainly associated with emphysema

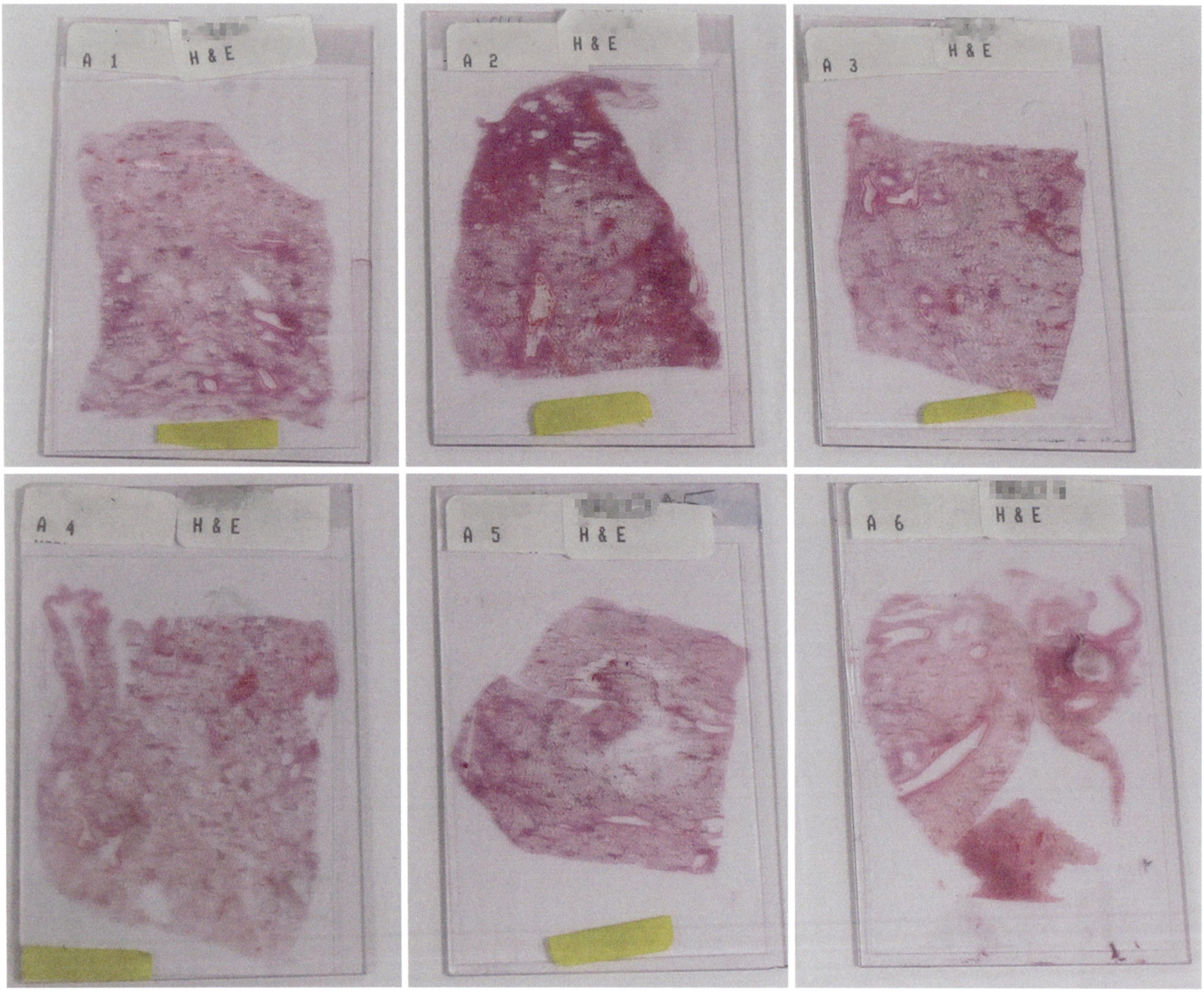

Fig. 4.106 The modern technique to assess lungs in a manner comparable to Gough-Wentworth slides uses large blocks of paraffin-embedded tissues

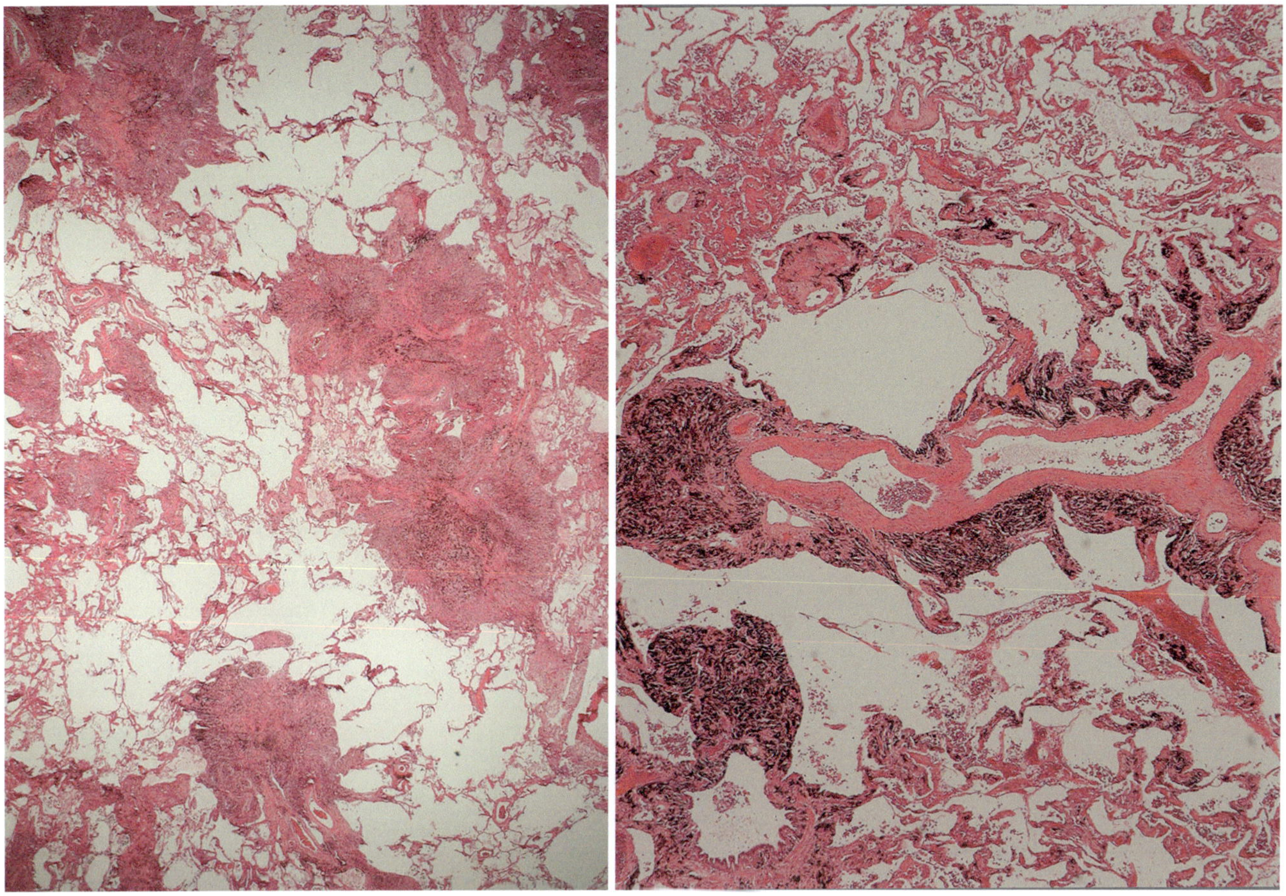

Fig. 4.107 Histological review of lung parenchyma allows assessment of the degree of dust deposition and any nodularity. *Left*. The size of any nodules should be assessed; those more than 10 mm in diameter are often functionally more important and are judged to represent complicated coal workers' pneumoconiosis. *Right*. Review of this lung shows emphysematous phenomena with dust accumulation in a centriacinar quality (dust-associated emphysema)

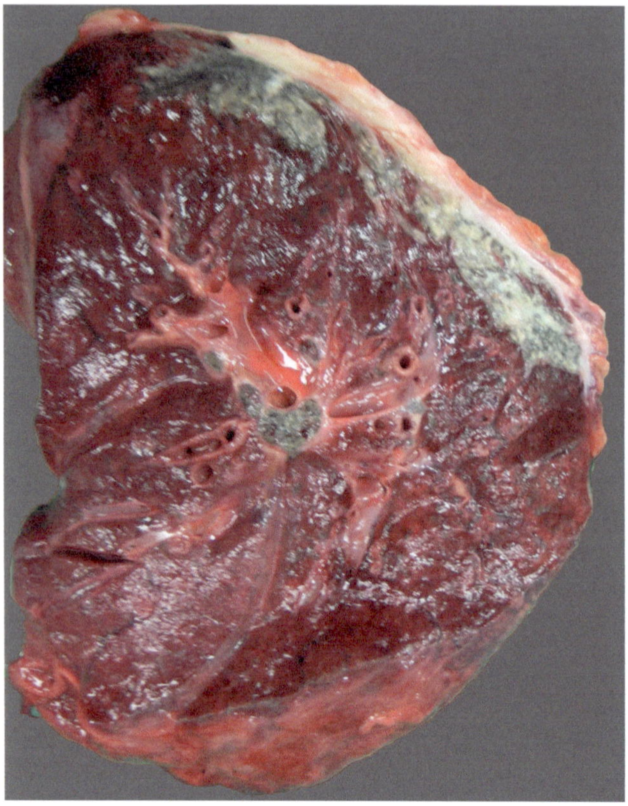

Fig. 4.108 The periphery of the lung tissues and some nodes centrally show an irregular grey/cream discolouration with nodularity. This is a case of silicotic change in the lung tissues, with the zones affected showing dense fibrosis and the characteristic stellate, irregular scars of this mineral dust accumulation

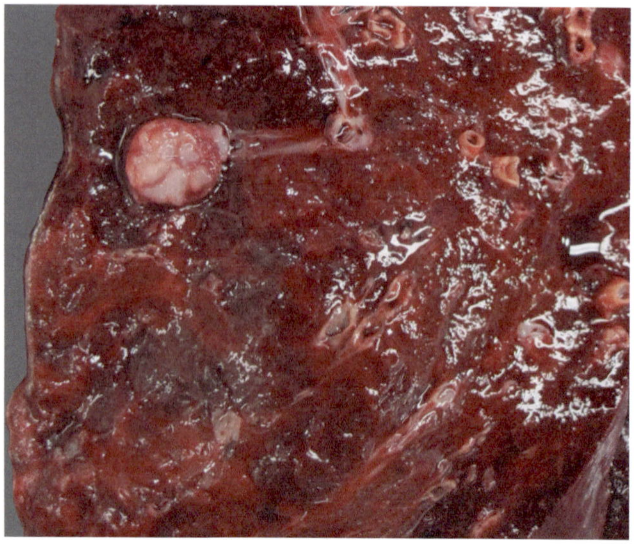

Fig. 4.109 Benign tumours occasionally can be found in lung tissues. This slice of lung shows a rounded hamartoma with unremarkable lung tissues adjacent

Thoracic Neoplasia

Lung cancer (Figs. 4.109, 4.110, 4.111, 4.112, 4.113, 4.114, 4.115, 4.116, 4.117, 4.118, 4.119, 4.120, 4.121, 4.122, 4.123, 4.124, 4.125, 4.126, 4.127, 4.128, and 4.129) is a major cause of morbidity and mortality, with these tumours being directly involved in the cause of death in many individuals. Secondary effects from chronic sepsis in the lungs are also well recognized, with disseminated disease being particularly important.

Lastly, issues with regard to the large airways and chest wall (Figs. 4.130, 4.131, 4.132, 4.133, 4.134, 4.135, 4.136, 4.137, 4.138, 4.139, 4.140, 4.141, 4.142, 4.143, 4.144, 4.145, 4.146, 4.147, 4.148, 4.149, 4.150, 4.151, 4.152, 4.153, 4.154, 4.155, 4.156, 4.157, 4.158, 4.159, 4.160, 4.161, 4.162, 4.163, 4.164, and 4.165) are noted.

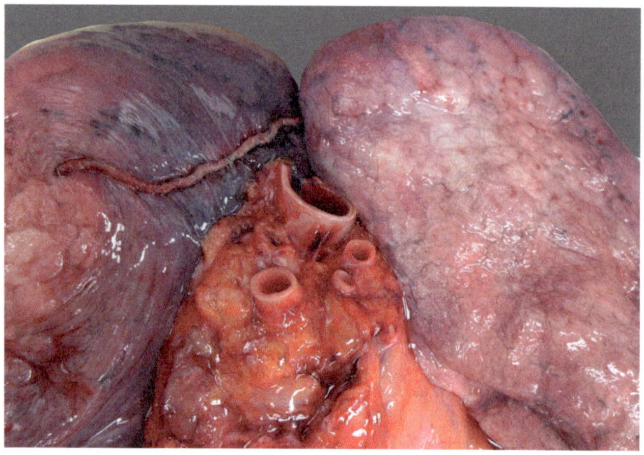

Fig. 4.110 Evidence of previous surgery to the lung tissues is seen in this case with a row of staples from a VATS segmentectomy. One notes the absence of tumour in the subsequent tissue review

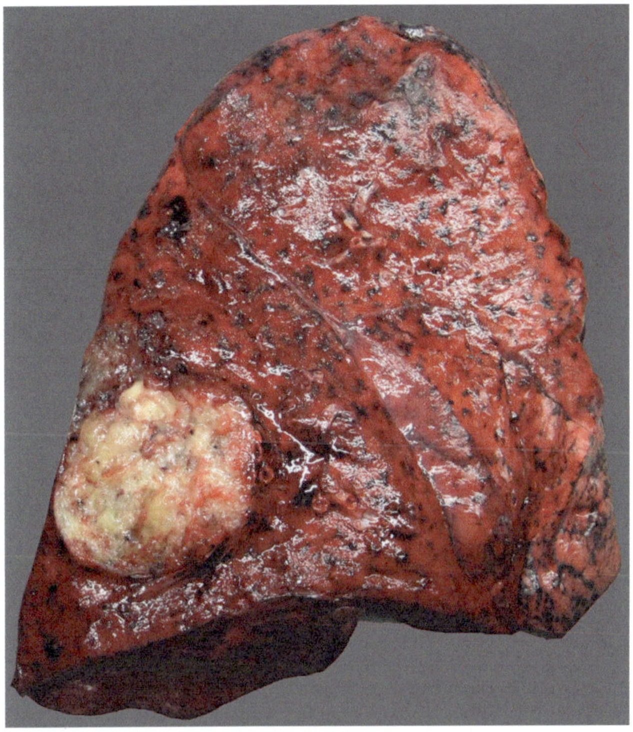

Fig. 4.111 Metastatic tumours are commonly found in the lung tissues. These tumour foci usually have a circumscribed, rounded profile with compression of the local tissues and little in the way of background lung alteration, unless there is airway obstruction. This was a case of disseminated colonic adenocarcinoma

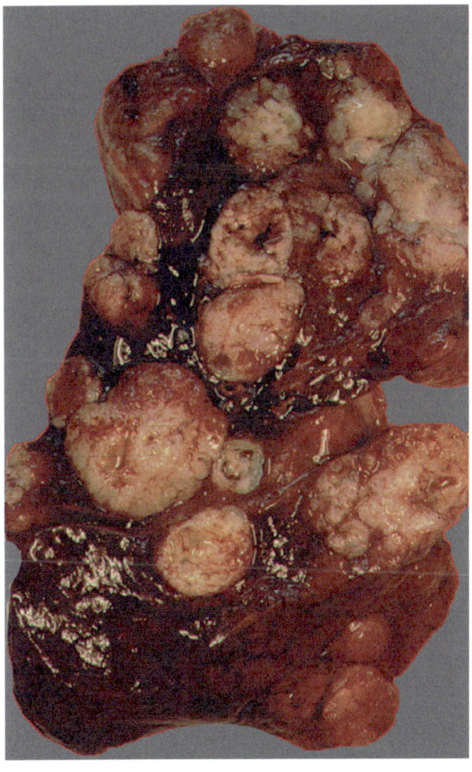

Fig. 4.112 Diffuse pulmonary metastases are often seen in sarcomatoid tumours. This is an example of metastatic chondrosarcoma

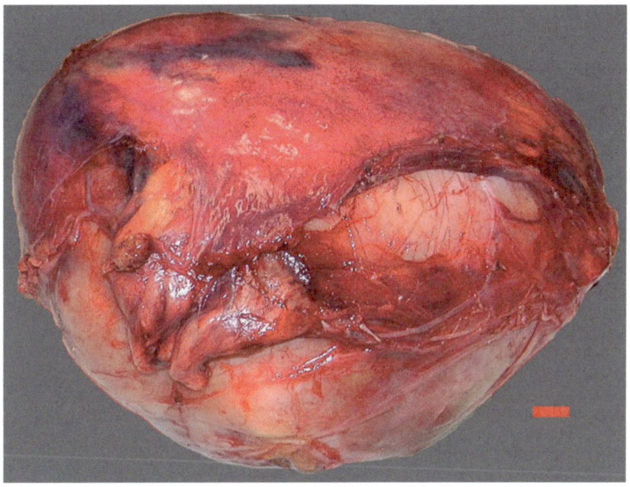

Fig. 4.113 Soft tissue tumours (occasionally of large size, as in this case of liposarcoma) can be found interacting with the lung within the thoracic cavity (*Bar marker* 10 mm)

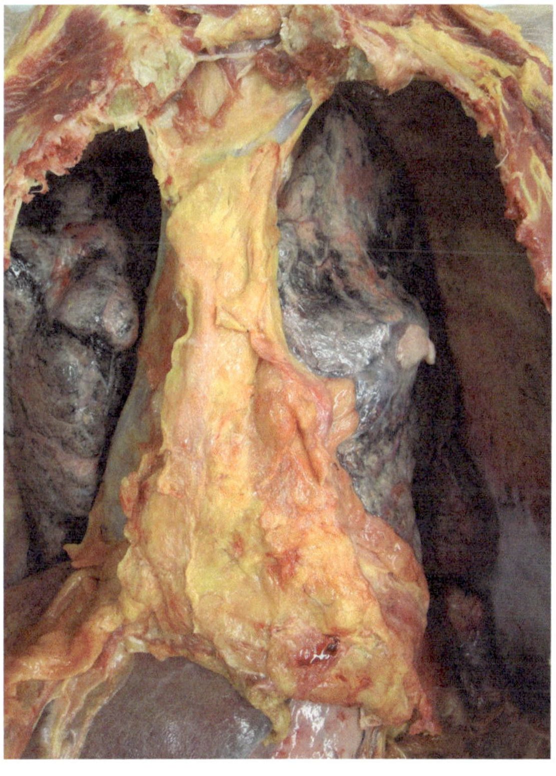

Fig. 4.114 Lung tumours are often primary carcinomas. This left upper lobe tumour clearly stands out from the adjacent lung tissues and is immediately apparent after opening the chest

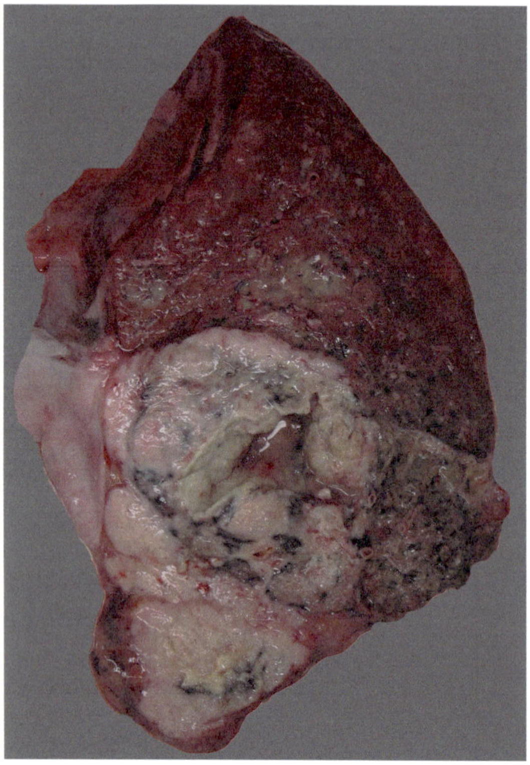

Fig. 4.115 Lung cancer is often associated with local or distal chest infection and collapse of the lung tissues, making precise assessment of the boundaries complex. This case shows a lower lobe tumour mass with central cavitation in this longitudinal section. This was a small-cell pulmonary carcinoma

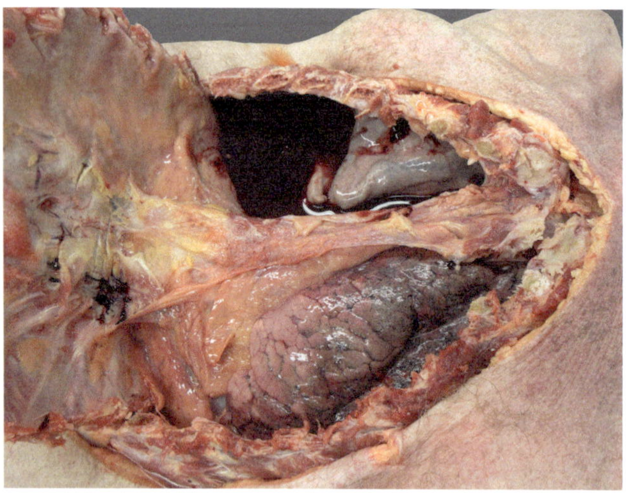

Fig. 4.116 This case of carcinoma of the lung is seen to have caused death with an acute on chronic pleural bleed. One notes the fibrosis and partial collapse of the right lung with subsequent massive haemorrhage as the final event into the right pleural cavity

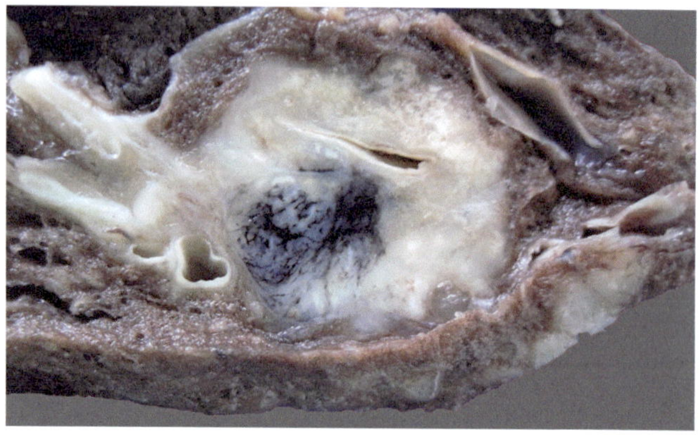

Fig. 4.117 Small-cell carcinoma rapidly disseminates to local nodes and the mediastinum, as seen in this view compressing the pulmonary vasculature. The tumour has surrounded and overrun a lymph node

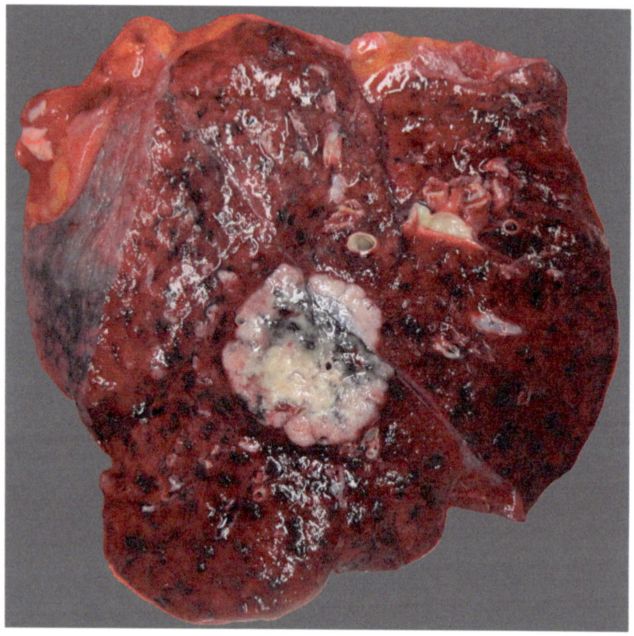

Fig. 4.118 A primary lung cancer is seen, with a relatively rounded periphery and a beige/black cut surface. The tumour crosses the interlobar fissure. It is often tempting to speculate as to the histological subtype (in this case, squamous carcinoma), but histology is required for confirmation

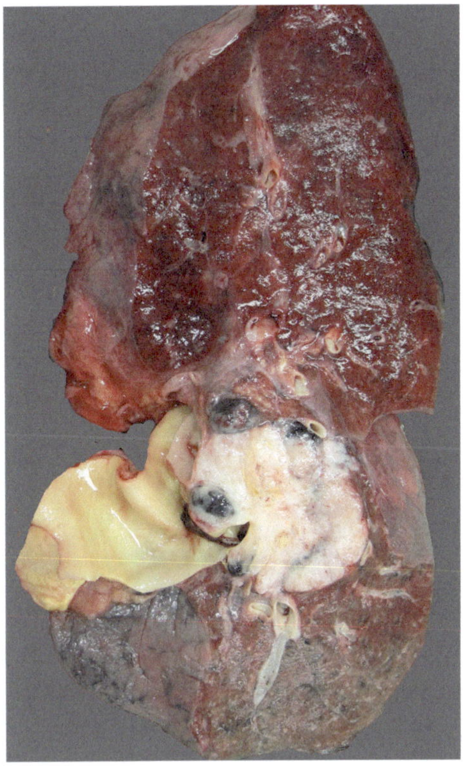

Fig. 4.119 The lung tissues have a central grey/cream tumour, clearly directly infiltrating the local nodes and interacting with the pulmonary vasculature in a case of primary squamous carcinoma of the lung

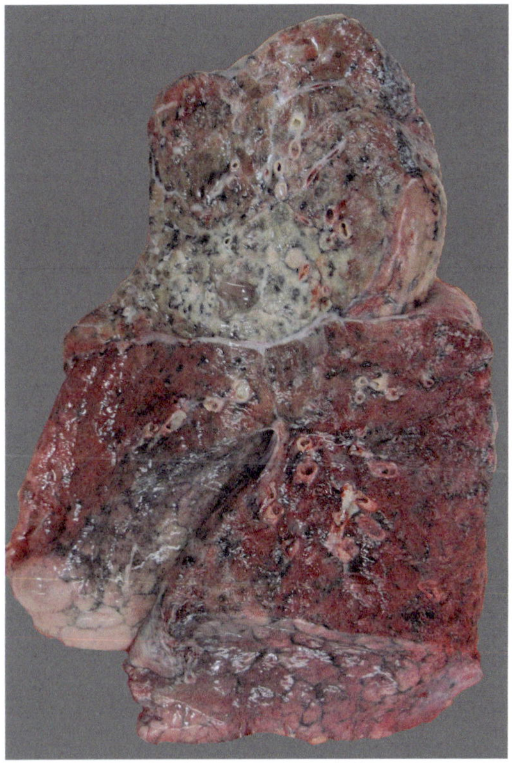

Fig. 4.121 Primary pulmonary adenocarcinoma is seen with infiltration of the interlobar fissure and upper lobe obstructive pneumonia

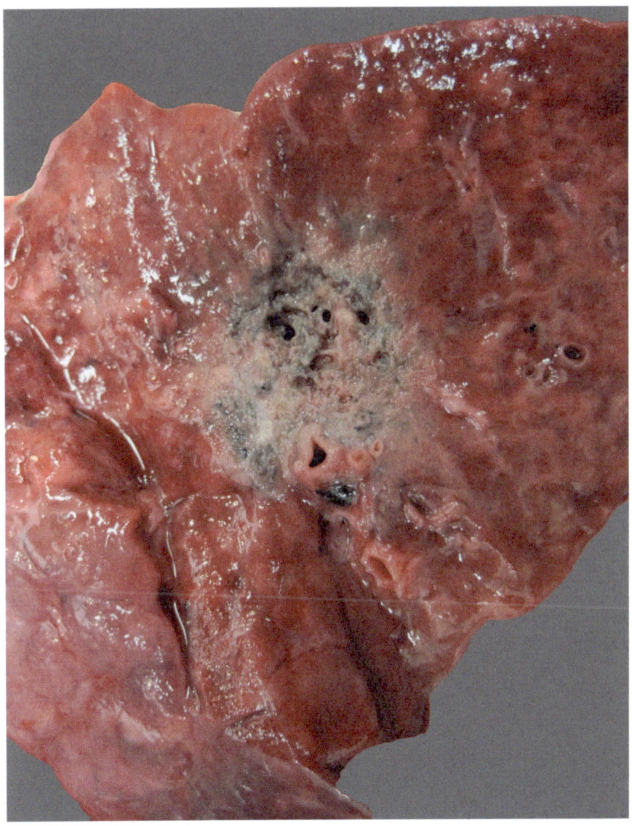

Fig. 4.120 A pulmonary adenocarcinoma is seen with some central degeneration and an irregular/infiltrating peripheral boundary. Local congestion and pneumonic change is present. Some central cystic degeneration is noted

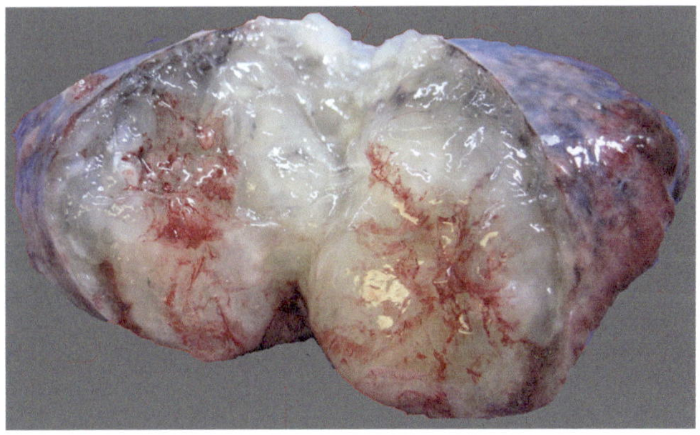

Fig. 4.122 The cut surface of some tumours is characteristic, such as this extensive mucoid material in a case of mucinous adenocarcinoma

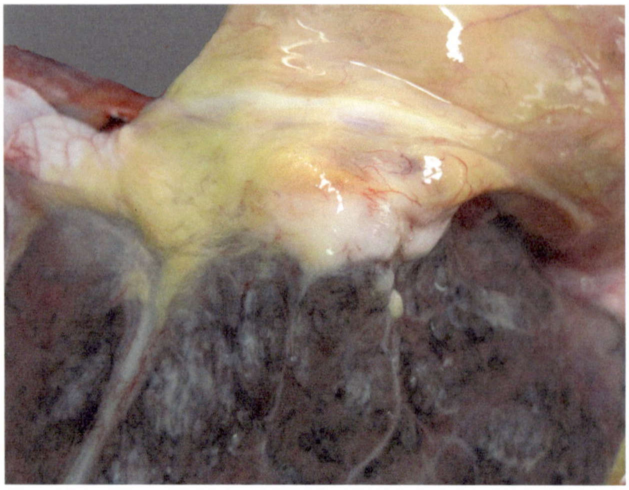

Fig. 4.123 Metastatic tumour is seen in the soft tissues around the hilar root at autopsy. Some grey discolouration of the surface pleural parenchyma is adjacent, representing lymphangitis

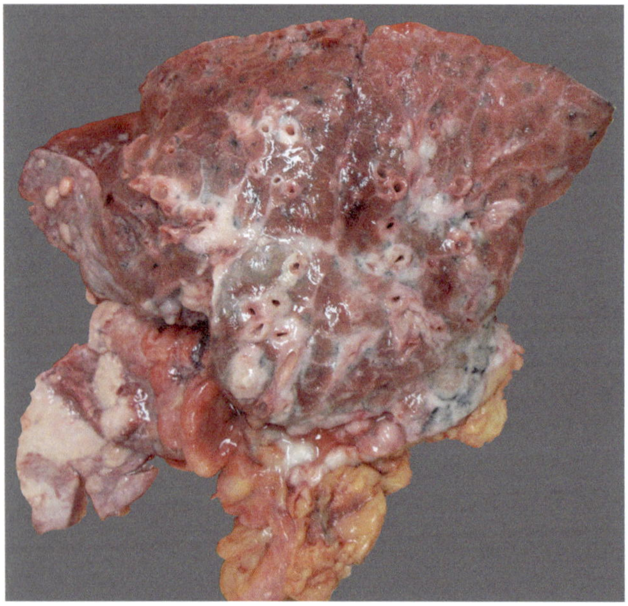

Fig. 4.124 Prominent channels noted macroscopically represent pronounced lymphangitis seen extensively involving this lung tissue with collapse and distortion of the parenchyma. Solid tumour is also noted

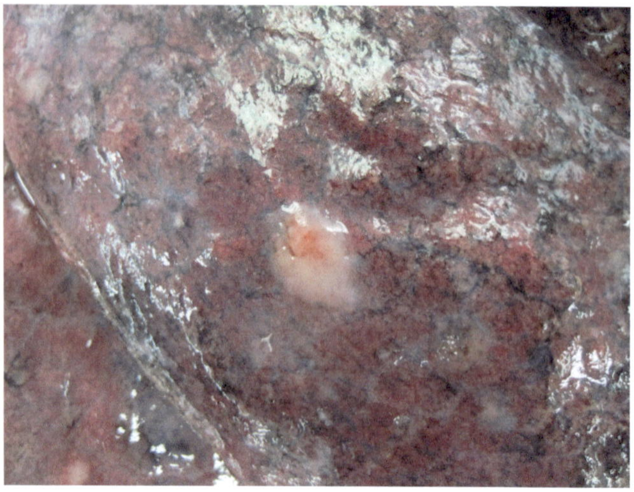

Fig. 4.125 The pleural surface is seen to be studded by small plaques of beige tissue with a somewhat lacy network of similar tissue running around the surface. This is the characteristic appearance of lymphangitis carcinomatosa involving the pleural surface

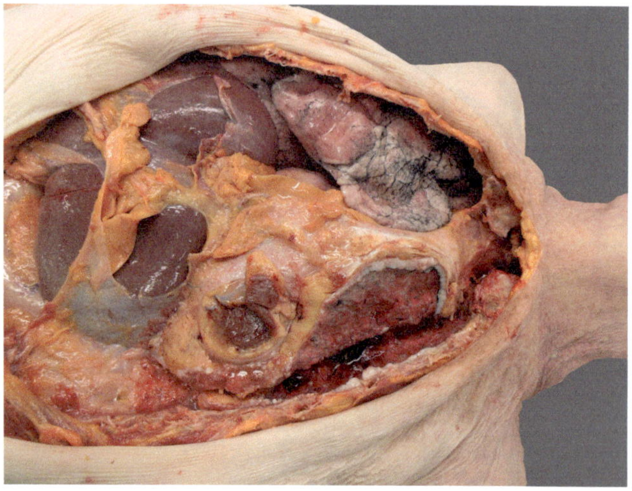

Fig. 4.126 Diffuse pleural infiltration is seen on the left side of this initial dissection, in keeping with the history of previously treated breast cancer

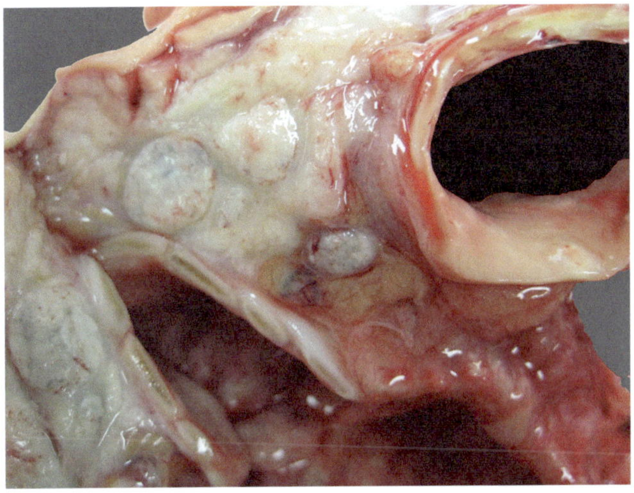

Fig. 4.127 A close-up view of the mediastinal content shows cream tumour widely occupying the mediastinal soft tissues and directly replacing local lymph nodes

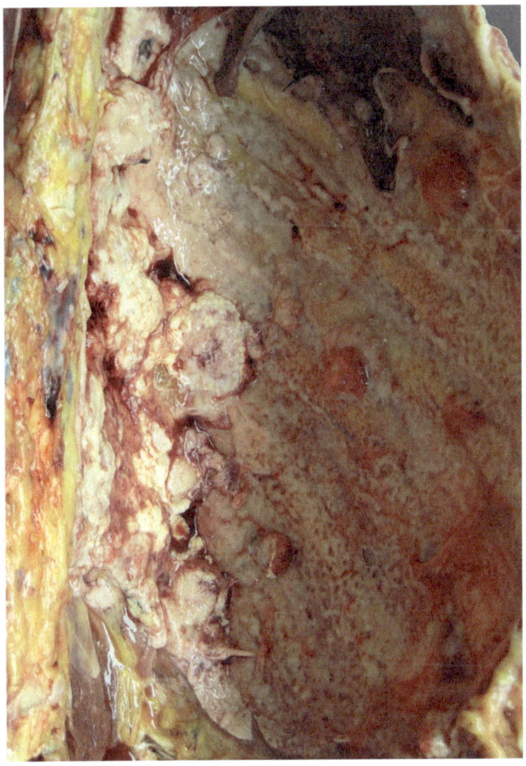

Fig. 4.128 Some lung cancers spread around the chest cavity, mimicking mesothelioma. This was a non-keratinising squamous carcinoma. The tumour is seen coating the parietal pleural tissues with nodularity

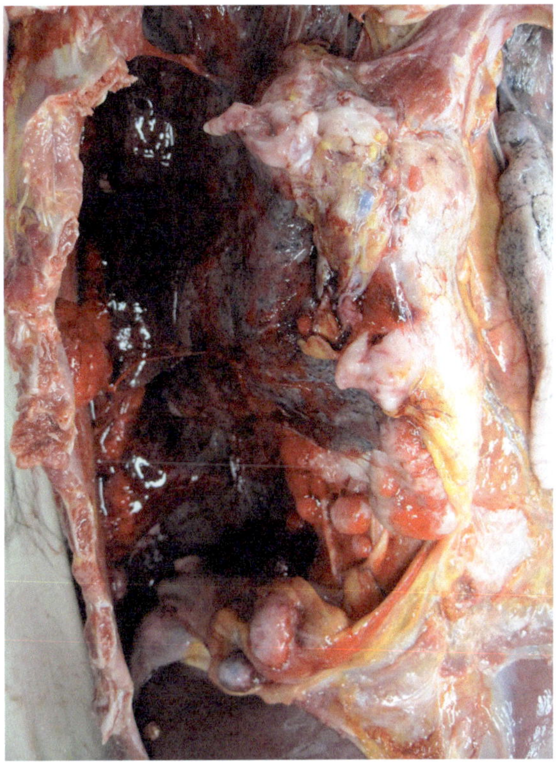

Fig. 4.129 Disseminated sarcomatoid neoplasia can be seen in a variety of forms, often mimicking mesothelioma. The right hemithorax in this case of spindle cell carcinoma shows widespread nodularity and distortion with some local haemorrhage

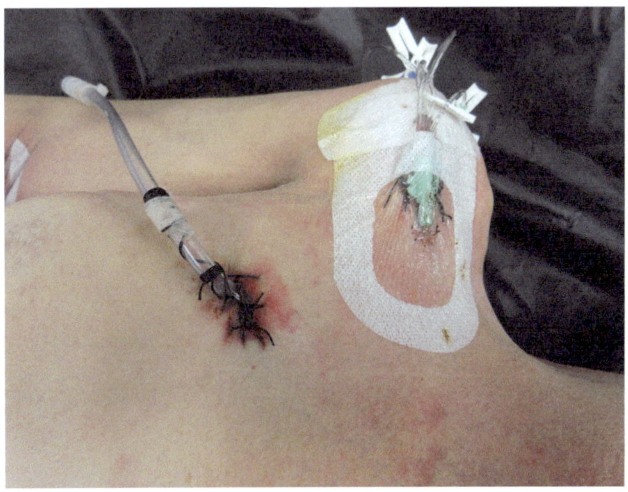

Fig. 4.130 The right upper chest has been cannulated for drainage purposes with a subclavian vascular line being seen immediately adjacent

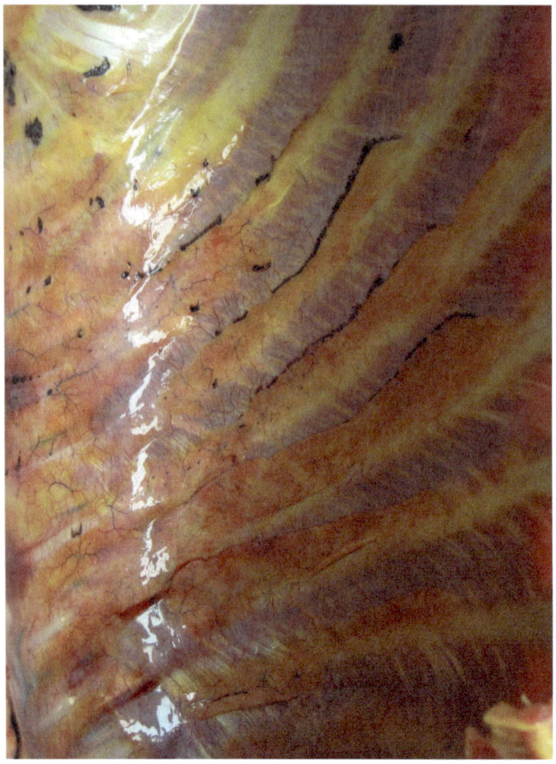

Fig. 4.131 The inner aspect of the hemithorax should always be considered, after removal of the heart, lungs, and mediastinal content. This chest wall shows the normal association of fat in relation to the musculature and ribs, with some anthracotic dust pigmentation (in this case reflecting coal dust exposure). The pleural surface is noted to be smooth, glistening, and without any fluid accumulation

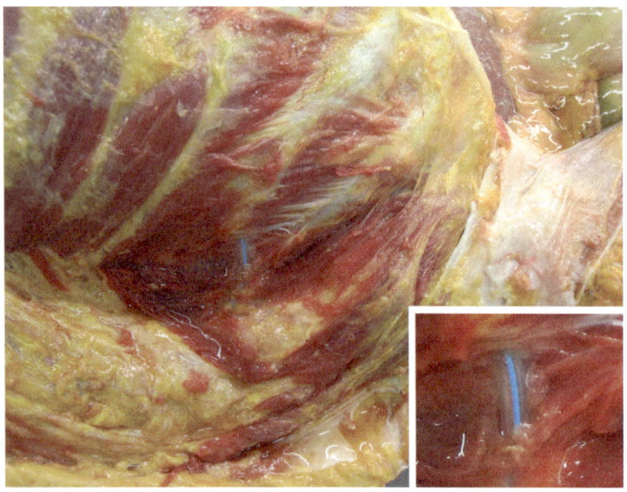

Fig. 4.132 In cases of chest disease with drains, assessment of the body requires identification of the drainage tube and assessment of its position within the hemithorax. Drains should not be pulled from the body until the assessment has taken place. In many cases, the drains are cut flush with the skin, and then pushed a small distance inwards. This allows dissection of the skin and soft tissues around the chest in the normal manner and preservation of the tube position. Here a chest drain is seen in the low lateral thorax, having been placed under radiology guidance. The *low right inset* shows higher magnification. The drain is highlighted by a bright blue band within the clear plastic tube

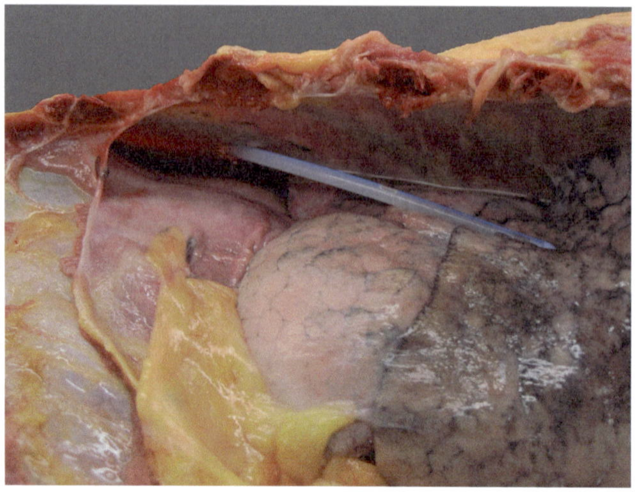

Fig. 4.133 A correctly positioned chest drainage tube is seen entering the low thorax and running up onto the outside aspect of the lung tissues. This targeted chest drainage was placed under radiological observation. Some fluid is still present behind the drain

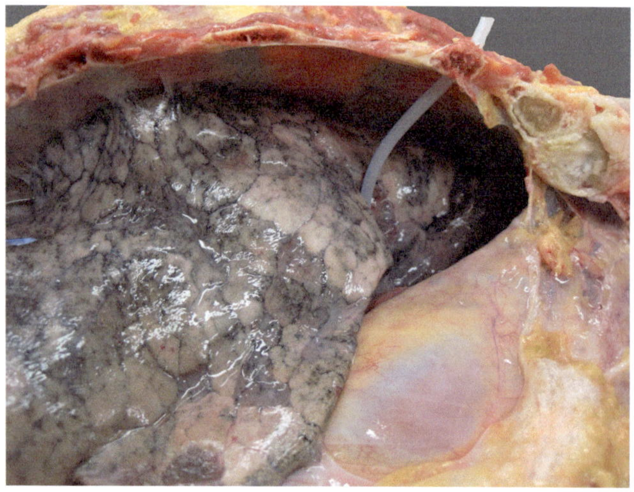

Fig. 4.134 Another example of a correctly positioned chest drain is seen to push into the chest wall and lie in the interlobar fissure rather than on the periphery of the lung tissues. Local adhesions are present, binding the visceral and parietal pleural tissues together

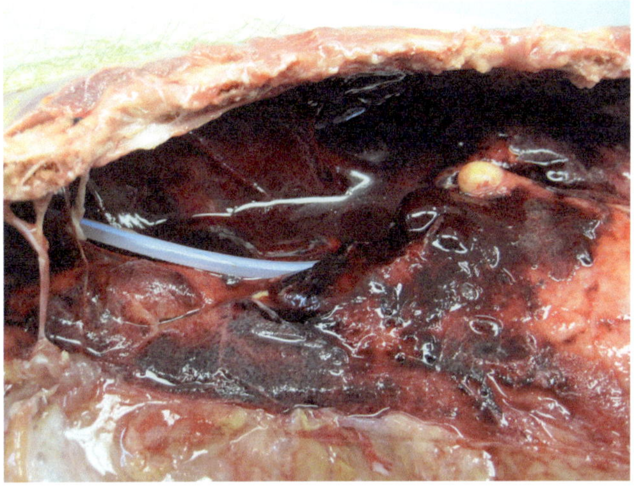

Fig. 4.135 Any chest drain device inserted into the thoracic cavity should always be assessed for position and for complications. In this case, massive haemorrhage was incurred due to direct lung trauma

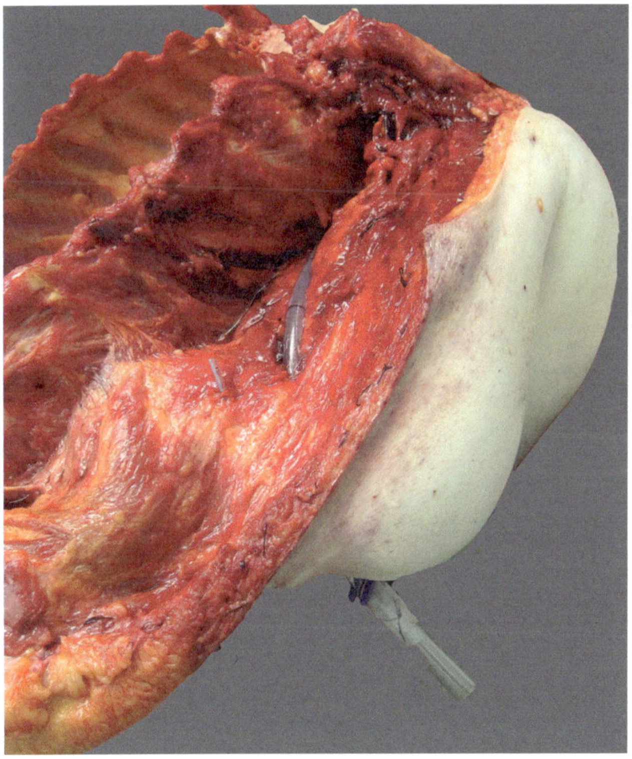

Fig. 4.136 This chest drain did not enter the pleural space, having been placed into the chest/axillary soft tissues. It clearly would not have improved the patient's situation and may be a factor in the cause of death

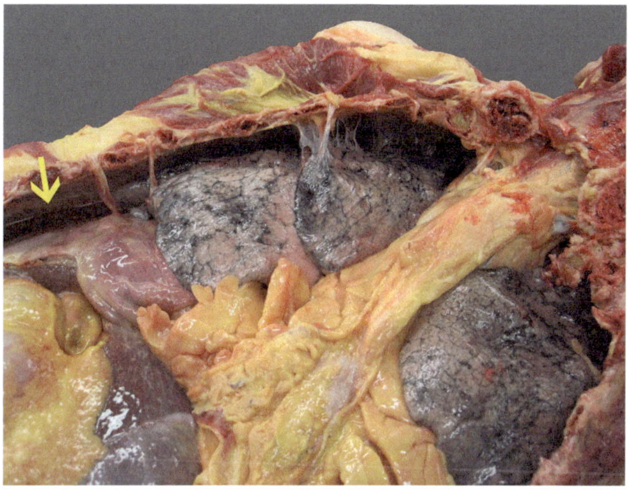

Fig. 4.137 After removal of the chest plate, adhesions and fluid collections should be assessed. It is possible to culture fluid collections if present, even small effusions (*arrow*), but some caution is needed, as post-mortem contamination of static fluids is not uncommon

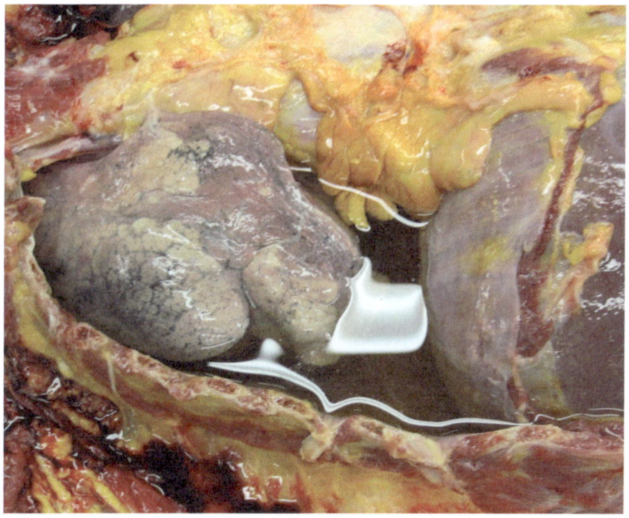

Fig. 4.138 Large pleural effusions often have a physiological impact in life. Their volume and character must be considered. Inspection of any fluid collection requires assessment of both the volume of fluid and the nature of the collection. Such collections should be described in general terms (*e.g.*, clear yellow fluid, turbid brown fluid)

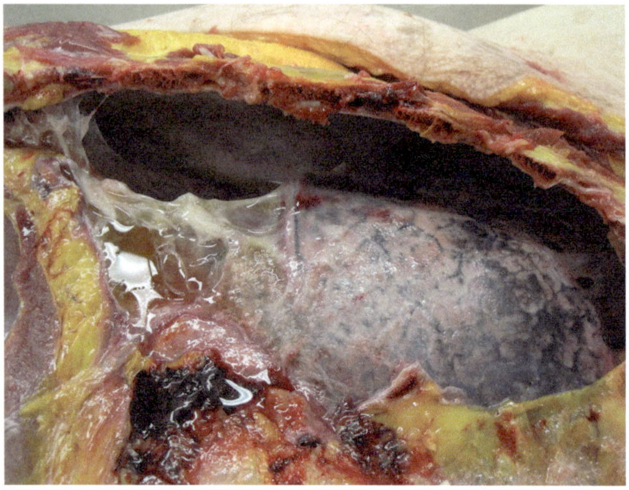

Fig. 4.139 Lung adhesions to the chest wall can become loculated. The encysted pools of effusion fluid potentially provide an ideal septic focus. Assessment of adhesions is important in cases of lung disease. Adhesions may reflect both reactive/reparative phenomena and tumour infiltration of the pleural cavity. The fibrous adhesions and some fluid in this case reflected persistent chest sepsis

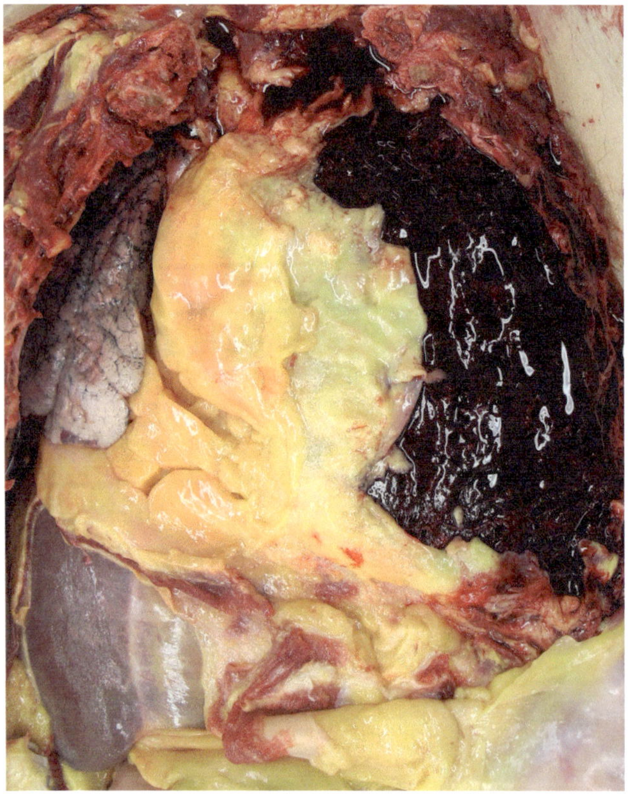

Fig. 4.140 Haemorrhage into the pleural cavity may also occur from tumours. The necrosis of a tumour involving the pleural cavity, in a patient with anticoagulant treatment, has resulted in a massive haemothorax, which was pertinent to the death of this individual

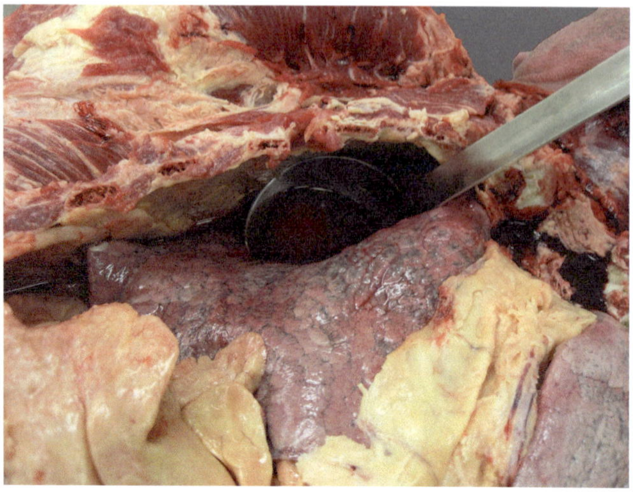

Fig. 4.141 Fluid collections can be assessed by ladling out the content into measuring jugs or by direct mechanical aspiration into fluid drainage devices

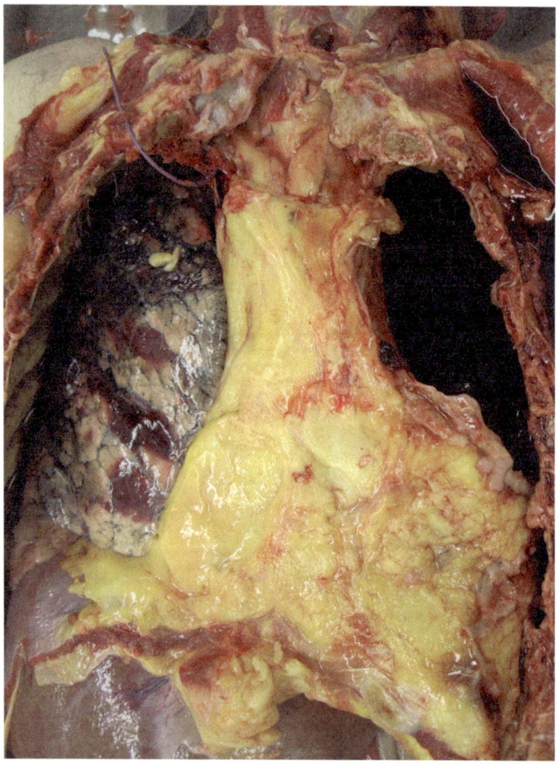

Fig. 4.142 Pneumonectomy, with complete removal of the tissues of the whole lung, leaves a potential space in the hemithorax. Part of this space is filled by expansion of the other lung and movement of the mediastinal content, but the chest space initially is normally occupied by fluid, with subsequent organization. This person died shortly after the surgical procedure, with evidence of significant haemorrhage into the chest space. This case involved systemic sepsis following the pneumonectomy

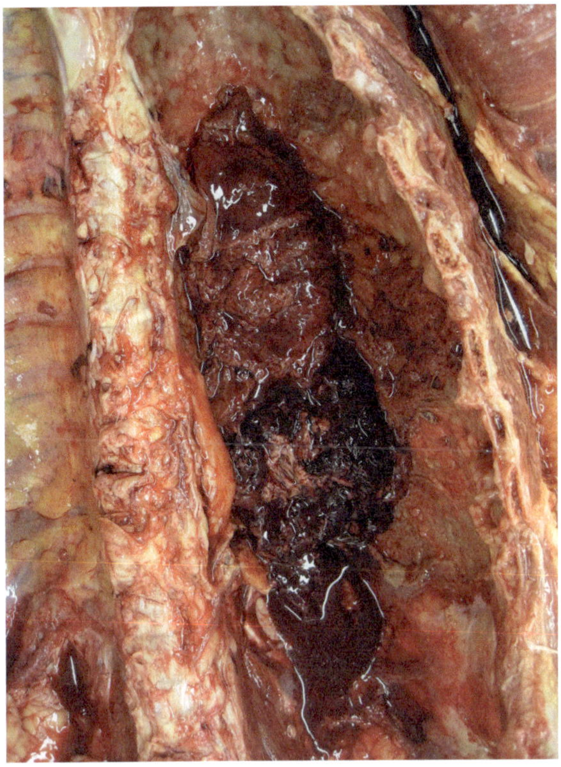

Fig. 4.143 Later stages of pneumonectomy (without sepsis) involve the organization of the proteinaceous and blood-stained material. A protein coagulum is seen on the posterior aspect of the chest. Histologically, this characteristically has a moderate mixed inflammatory infiltrate within it, although one can check for recurrent carcinoma

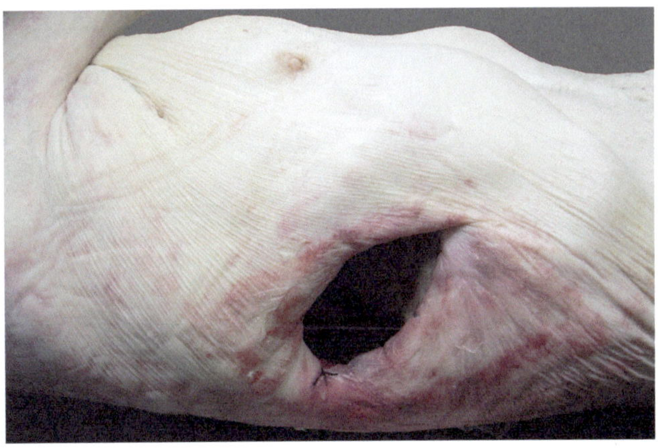

Fig. 4.144 This large thoracostomy was required for chronic sepsis following pneumonectomy. The persistent production and accumulation of septic material in the right hemithorax required a large drainage route. The object of such surgery is to permit complete drainage and treatment of any septic focus, with subsequent chest closure (if possible)

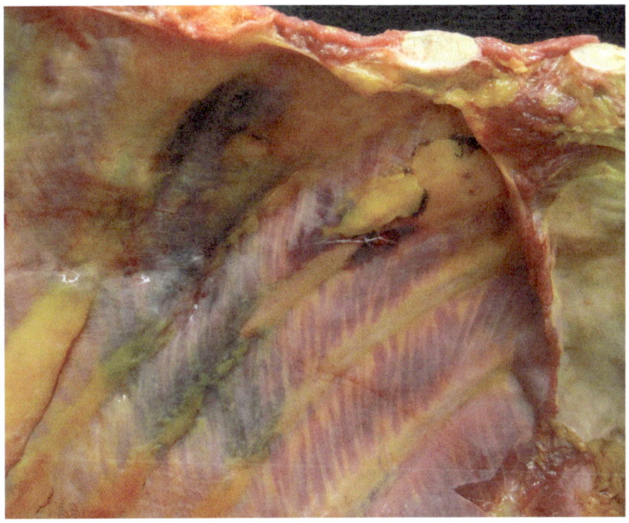

Fig. 4.145 Undisplaced fractures of the ribs are often apparent with local bruising, even if there is no penetration of the pleural cavity by the fracture itself

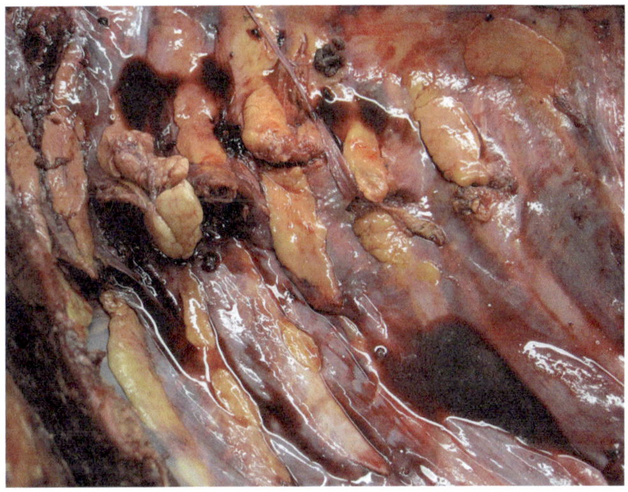

Fig. 4.146 Multiple fractures are seen in this chest, with clear evidence of local haemorrhage into the soft tissues and pleural compartment. If the ribs are broken on both sides, then the chest wall integrity is lost and it becomes a 'flail' chest, leading to paradoxical chest movements and subsequent respiratory failure

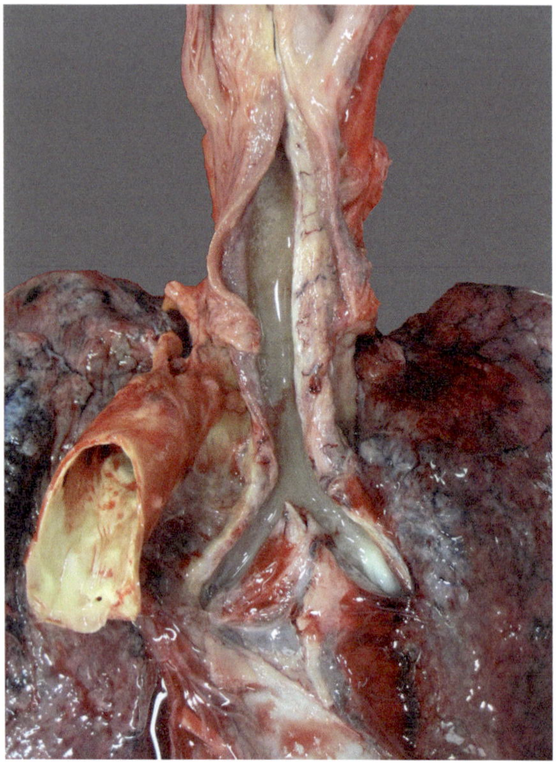

Fig. 4.147 Significant allergic reactions (anaphylactic shock) are classically associated with extensive tenacious mucoid secretions within the airways. These are best appreciated early in the thoracic dissection, as the trachea is opened with the cut extended towards the lobar bronchi. This is not to be confused with bronchopneumonia

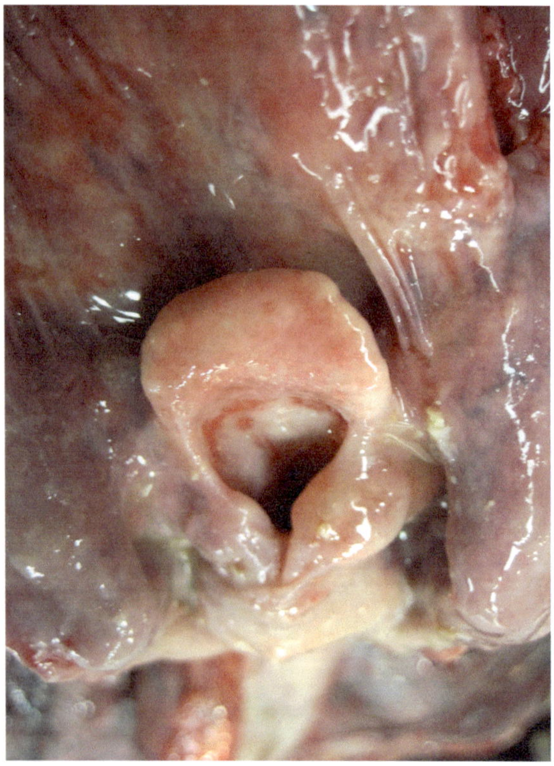

Fig. 4.148 Acute anaphylaxis is seen with laryngeal oedema in a case of drug-related allergy. The airway was closed, causing the death of this patient in a case of penicillin allergy

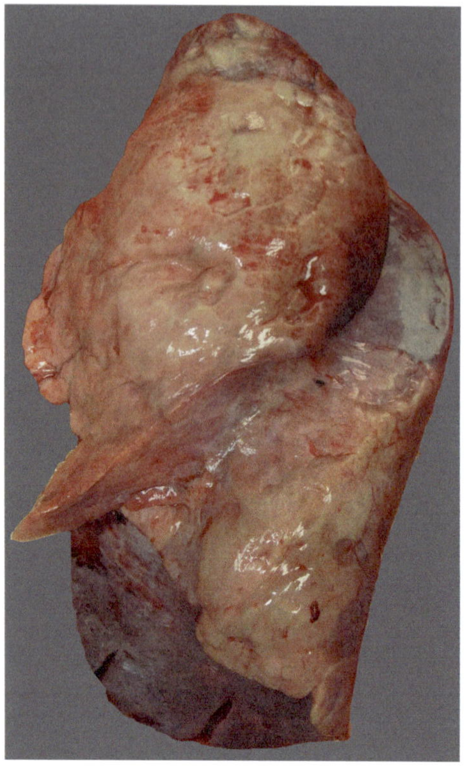

Fig. 4.149 In a case of acute asthma, hyperinflated lungs are often seen, remaining in their inflated form even after separation from the mediastinal content

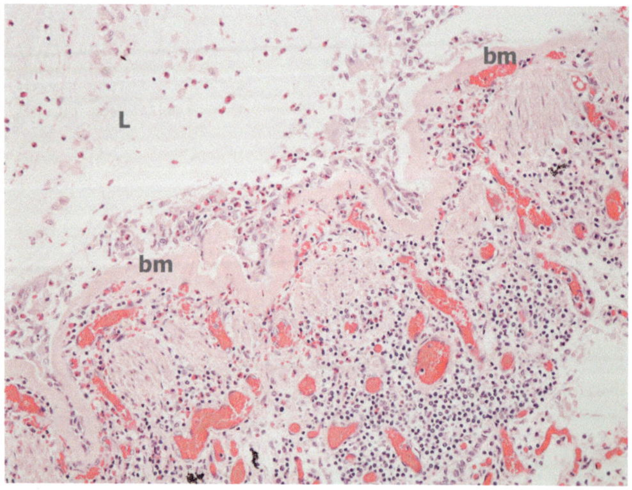

Fig. 4.150 Histological examination in a case of allergic lung reactions shows epithelial denudation with inflammatory cells and degenerate cellular material being seen within the bronchial lumen (*L*). The basement membrane (*bm*) is slightly corrugated but is clearly thickened and eosinophilic. The adjacent connective tissue shows pronounced vascular engorgement with a moderate inflammatory cell component containing many eosinophils

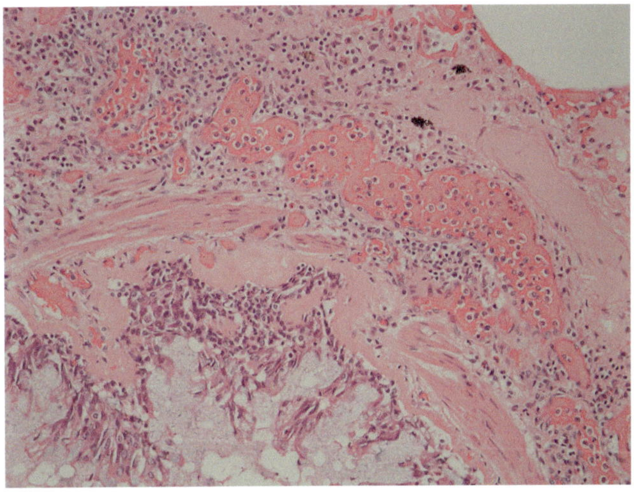

Fig. 4.151 The proximal airways in asthma cases often show hyperplasia of the epithelium with excess mucus secretion. There is widespread local inflammation with many eosinophils

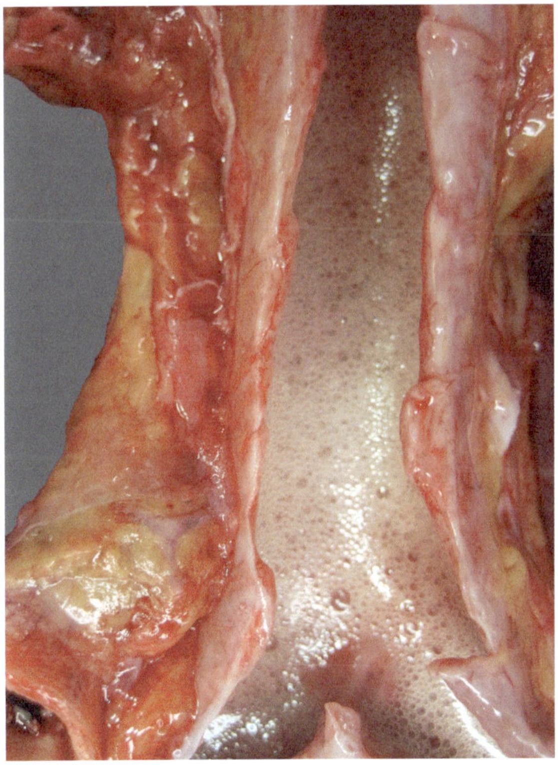

Fig. 4.152 In drowning, a plume of frothy material often extends from the mouth and nose, but this may be lost by the time of the autopsy. Foamy fluid can also be seen within the trachea, supporting this interpretation of drowning

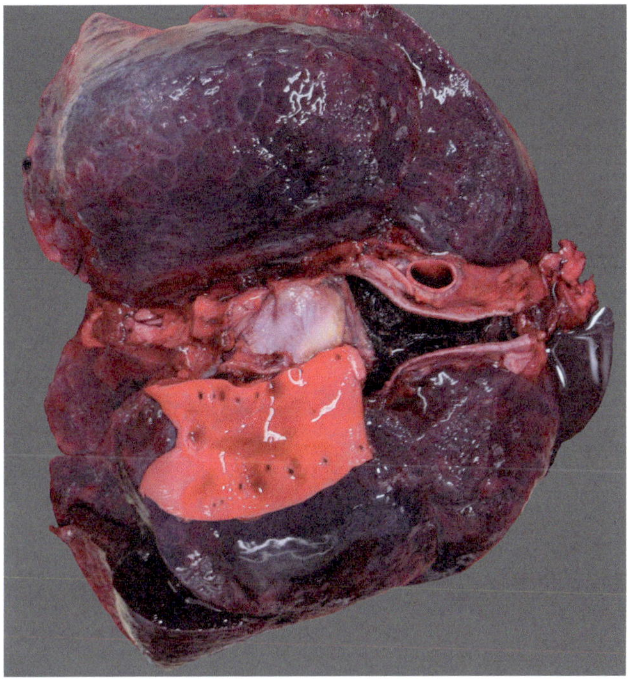

Fig. 4.153 The cherry-pink discolouration of the aortic wall tissues is noted in association with blackening of the airway surface in a case of an individual trapped within a fire and dying from the combined effects of carbon monoxide toxicity and smoke inhalation

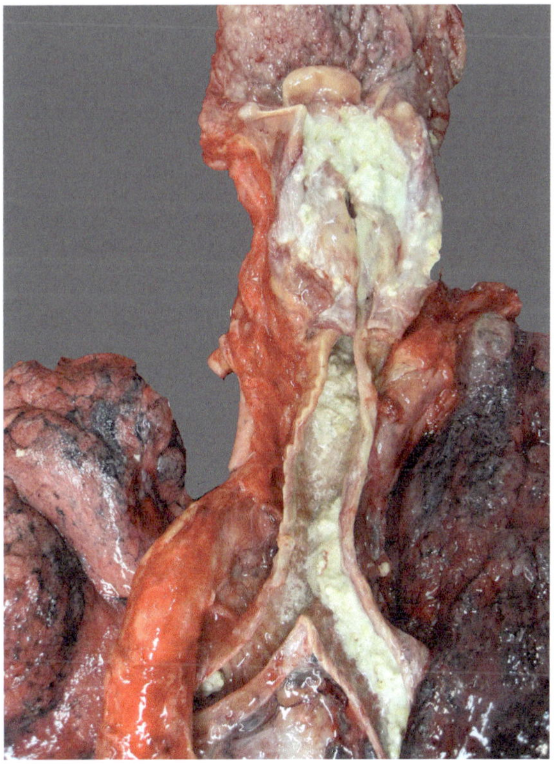

Fig. 4.154 This thoracic dissection, opening the trachea and bronchi as well as the larynx, shows a case of massive food aspiration, clearly occluding the proximal airway and causing death. Photographic evidence is of particular use in such cases with a medicolegal reality

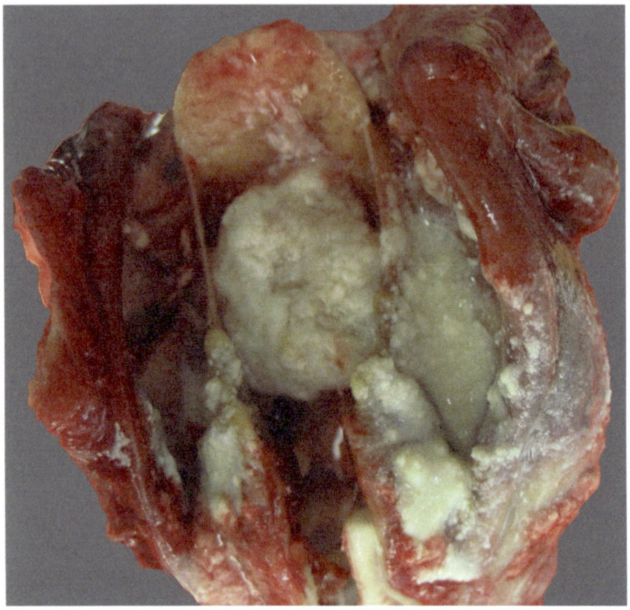

Fig. 4.155 A close-up view of the larynx with food material blocking the airway

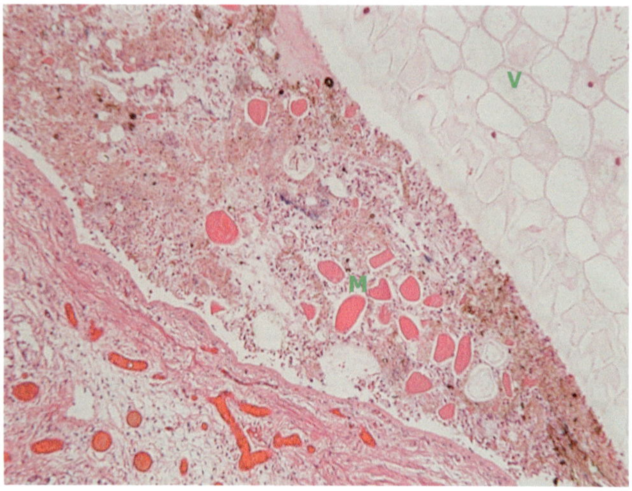

Fig. 4.157 Aspirated material is often best appreciated in the small airways by histology. Small fragments of meat (*M*) are present within irregular mucoid and degenerate matrix. Some vegetable (*V*) material is seen adjacent

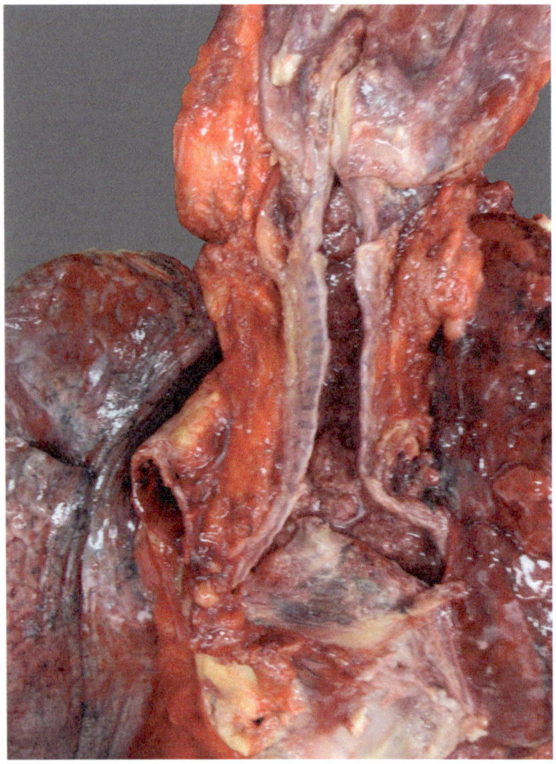

Fig. 4.156 The airway in this case is largely occluded by aspirated food content

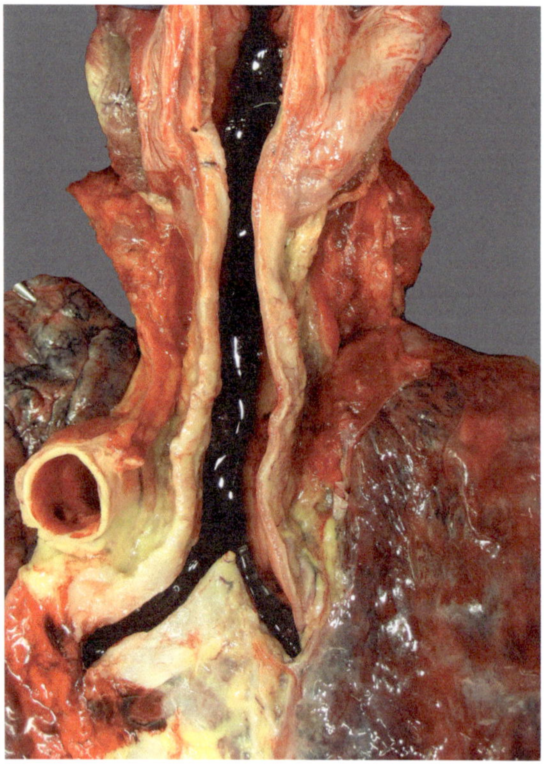

Fig. 4.158 Massive haemorrhage into the large airways has occluded the trachea, in a case of carcinomatous intrapulmonary haemorrhage due to bronchial artery rupture directly into the airway of one lobe

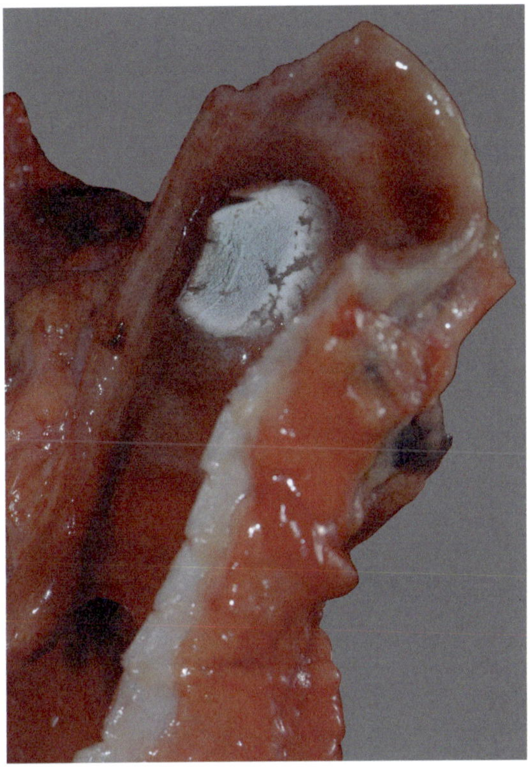

Fig. 4.159 An incidental, nonpathological feature seen in some autopsy cases is post-mortem growth of a fungal colony within the airways

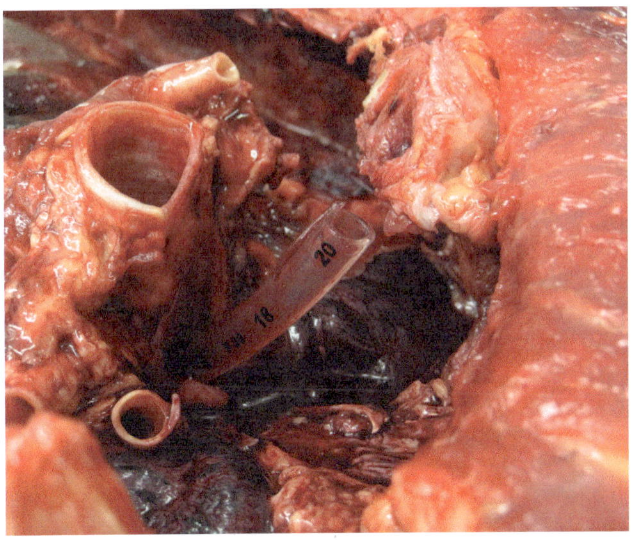

Fig. 4.160 Assessment of the pulmonary tissues will always involve the position of devices. In this case, the endotracheal tube is incorrectly positioned in the esophagus, behind the trachea. This positioning clearly would have a significant impact on the chances that the patient will survive a cardiorespiratory arrest

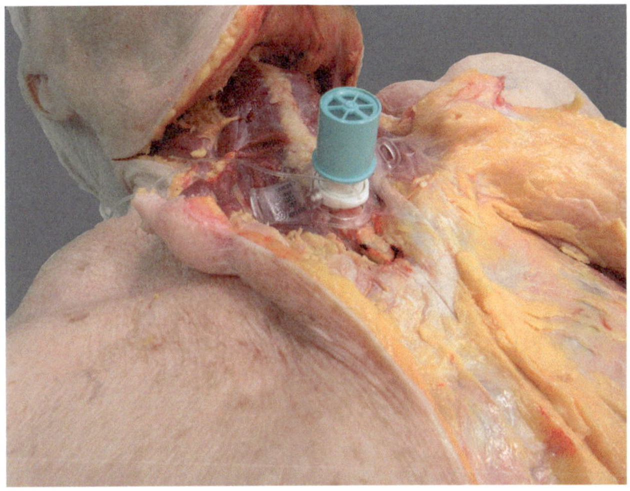

Fig. 4.161 This is a tracheostomy device used in cases of impaired respiratory function and with significant autonomic instability following high cervical cord injury. The question with regard to examination of these devices normally reflects whether the device is blocked, malpositioned or indeed incorrectly aligned. Slow and careful dissection with multiple static photographic images is recommended in order to assist case examination subsequently

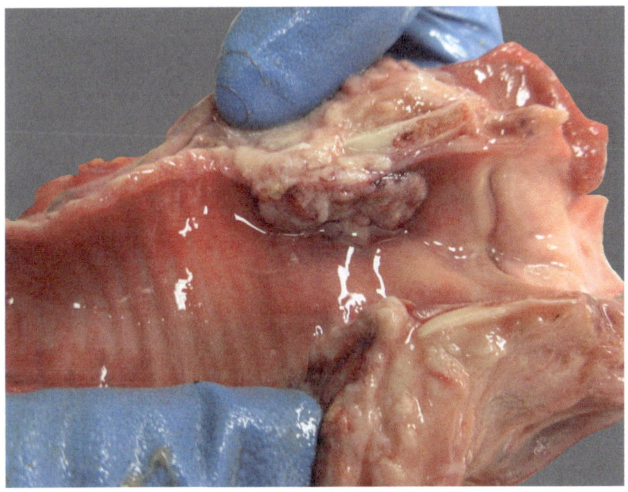

Fig. 4.162 An early squamous carcinoma of the larynx is seen below the vocal cords

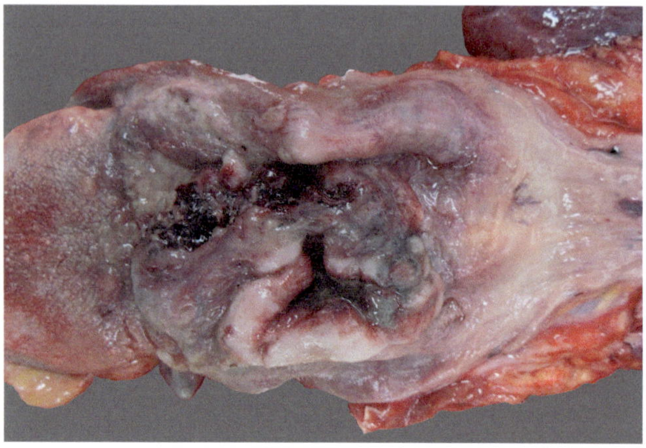

Fig. 4.163 Advanced laryngeal carcinoma is seen largely occluding the airway. The ulceration and haemorrhage in the tumour are noted with direct infiltration into the local soft tissues

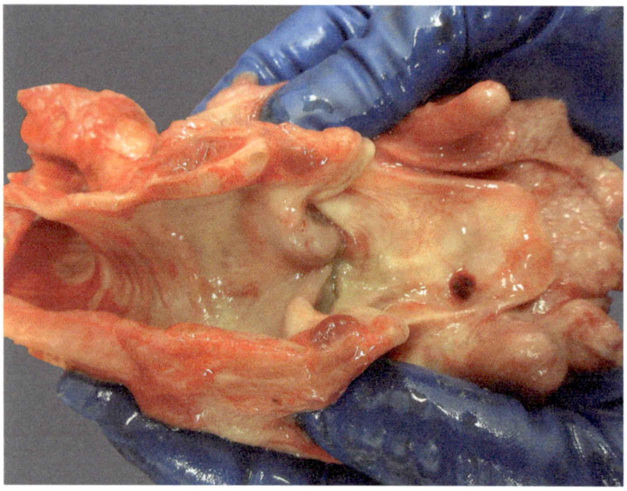

Fig. 4.164 This larynx is distorted and fibrotic with irregularity in keeping with the history of laryngeal carcinoma treated by radiotherapy

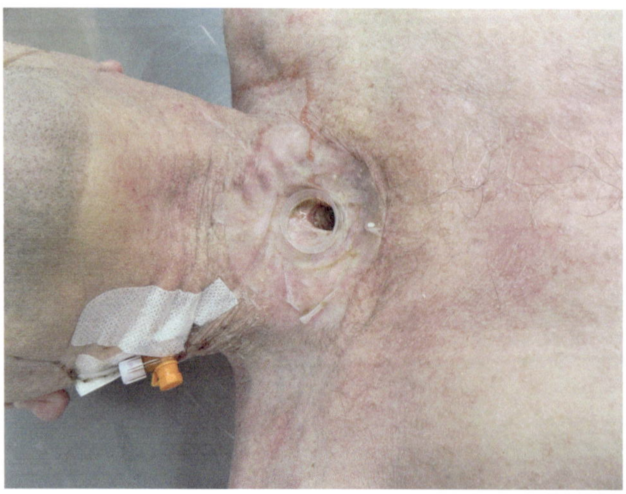

Fig. 4.165 This is a case of a previous laryngectomy, with evidence of surgery and scarring around the lower neck along with a vascular line present on the right side of the neck. The entrance to the tracheostomy site is marked by a plastic device with no evidence of obstruction or sepsis

Gross Cardiac Pathology

The cardiac tissues (Figs. 4.166, 4.167, 4.168, 4.169, 4.170, 4.171, 4.172, 4.173, 4.174, 4.175, 4.176, 4.177, 4.178, 4.179, 4.180, 4.181, 4.182, 4.183, 4.184, 4.185, 4.186, 4.187, 4.188, 4.189, 4.190, 4.191, 4.192, 4.193, and 4.194) are best assessed in terms of the gross anatomy, the coronary arteries, the myocardial tissue itself, and the valves. Given the architectural complexity of this dynamic organ, it is vital to examine the tissues in a stepwise fashion, as the disorders liable to be seen in the autopsy room merit judgement in turn. This order guides the observer to identify congenital lesions, degenerative and inflammatory disorders, infections and inflammation, and the cardiomyopathies.

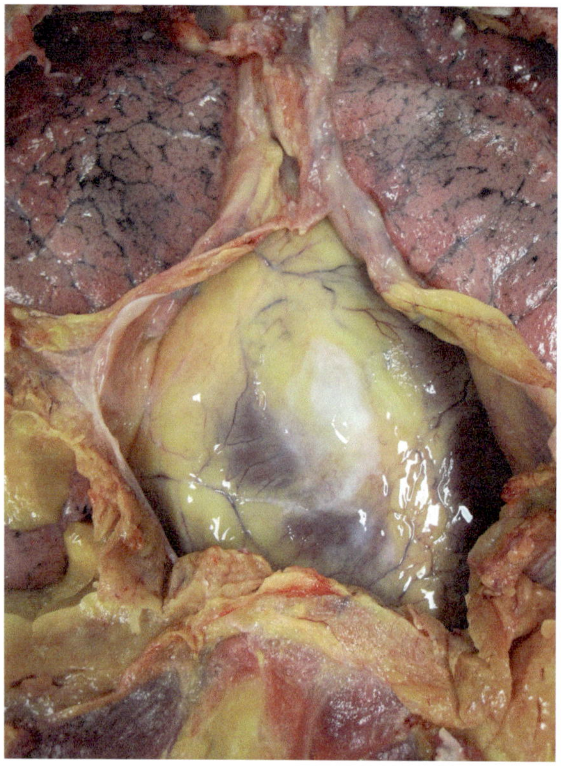

Fig. 4.166 The cardiac tissues initially may be examined in situ, just after the chest plate has been removed. In this view, the pericardium has been opened, with the local thoracic tissues still in situ. The heart is seen in its normal position, with some fibrous tissue on the anterior epicardial surface. This fibrous tissue plaque is a normal feature, reflecting the epicardial surface rubbing against the inner aspect of the anterior chest wall tissues

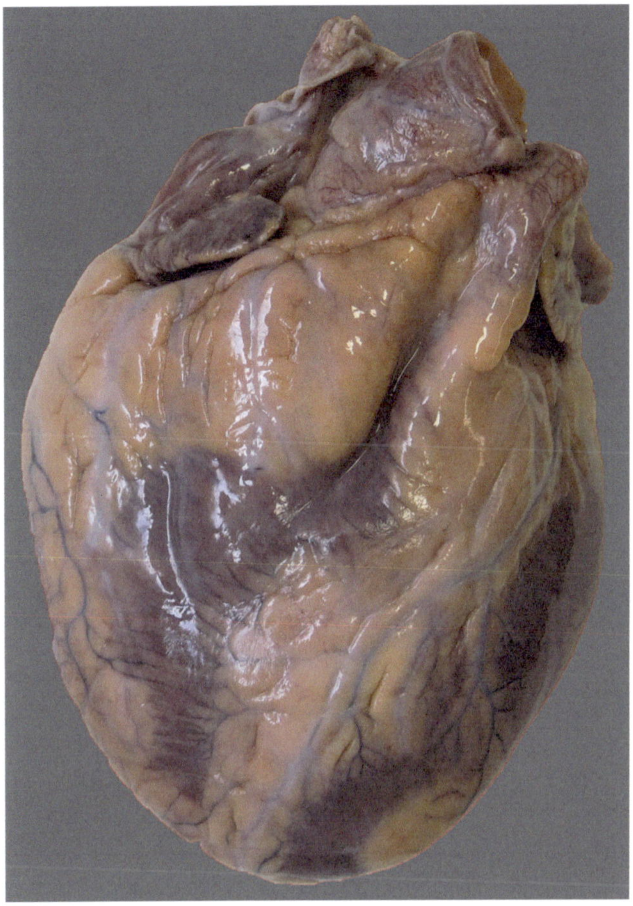

Fig. 4.167 This adult heart (fixed after extraction in this case) is seen from the anterior aspect. The auricular appendages can be seen, with the normal position of the great vessels. Also seen is the normal coronary tributary pattern and the usual amount of fat adjacent to the main coronary arteries and veins

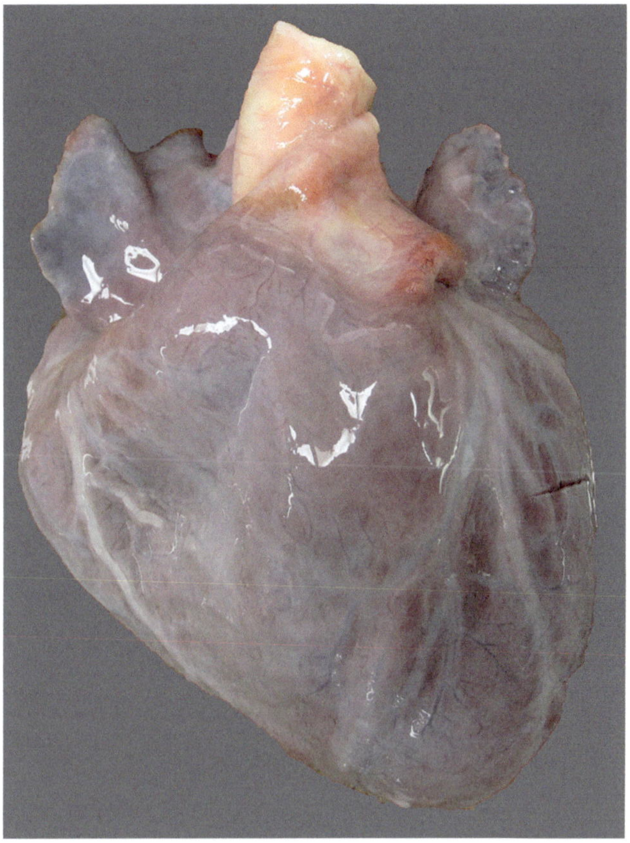

Fig. 4.168 This adult heart has no appreciable epicardial fat. This is a rare occurrence in Western society. The individual was of light build and was very undernourished. It is unusual to see no fatty tissue around the course of the coronary artery tissues on an adult heart

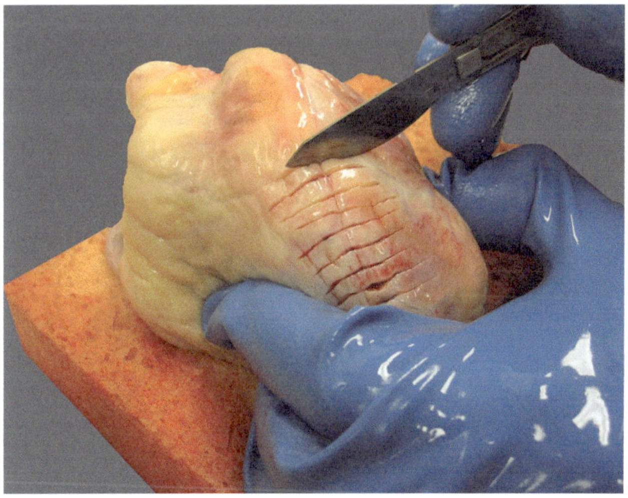

Fig. 4.169 The coronary arteries may be sectioned at intervals of 3–5 mm, with direct inspection of the lumens. This process is ideally performed with a sharp scalpel blade. Areas of high-grade atheroma, thrombosis, or both may be identified and scored (generally as a percentage occlusion remark, such as "*50% narrowed*"). The tissues are partly stabilized by holding the tissue on a sponge

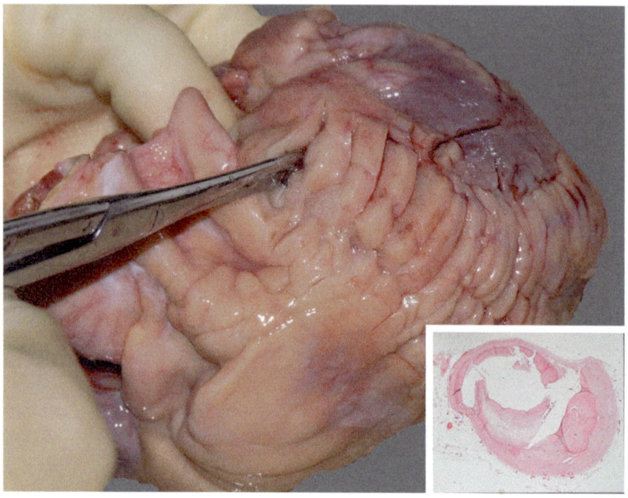

Fig. 4.170 Heavily calcified coronary arteries are difficult to cut with scalpels. They may be cut with scissors, but one must appreciate that the scissors may partly fragment any calcified plaque disease, as seen in subsequent histology (*inset*)

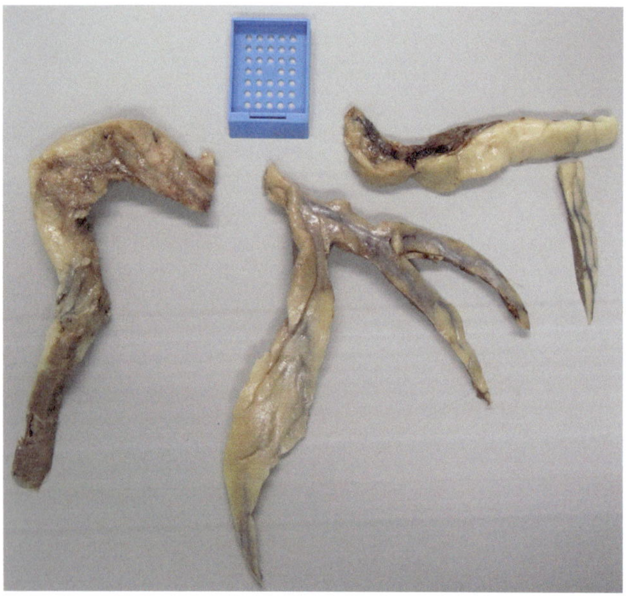

Fig. 4.171 Some coronary arteries can be very heavily calcified, significantly hindering examination of the vessels, but if they are dissected intact (en bloc), the arteries can be fixed (48 h) and then decalcified (48 h)

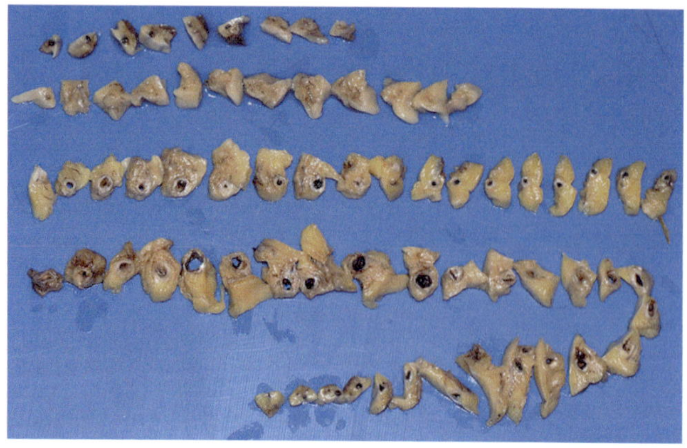

Fig. 4.172 After decalcification, the three main arteries, as intact vessels, are easy to transversely slice and examine in sequential format. Areas of heavy plaque disease may be selected for photography and/or histology. (Adapted with permission from Suvarna SK. National guidelines for adult autopsy cardiac dissection and diagnosis-are they achievable? A personal view. Histopathology. 2008;53:97–112)

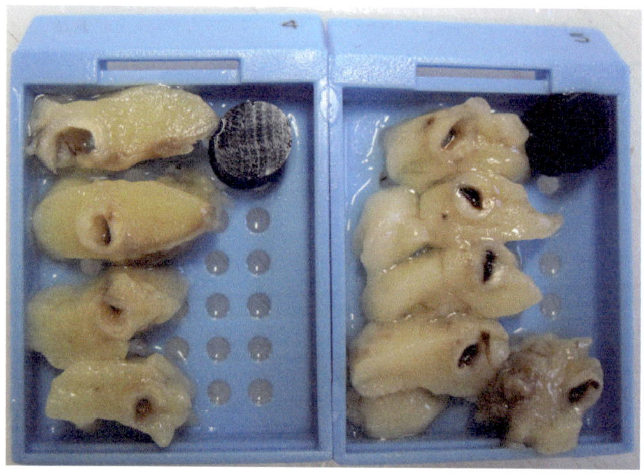

Fig. 4.173 The coronary arteries can be mounted into cassettes in small groups, allowing precise understanding of the degree of atheroma as each slice is a step along the coronary artery course

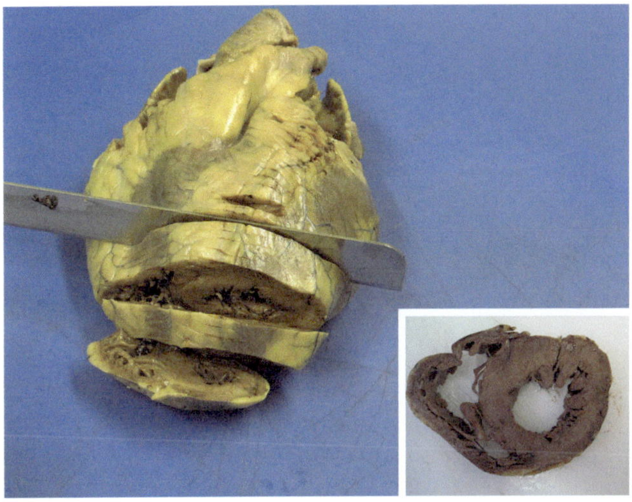

Fig. 4.174 The heart (following examination of the coronary arteries) is sectioned across the ventricles (usually in three slices), with the final cut at mid-ventricular level. The *inset* shows the view of the slice of ventricular tissues. The right ventricle is positioned on the left side of the image, with anterior tissues towards the base of the image. (Reproduced from Suvarna SK, editor. The heart at autopsy, including radiological autopsy of the heart, in Cardiac pathology: a guide to current practice. London: Springer-Verlag; 2013, with permission)

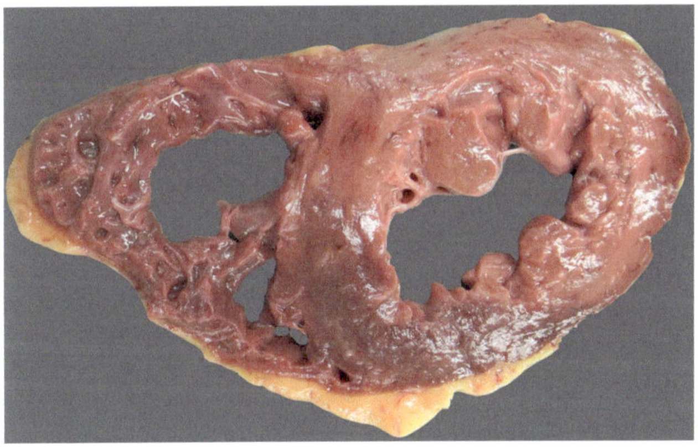

Fig. 4.175 The transverse sections of myocardium at mid-ventricular level provide information about the right and left ventricle walls and the septum, in relation to the chamber architecture. In this case, the colour of the otherwise normal ventricular tissues mapped to the position in which the individual was found (lying on the front/right side), with hypostasis being more marked in this position

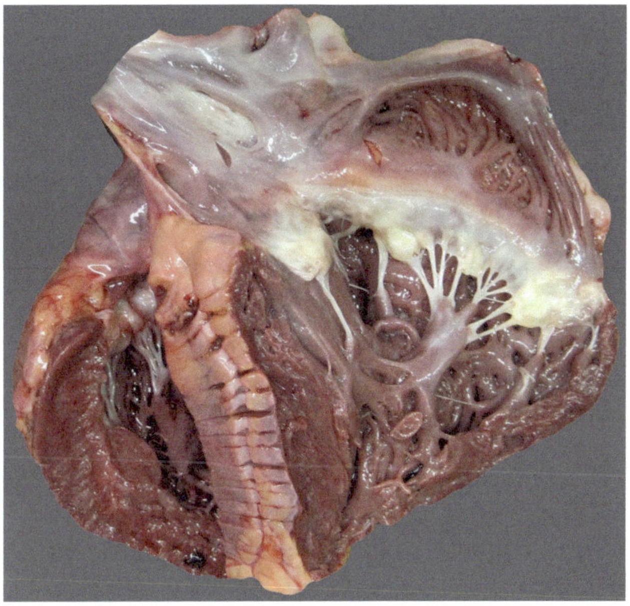

Fig. 4.176 The right atrium and ventricle in this intact heart have been opened by a cut running along the back of the right atrium (between the superior and inferior vena cava) and then across the tricuspid valve. The cut passes downwards into the right ventricle, about 10 mm to the side of the posterior interventricular artery. The three cusps of the tricuspid valve are seen; the anterior aspect of the atrium/auricle is notably trabeculated. This appendage can be inspected without further dissection. The right ventricle trabeculations are moderately coarse. The papillary muscles are seen with the chordae running upwards to the tricuspid valve tissues

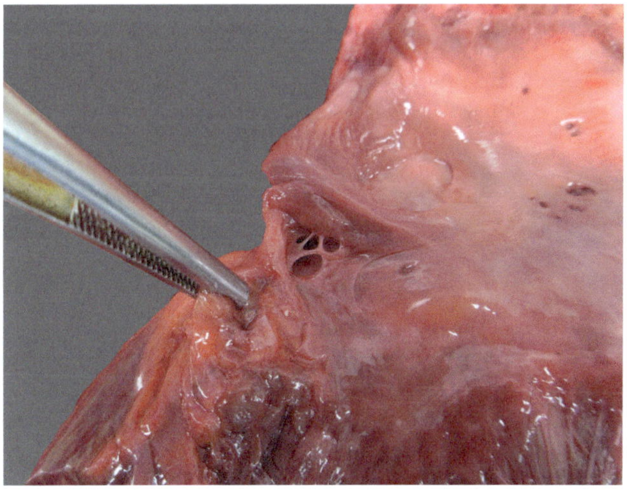

Fig. 4.177 The coronary sinus often has partially formed webs at its insertion point into the right atrium. These are of no functional significance

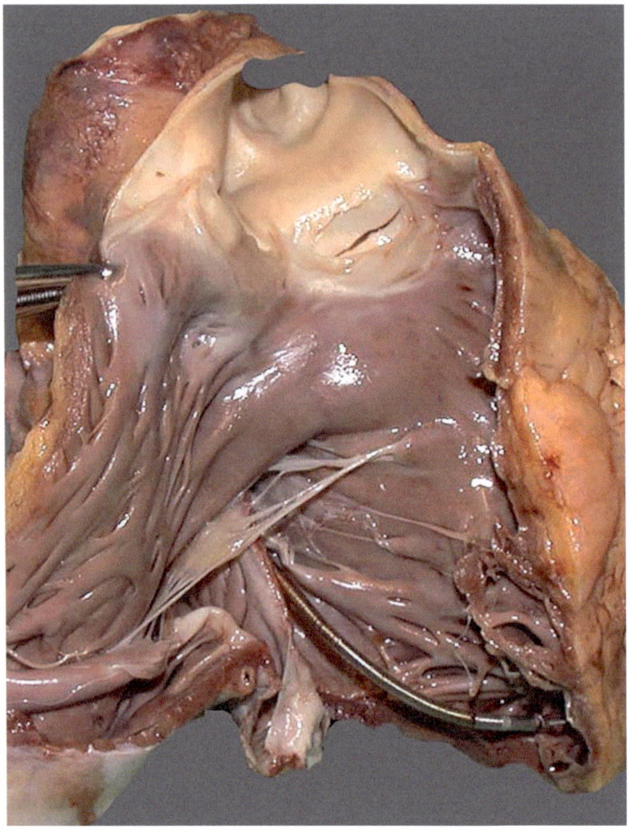

Fig. 4.178 Turning the heart onto the back allows one to cut along the anterior aspect of the right ventricle, across the pulmonary valve and into the pulmonary artery. This demonstrates the outflow tract of the right ventricle with three cusps of the pulmonary valve showing a normal semilunar architecture. Note the absence of coronary ostia. The outflow tract to the right ventricle is smooth, contrasting with the rest of the right ventricle tissue. An incidental pacemaker lead is seen running to a normal position in the tip of the right ventricle

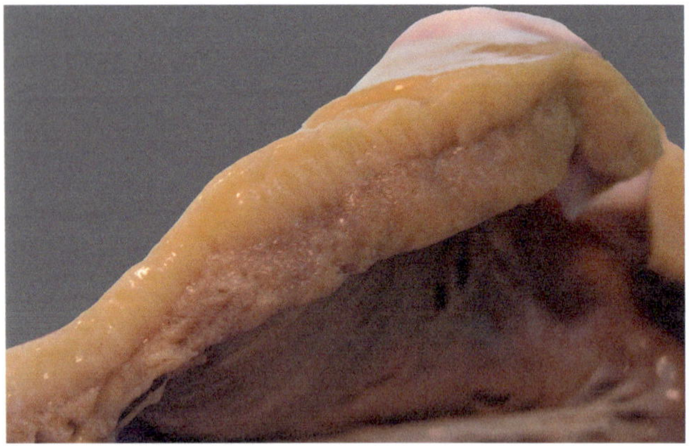

Fig. 4.179 Fatty tissue on the pericardial aspect of the right ventricle outflow tract is normal, but variable. In this view, the amount of fat is very pronounced, but not associated with wall thinning or overt fibrosis. This is a normal variant, seen in the general population; it is more common in females and the elderly. It should not be mistaken for arrhythmogenic right ventricular cardiomyopathy

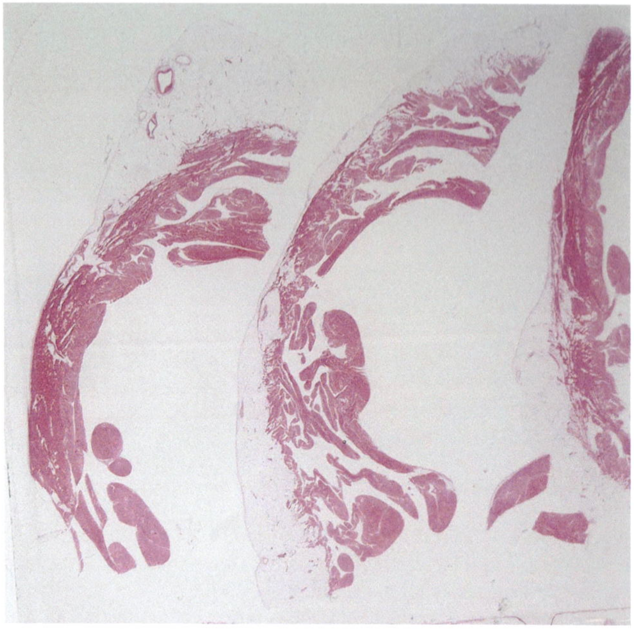

Fig. 4.180 Histological examination of the right ventricle tissues may confirm the presence of a large amount of fat. Without loss of muscular tissues and fibrosis, this should not be taken as indicating arrhythmogenic cardiomyopathy (ACM)

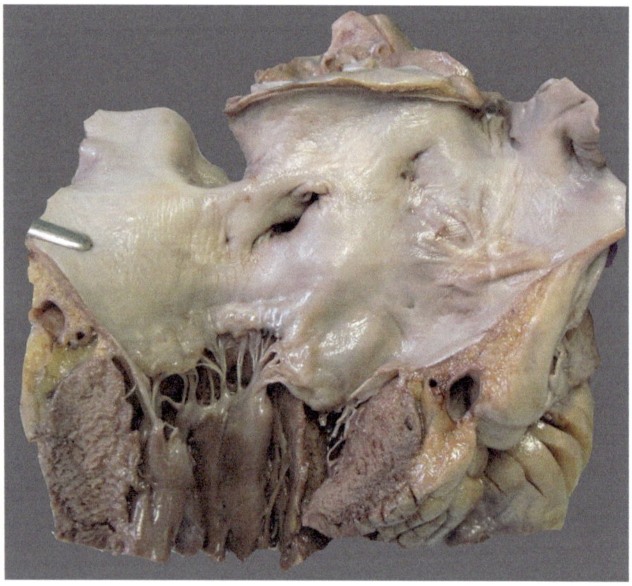

Fig. 4.181 The left atrial and upper left ventricular tissues are opened from the back in this view, with the mid and apical ventricular tissues having been removed beforehand by the three-slice technique. This view requires the orifices of the pulmonary veins to be opened at the atrium roof. Next, a cut passes from the right inferior vein orifice along the posterior wall of the left atrium, down across the mitral valve. The cut is extended down the back of the left ventricle (about 10 mm to the side of the posterior interventricular artery). The overall view shows that the left atrium is smooth compared with the right side. The auricle is usually smaller than that on the right side, but it can be inspected directly without further cuts being made. The left atrial view also shows the closed foramen ovale. The twin-leaflet mitral valve is thin, pliable, and attached to thin chordae and the papillary muscles

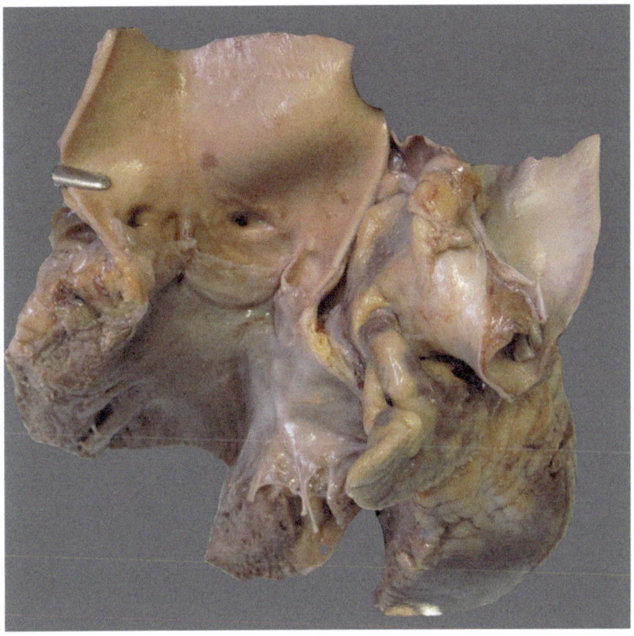

Fig. 4.182 Turning the heart onto the back allows one to run a cut alongside the course of the left anterior descending artery, up towards the bifurcation of the left main stem, into the left anterior descending and circumflex arteries. At this point, the cut turns inwards and towards the aortic root, passing transversely across the origin of the circumflex artery. In this view, the outflow tract of the left ventricle has been opened across the aortic valve. This shows that two cusps of the aortic valve are associated with coronary artery ostia. The third (noncoronary) cusp is seen to be positioned adjacent. The left ventricular outflow tract is notably smooth, as compared with the remainder of the trabeculated chamber. The left side trabeculations are generally finer than those on the right side. Note that there is no encroachment of the muscular part of the ventricular septum into the outflow canal

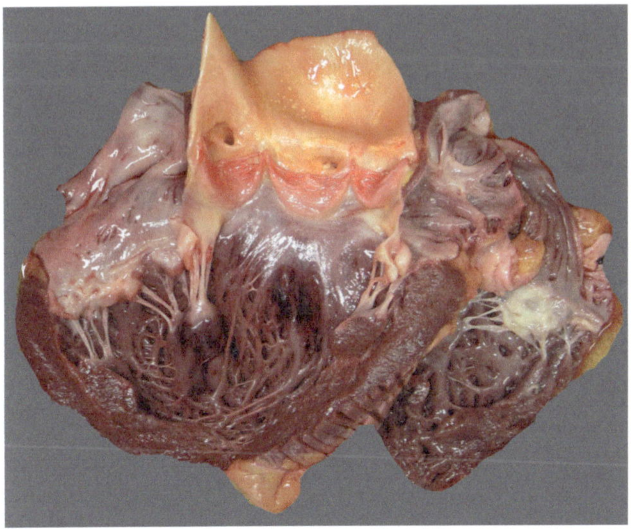

Fig. 4.183 The alternative opening of the tissues of the left ventricle is with a cut across the mitral valve and thereby into the aortic root. This cut naturally distorts the mitral valve by dividing it into two parts, but it is less complex than the cut passing alongside the left anterior descending artery, as described above. It may have some additional value in simplifying the cuts needed for the Fulton weights assessment (see Figs. 4.312 and 4.313)

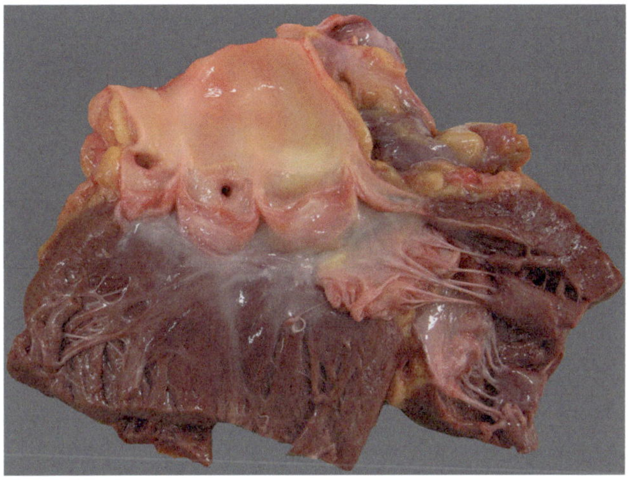

Fig. 4.184 The aortic root shows the normal coronary artery origins. There are three cusps: the left main stem, right coronary, and noncoronary cusps (from left to right). One should note the close arrangement of the aortic and mitral valve, explaining why disorders of one often affect the other. Note also how the chordae interact with the underside of the mitral valve, not just the edge. The ventricular trabeculations are finer than those of the right ventricle

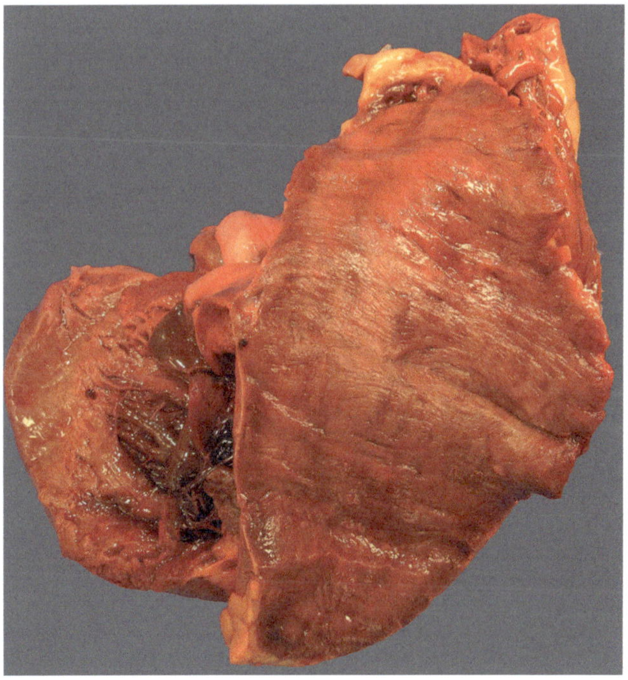

Fig. 4.185 Some practitioners slice the lateral wall and septum of the left ventricle along the midmural plane. This approach exposes a large amount of muscular tissue but distorts one's appreciation of the relationship of the wall and chambers. It is not recommended

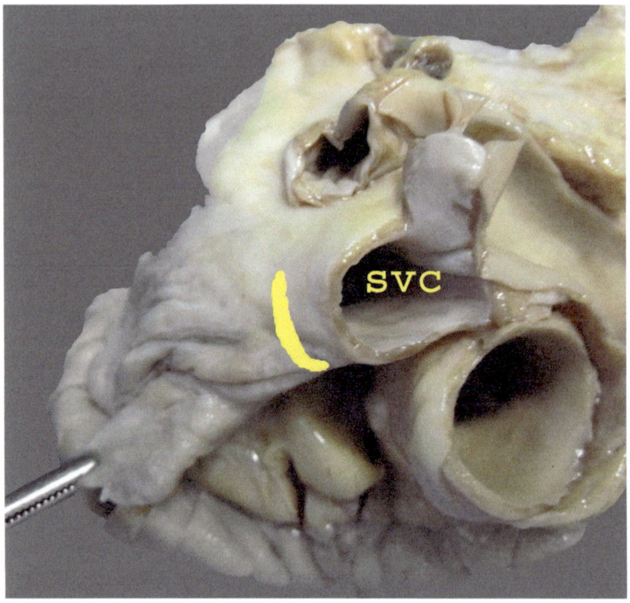

Fig. 4.186 The sinoatrial node is not apparent by naked eye inspection. With the heart seen from above the right atrium, its position (*yellow*) is found at the tip of the right atrium adjacent to the superior vena cava. (Reproduced from Suvarna SK, editor. The normal adult heart and methods of investigation, in Cardiac pathology: a guide to current practice. London: Springer-Verlag; 2013, with permission)

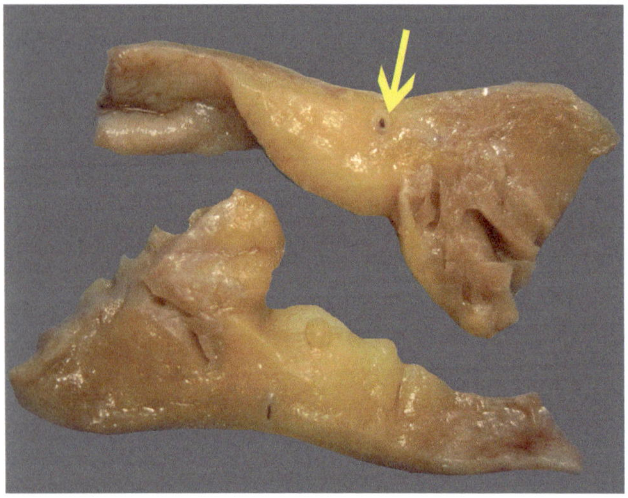

Fig. 4.187 A close-up view of the sectioned tissues at the top of the right atrium shows the small sinoatrial artery (*arrow*) at the interface between the atrial parenchyma and the superior vena cava. This is the landmark for the sinoatrial node, although the node itself cannot be discerned macroscopically

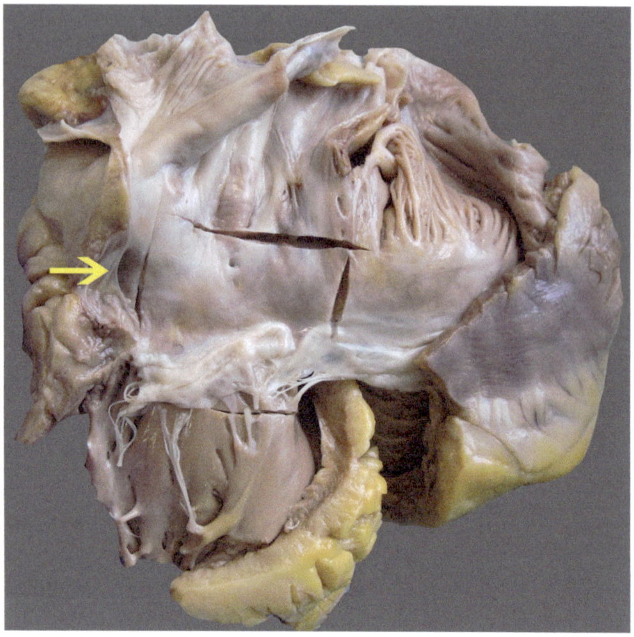

Fig. 4.188 For sampling of the atrio-ventricular node, a view of the right atrium and ventricle in a fixed heart is shown. The coronary sinus is seen immediately to the left of the view (*arrow*). Four superficial cuts have been made into the tissues, to define where one will then make deeper cuts. The deep cuts will allow removal of the centre of the heart parenchyma. The block of tissue will incorporate part of the tricuspid valve at the base, the membranous septum in the centre, and tissues from the atrium

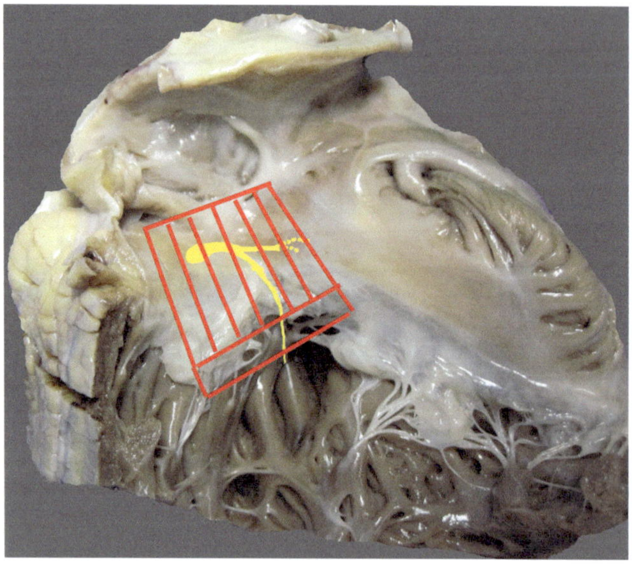

Fig. 4.189 Further sectioning of this square block of tissue involves initially removing a transverse slice from the base (*i.e.*, the septal tissues, with both the right and left side being evident). One then sections the remainder in a north-south direction, passing from the left to right side. Taking pieces at intervals of 2–3 mm allows the slices to go straight into cassettes. This protocol allows atrial, membranous septum and ventricular tissues to be assessed. It also allows histological evaluation of the atrioventricular node, the His bundle, and bundle branches. (Reproduced from Suvarna SK, editor. The normal adult heart and methods of investigation, in Cardiac pathology: a guide to current practice. London: Springer-Verlag; 2013, with permission)

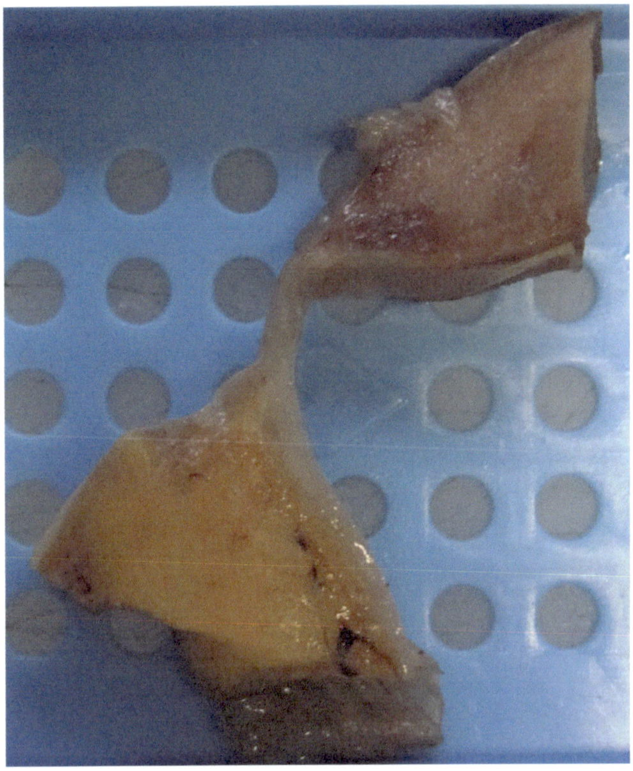

Fig. 4.190 As an illustration, one section of the atrioventricular node/His bundle system has been cut and placed in a cassette so that architectural integrity is maintained. The thin and pliable membranous septum spans between the fatty atrial tissues and the upper interventricular muscular parenchyma. It should be noted that the fat of the atrial septum (*lower left corner*) may be prominent, but it should not be confused with a lipoma or lipomatous hypertrophy of the septum, which usually shows a rounded tumour phenotype, as in Figs. 4.352 and 4.353

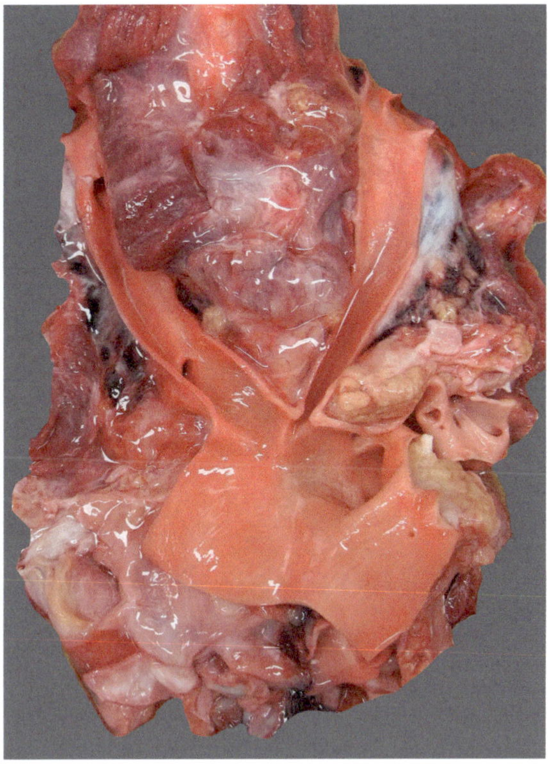

Fig. 4.191 The aortic arch has been opened, revealing the origin of the innominate artery, branching to the right subclavian and right common carotid artery. Next is the left common carotid artery, and beyond this is the origin of the left subclavian artery. Note the absence of atheroma

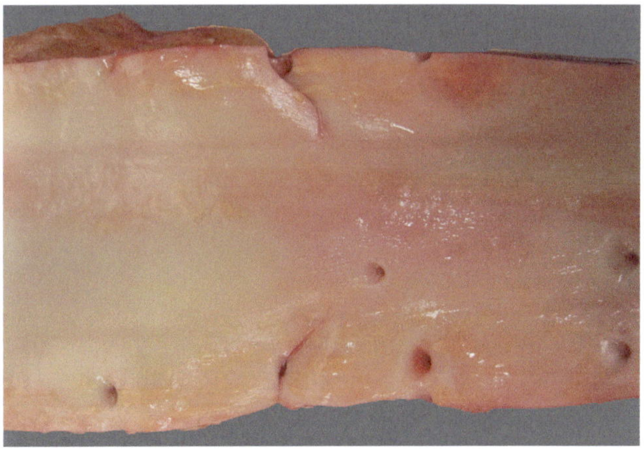

Fig. 4.192 The normal thoracic aorta is characterized by a smooth, yellow intimal aspect, patent arteries, and the absence of atheroma, dissection, or ulceration. This intimal appearance is normal for all major arteries

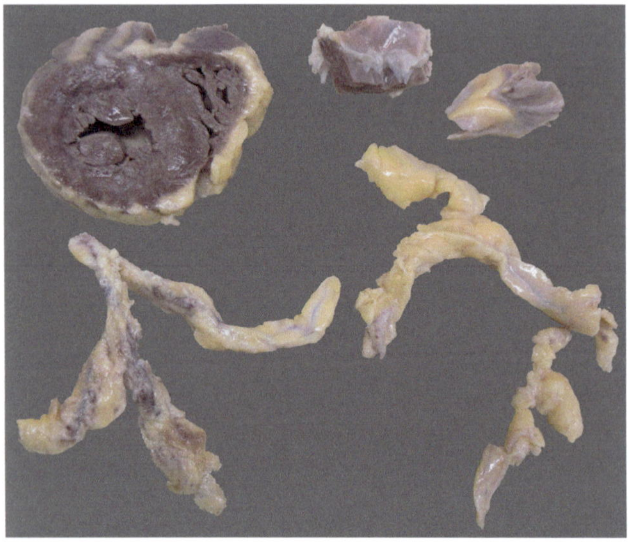

Fig. 4.193 There is often a balance required when retaining heart tissues for examination and considering the needs of the relatives. In this case, it was requested that the majority of the heart tissue was to be made available almost immediately following autopsy for burial purposes. It was agreed that the samples to be taken involved a transverse slice through the right and left ventricle including a septum, the main coronary arteries and the tissues around the atrioventricular node and sinoatrial node. This sampling protocol allows full assessment of coronary arteries, the myocardial tissue, the conduction pathway and indeed some reservation of tissue for possible electron microscopy and other tests

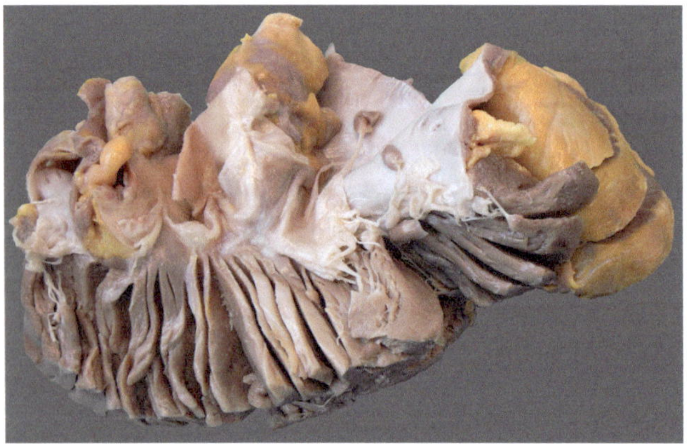

Fig. 4.194 Normally one expects cardiac tissues to be presented for review in the form of the transverse standard protocols given in most cardiac references. However, this does not prevent some pathologists indulging in quite unusual dissection patterns, as seen here. It is unclear whether this protocol has any particular benefit. It is clearly a situation which makes any subsequent assessment or review of the cardiac tissues very difficult

Ischaemic Heart Disease

Ischaemic heart disease (Figs. 4.195, 4.196, 4.197, 4.198, 4.199, 4.200, 4.201, 4.202, 4.203, 4.204, 4.205, 4.206, 4.207, 4.208, 4.209, 4.210, 4.211, 4.212, 4.213, 4.214, 4.215, 4.216, 4.217, 4.218, and 4.219), manifesting as coronary narrowing of varying degrees, possibly augmented by coronary thrombosis or dissection, is the primary player in terms of the cause of death in the developed world. Findings often can provide a cause of death just by macroscopy, but reservation of tissues for histology may also be relevant. Any devices placed for correction of arterial narrowings (*e.g.*, stents) should be assessed.

The impact of myocardial ischaemia is seen in the form of acute, subacute, and chronic myocardial infarction realities. Many of these have direct relevance to the cause of death, being potent drivers for cardiac dysrhythmias, as well as causing "pump failure". Sampling of these tissues may assist dating of the ischaemic events, but it must be recognised that modern therapeutics with revascularisation techniques and medicines does alter the basic pathophysiology of this natural disease.

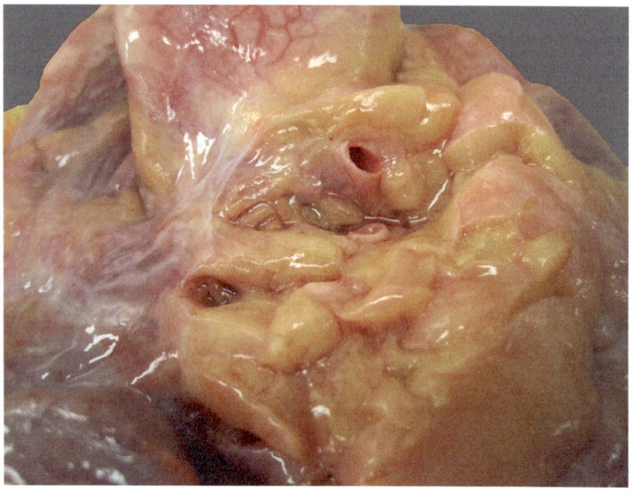

Fig. 4.195 This view of the proximal right coronary artery, next to the aorta, shows no appreciable atheromatous disease

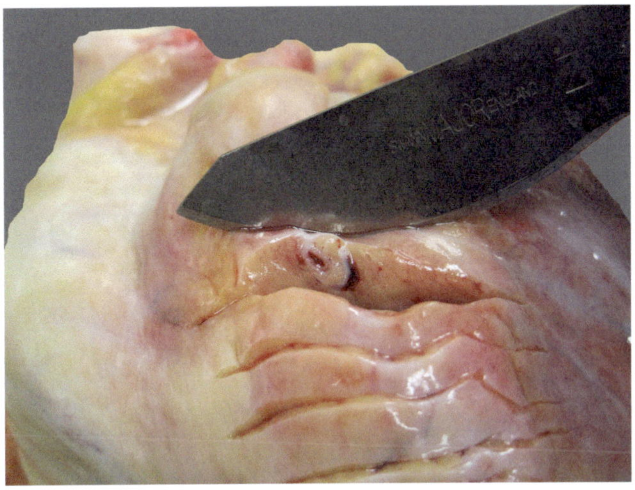

Fig. 4.196 The serially sectioned coronary vessels in most adults seen at autopsy have some atheromatous changes. As one progresses across the arterial tree with this slicing technique, it is important to examine the cut surface of the arteries and make a judgment about the degree of narrowing (reflecting low grade or high grade coronary artery disease)

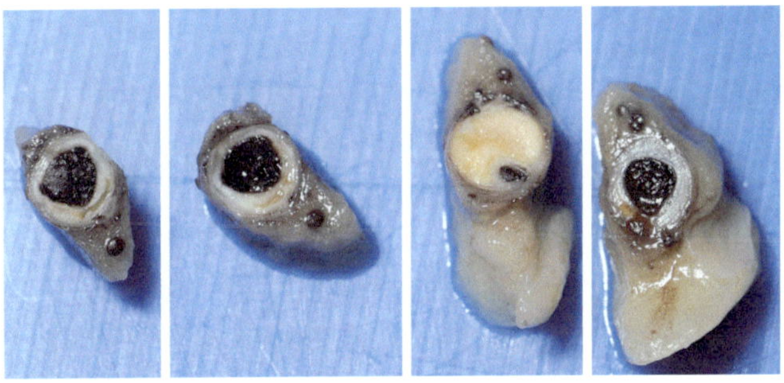

Fig. 4.197 Sequentially sliced coronary artery tissue often shows considerable variation in the degree of stenosis. This artery shows a focal, high-grade lesion with thrombotic change of an acute type in the segments adjacent

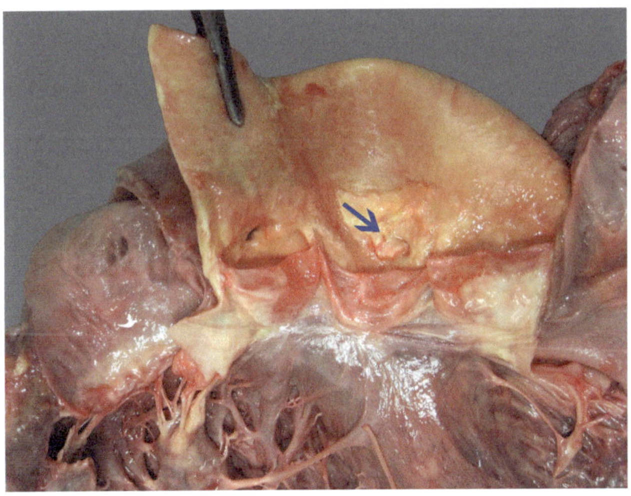

Fig. 4.198 The coronary arteries may have only mild or moderate disease in some cases of myocardial infarction. Review of the coronary ostia (in this case, the right coronary ostium) will occasionally point to the culprit lesion (atheromatous plaque, *arrow*) that has occluded blood flow along the entire length of the artery

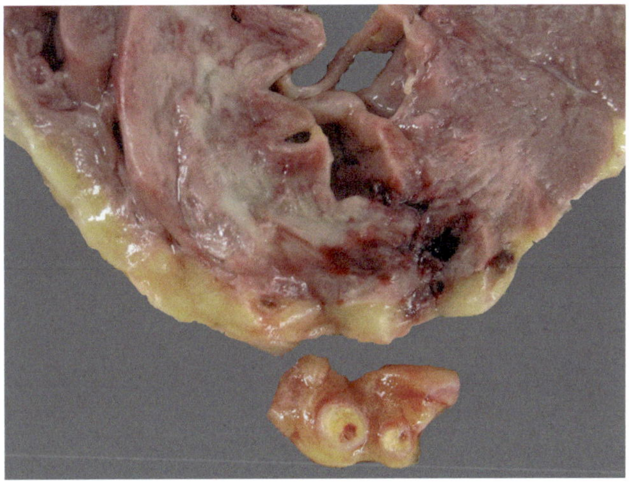

Fig. 4.199 High-grade coronary atheroma may be complicated by thrombosis. The consequence of thrombosis of main branches of the coronary artery is zonal myocardial infarction. This case of myocardial infarction was linked to the thrombosis of the left anterior descending artery, seen adjacent

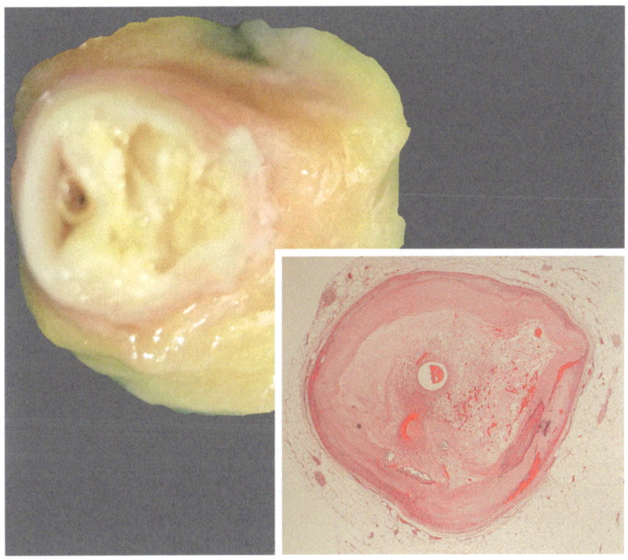

Fig. 4.200 High-grade stenosis (seen in histological and macroscopic views) is commonly encountered in cases of sudden death and clearly points to a causal link, but one should not forget that the individual had this degree of disease in the days and months beforehand, given the slow rate of disease progression. Histology of a high-grade stenosis lesion often provides the best understanding of the disease status

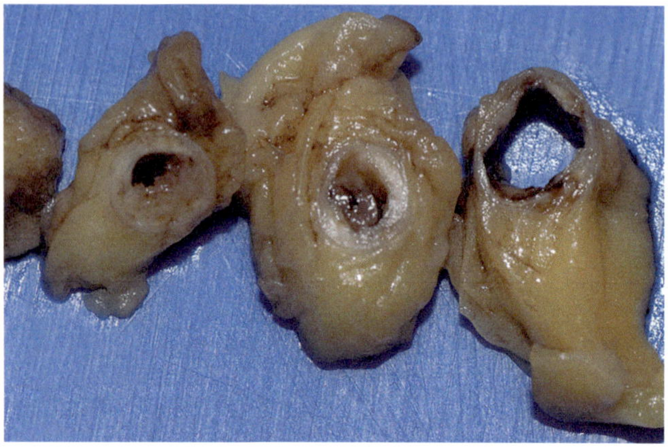

Fig. 4.201 Atheromatous disease may be complicated by thrombus that persists. It often has a grey-brown granular or solid quality. There may yet be a microscopic lumen through this area of narrowing, explaining why complete occlusion is not seen in the adjacent segments

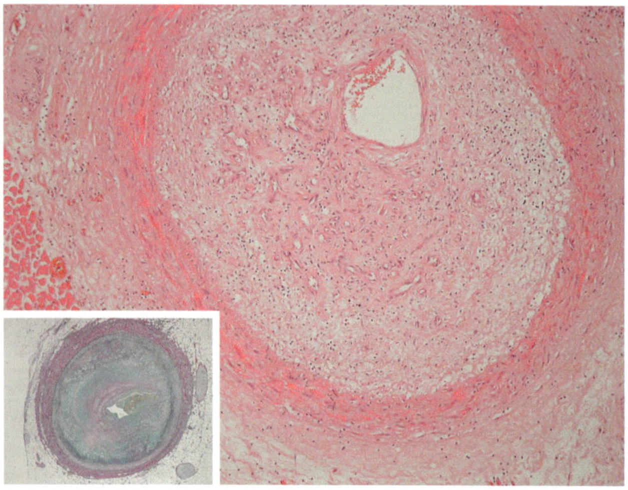

Fig. 4.202 Not all coronary narrowing is atheromatous. This case of myocardial ischaemic damage was caused by antibody-mediated rejection causing high-grade circumferential triple vessel narrowing of the arterial vasculature in a cardiac transplant. Abundant lymphoid cells need not be present. The standard histology can be augmented by a combined elastic van Gieson and Alcian blue stain (*bottom left*), highlighting the oedematous stromal background

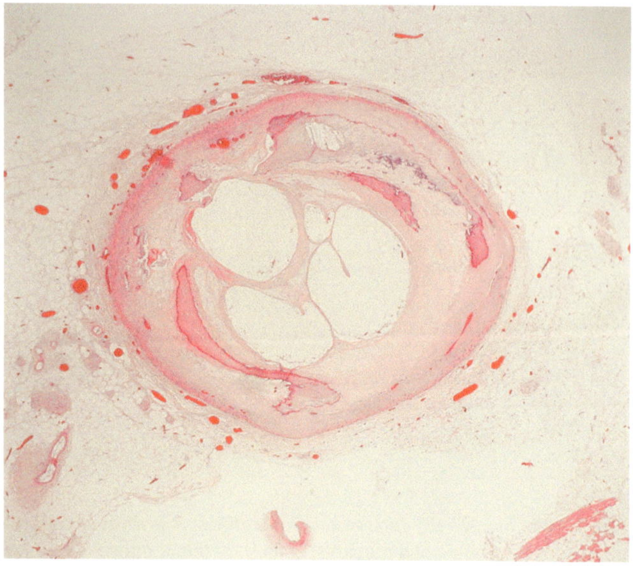

Fig. 4.203 Histological review of high-grade coronary artery disease confirms the presence of a recanalised artery lumen following a previous occlusive event

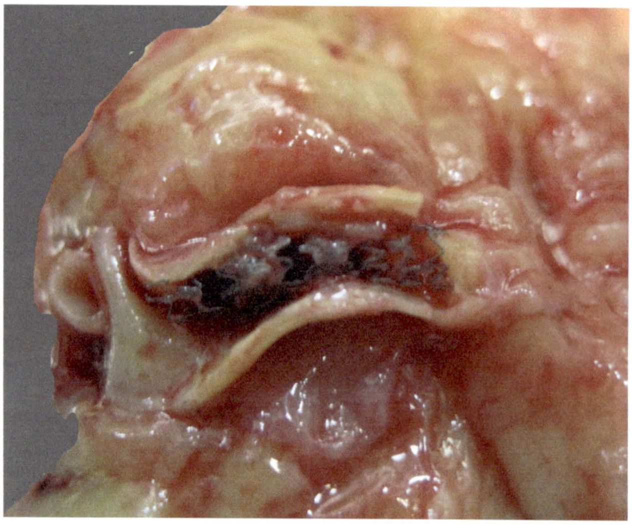

Fig. 4.204 Coronary artery stents can thrombose, particularly in the time immediately after implantation. This deroofed stent has no significant thrombus. This technique is good for demonstration purposes but is rather fiddly and is likely to damage the wire framework

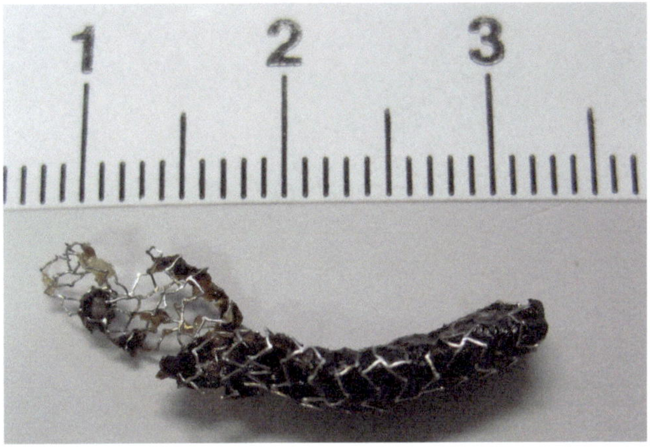

Fig. 4.205 Extraction of the stent in one piece allows confirmation of thrombus within the stent. An additional technique for assessing the stent sometimes is to pass fluid along the course of the coronary artery and confirm the lack of distal flow along the artery. (Reproduced from Suvarna SK, editor. The heart at autopsy, including radiological autopsy of the heart, in Cardiac pathology: a guide to current practice. London: Springer-Verlag; 2013, with permission)

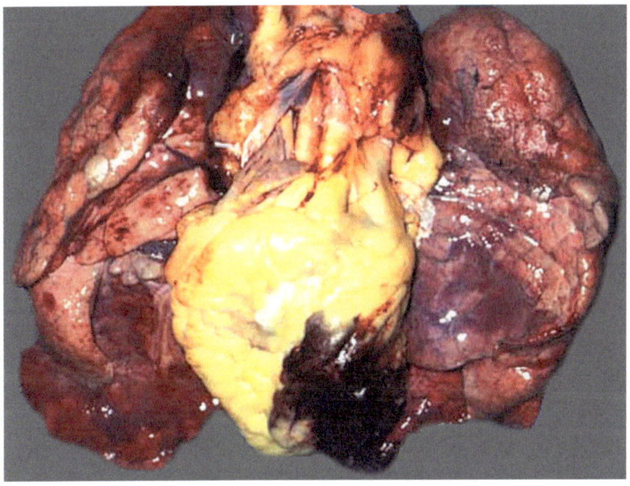

Fig. 4.206 Coronary stenting can cause rupture of the artery with secondary local haemorrhage and cardiac tamponade resulting in death. This case shows distal left anterior descending artery damage in a case of coronary artery disease stenting. (Reproduced from Suvarna SK, editor. The heart at autopsy, including radiological autopsy of the heart, in Cardiac pathology: a guide to current practice. London: Springer-Verlag; 2013, with permission)

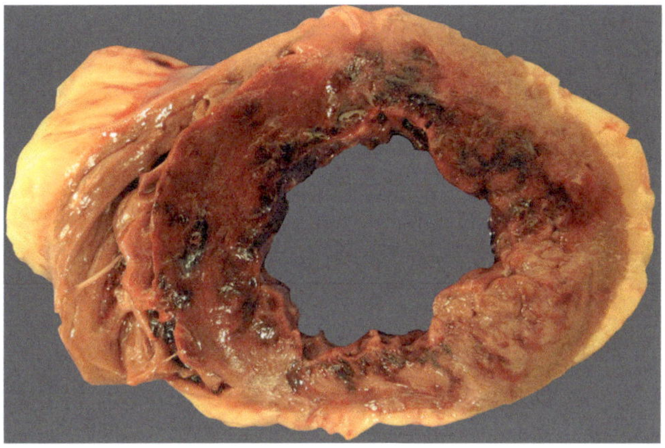

Fig. 4.207 Myocardial infarction is often zonal in distribution, representing just one coronary artery territory, but hypotension and widespread atheromatous disease tends to produce significant subendocardial infarction. In this case, the subendocardial infarction is almost global/circumferential. The demarcation between infarcted tissue and viable peripheral parenchyma is relatively easy to see but has been complicated by some haemorrhage, reflecting revascularization drug therapy. There is some chamber dilatation in keeping with cardiac failure

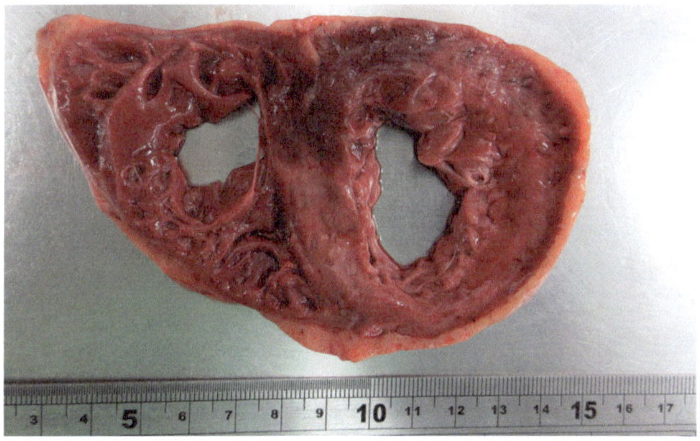

Fig. 4.208 This is a mid-ventricular transverse section of the right and left ventricle showing posterior infarction. The hyperemia (red/brown discolouration) noted in the posterior aspect of the interventricular septum, extending into the myocardium of the posterior left and right ventricle walls represents early myocardial infarction change (up to 48 h) and is indicative of right coronary artery occlusion

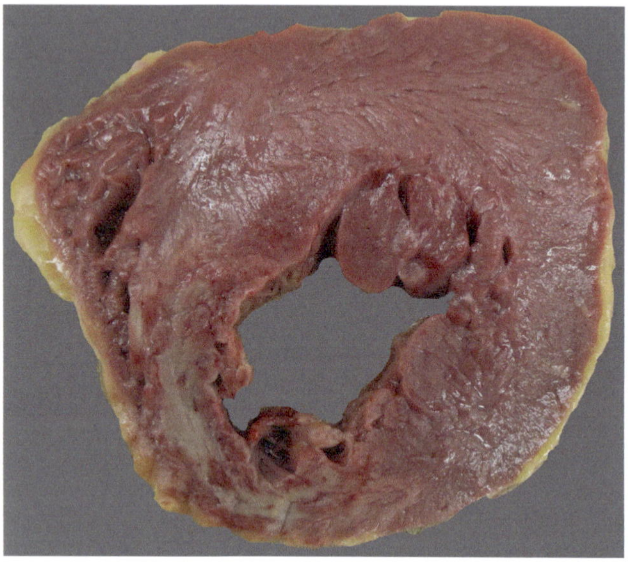

Fig. 4.209 This hypertrophied left ventricle has an anterior myocardial infarction visible. The yellow-grey discolouration indicates infarction 2–3 days prior to death. The anterior wall is thinned; this thinning may indicate previous (several months or more) infarction at this site

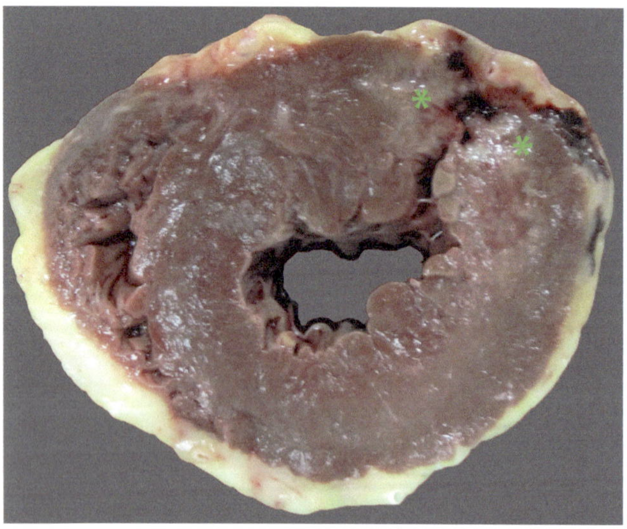

Fig. 4.210 Acute myocardial infarction of zonal type is capable of rupture after about 4–6 days, spilling blood into the pericardium (cardiac tamponade). At autopsy, this manifests as pale, necrotic tissue (*asterisks*) with a central haemorrhagic tract running through the ventricular wall

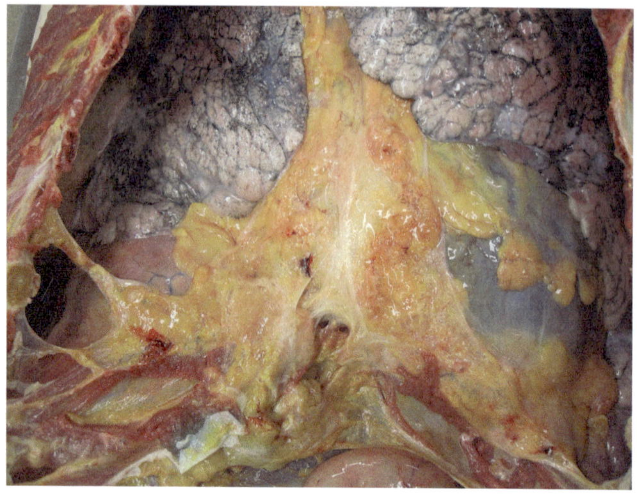

Fig. 4.211 A 'blue bag' in the case of acute cardiac tamponade. The pericardial sac is distended by a large amount of blood and clot. The features are evident after the chest wall has been removed at the start of evisceration

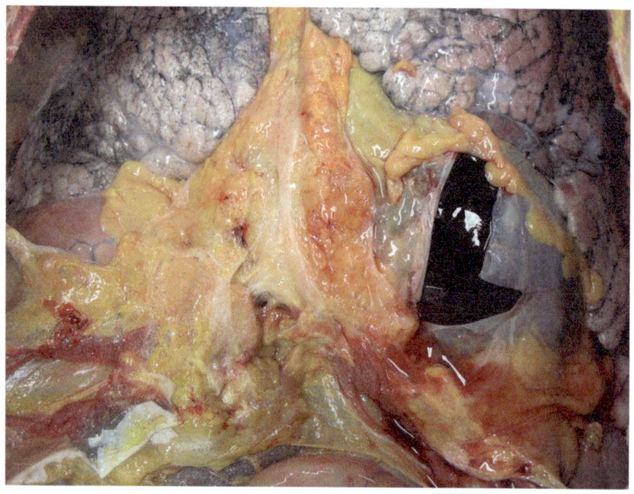

Fig. 4.212 The cardiac tamponade case has been opened to reveal the blood and clot that caused the tamponade surrounding the heart. The infarcted heart tissue is not visible until the blood and clot has been removed. The weight of the removed clot is recorded as part of the examination

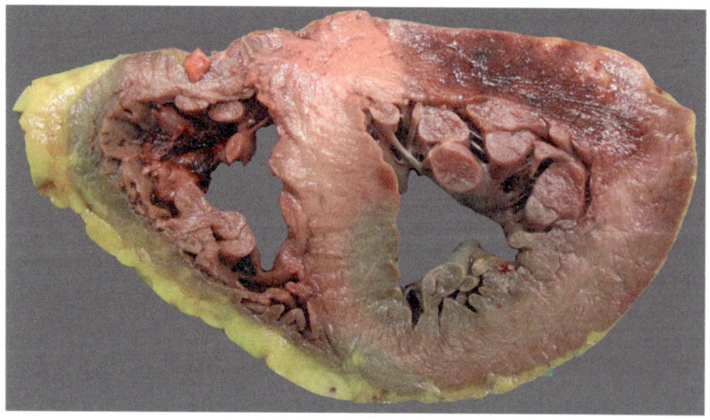

Fig. 4.213 Myocardial infarction is rarely left without treatment, commonly thrombolytic and/or other revascularization therapy. This therapy may cause secondary haemorrhage within the infarcted myocardium, as seen in the posterior left ventricle in this case

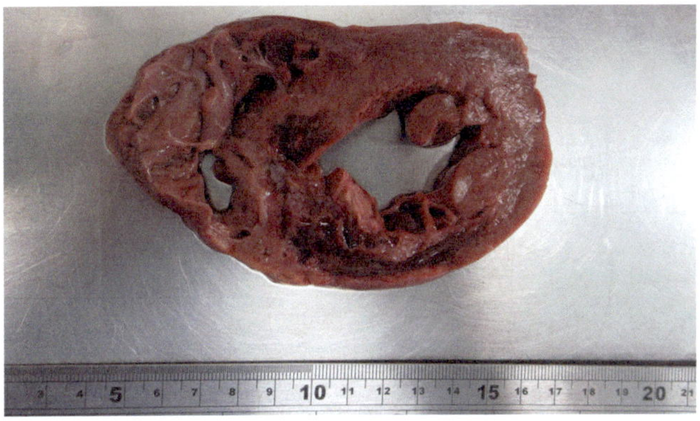

Fig. 4.214 Myocardial infarction is usually treated by modern medical therapy which restores blood flow and causes reperfusion injury in areas of previously undervascularised and hypoxic cardiac tissues. This is seen clinically as a poorly functional heart following the infarction and resuscitation procedures, and pathologically the heart tissue demonstrates extensive interstitial haemorrhage, myocyte loss and degenerative qualities of the surviving myocytes

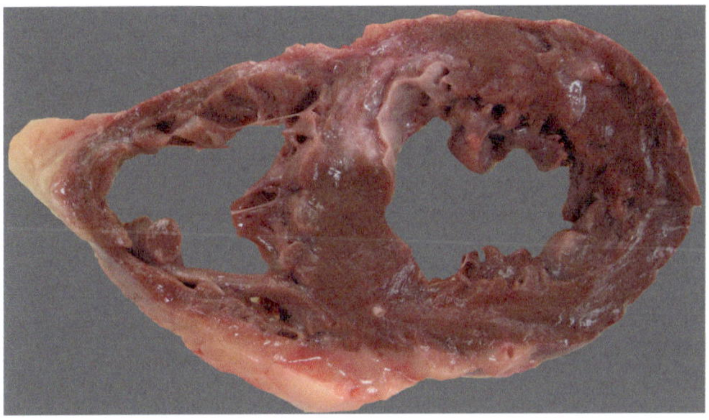

Fig. 4.215 Scarring fibrosis in the posterior septum and back wall of the left ventricle is indicative of previous (now healed) infarction damage

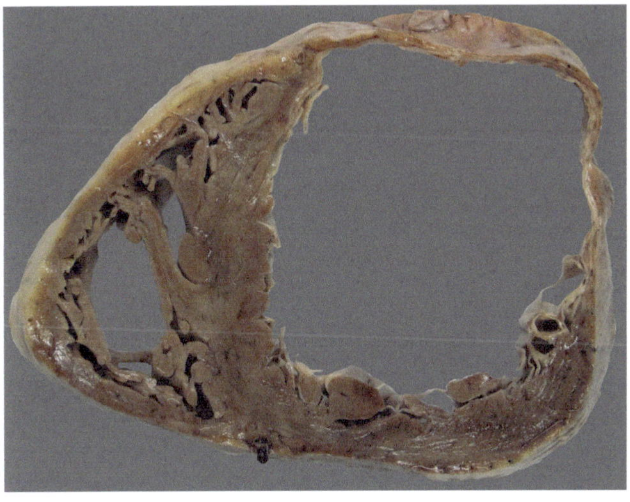

Fig. 4.216 Aneurysmal dilatation of the left ventricle is common in cases of extensive infarction. The secondary mural fibrosis and thinning allows the aneurysm to expand

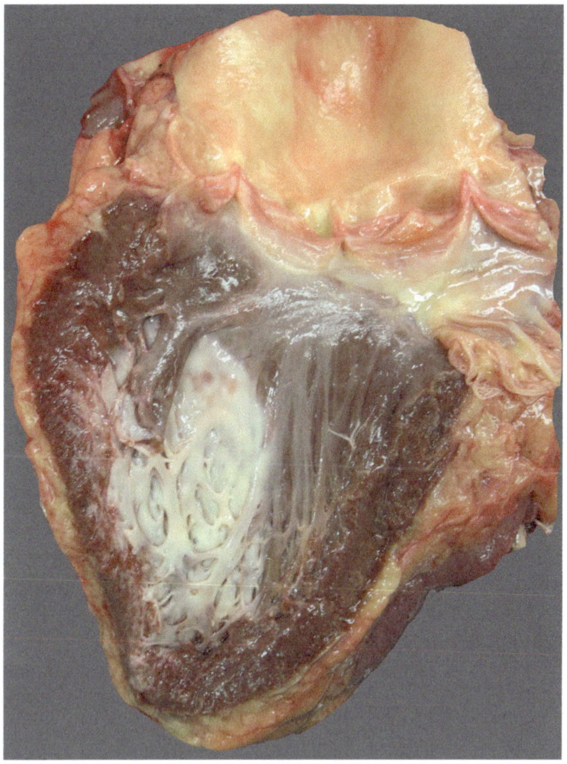

Fig. 4.217 A well-defined zone of infarction, with pronounced endocardial fibrosis, is seen in the low septal tissues. No acute changes are seen. This may cause a functional aneurysm bulging into the right ventricle or a risk for sudden dysrhythmic death

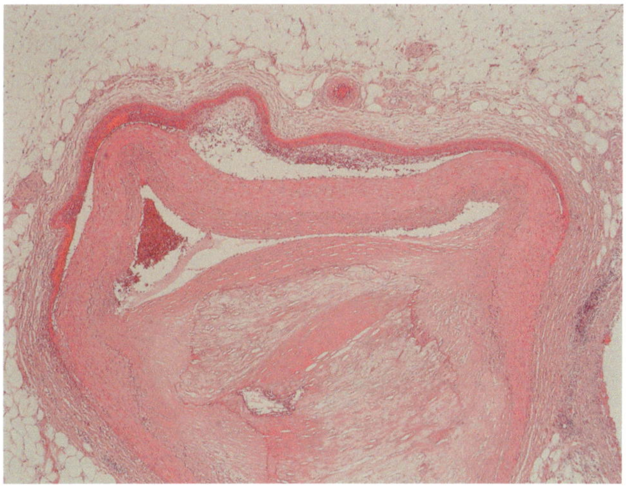

Fig. 4.218 Acute coronary occlusion may follow coronary dissection. Histology is helpful in confirming that the true lumen is occluded by the false lumen (running in the outer media), which fills with blood and blocks the normal luminal blood flow. Background atheromatous disease is present

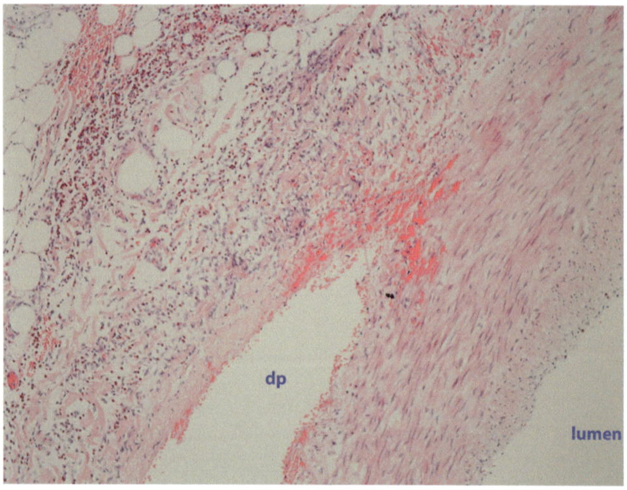

Fig. 4.219 Coronary artery dissection can occur as a consequence of localised vasculitis. This case had a pronounced eosinophilic component. The true lumen is seen in the bottom right of the image, with the dissection plane (*dp*) running across the tissue obliquely. There is some debate as to whether the eosinophils are a consequence of the dissecting artery or the cause for the dissection

Valvular Heart Disease

This group of disorders (Figs. 4.220, 4.221, 4.222, 4.223, 4.224, 4.225, 4.226, 4.227, 4.228, 4.229, 4.230, 4.231, 4.232, 4.233, 4.234, 4.235, 4.236, 4.237, 4.238, 4.239, 4.240, 4.241, 4.242, 4.243, 4.244, 4.245, 4.246, 4.247, 4.248, 4.249, 4.250, 4.251, 4.252, 4.253, 4.254, 4.255, 4.256, 4.257, 4.258, 4.259, 4.260, 4.261, 4.262, 4.263, 4.264, 4.265, 4.266, 4.267, 4.268, 4.269, 4.270, and 4.271) is principally degenerative in type, with associated stenosing and incompetent processes. Documentation of the ring circumferences of the valves may be of assistance alongside measurements of transverse chamber diameters and mural thicknesses. The presence of any thrombotic or septic process in relation to a valve is an important data item and likely pertinent to the cause of death.

Valve prostheses, both tissue and metal, are increasingly seen in autopsy practice. The same rules apply with regard to assessing valve function; careful inspection of the leaflet should be undertaken in order to test valve function. Any thrombus should be reserved for microbiology and histology to exclude sepsis.

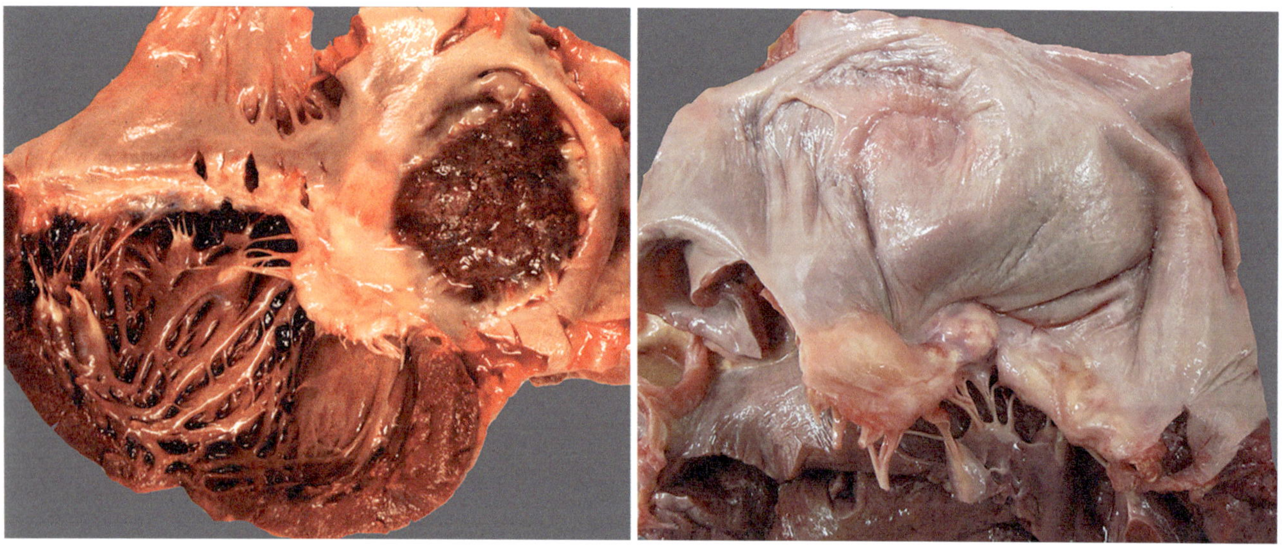

Fig. 4.220 Mitral valve stenosis can be difficult to define at autopsy. A particularly enlarged or ballooned left atrium (*right image*) often is supportive evidence for this process, but requires mapping to ante-mortem clinical data. A dilated atrium is often a potent driver for thrombosis associated with atrial fibrillation (*left image*) and a risk for systemic embolization

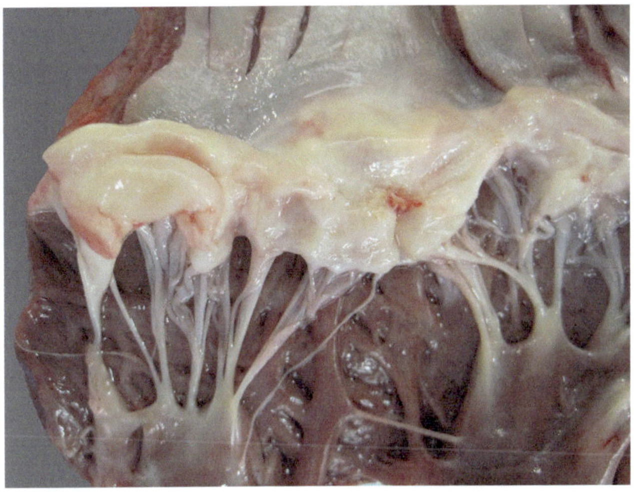

Fig. 4.221 A floppy mitral valve is seen. It demonstrates the thickened and mucoid quality of the valve tissue, with similar changes affecting the chordae tendineae

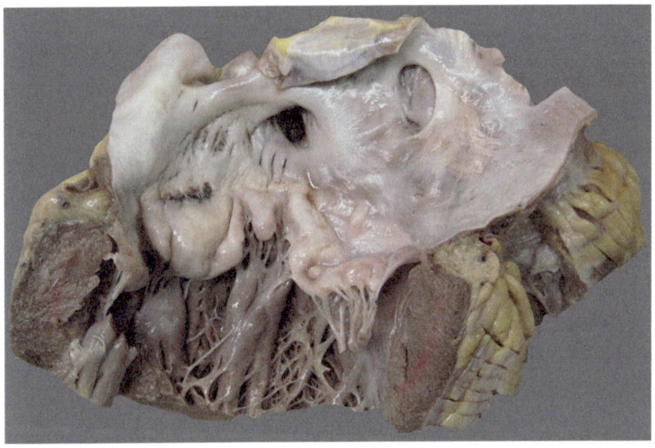

Fig. 4.222 A floppy mitral valve is seen with classic ballooning, 'parachute-type' deformity of the free margins

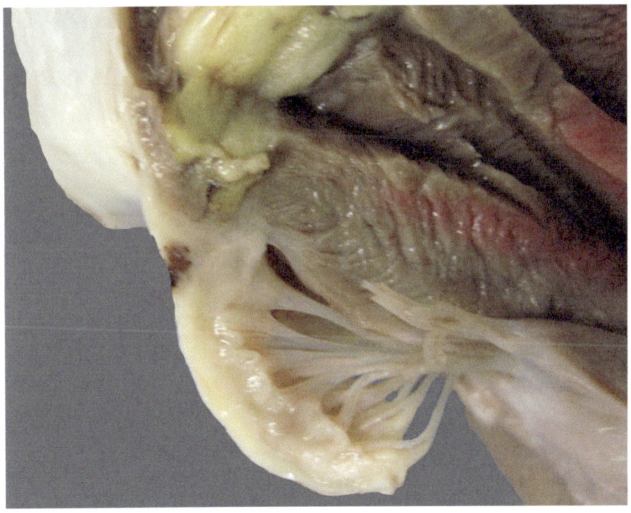

Fig. 4.223 Section through a markedly thickened and mucoid floppy valve. Note how the chordae extend from the free margin of the valve as well as from various points of attachment along the undersurfaces of the valve

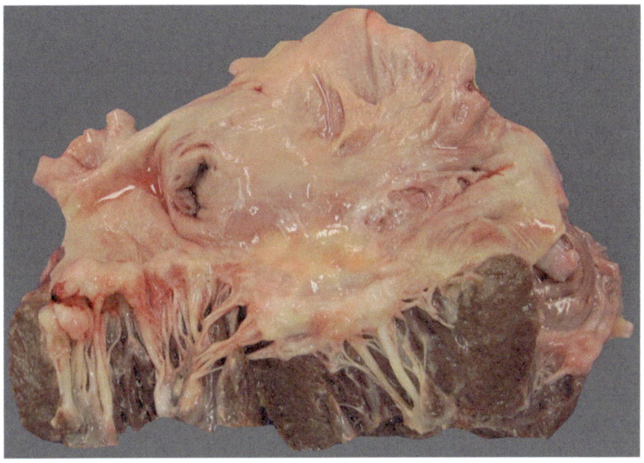

Fig. 4.224 Rheumatic mitral valve disease is still a common feature in the autopsy room. Thickening of the chordae and irregularity, distortion, and thickening of the valve cusps are common on the atrioventricular valves. Thickening and distortion of the semilunar valves in aortic and pulmonary roots also can be seen. It is important to consider whether there is a functional deficit of valve function in terms of opening and closure. One should also diligently search for features of infective endocarditis

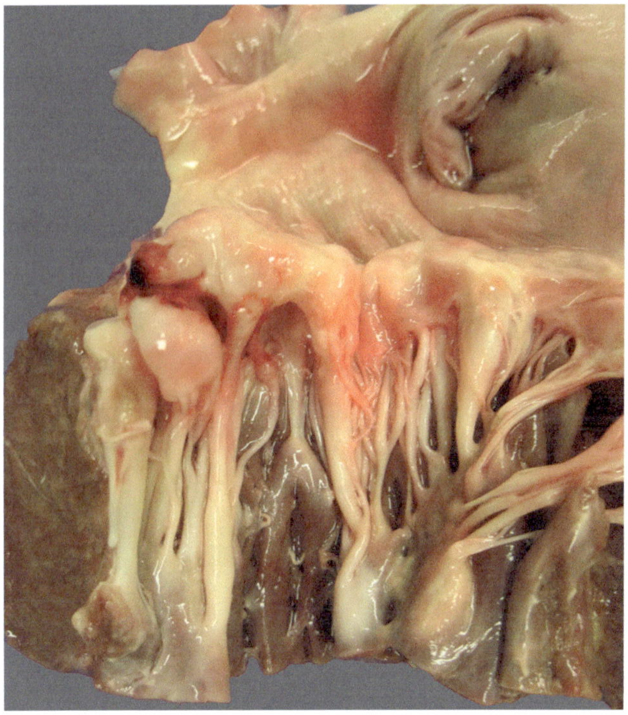

Fig. 4.225 Close-up magnification of the thickened chordae in a case of mitral valve stenosis secondary to rheumatic fever

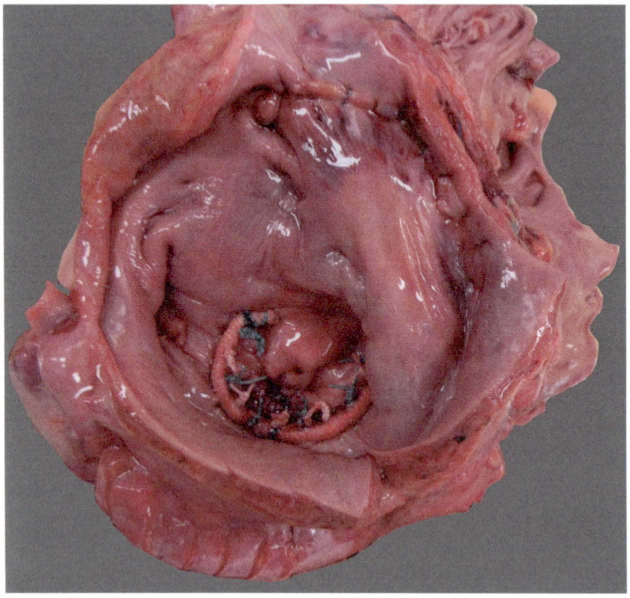

Fig. 4.226 This is an annuloplasty of the mitral valve showing the sutures holding the annuloplasty ring in position which have been tethered to the mitral valve tissues. There is no evidence of infective endocarditis

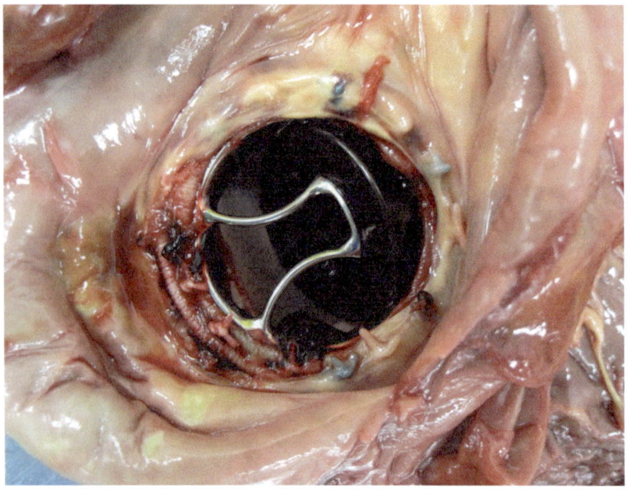

Fig. 4.227 In this case, mitral valve disease has been treated by metal valve replacement. The valve opens and closes with the central disc tilting back and forth. This type of device is no longer used but is still occasionally encountered in the autopsy room

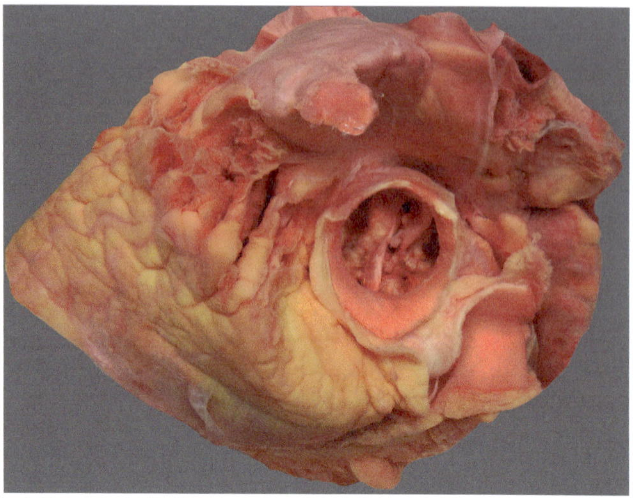

Fig. 4.228 The aortic root, seen from above, shows a tightly stenotic, bicuspid aortic valve. Nodular dystrophic calcification is present in the valve cusps. This case was photographed having been placed under water to aid and support the natural positioning of the cardiac tissues

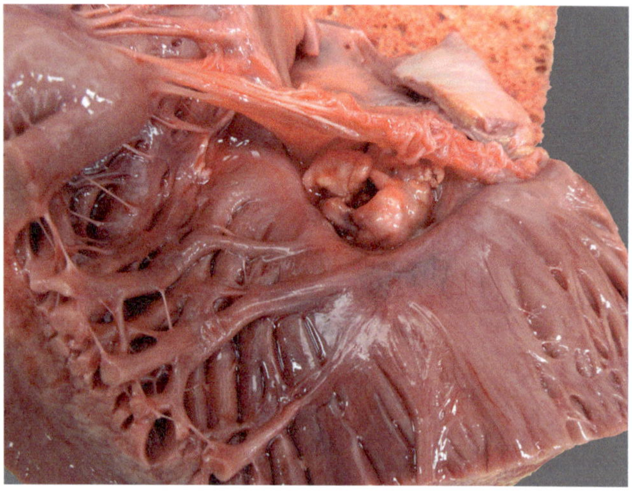

Fig. 4.229 This aortic valve dissection shows an irregular unicommissural architecture with heavy calcification and distortion. Note the mitral valve appears normal albeit stretched over the top of the aortic valve. No vegetations are present

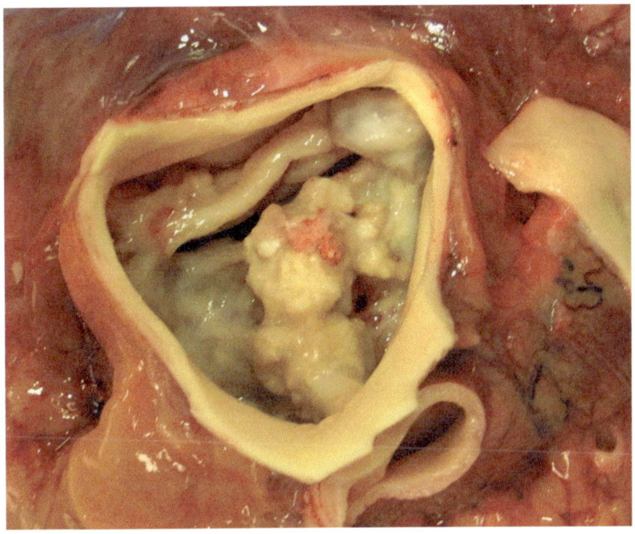

Fig. 4.230 A pseudobicuspid aortic valve is seen with heavy nodular calcification. One of the commissures is fused with nodular calcific deposits. The net result is tight occlusion of the valve orifice. No vegetations are seen on the valve tissue

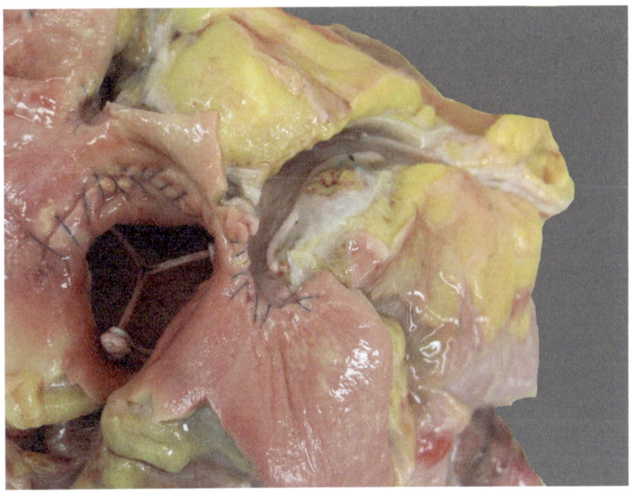

Fig. 4.231 Replacement of the calcified aortic valve has been accomplished by a tissue graft with vein bypass surgery. Exploring this reality at autopsy requires consideration of the surgery performed and then careful incisions to expose the operative solutions. The valve must be shown to be correctly positioned and without sepsis or thrombus. The vein graft should be free from thrombus. The suture lines from the surgery can also be inspected for leakage

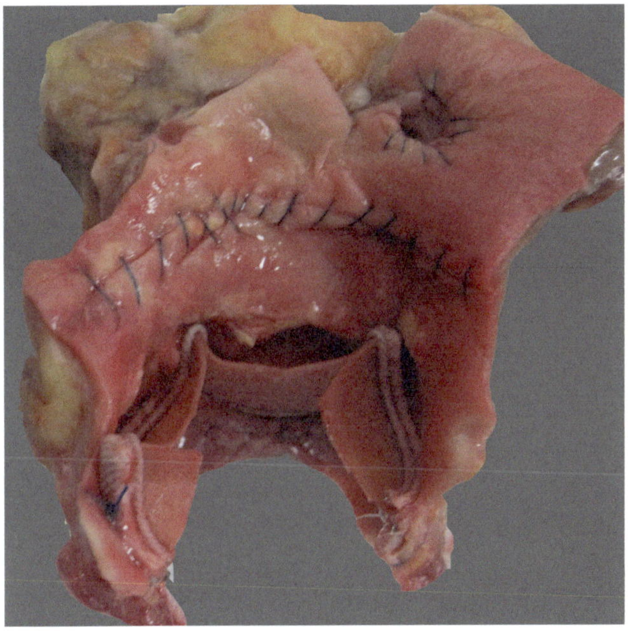

Fig. 4.232 The tissue graft has been removed, shown with local cardiac tissues. The valve ring is then cut open with metal pliers, as scissors will not be able to cut through the metal support rings. The valve is forced open to demonstrate the inner leaflets

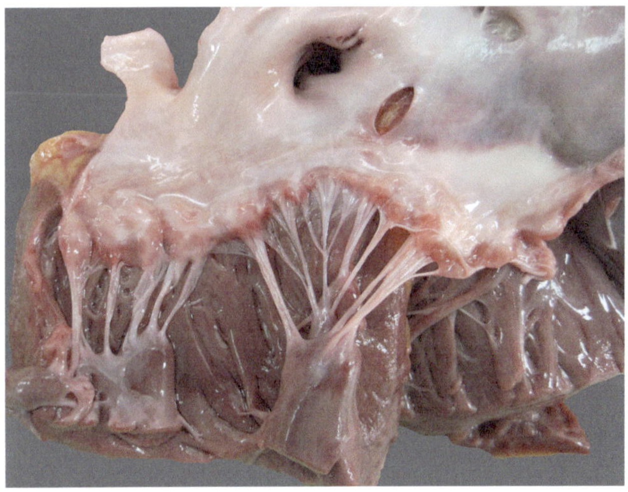

Fig. 4.233 Nonbacterial (noninfective) thrombotic endocarditis [NBTE] is often seen as a rather fleshy line of thrombotic matter at the free margin of the valves. It is not associated with valve tissue destruction and often appears to run in a complete ring around the mitral valve, as in this case. Note the preservation of the chordae. Histology and microbiology assessment to confirm the aseptic quality of the vegetations should follow

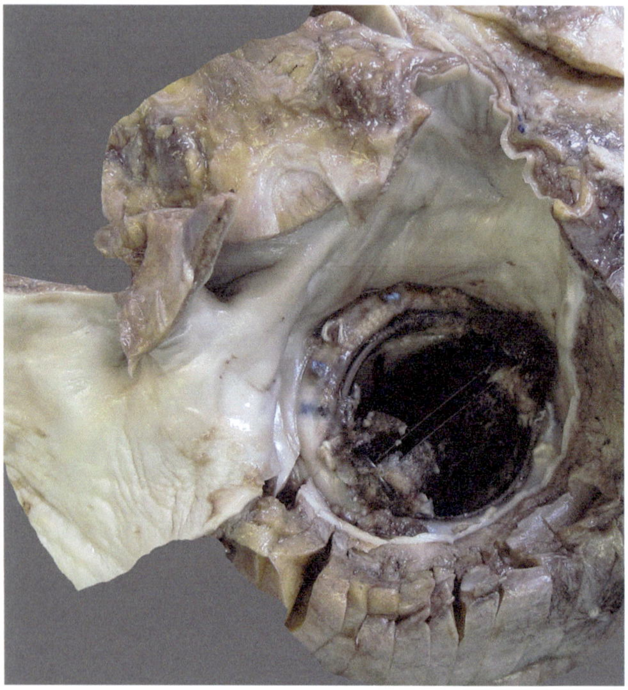

Fig. 4.234 A valve may show a marked degree of thrombus, often occluding valve leaflet excursion. Such tissues should be reserved for microbiological study and for histology in order to consider the possibility of infective endocarditis. This case proved to be streptococcal infective endocarditis

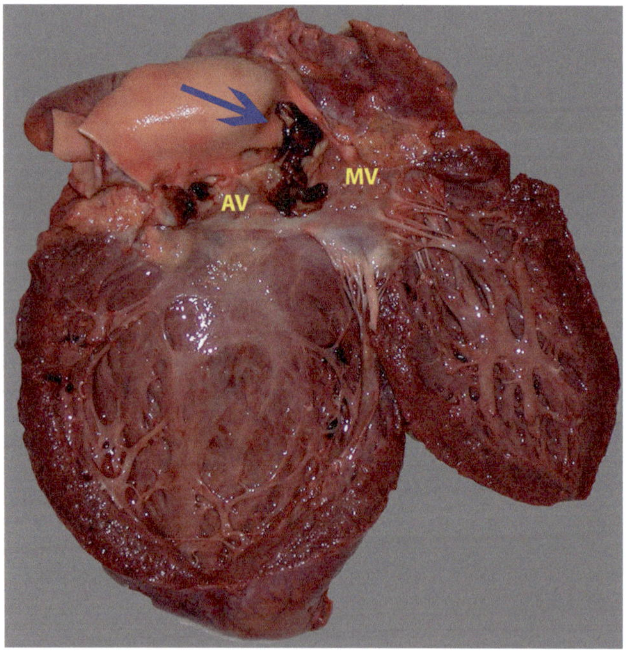

Fig. 4.235 Infective endocarditis (*arrow*) can involve any valve, although the mitral and aortic valves are most affected. This case of infective endocarditis reflected streptococcal sepsis, settling upon the aortic valve. No specific underlying valve defect was identified, but often the severe tissue destruction prevents accurate assessment of the possible drivers for infective endocarditis. Note the proximity of the aortic valve (*AV*) disease to the mitral valve (*MV*) parenchyma, explaining why dysfunction of two valves can occur readily

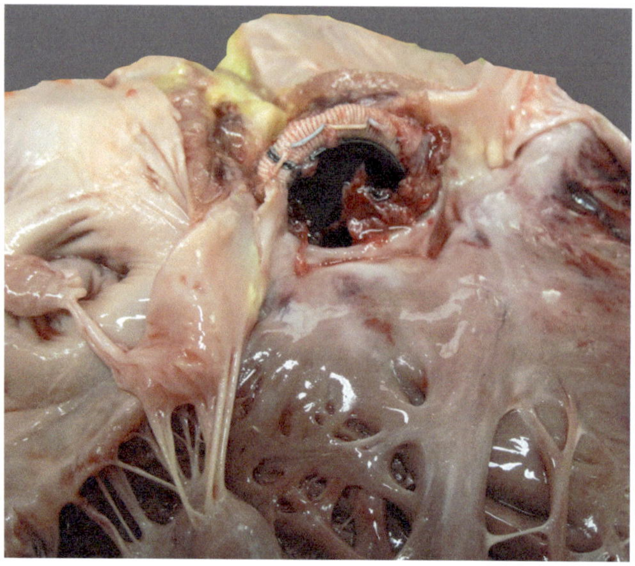

Fig. 4.236 A mitral valve prosthesis (twin-leaflet metal device) is seen with irregular vegetation around the rim of the valve and partially interacting with the valve mechanism. Histological identification of bacterial colonies confirmed infective endocarditis

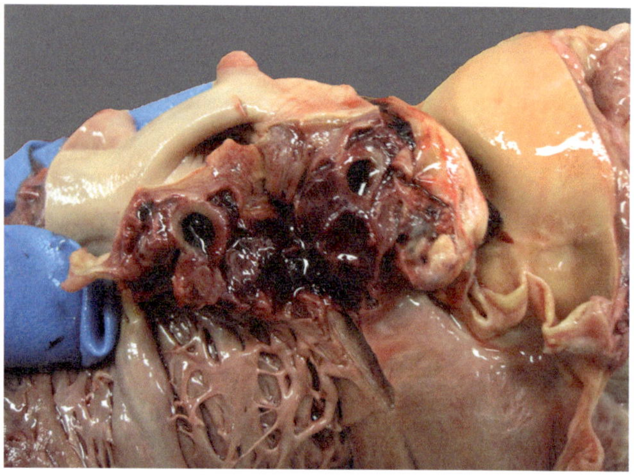

Fig. 4.237 The degree of tissue destruction in cases of infective endocarditis can be underappreciated when looking at the ventricular aspect of the valve. Slicing into the septic focus can expose significant haemorrhagic tissue destruction with cystic loculi, as in this case. Such tissue destruction often is associated with virulent bacteria, in this case staphylococci

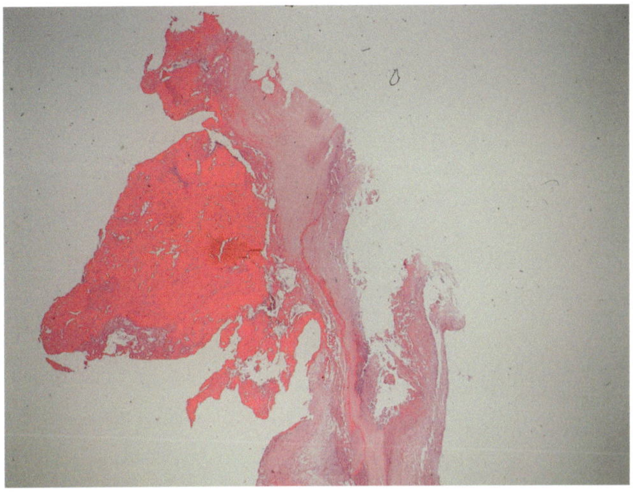

Fig. 4.238 Histology of infective endocarditis shows adherent thrombus and valve destruction

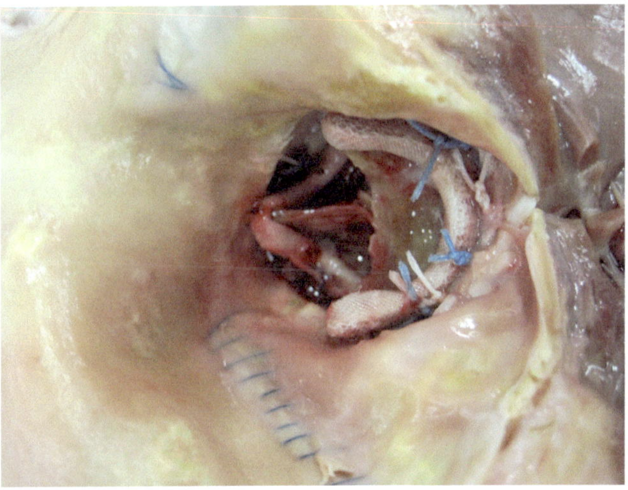

Fig. 4.239 One complication seen in tissue valve prostheses is that the leaflets degrade with time to become progressively less competent. These valves were thickened, discoloured, and partly fragmented

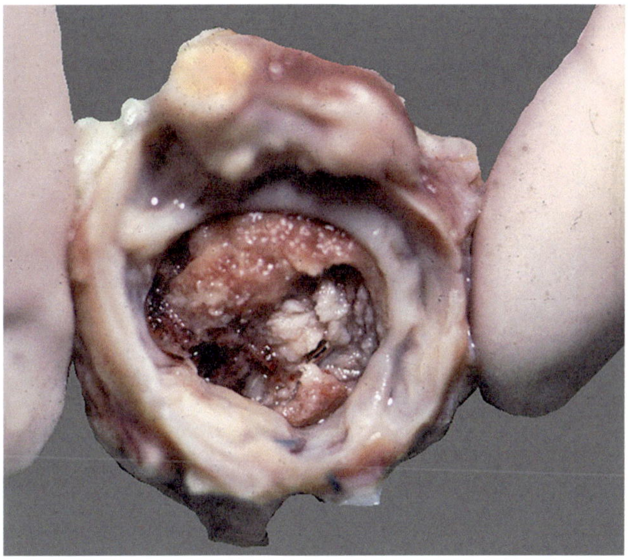

Fig. 4.240 Large amounts of thrombus forming on the valve prosthesis will occlude leaflet movement and put the individual at risk of infective endocarditis

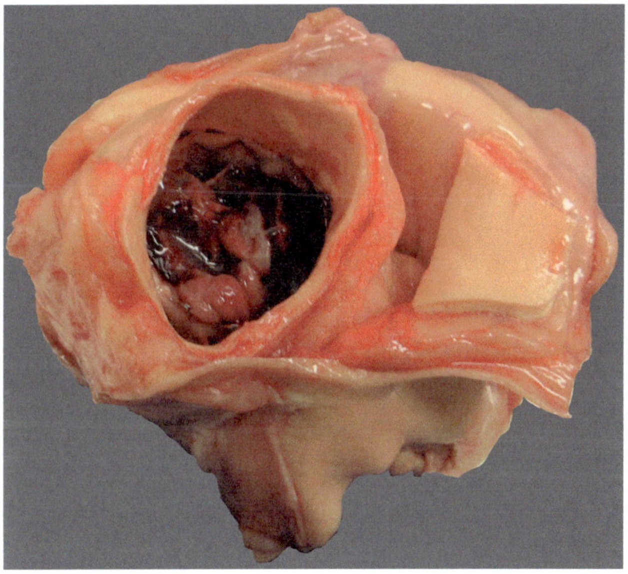

Fig. 4.241 This is a transcatheter aortic valve implantation (TAVI) valve procedure which has been complicated by dense haemorrhagic and thrombotic material occluding the valve leaflet movement. The case was confirmed as infective endocarditis by means of antemortem blood cultures

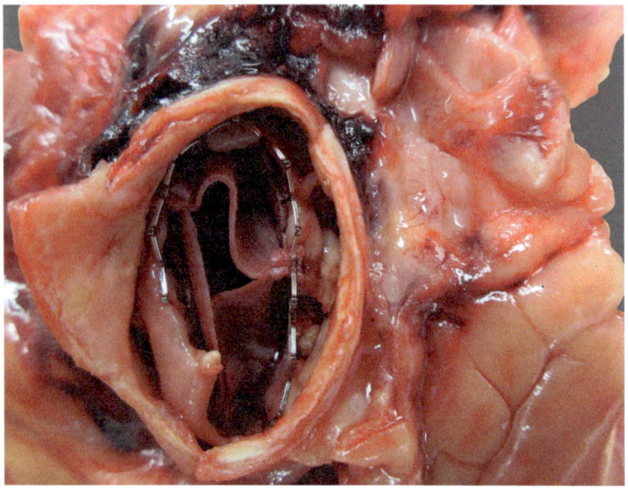

Fig. 4.242 This individual died during insertion/deployment of a TAVI device. The device is seen correctly positioned in terms of its location within the aortic root but clearly has not deployed fully. The extremely heavy calcification that was present at the aortic valve root prevented complete expansion of the metal frame

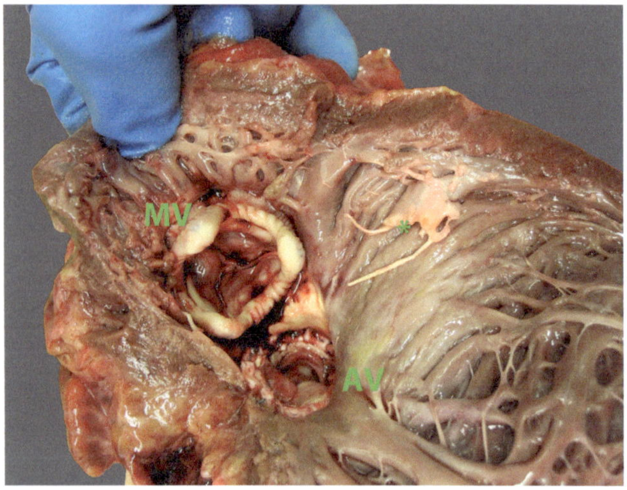

Fig. 4.243 Two tissue prostheses are seen replacing the mitral valve (*MV*) and aortic valve (*AV*). Both sides of the tissue prostheses can be seen in this view. Opening the ventricular tissues is hampered by the prostheses, blocking cuts made in the standard perpendicular fashion across the valves. One alternative is to cut around the ventricle at a high level and open the tissues outwards. This allows direct visualization of the valves and their movement (in effect looking upwards). Residual mitral valve chordal and papillary muscle elements (*asterisk*) are present

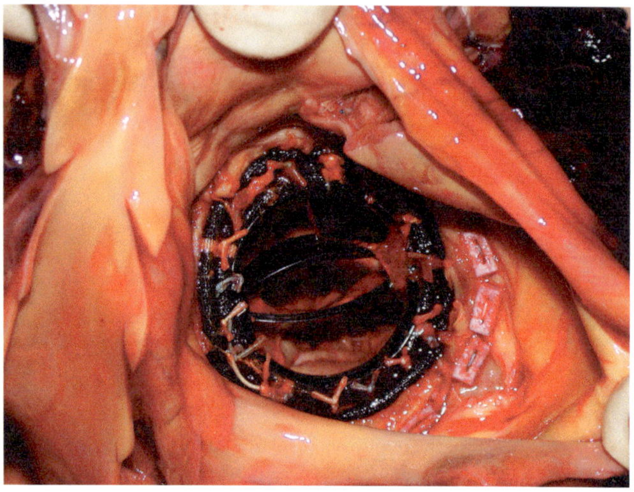

Fig. 4.244 The valve replacement here is a twin-leaflet tilting device. At autopsy, the leaflets should be checked to see if they open and close normally. As always, check for infective endocarditis and/or thrombus

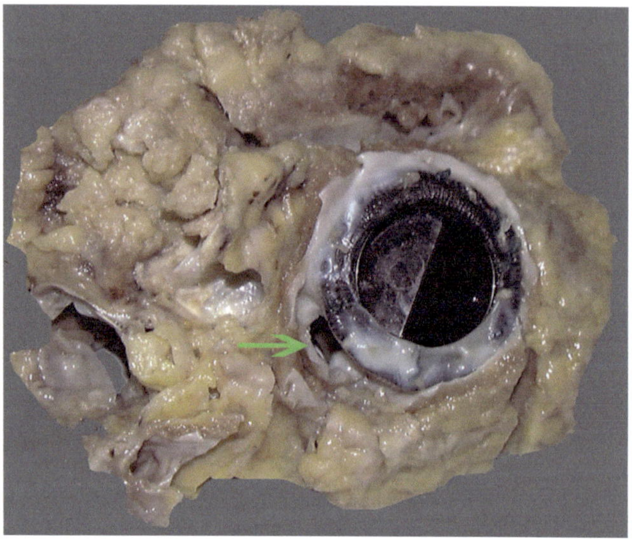

Fig. 4.245 Demonstration of paravalvular leak is often difficult in the autopsy room, particularly as the valve tissues are often fibrosed within somewhat distorted tissues. In this case, the entirety of the left atrium has been dissected free, exposing the mitral valve prosthesis and a leakage point (*arrow*) causing valvular inefficiency

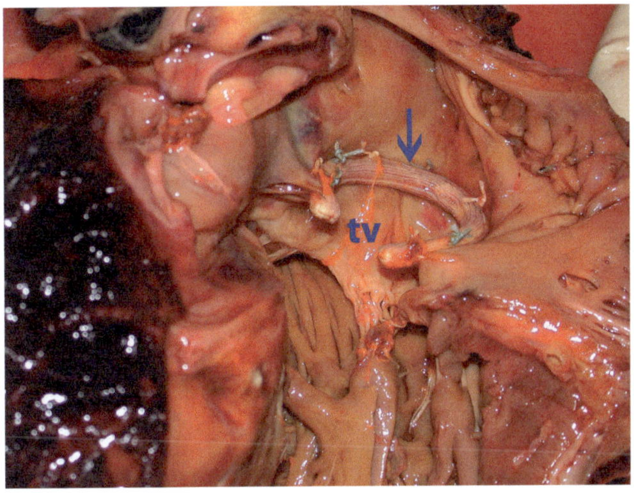

Fig. 4.246 The right atrium and ventricle have been opened from the posterior aspect to reveal a C-shaped annuloplasty device (*arrow*) at the root of the tricuspid valve (*tv*). The incompetent valve has been assisted to close normally, with the annuloplasty drawing the valve ring inwards. (Adapted with permission from Suvarna SK. National guidelines for adult autopsy cardiac dissection and diagnosis-are they achievable? A personal view. Histopathology. 2008;53:97–112)

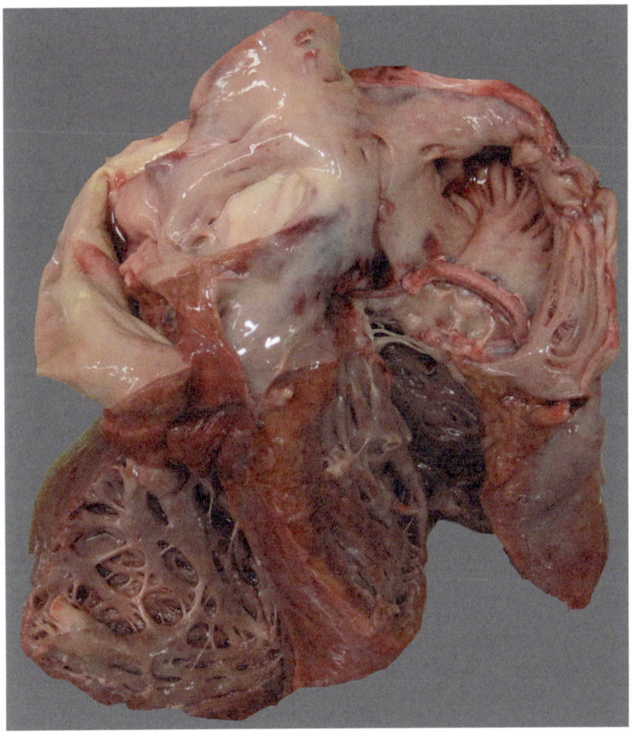

Fig. 4.247 Another annuloplasty is seen with local septal haemorrhage. This patient had also undergone a mitral valve replacement, which was accomplished by a transeptal approach

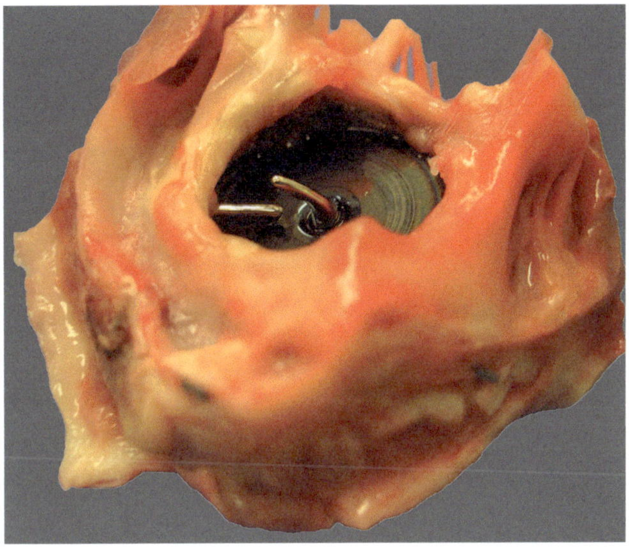

Fig. 4.248 Pannus is a fibrous tissue overgrowth that runs from the local paravalvular soft tissues onto the surface of the valve mechanism. If significant, it can partially or largely obstruct valve function and cause progressive cardiac failure

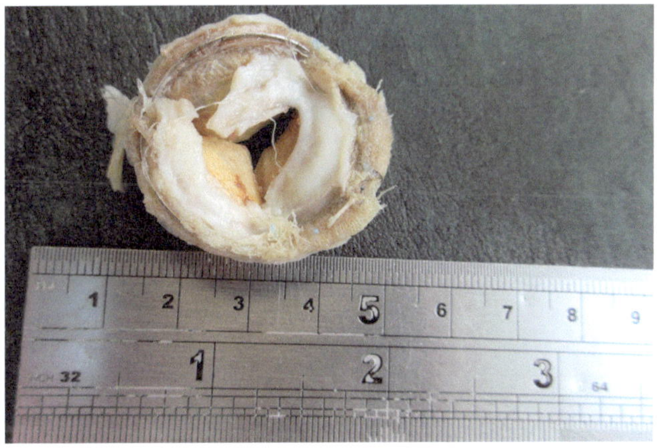

Fig. 4.249 Dense pannus is seen around the inner aspect of the aortic valve implant. It is partially occluding the orifice but was not complicated by infection

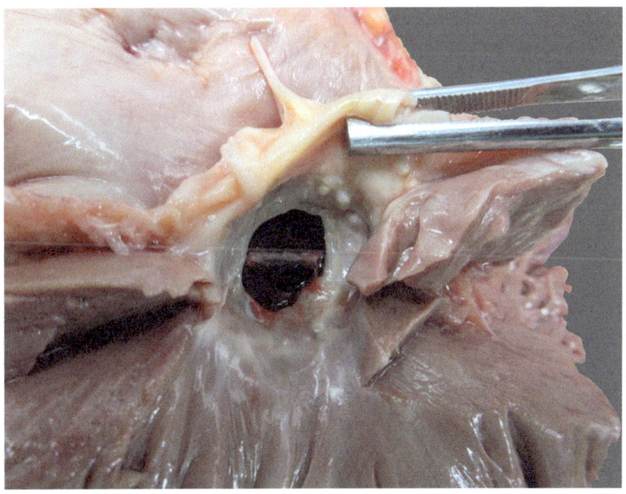

Fig. 4.250 Dense pannus is seen largely occluding the orifice of this aortic valve metal leaflet device. No infection was present

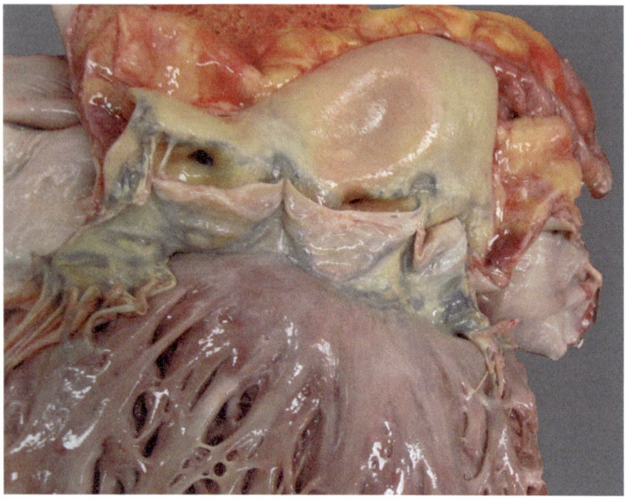

Fig. 4.251 Discoloured aortic valve tissues are seen in a case of ochronosis. The impact on valve function generally is minimal

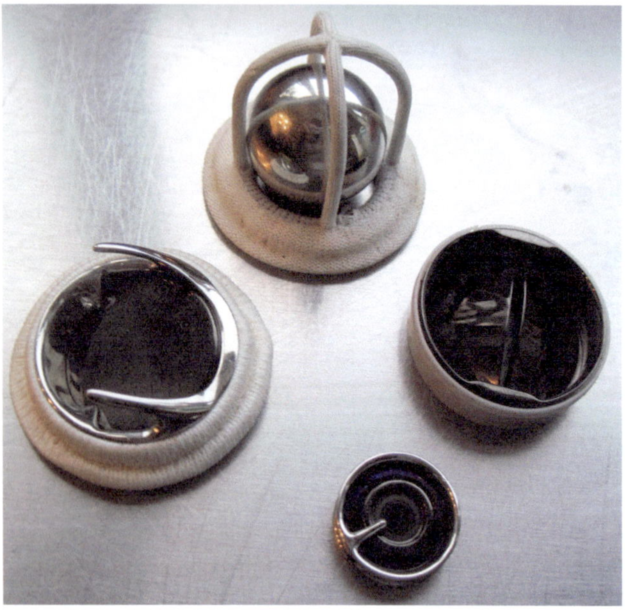

Fig. 4.252 A selection of metal cardiac valves, showing different designs over the years. The early types were ball-in-cage devices (*top*), which were associated with red cell haemolysis and thrombotic issues. Several tilting-disk devices are also shown (*left* and *bottom*). The favoured type of metal device (*right*) has twin metal leaflets set within a metal frame

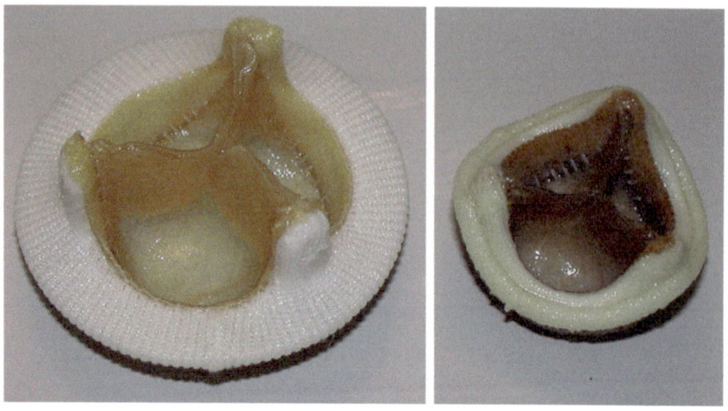

Fig. 4.253 Two tissue prostheses of different sizes are shown here. The tissue valve prosthesis generally comprises a plastic/fabric ring and strut mechanism, which allows the xenograft or homograft tissue valve to be hung on the support

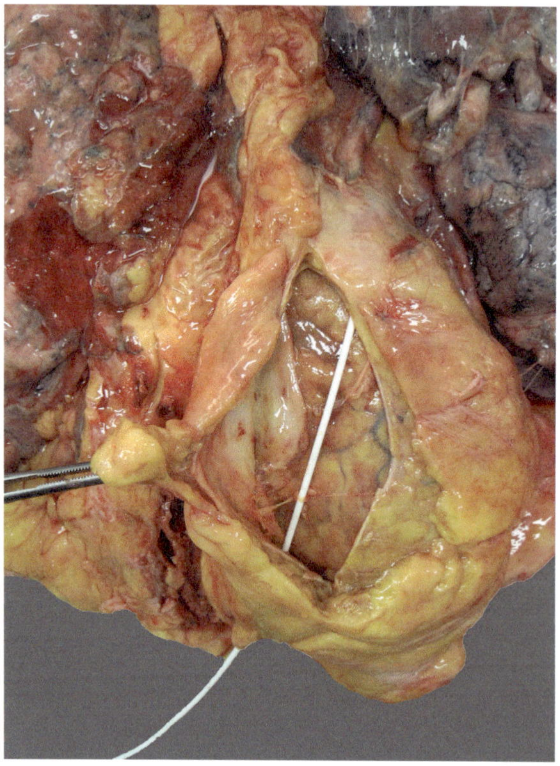

Fig. 4.254 The following set of images details the examination of a postoperative case (coronary bypass surgery and aortic valve surgery), in which the surgery complicates the tissue analysis. Part of the dissection will inevitably be altered, but part follows the usual dissection protocol. At the start, dissection of the pericardium demonstrates a correctly positioned pericardiocentesis drain, without damage to the underlying myocardium

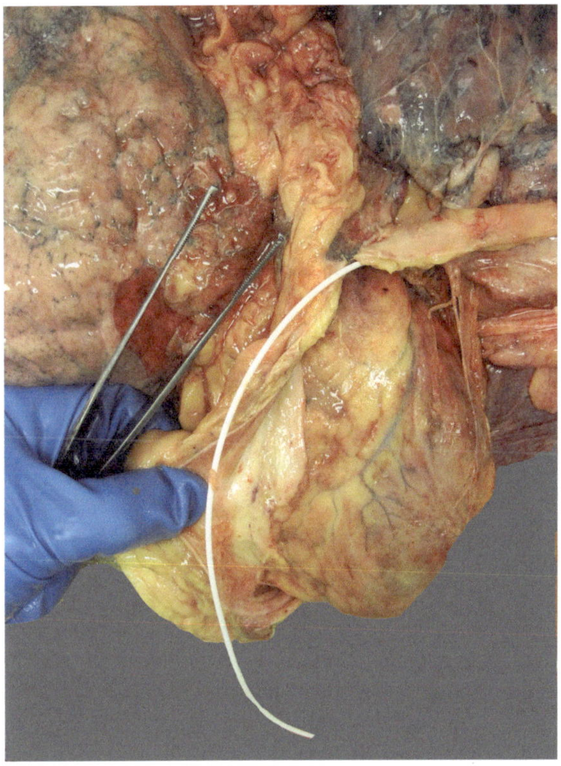

Fig. 4.255 The pericardial tissues are dissected free of the specimen

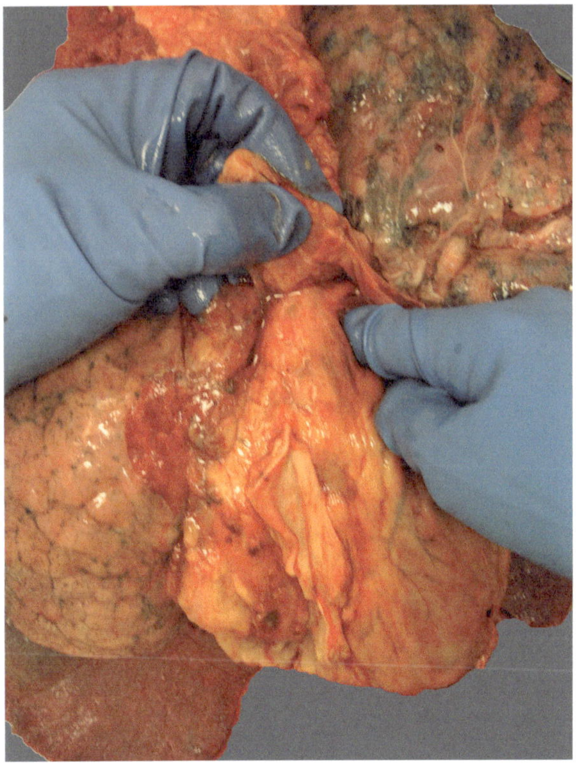

Fig. 4.256 The pulmonary artery is incised, and fingertip palpation for pulmonary embolism follows. This procedure may be complicated by the nature of the cardiac surgery, which prevents easy manipulation of the large vessels and upper heart tissues

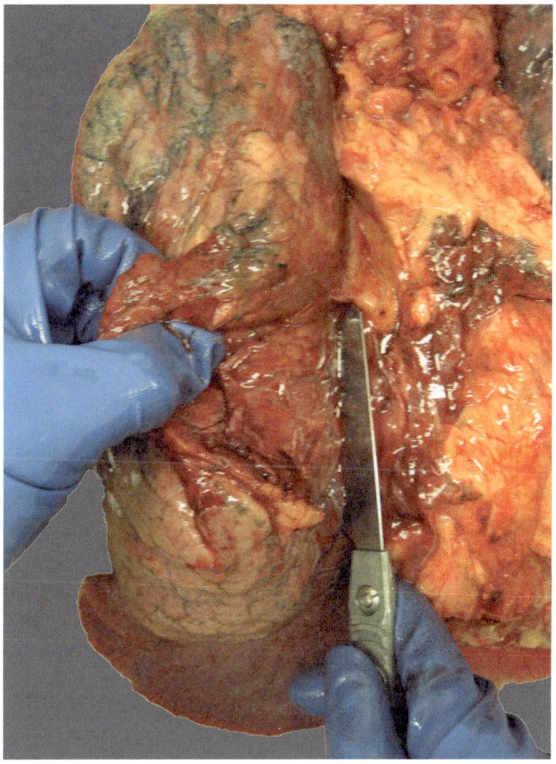

Fig. 4.257 It is recommended that the two lungs are removed at this point by direct transection of the pulmonary hilum on either side. The heart tissues are then available for study, paralleling the normal approach

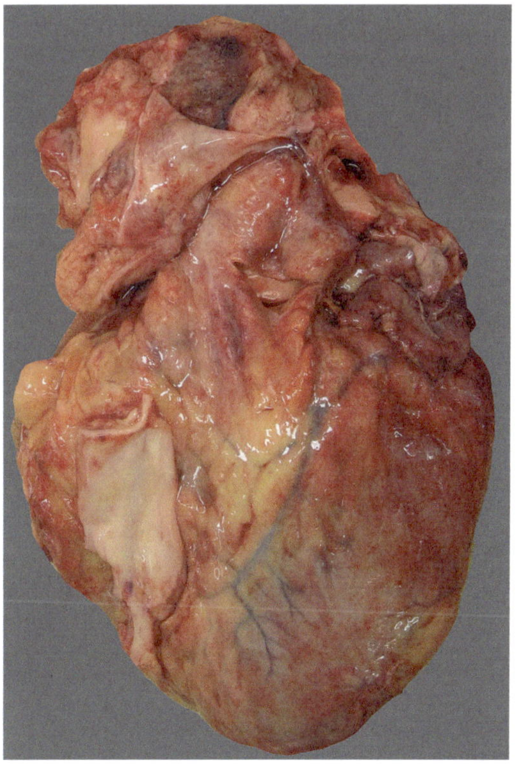

Fig. 4.258 The freely dissected cardiac tissues are now available for inspection. The front of the heart should be considered first

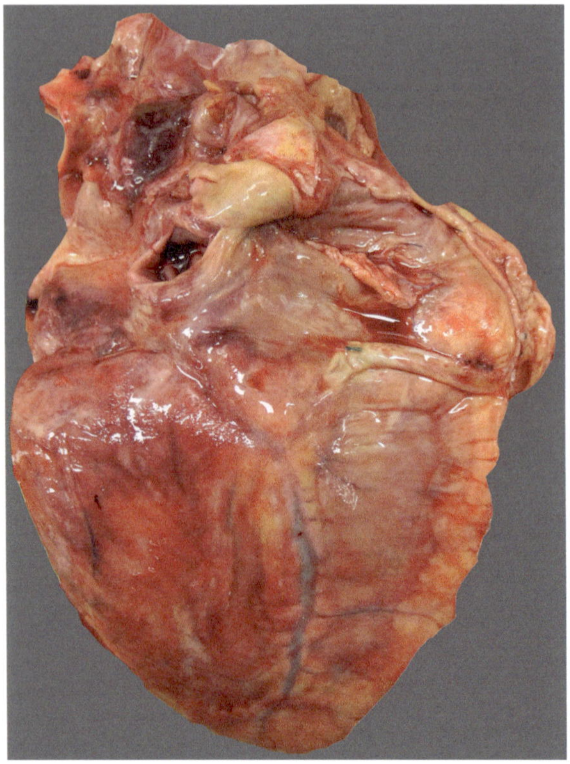

Fig. 4.259 The tissues at the back of the heart are likewise to be examined. Surgical suture lines should be considered. The insertion points of the coronary grafts should be also sought

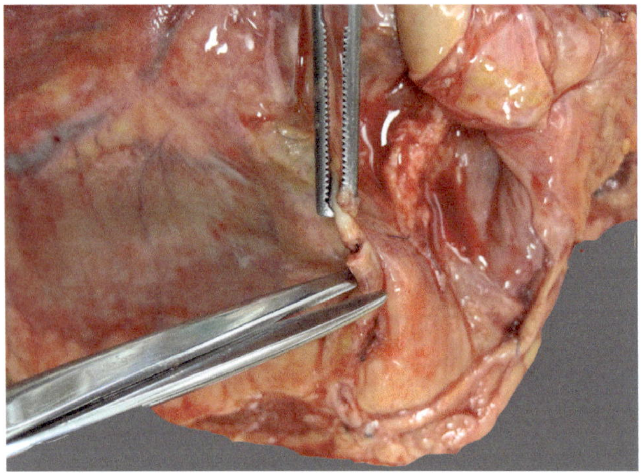

Fig. 4.260 Partial transection of the vein graft immediately above the insertion allows direct inspection and consideration of possible thrombus in the vessel at this point

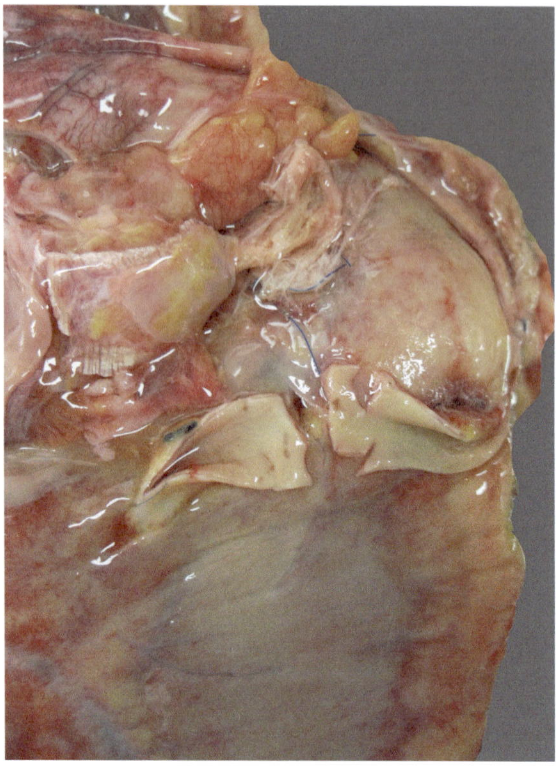

Fig. 4.261 If there is no thrombus, then the origin can likewise be partially transected and inspected. If there is no thrombotic obstruction at either end, then the artery can be opened longitudinally using the scissors along its length

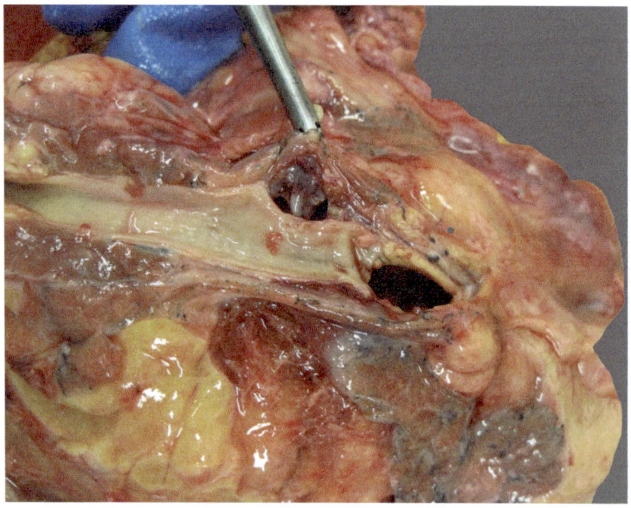

Fig. 4.262 Both ends of the graft were clear of thrombus. The scissor dissection runs upwards into the aortic root

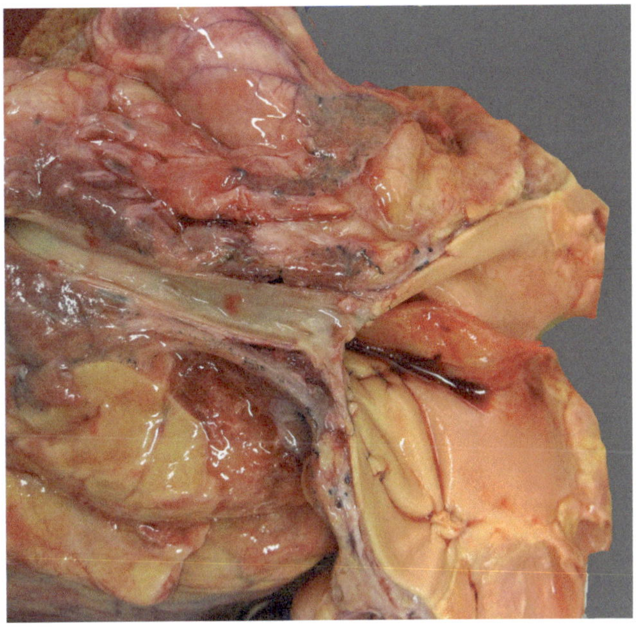

Fig. 4.263 The ostium of the vein graft shows no atheroma or stenosis. It is always advisable to look inside the aorta as one makes this cut, to be sure that thrombus is not being pushed out of the way

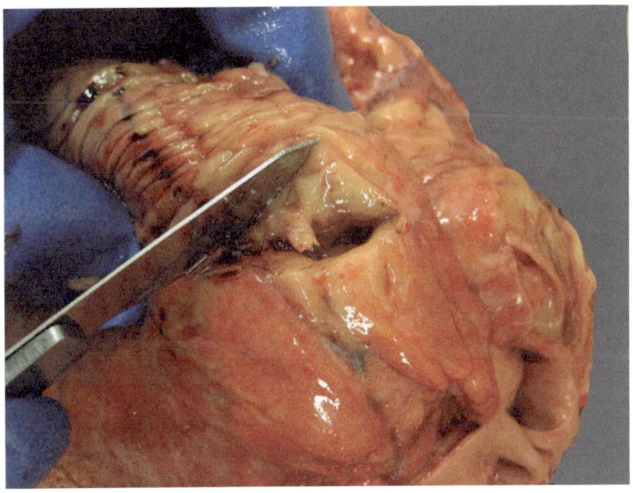

Fig. 4.264 The native coronary arteries are examined in the normal fashion, after the grafts have been examined. Heavily calcified vessels (seen here) may need to be taken off, decalcified, and then examined later (in sequence) by macroscopy and histology

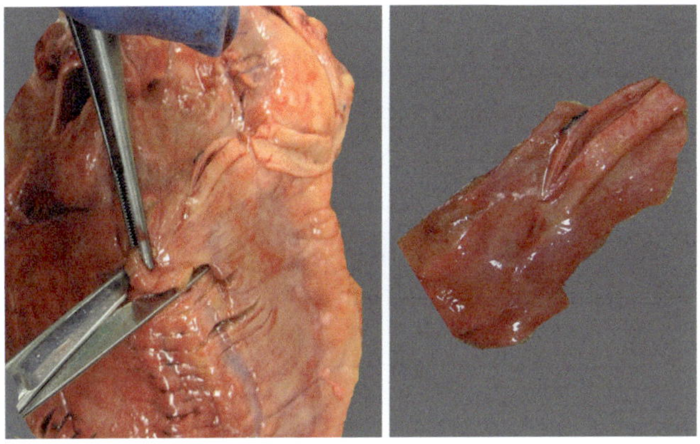

Fig. 4.265 If there is a suspicion or evidence of thrombus obstructing the origin or anastomosis point, the section of tissue must be taken out intact for histology (after fixation and decalcification). The insertion point of the graft should be fixed whole. It is recommended that the tissue is decalcified (48 h). After this, the tissue may be sliced transversely and processed for histology. The close-up image is a photo of the pre-decalcified specimen

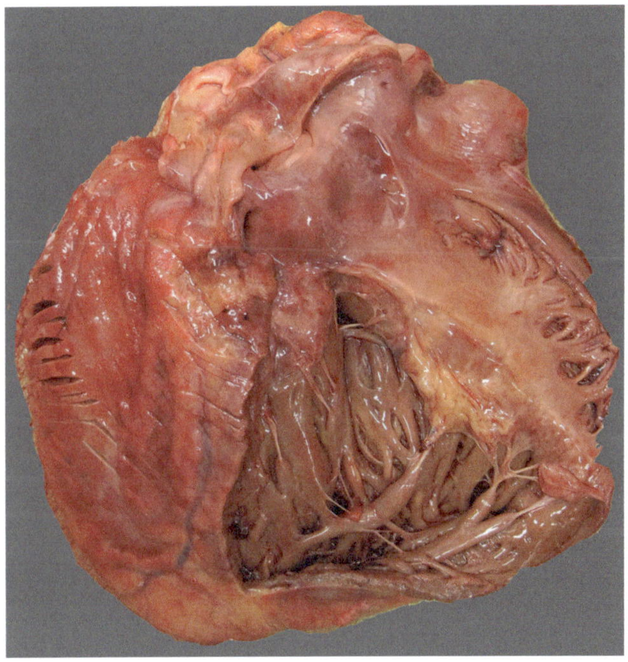

Fig. 4.266 Whilst it is possible to follow the transverse slicing of the ventricular tissues in cases of previous cardiac surgery, occasionally it can be beneficial to leave the specimen intact and open the back of the right ventricle down towards the apex

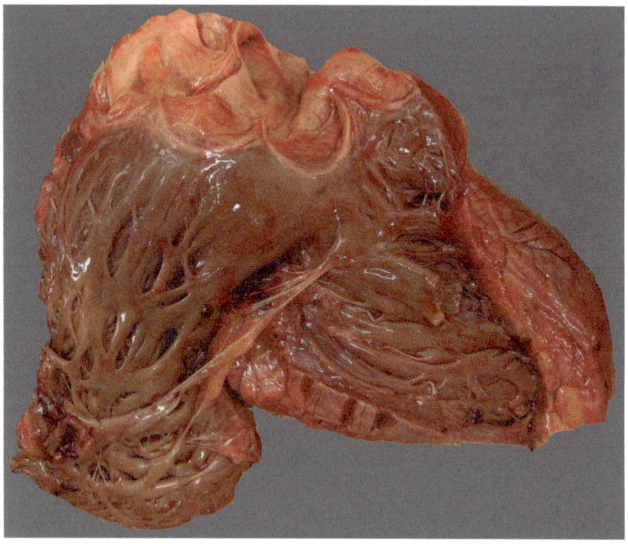

Fig. 4.267 The cut is then extended around onto the front of the heart and out through the pulmonary valve into the pulmonary artery root. The internal architecture of the right ventricle is now fully available for study

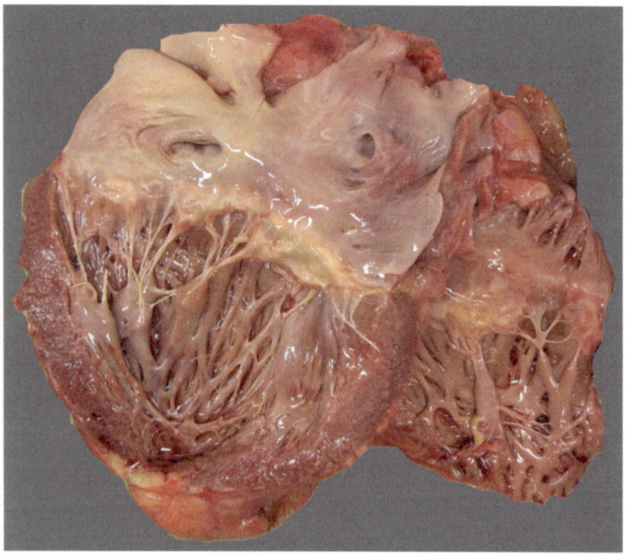

Fig. 4.268 The left atrium and ventricle are examined by opening the back of the mitral valve and then down along the left ventricular posterior free wall. Inspection of the atrial and ventricular tissues and valvular apparatus is accomplished with this technique

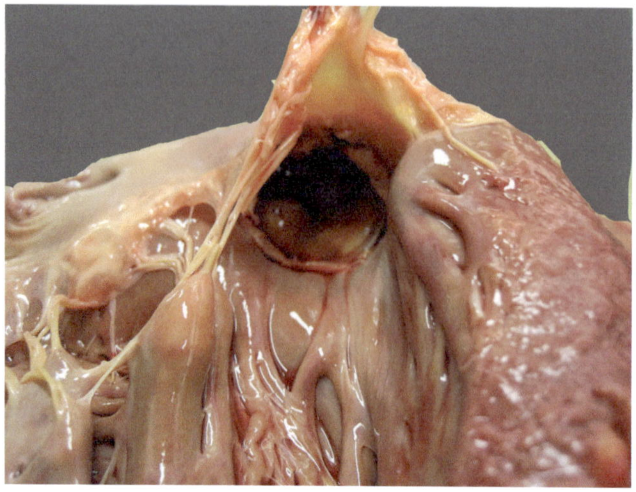

Fig. 4.269 In this case, an aortic valve replacement is evident. It can be inspected initially from below by lifting the mitral valve tissues upwards, thereby allowing direct inspection of the valve parenchyma

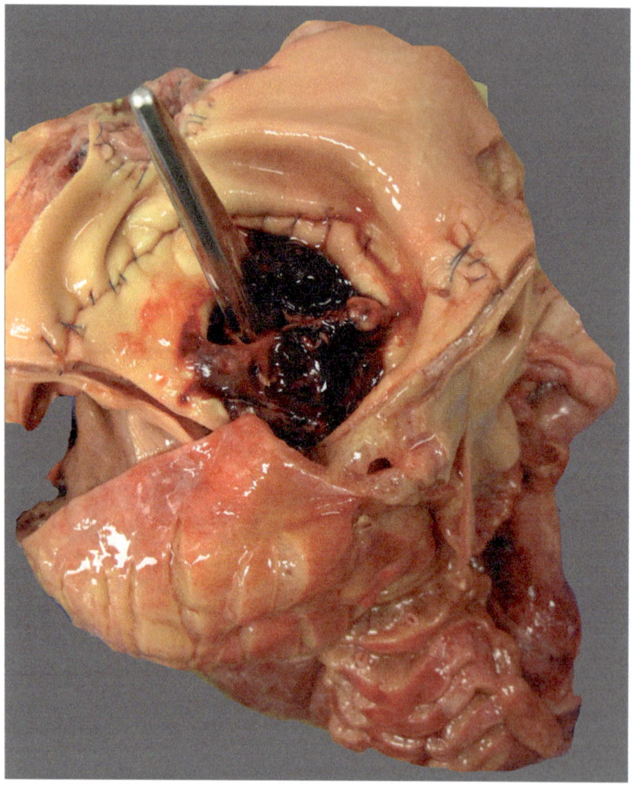

Fig. 4.270 The valve patency can be assessed gently, probing the valve prosthesis by a small finger or closed scissors. One should be careful not to dislodge any vegetations or adherent thrombus

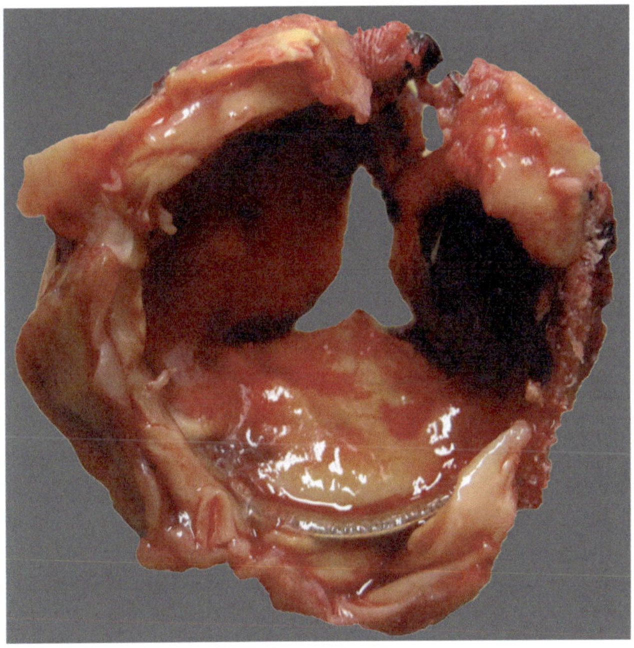

Fig. 4.271 The valve xenograft has now been dissected free and can be closely inspected from above and below

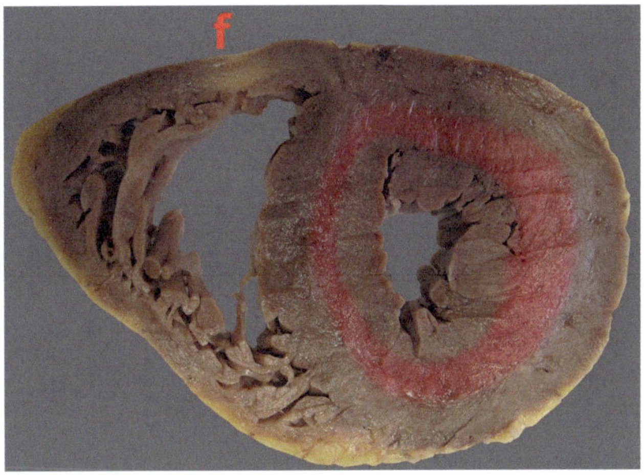

Fig. 4.272 The macroscopic appearance of arrhythmogenic ventricular cardiomyopathy (previously called arrhythmogenic right ventricular cardiomyopathy) is often first suspected using the transverse ventricular slice, which highlights an unusually large amount of fatty tissue (*f*) within the wall of the right ventricle

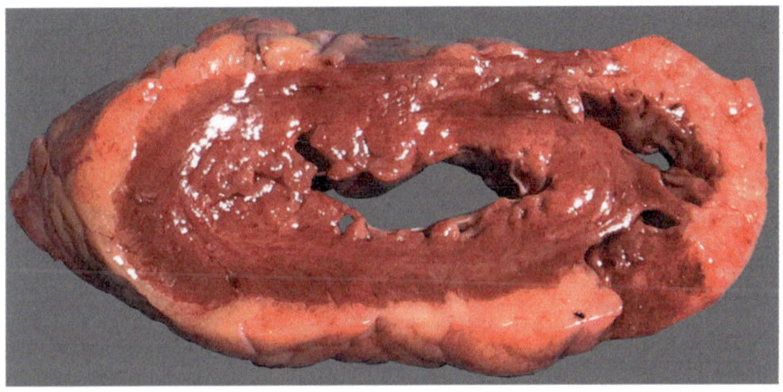

Fig. 4.273 This is a case of arrhythmogenic ventricular cardiomyopathy. One notes the right ventricle has a pronounced fatty component with little or no myocardium seen, apart from the very inner aspect of the ventricular trabeculations

Inherited and Congenital Heart Disease: The Adult Reality and Cardiomyopathies

Congenital cardiac diseases (*i.e.*, those one is born with) fall into two broad groups: structural anomalies (*e.g.*, septal defects, vascular or chamber anomalies) and cardiomyopathies (*e.g.*, hypertrophic or arrhythmogenic cardiomyopathies). These entities and some cardiac interventions are illustrated in Figs. 4.272, 4.273, 4.274, 4.275, 4.276, 4.277, 4.278, 4.279, 4.280, 4.281, 4.282, 4.283, 4.284, 4.285, 4.286, 4.287, 4.288, 4.289, 4.290, 4.291, 4.292, 4.293, 4.294, 4.295, 4.296, 4.297, 4.298, 4.299, 4.300, 4.301, 4.302, 4.303, 4.304, 4.305, 4.306, 4.307, 4.308, 4.309, 4.310, 4.311, 4.312, 4.313, 4.314, 4.315, 4.316, 4.317, 4.318, 4.319, 4.320, 4.321, 4.322, 4.323, 4.324, 4.325, 4.326, 4.327, 4.328, 4.329, and 4.330.

The most complex end of structural congenital heart disease tends to be fatal in early infancy, but adult survivors of structural lesions (whether treated or undiscovered) may find their way to the autopsy room—often to the surprise of surviving family members. Those surviving surgical therapies are often described as having 'grown-up congenital heart disease' (GUCH). Clearly, this text cannot be exhaustive in terms of presenting these diseases, but some common culprit lesions are shown.

Should one be faced with an adolescent with congenital heart disease, whether surgery has been performed or not, the standard rules of dissection will apply, along with photography and histological sampling.

The cardiomyopathies are a complex and diverse group of diseases. They are generally broken into those of primary nature (gene-related disorders) and secondary processes. Whilst some maintain that cardiomyopathy should be simply regarded as primary diseases of the heart (*e.g.*, hypertrophic cardiomyopathy, arrhythmogenic cardiomyopathy, mitochondrial cardiomyopathy), it is realistic to see that other disease processes also contribute to cardiac hypertrophy, dilatation, and distortion. Thus, amyloid heart disease and

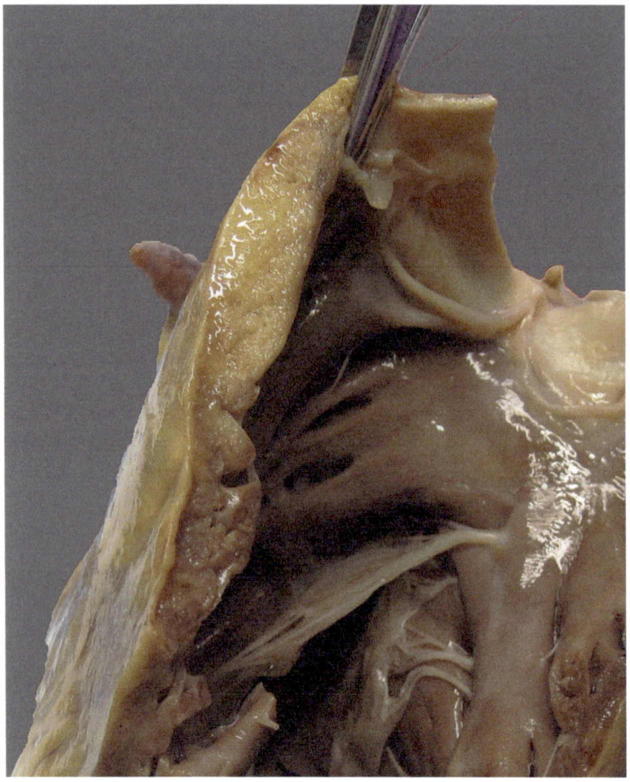

Fig. 4.274 Arrhythmogenic cardiomyopathy (ACM), showing pronounced fatty tissue replacement in the right ventricular outflow tract. This tissue appearance is often most marked in the outflow tract

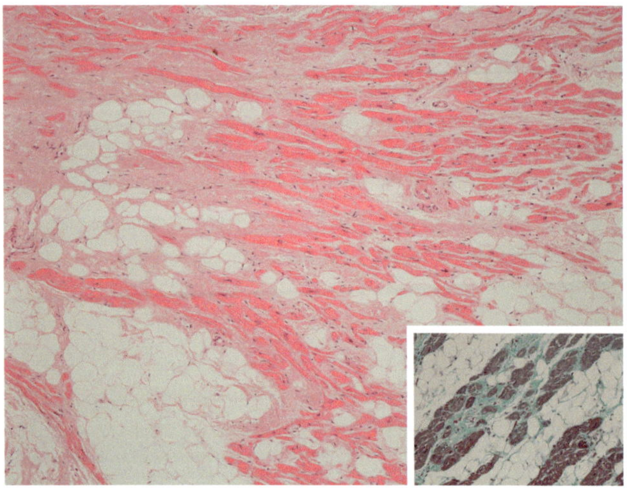

Fig. 4.275 The histology of arrhythmogenic cardiomyopathy shows pronounced fatty and fibrous tissue replacement of the cardiac myocytes. The inset at lower right shows the same features using the Masson trichrome stain to highlight the fibrosis

hypertensive heart disease may produce a 'myopathic' quality. The value of histology cannot be underestimated in this regard. It is also possible to perform electron microscopy, even from paraffin-embedded material, if required. In general, any case with even slight suspicion of an inherited disorder should have full histology, possibly with ultrastructural analysis of one section of myocardium (ideally fixed in glutaraldehyde, but formalin will suffice).

Among the inherited lesions are myogenic mutations, cytoskeleton mutations, and storage disorders. The more commonly identified in terms of the general autopsy examination are hypertrophic cardiomyopathy, arrhythmogenic cardiomyopathy, and dilated cardiomyopathy. Characteristic macroscopic and histological features may be readily seen in the heart, or the heart may be unremarkable, requiring comprehensive specialist tests to be undertaken in the context of an otherwise negative autopsy or clear history suggesting cardiac death.

The issue of channelopathies is complex. These often present in the autopsy room as sudden deaths with no positive findings, and they are histologically unremarkable. If such a disorder is considered to be present, the autopsy practitioner is advised to perform multiple tests, as described by specialist texts.

Suspected congenital myopathies, particularly of the children's type, may require fresh tissue to be snap frozen for enzyme assessment, although this procedure is usually not needed. It is also important to remember that a 2 cm cube of spleen should be reserved in cases of suspected cardiomyopathy, in order to assess any genetic mutations. The high nuclear content of the spleen makes this tissue ideal for the purposes, although technically any tissue could be used.

Often, these cases are examined and then referred to specialist centres for further commentary and analysis.

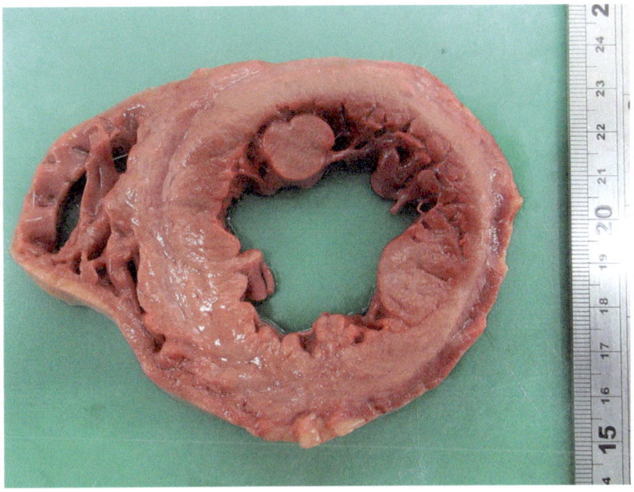

Fig. 4.276 This is an example of left ventricle variant arrhythmogenic cardiomyopathy. This is a subtle diagnosis but one can appreciate a variation in colour on the outer quarter of the wall thickness running anteriorly round and laterally. The degree of fatty tissue replacement may be not marked by naked eye appearances but can be quite pronounced histologically

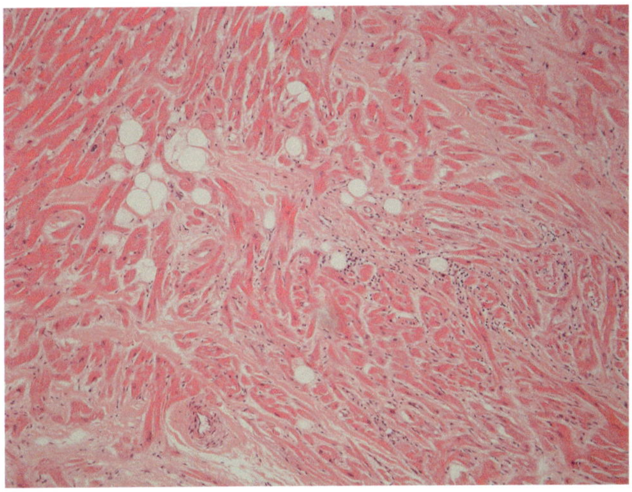

Fig. 4.277 It must be remembered that finding some fat and fibrous tissue in cardiac tissues is not automatically indicative of arrhythmogenic cardiomyopathy. This case showed some nonspecific features in a patient dying from metastatic neoplasia

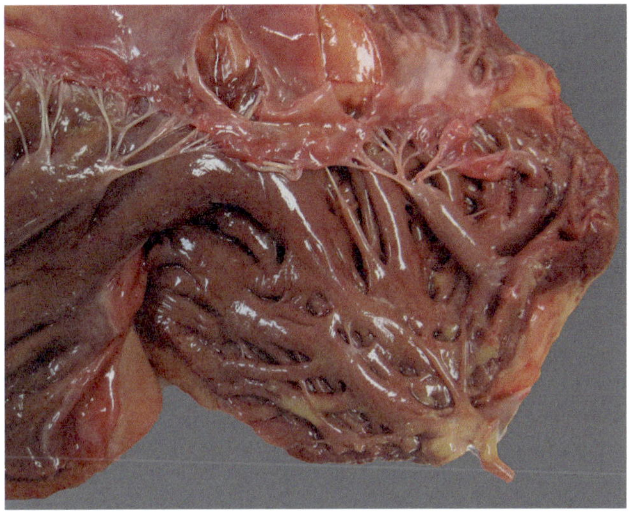

Fig. 4.278 The so-called 'tabby-cat' heart is characterized by yellow flecks of fatty tissue, particularly on the endocardial aspect of the ventricular parenchyma. This is a normal reflection of increased age, with a female sex bias. It is very mild in most cases. When marked, it can provoke consideration of arrhythmogenic cardiomyopathy

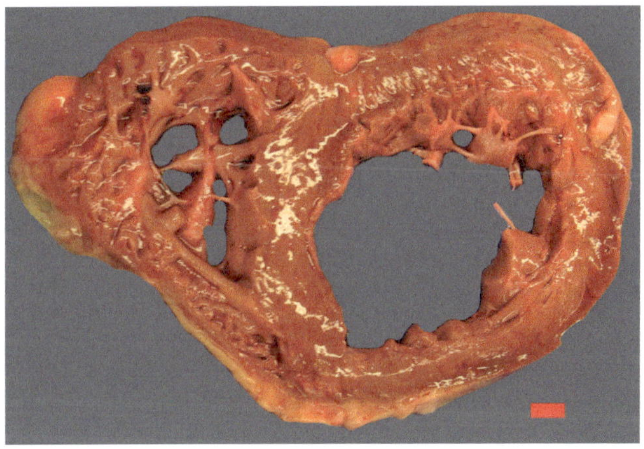

Fig. 4.279 Dilated cardiomyopathy is best perceived from the ventricular transverse slice, in which the transverse diameters of the right and left ventricles can be appreciated. It is possible to define a variety of different transverse diameters depending on the plane of measurement taken, but the largest should be used

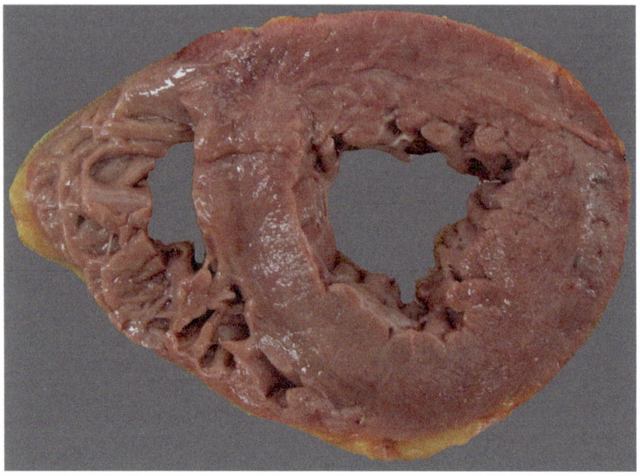

Fig. 4.280 Peripartum cardiomyopathy can occur in the peripartum and immediate postpartum period. This rare condition can be fatal owing to rapidly progressive dysfunction of the heart. The macroscopic and histological features are not specific. Correlation against the antemortem and maternal record is required, along with consideration of the family history. Exclusion of alternative causes of cardiomyopathy is paramount

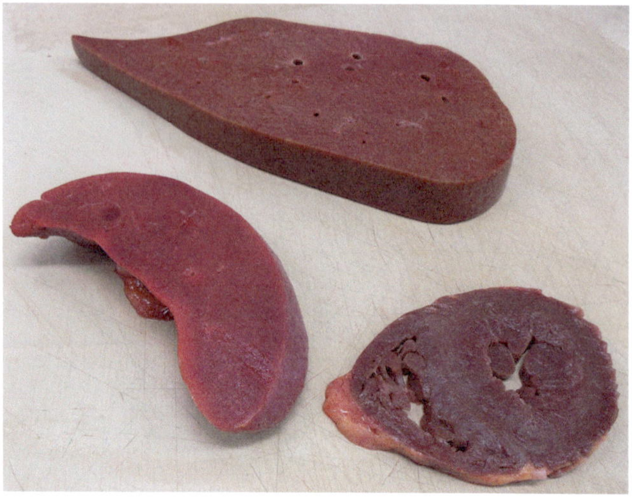

Fig. 4.281 This is a case of systemic amyloidosis affecting splenic, cardiac and liver tissues. These all have a well-defined edge on section when cut fresh at autopsy. The pronounced left ventricular hypertrophy is a clue for amyloidosis, as is the very firm and waxy quality of the spleen (lardaceous spleen)

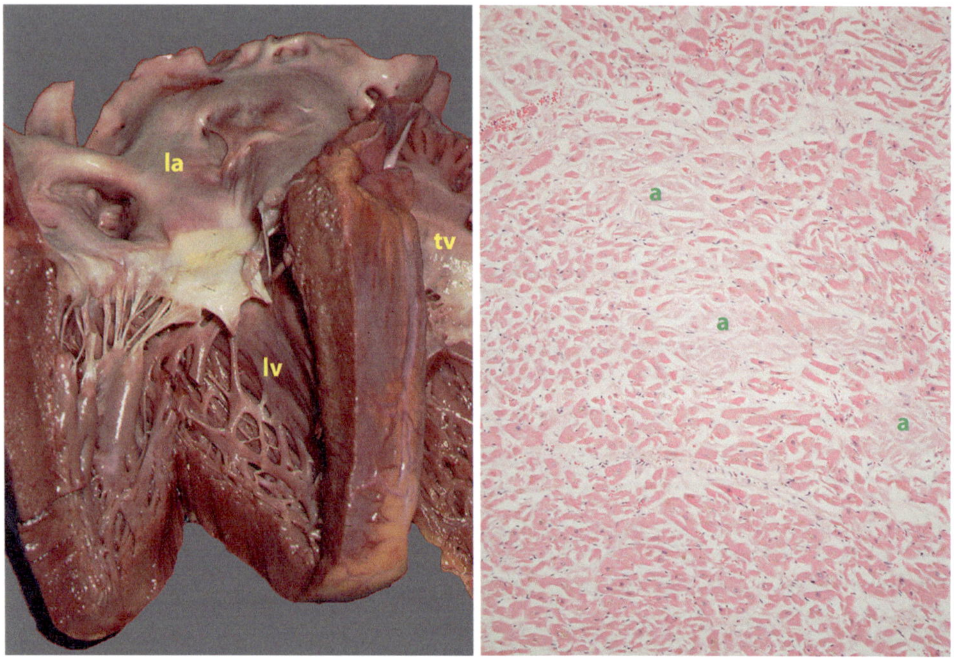

Fig. 4.282 *Left.* Cardiac amyloid often may be seen with enlarged, thick, and stiff ventricle tissues (*la*, left atrium; *lv*, left ventricle; *tv*, tricuspid valve). This fresh specimen shows the rigidity of the ventricular parenchyma, despite being sliced open. *Right.* Histologically, cardiac amyloid can be subtle or marked. The degree of eosinophilic matrix infiltrating around cardiac myocytes, in the interstitium (*a*), and (in other cases) around blood vessels varies. It is often suspected on standard haematoxylin and eosin (H&E) staining, but it is best visualized using special stains (Congo Red or Sirius Red), or potentially electron microscopy

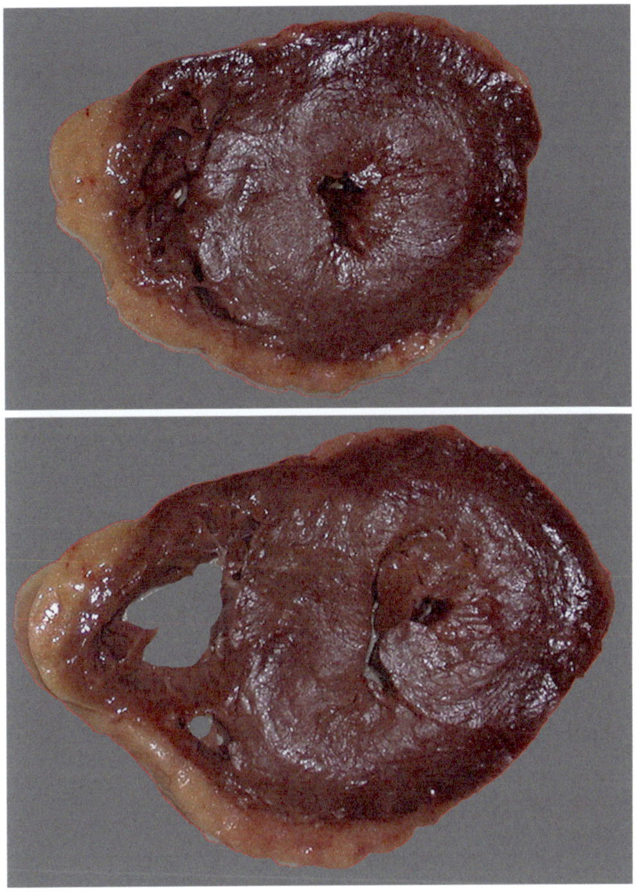

Fig. 4.283 Hypertrophic cardiomyopathy is often suspected by virtue of the macroscopic features. Transverse sections across the right and left ventricle may show the asymmetry that is suggestive of this condition

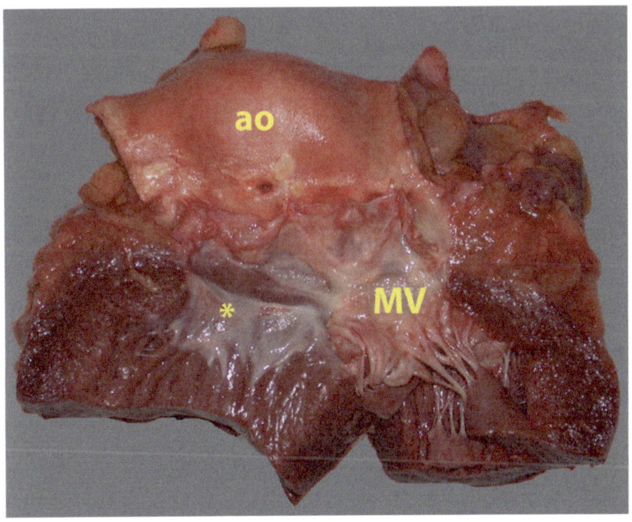

Fig. 4.284 Hypertrophic cardiomyopathy often shows an impact lesion (*asterisk*) on the endocardial surface adjacent to the anterior mitral valve (*MV*) leaflet. This is often the mirror image of the valve tissue itself, representing localised trauma to the endocardial tissues as the septal tissues are struck by the valve leaflet at the maximal excursion point. The aorta (*ao*) is seen above the left ventricular outflow tract

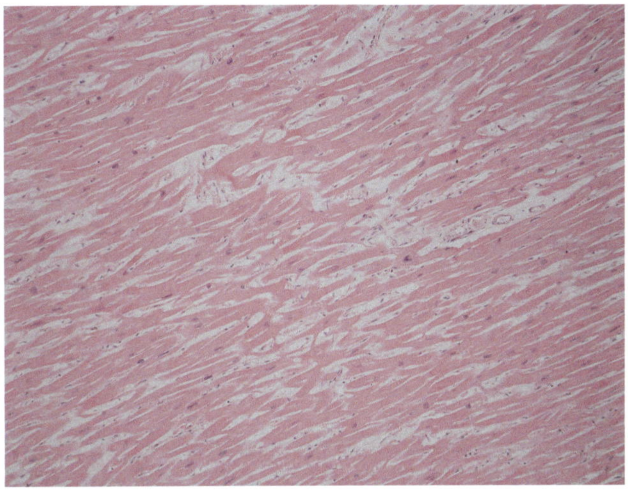

Fig. 4.285 Hypertrophic cardiomyopathy shows characteristic myocyte disarray histologically. A minor degree of disarray is often seen at the confluence of the right and left ventricle free walls, but finding disarray of this quality in most blocks diffusely across the myocardial parenchyma points towards hypertrophic cardiomyopathy

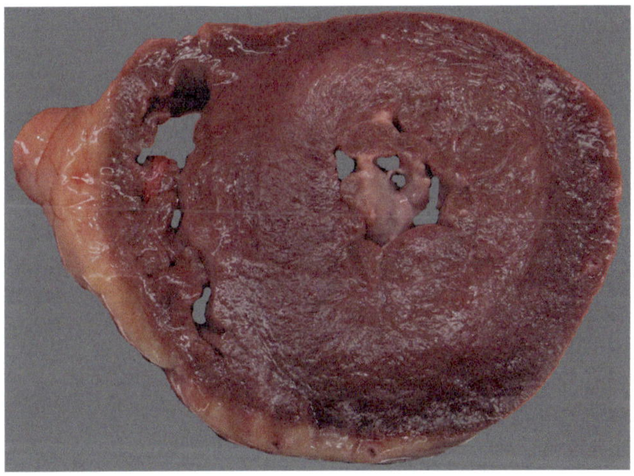

Fig. 4.286 Hypertension may produce significant left ventricle muscle bulking and mimics hypertrophic cardiomyopathy, but the hypertrophy is concentric. There will be little or no myocyte disarray histologically, but there does appear to be familial linkage in some cases. Idiopathic left ventricular hypertrophy might be considered if there is no evidence of hypertension

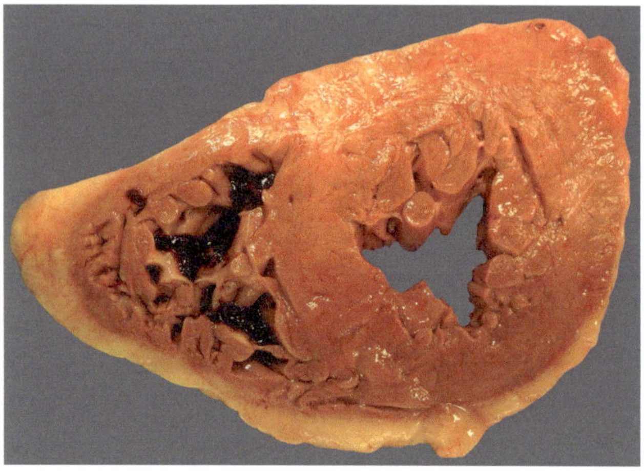

Fig. 4.287 Cases of inherited channelopathy, manifesting as unexpected sudden death, occasionally may appear in the autopsy room. The gross examination and histology are unremarkable. Ancillary tests (microbiology, toxicology, and serology) are negative. This case, in which the individual died suddenly while at rest, involved a known Brugada-type mutation, emphasising the need for reserving splenic or other tissue for subsequent DNA analysis

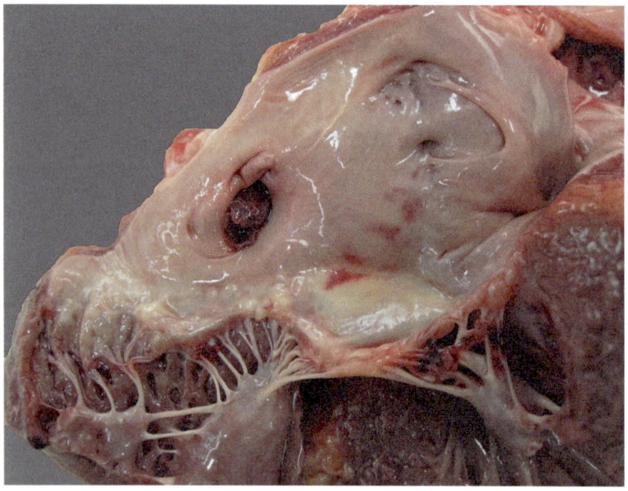

Fig. 4.288 Many cardiomyopathic conditions—and indeed secondary degenerative disorders of the myocardium—are often associated with atrial fibrillation. Thrombus in the appendages can be seen in such circumstances and provides a risk for systemic artery embolization

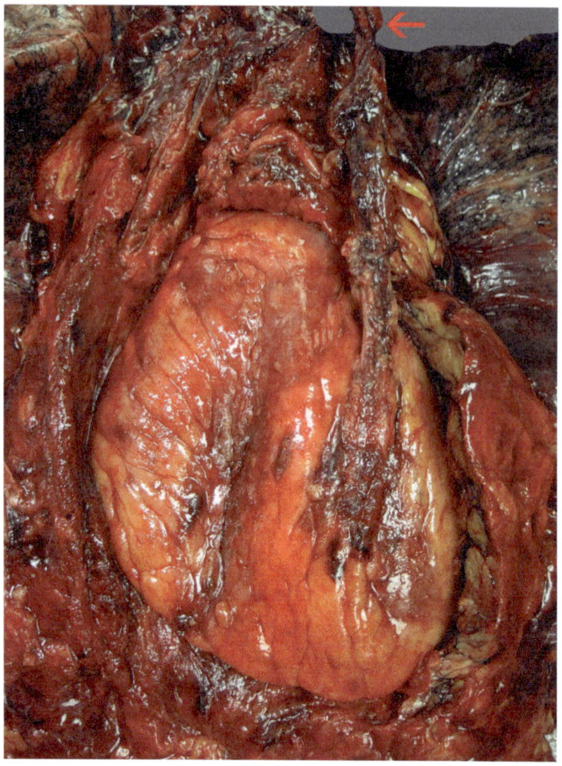

Fig. 4.289 Examining the heart in a death shortly after surgery often requires inspection of the connections in situ. This case demonstrates the left internal mammary artery (LIMA) branch running onto the left anterior descending artery from the undersurface of the sternum/chest wall. If one is to assess the patency of the bypass artery tissue, careful dissection of the ribs and sternum is required. Photography is essential to record steps of dissection

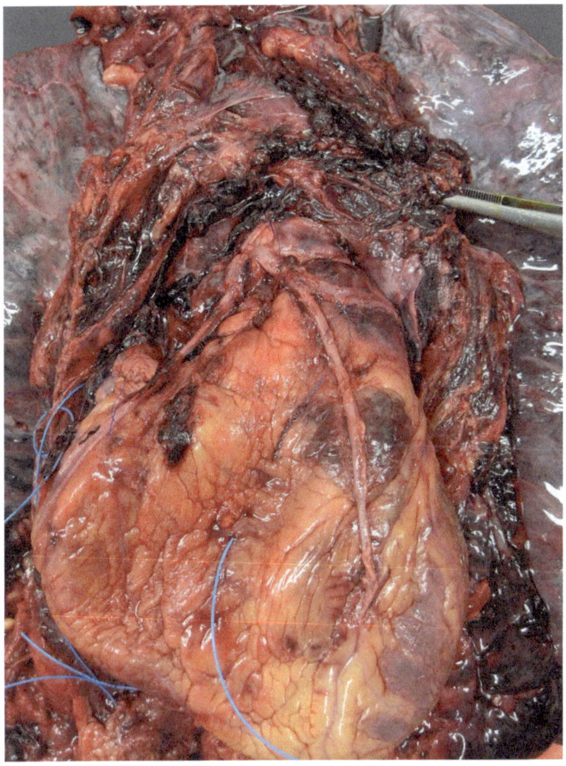

Fig. 4.290 This heart has had bypass surgery using vein grafts harvested from the leg. The patient had complications almost immediately after surgery, and fresh haemorrhage in the soft tissues is noted. Blue pacing wires are also present focally

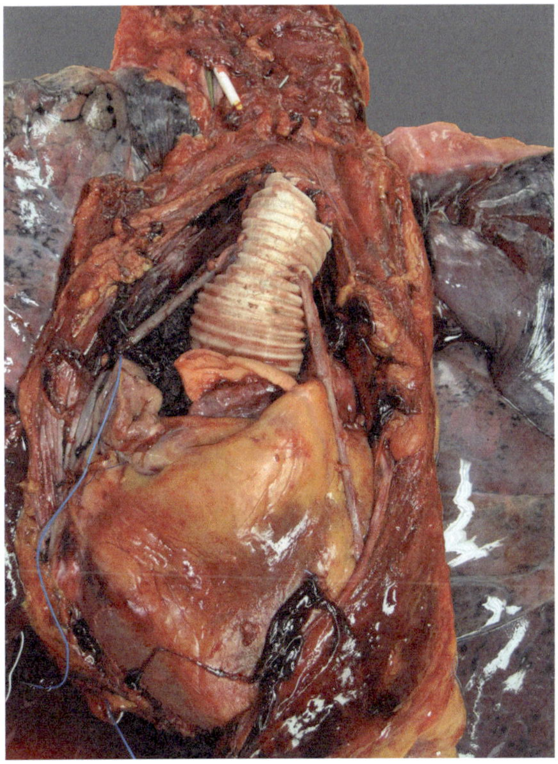

Fig. 4.291 Coronary bypass surgery has taken place, with an aortic valve/root replacement. Examination of the tissues before manipulation and evisceration is vital for full assessment of the vascular modifications

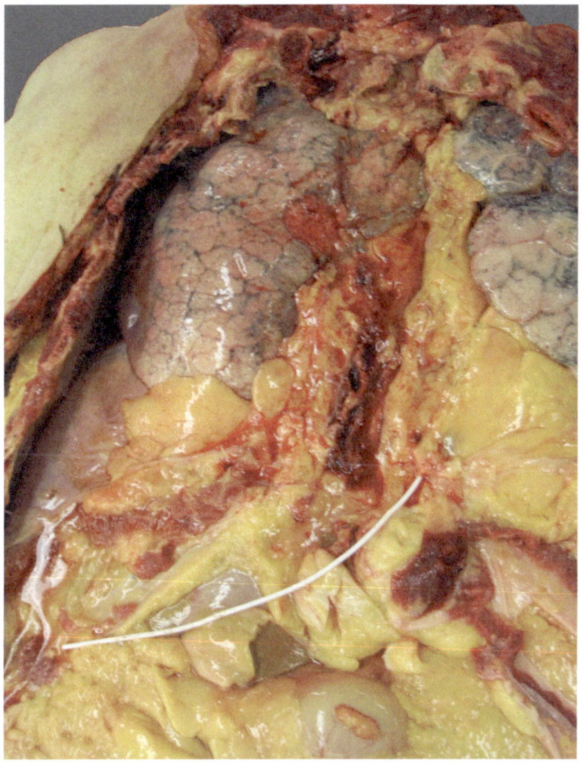

Fig. 4.292 Pericardial collections may need drainage, if there is tamponade. Various routes can be used to perform the drainage, but inserting such lines is not without risk. This image shows an anterior subxiphisternal approach. Tracing a pericardial drain is important if there is any possibility that the drain insertion has adversely affected the heart or other tissues. In such circumstances, it is recommended to cut the drain flush with the skin and push the device slightly inwards; then the drainage line is approached from inside the body in order to guarantee the correct alignment and position of any drainage tubes

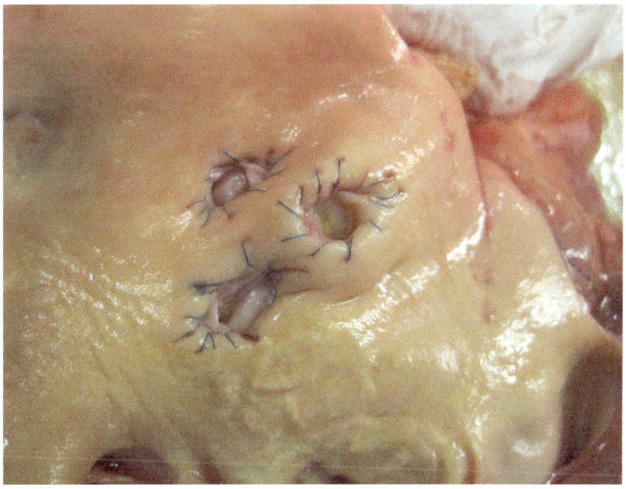

Fig. 4.293 The origin of vein bypass grafts in the aorta is seen with three closely placed buttonholes

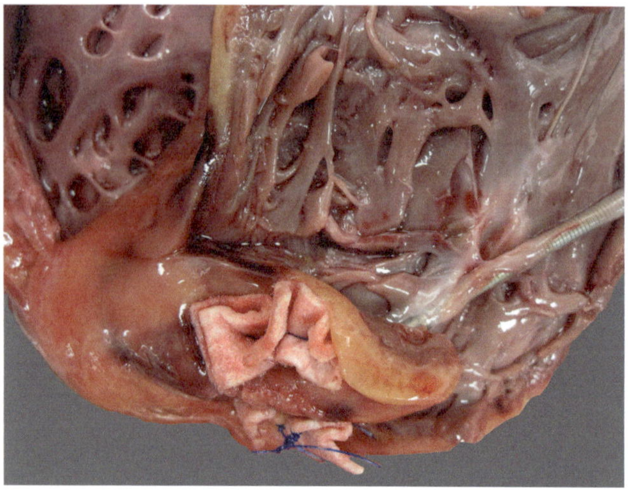

Fig. 4.294 This is a view of the tip of the right ventricle, which has required open surgical repair with pledgets following an attempt to remove the right ventricle lead. Tearing of the right ventricle at this point caused cardiac tamponade. Although the haemorrhage was stemmed to a large degree, the patient died during the procedure. Close examination of the position of the pledgets and careful probing of the site of perforation should occur in order to test whether any residual leak was present. It is stressed that over-pressure by the probe on the right ventricle wall will always create a false dissection tract, so only gentle probing should be used

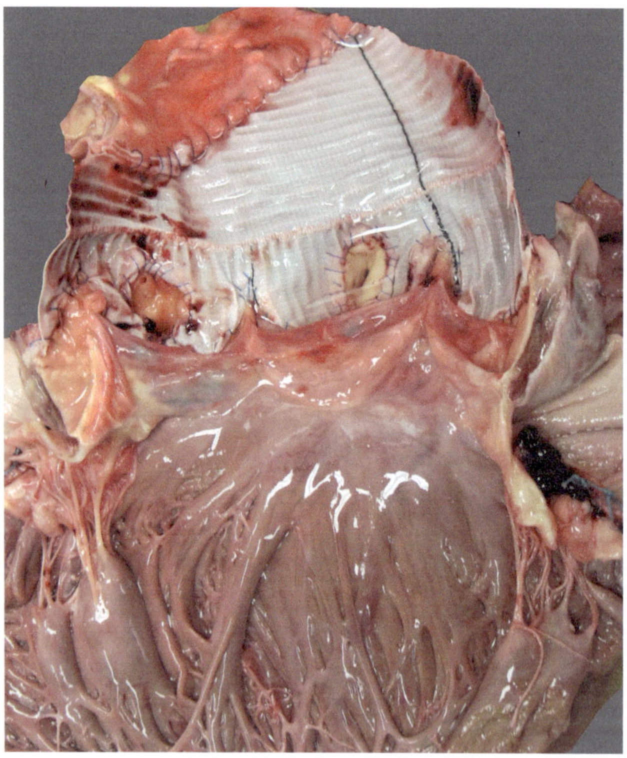

Fig. 4.295 An aortic root graft is seen with buttonholes for the coronary arteries. The Dacron root graft has intact suture lines. This patient died from complications outside the heart shortly after surgery. Autopsy examinations in such cases require careful consideration of the surgical materials, to exclude leak points and sepsis

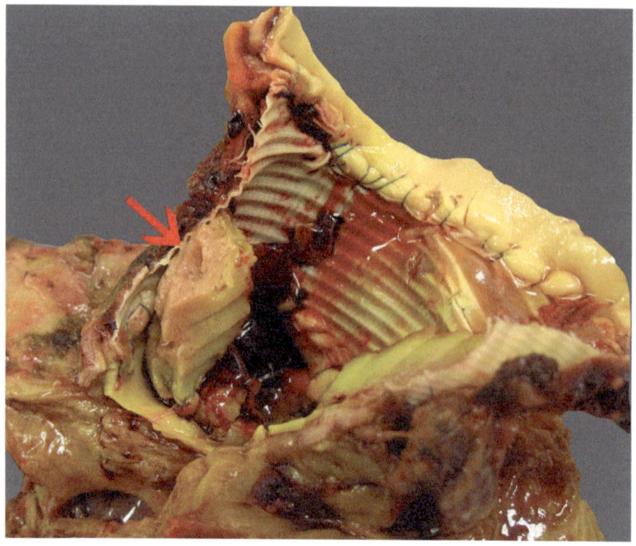

Fig. 4.296 This aortic root graft shows an infected yellow thrombus (*arrow*) on the luminal aspect of the Dacron graft

Technology and the Heart

The heart has become a common site for interventions such as vascular devices (*e.g.*, stents) and valve prostheses. Other devices of importance include Dacron structural grafts and septal closure devices.

Perhaps the most commonly employed device, which is regularly seen in autopsy practice, is the pacemaker. Single-lead, double-lead, and triple-lead pacemakers are increasingly common and used to treat a variety of cardiac disorders. The pacemaker needs to be considered as a unit, and if there is any suspicion of pacemaker dysfunction, then the pacemaker generator unit (box), the lead (wire from the box onwards), and the electrode (the tip of the wire) must be dissected without pieces being cut apart. In short, the device may need to be retained whole for detailed inspection. Examination of the pacemaker site may be relevant in terms of sepsis, and it is possible to send the pacemaker away for testing of the programme, battery life, and functionality.

The other common technology involving the heart is valve prostheses. These have evolved markedly over the past 50 years, with many poor designs. Modern replacement valves are implanted by open surgery or endovascular routes. They can radically improve cardiac function in the elderly, but anticoagulation may be required. Complications of sepsis are particularly important.

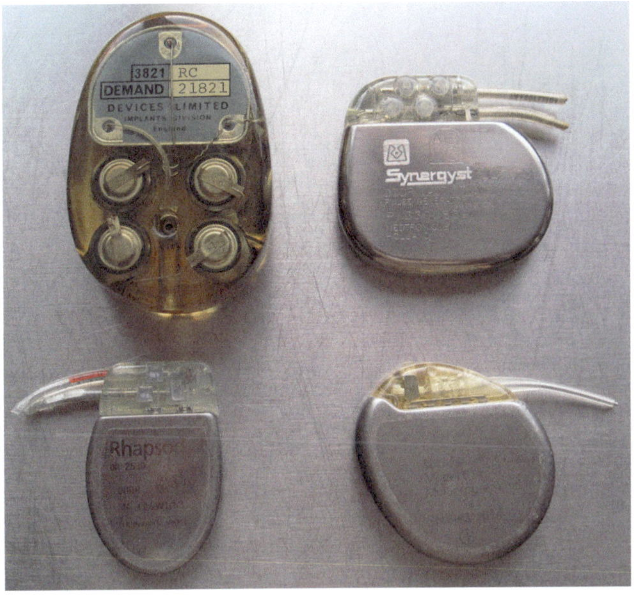

Fig. 4.297 Pacemakers have changed in design, shape, and complexity over many years. A variety of pacemakers are seen in this view, for comparison with an old design (*top left*). By contrast, modern devices are relatively thin and light. Most are designed simply to check for gaps in the cardiac cycle and fill in the necessary electrical stimulus, if missing. Examination of the pacemaker will show the device, manufacturer details, and a serial number. This information can be particularly useful in identifying a decomposed body. The leads emerge from one point on the device and pass onwards to the heart. At autopsy, most cases have the generator unit (box) cut free from the wires to allow easy extraction

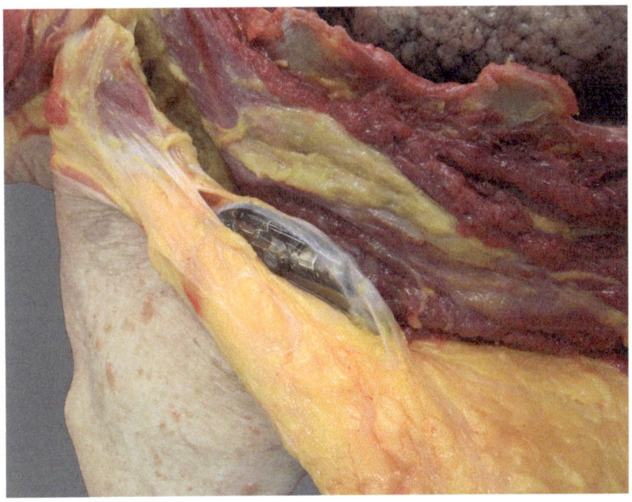

Fig. 4.298 A pacemaker is seen in its fibrous walled 'pocket' on the upper chest. There is no evidence of sepsis

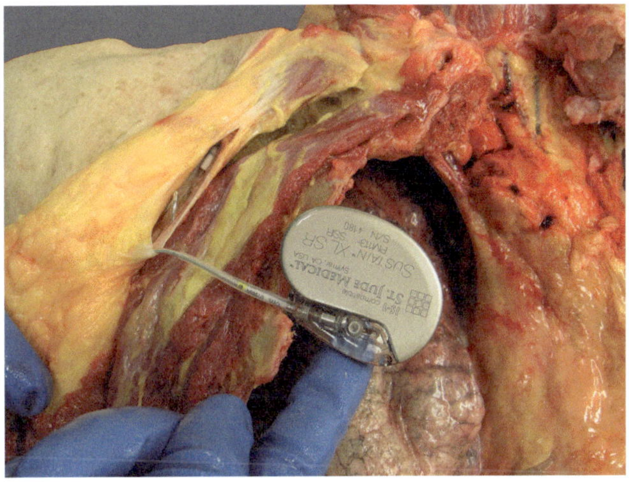

Fig. 4.299 The pacemaker generator unit has been pulled free, still with the leads attached. Pacemaker devices can come with one, two, or three leads. Most autopsy dissections simply cut the leads about 20–40 mm from the generator (box). It is important to remember that defibrillator pacemakers (ICDs) must be deactivated before wires are cut, in order to prevent accidental discharge of the device affecting mortuary staff

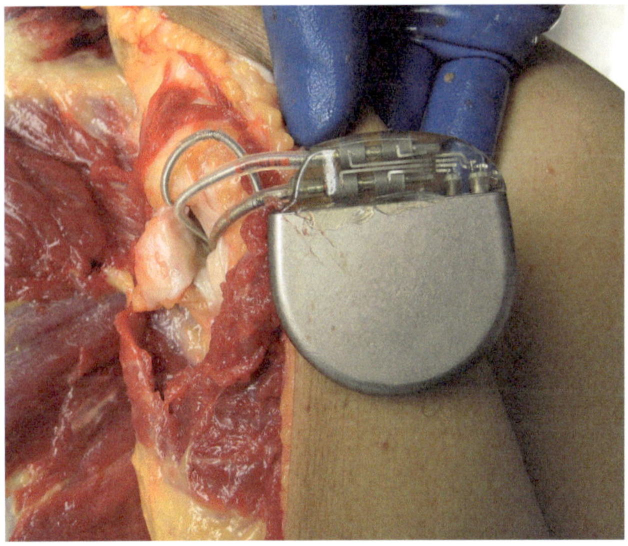

Fig. 4.300 A pacemaker unit ideally should be inspected in situ before any wires are cut. In this case, the soft tissues have been opened to show the pacemaker pocket to be free of infection. The pacemaker generator unit is seen with the three leads attached

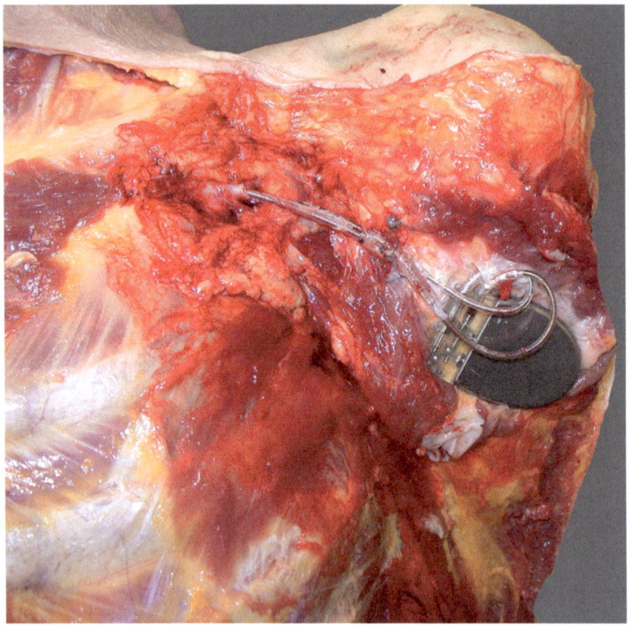

Fig. 4.301 There is marked fibrosis around the leads of this pacemaker, in keeping with the pacemaker insertion previously. The wires pass normally towards the venous system and may be dissected out without transecting any wires. If one wishes to dissect pacemakers in this fashion, it may be helpful to cut across the clavicle in order to maintain wire integrity before removing the sternum and rib sections

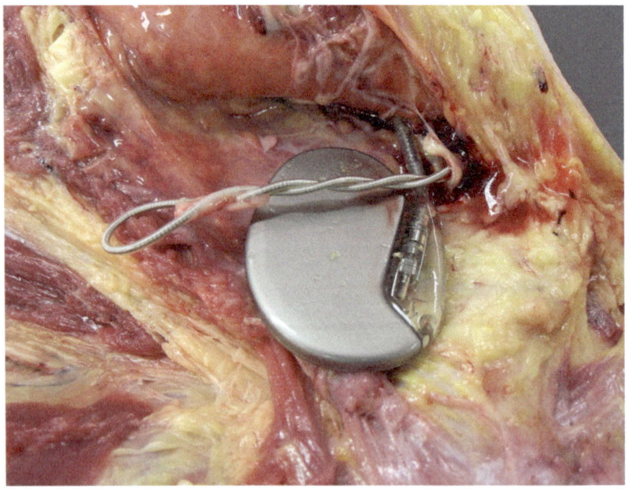

Fig. 4.302 Extensive twisting of pacemaker leads can be found in some individuals. It can occur naturally, but twisted wires may represent a 'pacemaker twiddler', an individual who fidgets with the pacemaker unit under the skin. The wires become twisted, even to the point of dislodging the electrodes from the cardiac attachment site. More importantly, in this case there was a light exudate present, which points towards possible active sepsis at the site. The exudate should be swabbed for microbiology, and histology of the pocket should follow

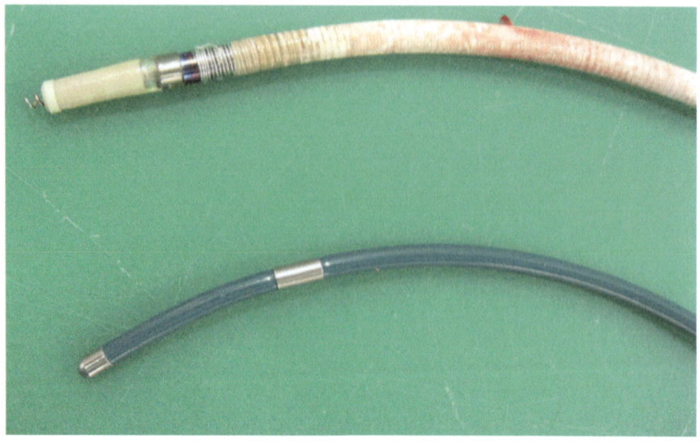

Fig. 4.303 A temporary (*lower*) and permanent (*upper*) pacemaker lead electrode. The temporary wire has two electrical connection points, seen by the metal parts; it can be withdrawn with ease from the patient. The permanent pacemaker has a screw insertion point to help anchor it to the endocardial substrate. It is noted that the insulation in this case has been partially pulled back during electrode handling, exposing the inner aspect of the lead

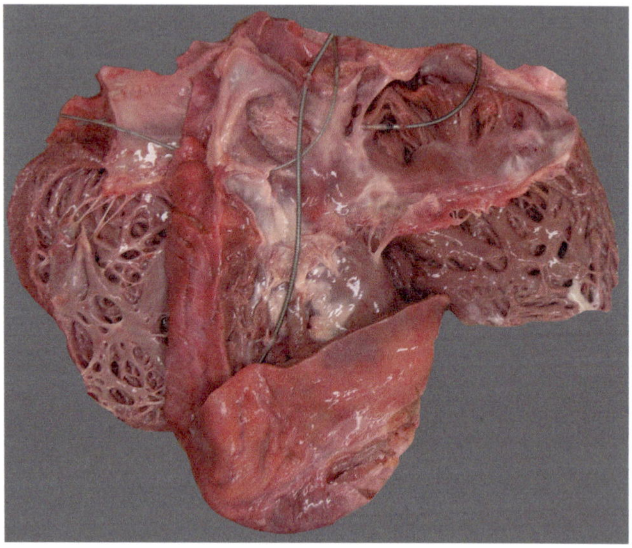

Fig. 4.304 A three-lead cardiac pacemaker device was present in this case. One lead proceeds to the right atrium. Another passes across the tricuspid valve and runs into the apex of the right ventricle. A third lead is noted to enter the coronary sinus and to run around the great cardiac vein to be attached over the tissues of the anterior left ventricle

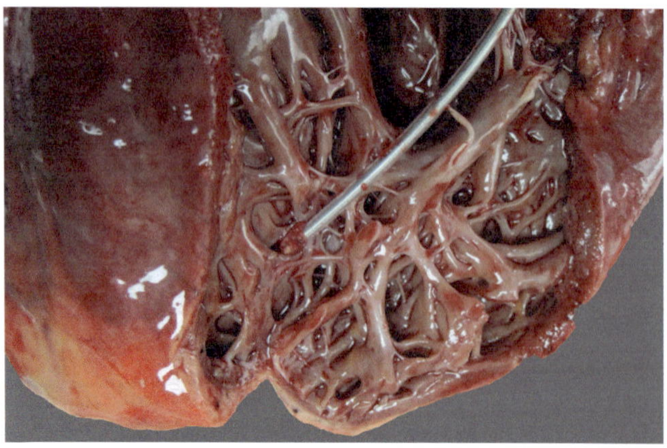

Fig. 4.305 The cardiac pacemaker lead is seen correctly embedded in the tip of the right ventricle

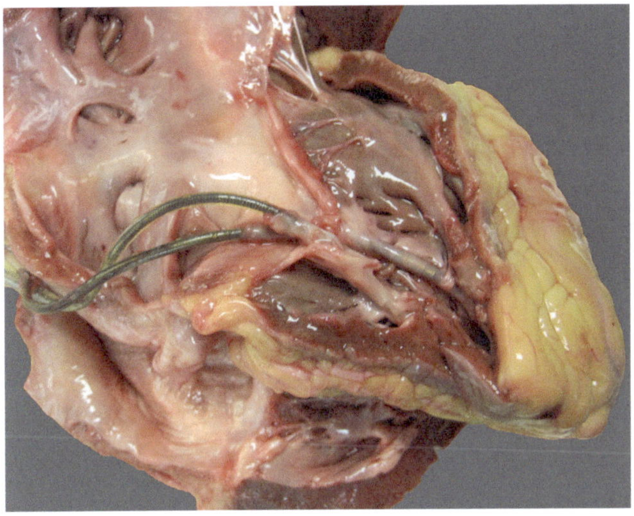

Fig. 4.306 Pacemaker generator units do need replacement with time, and on occasion the lead will need replacement, but sometimes it can be difficult to remove some pacemaker leads. Specialised tools to extract the leads exist, but some leads are simply left in situ. A second pacemaker lead has been inserted in this case, with the electrode embedded in the tip of the right ventricle. The first lead is noted to have extensive fibrosis binding it to the cardiac tissues

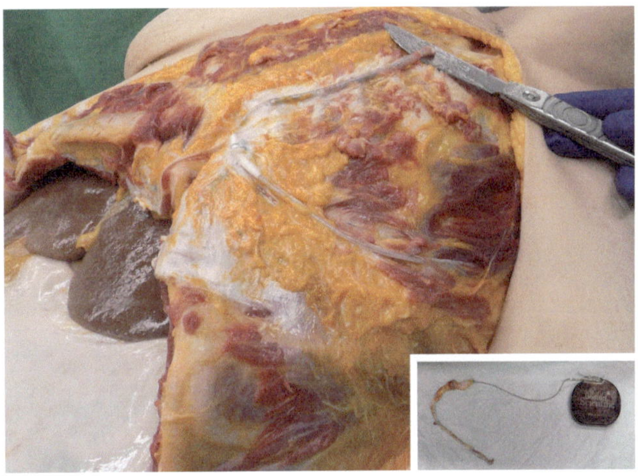

Fig. 4.307 This novel type of defibrillation device, a subcutaneous implanted cardiac defibrillator (S-ICD) comprises a generator unit in a subcutaneous pocket towards the axilla and a single lead which analyses and converts fatal dysrhythmias from outside of the chest wall. It can be used in patients with primary electrical or structural heart disease. The risk of infection is reduced compared to classical pacemaker devices as there is no intravascular component

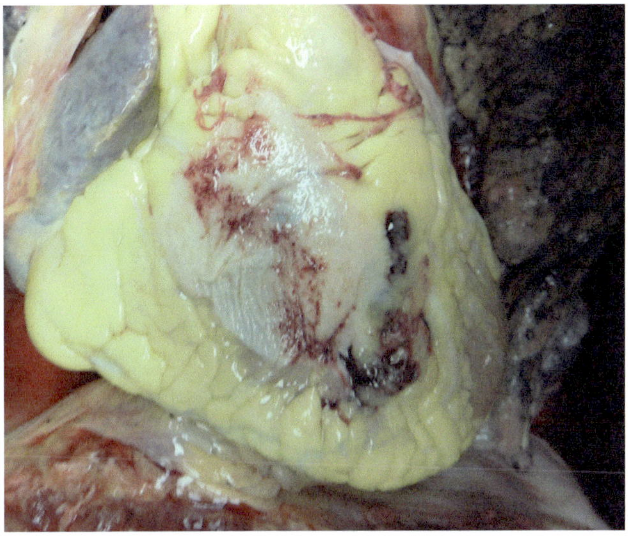

Fig. 4.308 Placement of a temporary cardiac pacemaker wire lead can be complicated by right ventricular perforation. This case had clear evidence of cardiac tamponade with evidence of haemorrhage and a dissection path close to the apex of the right ventricle

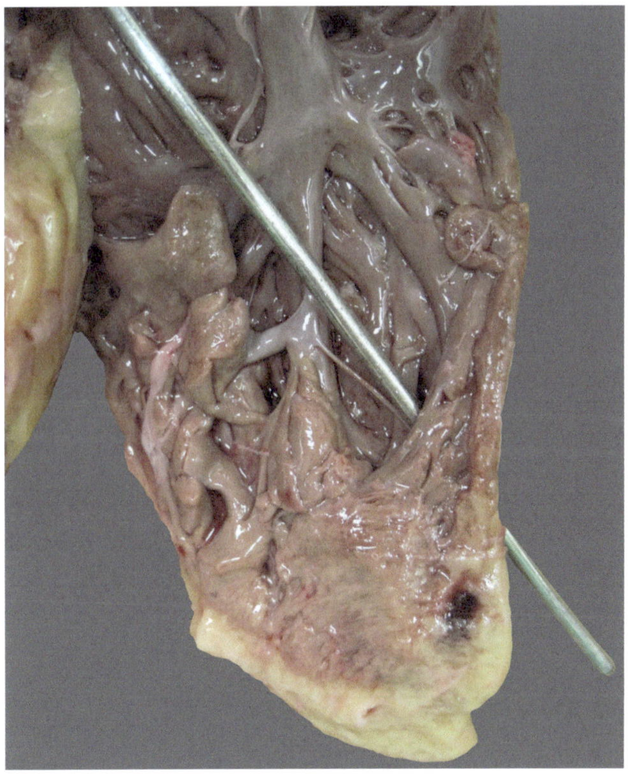

Fig. 4.309 Another case of temporary pacemaker lead penetration of the right ventricle wall. Transverse slicing of the ventricle should not take place, but dissection along the flow of blood is maintained with the heart intact, thereby preserving the wire connections. Here, the autopsy probe highlights the perforation pathway with some soft tissue haemorrhage adjacent. Right ventricular perforation is probably more common than appreciated, but because the right ventricle is a relatively low-pressure chamber, the perforation can seal relatively promptly with minimal blood loss

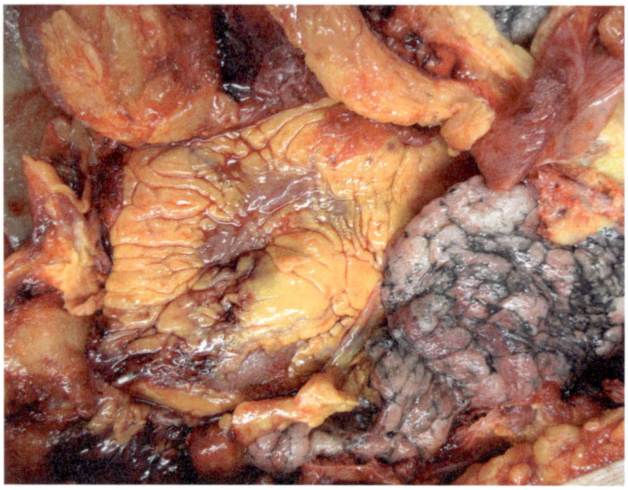

Fig. 4.310 The right ventricle in this case shows a focal perforation and the tip of the wire is visible, which is in keeping with the history of an acute deterioration and cardiac tamponade following pacemaker insertion. It is vitally important that very careful dissection of such cases is undertaken at the beginning of the autopsy with photographic records being kept during this procedure in order to confirm and preserve evidence of the events that took place

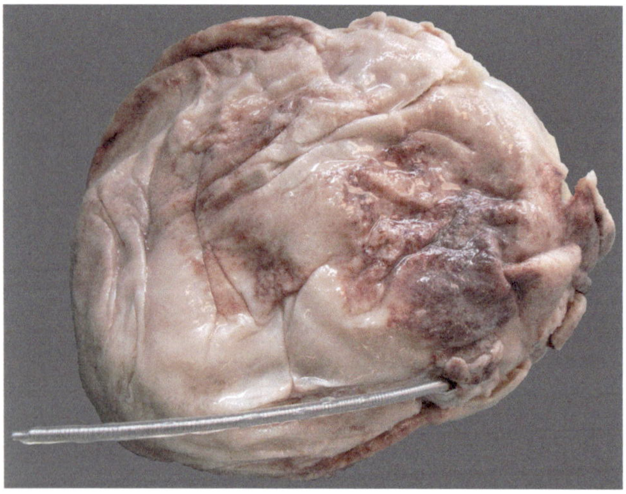

Fig. 4.311 Most cardiac pacemakers have electrodes inserted into the inner aspect of the ventricular and other tissues. This case involved an epicardial placed pacemaker, with the pacemaker unit otherwise performing exactly the same function as an endocardial device

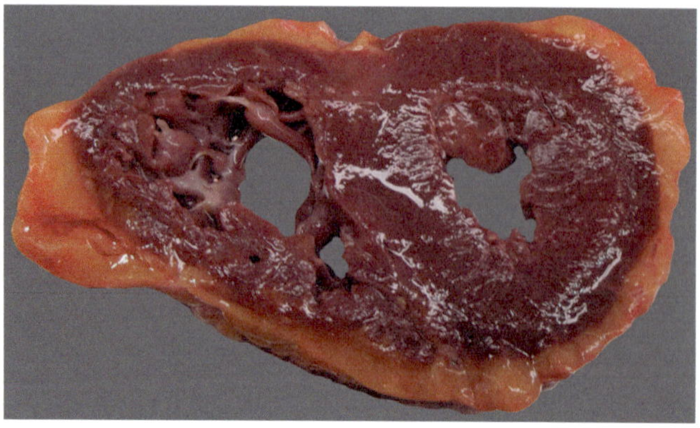

Fig. 4.312 Cardiac hypertrophy can occur in cases of lung disease, with the increased mass affecting the right ventricle. The comparison ratio of the right ventricle weight against that of the left ventricle and septum (Fulton index) provides an estimate of the degree of right ventricle overload

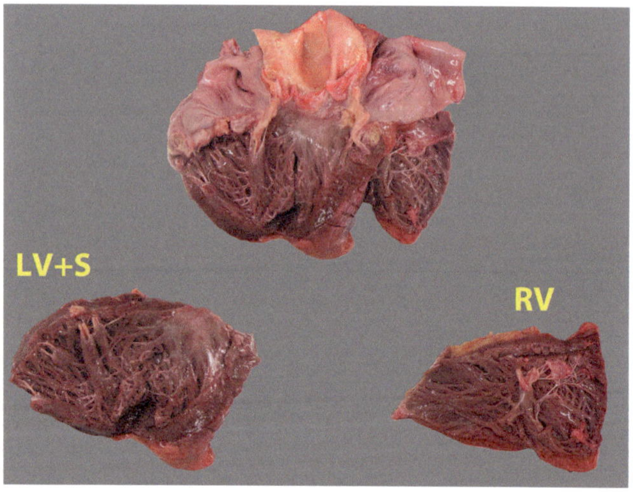

Fig. 4.313 The Fulton method uses the heart after dissection and coronary examination. Here, the dissection lays open the heart with the mitral valve bisected, thereby making this weighing protocol easier. The right ventricle (*RV*; without fat) is dissected free and compared with the left ventricle and septum (*LV + S*; without fat). A ratio of 2.3–3.3:1 for the LV + S:RV is normal

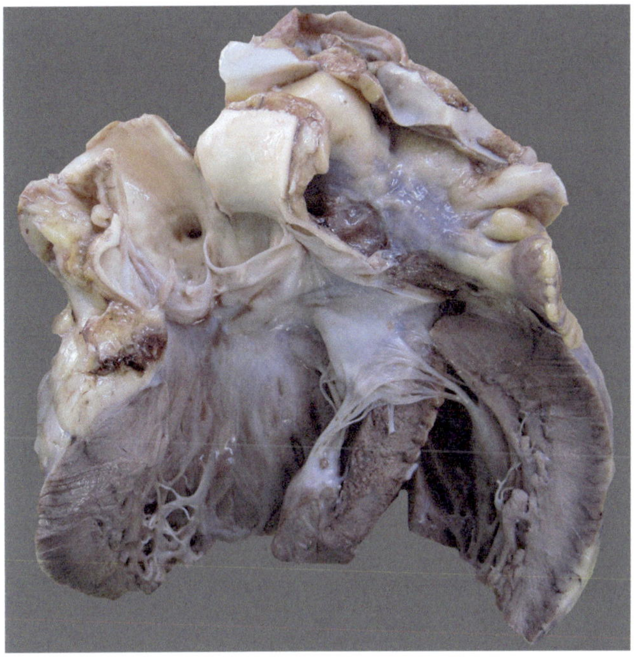

Fig. 4.314 A fixed heart specimen is seen with a coronary artery anomaly, with only one coronary ostium being present. This underwent bifurcation into the left anterior descending artery and right coronary artery branch, which continued around the back of the heart to supply the posterior wall and ultimately the lateral wall of the left ventricle. At this point, there was left ventricular fibrosis in a patchy fashion, indicative of ischaemic heart disease, explaining the sudden death of this individual

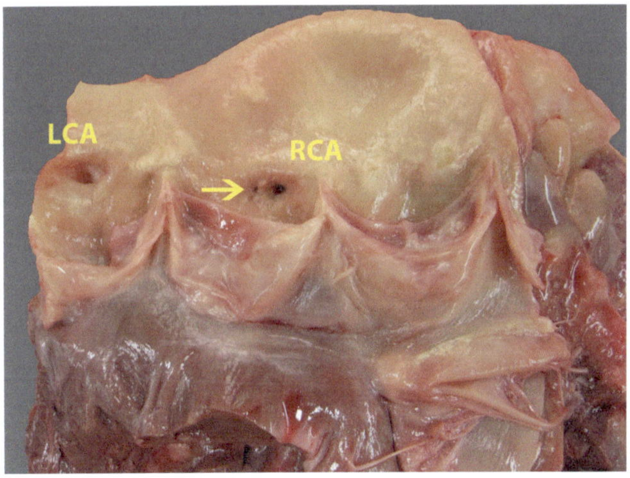

Fig. 4.315 This is an example of a conus artery. The aortic valve tissues have the normal arrangement of the origins of the right coronary artery (*RCA*) and left coronary artery (*LCA*). In addition, there is a small artery (*arrow*) next to the RCA. This is the conus artery—a normal variant, not a congenital coronary anomaly

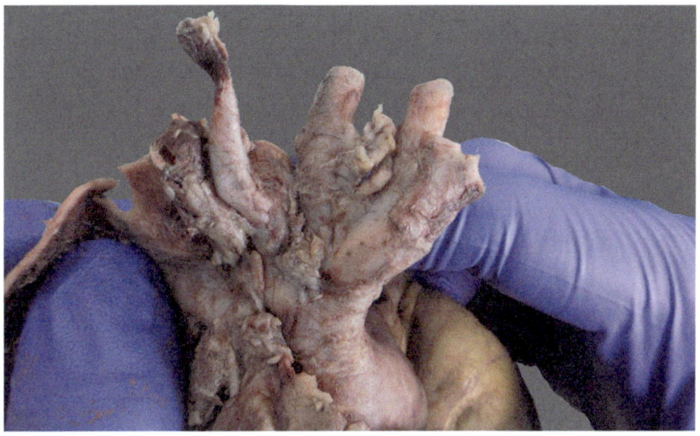

Fig. 4.316 Congenital heart disease can be seen in various formats. However, it is often easy to overlook major vessel abnormalities. In this case, there is sub-splitting of the right subclavian/internal carotid and the left subclavial internal carotid vasculature. In other respects, the major arteries are normal

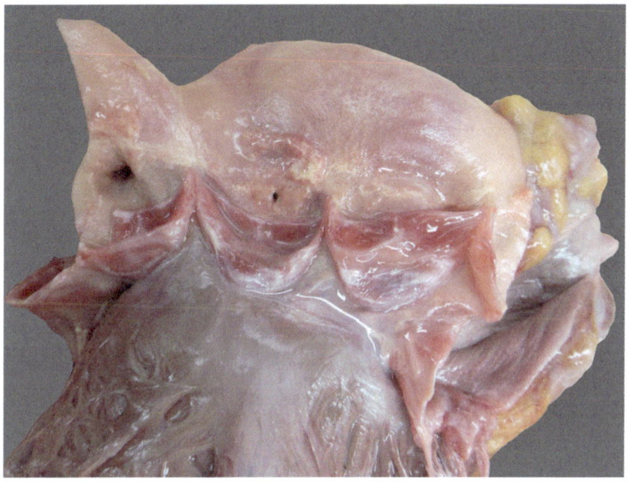

Fig. 4.317 The coronary vasculature in this case shows a normal architecture for the left main stem, supplying the circumflex and left anterior descending artery with the right coronary artery being of very small calibre/transverse diameter. The runoff of the right coronary artery is similarly small with disproportion of the vasculature

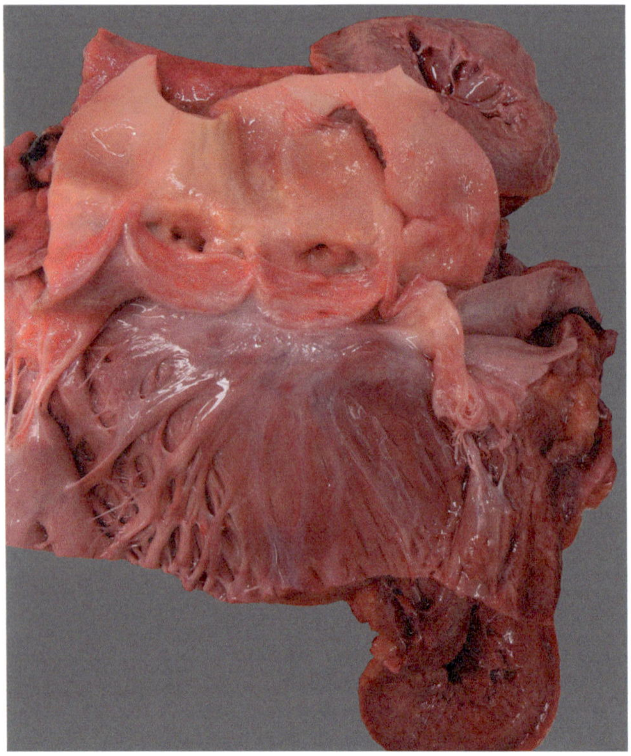

Fig. 4.318 The coronary vasculature can occasionally show individual origins for the three main arteries. This normally has no functional impact on the case concerns in terms of myocardial performance

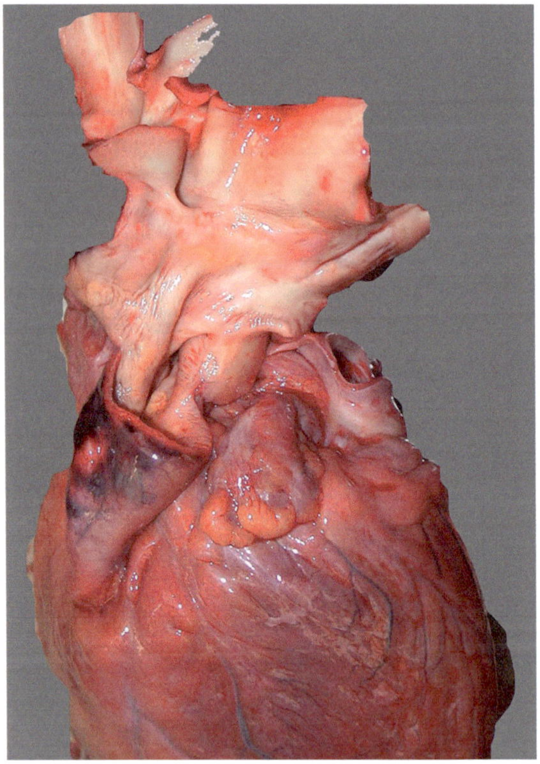

Fig. 4.319 This is a complex dissection showing both aortic and pulmonary artery tissues that have been opened anteriorly to demonstrate the small area of connection between the two circulation vessels. This is an example of patent ductus arteriosus, which has not been complicated by infective endocarditis

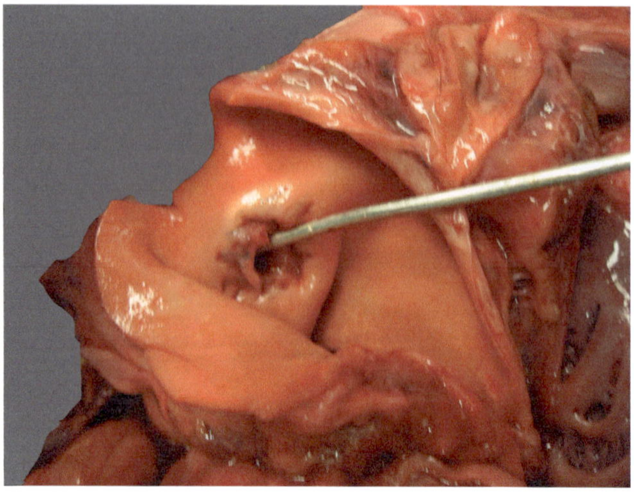

Fig. 4.320 Congenital disease of major significance is occasionally treated with a surgical fistula to offload the circulation problems. This view shows a connection between the aorta and pulmonary artery

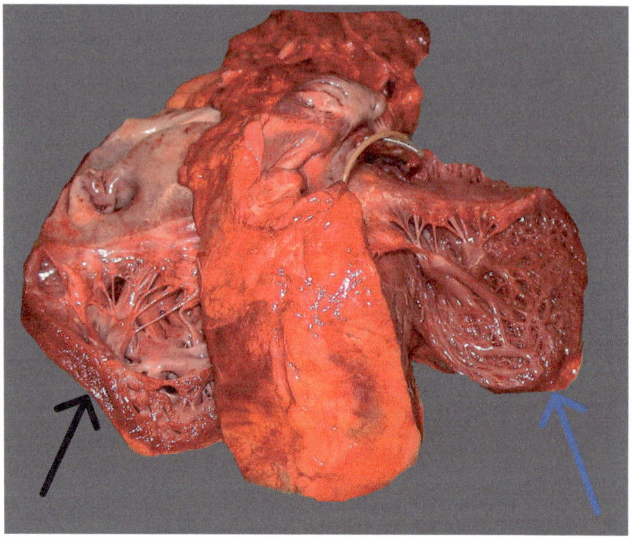

Fig. 4.321 The increase in successful congenital heart surgery means that patients often live to adulthood. This individual, with the heart viewed posteriorly, underwent an operation to treat transposition of the great arteries (TGA), in which the anatomical left ventricle shows morphological features more in keeping with the right ventricle, *i.e.* coarse trabeculations (*black arrow*). Conversely, the right ventricle shows morphological features more in keeping with the left ventricle with crisscrossing finer trabeculations (*blue arrow*)

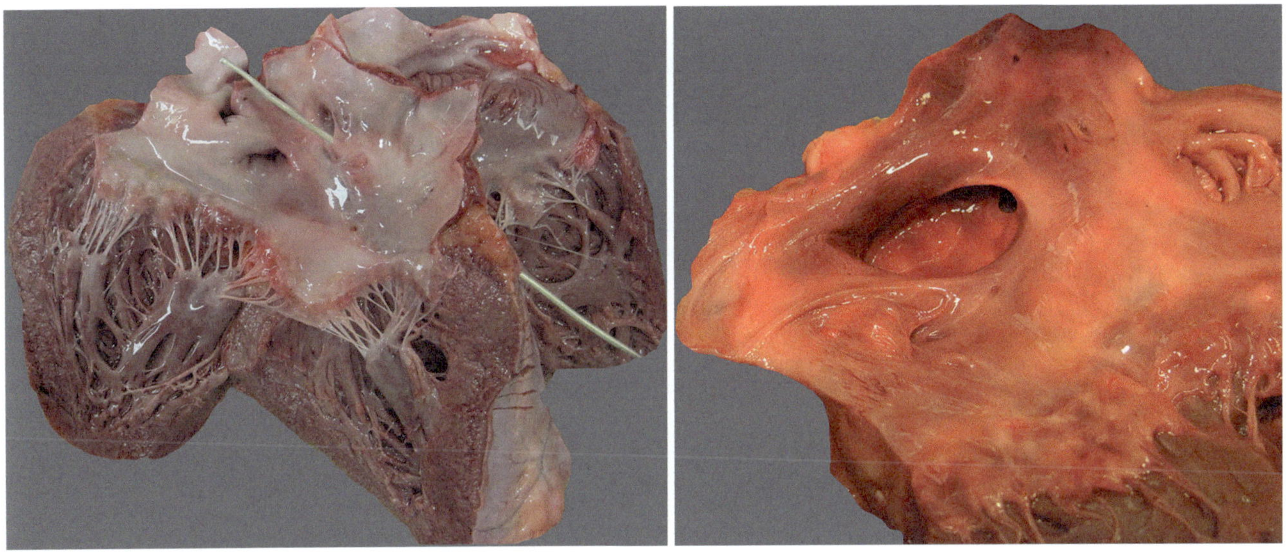

Fig. 4.322 A probe-patent foramen ovale (*left*) is not an uncommon feature, occurring in 15–20% of normal subjects. It generally has no functional significance, although there is a small risk of infective endocarditis. This view shows a probe passed from the right atrium into the left, highlighting the patency of the septal wall. If the natural closure of the foramen ovale has not been complete (*right*), a persistently open rounded defect can be found anteriorly. This defect may be relatively small, but it can have significant flow across it, capable of causing shunting that could end up with functional haemodynamic significance

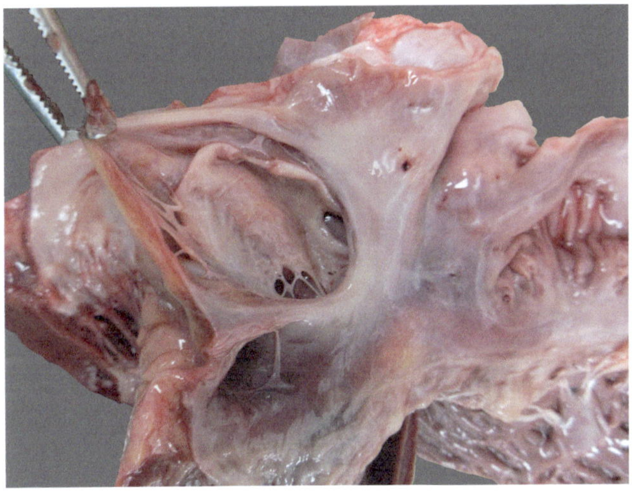

Fig. 4.323 A foramen ovale (primum) defect is seen with a somewhat web-like and fenestrated component. The size of the defect is large and significant functional deficit and sudden death is a likely end point of such cases, although there may have been minimal symptomatology beforehand

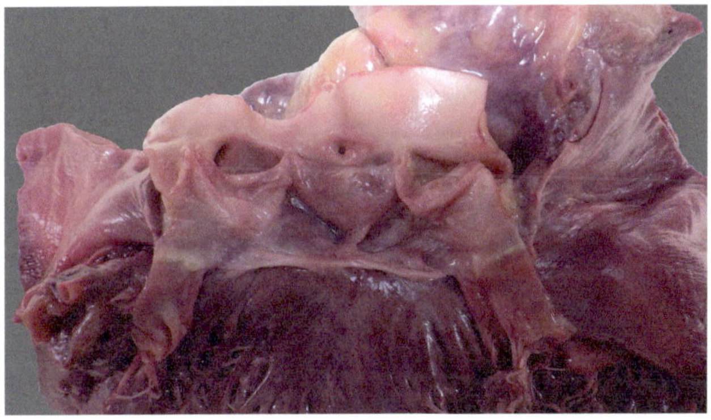

Fig. 4.324 This aortic valve was impeded by a dense constrictive subaortic band of fibrous tissue below the three normal aortic valve leaflets. The degree of impediment can vary quite significantly and is difficult to predict simply from direct observation of the pathology. Understanding whether this had significant impact clinically requires knowledge of the cardio-pulmonary status antemortem

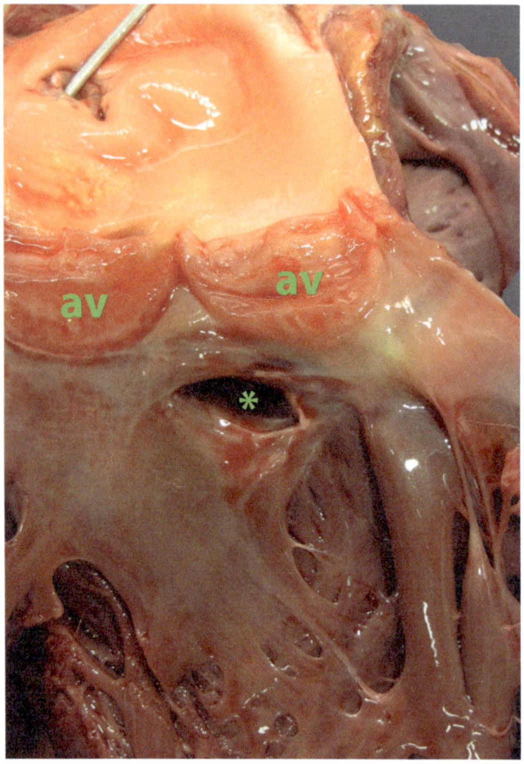

Fig. 4.325 A ventricular septal defect (*asterisk*) is seen centrally, below the aortic valve cusps (*AV*). No vegetation is present. A probe is seen entering the aortic root fistula created between the aorta and pulmonary artery in this treated case of heart disease. Sudden deaths in the second or third decades are common in such cases, even with apparent functional restoration of the congenital lesion

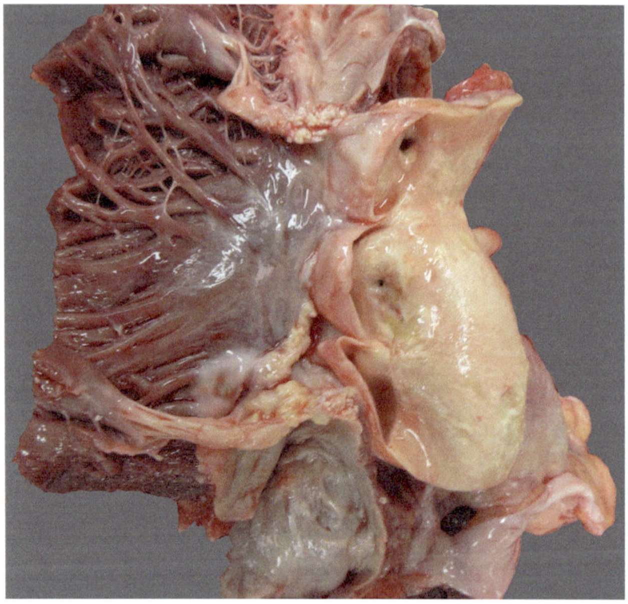

Fig. 4.326 This individual had a left ventricle septal defect which was closed operatively in early childhood. Note the irregular zone of fibrosis at the site of previous surgery without features of infection or other valvular dysfunction. The granular material is calcification of the valve annulus

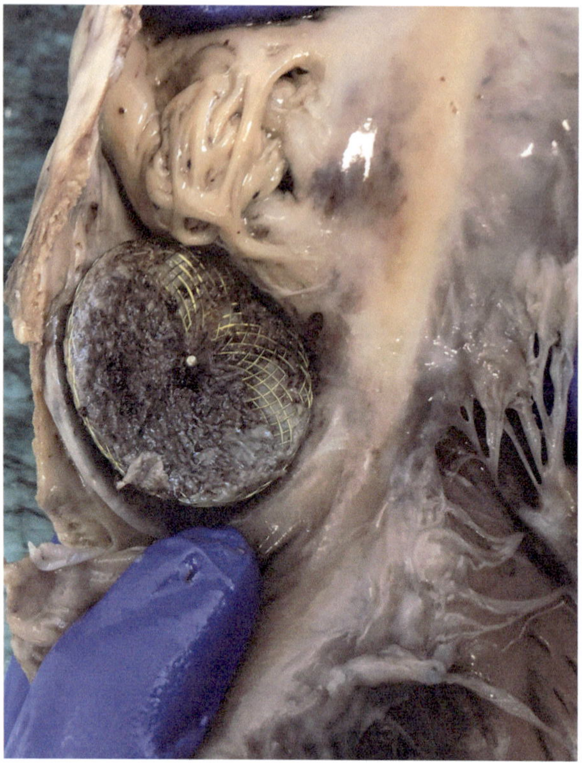

Fig. 4.327 Atrial septal closure devices (Amplatzer™ Septal Occluder) consist of two discs of meshed metal which sit either side of the atrial wall tissues. When the device is deployed, it extends outwards and then pulls the discs together, sealing the septal defect. The surgical route is a percutaneous, transcatheter approach and so it is unlikely there will be thoracic surgical scars to provide a clue to previous heart surgery

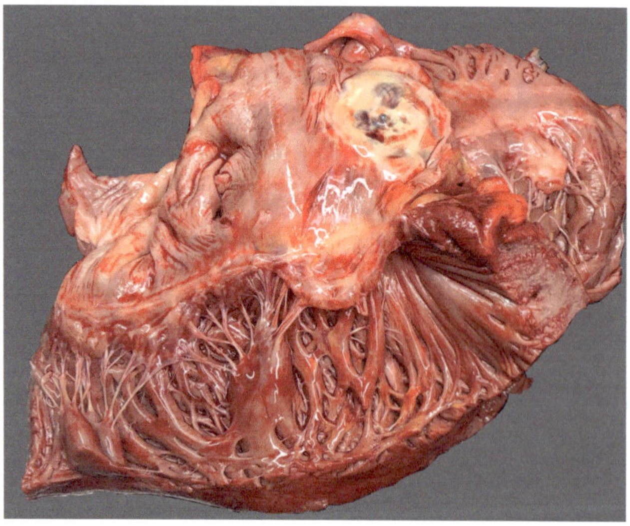

Fig. 4.328 This atrial septal defect repair has been in position for many years resulting in initial thrombosis and subsequent fibrosis around the metal mesh discs, thereby sealing the defect

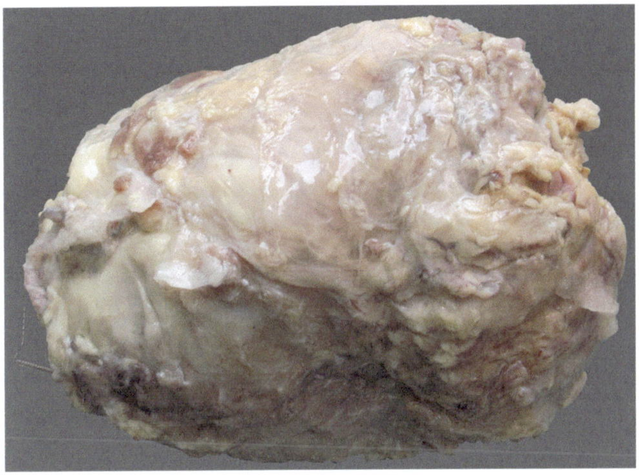

Fig. 4.329 It is often difficult to accurately consider and evaluate congenital heart cases, particularly if they have received numerous operative interventions beforehand. This individual died some 30 years after the first of his operative, pacemaker and valvular manipulations. The epicardium and pericardium appear tightly meshed within dense fibrous tissue and it is very difficult to make an initial assessment of the case without having a good knowledge of the preceding medical history. Indeed, one should not undertake dissections in such cases without appropriate previous medical history being available. Note the wire protruding though the apex of the heart

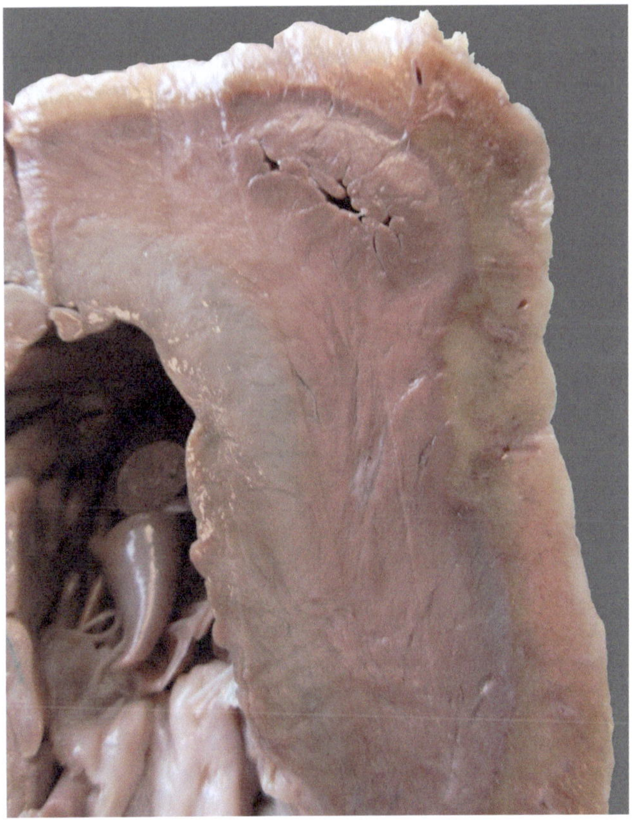

Fig. 4.330 This is the same case as Fig. 4.329, previously operated congenital heart disease. The case involved tricuspid atresia and right ventricle hypoplasia. The right ventricle remnant is seen in the wall of the left ventricle (univentricular case) with pronounced mural hypertrophy adjacent. The coronary arteries seen in the epicardium appear normal. No infection or other lesion was seen but clearly extensive remodeling surgical interventions have been required to allow some normality of life. Prior to congenital heart disease surgery, such cases used to die in early infancy

Infections and Inflammatory Conditions

Inflammatory conditions in the heart (Figs. 4.331, 4.332, 4.333, 4.334, 4.335, 4.336, 4.337, 4.338, 4.339, 4.340, 4.341, 4.342, 4.343, 4.344, 4.345, 4.346, 4.347, 4.348, 4.349, and 4.350) generally produce significant clinical effects with rapid-onset cardiac failure or sudden death. The presence of myocarditis should be specifically sought, with macroscopic analysis, histological sampling, and reservation of tissue samples (at least a 1 cm cube) for genetic and viral studies. Lymphocytic, eosinophilic, and granulomatous disorders are the most common forms of myocarditis. Direct sepsis from local infections may also be apparent, occasionally seeding from infected valves or being part of a more systemic bacteraemia.

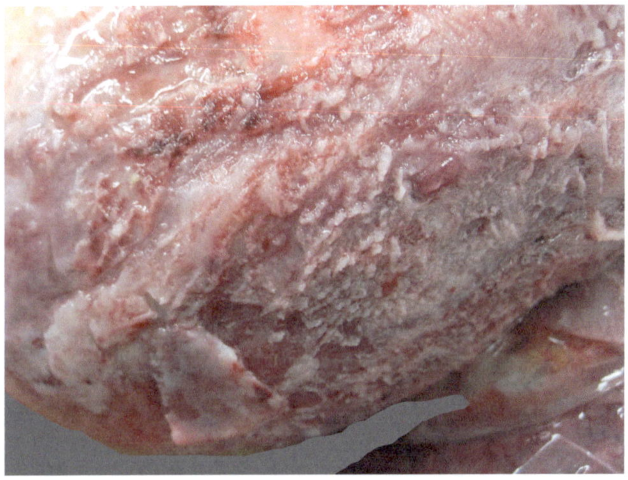

Fig. 4.331 Extensive pericardial roughening due to fibrin deposition is seen soon after valve replacement, described as bread-and-butter pericarditis

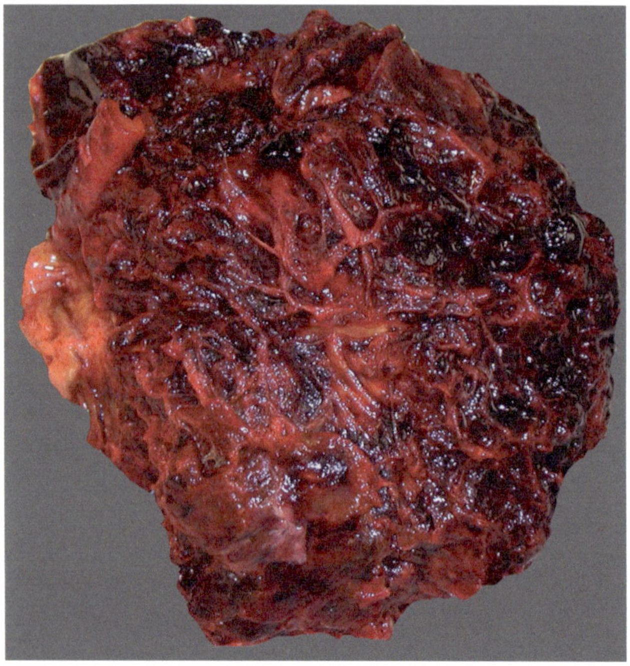

Fig. 4.332 Markedly heavy haemorrhagic pericarditis is seen shortly after complications following cardiac surgery. This pericarditis may have a tamponade effect and provide a locus for sepsis. In this case, the organising clot matrix completely obliterates the external view of the heart tissue. Carefully teasing this material away from the heart surface allows standard cardiac tissue examination to follow

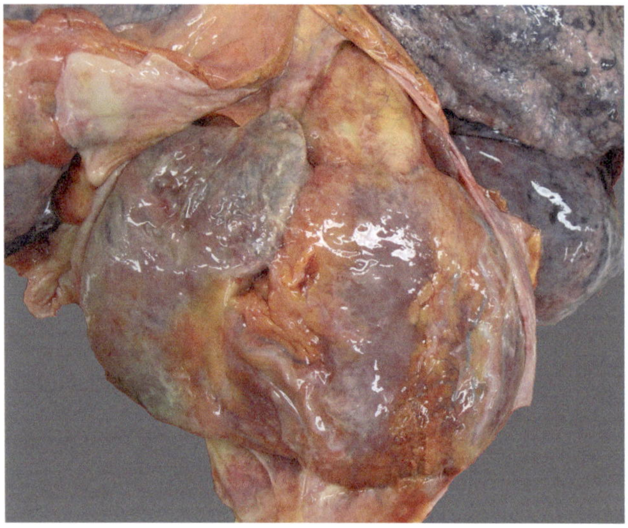

Fig. 4.333 This is a case of chronic fibrotic pericarditic change following coronary bypass surgery, performed about 1 year previously. The pericardial sac is bound to the epicardial surface. Note that the sac is adherent to the heart surface but can be separated with patience

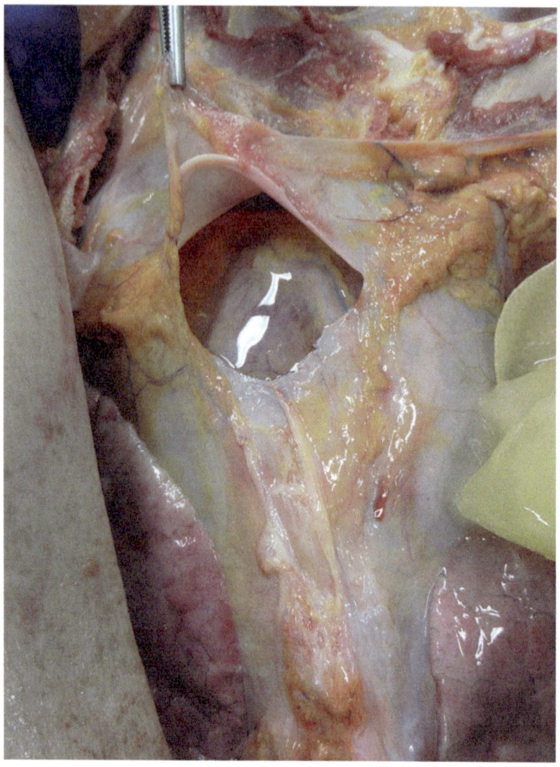

Fig. 4.334 The volume of pericardial fluid should be evaluated and assessed for its clarity and consistency during any autopsy protocol. Drawing up the fluid using a syringe without a needle, or draining the fluid into a jug are convenient ways to do this. This is a small volume, chronic pericardial collection of clear serous fluid consistent with the clinical history of heart failure

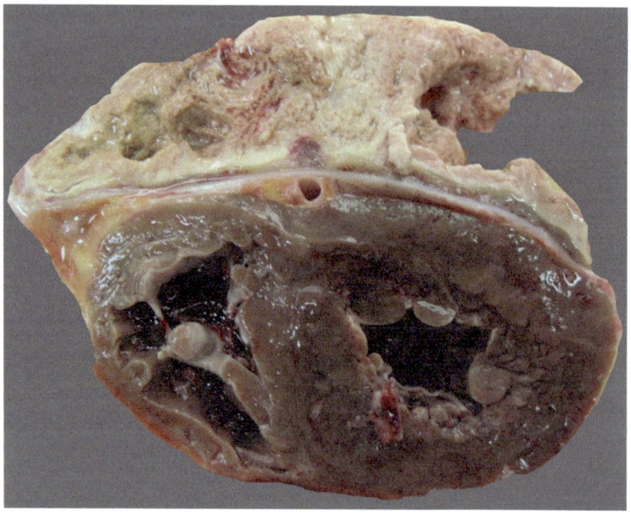

Fig. 4.335 Rheumatoid arthritis can cause a significant reaction in the pericardium. In this view, the right and left ventricles are covered by an adherent thick, spongy material. It was microscopically confirmed to be a florid, necrobiotic, granulomatous reaction, limited to the pericardial tissue. The remainder of this inflammatory material has been dissected free of the specimen, but clearly this inflammatory/fibrotic process caused significant tamponade

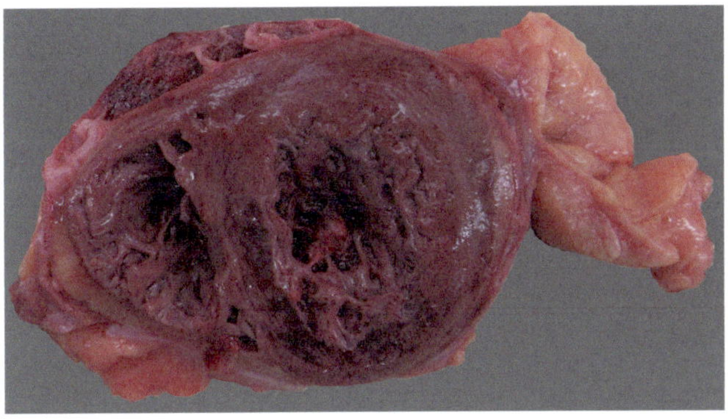

Fig. 4.336 This is a case of constrictive pericarditis. In most cases constriction of the pericardium and epicardium involves dense fibrosis which can be seen and palpated without difficulty. However, this case had very tight fibrosis but with only a thin rind of fibrous tissue being evident. Indeed, it is easy to miss such constriction if dissection is over hurried

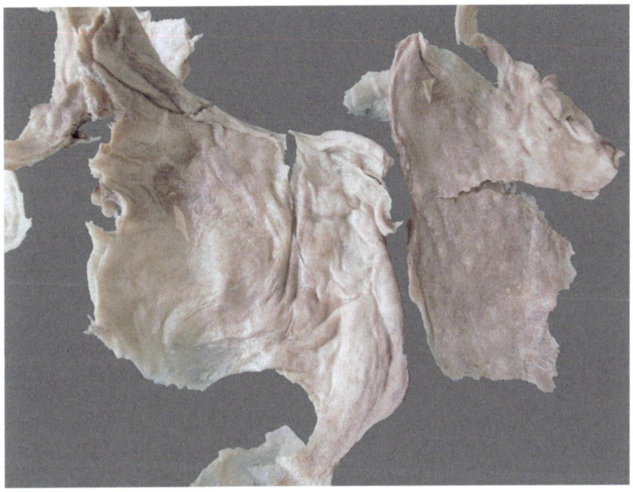

Fig. 4.337 Dressler's pericarditis/syndrome may follow recent myocardial infarction or other myocardial injury between 1 and 3 weeks after the event. These are sheets of fibrin exudate removed from the pericardial surface of the heart. Had the individual lived longer, then a degree of constriction of the cardiac tissues would be expected

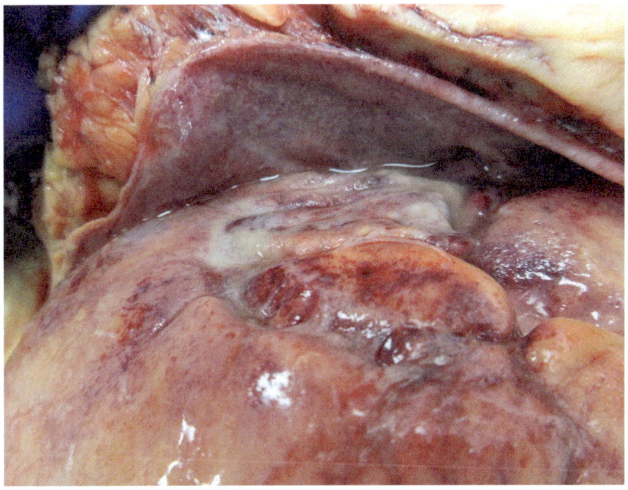

Fig. 4.338 Septic pericarditis can be easily overlooked during dissection. The surface of the parietal pericardium and visceral pericardial surface have an oedematous, erythematous appearance, and there is focal thick whitish/yellow exudate, which are clues to underlying sepsis. In this case the origin of infection was a pronounced semi-necrotic lobar pneumonia

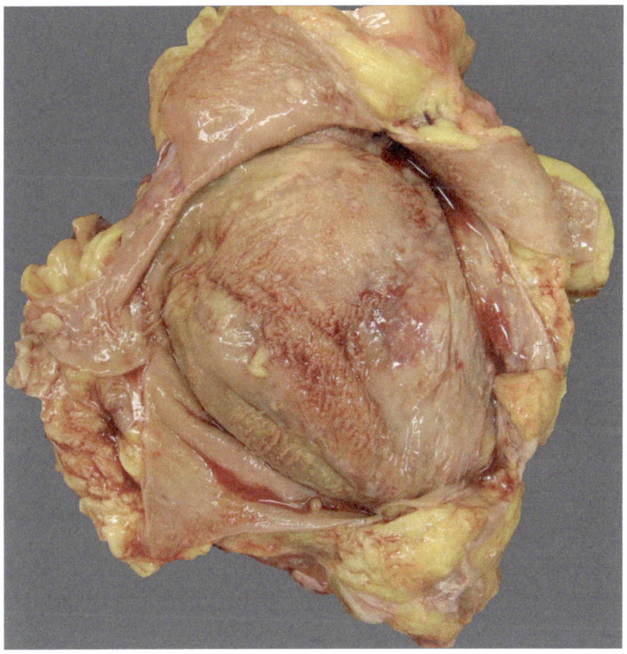

Fig. 4.339 The profound pericarditis in this case has heavy fibrin deposition (bread-and-butter appearance). The differential diagnosis would be disseminated neoplasia

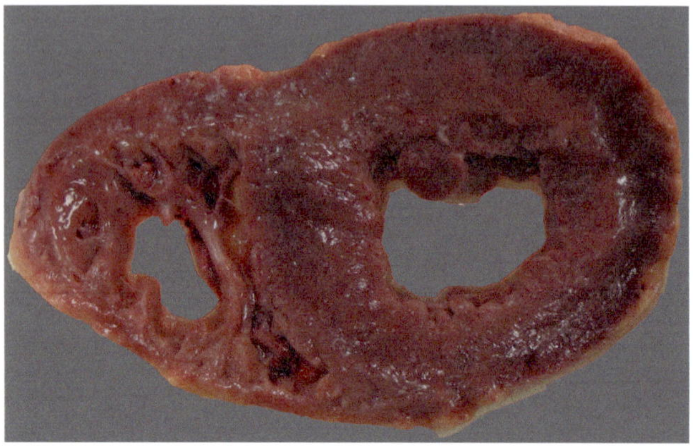

Fig. 4.340 The macroscopic features of myocarditis are often not evident, although histology will provide the diagnosis. This case of acute lymphocytic myocarditis shows some slight congestion of the myocardial parenchyma in transverse section but no clues as to the diagnosis. This case reflected viral infection

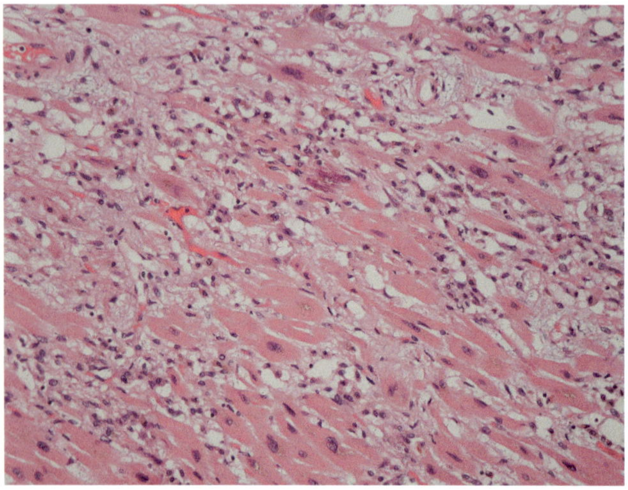

Fig. 4.341 Marked lymphocytic myocarditis with widespread disruption and damage to individual cardiac myocytes is seen in this histological section

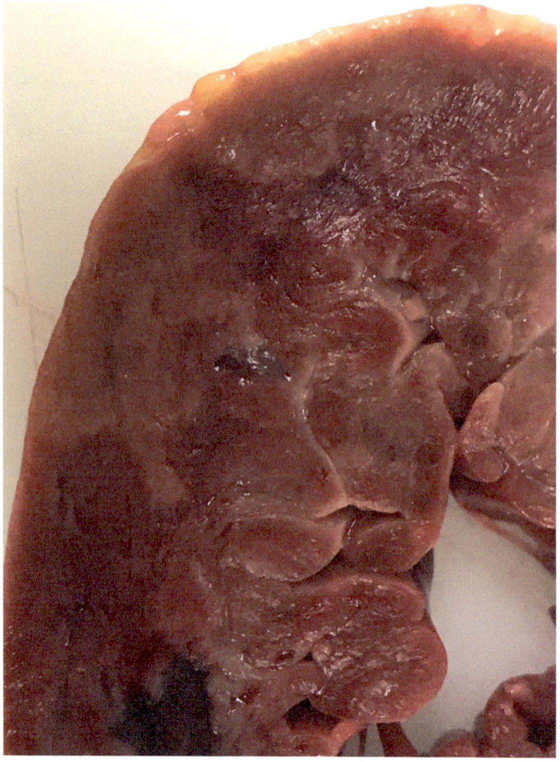

Fig. 4.342 In this case there is macroscopic mottling of the myocardium, along with endocardial fibrosis. Histologically, it was shown to have features of giant cell myocarditis

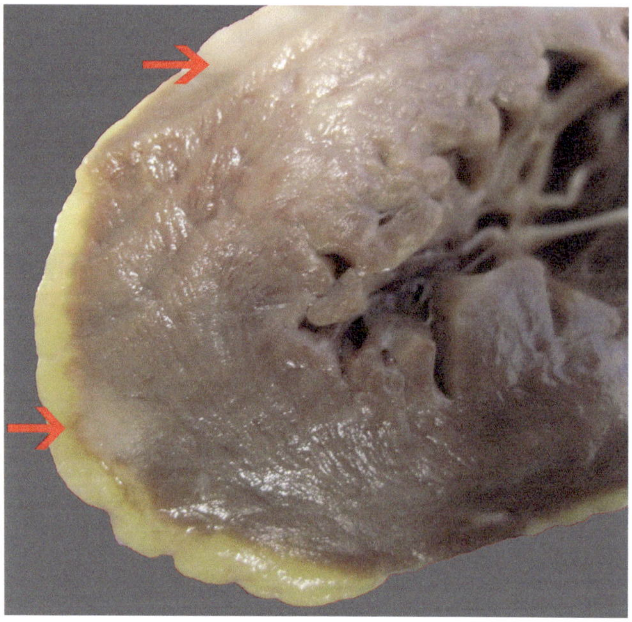

Fig. 4.343 Giant cell myocarditis in a primary presentation with sudden death is seen with flecks of congestion and fibrosis in the left ventricle wall

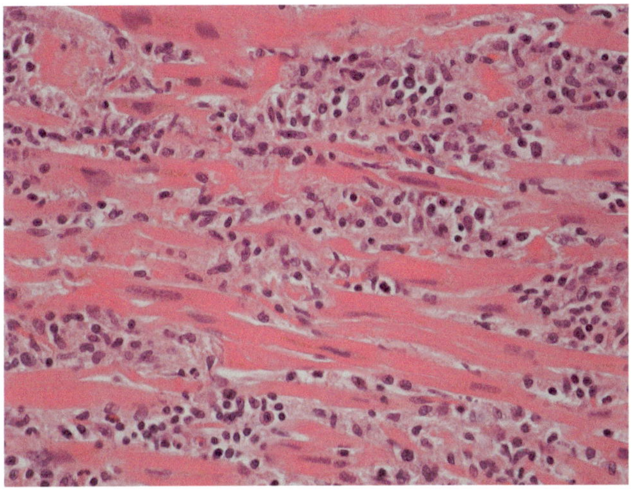

Fig. 4.344 Myocarditis can be variable in density within the heart tissues. There is infiltration of the interstitium by a variety of inflammatory cells, with separation and lysis of individual cardiac myocytes

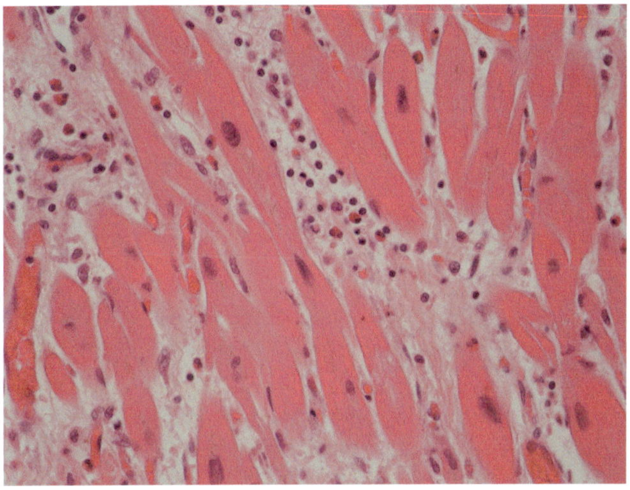

Fig. 4.345 Classically, lymphocytic myocarditis (associated with viral infections) can cause death, but this case shows a florid, eosinophil-rich myocarditis, which should prompt consideration of atypical infections and allergic phenomena

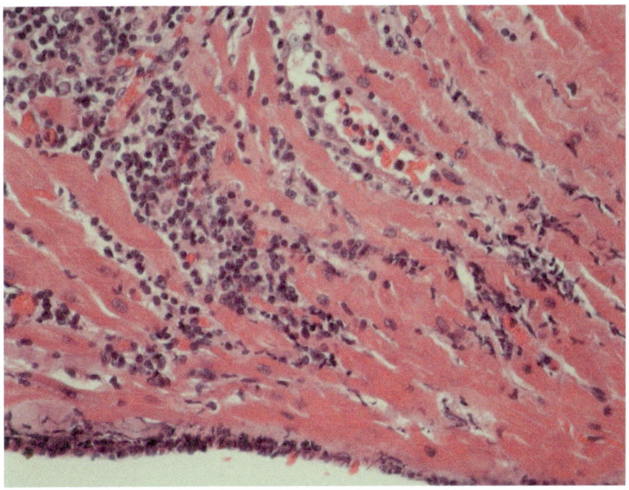

Fig. 4.346 To an extent, acute cellular cardiac rejection is a form of myocarditis. Significant graft infiltration by activated T cells will cause myocardial damage and potentially sudden death

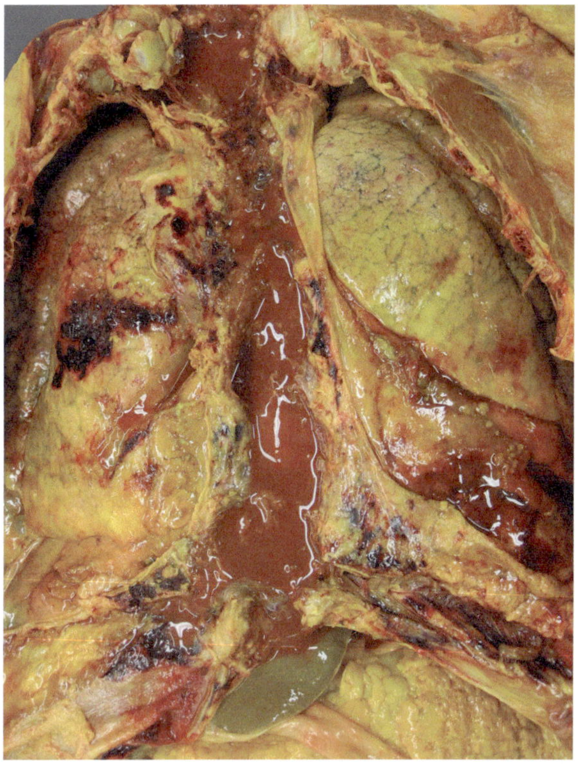

Fig. 4.347 Infections following surgery for coronary and/or valve surgery are generally bacterial, particularly staphylococcal. Atypical infections, such as *Aspergillus* in this case, can nevertheless complicate various surgical techniques. This case shows purulent collections around the site of prior surgery. Heavy jaundice was also present in this case because of right-sided cardiac failure causing acute hepatic necrosis

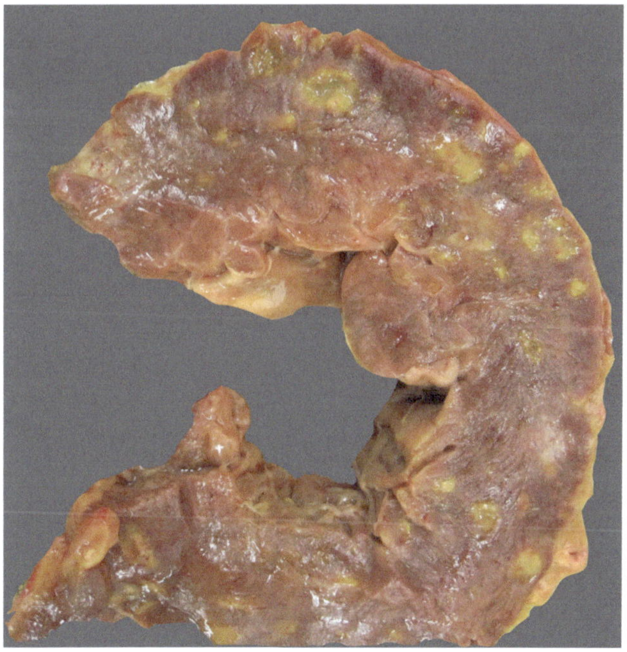

Fig. 4.348 Seeding of septic organisms into the coronary tissues causes a florid septic myocarditis. The *Aspergillus* infection in Fig. 4.347 was responsible for the fatal suppurative myocarditis

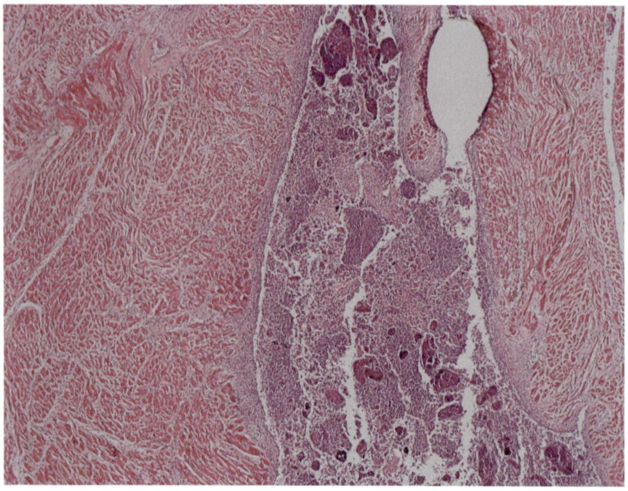

Fig. 4.349 A histology section of myocardium showing perimortem 'showering' of staphylococcal organisms into the coronary circulation (in a case of aortic valve infective endocarditis) leading to patchy bacterial myocarditis

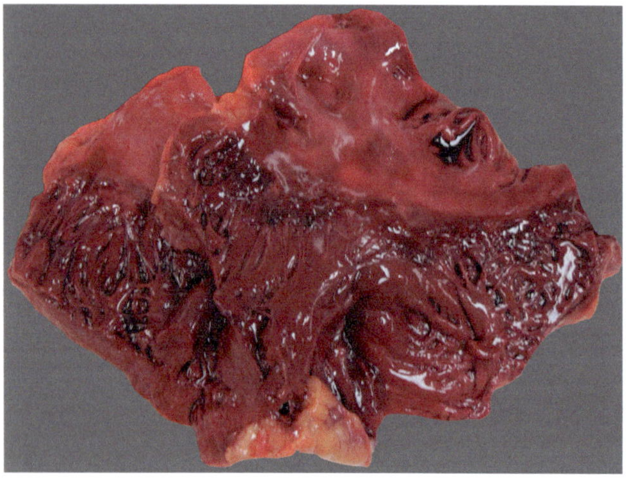

Fig. 4.350 Terminal bacteremia may cause significant haemolysis. Whilst not specific, the finding of brown staining of the endocardial and arterial intimal surfaces may suggest infection by a group A streptococcal or equivalent species

Cardiac Tumours

Cardiac tumours (Figs. 4.351, 4.352, 4.353, 4.354, 4.355, 4.356, 4.357, 4.358, 4.359, 4.360, 4.361, 4.362, 4.363, and 4.364) are comparatively rare, but disseminated neoplasia involving the heart is not uncommon; breast, thoracic, and melanomatous tumours are well documented. Primary neoplasms of the heart, aside from mesothelioma of the pericardium, generally reflect cardiac myxomas. Rare cardiac tumours such as lymphomas or sarcomas are unlikely to be encountered in routine practice unless one works close to a cardiac unit. Such tumours merit photography and histological sampling in order to confirm macroscopic features and to assist possible referral of the case to a specialist centre.

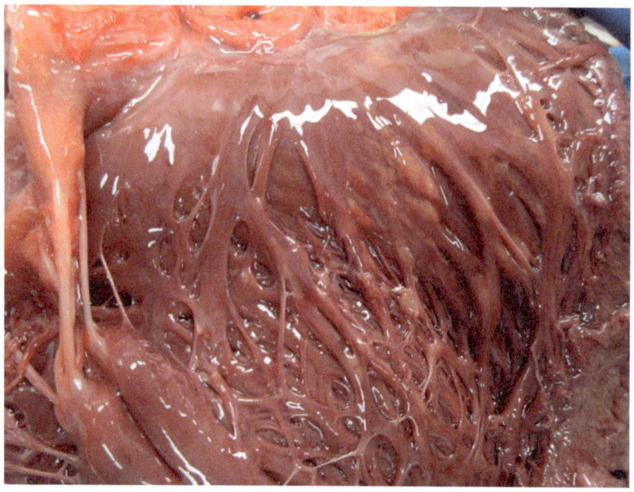

Fig. 4.351 A case of diffuse endocardial lipomatosis (fatty tissue infiltration) is seen. This is common in the elderly and particularly in women and has no functional deficit normally. It is colloquially described as 'tabby cat heart'

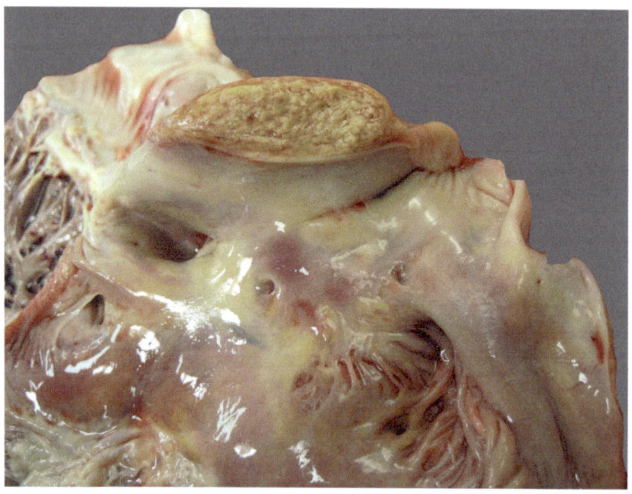

Fig. 4.352 Pronounced fatty tissue in the wall of the interatrial septum can be seen in cases of atrial lipoma and atrial lipomatous hypertrophy. This lipoma was composed entirely of adipocytes histologically, but the cells were largely of brown fat morphology and it was designated a cardiac hibernoma

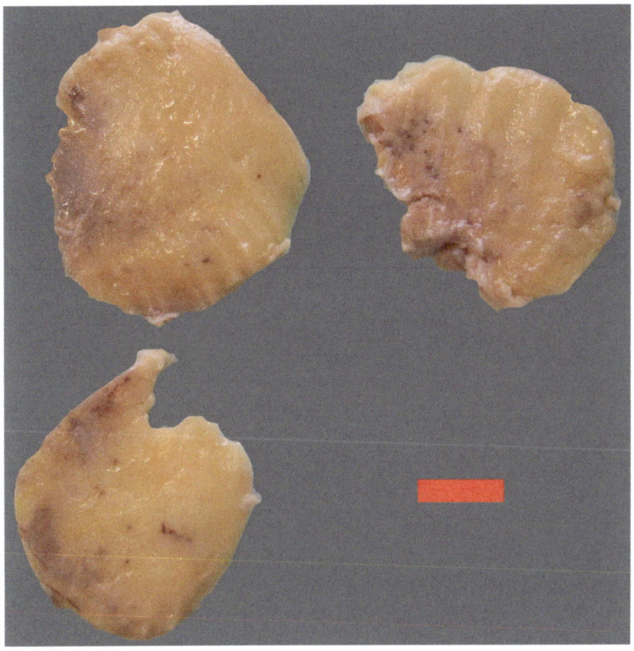

Fig. 4.353 This surgical specimen shows a standard area of lipomatous hypertrophy of the interatrial septum, which has been resected successfully. The fatty tissue appears uniform for most of the cut surface, although clearly there is more obvious myocardial parenchyma seen peripherally at several points (*Marker* 10 mm)

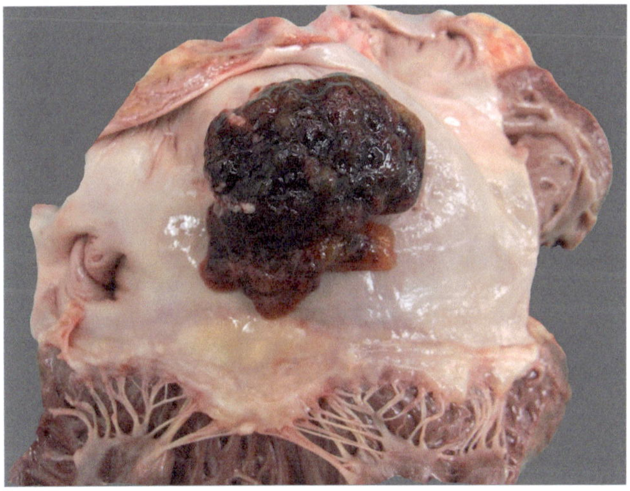

Fig. 4.354 A cardiac myxoma within the left atrium can be an unexpected finding in the autopsy room. These tumours classically occur on the interatrial septum, although they may be associated with other sites within the heart, including across the valves, within the ventricles, and occasionally in multiple sites. They are characterized by a soft, jellylike quality, and red/brown appearance due to intra-myxomatous parenchymal haemorrhage. Myxomas can be the source of systemic emboli, and appropriate confirmatory histology may be required (at other sites)

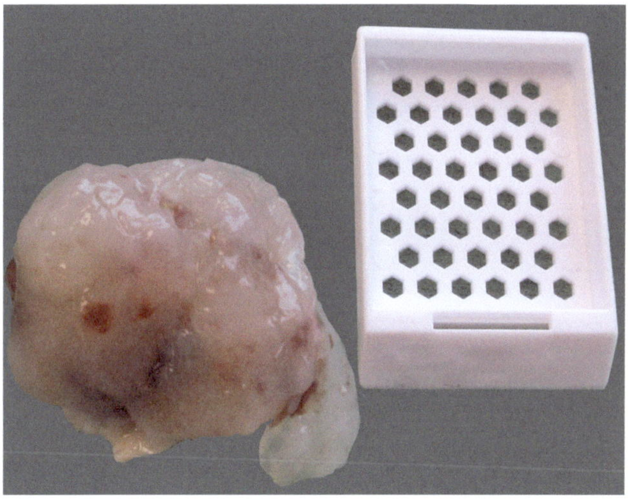

Fig. 4.355 A cardiac myxoma is seen with a thin myxoid stalk in this surgical case

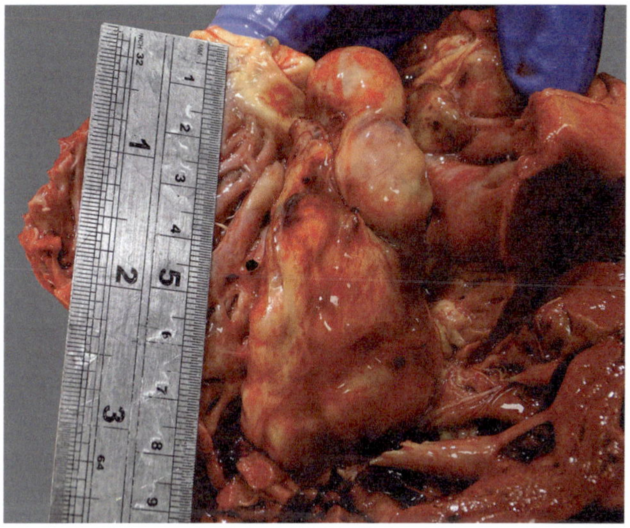

Fig. 4.356 A large irregular, multinodular, fleshy mass is apparent (although partly covered by blood). This involves both atrial and ventricular tissues and was confirmed to be a cardiac sarcoma

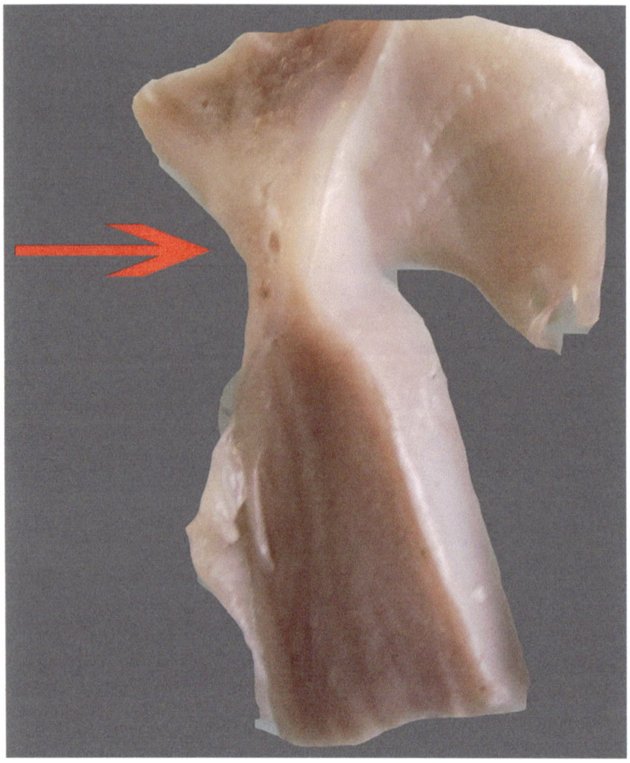

Fig. 4.357 This close-up view of the membranous septum of a young child shows the characteristic small, cystic spaces of the cystic atrioventricular node tumour. This is a rare cause of complete heart block and potentially sudden cardiac death, both in childhood and in adulthood. It is characterized by epithelial-lined spaces with variable cystic content (see Figs. 14.62 and 14.63). It has no malignant potential, but it may be functionally malignant by virtue of posing a risk for sudden cardiac dysrhythmias or death

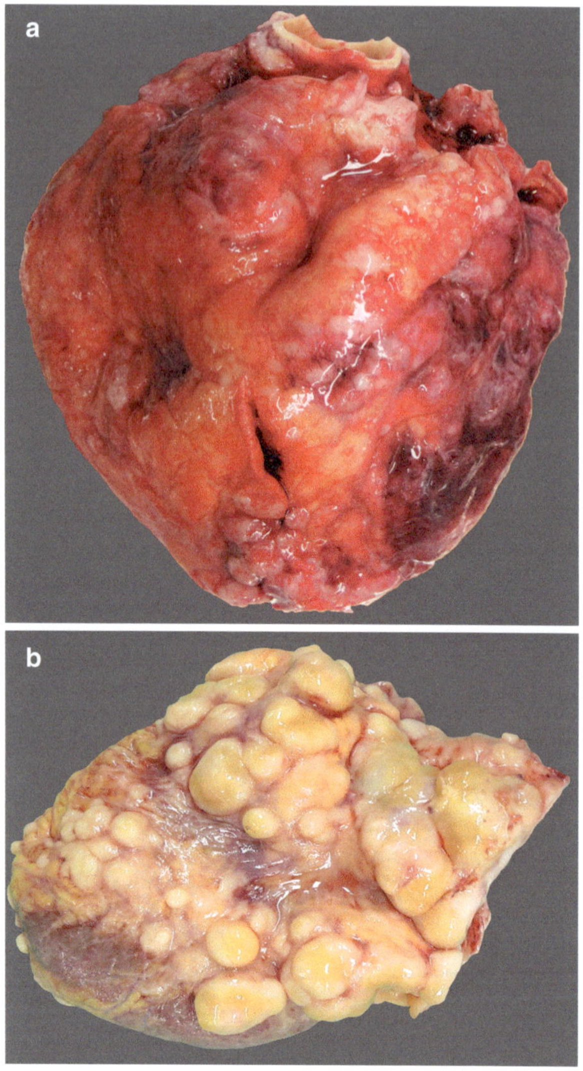

Fig. 4.358 (**a**, **b**) Mesothelioma of the pericardial sac is a recognised condition associated with asbestos exposure. It will behave exactly the same as pleural mesothelioma, but often it produces a more rapid decline and death, given the involvement of the cardiac tissues. Pleural mesothelioma can also directly invade the pericardial tissues or metastasize

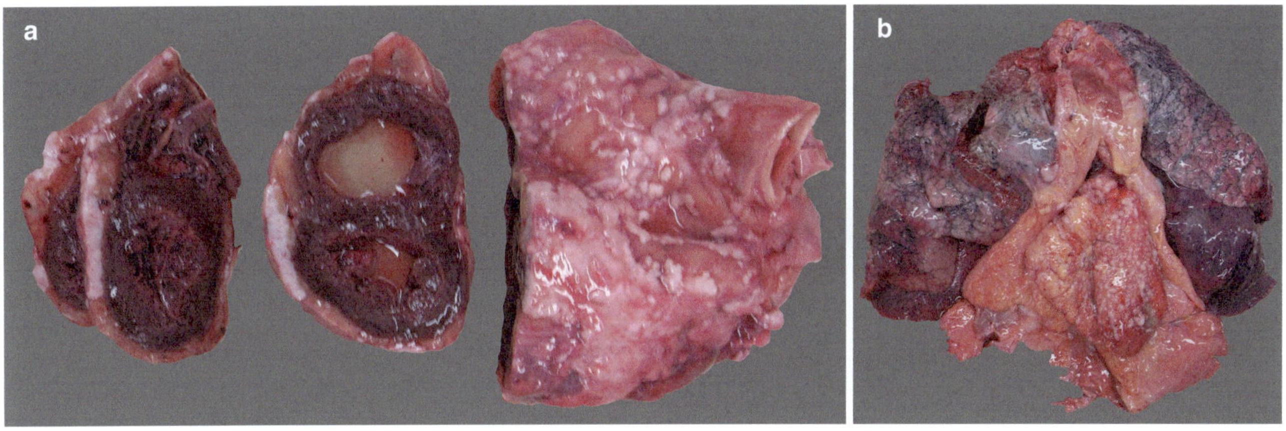

Fig. 4.359 (**a**, **b**) Metastatic tumour deposits in the pericardium. Potentially any malignancy can metastasise to the pericardial tissues, the most common being breast and lung carcinomas. Possible fatal consequences include constrictive cardiomyopathy and pericardial effusion leading to tamponade

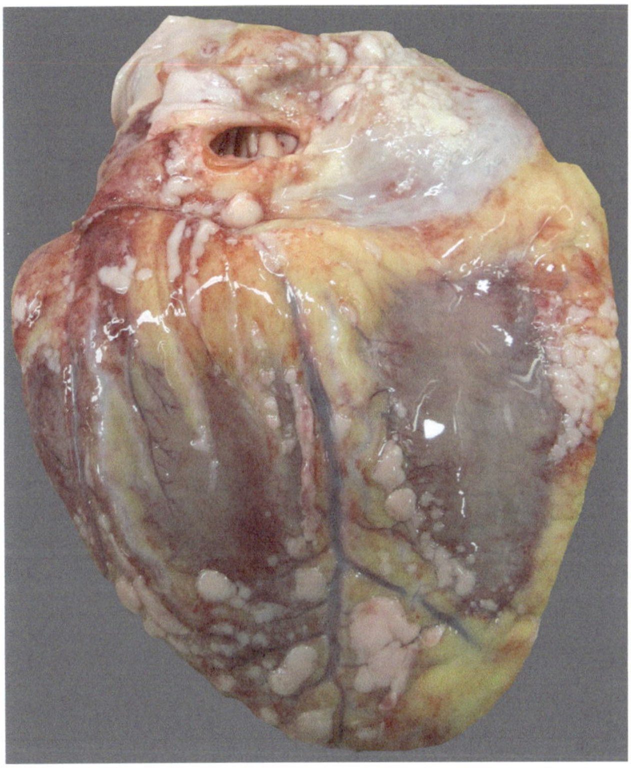

Fig. 4.360 The heart may be involved by metastatic disease on the epicardial surface. Widespread pulmonary carcinomatous metastases are most marked around the coronary tissues

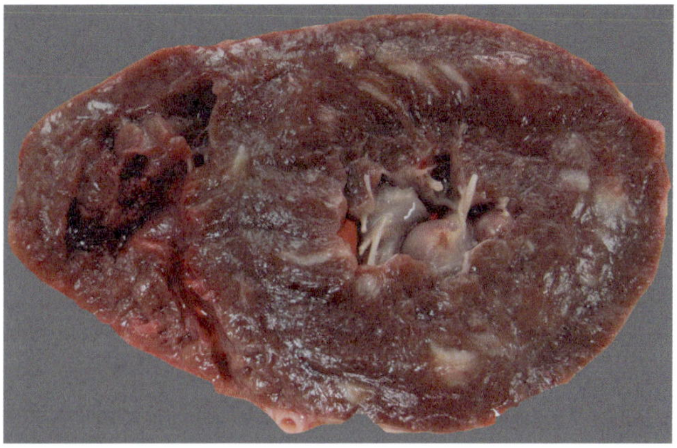

Fig. 4.361 The left ventricle wall (seen in transverse section) has multiple flecks of cream/grey tumour scattered throughout, in some places appearing to run alongside the branches of the penetrating arteries

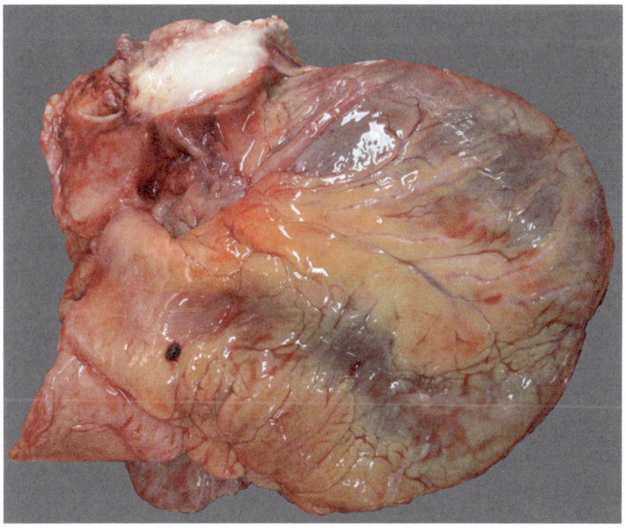

Fig. 4.362 Tumour can be seen to directly infiltrate the vasculature of the left atrium from the root of the lung in this case of small cell lung cancer

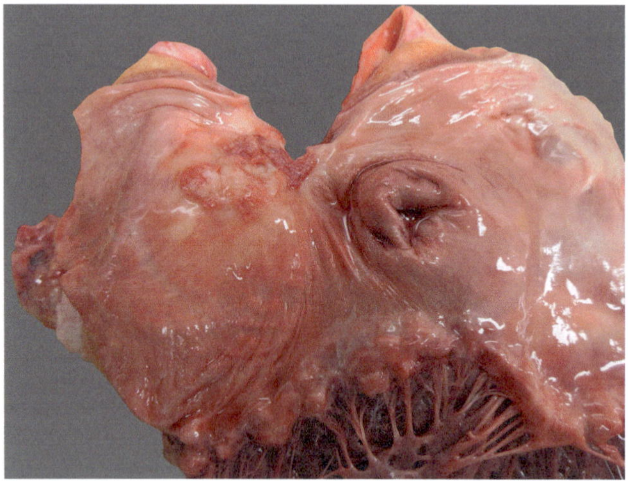

Fig. 4.363 There is irregular focal loss of the smooth atrial tissues, with a granular nodularity and possible ulcerated surface. This lesion was confirmed as small cell carcinoma metastasis eroding into the inner aspect of the left atrium

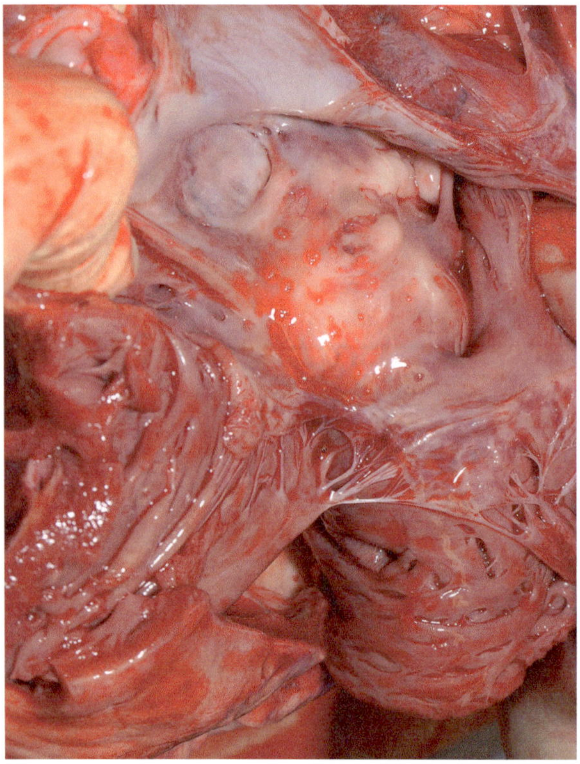

Fig. 4.364 There is a large tumour mass in this heart, which is not immediately obvious. Palpation of the heart tissue suggested an irregular mass lesion, which on closer inspection gives the right atrial wall a pale yellow/white appearance. This was a case of high-grade non-Hodgkin lymphoma. The proximity of the tumour to the conduction system explains the sudden dysrhythmic death

The Large Arteries

Whilst much of this vasculature exists outside the thorax, it is considered specifically in this chapter (Figs. 4.365, 4.366, 4.367, 4.368, 4.369, 4.370, 4.371, 4.372, 4.373, 4.374, 4.375, 4.376, 4.377, 4.378, 4.379, 4.380, 4.381, and 4.382). Vascular catastrophes, principally atheromatous in type, are commonplace and must be assessed and recorded accurately.

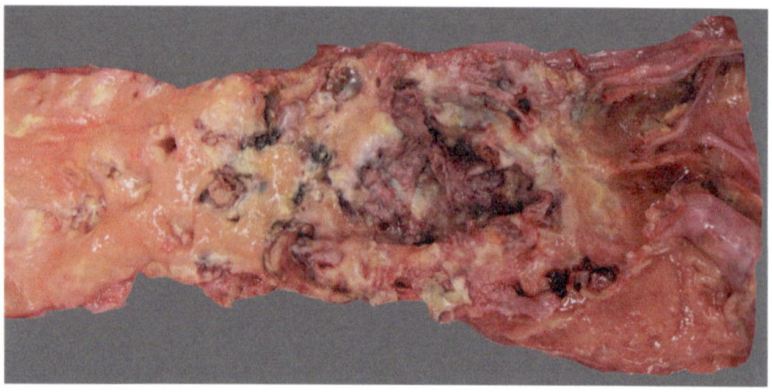

Fig. 4.365 The lower aorta is seen with extensive, ulcerated atheroma. This is a particularly vulnerable site with regard to fibrolipid plaque disease and aneurysmal change. It is noted that the more proximal part of the aorta is less affected

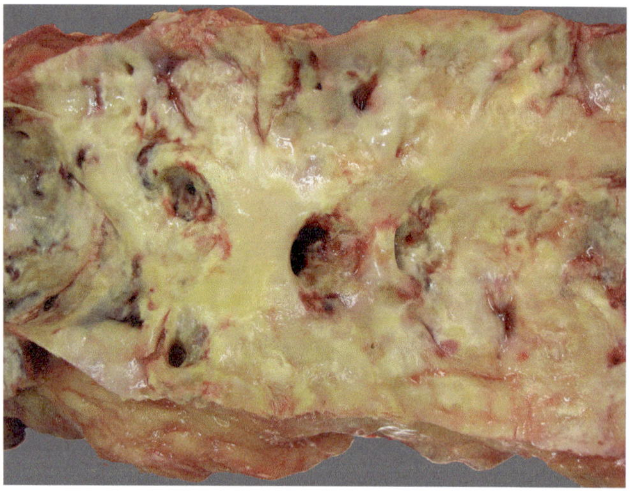

Fig. 4.366 Part of the abdominal aorta is seen with significant narrowing of the main artery branches that run off to supply the abdominal viscera and retroperitoneal tissues

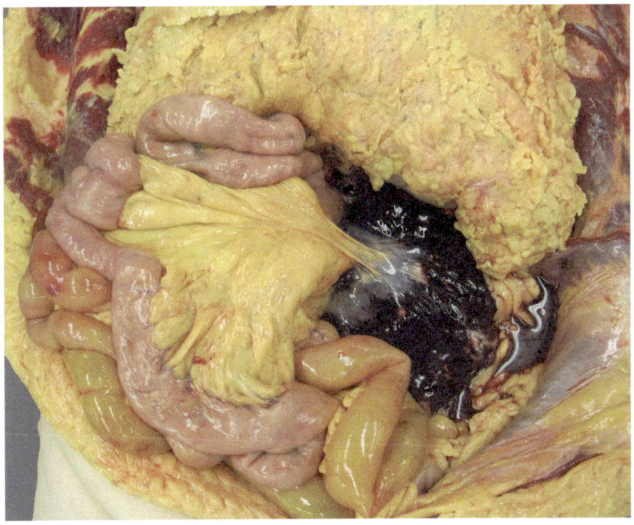

Fig. 4.367 Opening the abdomen shows a zone of massive haemorrhage in the retroperitoneal compartment from a burst aortic aneurysm

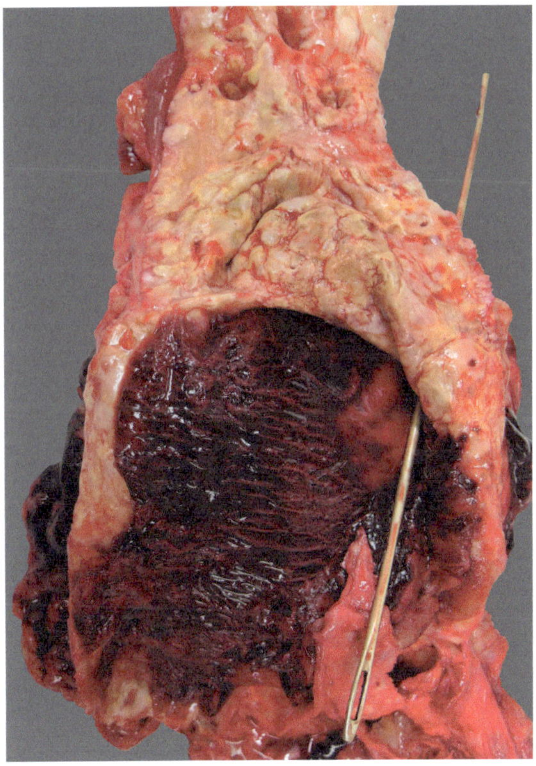

Fig. 4.368 An aortic aneurysm is seen with dilatation of the vessel and marked thrombus on the endoluminal aspect. The vessel had ruptured. The leak point is marked by a probe

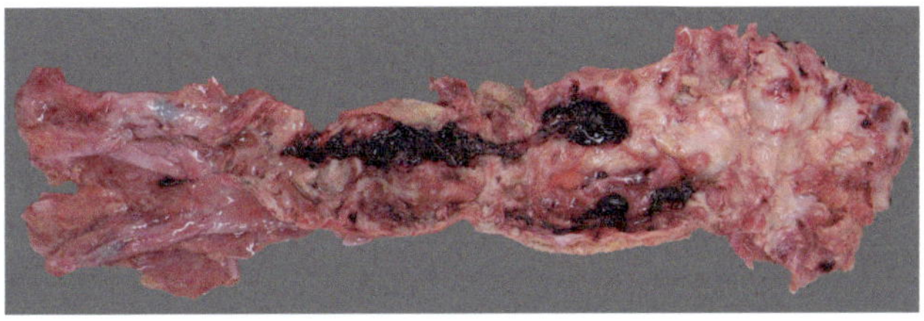

Fig. 4.369 This is heavily atheromatous aortic tissue with evidence of a dissection plane separating the mural layers

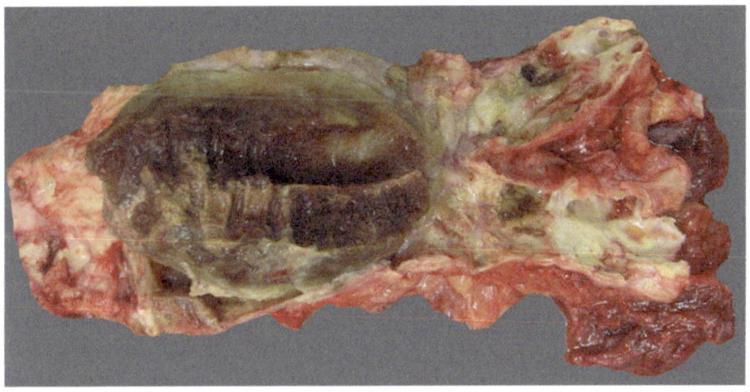

Fig. 4.370 Laminated thrombus is seen with the imprint of a synthetic graft running centrally. This patient had had a large aneurysm at risk of rupture, prompting endovascular repair

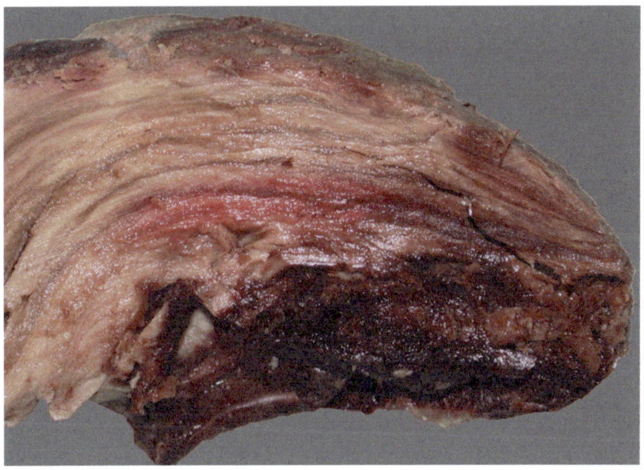

Fig. 4.371 The thrombus from an aneurysm has been removed. The sectioned material shows the lines of Zahn, comprising laminated thrombus with admixed blood components

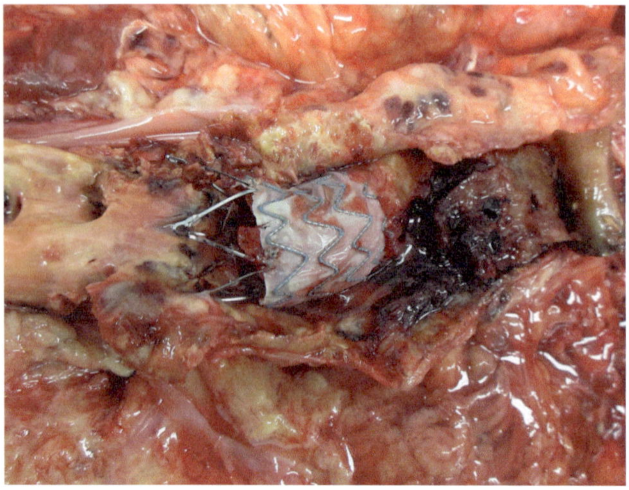

Fig. 4.372 Part of an endovascular graft device is seen here with the fabric and wire assembly in its deployed state. The device is correctly positioned but there appears to be extensive thrombus in and around the repair unit

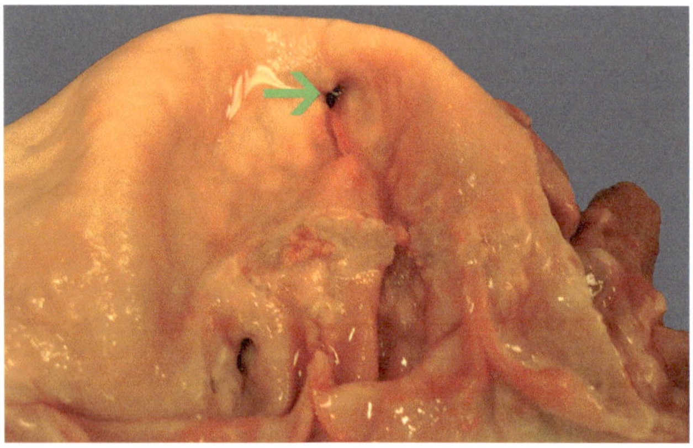

Fig. 4.373 The proximal aorta is seen with the aortic leaflets at the bottom of the view. One coronary ostium is present. The aorta appears largely normal and without high-grade atheromatous disease, but an irregular laceration/splitting of the intima and media gave rise to aortic dissection and cardiac tamponade. The aortic dissection (*arrow*) can be relatively small in terms of the entry point size but pronounced in terms of the amount of blood loss

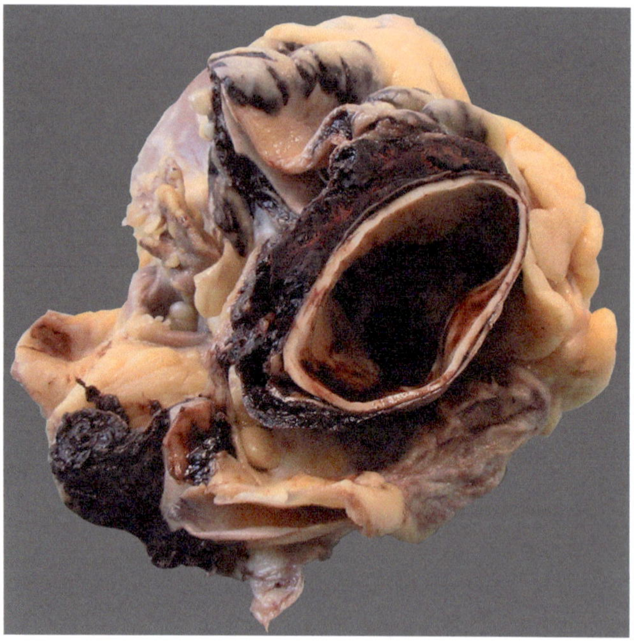

Fig. 4.374 Acute aortic dissection at the level of the aortic root, showing separation of the media and adventitial tissue planes and surrounding haemorrhage and thrombus formation

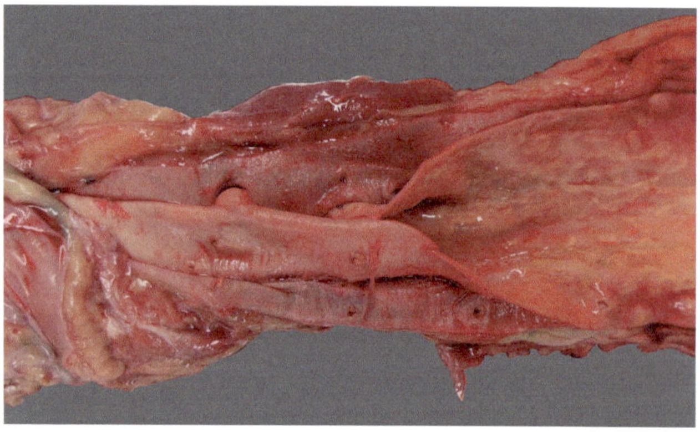

Fig. 4.375 This is an acute aortic dissection involving atheromatous aortic tissue. The intimal aspect of the aorta (towards the right side) shows the characteristic fatty and slightly wrinkled quality to the intimal surface. The dissection plane has run into the medial compartment and has pulled the medial inner tissues away from the outer such that one can see the plane of dissection running off towards the left side of the aortic dissection

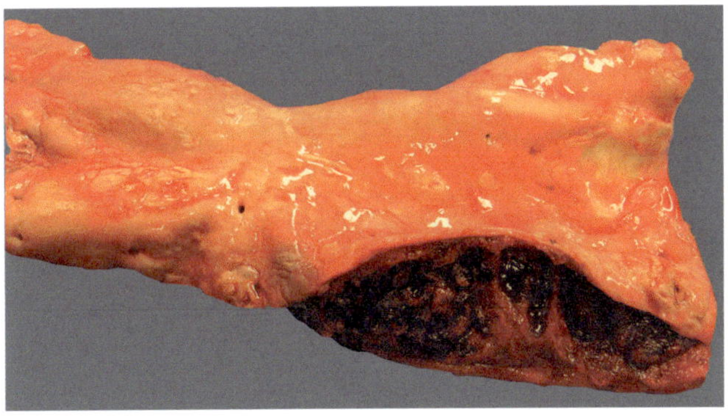

Fig. 4.376 An aortic dissection is present in the descending thoracic aorta. The intimal and medial tissues have been pushed forward into the lumen, and blood and fibrin are running in the outer media and within the adventitial tissues. This process will dissect and shear the vertebral arteries and others, causing ischaemic damage to various tissues

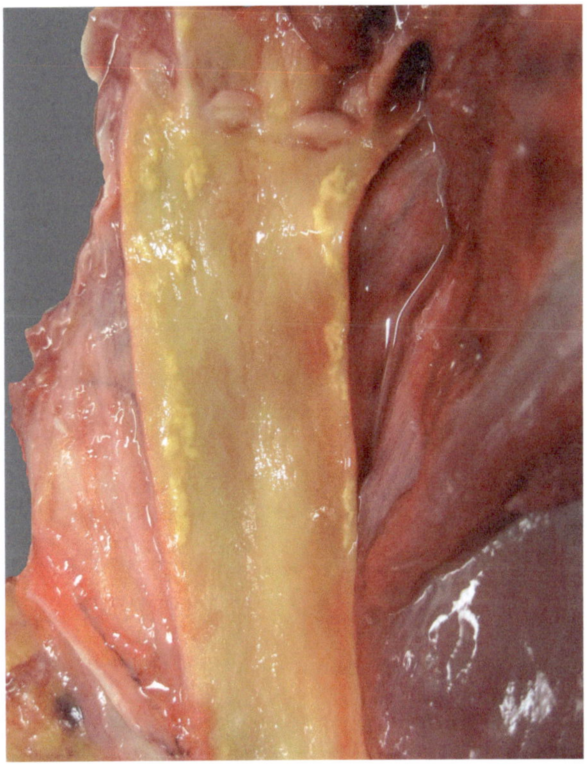

Fig. 4.377 This carotid artery bifurcation shows early-stage atheromatous disease with small fatty plaques. There is no occlusive disease

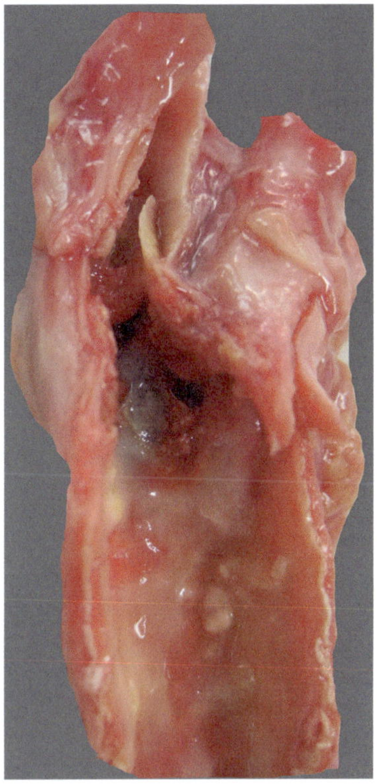

Fig. 4.378 High-grade atheromatous disease of the carotid bifurcation is relatively common. It may occlude the internal carotid artery and cause thromboembolic disease with secondary ischaemic and infarctive consequences in the brain, but can be clinically 'silent' in many individuals

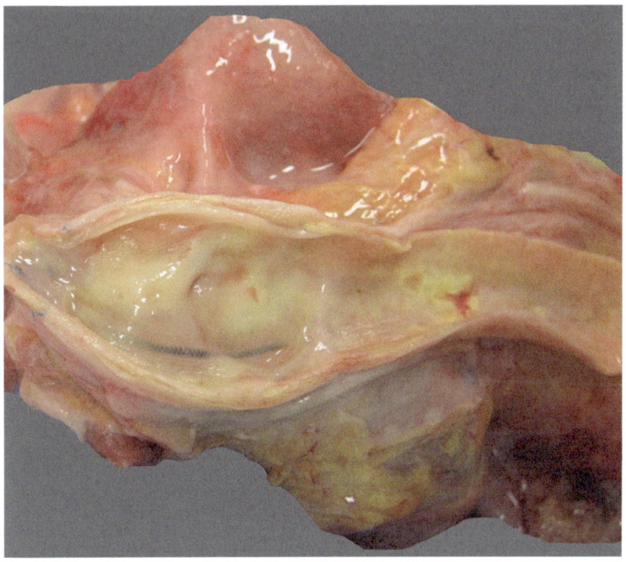

Fig. 4.379 Vascular grafts can be used at many sites in the arterial tree. Here is a largely incorporated Dacron graft at the carotid bifurcation. The blue marker in the synthetic matrix is seen running through the graft site. There is no obstruction, and the intimal surface is smooth and flat

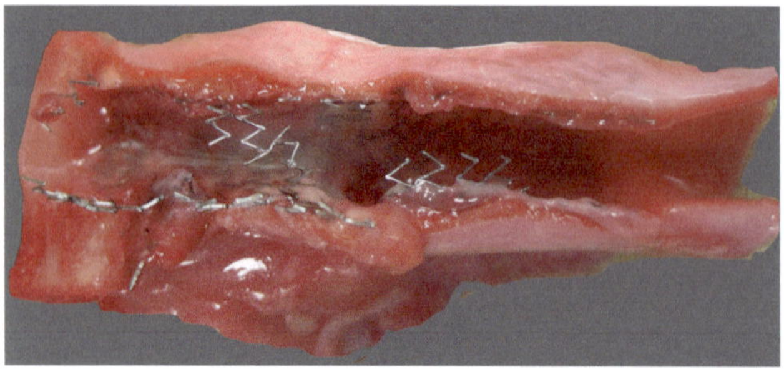

Fig. 4.380 High-grade stenosis is often treated by surgical excision of the plaque tissue (endarterectomy). Some individuals are not suitable for an open operation because of comorbidities. In such circumstances, a wire stent can be used to maintain the artery patency. This artery has been opened at autopsy using scissors, showing the metal from the stent. The endoluminal tissues appear smooth and without thrombus, indicating remodeling of the artery surface, in keeping with a good outcome for this endovascular repair

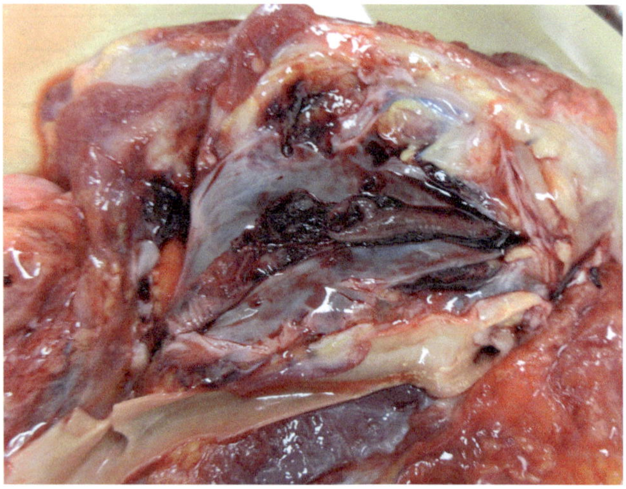

Fig. 4.381 The vasculature of the veins of the neck can contain extensive thrombosis in cases where internal lines have been positioned. Dense thrombus is seen around the site of a line insertion on the right side of this neck

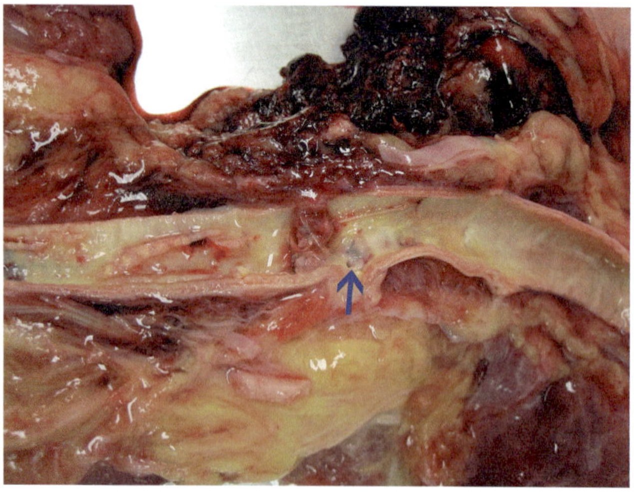

Fig. 4.382 Significant haemorrhage can occur at peripheral artery sites during angioplasty procedures. This external iliac artery underwent angioplasty. The grey fibrin plug (*arrow*), containing some suture material, is often difficult to discern. It appears that a dissection extended after the angioplasty procedure, causing rupture of the artery at this point. The intima is noted to have peeled off in part, and there is haemorrhage into the local soft tissues

Suggested Reading

Burton JL, Rutty G. The hospital autopsy. 3rd ed. London: Hodder Arnold; 2010. p. 136–58 and 262–76.

Clifton IJ, Ellames DAB. Respiratory medicine. In: Penman ID, Ralston SH, Strachan MWJ, Hobson RP, editors. Davidson's principles and practice of medicine. 24th ed. Edinburgh: Elsevier; 2023. p. 479–556.

Connolly AJ, Finkbeiner WE, Ursell PC, Davis RL, editors. Autopsy pathology: a manual and atlas. 3rd ed. Philadelphia, PA: Elsevier; 2016.

Cooke RA, Stewart B. Colour atlas of anatomical pathology. 3rd ed. Edinburgh: Churchill Livingstone; 2004.

Curran RC, Jones EL. Gross pathology: a colour atlas. Aylesbury, Buckinghamshire: HM + M Publishers; 1974.

Farrer-Brown G. Colour atlas of cardiac pathology. London: Wolfe Medical Publications; 1977.

Hasleton P, Flieder DB, editors. Spencer's pathology of the lung. 6th ed. Cambridge: Cambridge University Press; 2013.

Husain AN. The lung. In: Kumar V, Abbas AK, Aster JC, editors. Robbins & Cotran pathologic basis of disease. 10th ed. Elsevier; 2021. p. 673–730.

Ludwig J. Autopsy practice. 3rd ed. Ottawa: Humana Press; 2002.

Mitchell RN, Connolly AJ. The heart. In: Kumar V, Abbas AK, Aster JC, editors. Robbins & Cotran pathologic basis of disease. 10th ed. Elsevier; 2021. p. 527–82.

Mitchell RN, Halushka MK. Blood vessels. In: Kumar V, Abbas AK, Aster JC, editors. Robbins & Cotran pathologic basis of disease. 10th ed. Elsevier; 2021. p. 485–526.

Newby DE, Grubb NR. Cardiology. In: Penman ID, Ralston SH, Strachan MWJ, Hobson RP, editors. Davidson's principles and practice of medicine. 24th ed. Edinburgh: Elsevier; 2023. p. 385–478.

Suvarna SK, editor. Cardiac pathology: a guide to current practice. 2nd ed. London: Springer; 2019.

Yen-Ho S, Baker EJ, Rigby ML, Anderson RH. Color atlas of congenital heart disease. London: Mosby Wolfe; 1995.

Gastrointestinal and Hepatobiliary System

5

S. Kim Suvarna and Eu-Wing Toh

Introduction

The examination of the gastrointestinal organs is a major component of the autopsy. It takes in the examination of a large number of organs, and if done thoroughly can be time consuming. Often it is the case that pathology cannot be demonstrated in the gastrointestinal organs and sometimes it may not be inappropriate to perform an abridged examination. It may not be necessary in all autopsies to fully open the intestine, for example. However, in autopsies where there is a history suggestive of gastrointestinal disease, or where a cause of death is not immediately apparent in other organs, a thorough examination of the gastrointestinal organs is recommended.

Death caused by disease of the gastrointestinal system is not uncommon. The largest groups of these are cancer deaths, with the most common primaries being the colon, pancreas, esophagus, liver and stomach.

Non-neoplastic diseases form around one third of all deaths in the gastrointestinal tract with liver disease, particularly alcoholic liver disease, being very common. Alcoholic liver disease is one of the most common causes of death in younger patients.

Gastrointestinal deaths are most common in middle age, forming nearly a quarter of deaths in those in their 50s. This is because of a high prevalence of both alcoholic liver disease and malignancy in that group.

S. Kim Suvarna was deceased at the time of publication.

S. K. Suvarna (Deceased) · E.-W. Toh (✉)
Department of Histopathology, Sheffield Teaching Hospitals NHS Foundation Trust, Sheffield, UK
e-mail: eu-wing.toh@nhs.net

External Examination

The examination of the gastrointestinal system begins with the external examination of the body.

The eyes may show evidence of liver and biliary tract disease. Fingernail clubbing may be seen in chronic idiopathic inflammatory bowel disease and liver disease. The abdomen should be inspected for signs of natural disease and markers of medical intervention such as scars, stoma or drain sites.

External examination is not complete without an inspection of the anus, which may show evidence of malignant or inflammatory disease.

Internal In-Situ Examination

The abdominal cavity is entered in the manner described in Chap. 3, taking care not to damage the internal organs. On entering the abdominal cavity, one may notice fluid. There should usually be no more than about 20 mL. The omentum can be examined and then retracted to reveal the intestines and appendix beneath. Major pathology like intestinal dilatation, ischemia, volvulus, intussusception or adhesional scarring is usually better appreciated at this point, before evisceration.

The intestines may be manipulated to examine the mesenteries and peritoneum, as well as the bowels. The omentum can be gently retracted downwards to visualise the inferior aspect of the liver, the gallbladder, the spleen and the stomach. If indicated, the lesser sac can be inspected in-situ by cutting through the greater omentum where it joins the greater curve of the stomach.

The remainder of the examination will assume that the evisceration has been carried out in the method described in Chap. 3. However, if intestinal ischemia is encountered with in-situ examination, the usual technique of evisceration may be altered in order to consider the mesenteric vessels and preserve their relationship to the bowel.

S. K. Suvarna (represented by Grace Horne), A. K. Sharp (eds.), *Atlas of Adult Autopsy*,
https://doi.org/10.1007/978-3-031-72207-3_5

Dissection of the Tissues in Sequential Format

Omentum, Mesenteries and Peritoneum

The omentum is an apron of fatty tissue that is attached to the greater curve of the stomach and duodenum and hangs down freely to float over the intestines. The volume of adipose tissue varies between individuals and may be great.

Histologically it is characterized by lobulated adipose tissue with a mesothelial lining.

The small intestine, transverse and sigmoid colon have a mesentery which also carries a variable volume of adipose tissue.

The peritoneal lining envelopes the intestine and lines the abdominal wall, imparting a glistening appearance. Histologically it is characterized by mesothelium overlying a thin layer of loose connective tissue.

The omentum and peritoneum are usually inspected in situ, but the mesenteries can also be inspected in detail after evisceration.

Esophagus

The esophagus is a tubular muscular organ that extends from the pharynx to the stomach, traversing the diaphragm. It is approximately 20 cm in length.

The normal mucosa of the esophagus is a grayish white with vertically orientated mucosal folds. Histologically it is characterized by non-keratinized stratified squamous epithelium with submucosal mucinous glands.

It may be examined by opening it along its length, or by inverting it by pulling it through the gastro-esophageal junction with forceps.

Stomach

The stomach is a muscular lined expanded tubular reservoir lying in the upper left quadrant of the abdomen. When full it holds approximately a litre of food.

Like many of the luminal digestive organs, the mucosa of the stomach often shows a marked degenerative appearance on histology, but it is usually possible to distinguish between the body with oxyntic epithelium and the pylorus with foveolar epithelium.

The mucosa can be inspected by cutting along the greater curve. Care should be taken to preserve the stomach contents, if indicated.

Duodenum

The first part of the small intestine is broadly C-shaped and curves around the head of the pancreas, accepting the opening of the pancreatic ducts at the ampulla of Vater. Histologically, it has a villous architecture with distinctive submucosal glands in its proximal portion.

The duodenal mucosa can be examined by continuing the stomach incision through the pylorus. The ampulla may be identified by applying pressure to the gallbladder and observing bile extrude through.

Pancreas

The pancreas normally has a creamy salmon pink color, best appreciated on its anterior peritonealised surface. It is an approximately 15 cm long tongue of glandular tissue with a distinctive uncinate process that reflects back on itself, wrapping around the superior mesenteric vessels.

It usually shows marked autolytic change on histology, though some residual acinar glandular and islet structure may be appreciated.

The pancreas can be examined by serially slicing through its long axis or opening it up along its main duct, either from the tail or head end.

Gallbladder and Biliary Tract

The gallbladder is a blind-ended reservoir for bile lying underneath the liver and measuring approximately 8 cm in length. It is usually thin-walled with a mucosa pigmented green from the bile within. On opening it is not uncommon to identify calculi. Because of the spiral valve (of Heister) it is difficult to continue the gallbladder incision into the cystic duct. The rest of the biliary tract can be opened at the free edge of the lesser omentum if indicated and explored up and down. The common bile duct is normally no greater than 10 mm in maximum diameter.

Liver

The liver is a large organ that occupies much of the right upper quadrant of the abdomen. From the front it is broadly triangular and divided into two lobes by the falciform ligament. Histologically it tends to be relatively well preserved compared to the luminal structures, showing characteristic acini and portal tracts. It should be cut into sections no greater than 10 mm in width to maximize the chance of identifying small lesions internally.

Small Intestine and Appendix

This is usually presented for examination in a separate block of tissue containing the small intestine from the duodeno-jejunal flexure onwards, the appendix and colon. The small intestine is up to 7 m long and no greater than 3 cm in maximum diameter. Grossly the mucosa is pink with transverse plicae circulares.

Histologically it is characterized by a villous architecture, without submucosal glands. The intestine may be cut along its length to examine the mucosa. Alternatively, small incisions may be made at intervals along its length in order to examine its contents.

The appendix is a narrow, blind-ended muscular tube with a mesentery. Its size may range from 2 to 20 cm but is usually around 10 cm long and around 1 cm in maximum diameter. It can be found by tracing proximally the transverse taenia coli of the colon.

Colon

The colon makes a clockwise circuit of the lower abdominal cavity, starting in the lower right quadrant. It is approximately 150 cm in length. The caecum may be up to 9 cm in diameter, but the colon distal to the hepatic flexure should be no more than 6 cm. Much of the colon is attached directly to the posterior abdominal wall but the transverse and sigmoid parts have a mesentery. Like in the small intestine there should be a clear division between the fatty mesentery and the intestinal wall, with no encroachment of fat onto the serosa. Lobules of fat called appendices epiploica are typically seen on the transverse and sigmoid parts. The mucosa is normally featureless and histologically shows a characteristic "row of test tubes" appearance.

Rectum and Anus

The rectum is usually separated from the colon on evisceration and examined as part of an organ block with the other retroperitoneal organs. It is thin walled with a featureless mucosa and surrounded by a layer of fatty mesorectal tissue. It is usually around 15 cm long. The rectum is usually ligated at the level of the pelvic floor, leaving the perineal anus in situ in the body. The anus can be safely digitally examined after evisceration. Occasionally it may be appropriate to perform an exenteration-type excision of the anus in order to closely examine these tissues.

Figures 5.1, 5.2, 5.3, 5.4, 5.5, 5.6, 5.7, 5.8, 5.9, 5.10, 5.11, 5.12, 5.13, 5.14, 5.15, 5.16, 5.17, 5.18, 5.19, 5.20, 5.21, 5.22, 5.23, 5.24, 5.25, 5.26, 5.27, 5.28, 5.29, 5.30, 5.31, 5.32, 5.33, 5.34, 5.35, 5.36, 5.37, 5.38, 5.39, 5.40, 5.41, 5.42, 5.43, 5.44, 5.45, and 5.46 illustrate the dissection protocol described above. Examples of gastrointestinal pathologies are shown in Figs. 5.47, 5.48, 5.49, 5.50, 5.51, 5.52, 5.53, 5.54, 5.55, 5.56, 5.57, 5.58, 5.59, 5.60, 5.61, 5.62, 5.63, 5.64, 5.65, 5.66, 5.67, 5.68, 5.69, 5.70, 5.71, 5.72, 5.73, 5.74, 5.75, 5.76, 5.77, 5.78, 5.79, 5.80, 5.81, 5.82, 5.83, 5.84, 5.85, 5.86, 5.87, 5.88, 5.89, 5.90, 5.91, 5.92, 5.93, 5.94, 5.95, 5.96, 5.97, 5.98, 5.99, 5.100, 5.101, 5.102, 5.103, 5.104, 5.105, 5.106, 5.107, 5.108, 5.109, 5.110, 5.111, 5.112, 5.113, 5.114, 5.115, 5.116, 5.117, 5.118, 5.119, 5.120, 5.121, 5.122, 5.123, 5.124, 5.125, and 5.126.

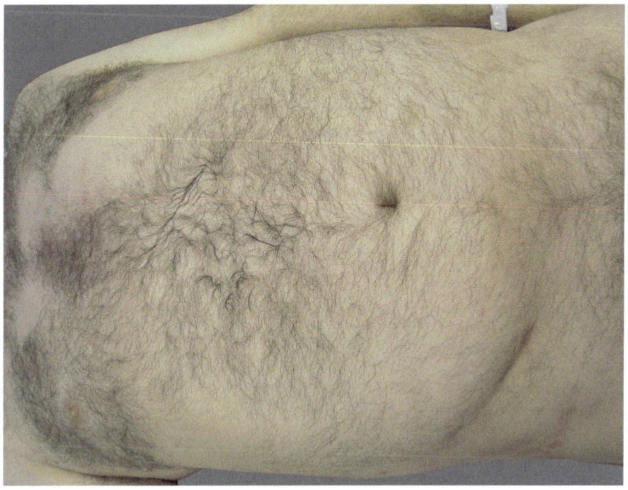

Fig. 5.1 Even before internal examination, there are clues regarding gastrointestinal disease to be seen in the external appearance of the body. Here, there is an oblique scar in the right iliac fossa consistent with a history of appendectomy. Also note the areas where hair has been removed on the chest, a sign that ECG electrodes were used during resuscitation attempts

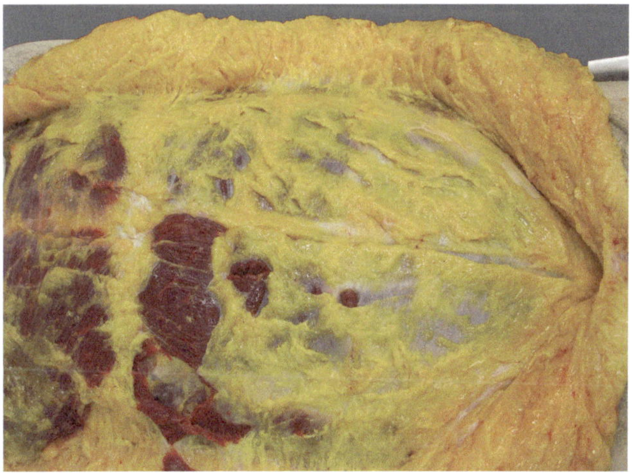

Fig. 5.2 The adipose tissue of the abdominal wall can be removed to reveal the underlying muscle. This dissection is not a standard part of the autopsy but may help in looking for hernias and assessing abdominal wall injury

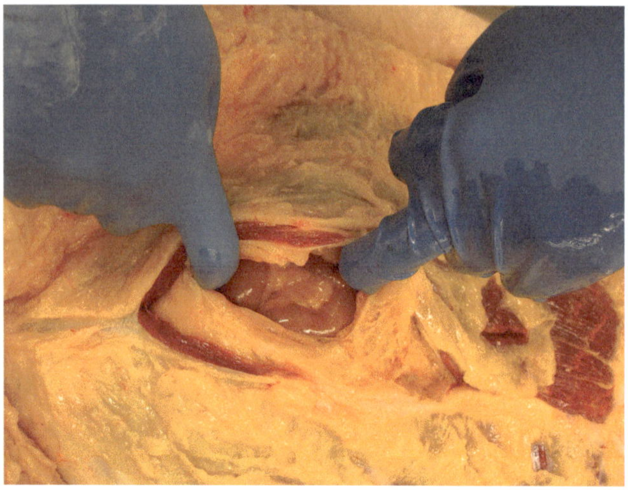

Fig. 5.3 The abdominal cavity is opened in the upper midline between the rectus muscles. Beneath the muscles is usually a pad of fat that can be swept away with the finger to reveal the abdominal cavity. This will give immediate clues regarding abdominal disease (e.g. peritonitis, neoplasia)

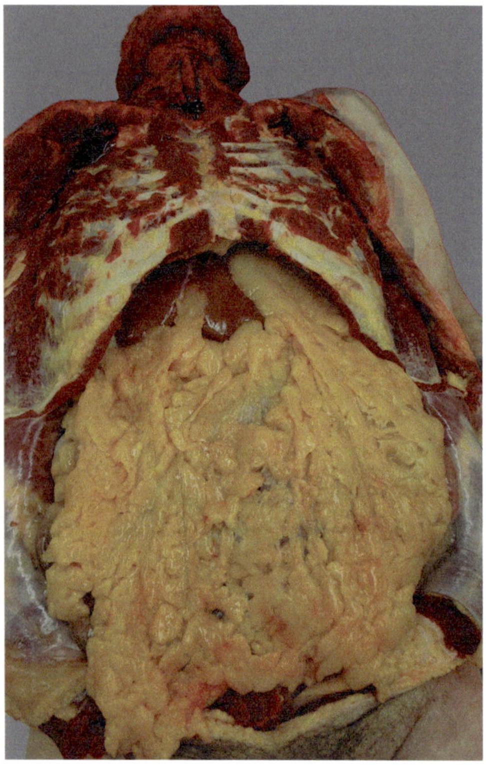

Fig. 5.4 The omentum is often overlooked in terms of gastrointestinal disease. It provides an assessment of the nutritional status of the individual. The omentum is usually thin but may be bulky with excess adipose tissue in those who have a raised body mass index. The omentum may become adherent to inflamed peritoneum, forming an abscess. The omentum, or part of it, may have been removed previously as part of surgical treatment for intraabdominal neoplasia, usually of the ovary, endometrium, appendix or colon

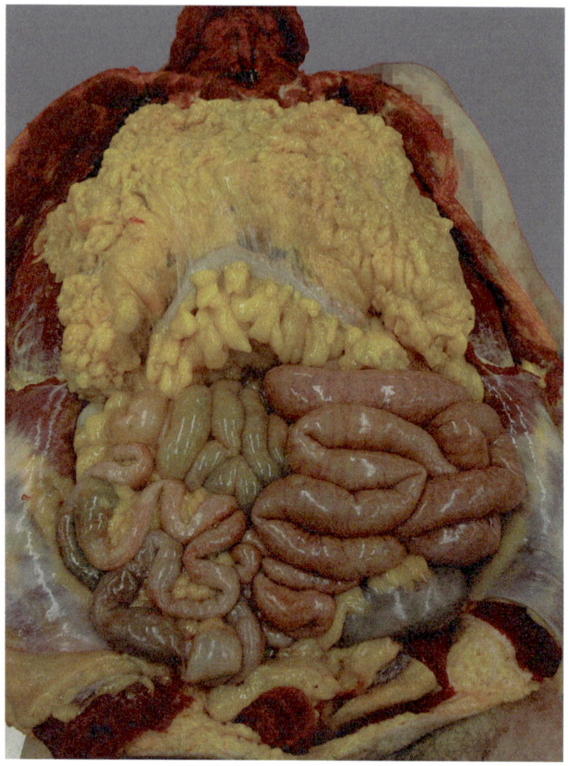

Fig. 5.5 The assessment of the intestines starts even before evisceration. The intestines appear to zig-zag back and forward, winding their way down to the lower right quadrant. The proximal intestine appears larger than on the left side of the body. This is the normal appearance, although the amount of gas distension of the bowel varies on a case-by-case basis

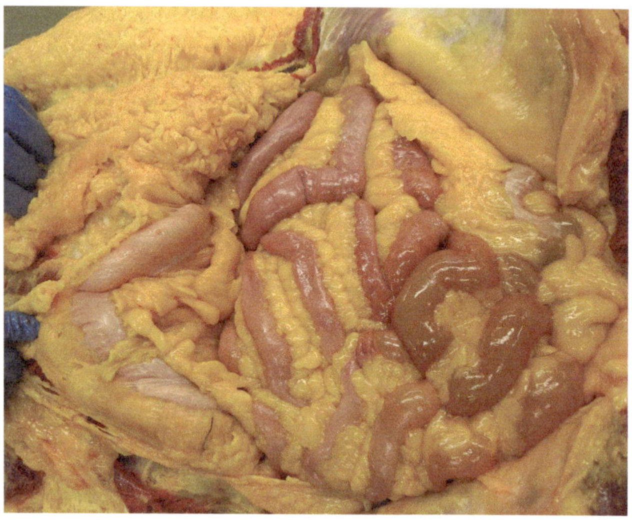

Fig. 5.6 This abdominal cavity shows a marked amount of fat around the bowel mesenteries

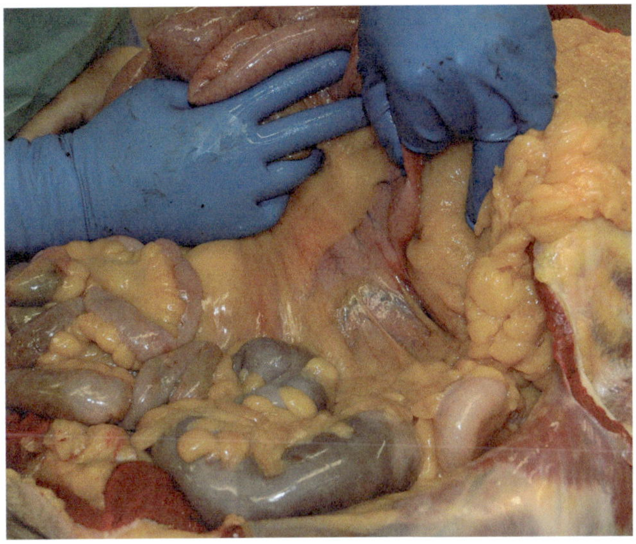

Fig. 5.7 The duodenojejunal flexure is the landmark used for evisceration of the bowels. Before cutting into these tissues to start removing bowel, it is worth considering the stomach, pancreas, spleen and local mesenteries for any overt disease

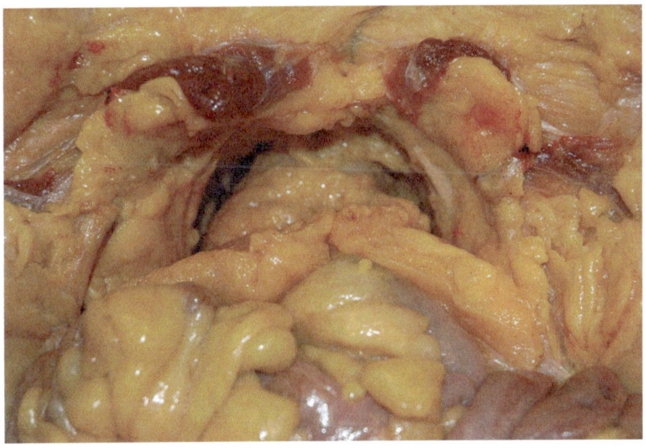

Fig. 5.8 In the same way, it is worth considering other parts of the peritoneal cavity and bowels at this stage. The view (looking down into the pelvis with the pubic ramus at 12 o'clock) shows no pathology. Note the mesorectal tissues have been dissected bluntly from the pelvic wall

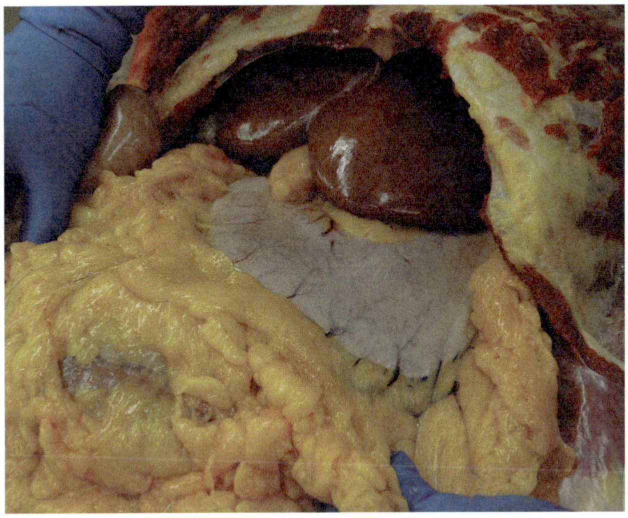

Fig. 5.9 Limited views of the liver and gallbladder may be obtained by retracting the omentum and stomach downwards. One should note any fluid collection around the liver. The anterior surface of the stomach can be seen

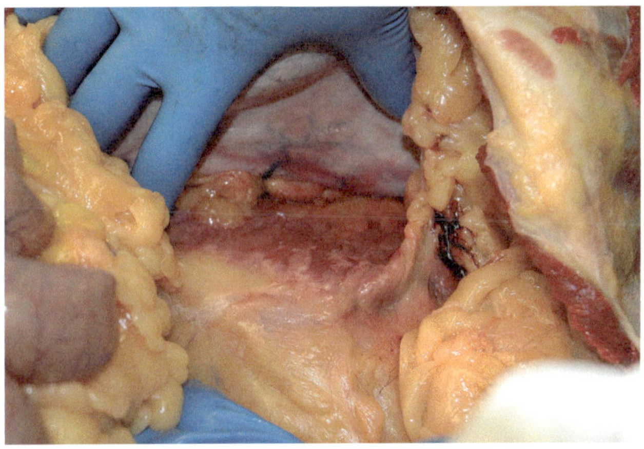

Fig. 5.10 Opening the omentum, below the stomach, allows one to look into the lesser sac. The bowels have been pushed to the right to facilitate the view

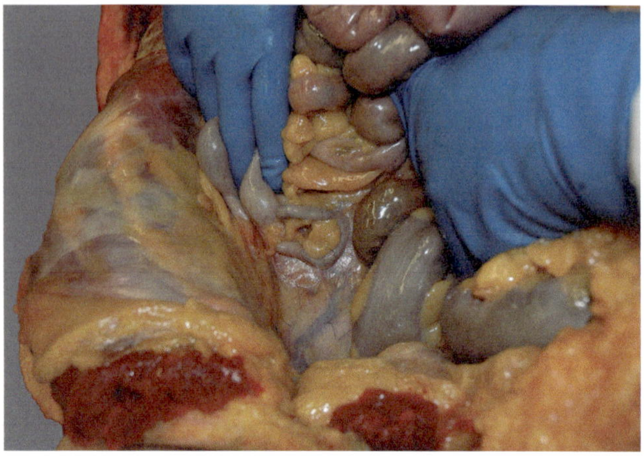

Fig. 5.11 The appendix can be seen in the right lower quadrant of the abdomen after retracting the intestines and colon. In addition, at this stage with the small intestine reflected, the nonmesenteric/retroperitoneal parts of the bowel can be inspected. This includes the paracolic gutters, which are often sites of fluid collection. These gutters may channel fluid from intraabdominal sepsis

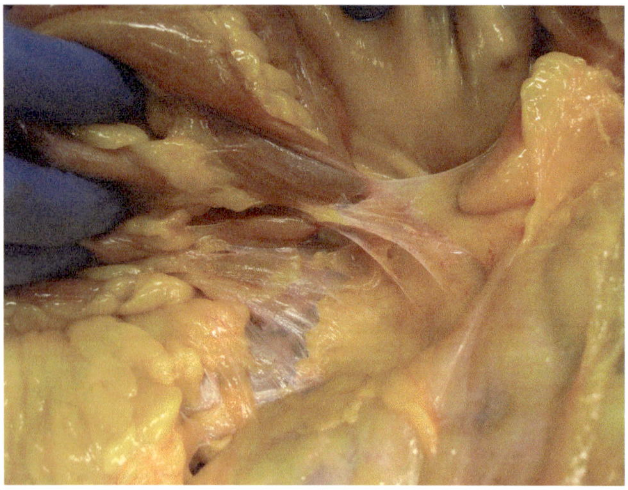

Fig. 5.12 Normally the peritoneum is smooth, thin and glistening. Where there has been previous inflammation or surgery, scarring can occur between organs and the abdominal wall. In this example the appendix has been removed, and as a result the caecum is now stuck onto the abdominal wall

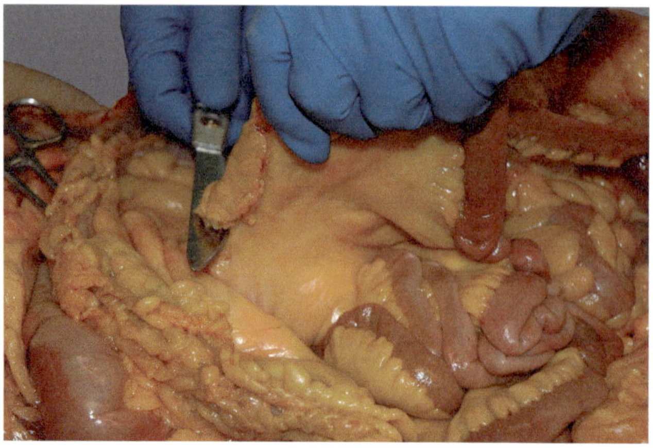

Fig. 5.13 The small intestine may be removed by cutting through the mesentery, at the mesenteric root in this view. This has the advantage of keeping the vessels and bowel together as a single block. However, it can be more difficult to open the small intestine or remove it from the mesentery later

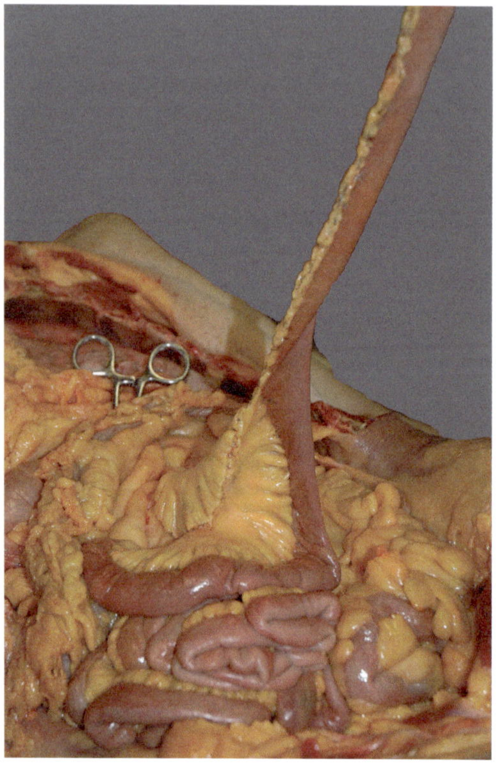

Fig. 5.14 The bowel can also be removed by cutting along the inner/mesenteric aspect of the small and large bowel. Whichever method is used, the evisceration protocol (see Chap. 3) continues, and the bowel from duodenojejunal flexure down to the upper rectum is resected steadily. Attention is paid throughout in order to palpate the bowels. Key elements include the identification of perforations and or tumors

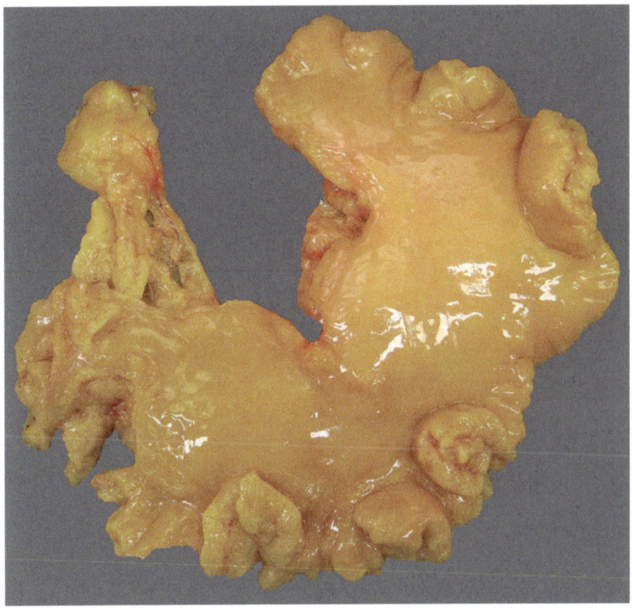

Fig. 5.15 Dividing the mesentery from the intestine after it has been removed en bloc with the intestine may simplify its examination. However, the lost sense of continuity with end organs may make evaluation of bowel ischaemia more complex

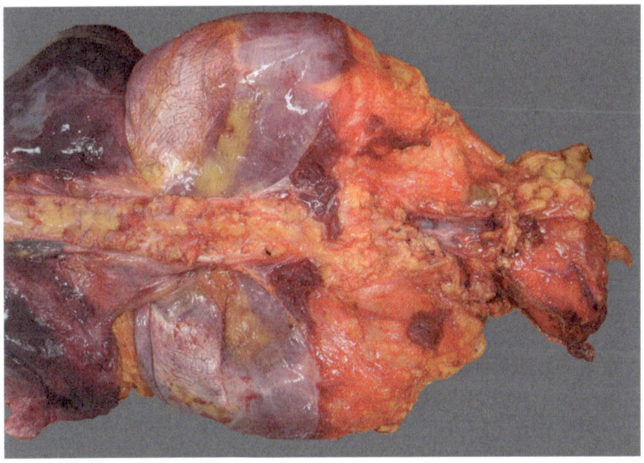

Fig. 5.16 Complete evisceration has occurred (see Chap. 3), and one is left with abdominal and retroperitoneal tissues below the diaphragm and also tissues above this landmark. The diaphragms, kidneys, adrenals, bladder and great vessels should be removed for later examination (see Chaps. 6 and 8)

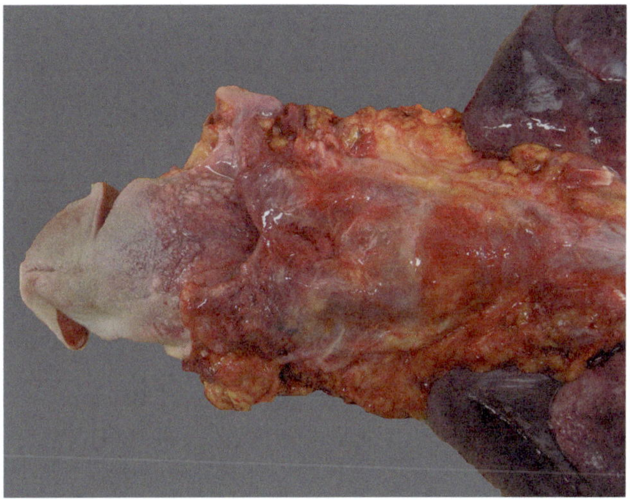

Fig. 5.17 The proximal part of the esophagus can be identified here posterior to the larynx. One should always check the tissues of the oropharynx for disease. One is also able to inspect the tongue. Areas of squamous mucosal change to the tongue should be sampled for histology. In addition, one may consider sampling of salivary gland tissues and inspecting the rest of the mouth

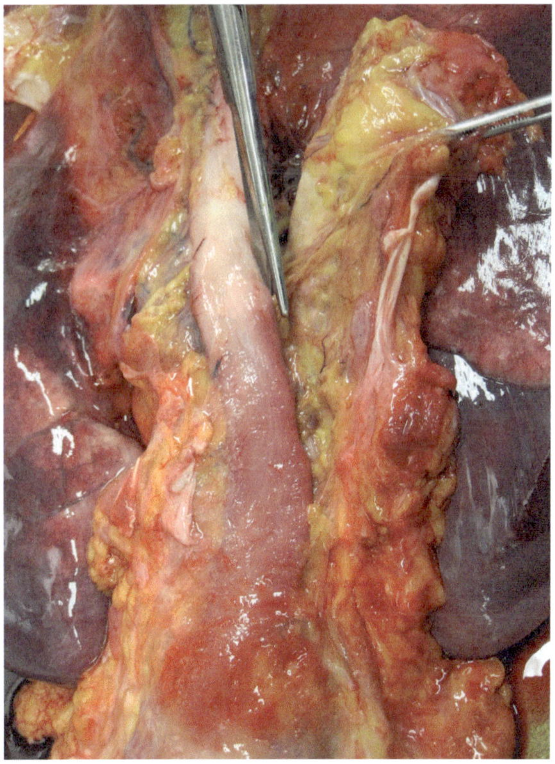

Fig. 5.18 It is possible, at this juncture, to open the esophagus and examine the esophageal mucosa, but often to simplify examination in continuity with the stomach it can be freed and left intact with the stomach. It should be easy to find a plane of dissection between the esophagus and the other thoracic organs. One should take care to avoid opening the trachea and the pericardium

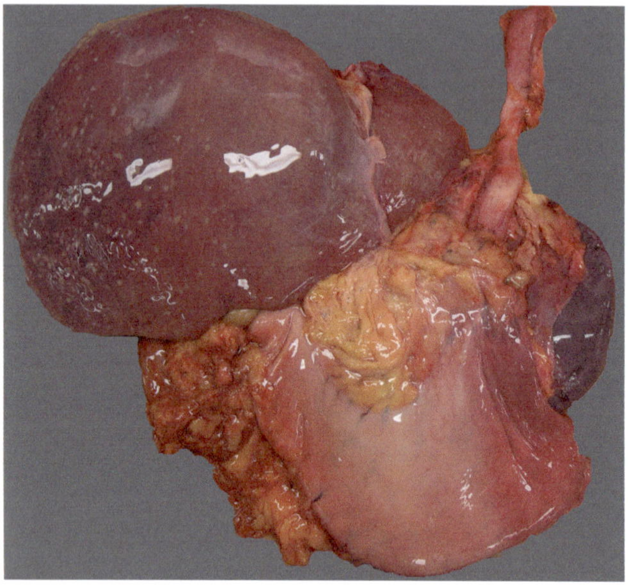

Fig. 5.19 The view of the upper gastrointestinal organ block shows the esophagus, stomach, liver and spleen anteriorly. The gallbladder, pancreas and biliary tree are not seen in this view

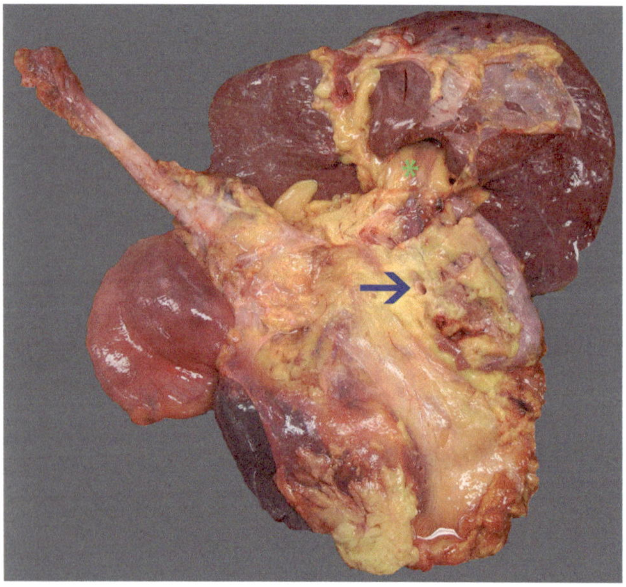

Fig. 5.20 Posteriorly, much of the detail is obscured by retroperitoneal fat. The portal vasculature and biliary structures (asterisk) may be seen at the hilum of the liver. The portal vein should be available for inspection at this point, but the pancreas is still obscured. The superior mesenteric artery (arrow) is seen open, heading underneath and anterior to the pancreatic uncinate process

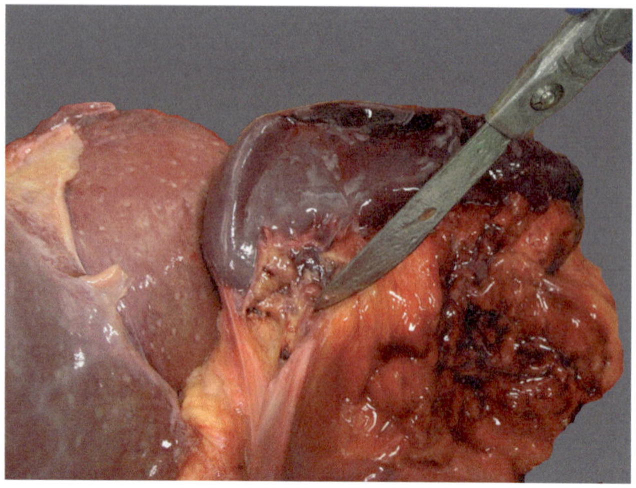

Fig. 5.21 At this point, one may separate the spleen, by cutting through the gastrosplenic ligament and splenic vessels. The biliary tract, pancreas and luminal structures stay connected

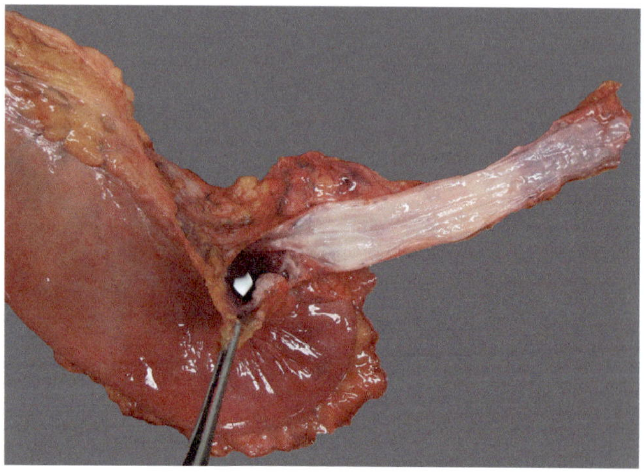

Fig. 5.22 Here the esophagus has been opened along its length to show its normal appearance. Common pathological findings to look for are strictures, tumors, ulcers and varices. Note the stomach contains some fluid, which may be sampled if toxicology issues are pertinent

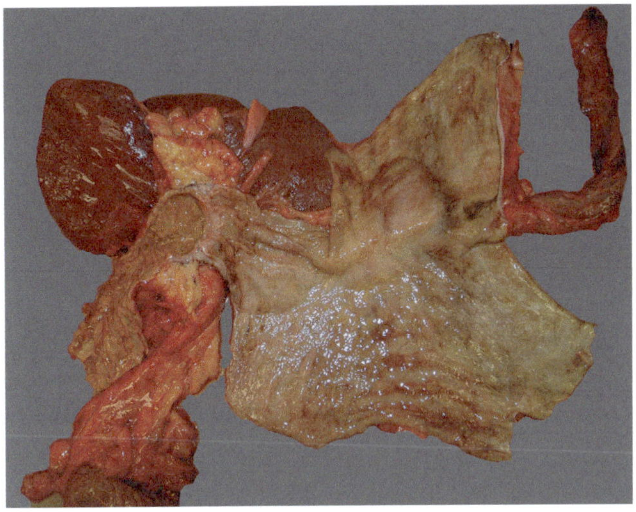

Fig. 5.23 Alternatively, the stomach and duodenum may be opened first along the edge of the stomach greater curve to the pylorus and then crossing to the small bowel outer aspect/greater curve. This has revealed the normal appearance of the gastric and duodenal mucosa. The gastric rugae seen here are mucosal folds. Note the transverse folds and biliary staining in the duodenum. Ulcers, tumors, and points of bleeding are not present in this case. Note also that this dissection has not opened the esophagus (see Fig. 5.24)

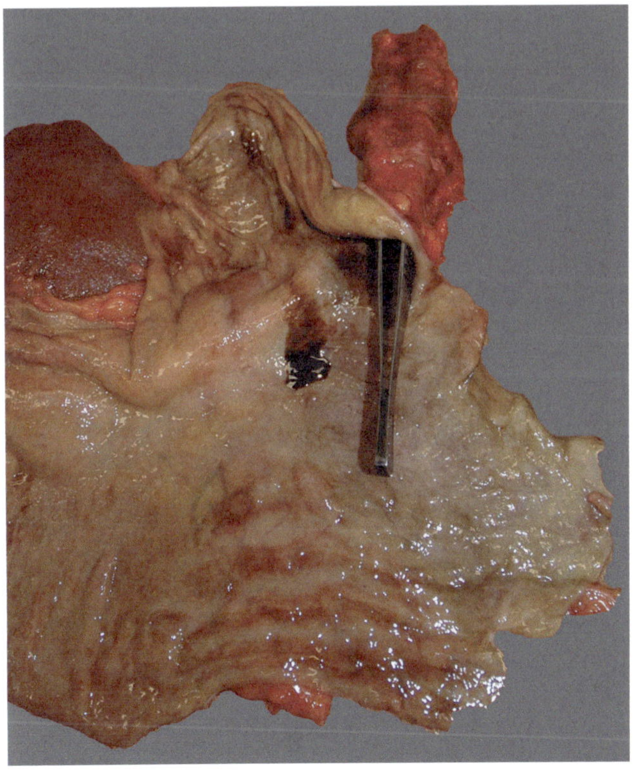

Fig. 5.24 An alternative to cutting open the esophagus is to pull it inside out through the stomach, having previously tied off the proximal end. This technique may assist in preserving engorged variceal vessels

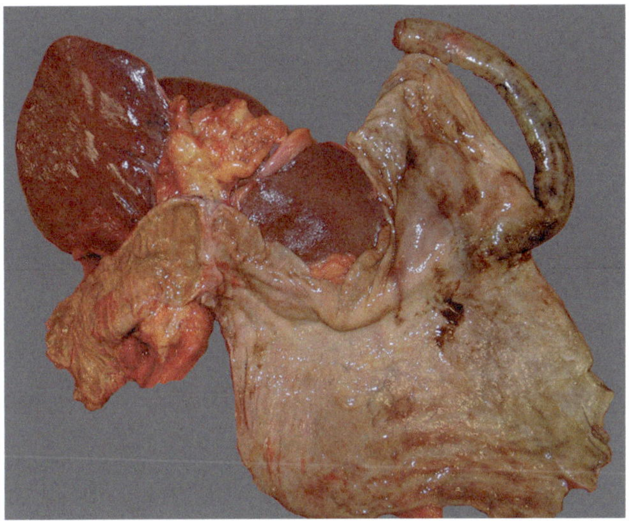

Fig. 5.25 The inverted esophagus is seen with the local stomach mucosa

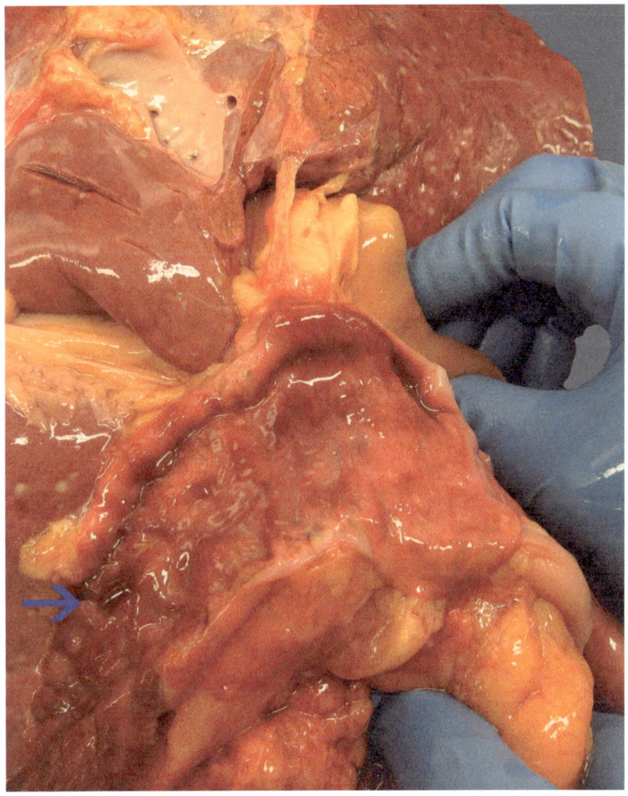

Fig. 5.26 Gently squeezing the gallbladder will often cause bile to extrude through the ampulla, allowing it to be identified (arrow). However, this cannot be relied on as an absolute test of obstruction or patency

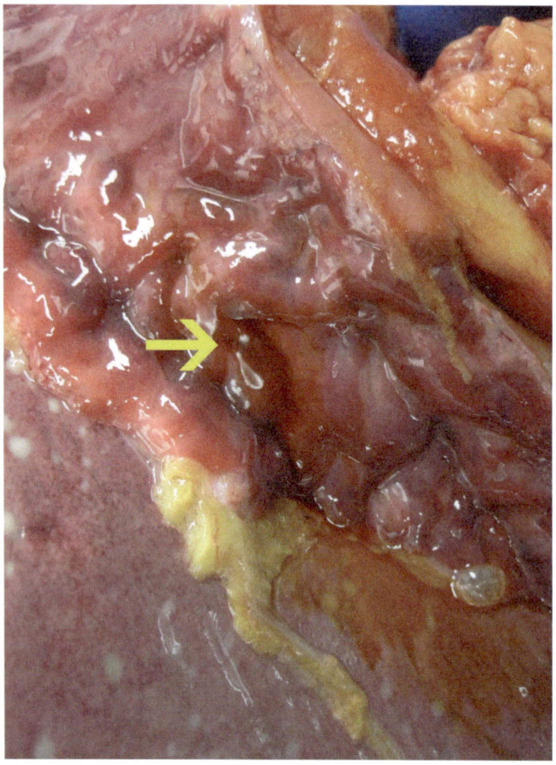

Fig. 5.27 The ampulla shows the flow of bile (arrow). If one wishes, one can explore the bile and pancreatic ducts upwards, having gently placed a probe into the ampulla

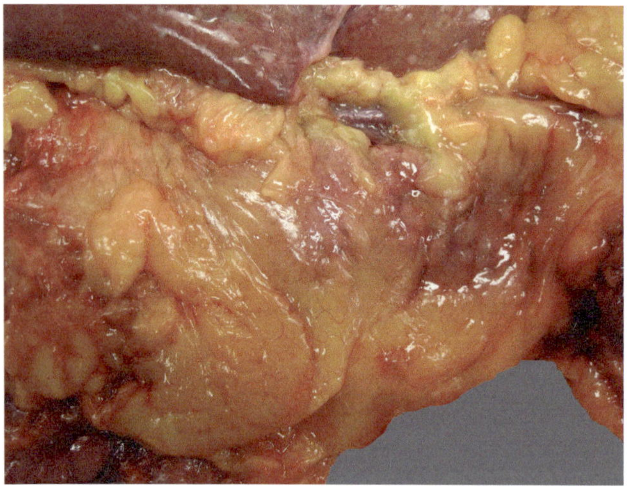

Fig. 5.28 The normal appearance of the anterior surface of the pancreas can be seen. Note the slightly nodular surface appearance and intimate association with the retroperitoneal fat. The splenic artery and vein run along the superior aspect

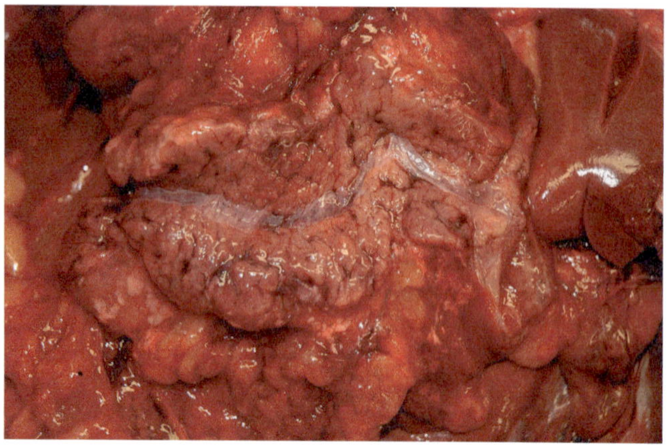

Fig. 5.29 One can open the pancreatic duct along its length. This should readily show any tumors or stones, or tumors within the adjacent acinar/endocrine tissues

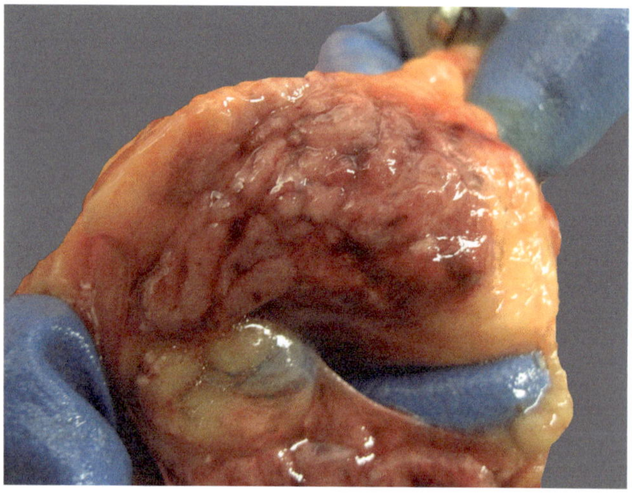

Fig. 5.30 Alternatively, one may opt to serially section in transverse fashion (10 mm intervals) along the body of the pancreas, starting at the tail. This has the advantage of showing the parenchyma at multiple points (helpful in looking for neoplasia) and also shows if there is any duct dilatation in cross-section format. This view shows one of the common issues with pancreatic parenchyma: softening and dissolution of the tissues

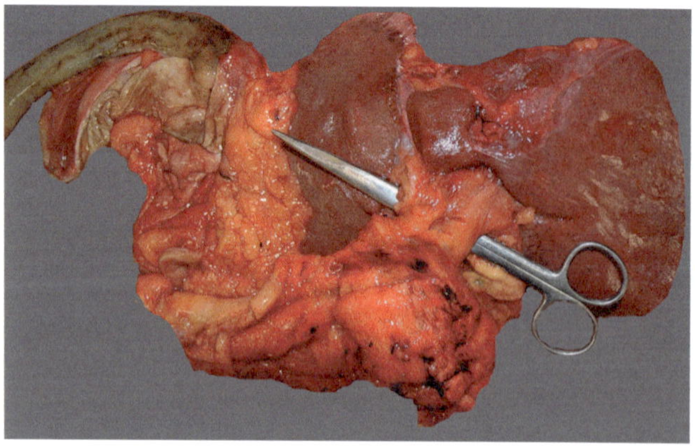

Fig. 5.31 The portal vasculature with the adjacent pancreas, stomach and spleen can be examined early if there are ante-mortem issues of obstruction. Here the portal vessels and common bile duct are supported by scissors. A cut into the tissues at this point assesses these conduits. They may be followed along their length or in transverse format

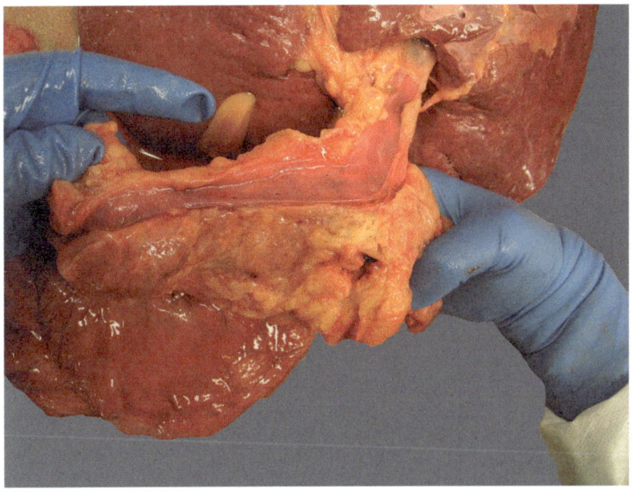

Fig. 5.32 This view shows the opened portal vein and its tributary, the splenic vein, running up to the liver. The splenic and superior mesenteric vein may be probed or opened if desired at this point

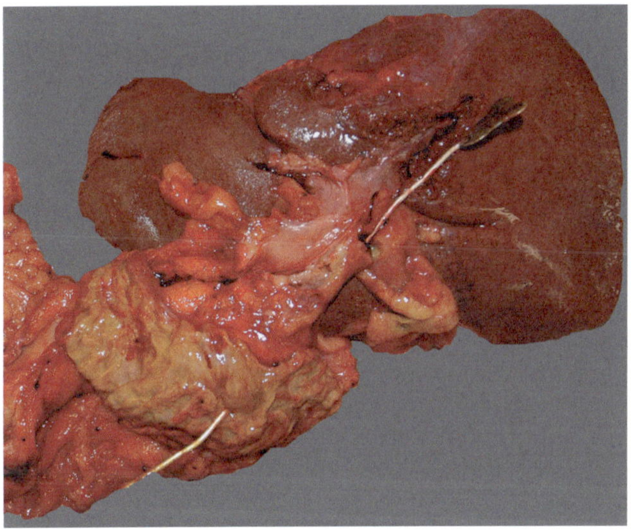

Fig. 5.33 Here a probe has been inserted into the common bile duct, below the spiral valve of the gallbladder, and passed into the duodenum

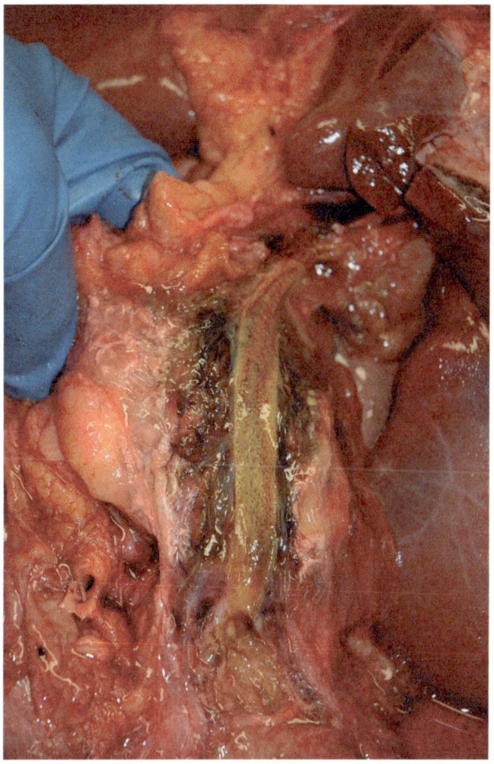

Fig. 5.34 One may use the probe to guide opening along the duct, if desired. This view shows the green mucosal surface without obstructive lesion

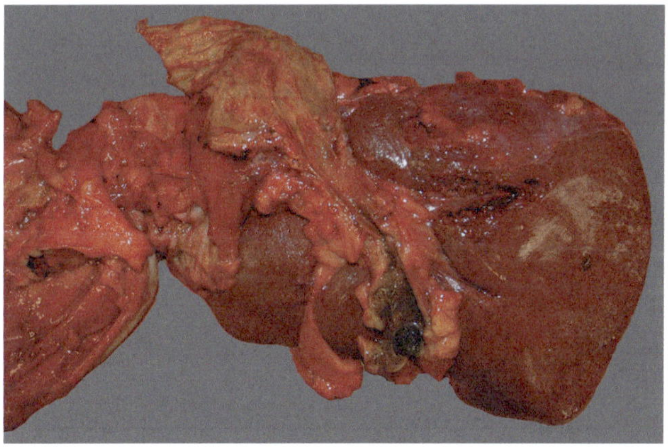

Fig. 5.35 The gallbladder and cystic duct have been opened, continuous with the common bile duct. Note the black calculus in the gallbladder

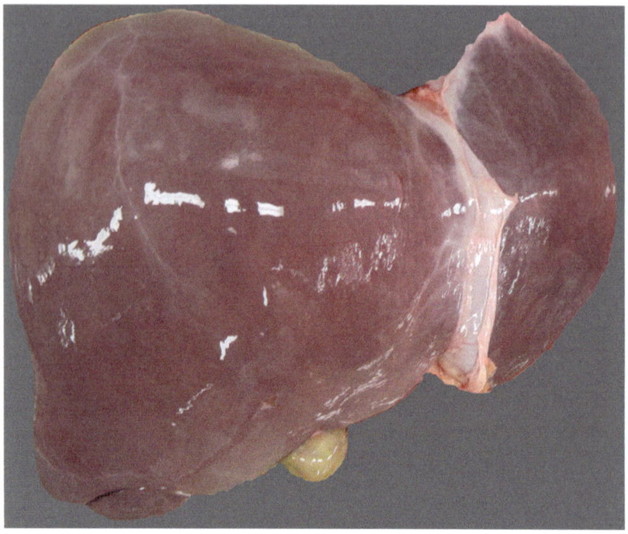

Fig. 5.36 Here the external anterior appearance of the liver can be seen, with the left and right lobes clearly evident

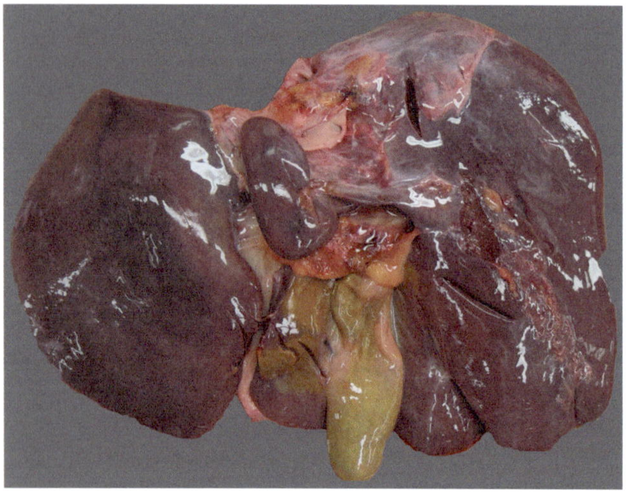

Fig. 5.37 Posterosuperiorly, the liver shows the caudate lobe, which can be seen above the gallbladder, and the quadrate lobe between the gallbladder and the ligamentum teres

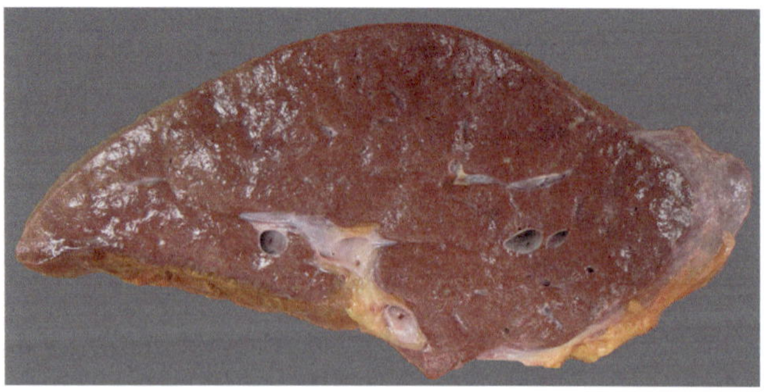

Fig. 5.38 On section, the normal red-brown color and smooth surface of the liver can be seen. The cuts are made, 10 mm apart from right to left conventionally, to help identify tumors and fibrosing processes

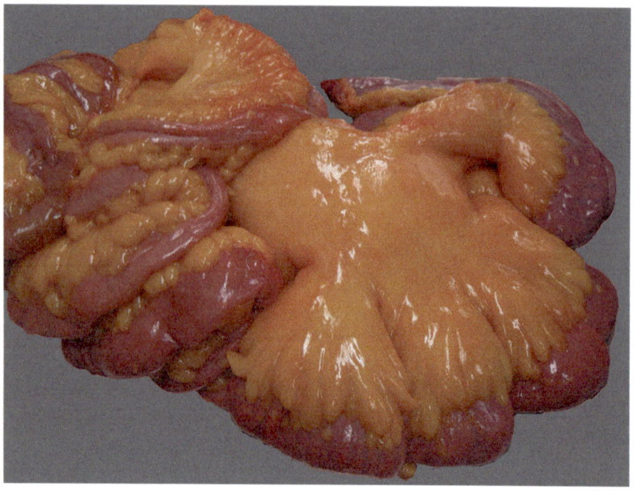

Fig. 5.39 A section of small intestine is seen with local fatty mesentery. Here there is some encroachment of fat onto the serosa of the bowel, but this is within normal limits. The mesentery, like the omentum, can contain abundant adipose tissue

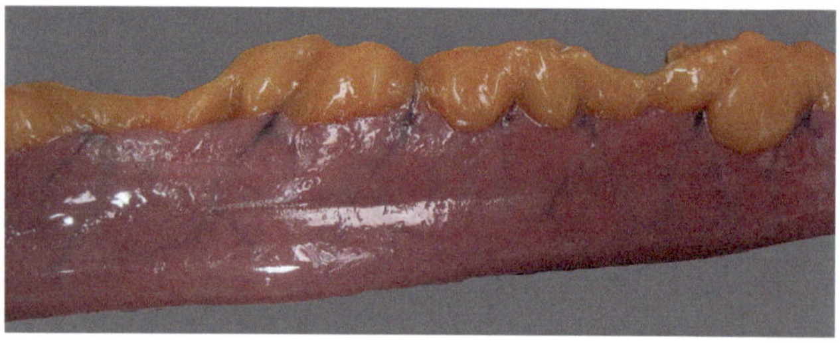

Fig. 5.40 The small bowel (largely stripped of local mesentery) may be laid out relatively flat. Any masses of significance can be readily seen, often in association with obstructive phenomena. Note the normal and smooth serosal surface. Often, if the case pathology lies elsewhere, the bowel is examined no further. However, the opportunity to open and washout the bowel exists at this point

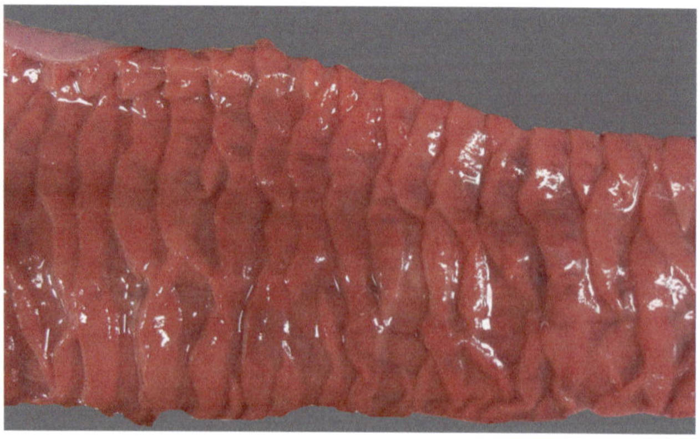

Fig. 5.41 The small intestinal tissues can be opened along their length. The intestinal mucosa does autolyse fairly fast, but one often sees the normal circumferential folds. These are permanent and fixed folds, unlike the rugae of the stomach

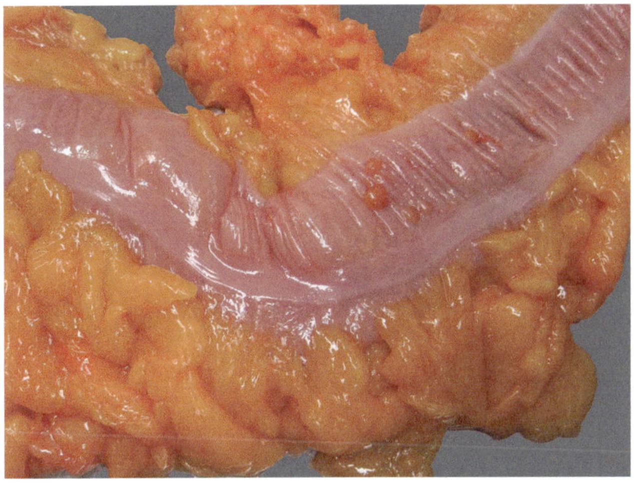

Fig. 5.42 The large intestine can be similarly examined, firstly from the outside, revealing normal fat and serosal tissues. The longitudinal taenia coli can be seen here on the surface of the sigmoid colon. Note the appendices epiploicae (fatty nodules). One should be aware that many individuals die with a variable amount of fecal matter within the lumen. Simple palpation and observation of obstruction may indicate pathology, but one should have a low threshold for opening the large bowel along its length

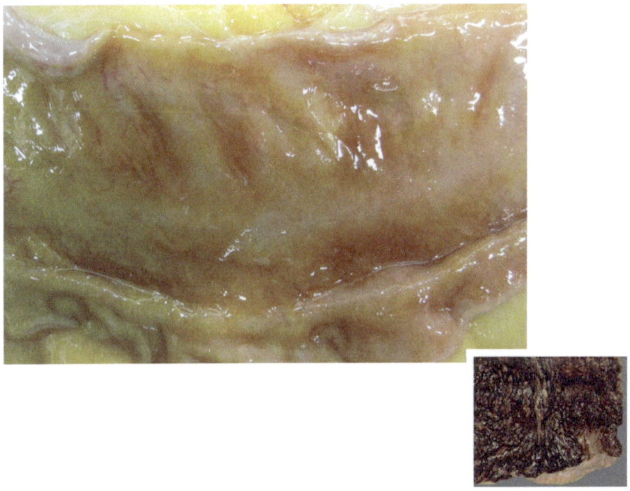

Fig. 5.43 Once emptied of content and with the mucosa washed, the large intestine mucosa is relatively featureless. Here it has been discolored minimally by the bowel content. Note the normal vascular markings. There may be extensive melanosis (brown discolouration), particularly in the elderly, due to lipofuscin deposition in the mucosa (inset)

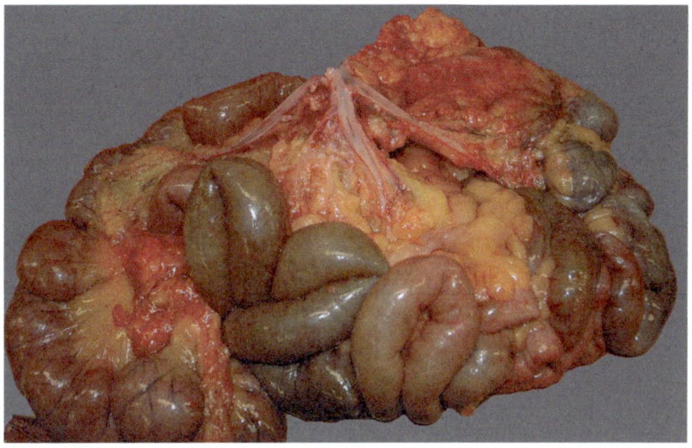

Fig. 5.44 The superior mesenteric artery and its branches have been dissected within the omentum adjacent to the normal small intestine. Examining the vasculature in this way can help relate vascular lesions to end organ changes

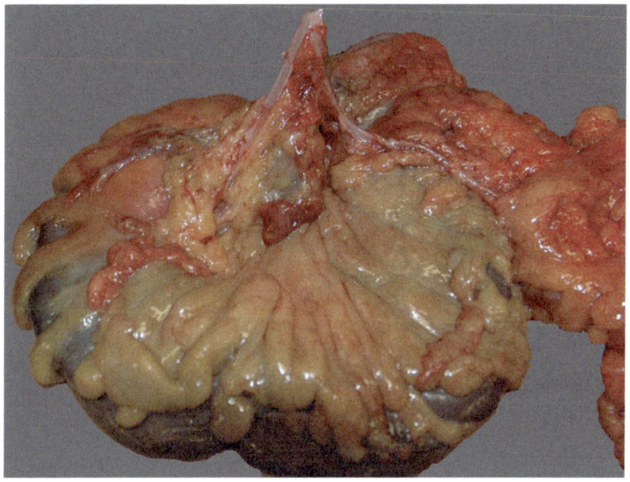

Fig. 5.45 The inferior mesenteric artery is less frequently involved in bowel ischaemia. Here it can be seen opened up along its branches in relation to a normal sigmoid colon

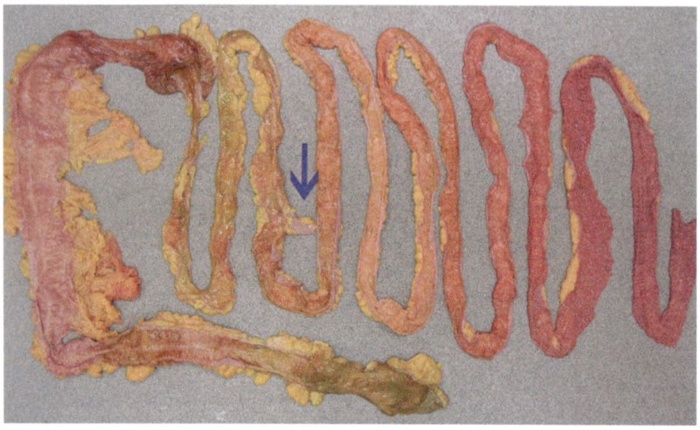

Fig. 5.46 Displaying the whole intestine is difficult. However, this is useful, particularly if one wishes to demonstrate regional pathology (e.g., inflammatory bowel disease, carcinomas, necrosis). Here the bowels were emptied, cleaned and photographed (from a position well above the tissues). The mucosa is normal in this case, but an incidental Meckel's diverticulum can be seen in the usual position, approximately 50 cm from the ileocaecal valve

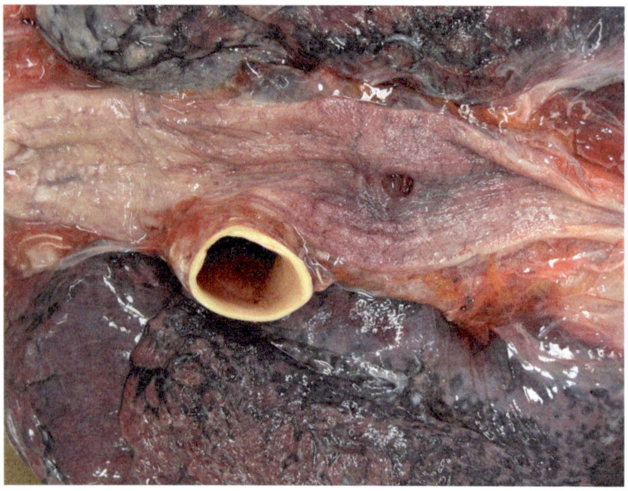

Fig. 5.47 Peptic ulceration can occur at any point in the esophagus, often related to acid reflux or drug therapy, or both. The significance will depend upon whether bleeding has occurred from the ulcer bed, or if the ulcer interfaces with the mediastinal tissues. On occasion, a large abscess can form adjacent (not seen here)

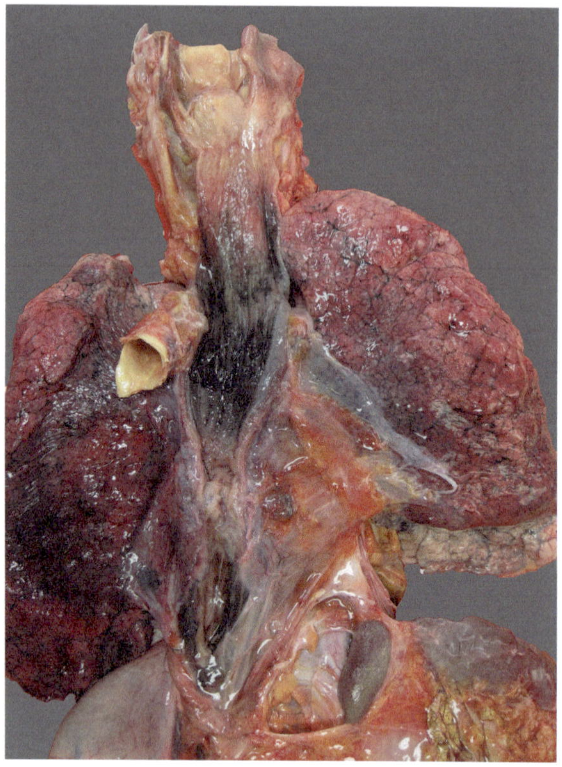

Fig. 5.48 This esophagus shows lower zone scarring and sclerosis, resulting in a stricture. The cause for this may include acid-reflux or possibly neoplasia. Histology is important in reviewing such lesions

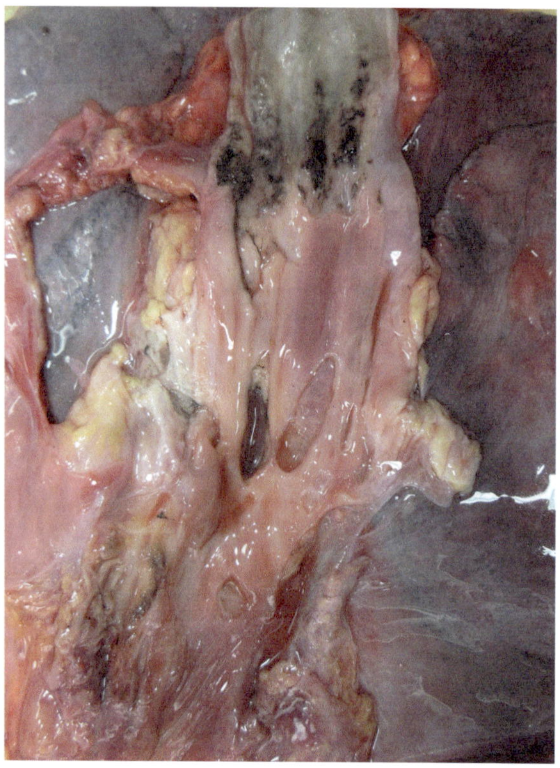

Fig. 5.49 This view of the lower esophagus shows a chronic ulcer just above the stomach inlet, with pronounced fibrosis locally. Immediately above the ulcer is a variegated grey/pink mucosal architecture, in keeping with Barrett's esophagus. The lower ulcer has a hard and sharp edge, pushing into the local soft tissues, without active bleeding or mediastinitis

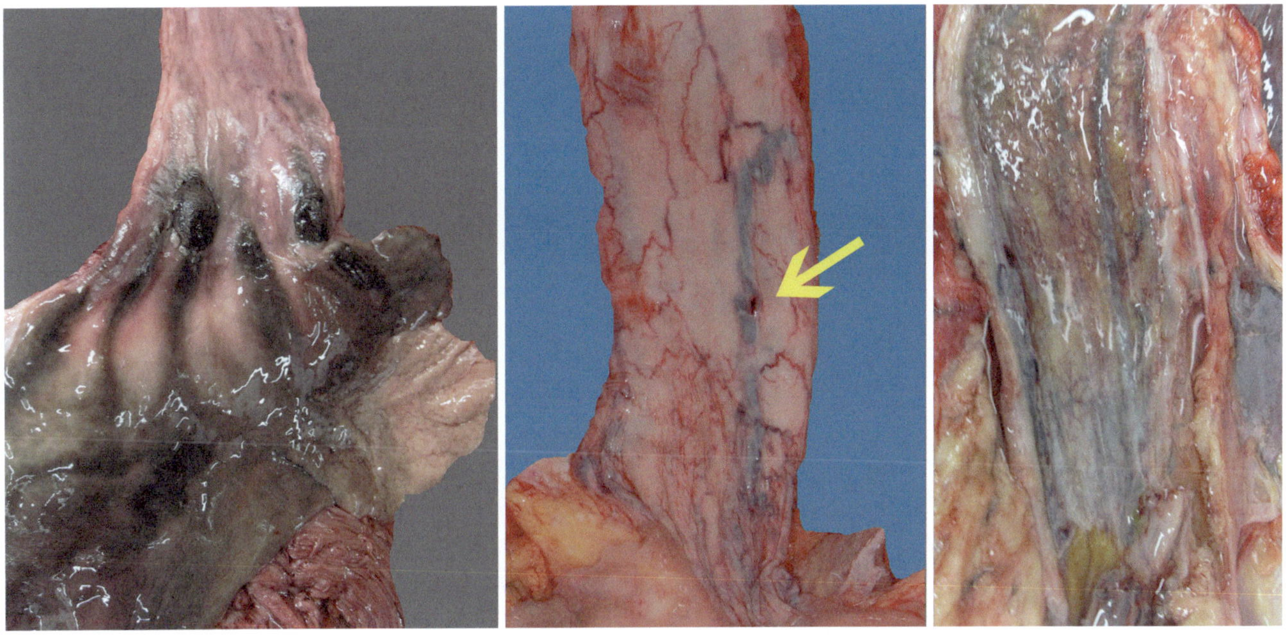

Fig. 5.50 Esophageal varices may have varying appearances, including following spontaneous thrombosis, or after sclerotherapy (left). In another case (middle), death followed a single vessel bleed (arrow). The right image shows pronounced, non-bleeding varices

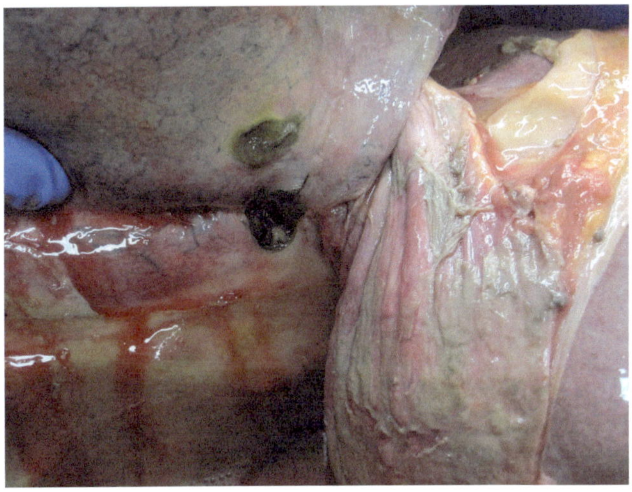

Fig. 5.51 This esophageal tumor has perforated into the right thorax cavity. It was associated with direct involvement of the inflammatory process onto the adjacent lung tissue with a resultant active pleuritic reaction (seen with purulent material covering the diaphragm)

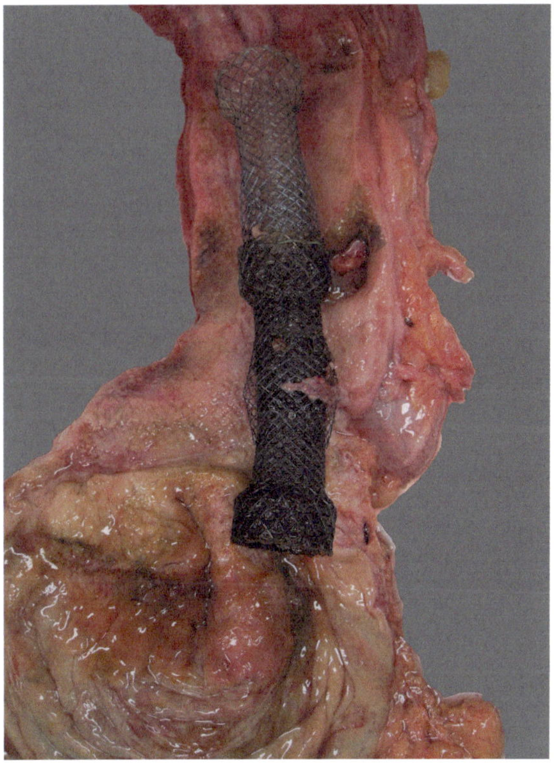

Fig. 5.52 This esophageal carcinoma has been treated by means of metal stent insertion to preserve esophageal lumen integrity. The stents can be positioned in multiple segment format so that a longer zone of protection is offered. In this case, the junction point between two stents is associated with an area of ulceration. It is important to consider the stent integrity as well as the lumen when examining tumor tissues. Careful dissection down on to the stent with a sharp scalpel is recommended

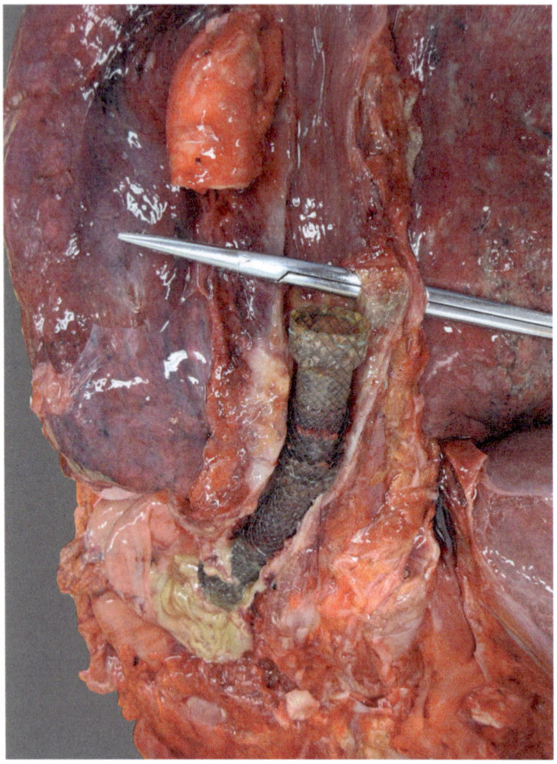

Fig. 5.53 An ulcer is demonstrated proximal to a stented esophageal tumour

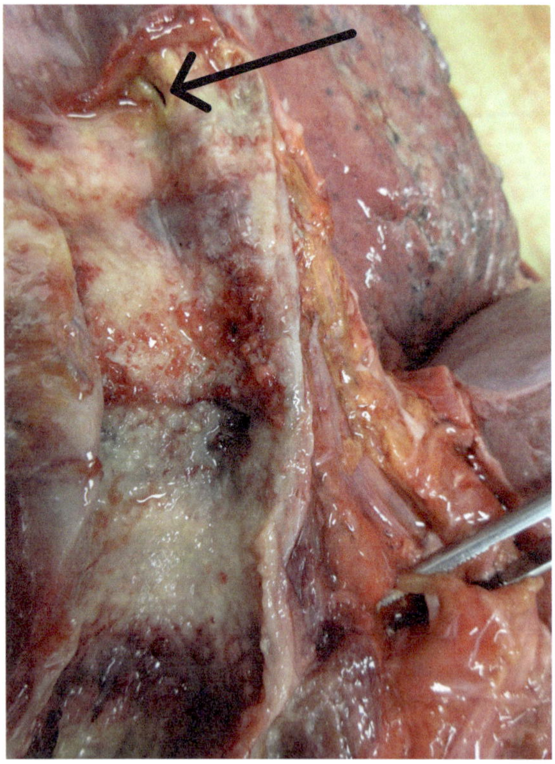

Fig. 5.54 The esophageal tumour shown in Fig. 5.53 with the stent removed. The ulcer can be seen towards the top of the picture (arrow)

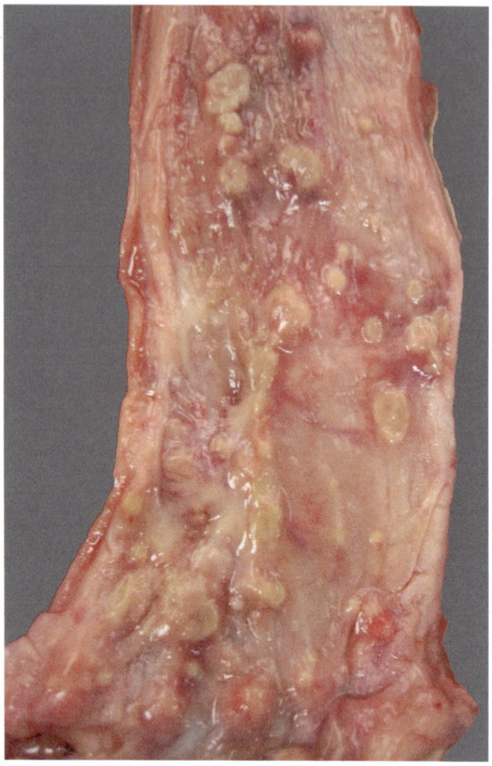

Fig. 5.55 Here, the esophageal tumor is seen to be spreading widely in lymphatics, with multiple nodules on the mucosal surface. This case was relatively early in stage, with the individual dying from another disease

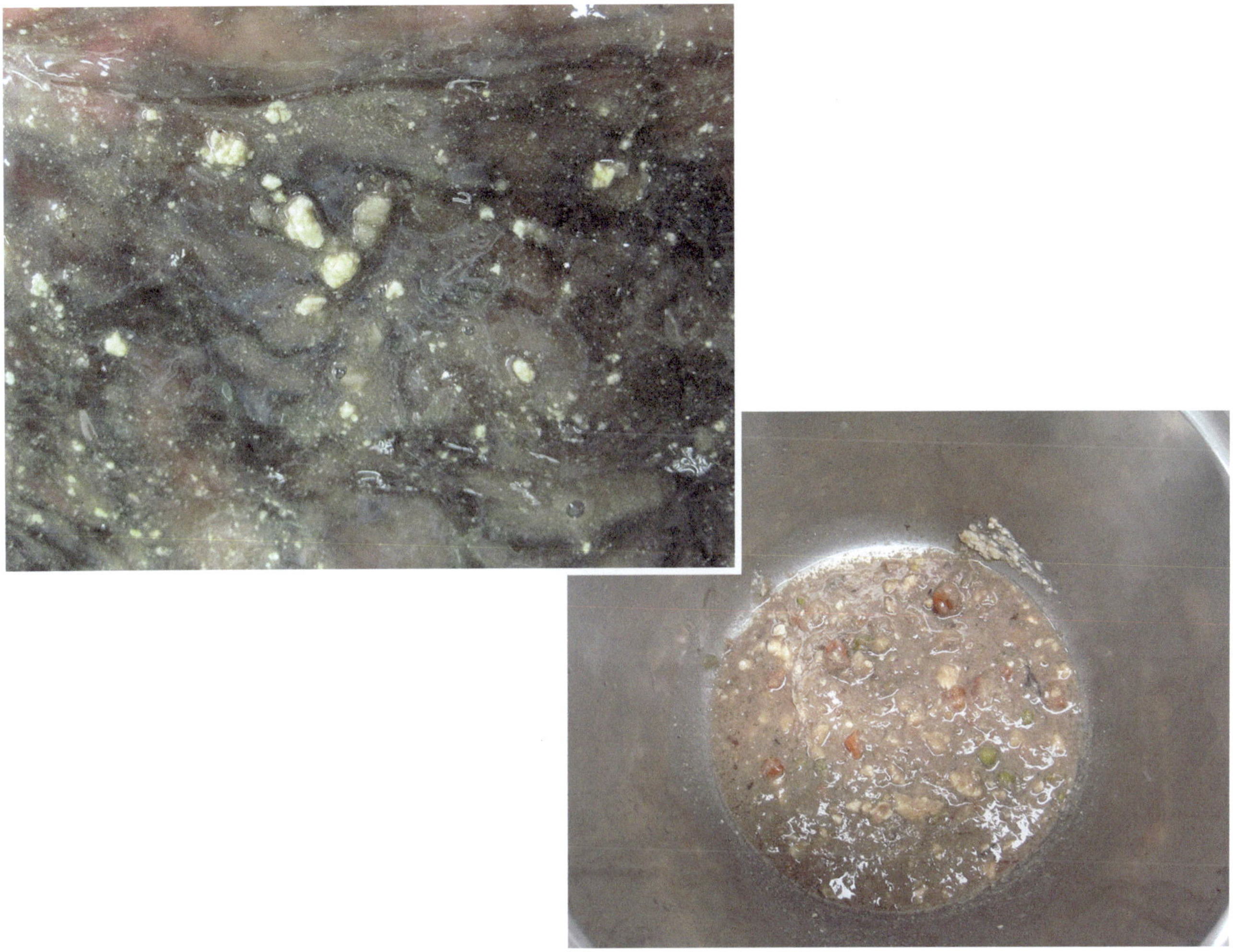

Fig. 5.56 The stomach mucosal surface (upper left) shows widespread granular debris, in keeping with tablet residue. In suspected cases of drug overdose, the stomach contents (food and tablet residue) should be reserved, weighed and measured in terms of mass and volume, with a portion being reserved for testing

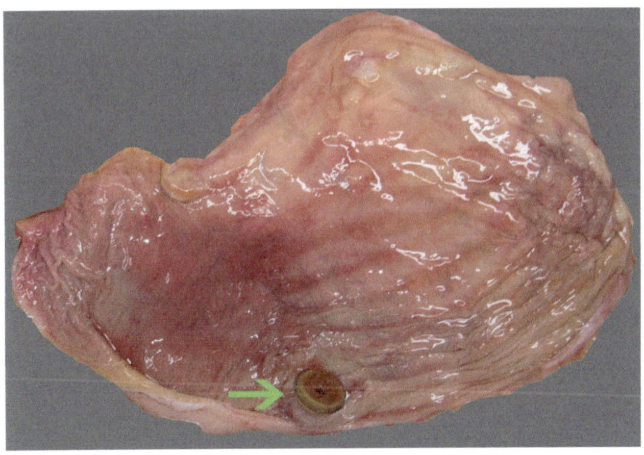

Fig. 5.57 The inner aspect of a PEG tube (used for feeding purposes) is seen on the mucosal aspect of the stomach

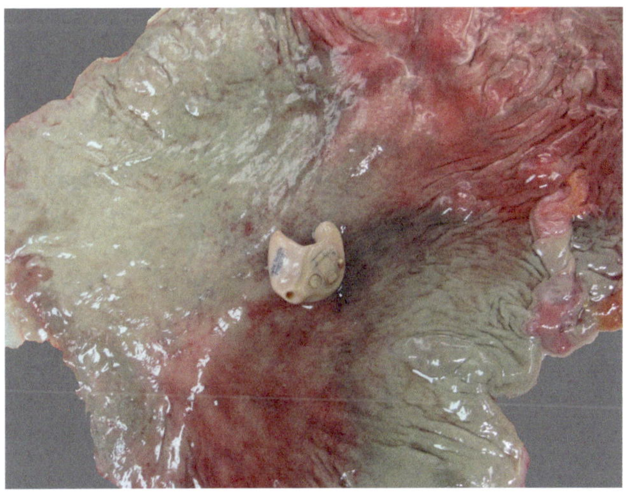

Fig. 5.58 Unusual items can be found in the stomach. In this case, a hearing aid was found in the stomach of a patient with dementia

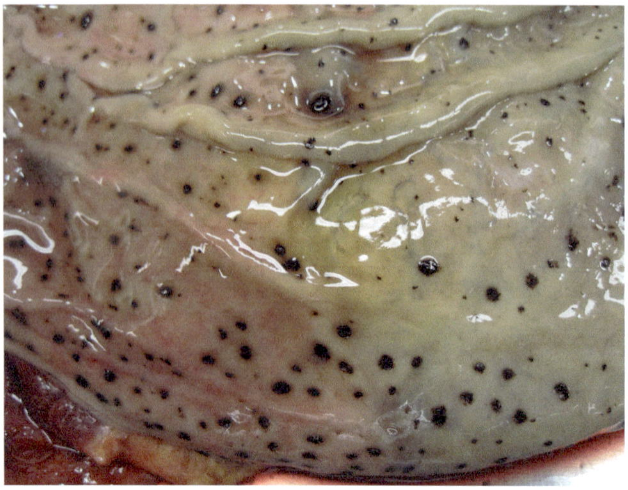

Fig. 5.59 Multiple black mucosal patches are often seen on the stomach surface in terminal stress-related conditions. They represent microscopic areas of ante-mortem ulceration and hemorrhage

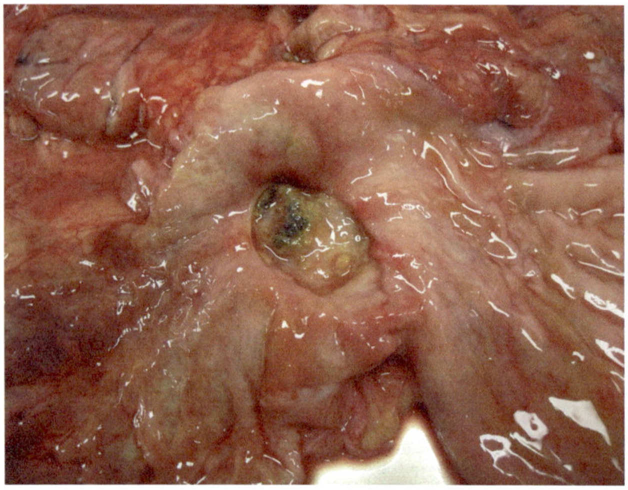

Fig. 5.60 This benign gastric ulcer is seen to have a relatively sharply defined edge, together with black areas of discoloration around the base. These are blood vessels with some thrombus. They can be associated with significant hemorrhage

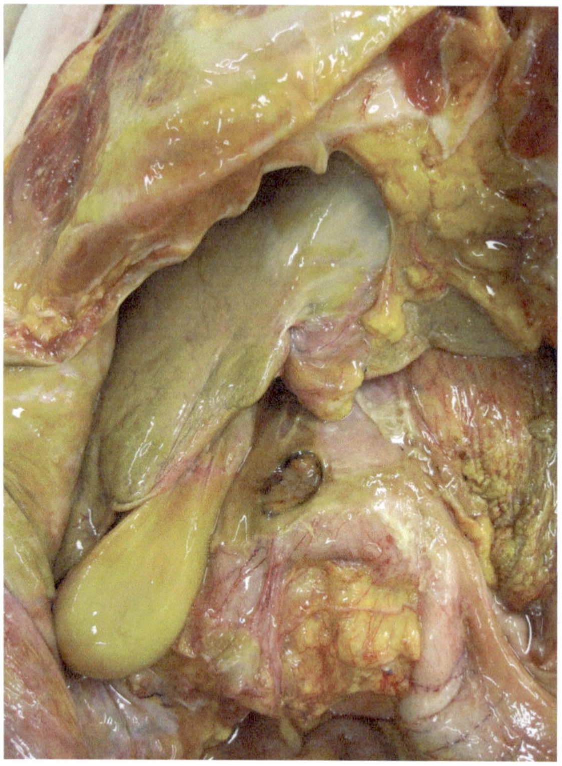

Fig. 5.61 This view shows a pyloric peptic perforation with associated peritonitis in a case of chronic peptic ulceration. There is a zone of black tissue around the edge of the ulcer where it interfaces with the serosal surface, in the form of coagulated blood and necrotic debris

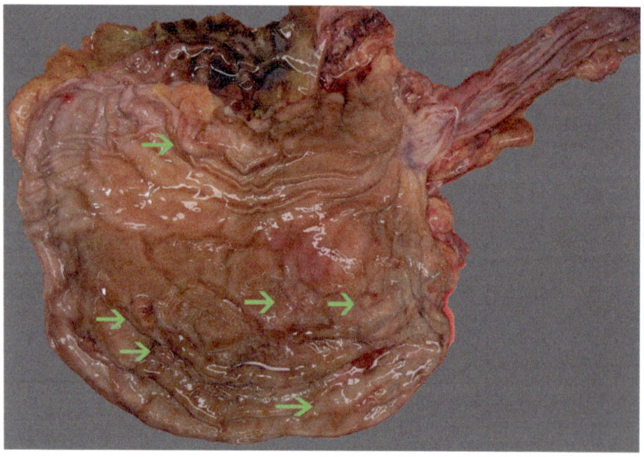

Fig. 5.62 Multiple small nodules (arrows) are seen on the mucosal aspect of the stomach in this case of neuroendocrine cell hyperplasia with evolving neuroendocrine tumors

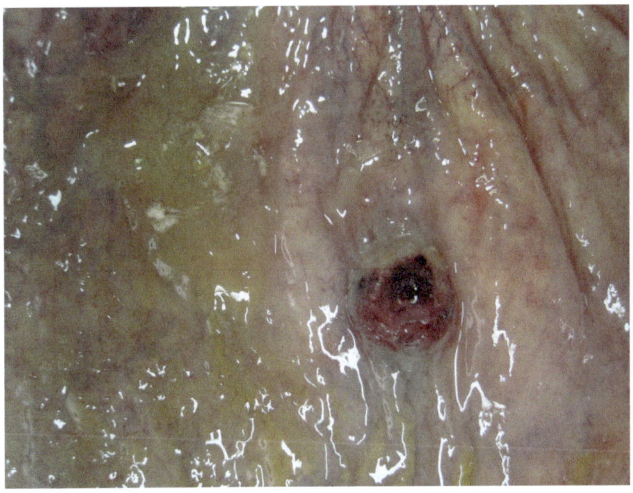

Fig. 5.63 Stomach tumours vary in their architecture and appearance. Some are very bland and nodular, with relatively shallow ulcers. This stomach carcinoma showed notable hemorrhage and firmness in association with relatively little local mucosal infiltration

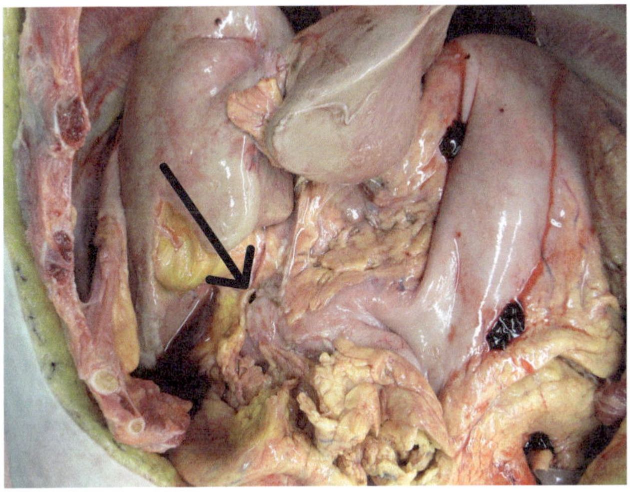

Fig. 5.64 A perforated duodenal ulcer (arrow), seen within the first part of the duodenum, has caused peritonitis. The liver has a pale external surface indicative of fatty liver disease

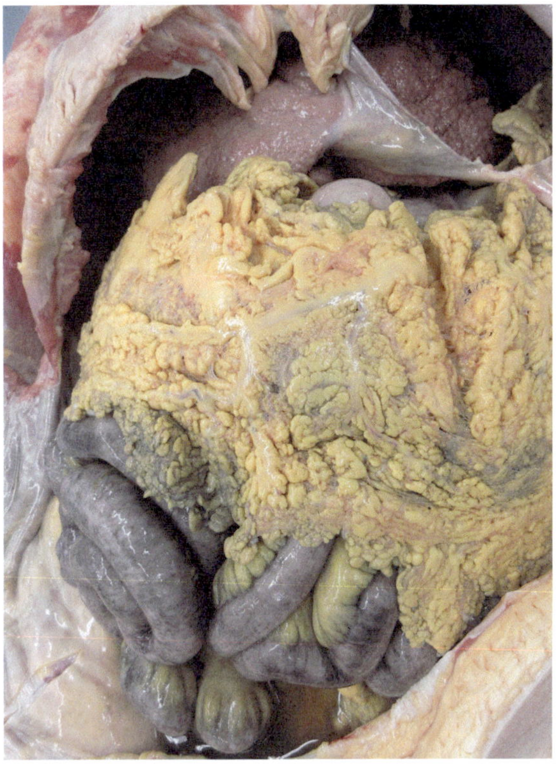

Fig. 5.65 The small bowel in the image is dark in colour. It contains blood following a significant upper gastrointestinal bleed. Note the nodularity of the liver indicating cirrhosis, in keeping with this sequence of pathology

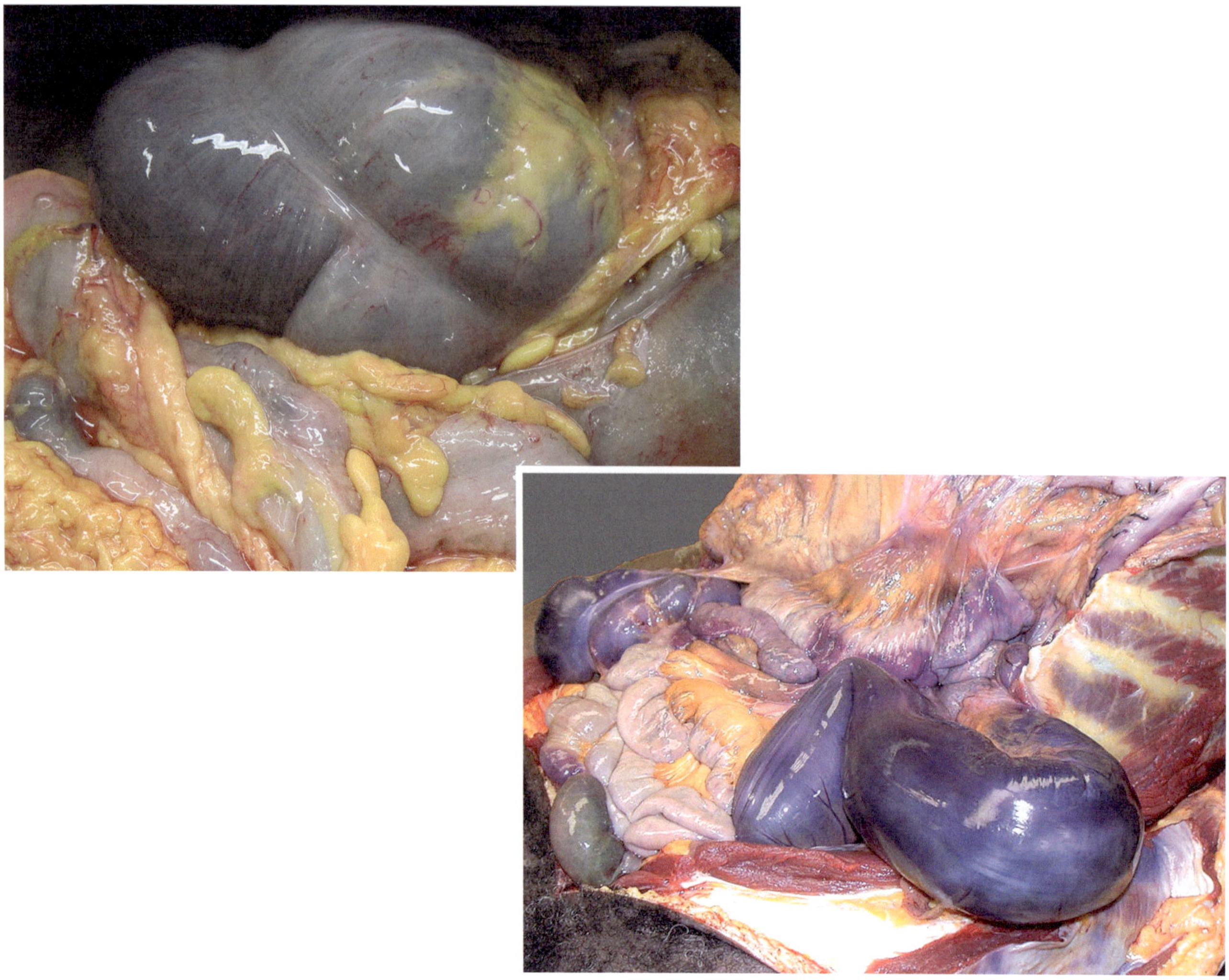

Fig. 5.66 The colour of bowel tissues may be markedly altered by contents, as in this case of an individual with pronounced dietary intake of beetroot (lower right). The dark grey/black colour (upper left) was initially considered to be evidence of malena, but there was no gastrointestinal bleeding. These tissues were discoloured by oral iron (ferrous sulfate) therapy

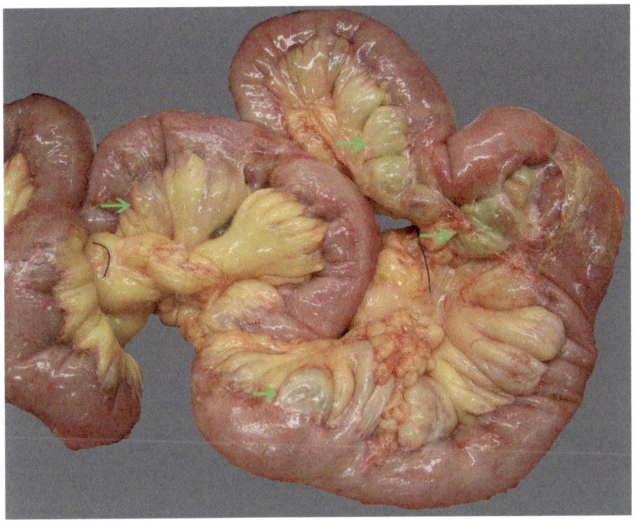

Fig. 5.67 Jejunal diverticulosis is seen as thin-walled outpouchings of the small bowel (arrows). This condition is often silent but may be associated with malabsorption conditions

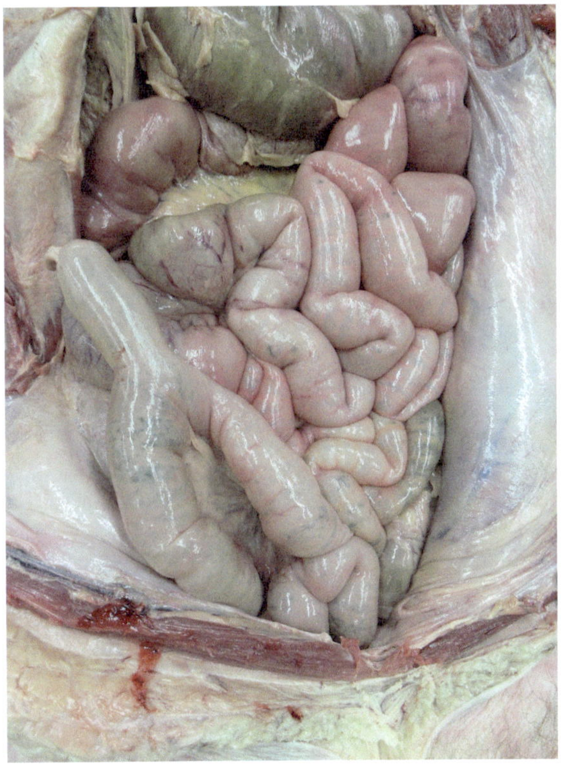

Fig. 5.68 Shown here is an incidental finding of a Meckel's diverticulum within the small bowel

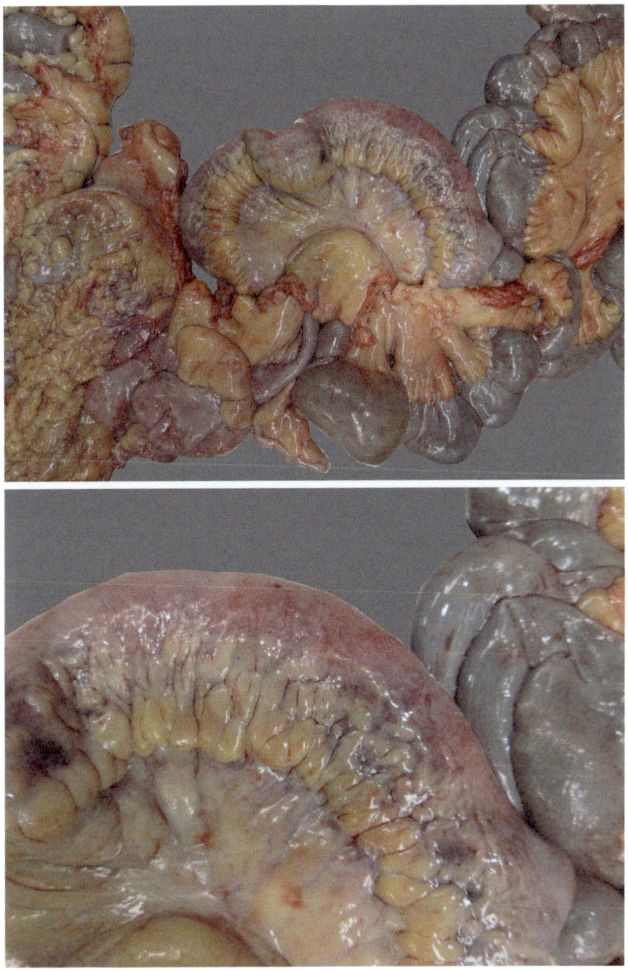

Fig. 5.69 These images show the typical fat wrapping seen in Crohn's disease. The adipose tissue of the mesentery extends around the circumference of the small bowel

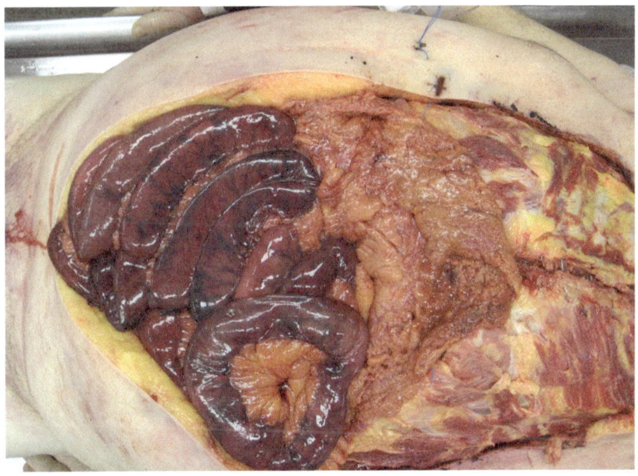

Fig. 5.70 The small bowel is particularly vulnerable to hypoxia in cases of hypotension. This individual suffered a profound drop in blood pressure following myocardial infarction, resulting in secondary small bowel mucosal necrosis and hemorrhage. This situation worsens the hypotension by virtue of blood loss, fluid loss and toxaemia. It may also result in small bowel perforation and peritonitis

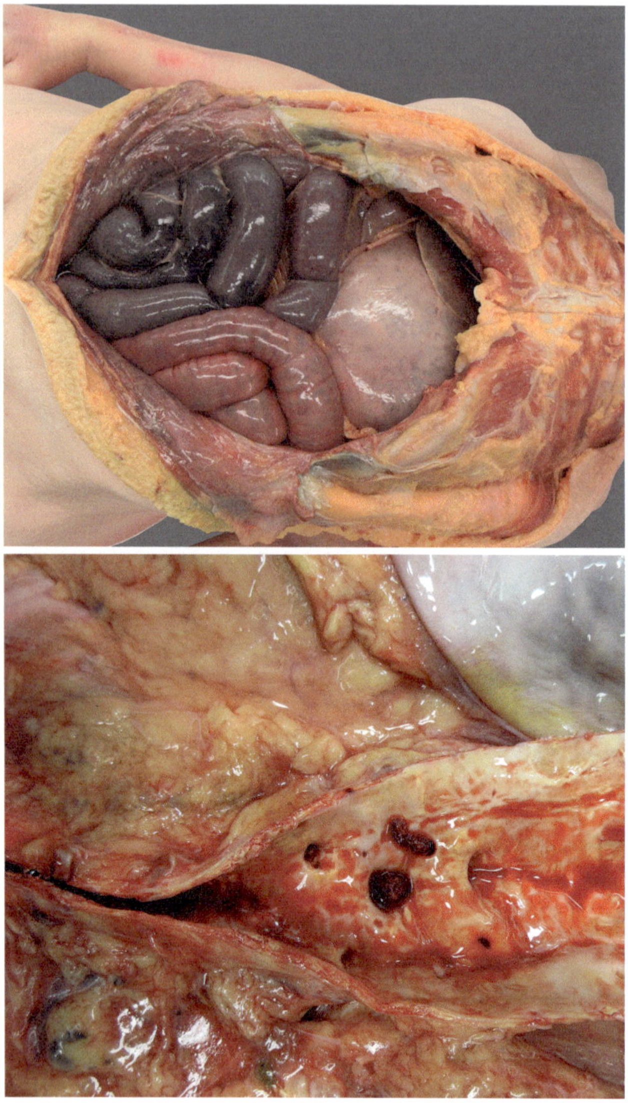

Fig. 5.71 This is an example of small bowel ischaemia secondary to mesenteric thrombus. The picture of the whole abdomen shows a sharp demarcation between the ischaemic and viable small bowel, seen early in the examination process. This view of the aorta from the posterior aspect shows a thrombus within the orifice of the superior mesenteric artery. This accounts for the ischaemic bowel seen

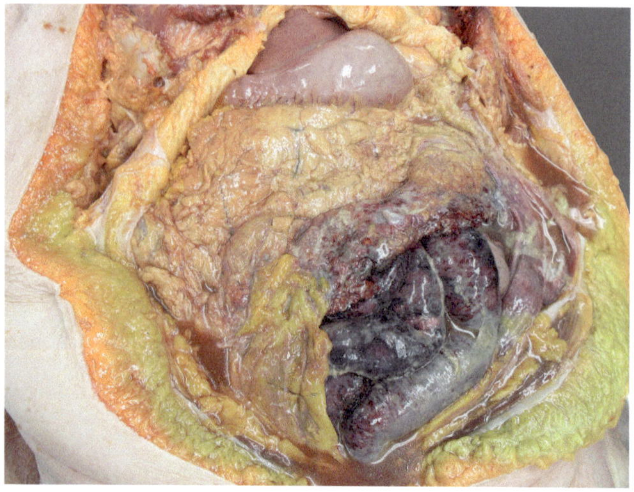

Fig. 5.72 A case of localized peritonitis arising from a perforated, infarcted small bowel

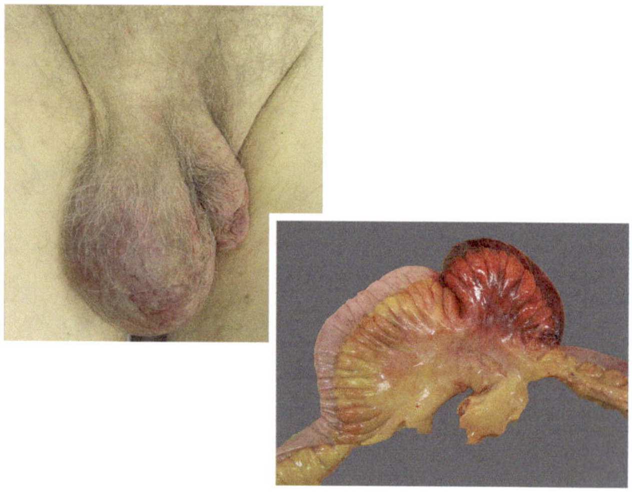

Fig. 5.73 This is a segment of small bowel that had been incarcerated in a hernia sac, leading to mucosal necrosis with secondary toxaemia and bacteraemia

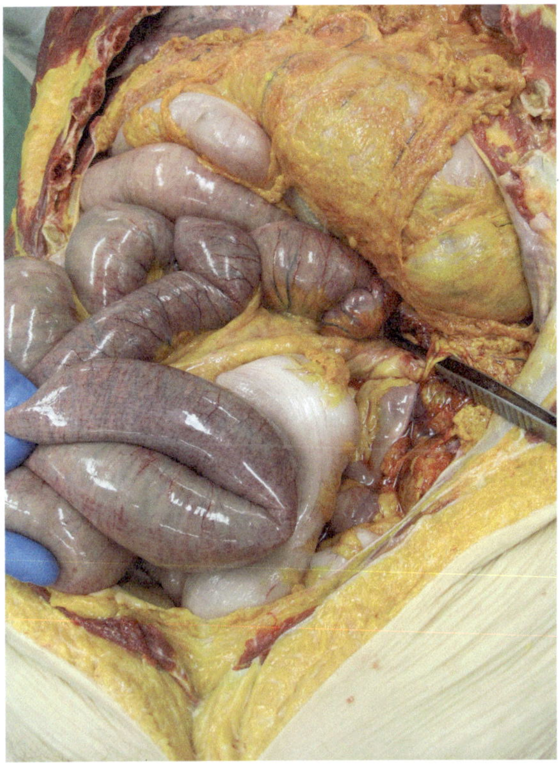

Fig. 5.74 Fibrous adhesions and bands are often consequences of previous surgery or instrumentation of the abdominal cavity. On occasion, these can obstruct the bowel tissues

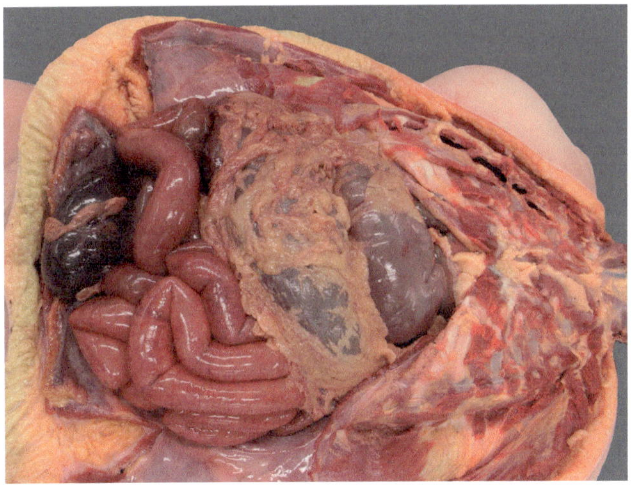

Fig. 5.75 Here is a case of small bowel ischaemia secondary to an internal band adhesion. There is a dusky segment of small bowel seen inferiorly with prominent and dilated proximal loops. The stark contrast between the infarcted small bowel and viable small bowel is pronounced

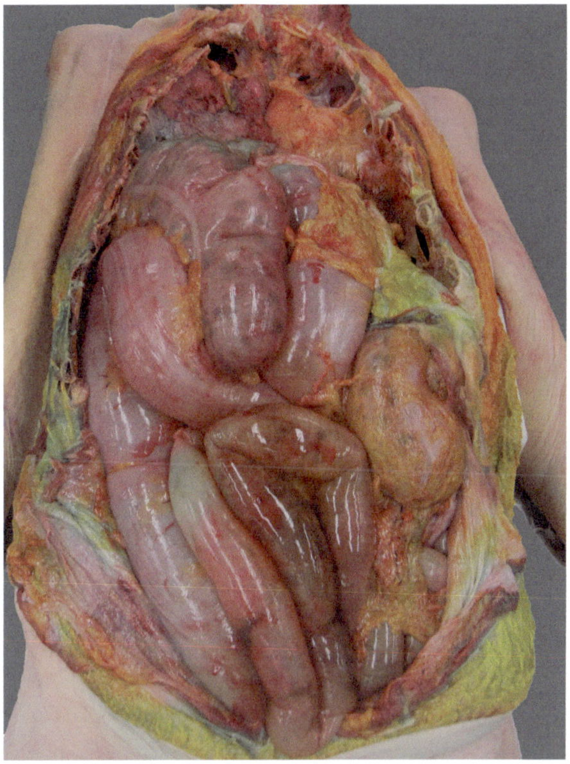

Fig. 5.76 Post-operative complications may include significant ileus. This individual showed pronounced gaseous dilatation of the small and large bowel in association with intestinal pseudo-obstruction. Nevertheless, an anatomical or pathological reason for the obstruction should be sought in all cases by opening of the bowel

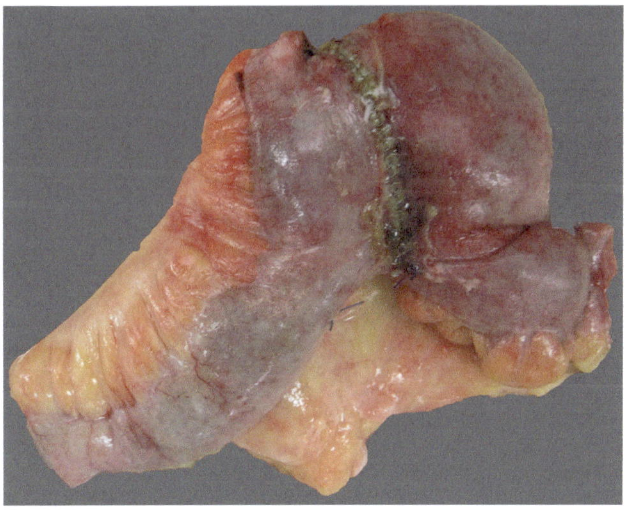

Fig. 5.77 Inflammation and necrosis around a poorly vascularized anastomosis can lead to significant bacteremia or peritonitis and thereby death. The postoperative status of all gastrointestinal surgical cases needs to be checked for possible leakage and mural necrosis. Histology may also be of benefit in these cases

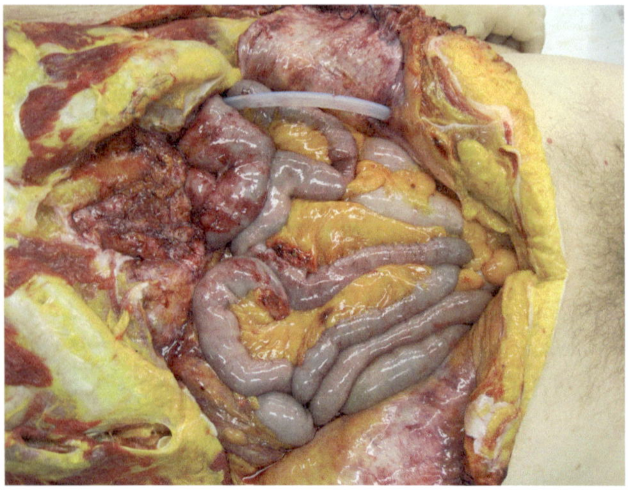

Fig. 5.78 In a further postoperative case shown here, there is pronounced haemorrhage around the site of previous closure of a perforated peptic ulcer by means of oversewing. One needs to consider the placement of any drains (entering through the left lower abdomen) and evaluate any collections, blood loss or further pathology

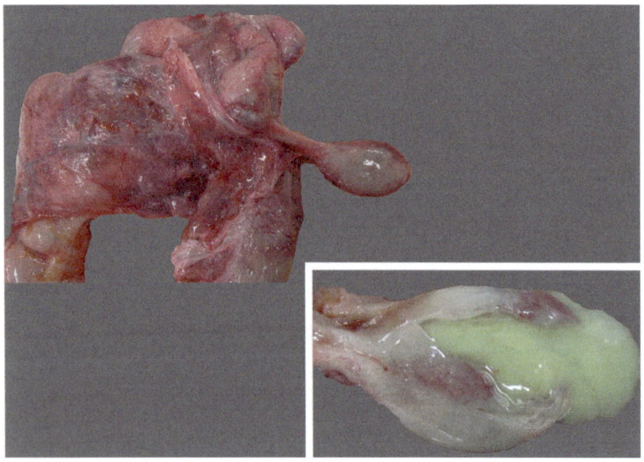

Fig. 5.79 An acutely inflamed, but not ruptured, appendix is seen. The fluctuant and dilated tip of the appendix is noted to be discolored. When incised (right lower inset), the same appendix contained purulent content

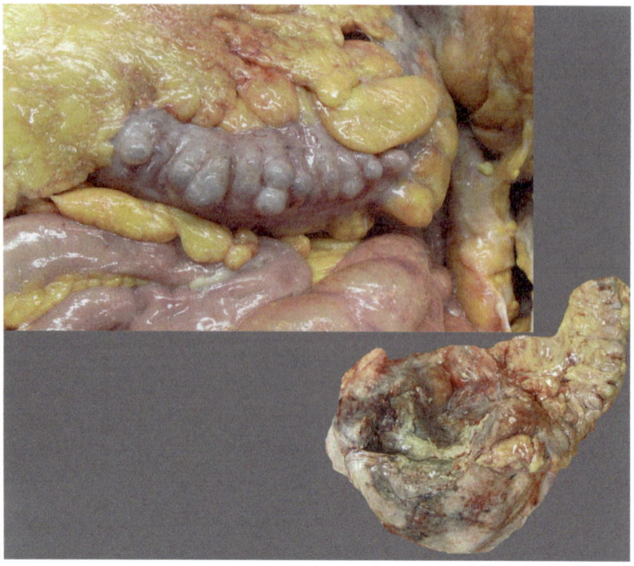

Fig. 5.80 Diverticular disease of the colon (upper left) is seen with pronounced saccular dilatations on the serosal surface. These are common findings at autopsy and rarely of significance unless there is rupture and associated peritonitis (lower right)

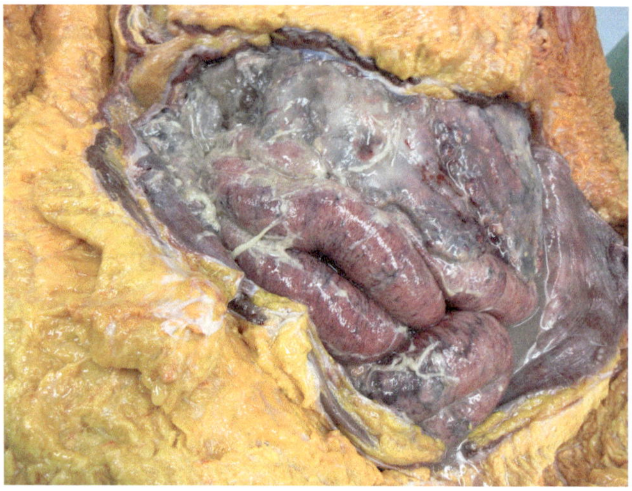

Fig. 5.81 Generalised peritonitis is seen arising from perforated diverticular disease of the sigmoid colon

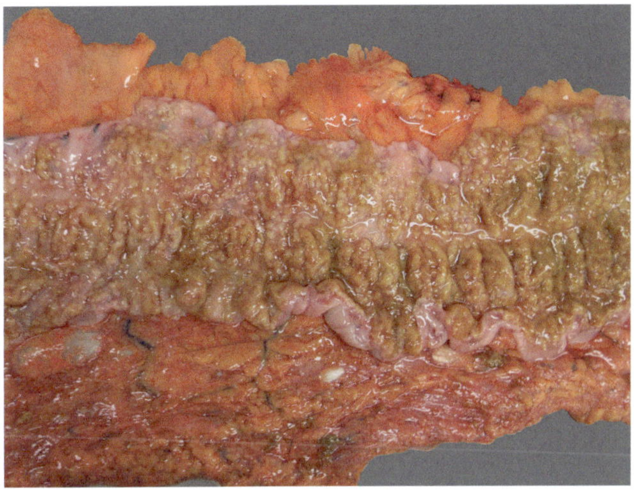

Fig. 5.82 Clostridium difficile colitis. There are small areas of ulceration, mucosal necrosis and exudative change represents the pseudomembranes. At autopsy they are often darkly stained due to fecal material

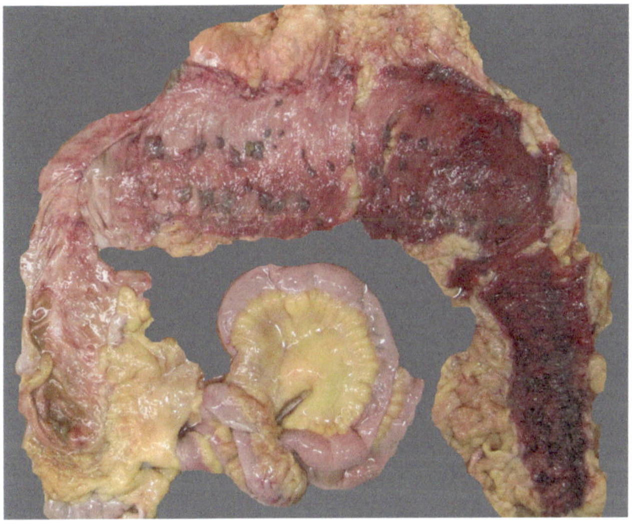

Fig. 5.83 An acute on chronic case of ulcerative colitis, showing classic inflammation and ulceration, particularly towards the left side. Note that the small bowel is spared

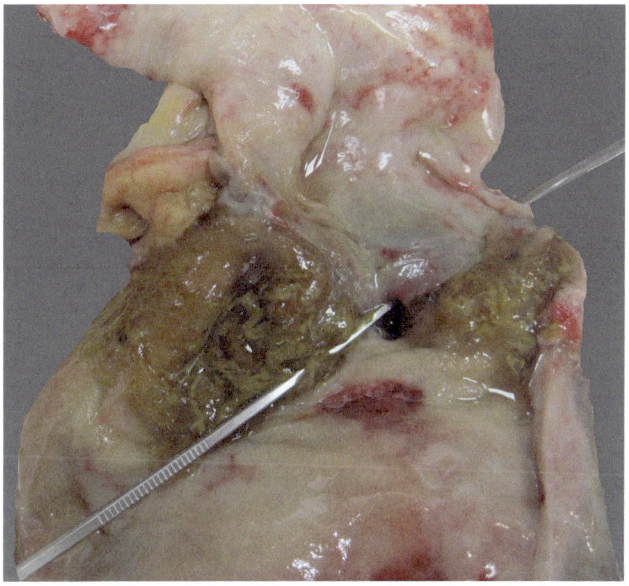

Fig. 5.84 Focal large bowel ulceration and perforation in a case of vasculitis

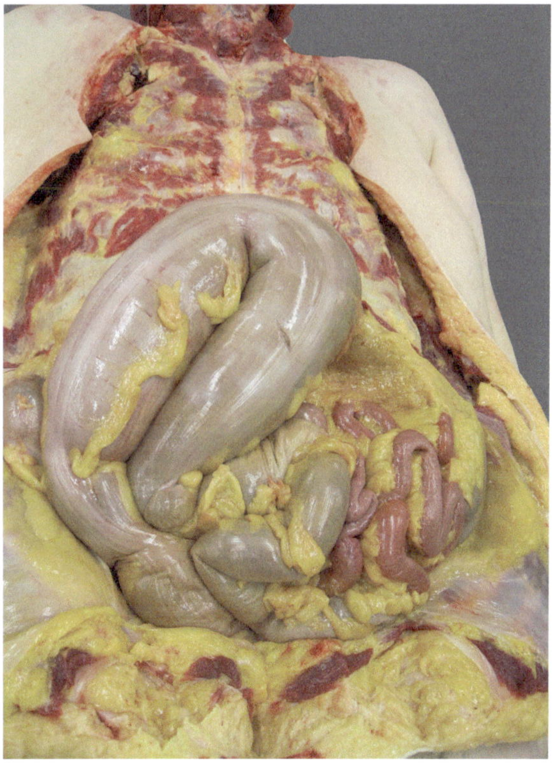

Fig. 5.85 A sigmoid volvulus is present with dilated, gas-filled content pushing the sigmoid tissues up and towards the liver. This is associated with a twisting of the mesenteric tissues, which can result in not only bowel stasis or obstruction but also bowel necrosis and peritonitis

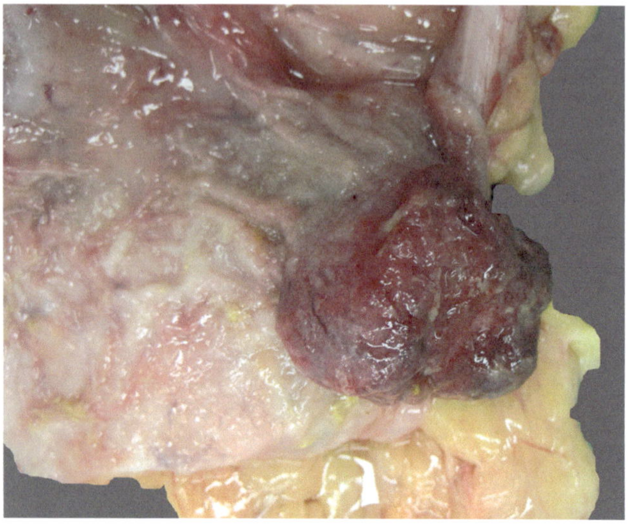

Fig. 5.86 Colon adenomas are commonly seen at autopsy. They have no significance unless they are obstructive or bleeding

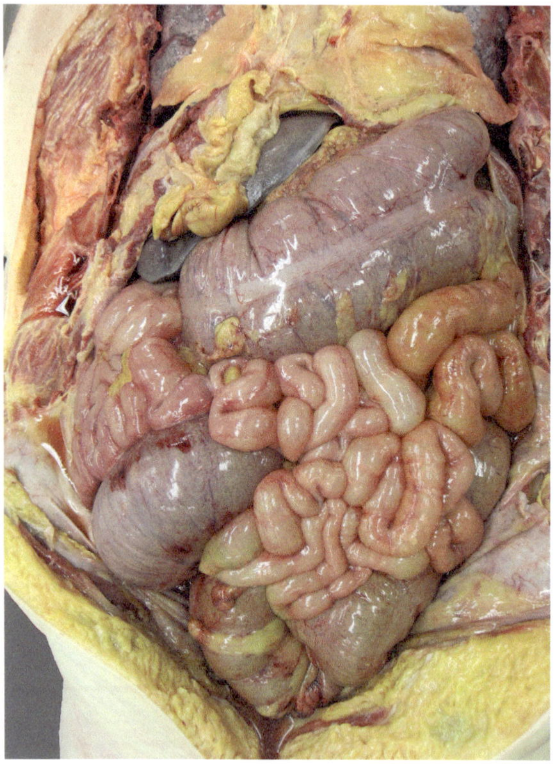

Fig. 5.87 Large bowel obstruction is seen, suggesting a rectal or sigmoid obstructing lesion

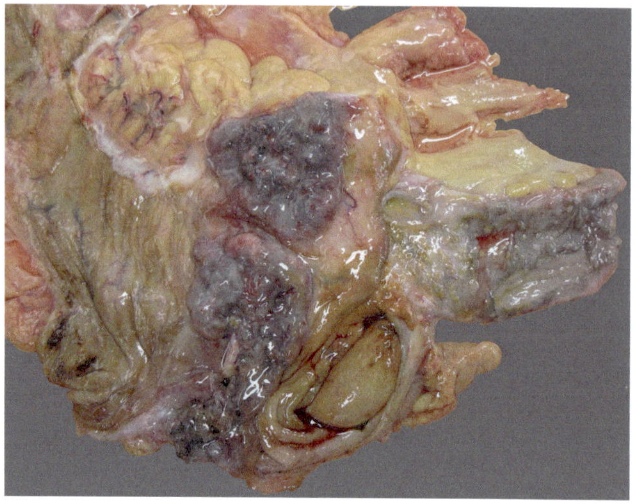

Fig. 5.88 In a different case, a circumscribed and obstructing tumour is present at the caecum

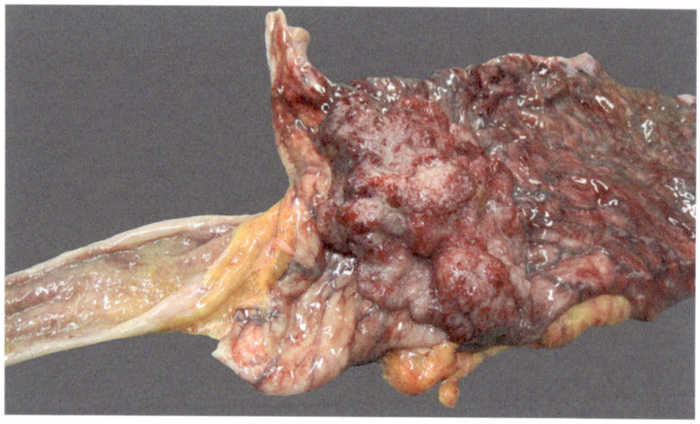

Fig. 5.89 Carcinoma of the colon can be the cause of death in some individuals with bowel obstruction and or perforation. Disseminated bowel cancer is relatively common in terms of autopsy analysis, but incidental findings of unsuspected adenocarcinoma can be identified by careful palpation of the bowel tissues during evisceration as well as opening the bowel at suspect sites

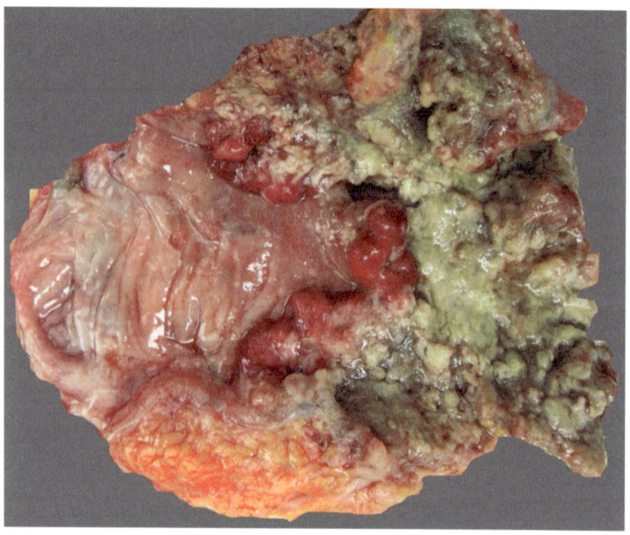

Fig. 5.90 Some cases of advanced rectal cancer are occasionally found at autopsy. They need to be staged in the same manner as ante-mortem cases

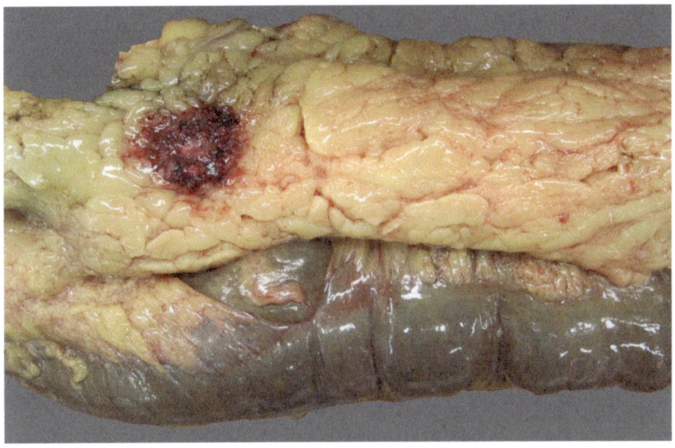

Fig. 5.91 Metastatic tumors to the bowel can be part of disseminated cancer cases. This image shows the serosa adjacent to the colon in a case of disseminated lung cancer

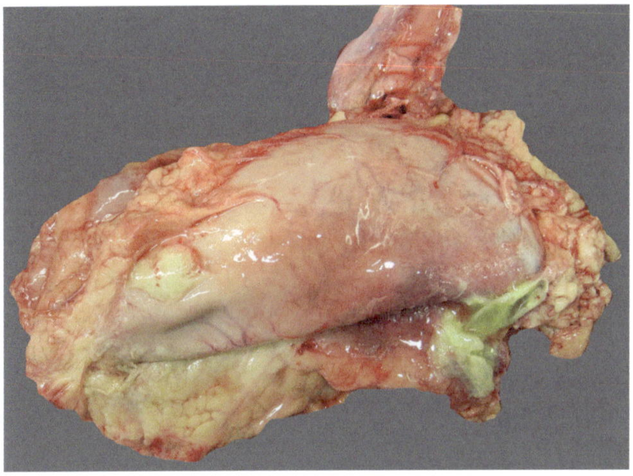

Fig. 5.92 The stomach has been pushed upwards in this case, revealing focal early acute pancreatitis

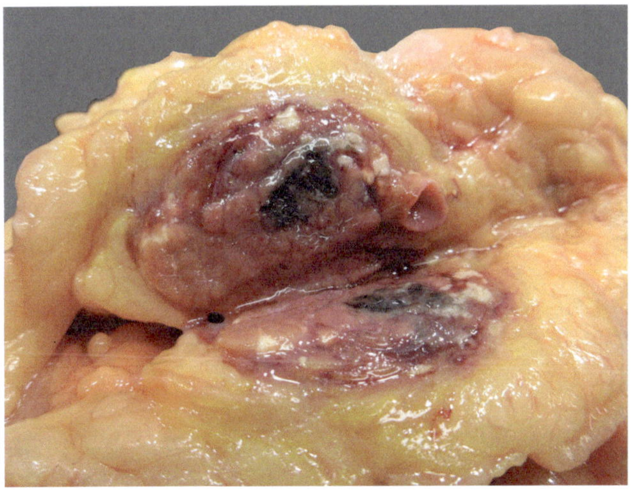

Fig. 5.93 A cross section of the pancreas displays haemorrhage and necrosis, in keeping with acute pancreatitis

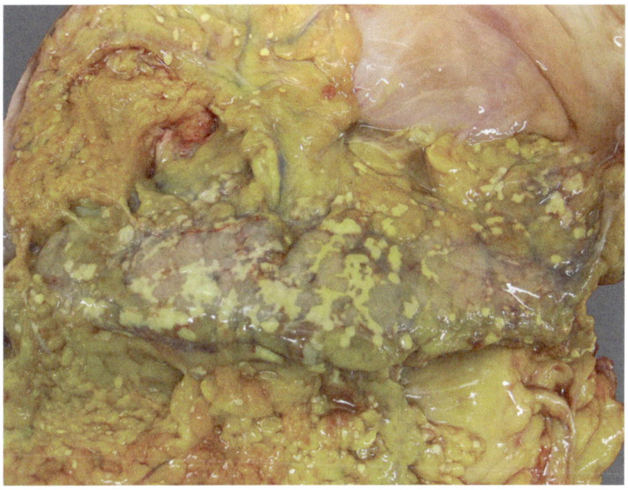

Fig. 5.94 Pancreatitis can be suspected on occasion in cases of peritonitis. This mottled fat necrosis change was present only on the pancreatic serosal surface. No deep parenchymal disease was present

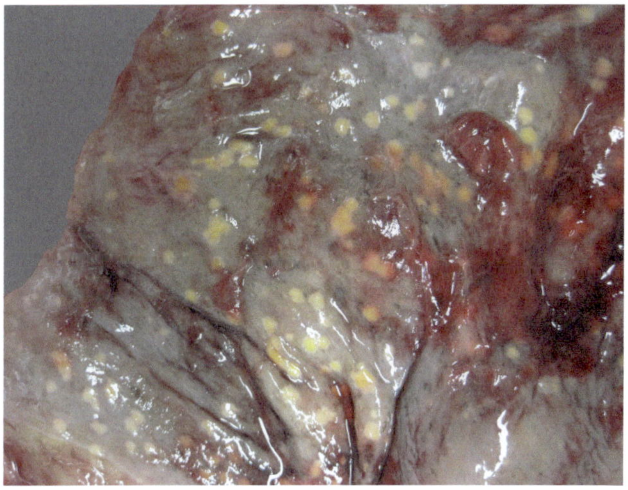

Fig. 5.95 The peritoneal surface is seen to be inflamed and congested, with areas of fat necrosis in this case of pancreatitis. These findings represent liberation of pancreatic enzymes into the peritoneal cavity, with patchy saponification of tissues

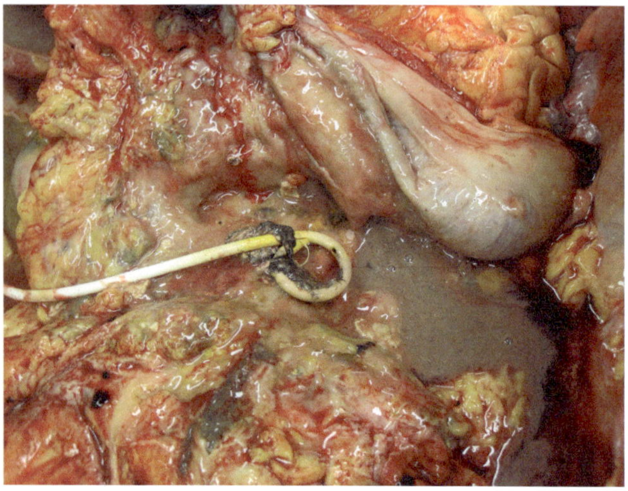

Fig. 5.96 A large pancreatic pseudocyst with associated semi-necrotic fatty residue in a case of acute on chronic pancreatitis. A pigtail catheter was being used to drain out the collection via the anterior abdominal wall. Despite this, the patient was overwhelmed by the pancreatitis

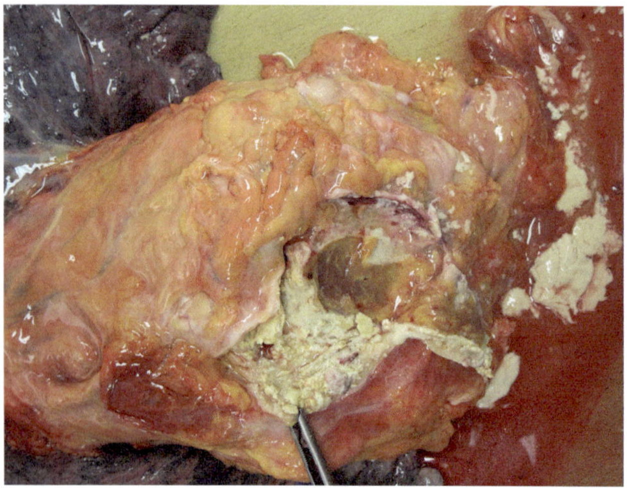

Fig. 5.97 A pancreatic pseudocyst is seen with inflammatory content and marked local fat necrosis. The stomach has been lifted upwards and the omentum has been cut to facilitate the view of the pathology

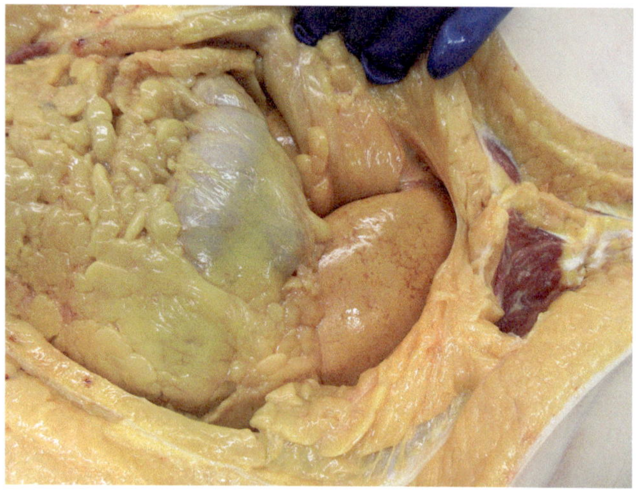

Fig. 5.98 Fatty change in the liver is suggested by a yellow/orange discoloration of the liver parenchyma. The liver itself often is enlarged

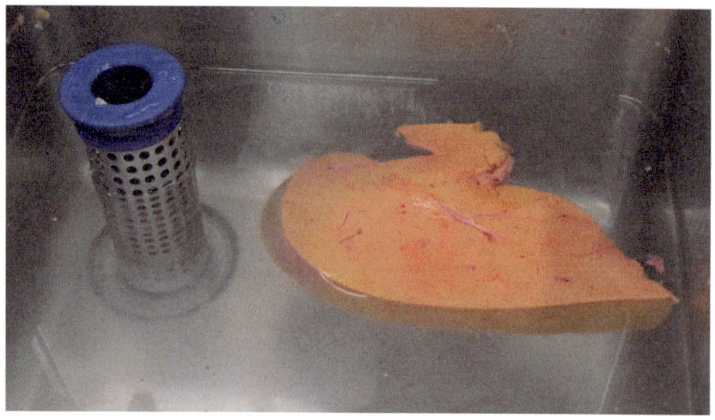

Fig. 5.99 Fatty livers tend to have a greasy cut surface, but in extreme cases the fatty liver tissue is capable of floating, as displayed here within a sink of water

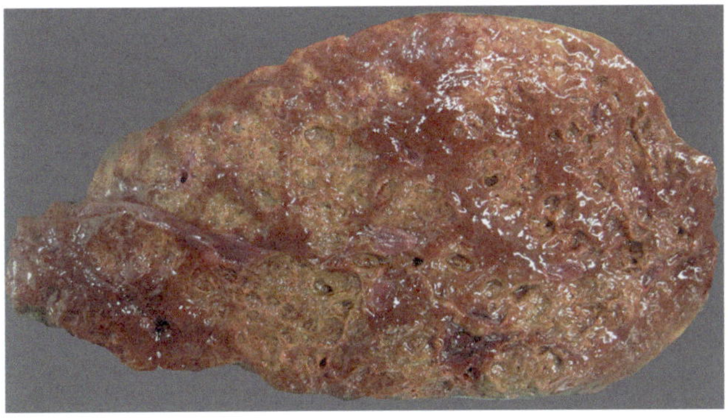

Fig. 5.100 Decomposing bodies often present gas collections in the liver. This 'Swiss-cheese' effect with softening/liquefaction change may indicate terminal bacteraemia or may just be part of general decomposition

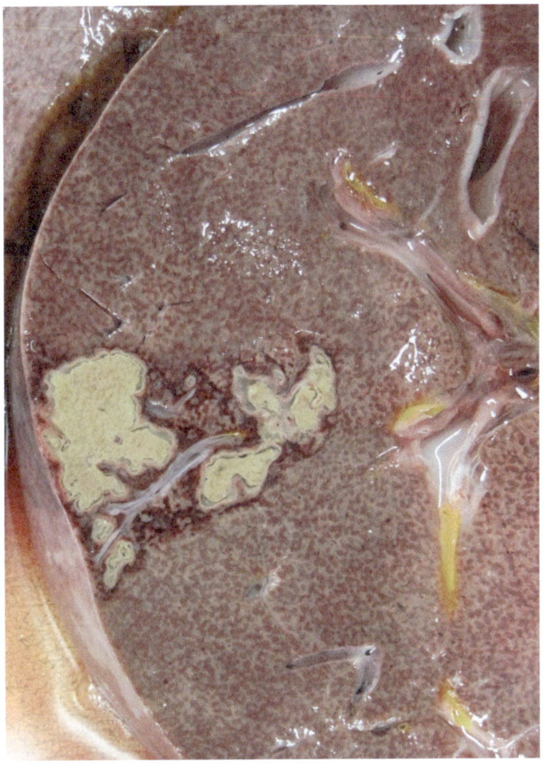

Fig. 5.101 A wedge-shaped infarct is seen in a case of infective endocarditis. Yellow discoloration is present, with associated moderate congestion and hemorrhage

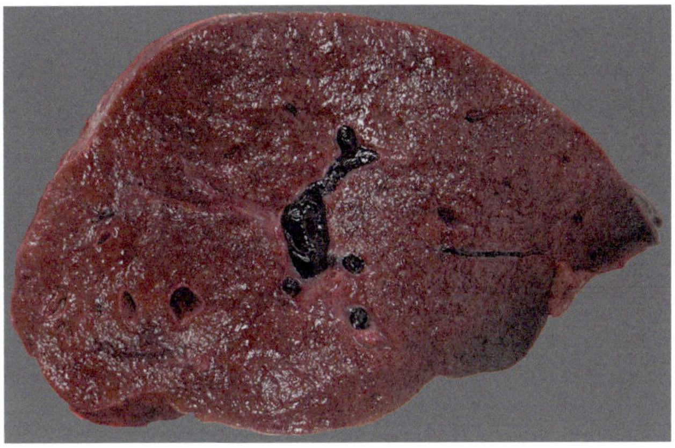

Fig. 5.102 Exacerbations of liver function can be associated with coagulopathies. Central venous congestion and then thrombosis has occurred in this case with an acute deterioration of liver function as a terminal event

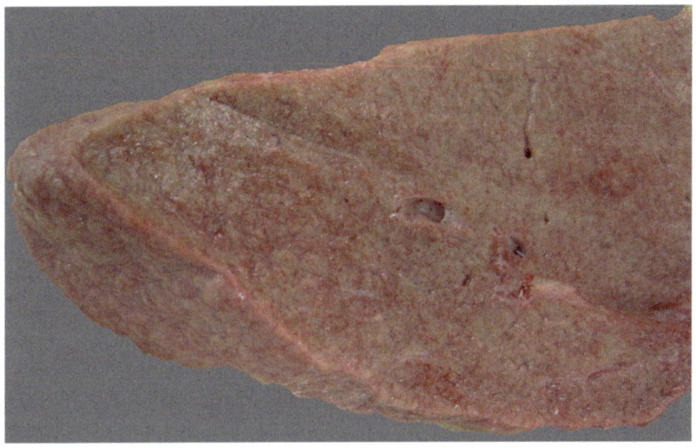

Fig. 5.103 The liver can show pronounced fibrosis, bordering on micronodular cirrhosis. In such circumstances, any cuts made into the liver tend to hold their shape and the cut surface of the liver also shows slight granularity. Histological review of such cases is important as the full criteria for cirrhosis may not be present

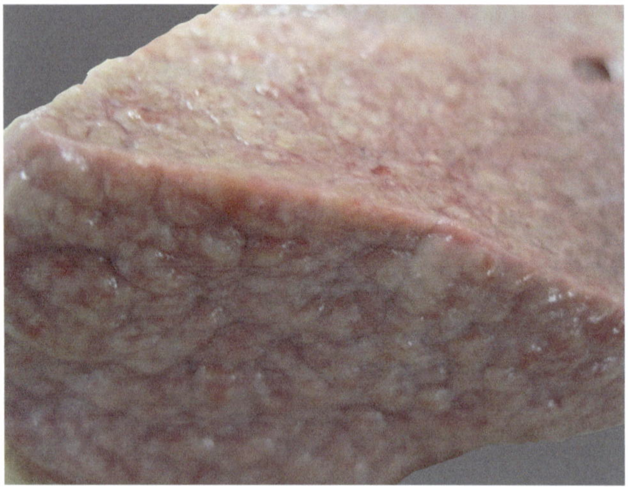

Fig. 5.104 Liver cirrhosis is characterized by nodularity not only on the surface of the tissue but also that extending into the deep parenchyma. Nodules vary in size from a few millimeters up to a centimeter or more

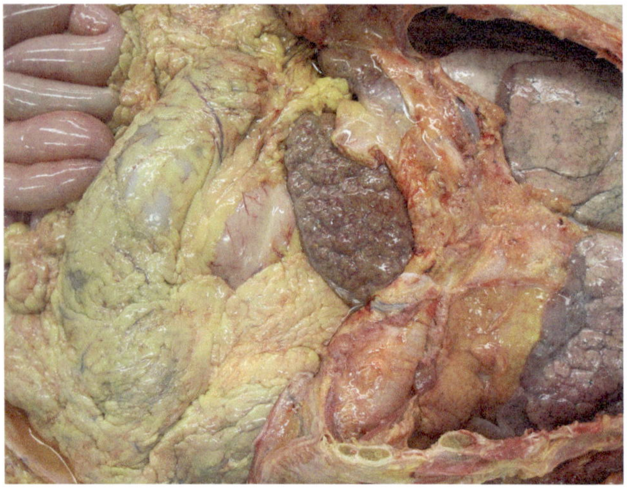

Fig. 5.105 Liver cirrhosis can be identified often at the beginning of the autopsy examination with the liver edge being clearly seen to have adjacent nodularity and fibrosis. One should be aware of the need to check for other lesions such as esophageal varices and other features of liver failure

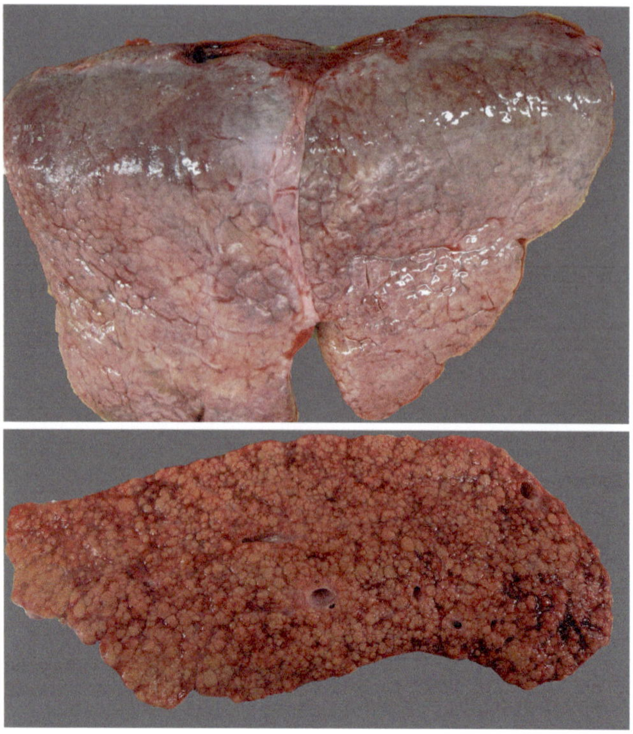

Fig. 5.106 Macronodular cirrhosis may be encountered in many different pathologies that end with cirrhosis

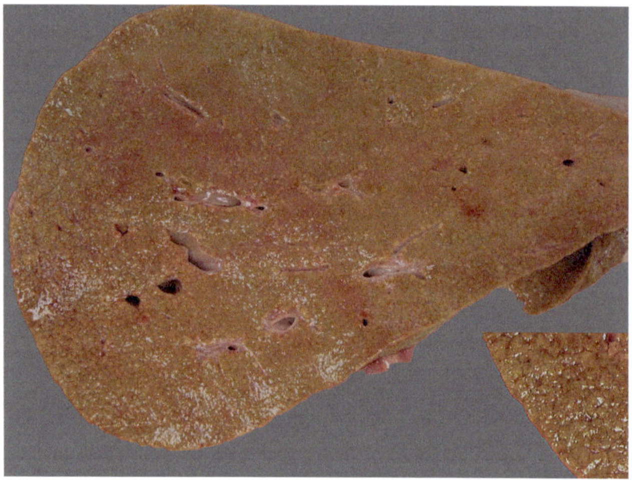

Fig. 5.107 Micronodular cirrhosis is classically associated with excess alcohol intake, but is not specific in this regard. The pronounced yellow/green color points to fatty change in surviving parenchyma and some bile stasis. The inset shows the fine nodularity

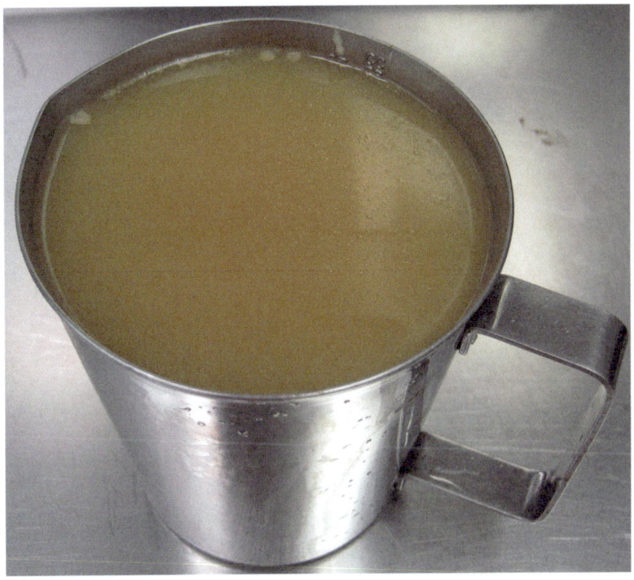

Fig. 5.108 Cirrhosis is often accompanied by clear, yellow ascites, as a feature of altered blood flow through the liver and a hypoproteinemic state. Should the fluid be opaque or turbid, then one may suspect spontaneous bacterial peritonitis, which can significantly aggravate any case of cirrhosis and can be fatal

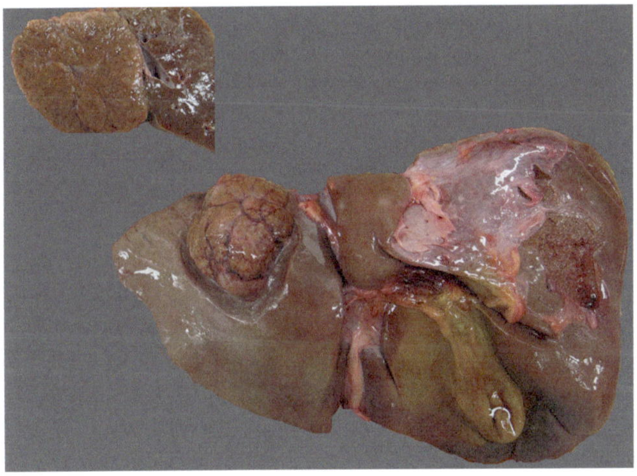

Fig. 5.109 A rounded liver tumor is seen on the undersurface of the left lobe. This has a characteristic bosselated and folding architecture. On section (top left), there is central fibrosis and distortion, in keeping with a hepatocellular adenoma

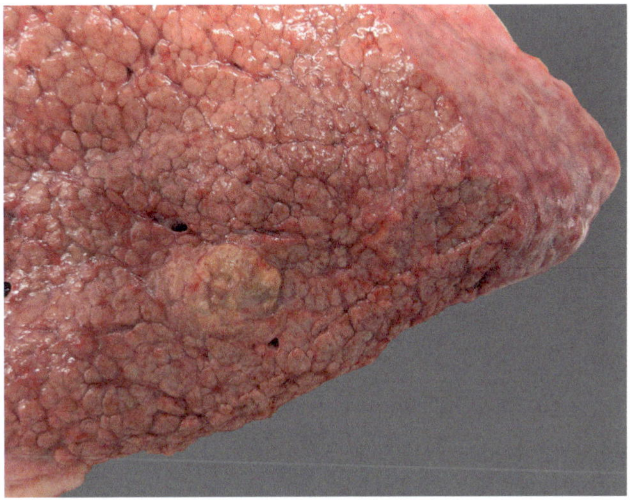

Fig. 5.110 A case of hepatocellular carcinoma in a cirrhotic liver

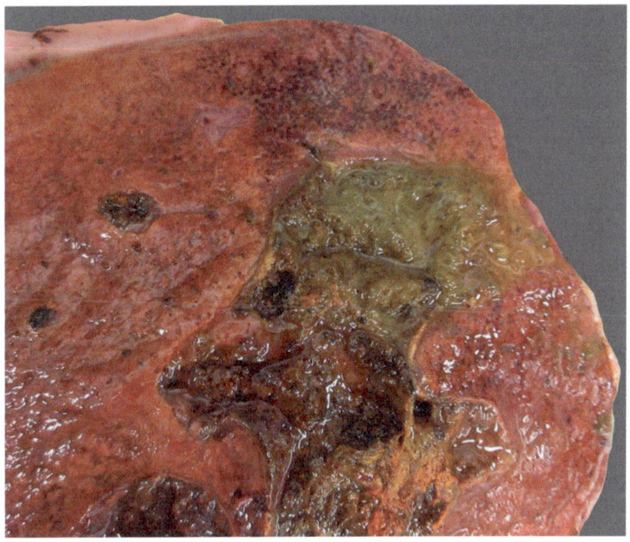

Fig. 5.111 A focus of infection and biliary obstruction is seen within a liver segment, secondary to a necrotic tumour proximal to this focus

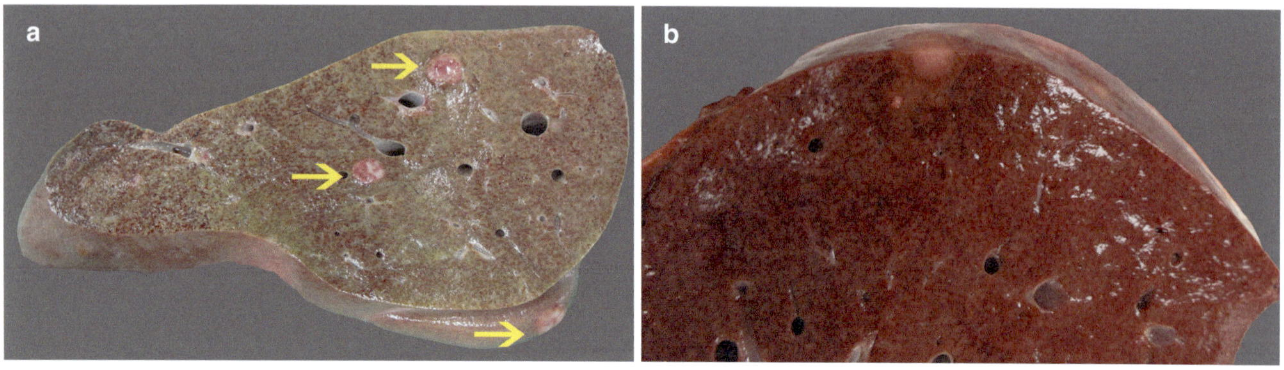

Fig. 5.112 Metastatic disease to the liver is commonplace at autopsy. Multiple lesions (arrows) are present in the first image. A single rounded deposit is seen at the liver surface in the second image. In such cases, a rigorous search for the primary should be undertaken with consideration of the prior medical history. Sampling for histological confirmation is often required, unless the tumour was documented before death

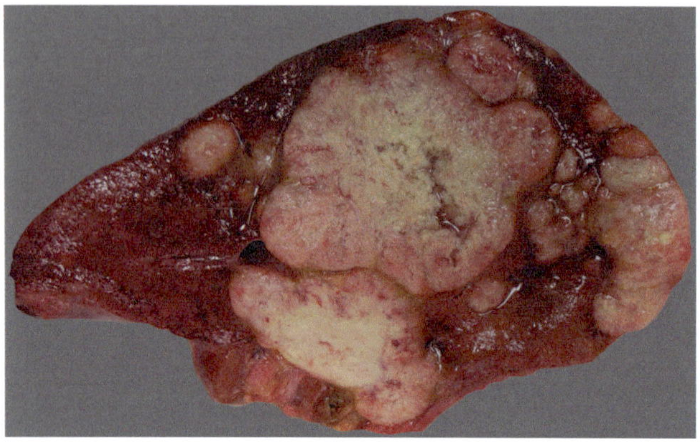

Fig. 5.113 The degree of carcinomatous infiltration of the liver can vary. Indeed, widespread infiltration of the liver can be associated with normal liver function. This individual had squamous carcinoma of the cervix with widespread bone, liver and lung metastases. The ultimate cause of death was in fact pulmonary embolism

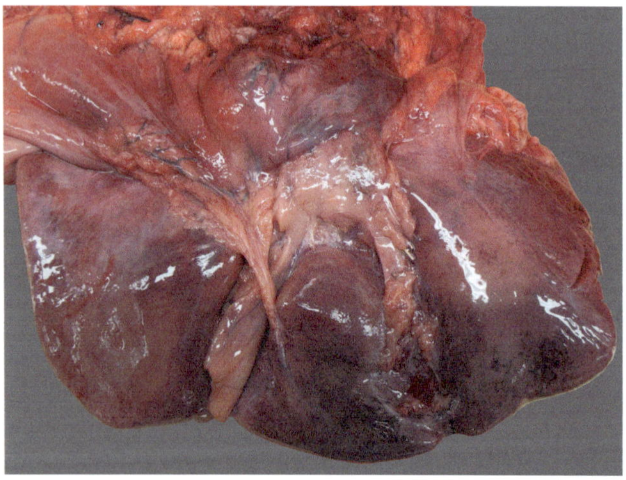

Fig. 5.114 This is the posterior aspect of a liver without a gallbladder following a laparoscopic cholecystectomy. The previous site of the gallbladder can be seen with some scarring

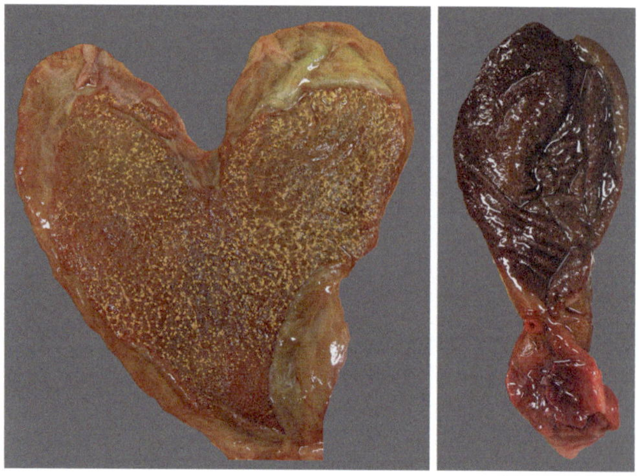

Fig. 5.115 Cholesterolosis of the gallbladder is characterized by small yellow foci of discoloration on the mucosal surface (left). These foci represent macrophages with abundant fat and are commonly seen in association with gallstones. The features are contrasted with the normal gallbladder seen (right)

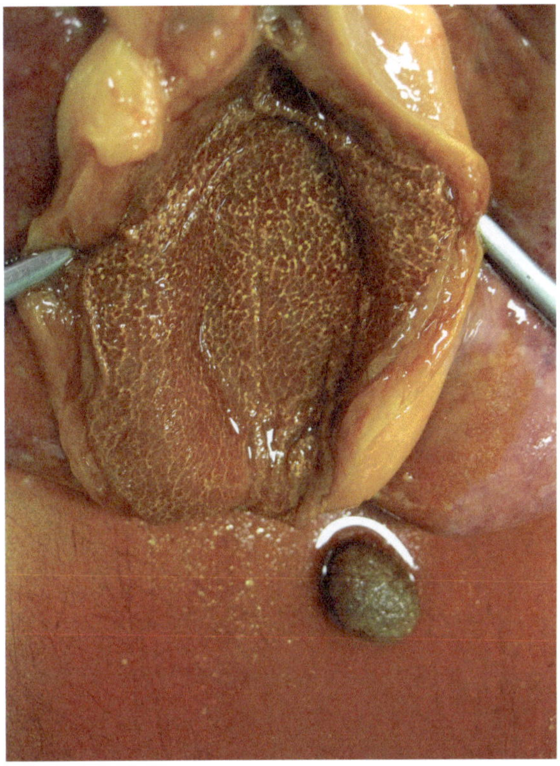

Fig. 5.116 This gallbladder has been opened to reveal a calculus and mucosal cholesterolosis. Note the yellow reticulate pattern of the mucosa, which is caused by cholesterol within macrophages in the tips of villi in the mucosa. The gallbladder wall is also thickened

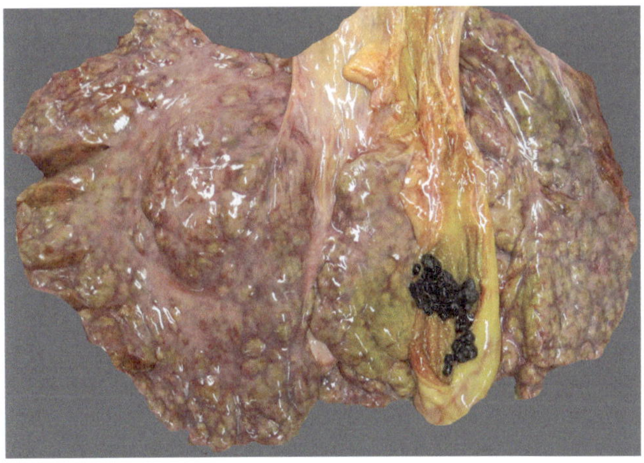

Fig. 5.117 A case of liver cirrhosis is seen in association with gallstones. The gallstones were incidental to the background liver disease, as is the case in many autopsy examinations

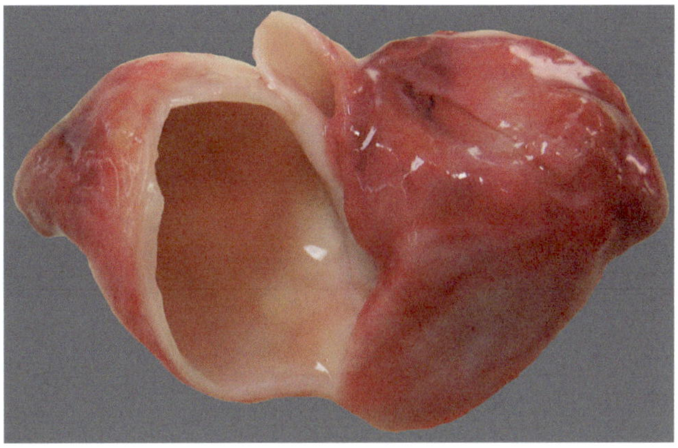

Fig. 5.118 Gallstones impacted at the neck of the gallbladder may cause chronic changes that end with a mucocele. The gallbladder content will be clear fluid

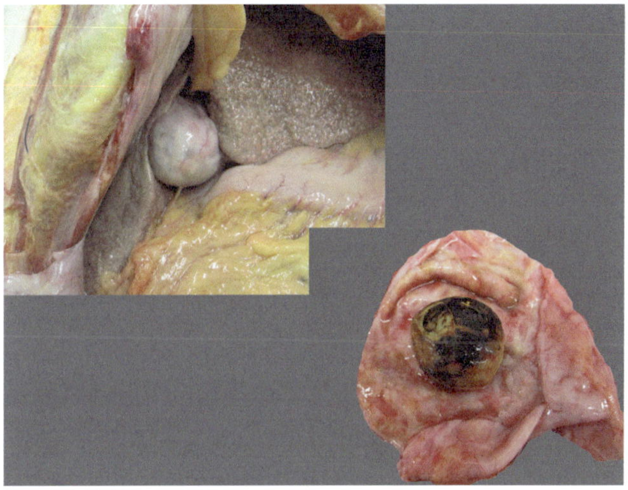

Fig. 5.119 The top left gallbladder is clearly visible at the point of opening the abdomen, with a single rounded stone filling the lumen. There is local fibrosis. The adjacent liver is noted to be finely granular and cirrhotic. These findings can represent either a hepatic inflammatory or degenerative condition or gallstone disease may have previously obstructed the bile ducts. The lower right image shows a rounded and pigmented stone is present in the gallbladder. Note the pale pink/beige mucosal surface in a case of chronic cholecystitis

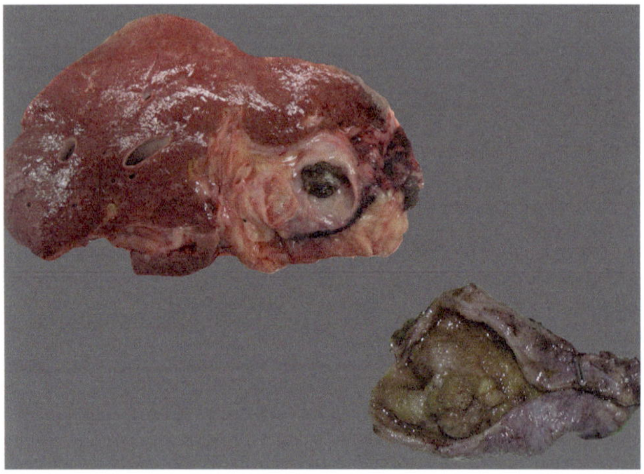

Fig. 5.120 Gallbladder carcinoma is often associated with gallstone disease. The autopsy may demonstrate widespread tumor infiltration of the liver, but on occasion (top left), the gallbladder will show simply more marked fibrosis and firmness around the gallbladder bed. The lower right image shows a surgical pathology (fixed) gallbladder with mucosal irregularities in a case of adenomatous disease transforming to carcinoma

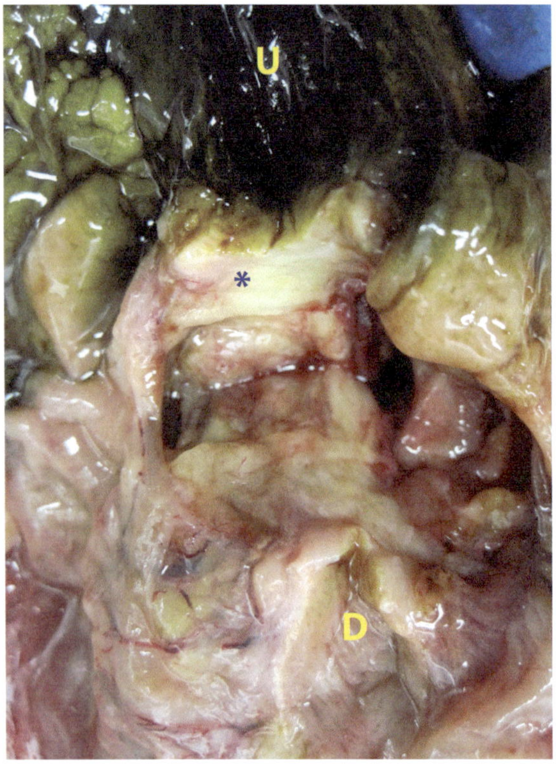

Fig. 5.121 This is a close-up view of the common bile duct. On section, there is a firm cream-colored tumor present (asterisk). On one side there is intense bile discoloration within the upstream dilated duct (U), with the duct carcinoma present blocking further flow of bile. The downstream duct (D) is smaller in transverse section and less bile stained

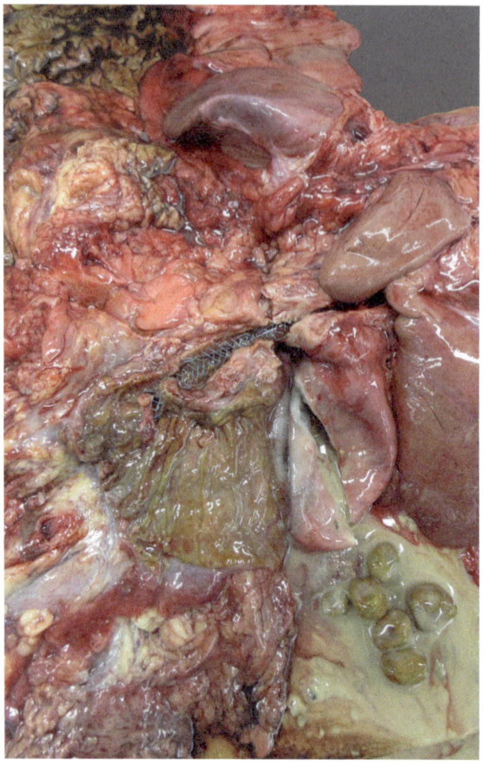

Fig. 5.122 Seen here is an extrahepatic cholangiocarcinoma requiring a stent within the common bile duct. There is purulent material seen spilling from the gallbladder that also contained multiple gallstones, indicating gallbladder empyema and biliary sepsis as complications of the tumour

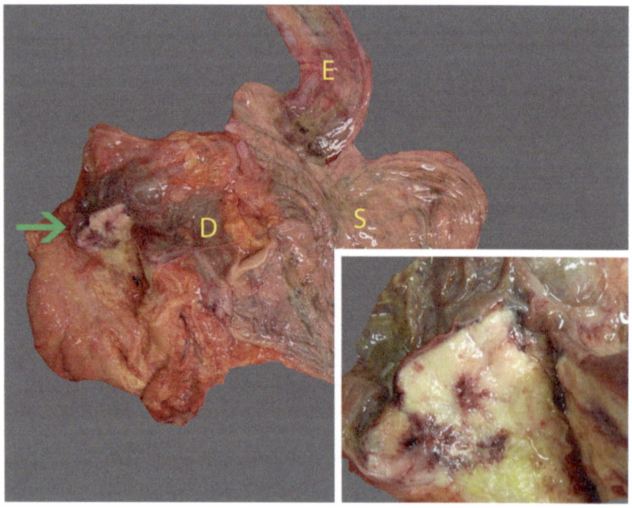

Fig. 5.123 This is a tumor at the end of the bile duct, seen in a patient suspected of having carcinoma of the bile duct, but with histology more in keeping with carcinoma of the pancreas. Such cases can be the source of disseminated neoplasia and one needs to dissect the tissue carefully to confirm that the pancreas is the source of the neoplasia. Here, a firm, cream-colored tumor (arrow) is present adjacent to the proximal duodenum (D). The stomach (S) and esophagus (E) are unremarkable. At higher magnification (inset), the tumor is lifting the duodenal mucosa upwards and extending into the adjacent soft tissues

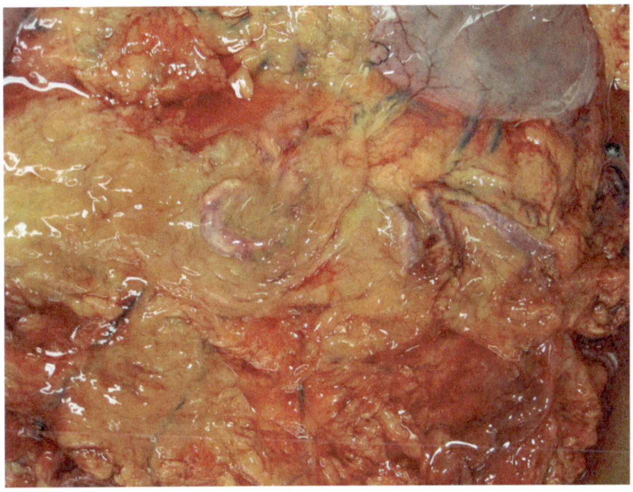

Fig. 5.124 Calcification of the splenic artery is common. It is rarely associated with pathology but is a marker for generalized arterial disease

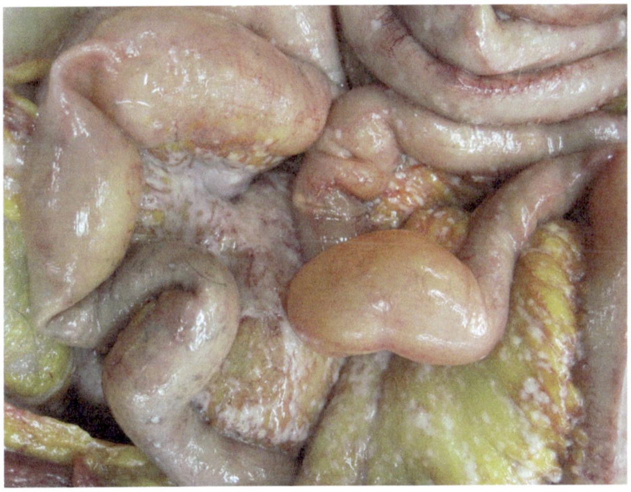

Fig. 5.125 Pronounced serosal surface contamination by disseminated tumor is seen in this case. It is not possible to identify such tumors simply on morphology, although peritoneal carcinoma should be suspected in women. Mesothelioma may be more commonly suspected in men with an appropriate occupational history

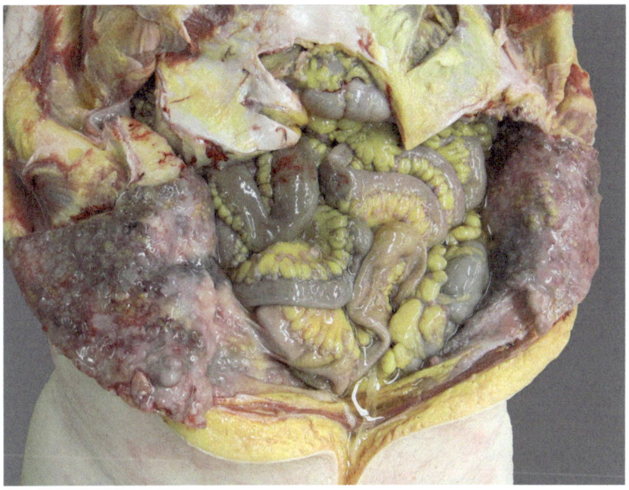

Fig. 5.126 A case of advanced diffuse peritoneal mesothelioma is seen with widespread infiltration of the abdominal wall and associated fluid collection

Acknowledgement The authors would like to acknowledge the significant contribution of Dr. Stuart Brown for provision of the images and text in this chapter from this book's first edition.

Suggested Reading

Bateman AC, Greenson JK, Lauwers GY, Loughrey MB, Novelli MR, Sheahan K, Shepherd NA, editors. Morson & Dawson's gastrointestinal pathology. 6th ed. Wiley-Blackwell Science; 2024 (Due 2024).

Burton JL, Rutty G. The hospital autopsy. 3rd ed. Hodder Arnold; 2010.

Connolly AJ, Finkbeiner WE, Ursell PC, Davis RL, editors. Autopsy pathology: a manual and atlas. 3rd ed. Philadelphia: Elsevier; 2016. p. 186–319.

Cooke RA, Stewart B. Alimentary system; pancreas, biliary system & liver, in color atlas of anatomical pathology. 3rd ed. Edinburgh: Churchill Livingstone; 2004. p. 59–130.

Curran RC, Jones EL. Alimentary tract; liver, gallbladder & pancreas. In: Gross pathology: a colour atlas. Harvey Millar HM + M Publishers; 1974. p. 27–46.

Gill RM, Kakar S, Maitra A. The gastrointestinal tract, liver and gallbladder, the pancreas. In: Kumar V, Abbas AK, Aster JC, editors. Robbins & Cotran pathologic basis of disease. 10th ed. Elsevier; 2021. p. 753–894.

Goldblum JR, Lamps LW, McKenney JK, Myers JL. Gastrointestinal and hepatobiliary tract. In: Rosai and Ackerman's surgical pathology. 11th ed. Edinburgh: Elsevier; 2018. p. 502–935.

Ludwig J. Autopsy practice. 3rd ed. Ottawa: Humana Press; 2002.

Srivastava A, Allende DS, editors. Gastrointestinal and liver pathology. Goldblum JR, series editor. Foundations in diagnostic pathology series. 3rd ed. Elsevier; 2023.

Genitourinary and Breast Tissues, Including Pregnancy

6

S. Kim Suvarna and Abigail K. Sharp

Introduction

This chapter deals with a variety of tissues which are both common and different between the sexes. The common elements include the kidneys, ureters and the bladder. These items are covered first, with gender-specific and pregnancy matters described later.

Genitourinary pathology is relatively commonplace in autopsy practice. Common themes include sepsis of the urinary tract (commonly called urosepsis), which can be acute as well as subacute/chronic. Chronic damage (from many causes) can have significant effects on the kidneys, in particular with secondary systemic effects. Common lesions to consider include scarring processes related to cortical damage and glomerular loss as can be seen in hypertension, diabetes and glomerulonephritis, among other conditions. Obstructive realities may also be pertinent to the cause of death in that renal outflow obstruction is a ready cause of renal decompensation and failure. These tissues are also involved by a variety of tumours, both primary and secondary. Metastatic disease is common to the kidney, although primary kidney cancers can be widely disseminated and may account for surprise findings at autopsy examination.

Pathology of the female genital tract principally reflects tumours, although sepsis is sometimes encountered in examinations. The female genital tissues to be covered include vulval and vaginal tissues. The uterine corpus and cervix will be considered with the tubes and ovaries.

The breast tissues are also discussed in this section, reflecting their role in pregnancy and reproduction. The breast tissues are rarely a significant factor in terms of the cause of death, aside from breast tumours with disseminated disease.

Specialist examination protocols and techniques are required for cases of maternal deaths which inevitably require a wide ranging investigative protocol.

The male genital tissues comprise the external genitalia (penis, scrotum and testes) and prostate. These are considered in turn. Aside from incidental findings of sexually transmitted disease, the male genital tract pathology at autopsy largely concerns tumours. These may be locally aggressive or disseminated at autopsy. Their impact will depend upon the secondary sites involved.

Kidney and Ureter

The kidneys exist as a pair of glands with an average weight of 100–150 g each. They are found in the retroperitoneal, paravertebral tissues. Looking at the Rokitansky block dissection they are often examined early in the autopsy protocol and may be removed intact with the ureter, bladder and associated pelvic tissues, or may be taken separately. Traditionally, if removed separately, the left side ureter is left longer than the right to allow identification of sidedness later in the examination.

The initial dissection and examples of kidney pathology are shown in Figs. 6.1, 6.2, 6.3, 6.4, 6.5, 6.6, 6.7, 6.8, 6.9, 6.10, 6.11, 6.12, 6.13, 6.14, 6.15, 6.16, 6.17, 6.18, 6.19, 6.20, 6.21, 6.22, 6.23, 6.24, 6.25, 6.26, 6.27, 6.28, 6.29, 6.30, 6.31, 6.32, 6.33, 6.34, 6.35, and 6.36. The kidney tissues can be involved by a variety of processes, falling into three principal groups. Firstly, degenerative and scarring processes are common kidney diseases in adult autopsy. The prime pathology of renal scarring is characterised by a roughening of the cortical tissues and thinning of the cortical parenchyma. Whilst there is some value in measuring the cortical thickness, the

S. Kim Suvarna was deceased at the time of publication.

S. K. Suvarna (Deceased) · A. K. Sharp (✉)
Department of Histopathology, Sheffield Teaching Hospitals NHS Foundation Trust, Sheffield, UK
e-mail: abigail.sharp@nhs.net

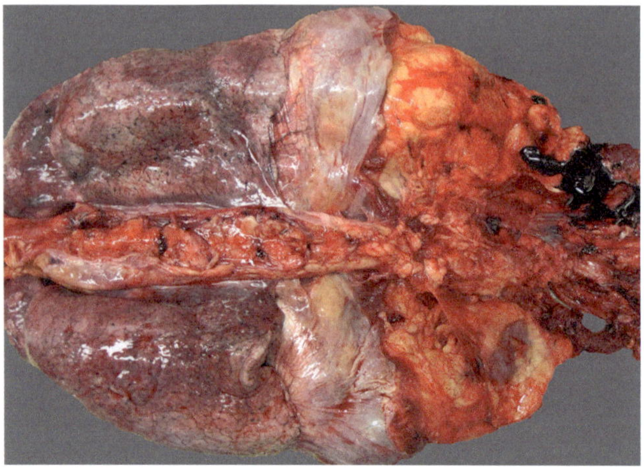

Fig. 6.1 The posterior aspect of the eviscerated tissue provides the start point for examination of the genitourinary system, focusing on the kidneys. The initial examination is complicated since the kidneys, the ureters and other tissues are often partially encased within fatty parenchyma. This must be sequentially and carefully incised to examine the tissues

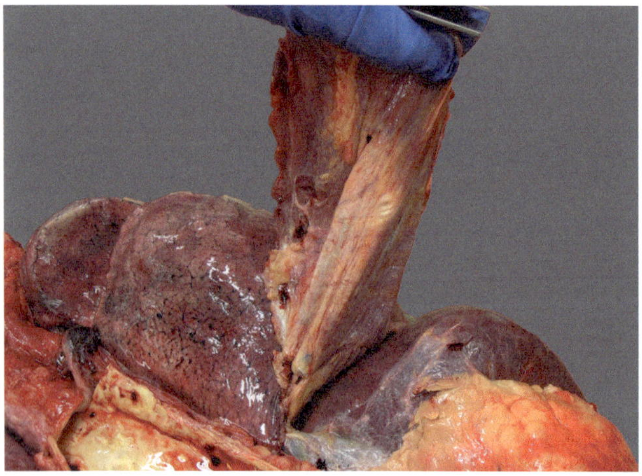

Fig. 6.2 The diaphragm tissues are removed, folding this muscular parenchyma up and away from the liver and upper abdominal tissues on both sides

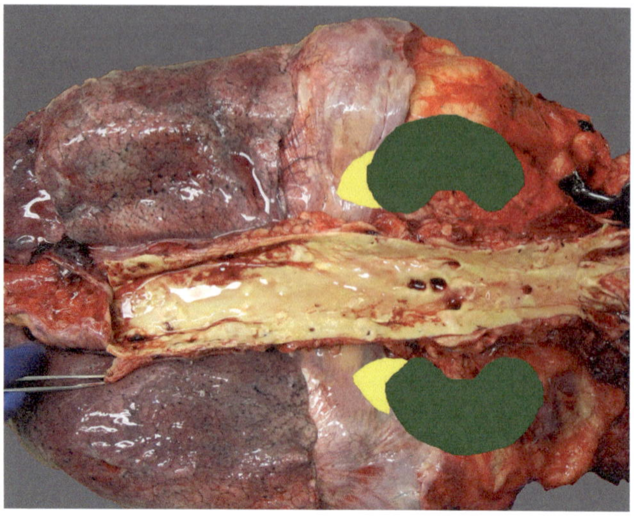

Fig. 6.3 When faced with an organ block with a fatty retroperitoneum it pays to be thinking about the likely position of the kidneys. These are marked on the overlay map in green, with the adrenals also marked in yellow

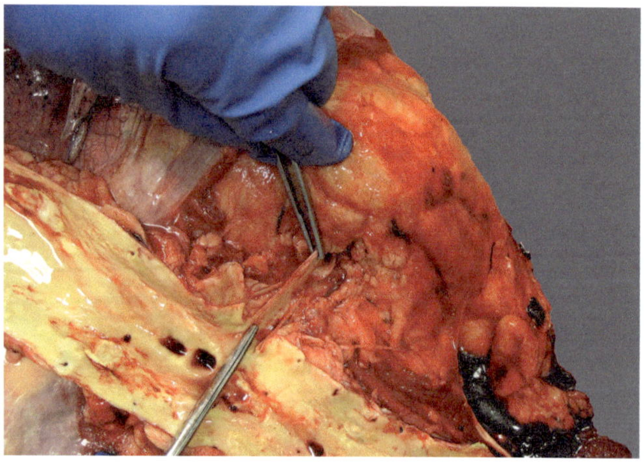

Fig. 6.4 To assist with identifying the kidneys, one can trace the renal artery on both sides, as it will point towards the kidney. Here the aortic tissue has been opened and residual blood content removed. The renal arteries should be explored on both sides to check for stenosis as part of the general autopsy. If one frees and folds the aorta down towards the pelvic tissues, then the same can be performed for the renal veins

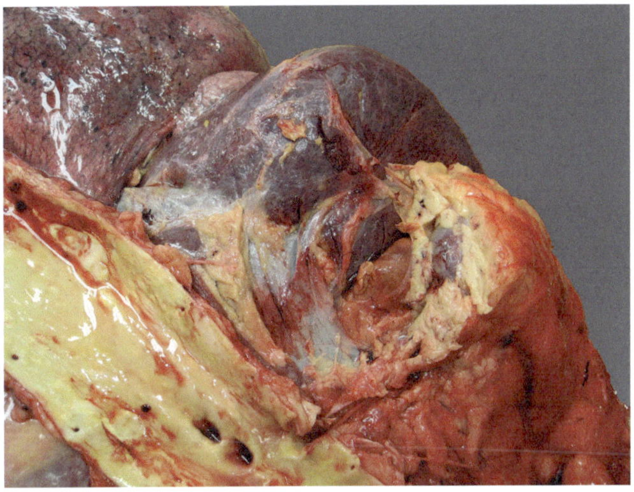

Fig. 6.5 This view of the upper retroperitoneal tissues has had the fatty tissue and adrenal parenchyma removed. The top part of the kidney is now open for inspection, but the remainder of the kidney is still hidden from view, encased within the perinephric fat and fascia

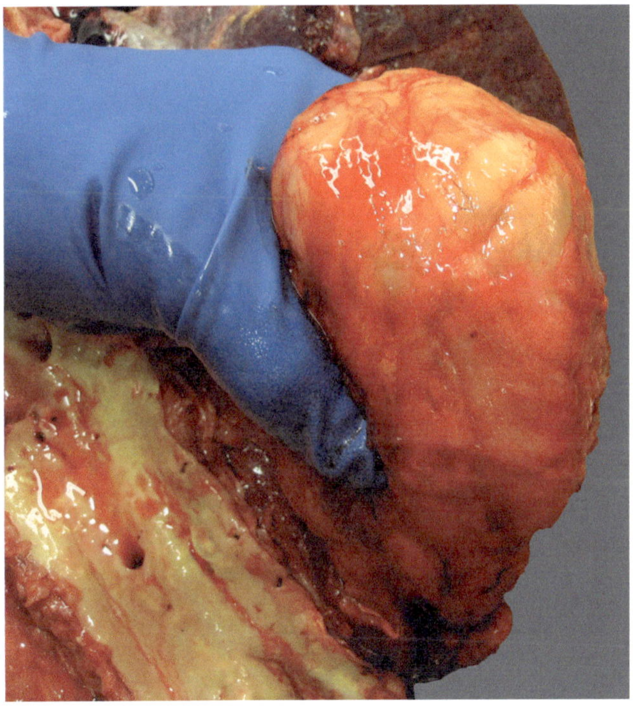

Fig. 6.6 Grasping the soft tissue and fat around the kidney one holds the outer aspect (anti-hilar) upwards, perpendicular to the cutting board or bench surface

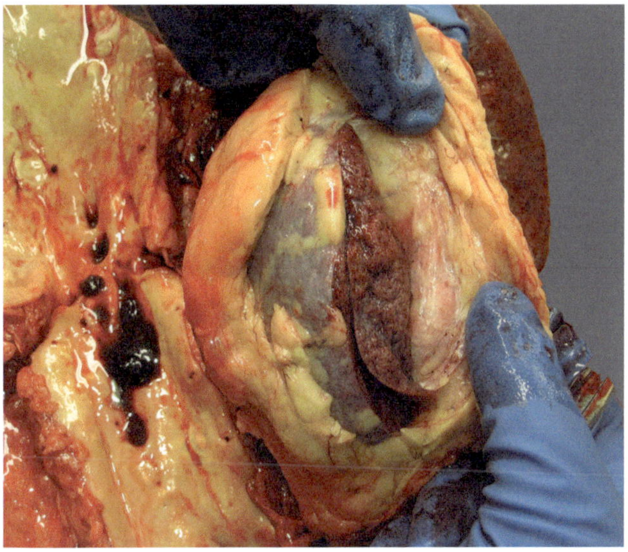

Fig. 6.7 A knife (PM40 type) has been used to incise a few millimeters into the kidney from the anti-hilar aspect. The kidney fat and capsule have been pulled from the surface of the kidney by grasping the capsule with toothed forceps to facilitate examination of the kidney and its removal. Here, the surface of the kidney is noted to be granular and pitted, in keeping with chronic kidney disease and hypertension. It does not matter at this stage whether the cut has gone deeper into the kidney, as this cut will be extended more deeply later

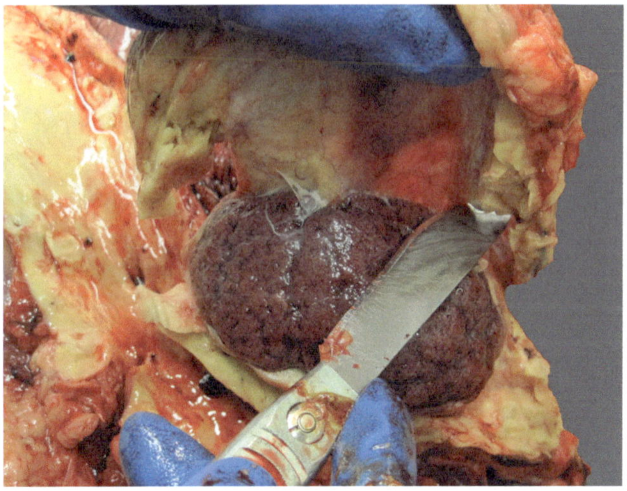

Fig. 6.8 The kidney is now laid flat. Holding the perinephric fatty tissue up at 90° away from the kidney surface/hilar blood vessels, ureter and soft tissue interface, one may now resect the plate of fat and capsule, being confident that no kidney damage will occur. This will simplify examination of the tissues and subsequent dissection

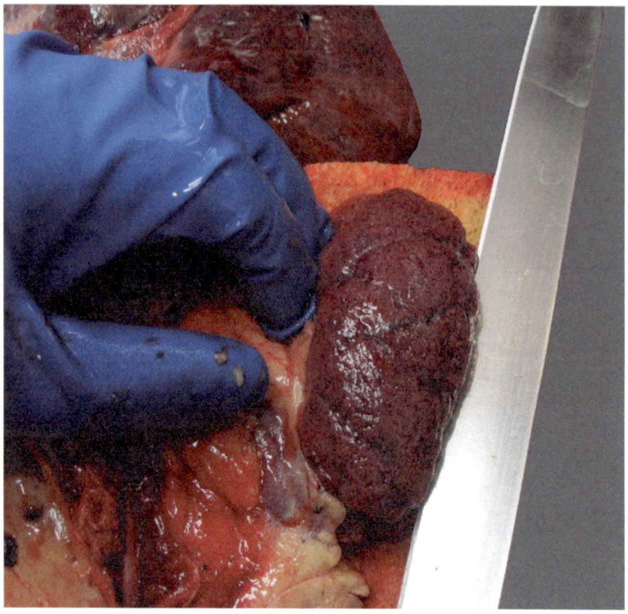

Fig. 6.9 Once the kidney has been dissected free of the fat, fascia and capsule, the entire cortical external surface can be seen. The granularity and scarring are noted here. The next step is to lay the kidney on a sponge or other support and to extend the initial cut made into the outer cortical plane. A long knife slices towards (but not through) the hilum, thereby opening into the pelvis. The cut surface of the renal medulla parenchyma and the cortex will be easily seen

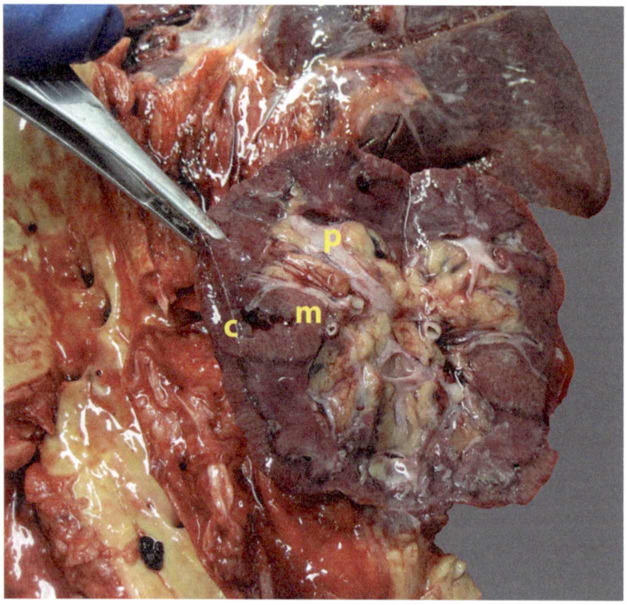

Fig. 6.10 The cortex (c), medulla (m) and renal pelvis (p) are now displayed. Note the tissues are still attached to the vasculature and ureter. The cortex and medulla are well demarcated from one another

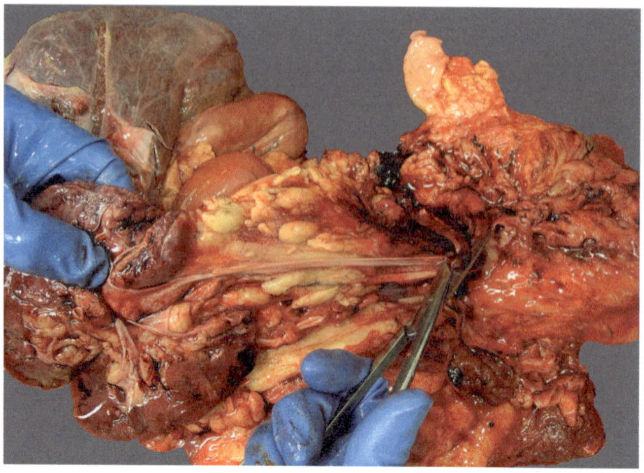

Fig. 6.11 By passing one blade of the scissors into the renal pelvis one can dissect steadily down along the ureter towards the bladder. This dissection should not be rushed to avoid tearing the ureter. This procedure keeps the ureter, kidney and vascular tissues still in one piece

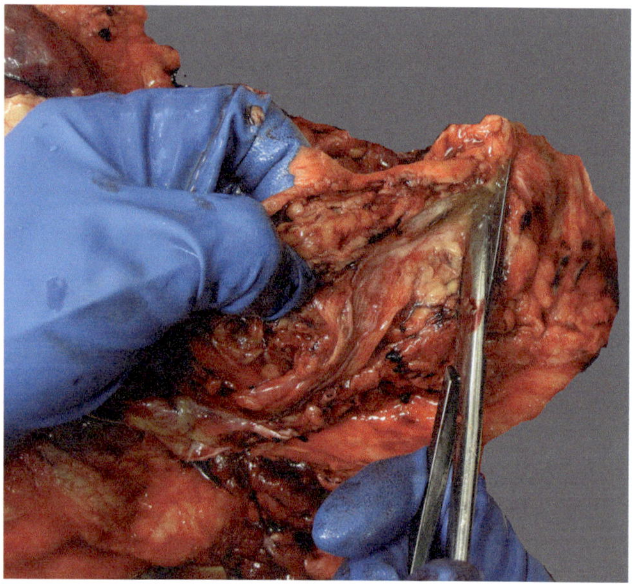

Fig. 6.12 There is a small gain to be made by rotating the pelvic tissues one quarter turn towards the contralateral side, which keeps the ureter and bladder alignment in a straight line. Any cut through the ureter/bladder interface will be made easier. The blade of the scissors can now be passed into the bladder with the ureter orifice being available for study

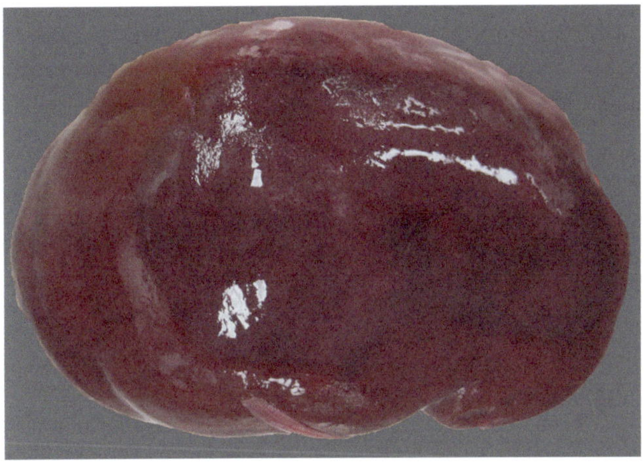

Fig. 6.13 The normal kidney has a smooth cortical surface

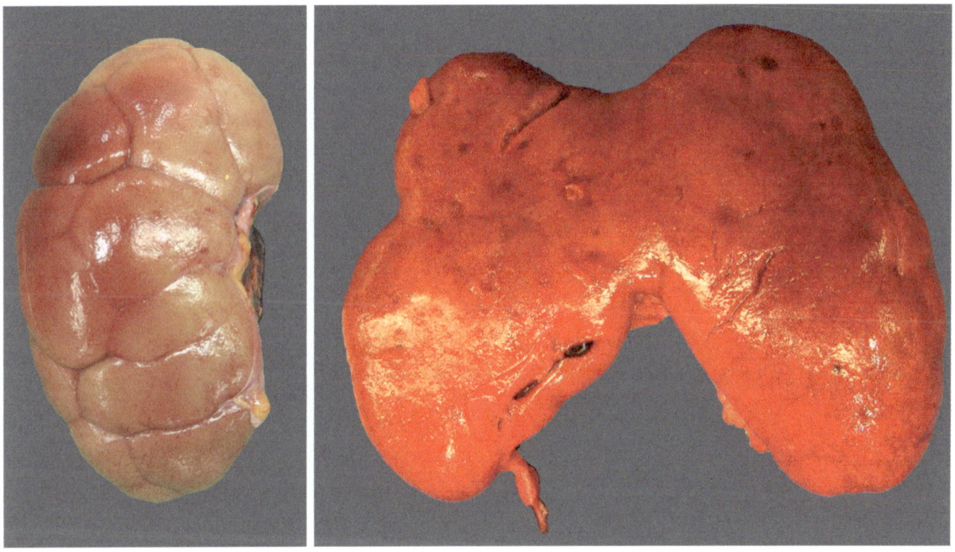

Fig. 6.14 Left side: On occasion, there is some lobulation evident, akin to that of fetal development. This is of no consequence and the cortical surface should be smooth and shiny, as in the normal kidney. Right side: A congenital variation with normal renal function is the 'horseshoe' kidney, where central/midline fusion of renal elements occurs and a single kidney is formed in utero

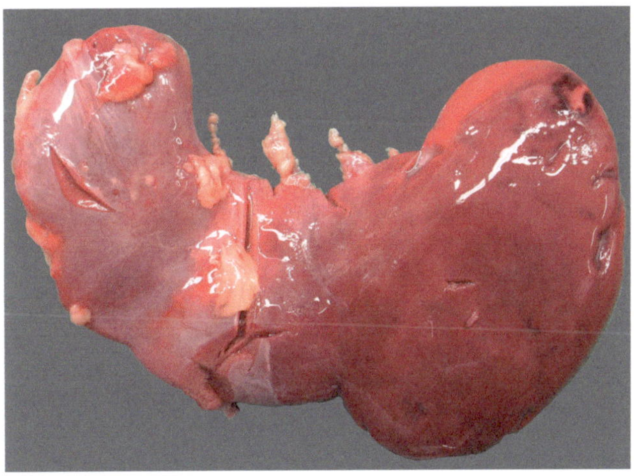

Fig. 6.15 This example of a horseshoe kidney is complicated by a small focal infarction (top right of the picture)

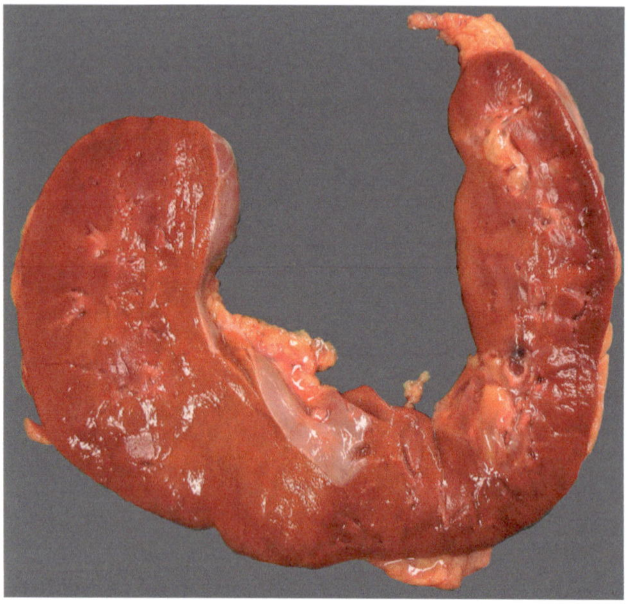

Fig. 6.16 This is another example of a horseshoe kidney, following sectioning. The typical cortical and medullary tissues of the cut surface are seen. These variant kidneys are usually asymptomatic, however, complications with stones, infection or obstruction can occur. Anatomically, they may reside lower in the abdomen, increasing the risk of injury from blunt force abdominal trauma

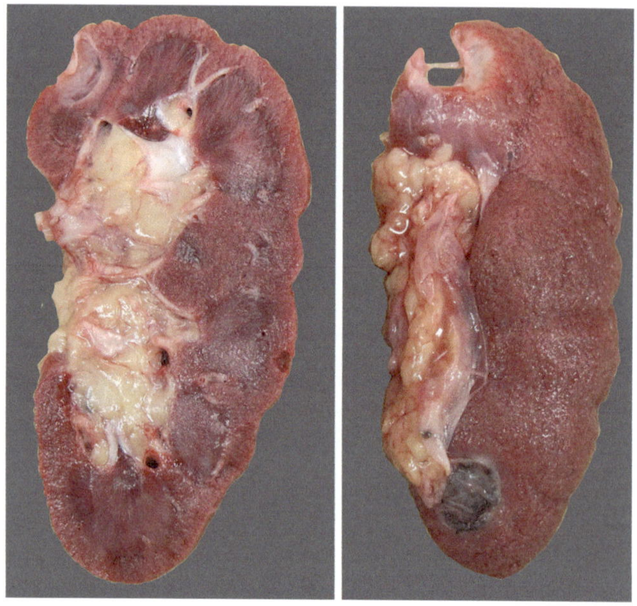

Fig. 6.18 Many kidneys seen at autopsy show granular surfaces and some reduction in the cortex thickness. As a general rule, the cortex and medullary parenchyma should be roughly equal in terms of thickness. Diminished cortical thickness and granularity may indicate a background of hypertension, although diabetes and glomerulopathies may also be pertinent. An incidental cyst is noted here

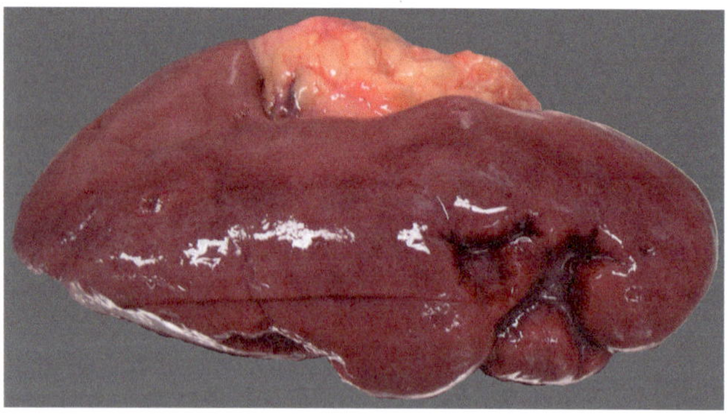

Fig. 6.17 This kidney, dissected free from the vasculature and ureter, has a partly normal surface. However, there is a focus of depressed scarring and distortion, in keeping with previous pyelonephritis or ascending infection. Note, there is a thin cut evident on the outer cortical plane which is in keeping with the dissection described above

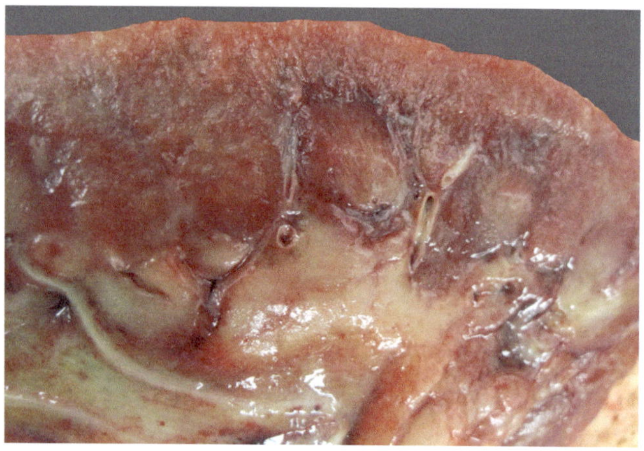

Fig. 6.19 The renal parenchyma shows the medullary tissues to be slightly thicker than that of the cortex. There is a moderate amount of fat in the peri-pelvic compartment. The renal pelvis is seen in part, with some congestion of the surface tissues. The corticomedullary junction in this case is somewhat blurred, mapping to a period of hypoxic injury in this patient, who was treated on the intensive care unit

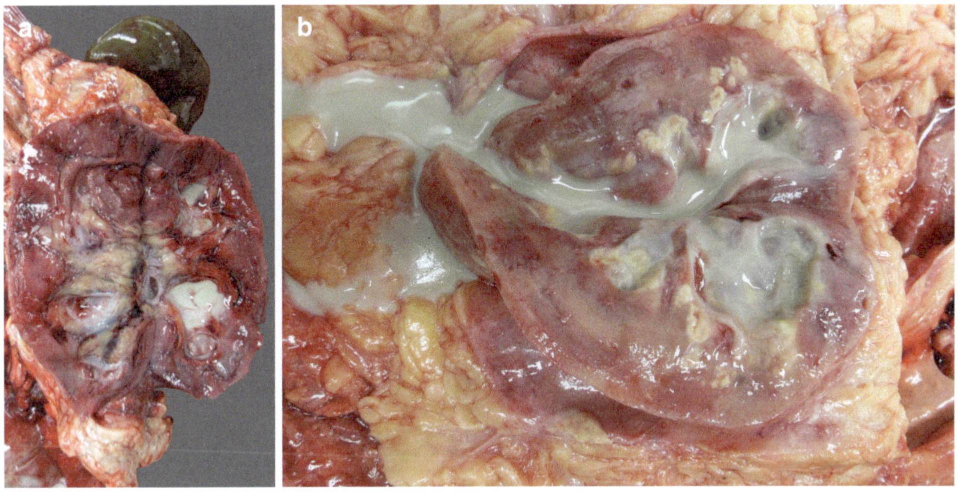

Fig. 6.20 The kidneys can become involved by infection via various routes, including ascending infection from the lower urinary tract and impaction of renal stones. In severe cases, pus builds up in the pelvicalyceal system, causing pyelonephritis. (**a**, **b**) This is demonstrated in the examples shown here. Image (**b**) is further complicated by granulomatous inflammation, diagnosed microscopically and found to be due to mycobacterial infection

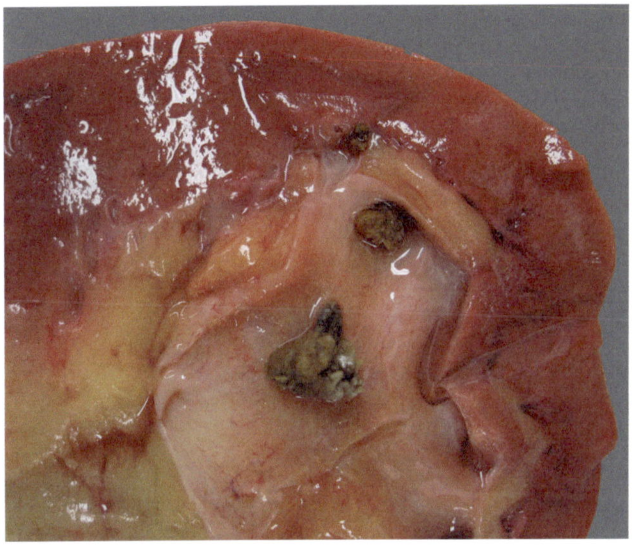

Fig. 6.21 Renal stones are often found as incidental findings at autopsy. This somewhat fragmentary stone was present in the pelvis and calyx. It broke during dissection. Stones can be associated with sepsis, obstruction, inflammation and ulceration, as well as neoplasia. However, in many cases they cause no significant abnormality and are incidental findings at autopsy

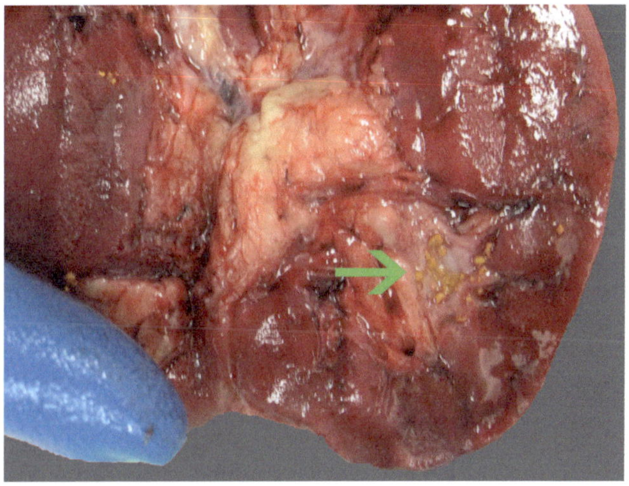

Fig. 6.22 Small kidney stones can be seen in the renal pelvic tissues (small, yellow, gravel-like material, *arrow*). This type of stone is prone to pass into the ureter and cause obstruction. When they are found in the renal pelvis, careful inspection of the ureters is recommended

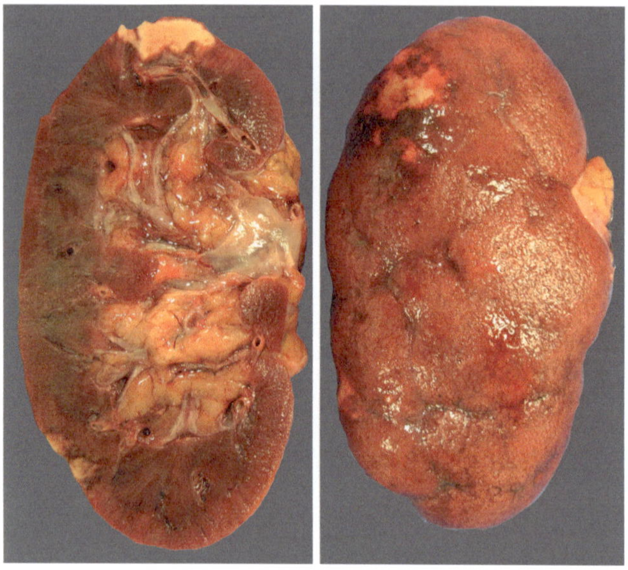

Fig. 6.23 Systemic embolic disease from the cardiac valves can embolise into the kidney. This will produce peripheral, cortical, wedge-shaped infarcts in the kidney parenchyma. Several are seen in this opened kidney, with lesions extending deeper into the renal parenchyma. Histology is recommended to investigate for tumour or septic emboli

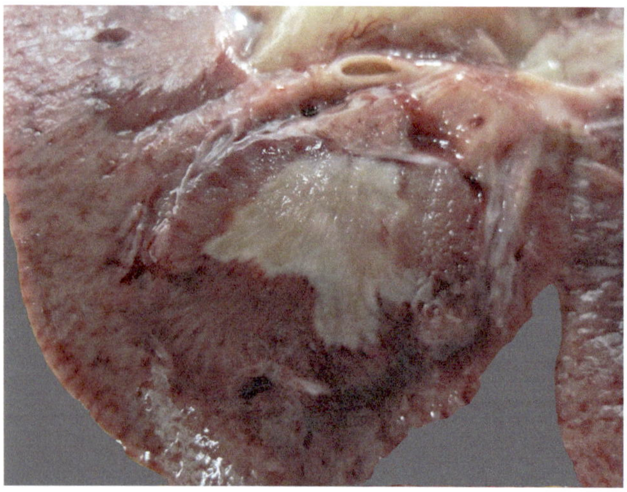

Fig. 6.24 Renal papillary necrosis can commonly be seen in patients with diabetes. The necrotic tissue often has a slight hyperaemic boundary with the normal parenchyma. One should always consider local sepsis as a compounding factor, particularly in those with diabetes

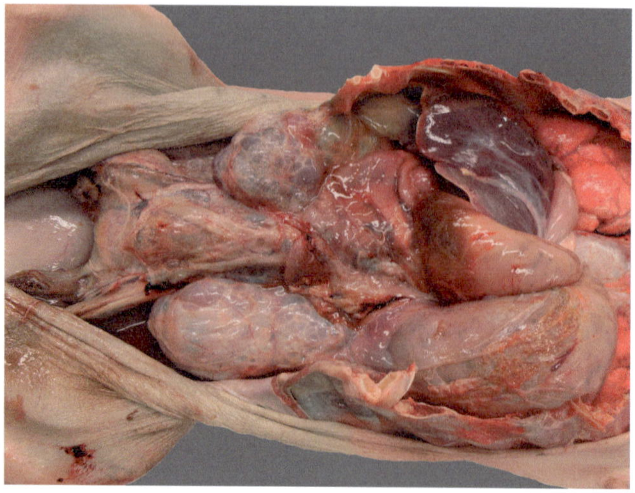

Fig. 6.25 Cystic change is common in adult kidneys seen at autopsy, usually as single, simple cysts (e.g. Fig. 6.18), with no sinister potential. Adult polycystic kidney disease (APCKD) is a hereditary non-neoplastic degenerative process, that is sometimes responsible for kidneys weighing 1.5 kg. Such kidneys can be seen here in situ, prior to removal

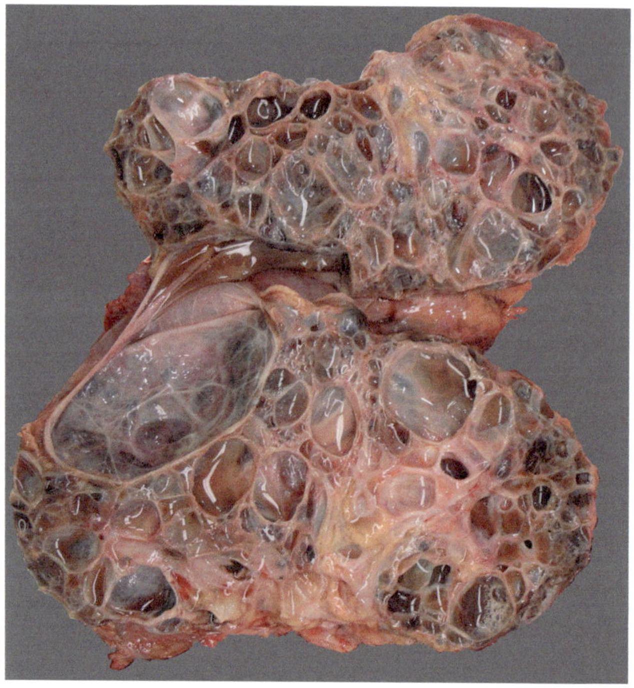

Fig. 6.26 Kidneys in APCKD show multiple cysts when opened. The main problem in APCKD is hypertensive disease and its consequences, alongside the realities of renal failure

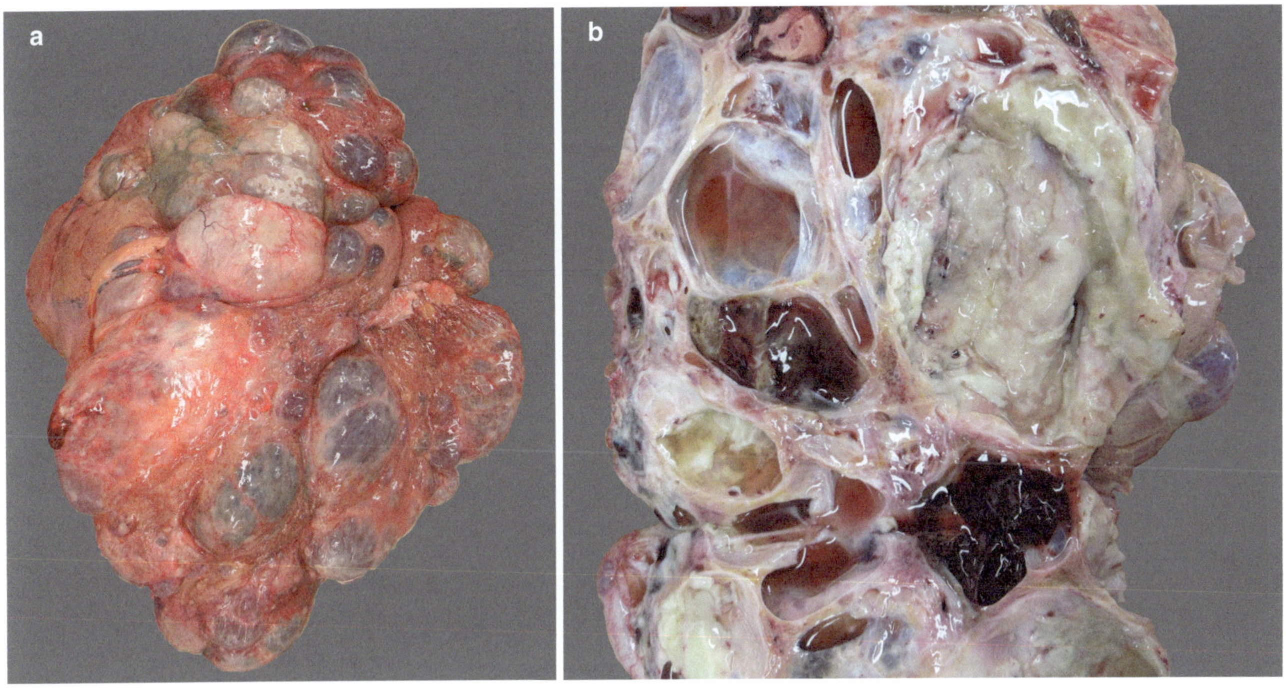

Fig. 6.27 The cysts in APCKD may enlarge with progression into adult life, with a risk of haemorrhage and/or sepsis. (**a**, **b**) These images show another example of APCKD, with complication in the form of pyonephrosis in some of the enlarged cysts on the cut section (**b**)

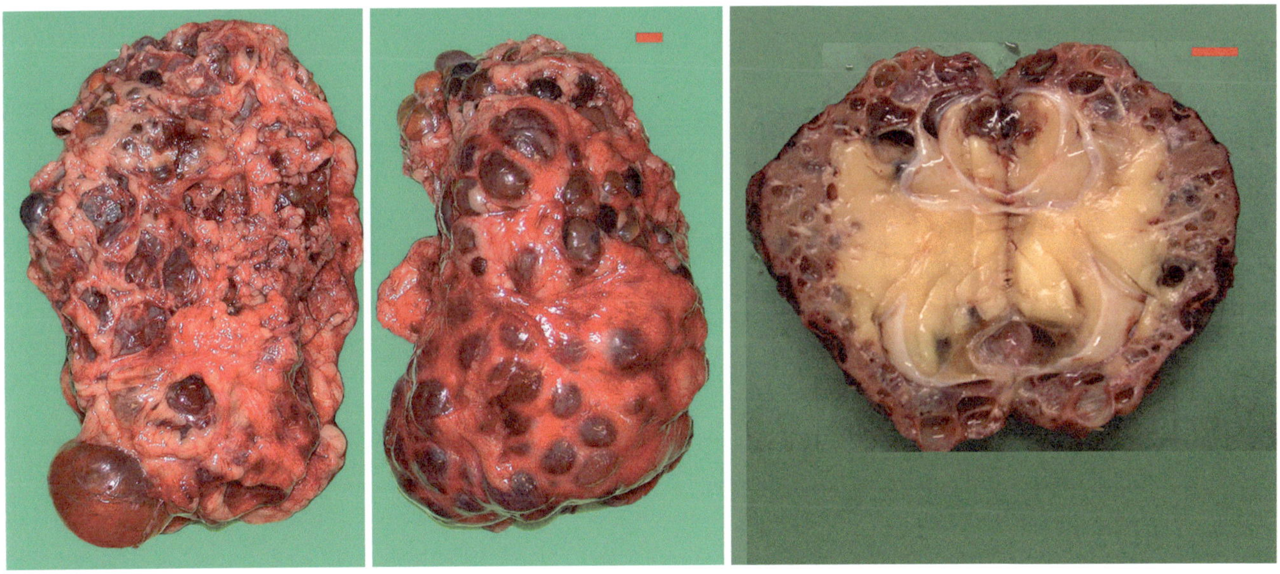

Fig. 6.28 A further example of APCKD is seen on the left. By contrast, acquired polycystic kidney disease (right image) often follows renal failure and dialysis. This is associated with a risk of renal cell carcinoma. Bar marker = 10 mm

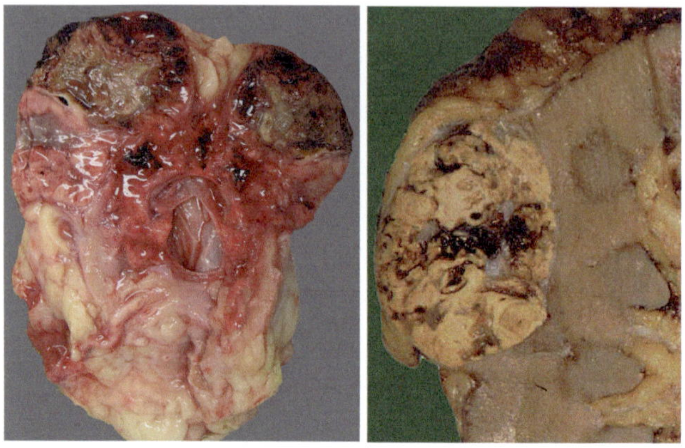

Fig. 6.29 Primary kidney cancer is not uncommon at autopsy. The commonest type, renal cell carcinoma, may present as an incidental mass, or as advanced and disseminated disease. The classic format (in the fixed sample, right side image) shows a yellow cut surface. Often at autopsy (left side), these tumours appear haemorrhagic and partly necrotic

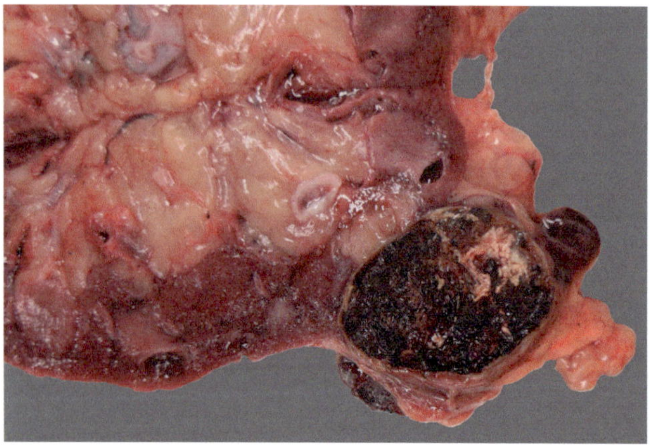

Fig. 6.30 Another example of renal cell carcinoma is shown here, with a haemorrhagic surface

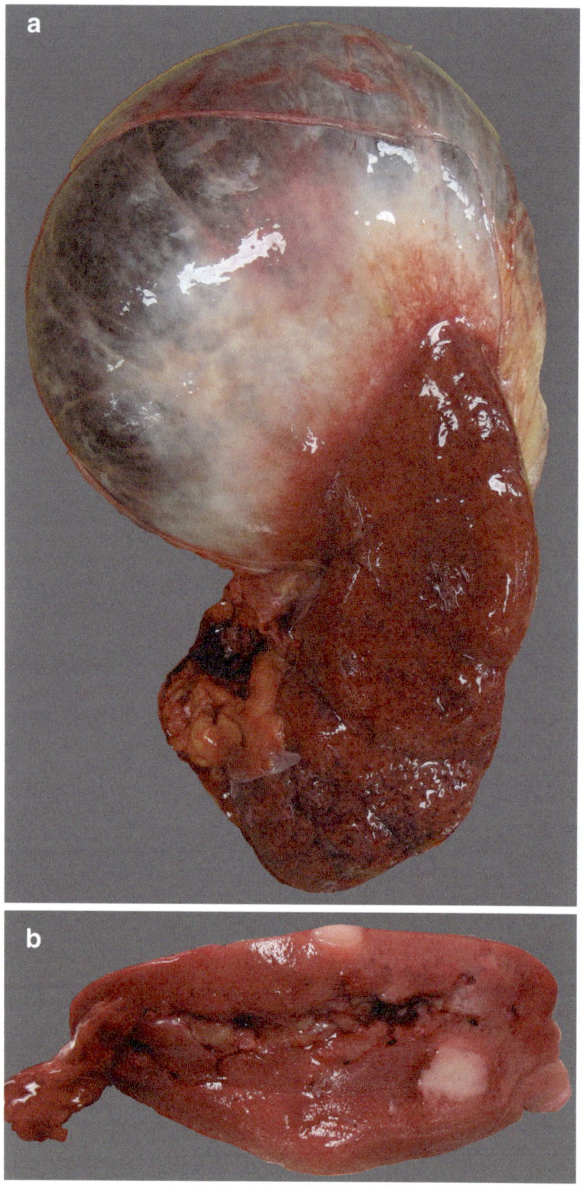

Fig. 6.31 Renal cell carcinoma can present as a cystic lesion, seen here in image (**a**). The turbid and haemorrhagic content and minor yellow/brown lining was the clue that this was a carcinoma, which was confirmed by histology. By contrast, image (**b**) is a kidney with multifocal metastatic tumours from primary lung cancer

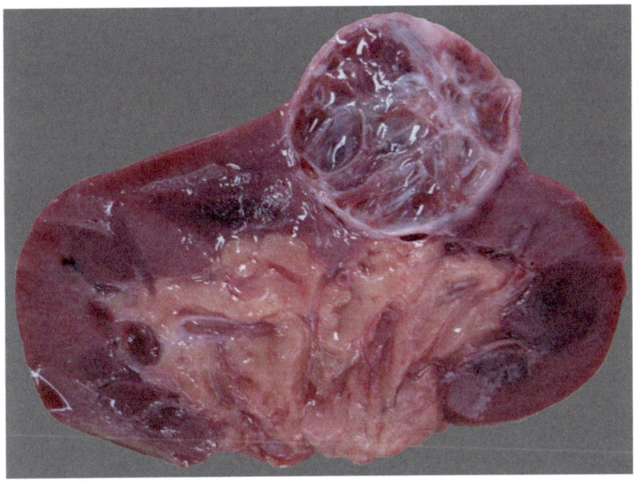

Fig. 6.32 Another example of a cystic renal cell carcinoma is shown here, in this case without the typical yellow/brown areas. Histology was required to diagnose this as a renal cell carcinoma

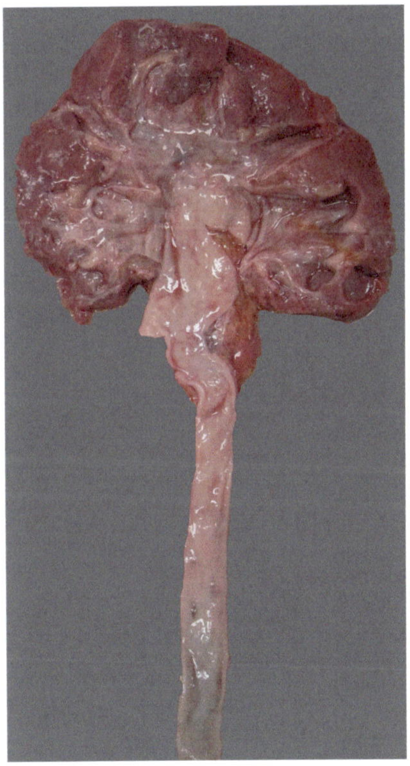

Fig. 6.33 Ureteric obstruction is seen with a dilated ureter and dilated pelvicalyceal system. The source of the obstruction should be considered with extension of the dissection into the lower ureteric parenchyma and down to bladder

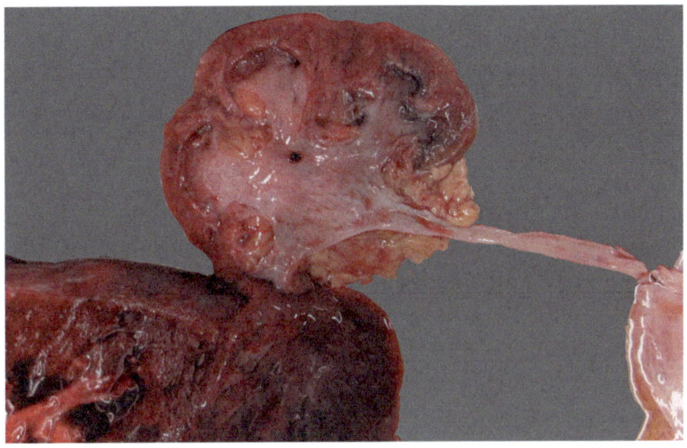

Fig. 6.34 A further example of pelvicalyceal dilation due to obstruction is shown here

cortex will vary according to the body-frame of the individual. Crudely, the cortical thickness should be the same as the thickness of the medulla (on average). Thinning of the cortex in relation to the medullary tissues is a marker for fibrosing processes and cortical tissue loss. Common pathologies underlying this process include hypertension, glomerulopathies (particularly immune complex glomerulonephritis), diabetes and various tubular injuries (caused by infections, drugs etc.). These processes often do not provide the prime cause of death but are commonly contributory factors. Indeed, this pattern of renal disease is often associated with hypertension which may be the driving force behind the cause of death.

The next group of disorders to characteristically affect the kidney is infection. Acute infections, whether blood derived or (more commonly) ascending in type (i.e. along the ureter and pelvis) can rapidly debilitate an individual and potentially cause death. This is particularly problematic for the elderly. Urinary samples should be considered if one suspects an unusual septic process. It should be remembered that tuberculosis can also affect the kidneys and consequently some caution is required when examining these tissues. Acute-on-chronic sepsis, or previous sepsis, can produce significant renal scarring and loss of function and may be a driver for renal impairment (chronic kidney disease).

Finally, renal tumours are not uncommon in autopsy practice. Primary renal cancers are mainly those of renal cell carcinoma (often an incidental or unexpected finding). Other tumours include transitional cell carcinomas of the pelvis and metastatic cancer, which is often seen in cases of disseminated carcinomatosis.

Obstructions of the upper urinary tract occur, with consequent ureteric and pelvic dilatation. If this is present, the source of obstruction should be sought, with features of hydronephrosis visible at initial examination. In such cases, it is important to dissect down the ureteric pathway towards the bladder prior to removing the kidney. Obstructions can

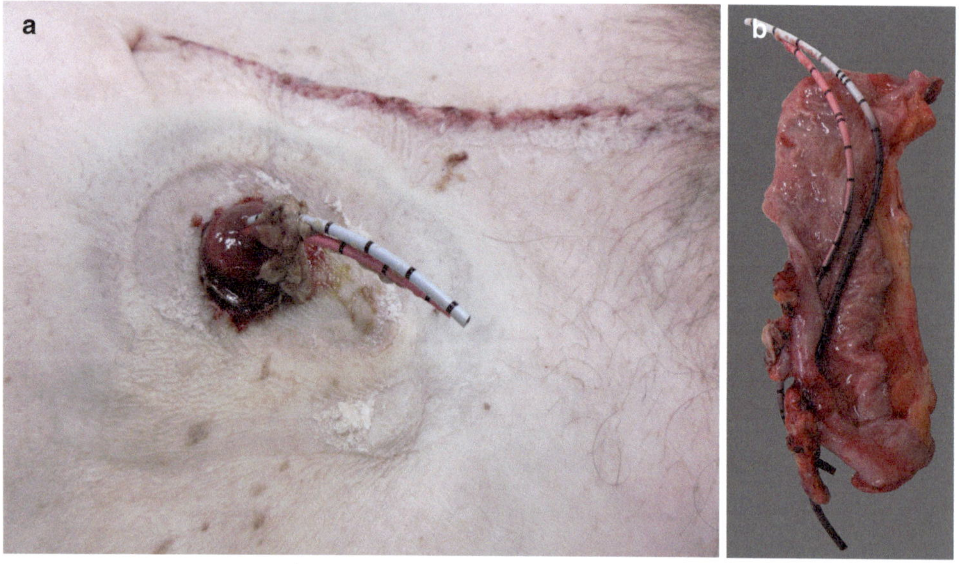

Fig. 6.35 Treatment for urinary obstruction below the kidney includes diversion of the urine flow away from the ureters, which can be temporary or permanent, depending on the clinical circumstances. Shown here is an example of a urostomy via an ileal conduit in a cystoprostatectomy case. Seen is the external appearance (**a**) and the tissues following removal (**b**) showing the small bowel reservoir created surgically. An example of a nephrostomy is included in Chap. 11

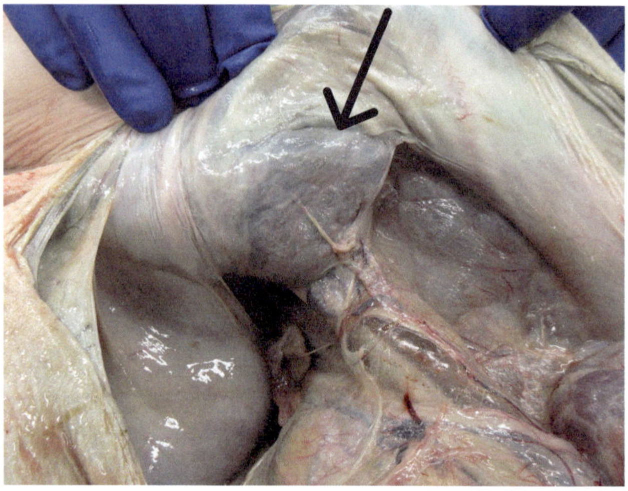

Fig. 6.36 In cases of renal transplantation, the transplanted kidney is commonly found on the anterior abdominal wall, as shown here and indicated with an arrow. Due diligence should be given to examine the transplanted kidney as well as the native kidneys, if they remain in situ

be wall-based in quality in terms of the junction of the pelvis and the ureter as well as at the ureter/bladder interface. Stones and tumours can also cause obstructive pathologies. There is often sepsis associated with obstructive conditions.

Bladder

The bladder (Figs. 6.37, 6.38, 6.39, 6.40, 6.41, 6.42, 6.43, 6.44, 6.45, 6.46, 6.47, 6.48, and 6.49) is of particular interest in autopsy practice, as a source of urine for toxicology testing. However, the bladder should always be inspected internally to assess for inflammation, infections and neoplasia. Urinary sepsis, in the form of cystitis, is not uncommon in adults, particularly in the setting of urinary catheterisation.

Post-mortem shedding of the urothelial surface occurs soon after death and one should remember that some turbidity of urinary content does not automatically imply sepsis. Sampling of urine for cytological assay and for infective agents may be relevant, but bacterial overgrowth in the post-mortem setting can create difficulty.

Bladder neoplasms are principally transitional cell carcinoma in nature and may be associated with features of urinary stasis and/or calculus disease. In these cases, careful examination of the pelvic soft tissues should be undertaken, looking for involved lymph nodes. Metastatic tumour from the bladder often also involves bony and lung tissues.

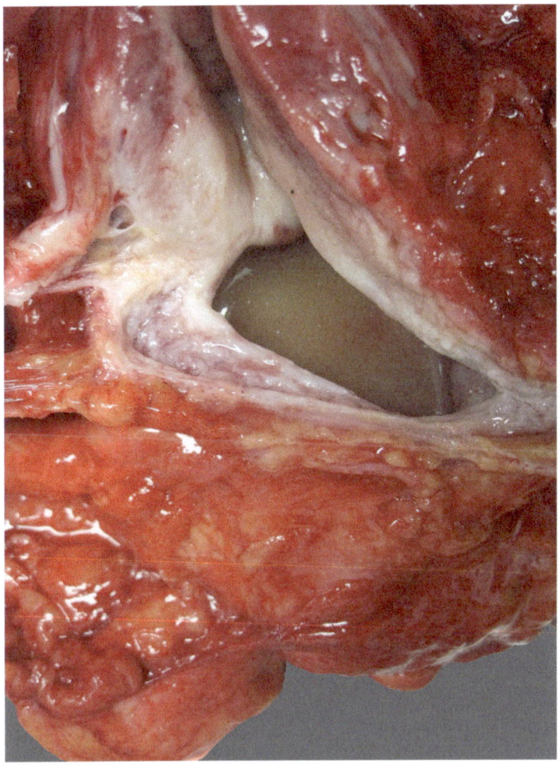

Fig. 6.37 As one examines the pelvic tissues, the bladder is often opened either from the roof or from the vesicoureteric junction. The urine may appear turbid at autopsy, but this appearance is likely to reflect sloughing of tissues from the urothelial surface mixing with the clear urine content

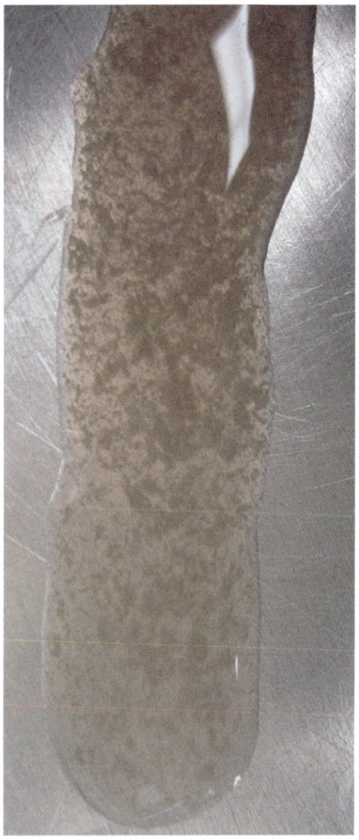

Fig. 6.38 Urine from the bladder often contains sloughed epithelial cells, as is evident in this sample spread onto a stainless steel surface. This material, whilst opaque in the bladder, should not be regarded as urinary sepsis, unless there are other supportive factors. It should be remembered that culture of urine at post-mortem examination is often a less than ideal exercise, as post-mortem colonisation is common

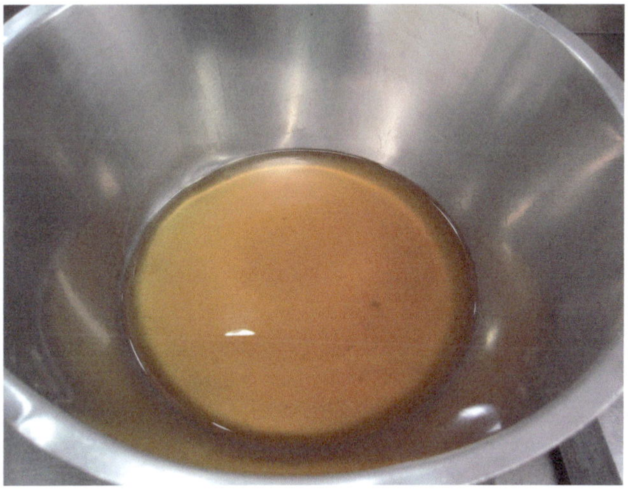

Fig. 6.39 Urine is generally clear at autopsy particularly in the recently deceased. Some urine should ideally be retained in cases of suspicious deaths or in those with likely drug abuse. The amount of sample required may be quite large, for example when considering steroids. One should contact the toxicology department to check the volume of urine required when seeking testing for unusual drugs

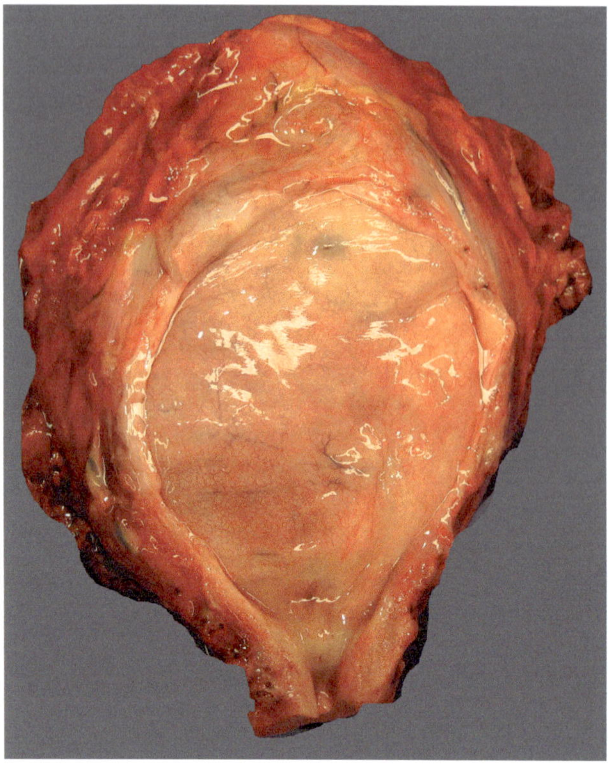

Fig. 6.40 The normal bladder has a smooth beige surface with only very mild vascular marking. The bladder wall should be soft and pliable

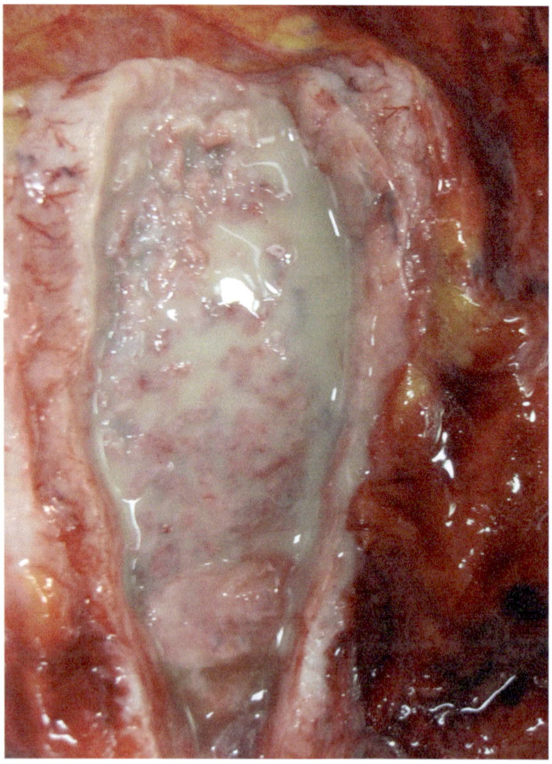

Fig. 6.41 This bladder shows a somewhat congested and discoloured surface. The light green and opaque material on the surface suggests active infection. However, one must be aware of post-mortem overgrowth as a potentially complicating factor when considering microbiology sampling

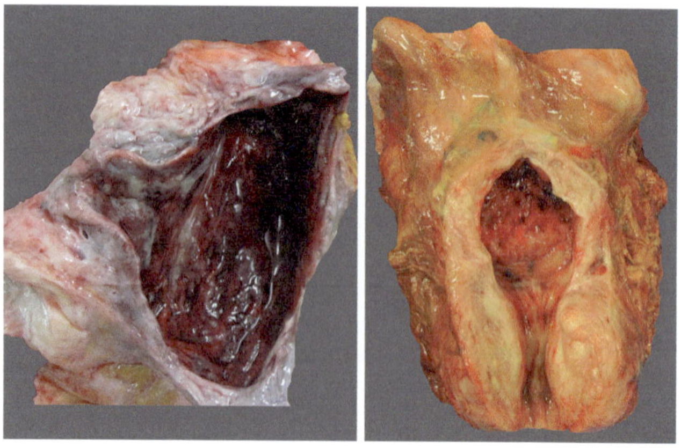

Fig. 6.42 Two views of inflamed bladders are seen. On the left, is an example of frank bladder sepsis with an inflamed surface lining and grey/green purulent material. Variable ulceration of the bladder lining may be present and the bladder itself appears intensely haemorrhagic/congested. On the right side, the bladder of a patient with a chronic catheter showed cystitis affecting the entirety of the internal surface with associated mural thickening and fibrosis. In such circumstances, sampling of the bladder wall for histology may be required to exclude dysplasia and neoplasia

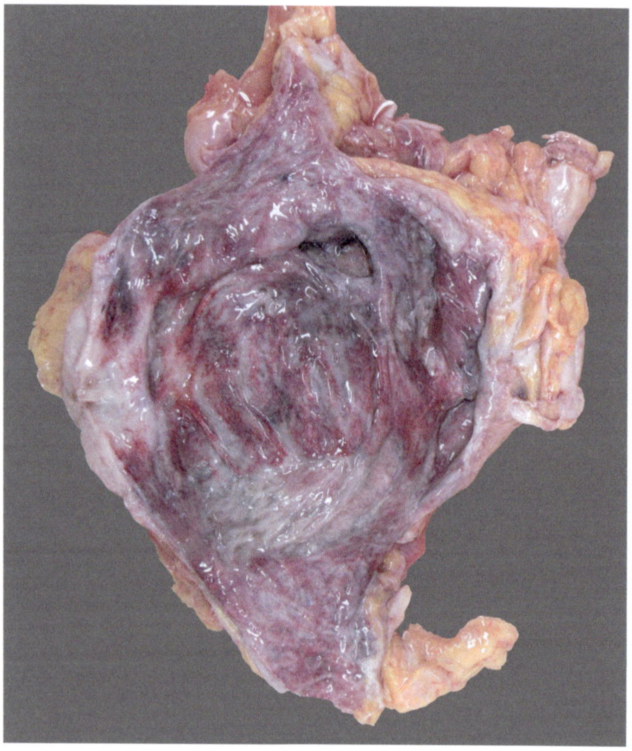

Fig. 6.43 Bladder diverticula can be seen here, with an associated haemorrhagic/congested lining. The green/grey material is, again, suggestive of an infectious process in this case of cystitis

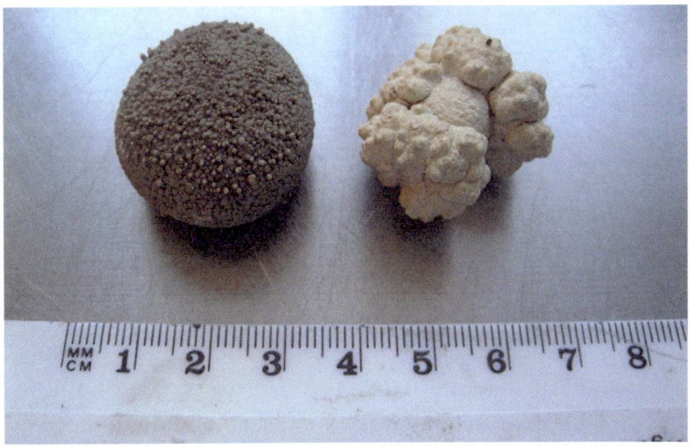

Fig. 6.44 Urinary stones vary in shape and size. They can be small and gravel-like (as seen in Fig. 6.22), but others can be quite large with rounded or irregular surface profiles

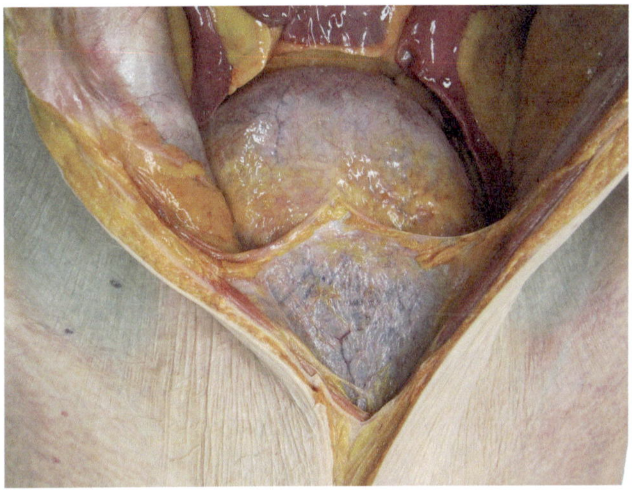

Fig. 6.45 A distended bladder seen when opening the abdomen may reflect significant obstruction of urine outflow, particularly in males. It may be prudent to deflate the bladder, measuring the total urine volume before proceeding to further tissue evisceration. Due diligence should be exercised to consider the cause of the urinary obstruction, by means of careful dissection and histology

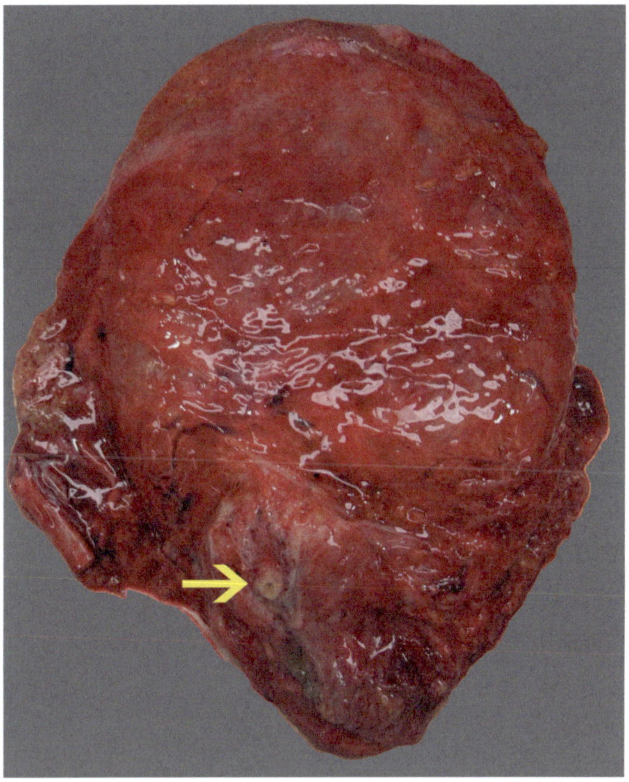

Fig. 6.46 A full bladder can be resected intact, although dissection of the tissue is more complicated if it is full of urine. The urethra at the prostate outflow is indicated with an arrow

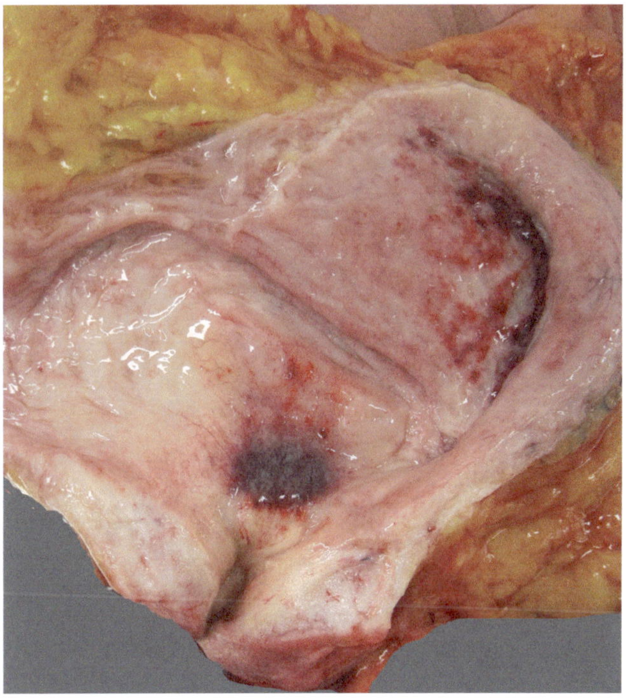

Fig. 6.47 The bladder in men is normally resected together with the prostate. Here, the prostatic outflow tract and urethra are seen in association with a focally inflamed bladder. The bladder has a thickened wall and focal bladder irritation, in keeping with a common complication of urinary catheterisation

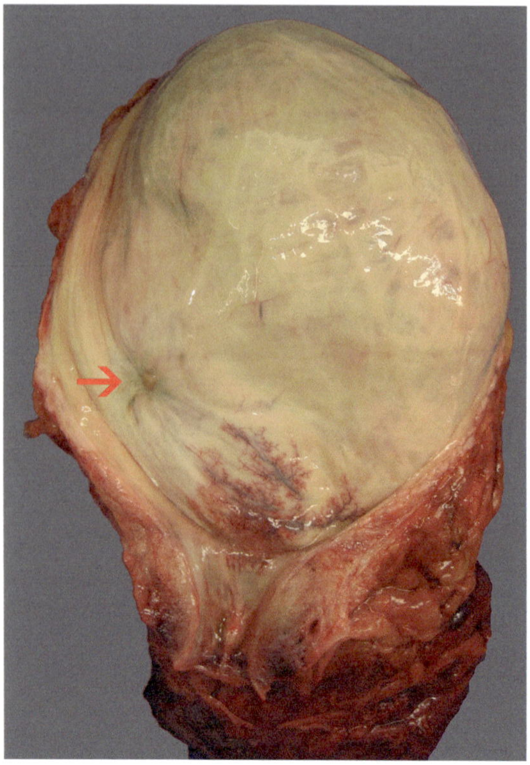

Fig. 6.48 This case of treated bladder cancer shows an area of telangiectasia towards the base of the bladder/trigone. Towards one side (arrow) is an irregular yellow/grey nubbin of tissue, representing a treated bladder carcinoma. This patient had been treated with external beam radiation for bladder cancer

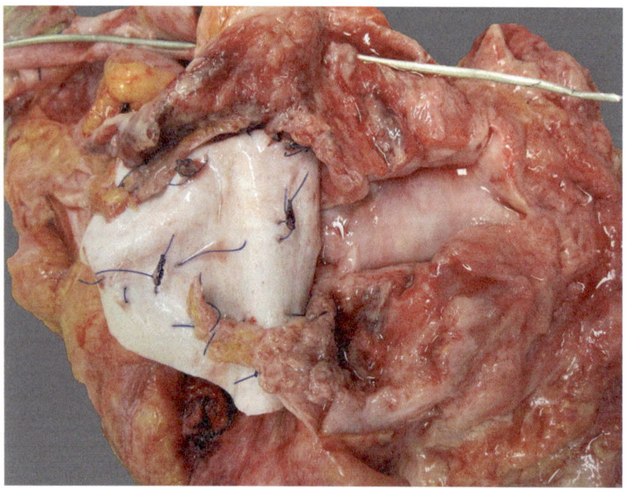

Fig. 6.49 Bladder tissue can be augmented by small intestine and other patches. In cases that are examined shortly after such augmentation procedures one should pay attention to features of local sepsis, dehiscence and local infective pelvic complications

Prostate

At autopsy, the prostate gland is considered from two main perspectives. Firstly, an assessment of size and nodularity is often relevant in terms of benign nodular hyperplasia. This is the normal reality for males with increasing age. This 'benign' process is linked with urinary outflow obstruction from the bladder, with a potential risk of backpressure onto the kidneys and sepsis. It may also provide a setting for the formation of stones. The size of the prostate can be measured in terms of its maximum dimension or by its weight, following dissection of the gland from the surrounding tissues.

The prostate is a common site of malignancy, almost entirely comprising prostatic adenocarcinoma. Whilst these tumors may be large, it is disseminated disease that is most likely to be relevant to the cause of death.

The seminal vesicles rarely contain significant pathology in autopsy examination and are rarely sought specifically. Likewise, the urethra and its passage into the penis is not usually a source of major pathology. Unless there is antemortem evidence of significant disease at this site, detailed dissection is rarely needed.

Male Genital Tissues

It is rare for the cord to be involved in significant autopsy pathology, although various degrees of lipomatous/fatty hypertrophy are often seen in elderly patients. The main pathology involving the cord often relates to local hernia realities with compression of the cord elements and subsequent testicular tissue atrophy.

By contrast, the testes may be involved by tumours, with the commonest being germ cell neoplasms. Metastatic neoplasia (mostly from the prostate) is possible, but rarely sought or identified.

The remaining external genital male tissues comprise the penis and scrotum. The external genitalia (Figs. 6.50, 6.51, 6.52, 6.53, 6.54, 6.55, 6.56, 6.57, 6.58, 6.59, 6.60, 6.61, 6.62, 6.63, 6.64, and 6.65) are commonly ignored during autopsy practice but some inspection is required, even in the elderly. These structures are mostly uninvolved by pathology at autopsy, apart from occasional incidental sexually transmitted disease (e.g. viral warts, condylomata, ulcers, etc.). Nevertheless, there may be sepsis in relation to genital studs, rings and implants.

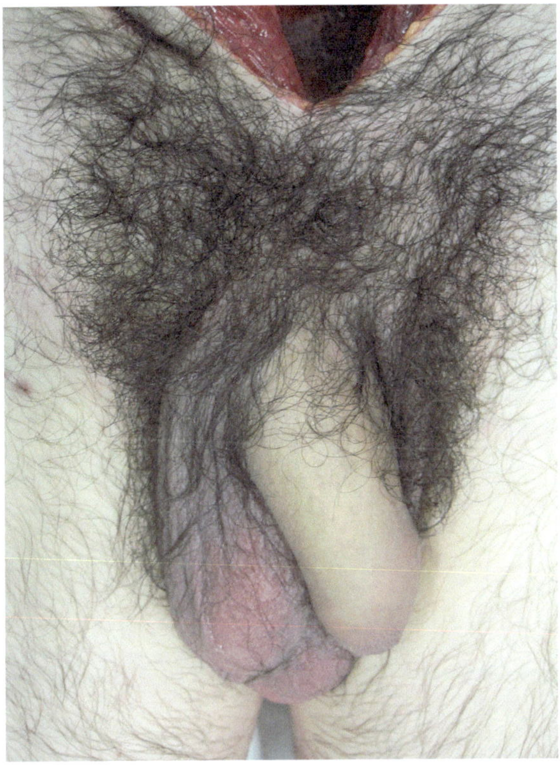

Fig. 6.50 The normal male genitalia are seen with pubic hair, penis and the scrotum (containing two testes)

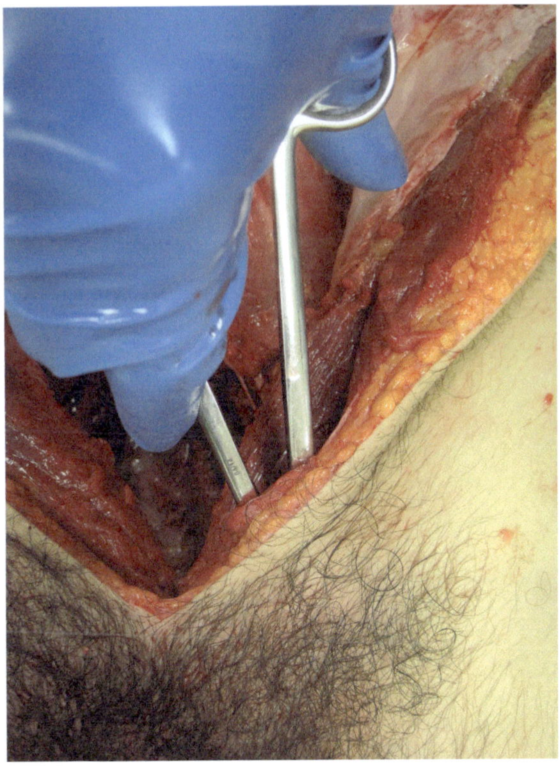

Fig. 6.51 Rather than directly dissecting through the scrotum, examination of the testes requires a dissection plane to be opened at the pelvic rim, running into the superficial soft tissues outside the pelvis and down towards the scrotum

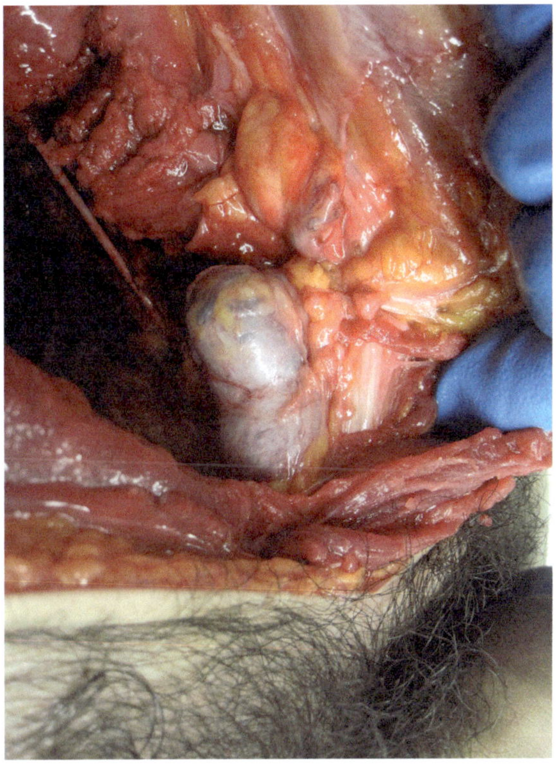

Fig. 6.52 Having bluntly dissected down alongside the cord, the testis can be mobilised. By pushing the testis upwards (from outside the scrotum) it is possible to extract the testes through the plane of dissection made and to remove it at the pelvic brim

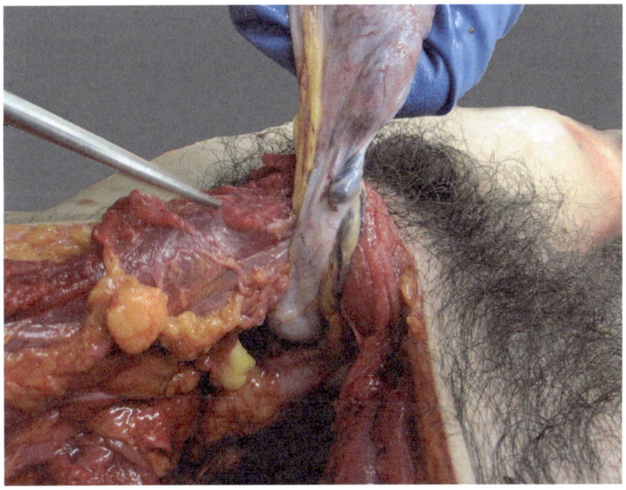

Fig. 6.53 The testis and cord are pulled free and upwards at 90°. The testis is seen with the cord and local soft tissues adjacent

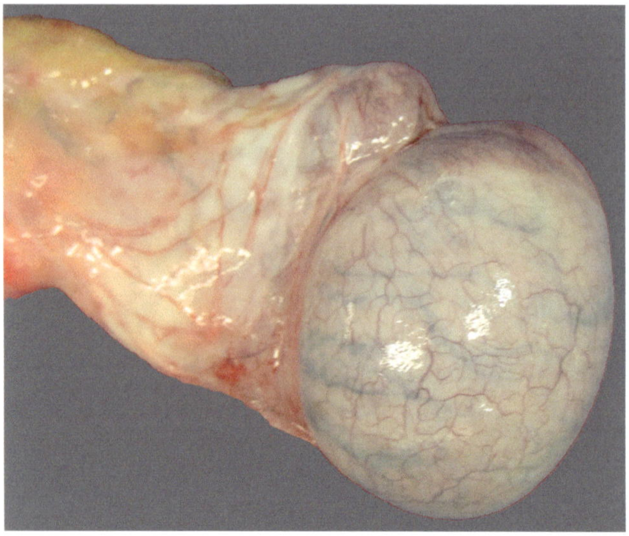

Fig. 6.54 The testis has a smooth and shiny external surface. The normal testis should be soft, without nodularity or fibrosis

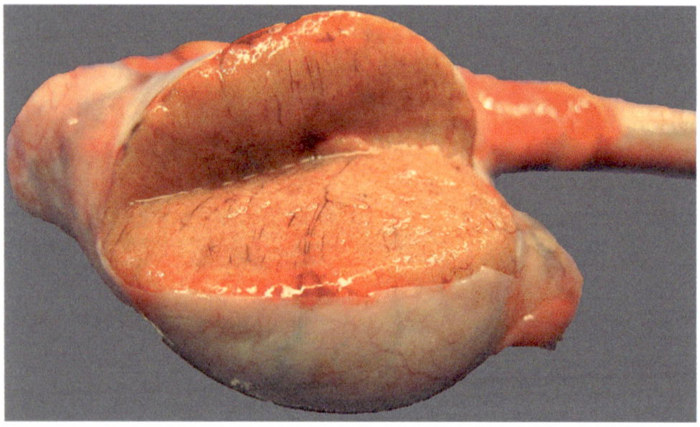

Fig. 6.55 The testis can be sliced open, revealing a congested parenchyma, which often has a yellow/orange colour

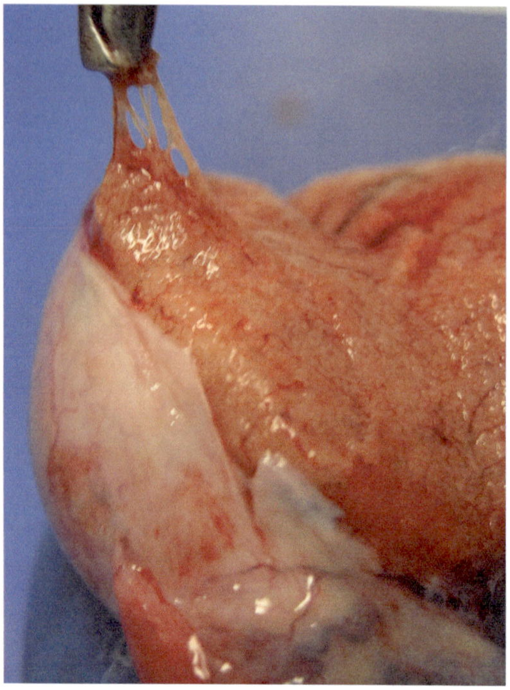

Fig. 6.56 The individual tubules can be grasped with toothed forceps and pulled upwards to demonstrate the highly folding quality of the testicular tissues

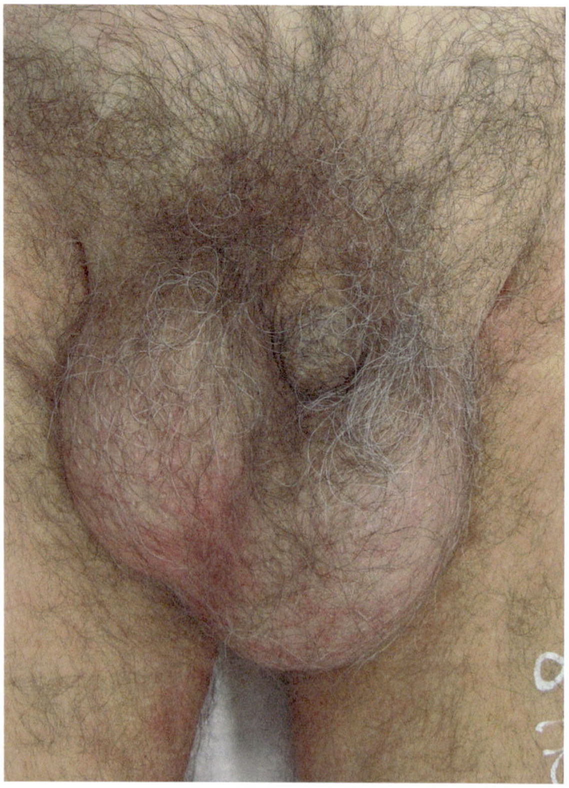

Fig. 6.57 Variation in size of the two sides of the scrotum may point towards testicular tumours or, more commonly, fluid collections around the testes

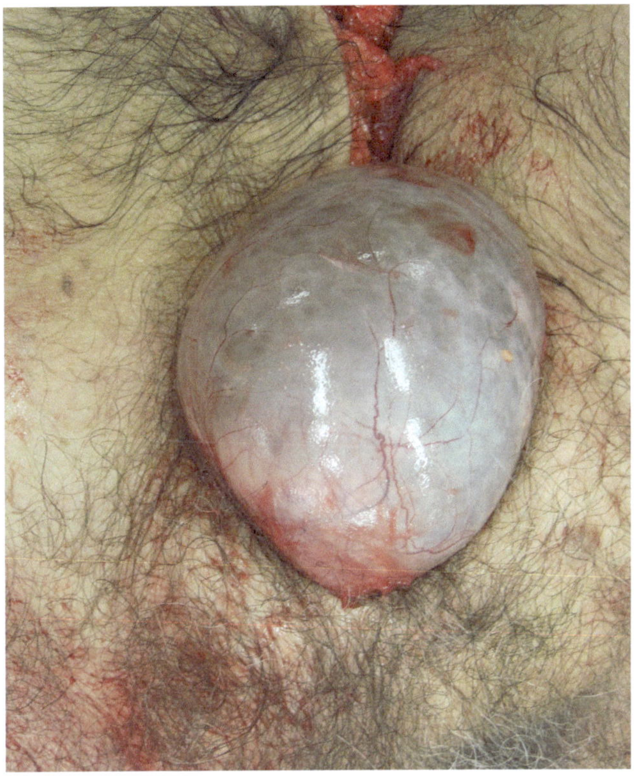

Fig. 6.58 When extracting the testis, the sac may be removed at the same time if there is a significant fluid collection

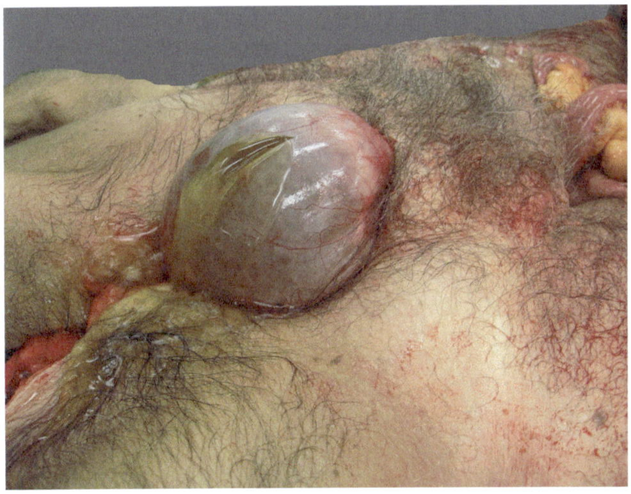

Fig. 6.59 Looking from the side, the sac is then incised to check the nature and volume of the fluid. Here, there is clear yellow fluid released from the cut surface, indicative of a hydrocele

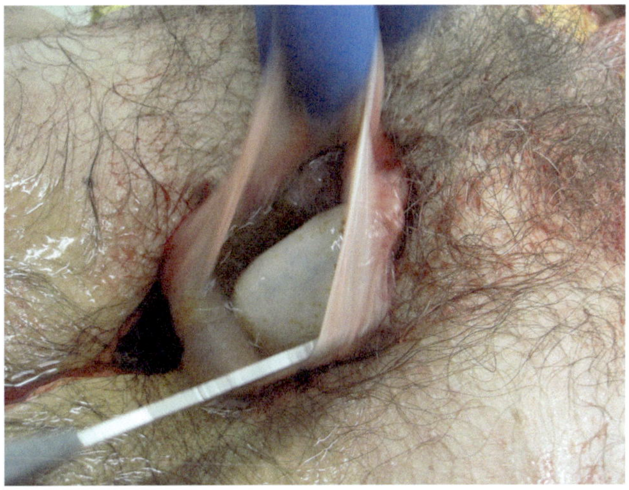

Fig. 6.60 Inside the hydrocele sac is a testis with normal shape and architecture

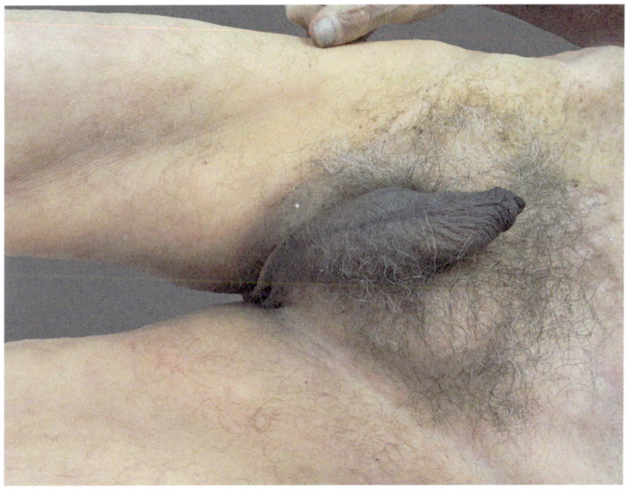

Fig. 6.61 Patients with hormonally driven prostate cancer may benefit from a bilateral orchidectomy procedure. The testes have been removed in this case to stunt prostate cancer growth by way of a reduced testosterone level. Other reasons for bilateral orchidectomy include male breast cancer and gender reassignment surgery

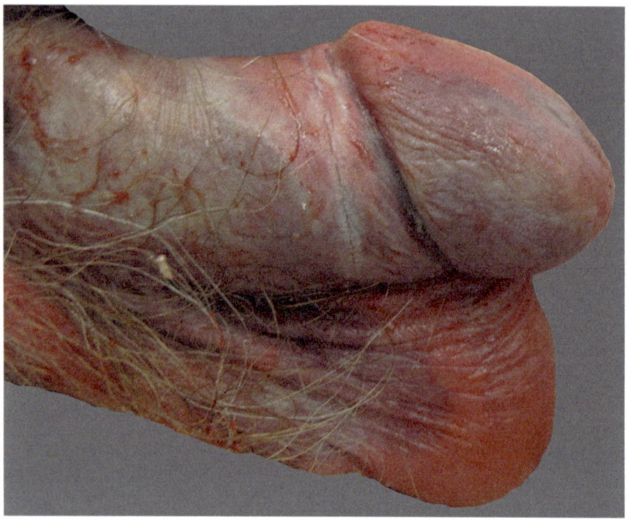

Fig. 6.62 There are a plethora of indications for surgical intervention of the penis, including, but not limited to, congenital variations, erectile dysfunction and neoplastic processes. A scar such as this is most likely from a procedure unassociated with the cause of death, unless the clinical circumstances point to a specific local pathology or complication

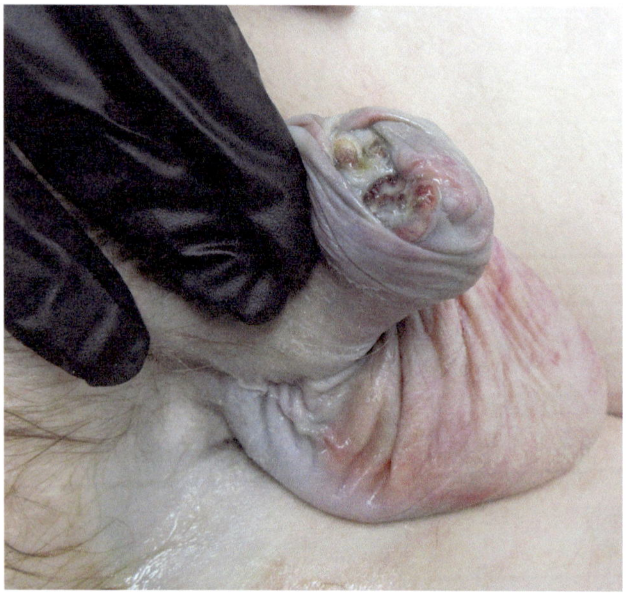

Fig. 6.63 Malignancy involving the penis is most commonly primary squamous carcinoma, as demonstrated here. An ulcerated lesion has largely replaced the penile shaft tissue, with associated foci of probable infection

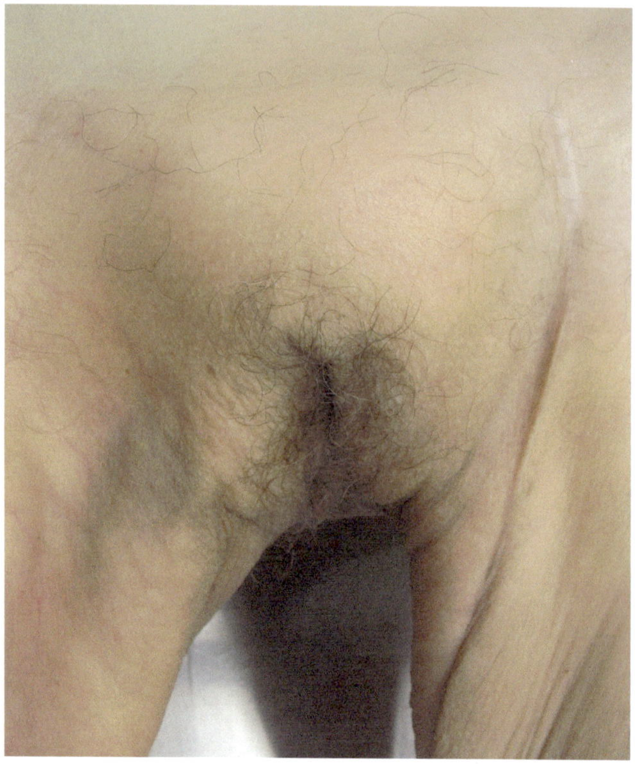

Fig. 6.64 Such penile malignancies may require resection of the external genitalia in the male. This procedure had been carried out on this man with a pseudo-female genital architecture

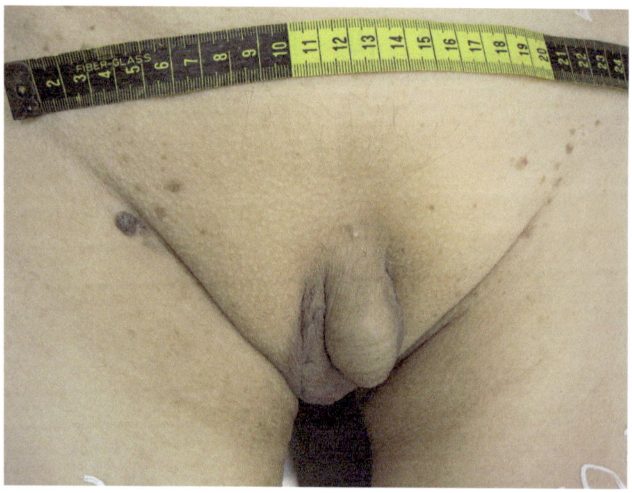

Fig. 6.65 Atrophy of the penis and loss of secondary sexual hair pattern is characteristic of patients who have been treated with orchidectomy for prostate carcinoma. Such external findings should prompt consideration of disseminated prostate cancer

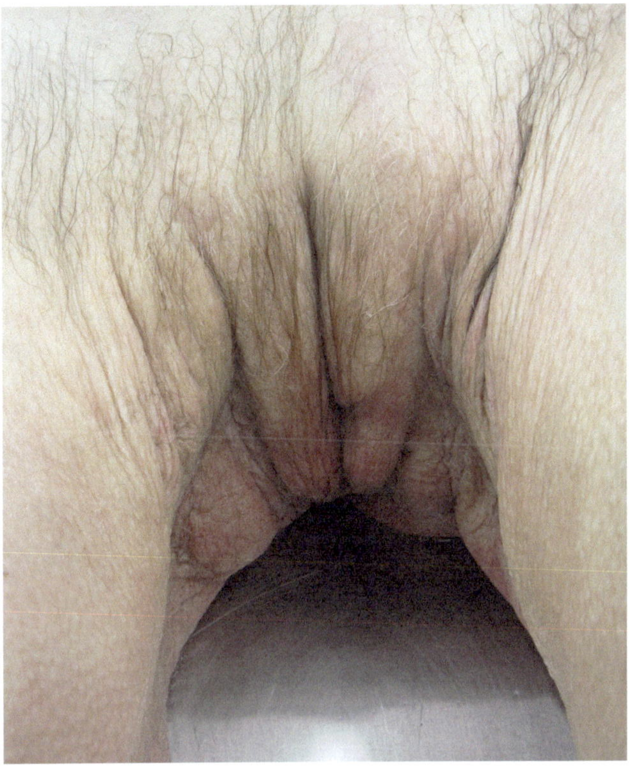

Fig. 6.66 The normal female genitalia are seen with vulval and pelvic tissues. The general autopsy will not have issues of sexual activity or assault as part of the routine screen, but one should always be aware of this possibility

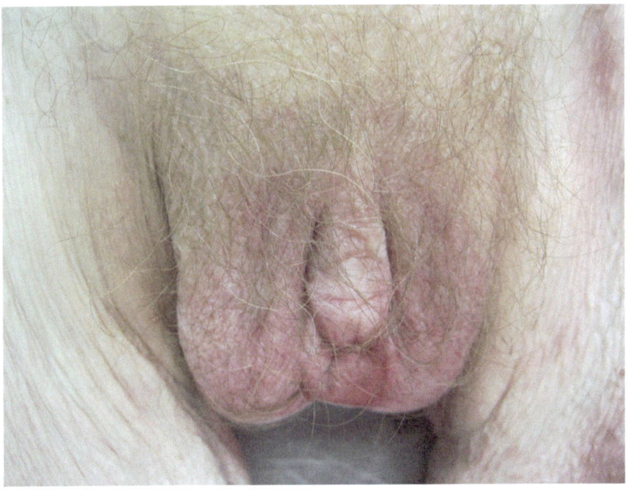

Fig. 6.67 Pronounced oedema of the female genital tract can produce a distorted vulval appearance and should not be mistaken for neoplasia

Female Genital Tissues

The vulva and vagina (Figs. 6.66 and 6.67) are intermittently involved in disease ante-mortem, but often have minimal attention focused upon this area at autopsy. Nevertheless, these sites may have common infections (e.g. candida), but exclusion of sexually transmitted diseases should be considered, particularly in the young. As with males, the fashion for genital jewellery (rings, studs, etc.) means that standard skin commensal sepsis may be significant in the groin area. Identification of genital sepsis with standard infections or sexually transmitted infections is important, as the infection may be easily overlooked and yet the disease may have generalized/systemic effects.

The uterus (Figs. 6.68, 6.69, 6.70, 6.71, 6.72, 6.73, 6.74, 6.75, 6.76, 6.77, 6.78, 6.79, and 6.80) is best considered as the uterine corpus and cervix (i.e. as one combined piece of tissue). In general terms, in the non-pregnant state the uterus is rarely of significance, showing variable endometrial features in relation to the standard monthly hormone cycle in pre-menopausal females. However, it is not uncommon to find a degree of mucus inspissation within the endometrial cavity, a benign polyp, or a contraceptive device. These devices may be associated with sepsis. The uterine body

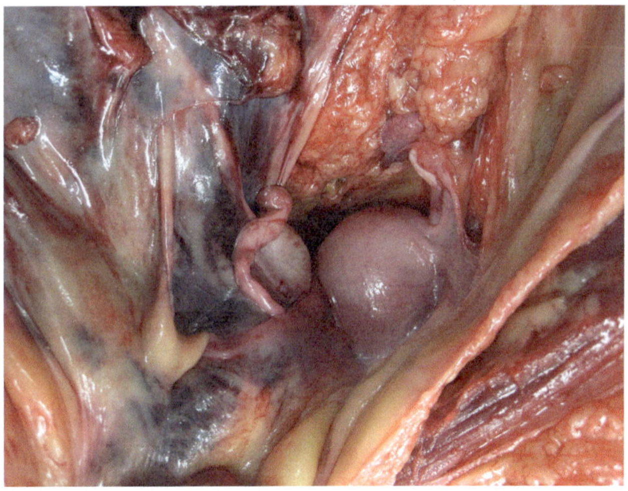

Fig. 6.68 During evisceration, looking downward from the pelvic brim, one can see the uterus, tubes and ovaries during examination of the pelvic content. The internal female genital tract tissues are removed during evisceration at the same time as resection of the rectal and bladder tissues

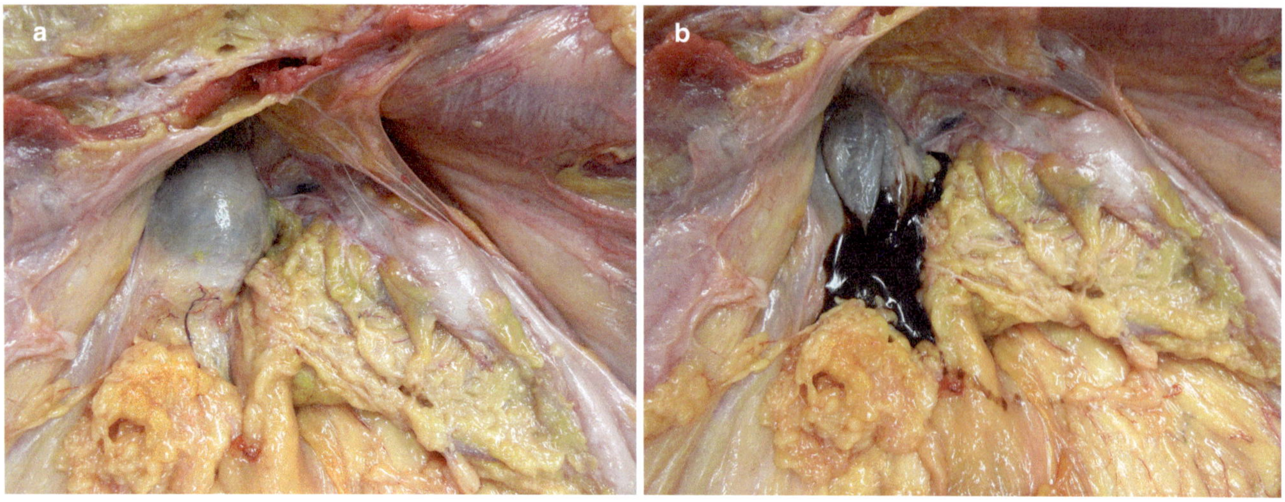

Fig. 6.69 A blue-tinged sac at this stage of dissection may indicate a collection of blood. In this case, an endometriotic cyst is seen within the pelvic cavity, photographed unopened (**a**) and after incision (**b**), displaying the brown content of old blood

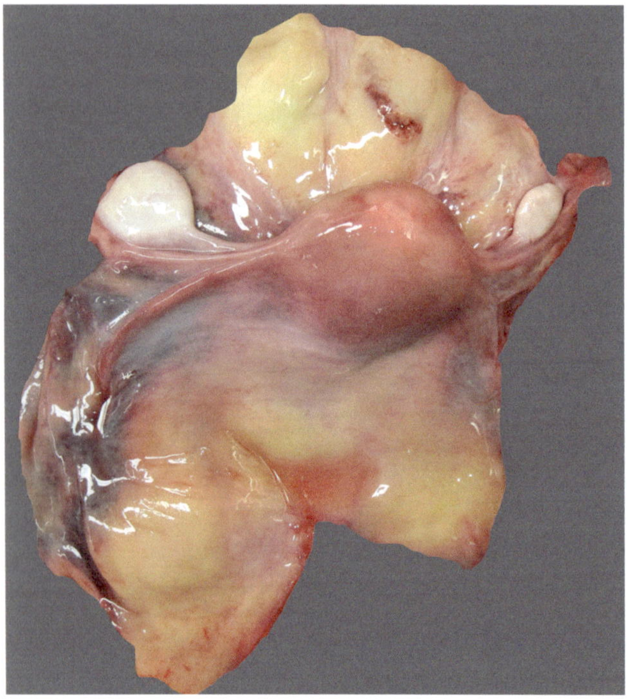

Fig. 6.70 The uterus, both tubes and both ovaries are seen with local soft tissues, prior to dissection in this postmenopausal case

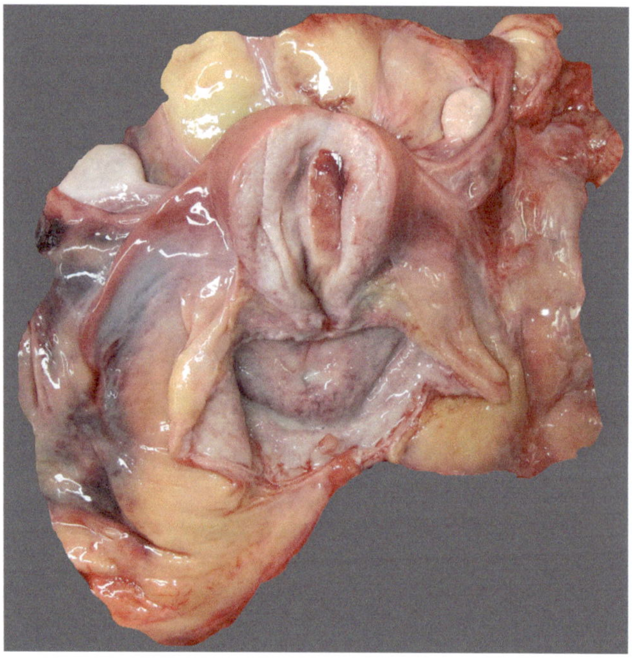

Fig. 6.71 The female genital tract tissues can be examined with different techniques. Here, the uterus and cervix have been opened anteriorly in association with the cut passing across the roof of the vagina anteriorly. The ovaries and tubes are seen in a normal position

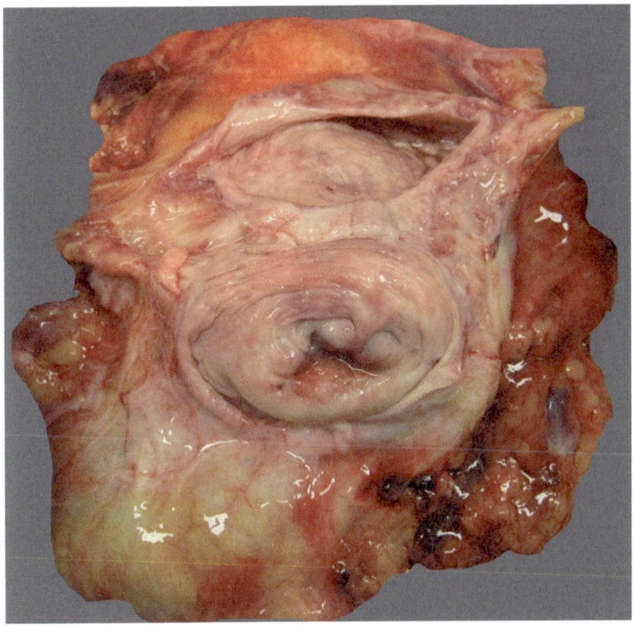

Fig. 6.72 The bladder has been opened (in front of the uterus) and the cervix is seen from below, looking towards the fundus. The os is ovoid/transverse, in keeping with prior gestation (i.e. multips os)

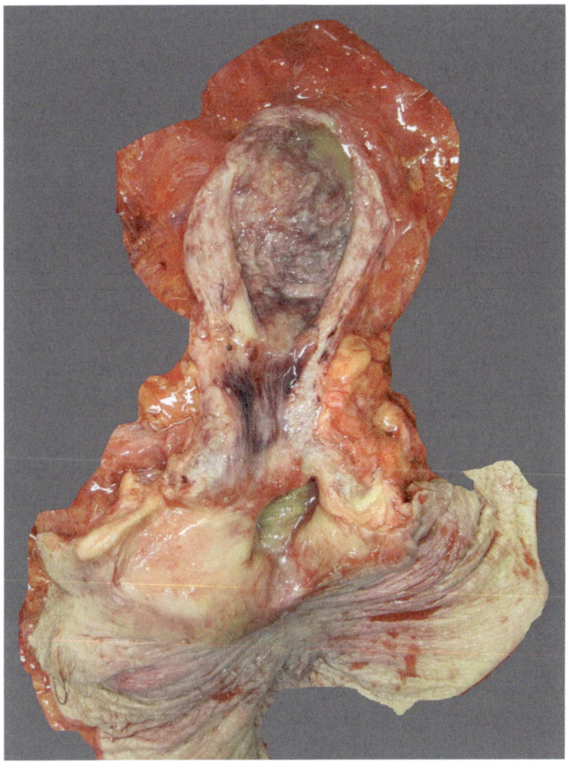

Fig. 6.74 The bladder has been opened longitudinally through the urethra. Some inflammatory changes are noted

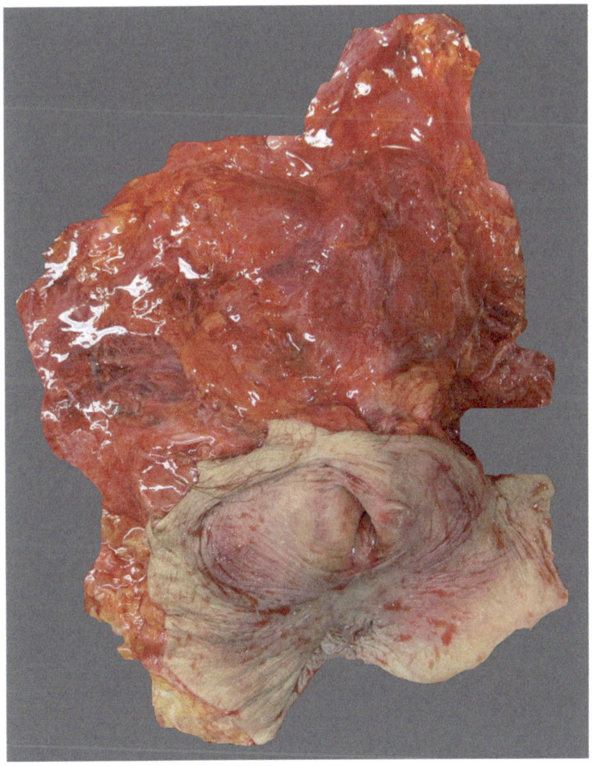

Fig. 6.73 One may wish to examine the entirety of the perineum, vulva, vagina, internal genital organs and anorectal tissues in one piece. These are removed in the style of an "apple core" around the inner pelvic walls and then the incision runs around the perineum. This encloses all the tissues under consideration. If sexual assault is a consideration, a wider pelvic-perineal resection margin may be needed, with a more detailed forensic examination. Here, one can see the vulva/vaginal tissues and fatty tissue around the internal genital block

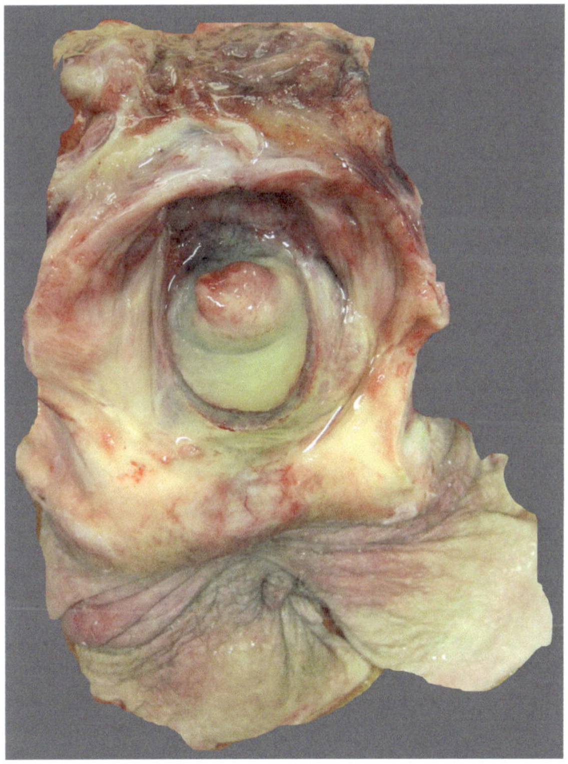

Fig. 6.75 The vagina is visualised longitudinally and the cervix is seen at the end. Swabs for microbiology and DNA analysis may be taken

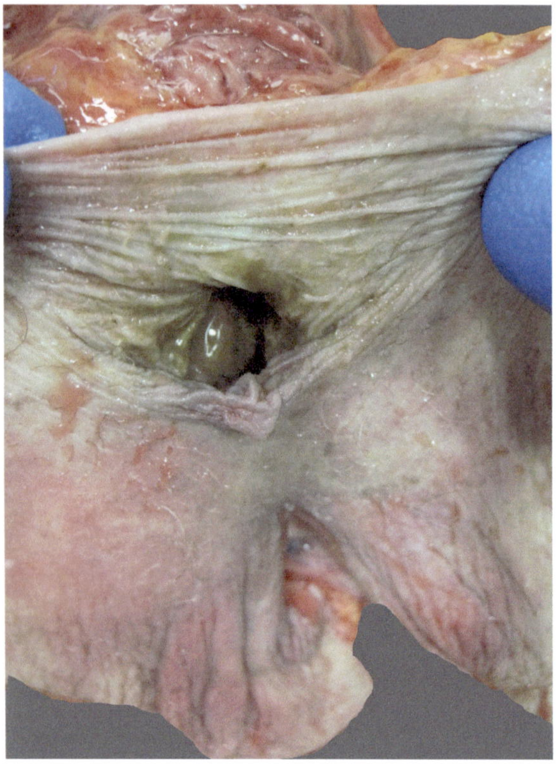

Fig. 6.76 Turning the tissues around so the rectal tissues are uppermost allows the external features of the anus and rectum to be inspected with the anal orifice. Any fecal matter can be sampled and swabs taken

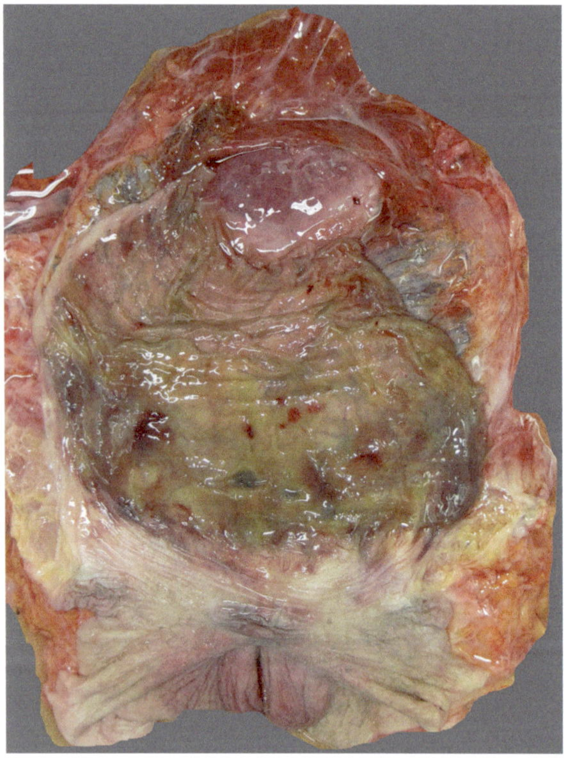

Fig. 6.77 Keeping the rectal tissues uppermost, the rectum is opened along its length in the posterior midline, allowing a full review of the mucosa and anorectal interface

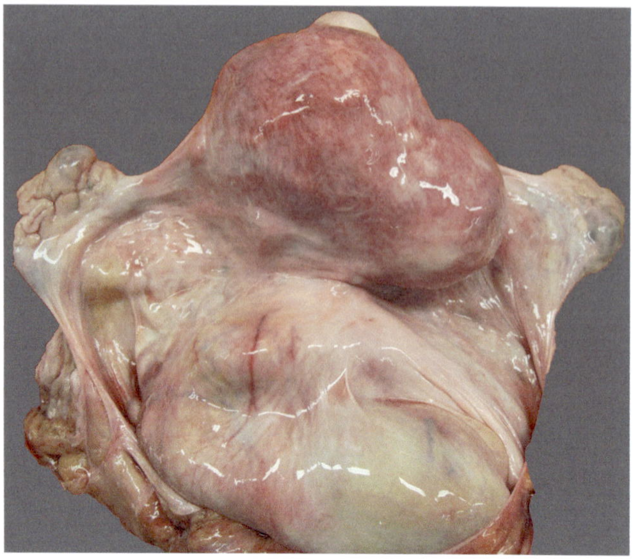

Fig. 6.78 This uterus, with tubes and ovaries, is nodular and distorted, in keeping with fibroid change. This is a common finding at autopsy. It usually has no significance unless the fibroids are sufficiently large to cause pelvic obstruction

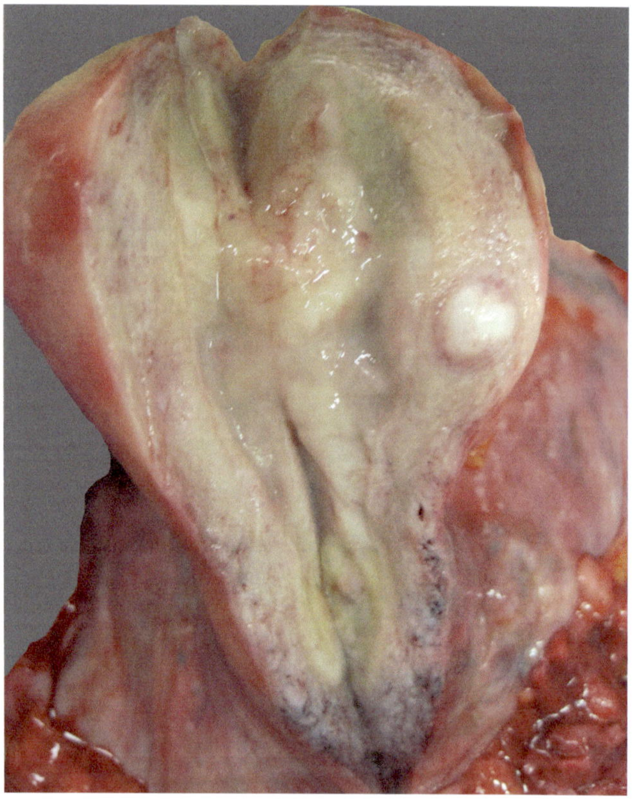

Fig. 6.79 This uterus has been opened longitudinally revealing a largely normal myometrium and endometrium. However, a rounded leiomyoma/fibroid is present in the mid-mural position focally

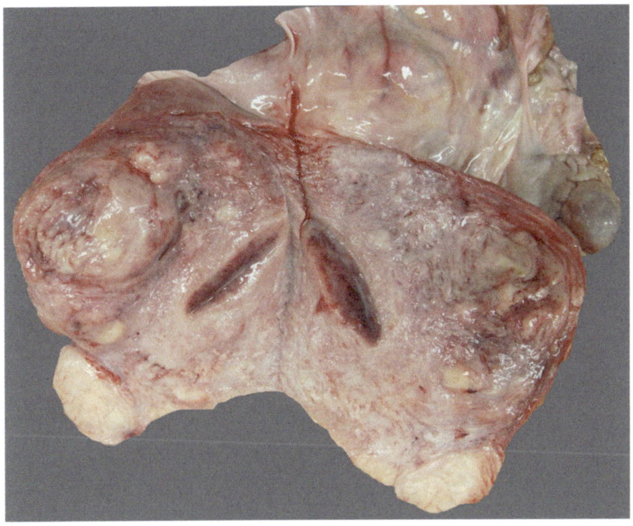

Fig. 6.80 This uterus and the endometrial cavity are significantly distorted by multiple fibroids (leiomyomas) of varying sizes, making the section down through the cervix difficult

itself has perhaps the commonest genital tract pathology in the form of fibroids. Rarely, other uterine neoplasia may be found. The cervix, likewise, can be involved by carcinoma and, if so, tumour spread to the pelvic tissues will need to be considered.

The fallopian tubes are rarely involved by pathology at autopsy, although cysts are intermittently found. Ties and clips from sterilization procedures should be documented as part of the routine examination.

The ovaries (Figs. 6.81, 6.82, 6.83, 6.84, 6.85, 6.86, 6.87, and 6.88) will vary in terms of architecture depending on the age of the individual. The presence of follicle cysts of various stages, corpus lutea and various scars may be relevant but generally one accepts these as normal. The presence of such elements in maternal death cases is, of course, an important description component.

The commonest pathology seen in the ovaries at autopsy is that of cystic tumours, ranging from small to very large. These are principally mucinous or serous adenomatous process, although carcinomas can present with cystic change. Rarely, germ cell tumours can be seen, the commonest being mature teratomas (dermoid).

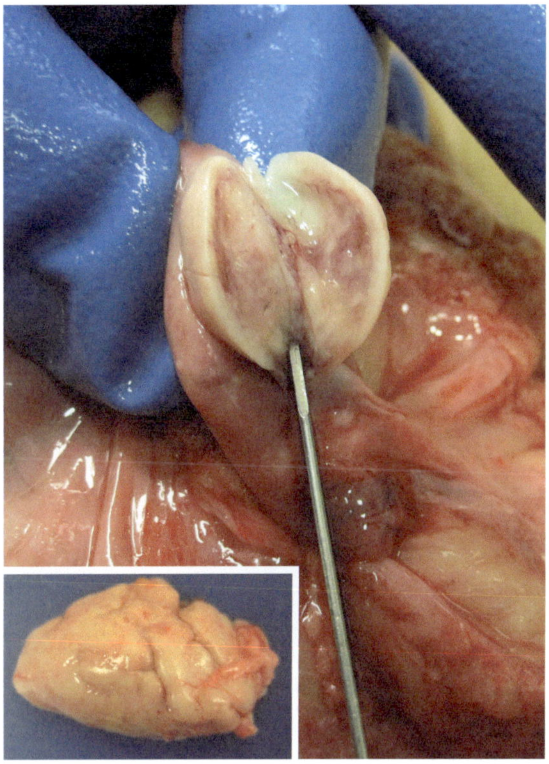

Fig. 6.81 Ovaries are best examined while still attached to the genital tissue block by slicing them along the long axis. The inset shows the slightly folded external surface often seen in ovaries

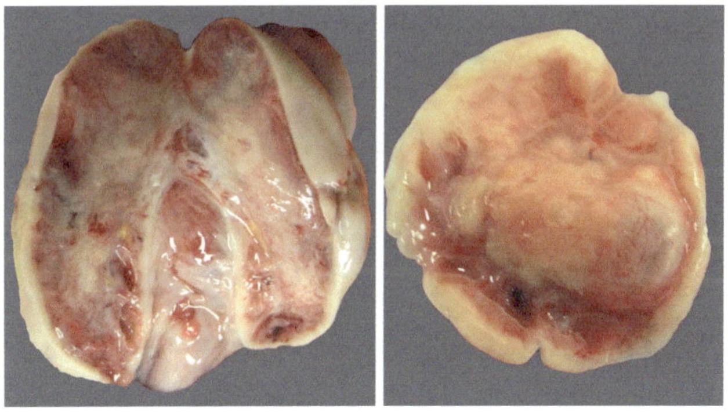

Fig. 6.82 Two ovaries are seen with small follicles and a bland pink/grey stroma

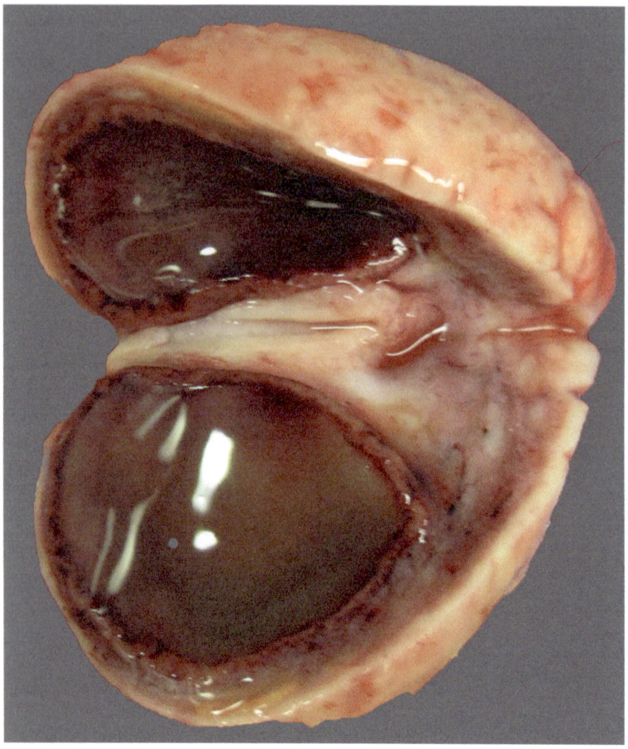

Fig. 6.83 The ovary shows a corpus luteum cyst, as part of early pregnancy

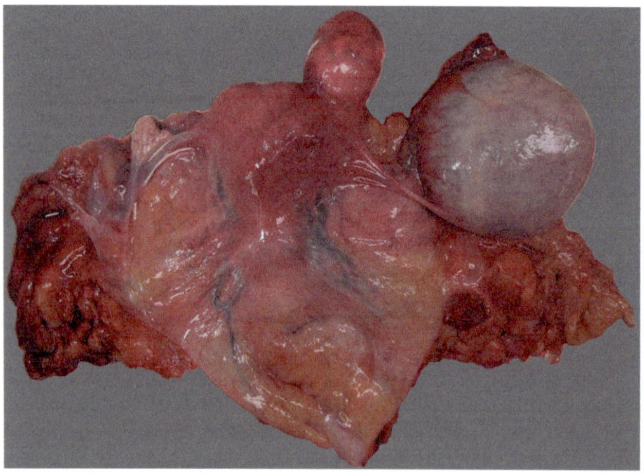

Fig. 6.84 This ovarian cystadenoma was an incidental finding during evisceration and had no bearing on the cause of death. The tube is stretched around the cyst

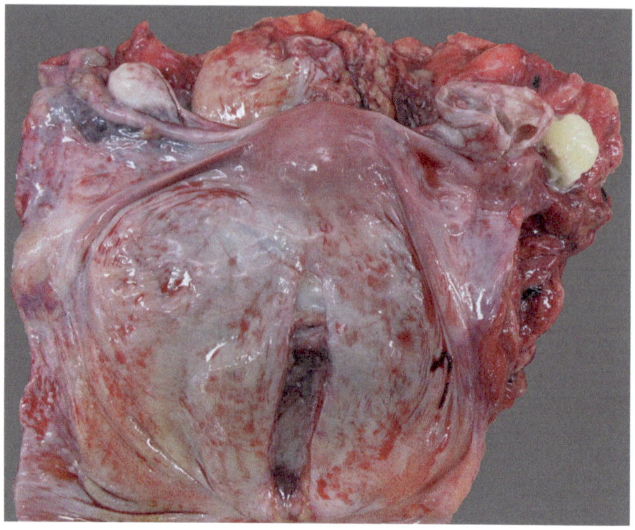

Fig. 6.85 Here is another incidental ovarian cyst identified on the left side. The yellow mucinous cyst content can be seen extruding to the right of the multiloculated cyst. This mucinous cyst did not contribute to death. The right ovary appears normal, although there are multiple paratubal cysts on the right fallopian tube

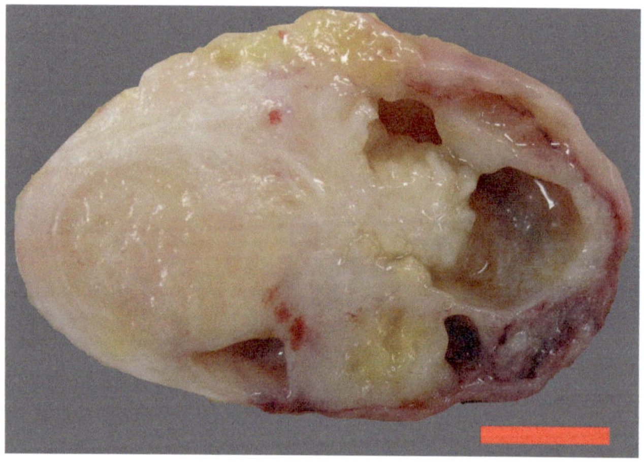

Fig. 6.86 Features of malignancy in an ovarian cyst are suggested by the presence of solid and papillary lesions. This ovarian carcinoma was found incidentally and disseminated disease was not identified. (Marker 10 mm)

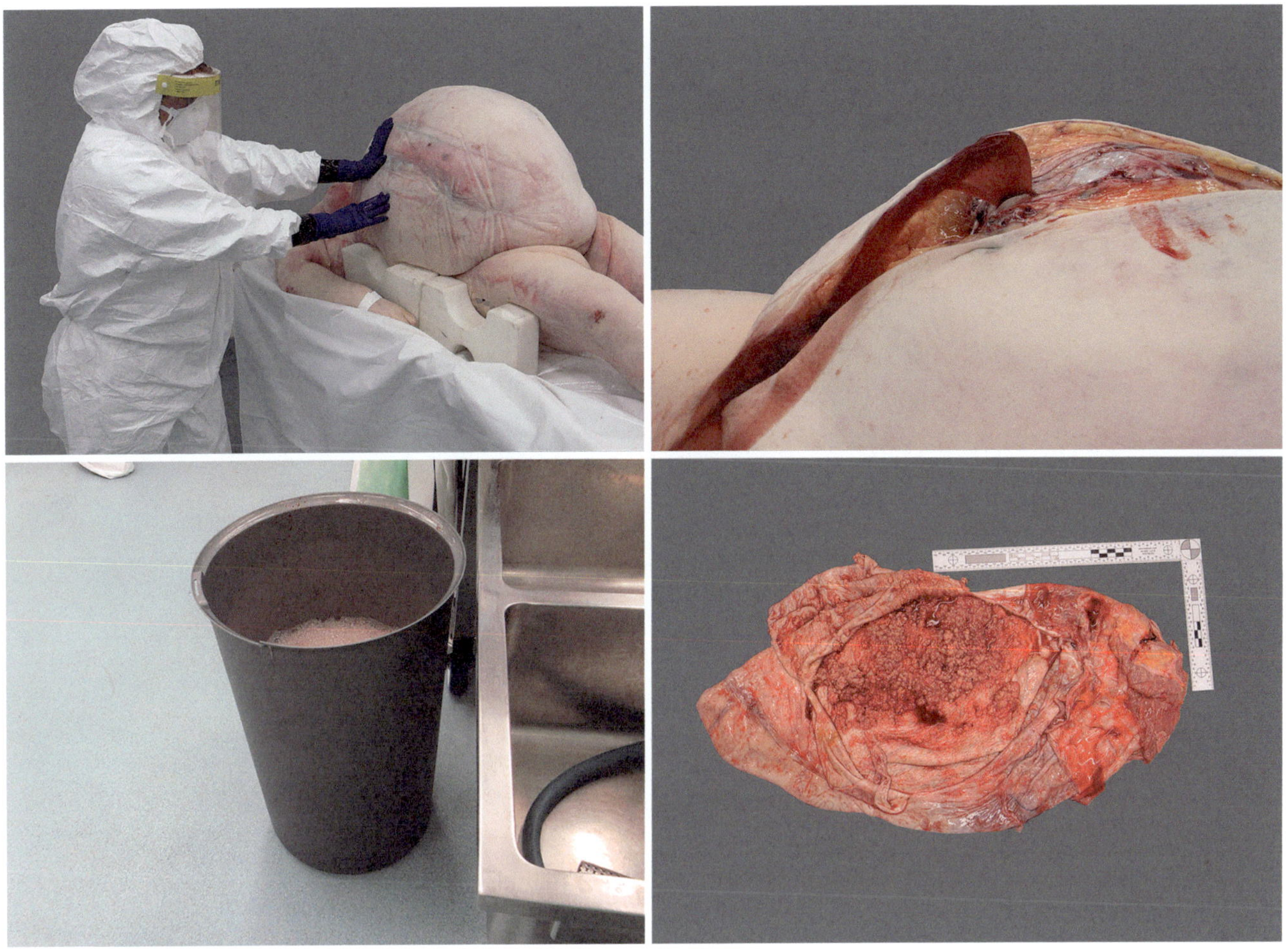

Fig. 6.87 Ovarian malignancy may cause significant abdominal distension, as is demonstrated in the first of this series of pictures. Many litres of blood stained fluid were released early in the autopsy, half-filling the bucket, as shown. When removed from the body, the cyst comprised a thin-walled unilocular sac measuring 600 mm in maximum dimension. There were internal papillary excrescences suspicious for (and confirmed by histology to be) a serous borderline ovarian tumour

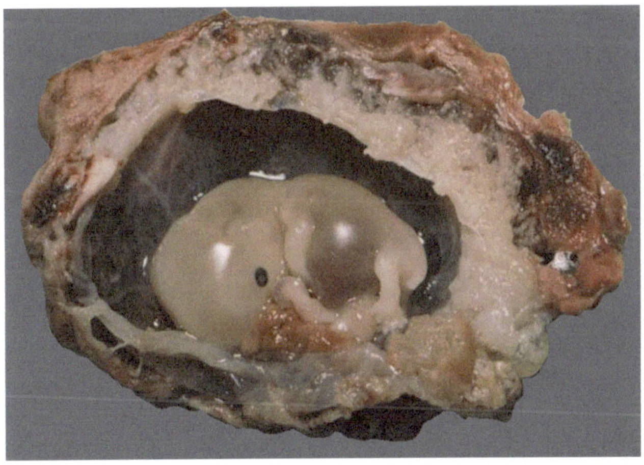

Fig. 6.88 Other cystic lesions adjacent to the ovary may include cysts of the tubes. These are mostly benign and of no consequence. However, pronounced bleeding and death may follow ruptured tubal ectopic gestation. This fixed surgical sample shows an ectopic early-stage pregnancy, without rupture of the tube

Pregnancy

The maternal death autopsy (Figs. 6.89, 6.90, 6.91, 6.92, 6.93, 6.94, 6.95, 6.96, 6.97, 6.98, 6.99, 6.100, 6.101, and 6.102) is a specialist autopsy analysis. It must cover antemortem matters in detail, alongside aspects of the pregnancy and potentially the delivery. Often, the concept of the maternal death autopsy may be invoked for up to a year following the birth of the child.

Particular emphasis upon the genital tract tissues will be required in maternal autopsy with close inspection of the entire female genital tract. Identification and sampling of any septic focus (uterine swabs, blood cultures, spleen swabs, etc.) is a priority and it is important to widely sample these tissues.

Likewise, histological assessment of the genital tract is important. In cases where delivery has recently taken place, an attempt to secure the placenta and membranes should be made. If the gestation is still in situ, then gross examination

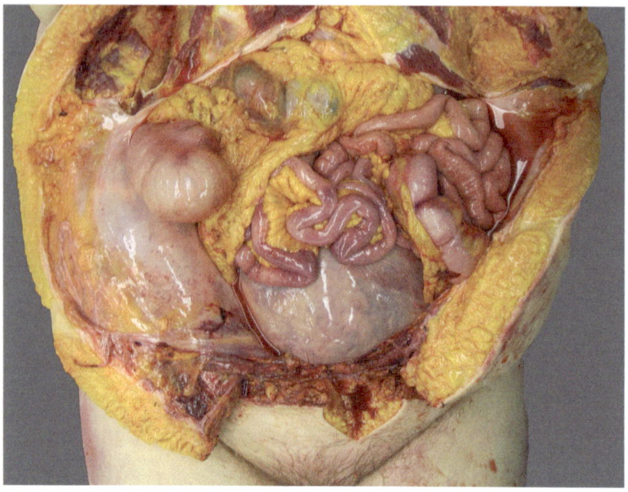

Fig. 6.89 Autopsy cases involving pregnancy require special consideration and examination. Where the fetus is still in situ then it is important to examine the genital tissues with particular care to exclude structural problems and sepsis pathology associated with the fetus. The uterus may appear enlarged, with the size reflecting the stage of gestation. One starts with the general overview as the abdomen is opened

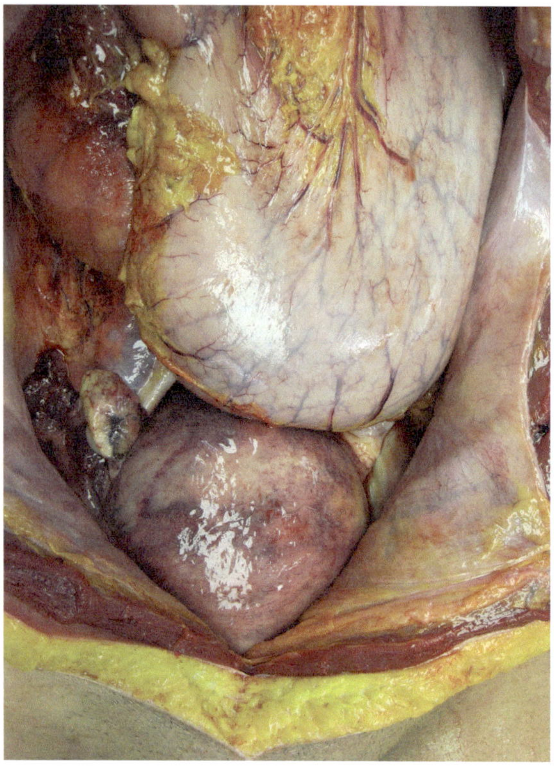

Fig. 6.90 The gravid uterus should be considered beforehand in terms of the anatomical position, the other abdominal viscera and the local vasculature

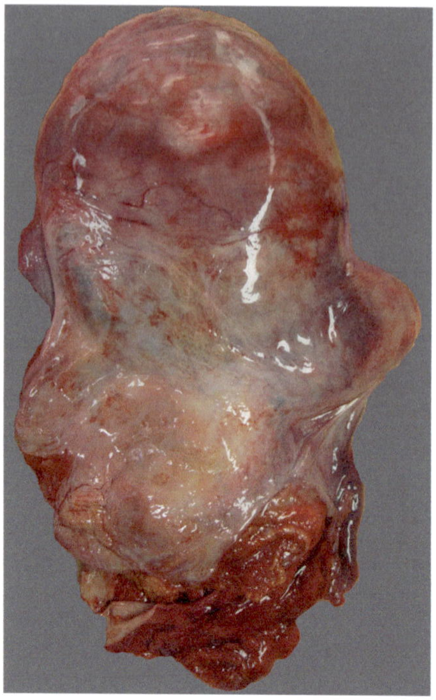

Fig. 6.91 Pregnancy-associated uterine enlargement needs to be carefully considered in terms of uterine content as well as possible sepsis or significant bleeding (neither was present in this case)

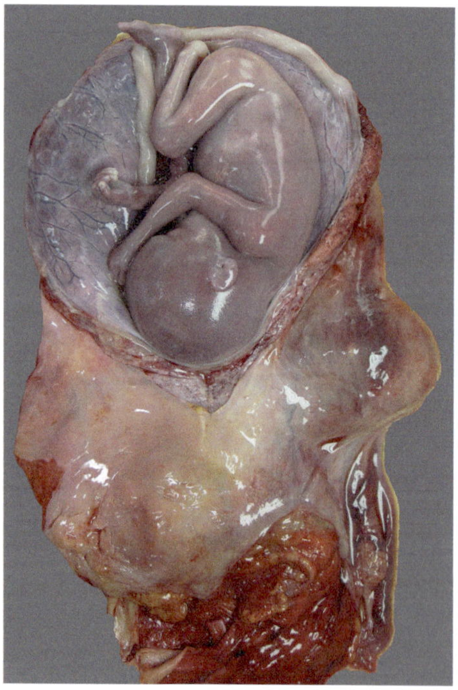

Fig. 6.92 Opening the uterus (done carefully to avoid damage to the placenta and fetus) will allow direct inspection of the uterine cavity, the membranes and the placental tissues. In most cases, the fetus has no abnormality and is not examined beyond recording standard measurements (foot length, crown rump length, crown heel length, head circumference and weight parameters). Examination to determine sex and appropriate development is required. Exclusion of congenital abnormalities is recommended. The cord length should be measured and sectioned to confirm the presence of three normal vessels. The placental surface and membrane should be clear and translucent. The presence of plaque or discoloured membranes suggests sepsis. Swabs should be taken when the gestational sac is open, to exclude sepsis

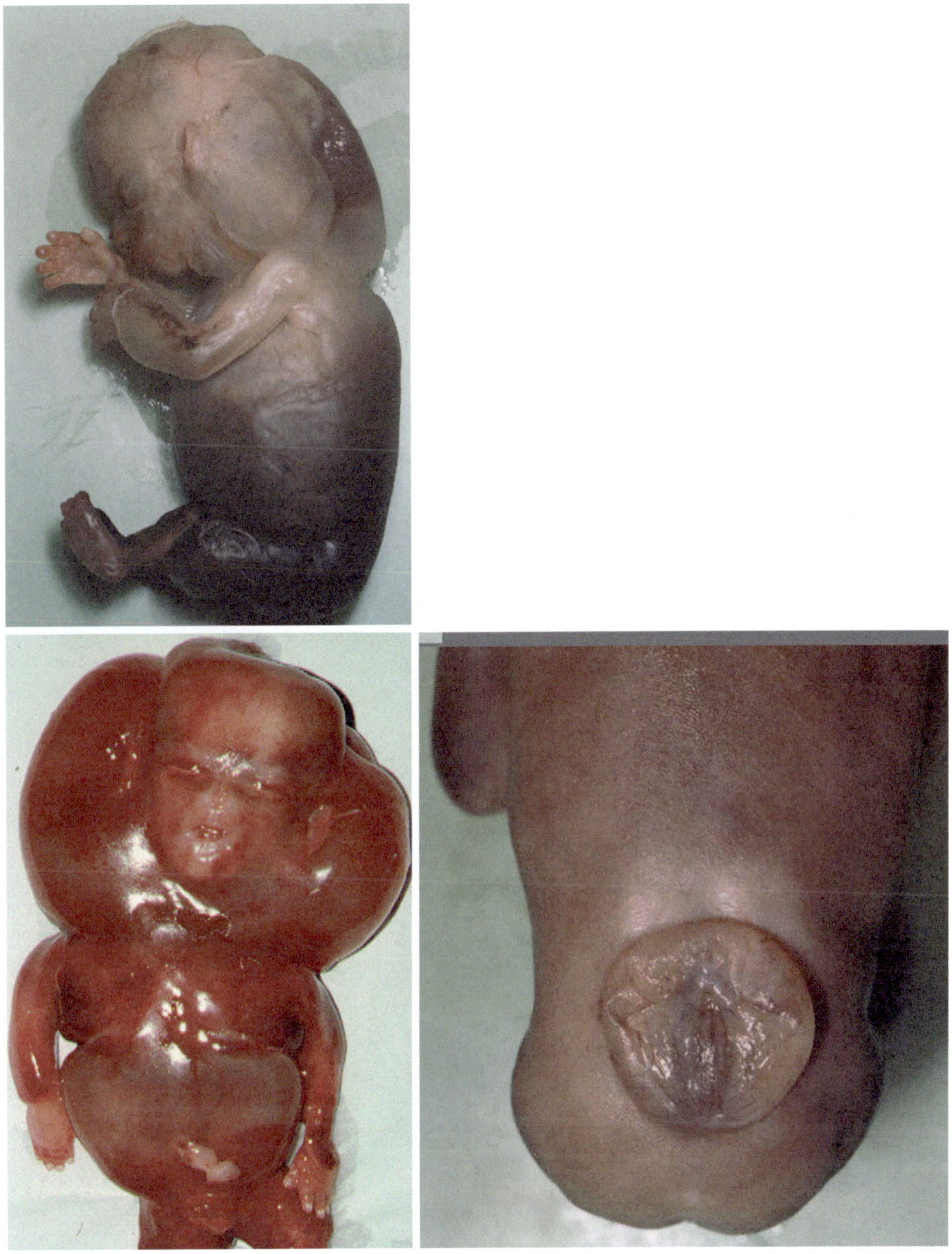

Fig. 6.93 A fetus may have various pathology. Nuchal oedema (upper left), generalised hydrops (lower left) and neural canal defects (lower right) should be noted. There may be a case for fetal tissue review by a pediatric pathologist, but this will need consideration on a case-by-case basis

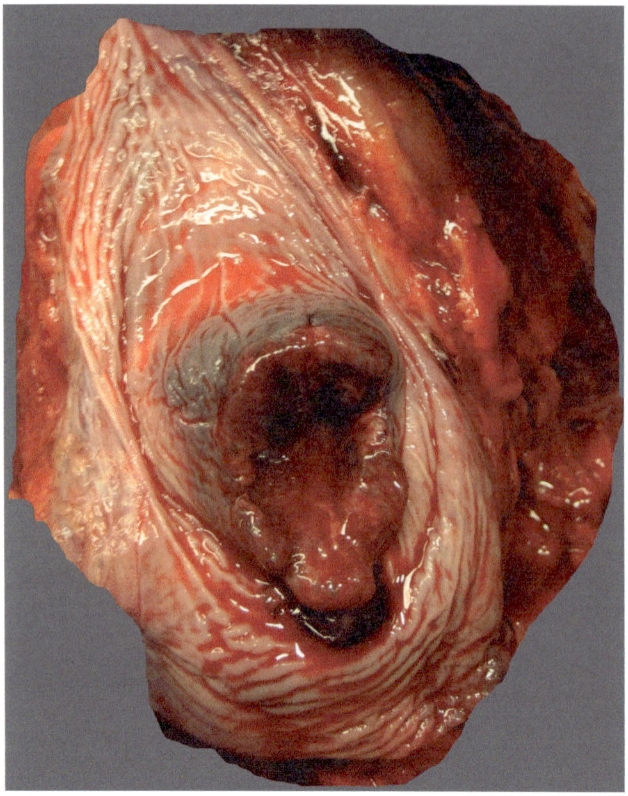

Fig. 6.94 If vaginal delivery has occurred, the uterus will be empty. Examination of the cervix may show an open and somewhat patulous cervix with variable degrees of congestion and haemorrhage, consistent with the delivery process

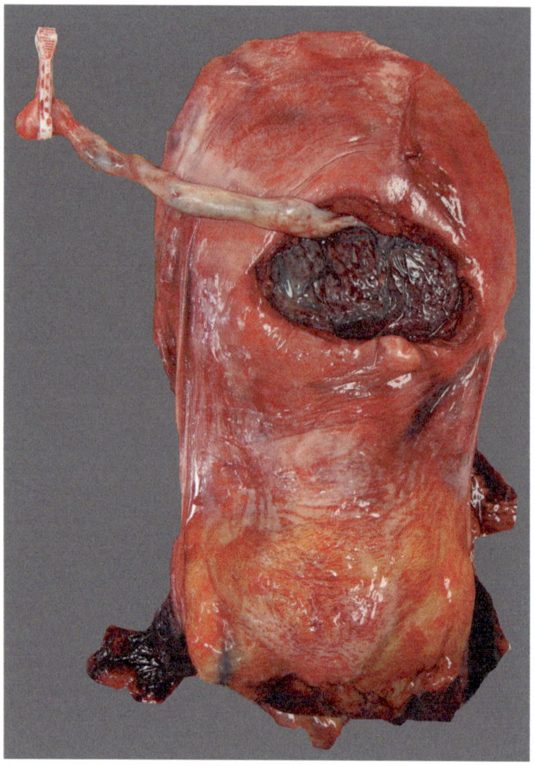

Fig. 6.95 Deaths occurring in late-stage pregnancy often have had emergency caesarian section performed. In these situations, the uterus will be empty of the fetus, but may still contain the umbilical cord and placental parenchyma. The same approach applies, whereby the cord length is measured and confirmed as to whether it has three normal vessels. The placenta may be examined in terms of gross anatomy and there may be a need for histology

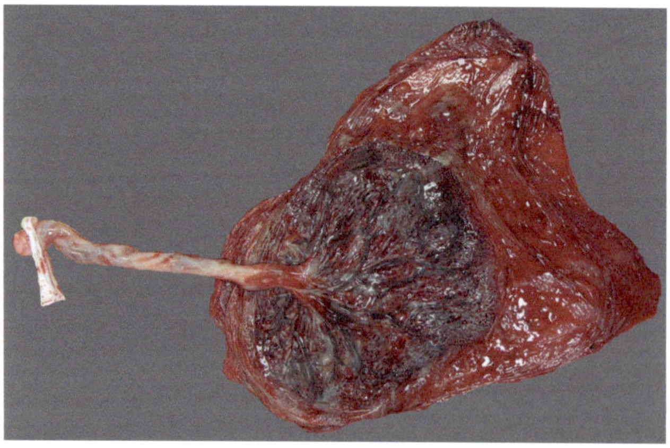

Fig. 6.96 The placenta can be removed from the uterus, usually without any difficulty. It should be examined in terms of size and weight. The placental tissue should be sliced to exclude infarction or frank sepsis. The membranes must be examined and the cord details checked

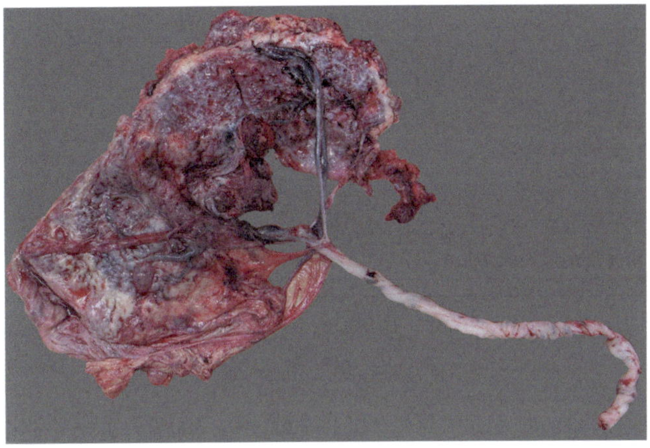

Fig. 6.97 After delivery of the placenta, through vaginal or caesarian section modalities, a non-empty uterus is of concern because retained products of conception can act as a nidus for infection with potential to cause sepsis and death, if not treated promptly. The internal uterine surface may show irregularities representing areas of retained placental tissue. The corresponding placenta in these cases should be examined. Such a placenta is shown here, with a roughened and incomplete placental disc

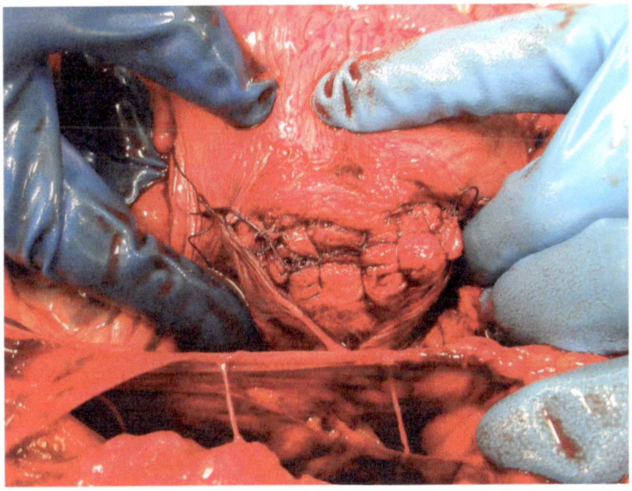

Fig. 6.98 Following caesarian section there may be signs of the operation at autopsy, such as the incision in the lower uterine segment which has been sutured closed here

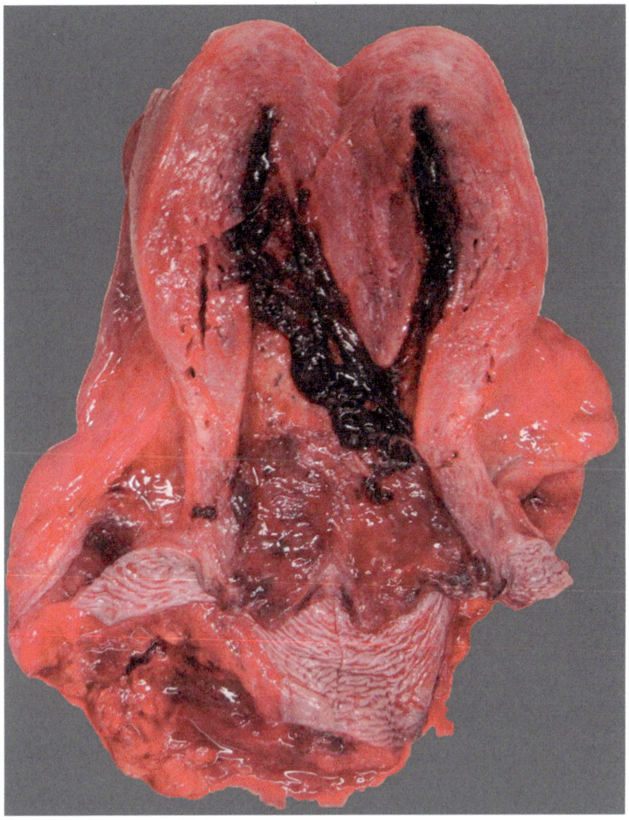

Fig. 6.99 This sample, with pronounced endometrial surface haemorrhage, represents an emergency caesarian section undertaken shortly after the death of the mother. The degree of haemorrhage is entirely in keeping with the emergency procedure, but samples for microbiology and histology may still be of value

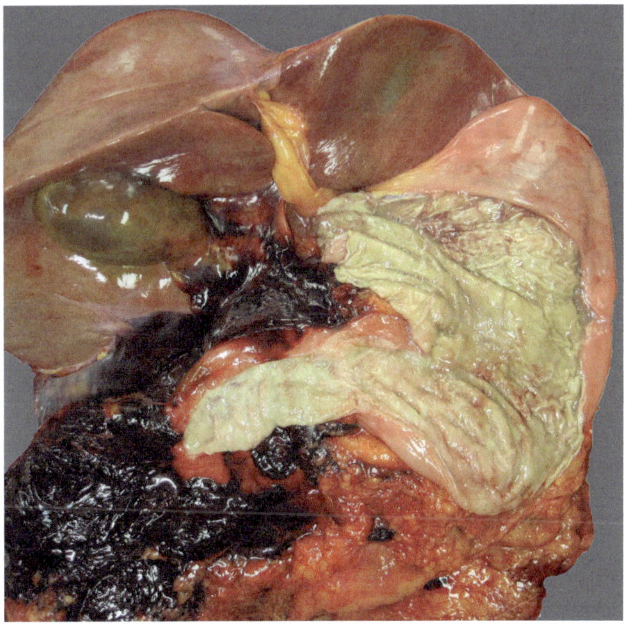

Fig. 6.100 This is a rare case of sudden death in mid-late pregnancy. There is isolated arteritis/aneurysm rupture with catastrophic abdominal bleeding. This case, showing the upper abdominal tissues, involved a small branch of the celiac artery. The etiology is unclear, but diligent search for the bleeding point is advocated

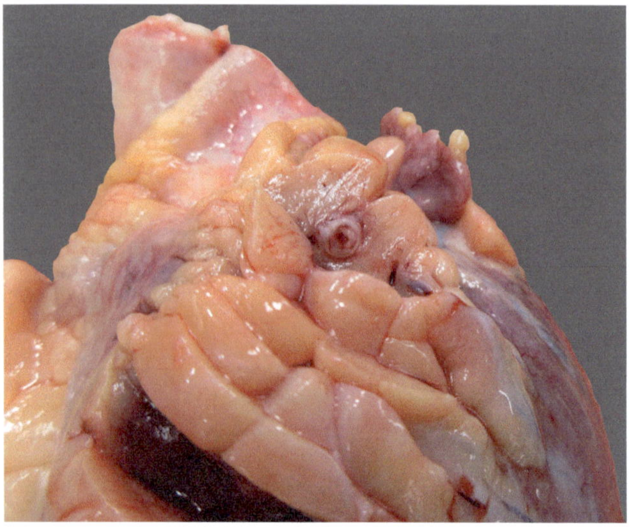

Fig. 6.101 Another example of sudden death in an otherwise healthy woman in the peri-partum period with pathology away from the uterus is shown here. The section of coronary artery shows dissection whereby creation of a false lumen is seen compressing the true lumen. Histology would be helpful in this case. Coronary artery dissection in these circumstances is a rare but well-recognised entity

of the fetus is often all that is required. This examination confirms normality in most cases.

It is recommended that a digital photograph of the genital tract tissues is undertaken for record purposes, but an image of the child may be helpful to the family at a later date. At least one image should be taken with a non-autopsy station background, such as an image akin to a sleeping child in blankets.

A fetal autopsy is rarely needed unless there is some specific issue regarding development. It should be remembered that, on occasion, a small amount of fetal or placental tissue should be retained for paternity tests. The fetal autopsy is beyond the scope of this text and the reader is advised to consult specialist texts accordingly or to seek advice or input from local paediatric pathologists.

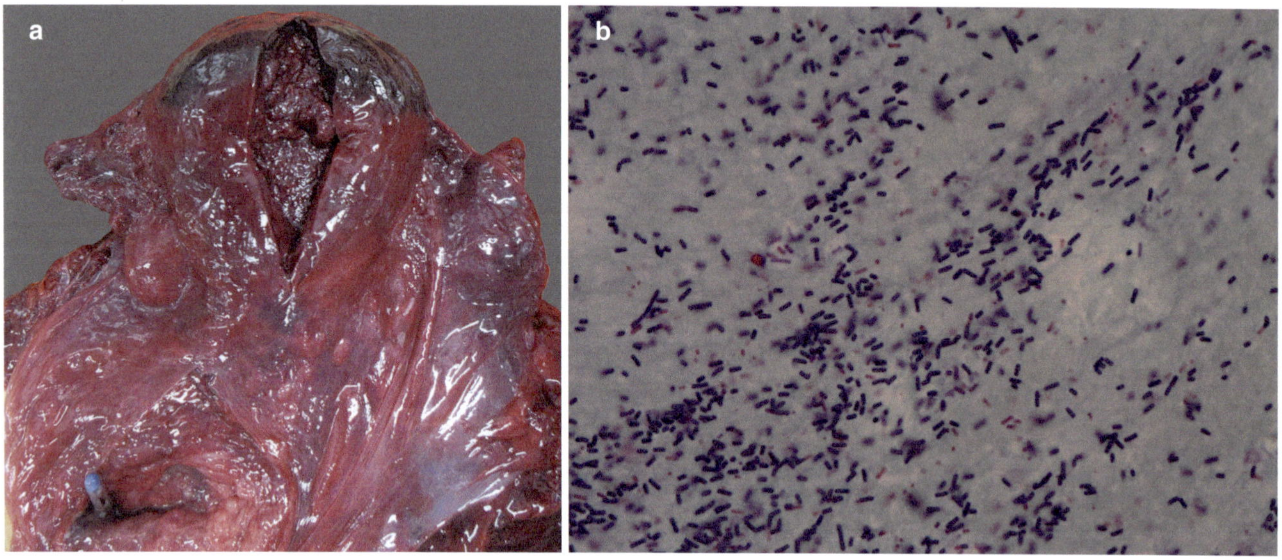

Fig. 6.102 Complications of miscarriage can occasionally lead to death. This is the diffusely congested uterus of a young female following surgical management for first trimester miscarriage whereby foul-smelling products of conception were removed. She later collapsed and could not be resuscitated. The endometrial cavity was haemorrhagic and contained friable material (**a**). Post-mortem microbiological sampling grew Clostridium perfringens pathogens from multiple sites. Histological review of the uterine tissue showed considerable gram-positive rods (**b**), in keeping with a genital tract source of sepsis, commensurate with the microbiology. Clostridium infection, specifically Clostridium perfringens, remains unfortunately a recognised significant human pathogen traditionally associated with contaminated limb injuries producing gas gangrene with subsequent septicaemia and death

Breast Tissue

The breast tissues (Figs. 6.103, 6.104, 6.105, 6.106, 6.107, 6.108, 6.109, 6.110, 6.111, 6.112, 6.113, 6.114, 6.115, 6.116, and 6.117) are rarely an important matter at autopsy. They are covered initially as part of the external examination. In most cases, simple palpation of the breast tissue will suffice. Breast implants are not uncommon, and care not to damage these is advised during evisceration. Rarely, breast implants

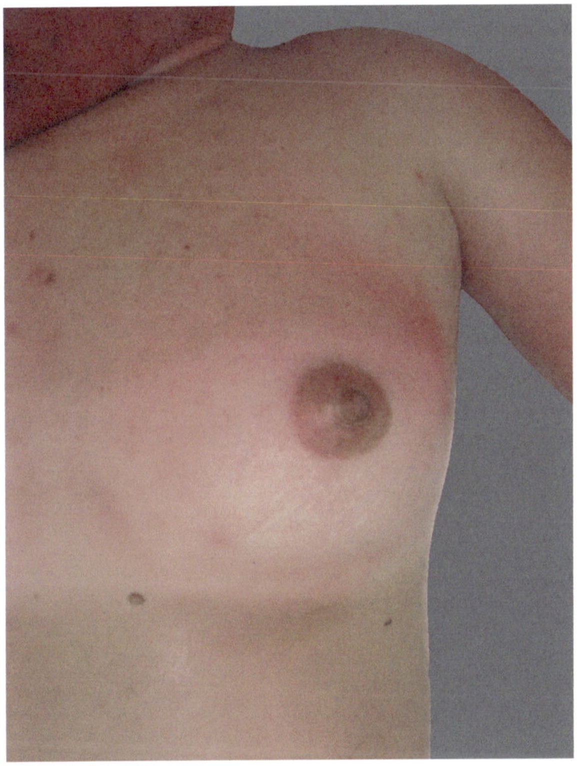

Fig. 6.103 Normal breast tissue is normally confirmed by visual inspection prior to the start of the invasive autopsy. Palpation of the axillae, to exclude nodal enlargement, and the breast parenchyma can be undertaken

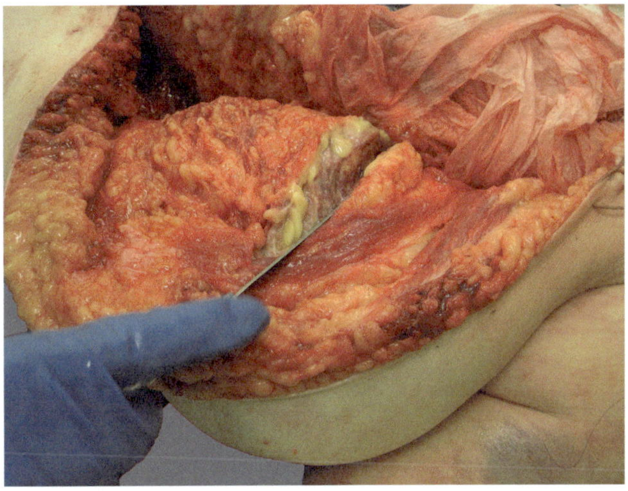

Fig. 6.104 If there is concern about the breast tissue, serially slicing the parenchyma on the internal aspect (i.e. without damaging the external breast skin) can be undertaken to search for focal lesions. Shown is some wadding around the sharp cut ends of the rib cage

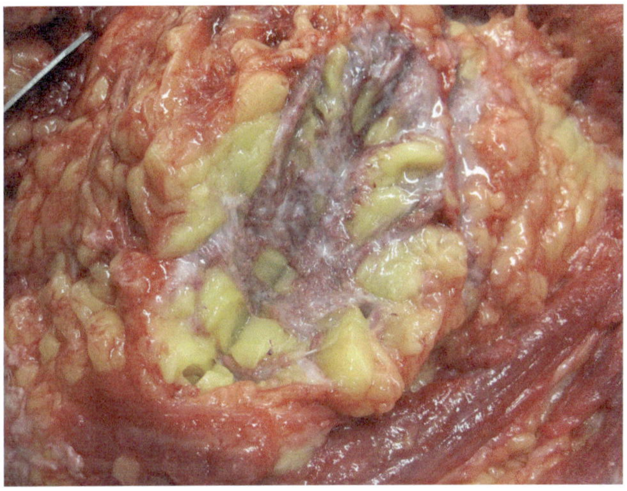

Fig. 6.105 Breast tissue can change significantly during pregnancy, with the acinar parenchyma being particularly prominent. Significant secretory development occurs towards the end of pregnancy

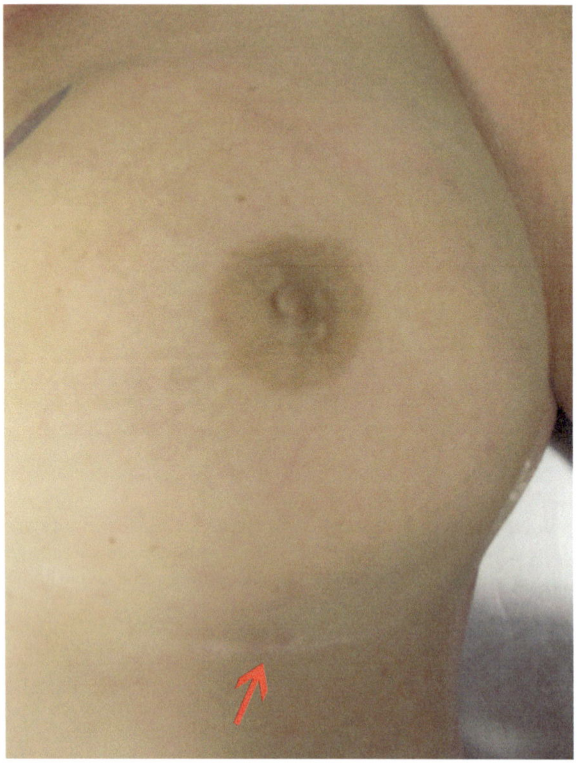

Fig. 6.106 Breast implants are increasingly seen in the autopsy room. This apparently normal breast tissue is seen to have scarring under the breast, in keeping with prosthetic breast enlargement. Characteristic sites include centrally below the breast and high in the axilla. The scar (arrow) often gives the first indication of an implant

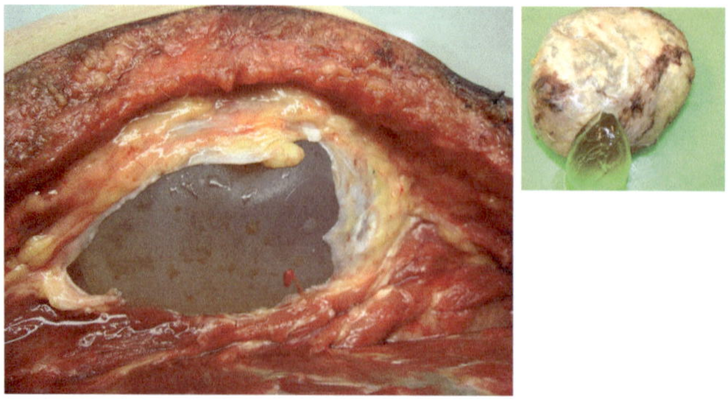

Fig. 6.108 Opening the body during evisceration may demonstrate the prosthesis (left). It is important not to damage the prosthesis during evisceration so that body reconstruction can proceed without significant change to the anatomical boundaries seen ante mortem. Modern implants have less associated fibrosis than those used previously (right) and are no longer filled with silicone materials

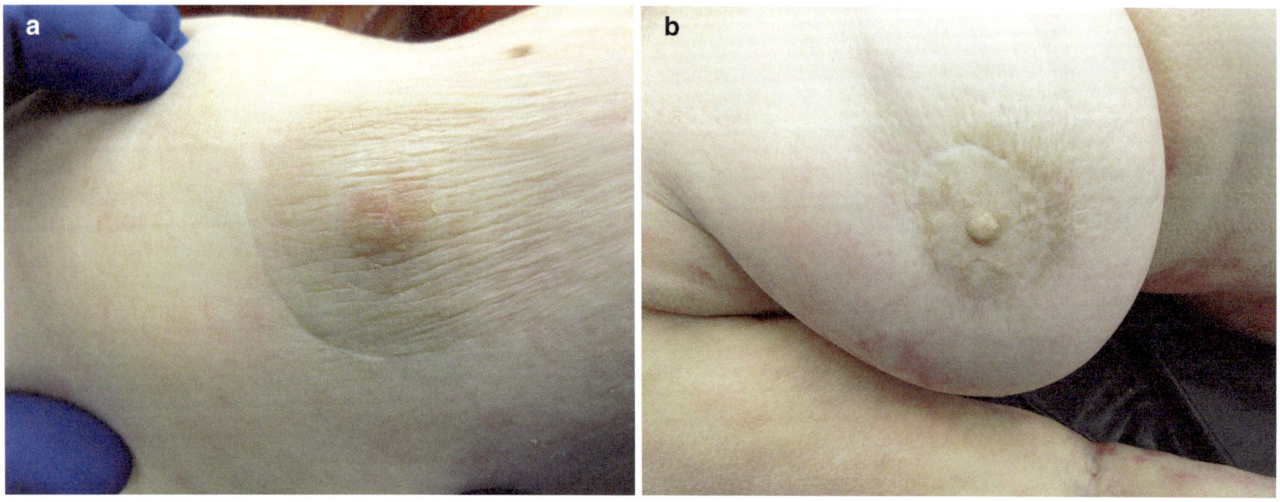

Fig. 6.107 Scars pertaining to breast surgery may be intentionally subtle, hidden within skin lines of tension, where possible surgically. This can make them difficult to appreciate on first look. The nipple can be relocated or manipulated surgically during cosmetic or reconstructive surgery. (**a**, **b**) The scars seen in these pictures are on the areola edge and would be easy to overlook without careful examination

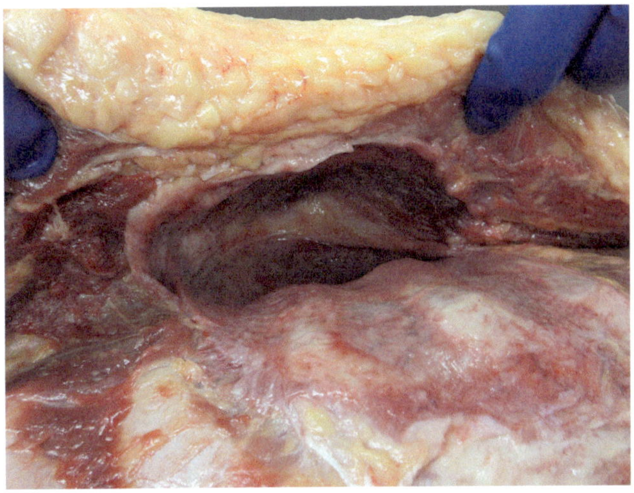

Fig. 6.109 The soft tissues of the chest wall have been lifted to reveal the cavitary defect in which a breast implant was sited, without complication. The anterior ribs are seen beneath the smooth-walled cavity

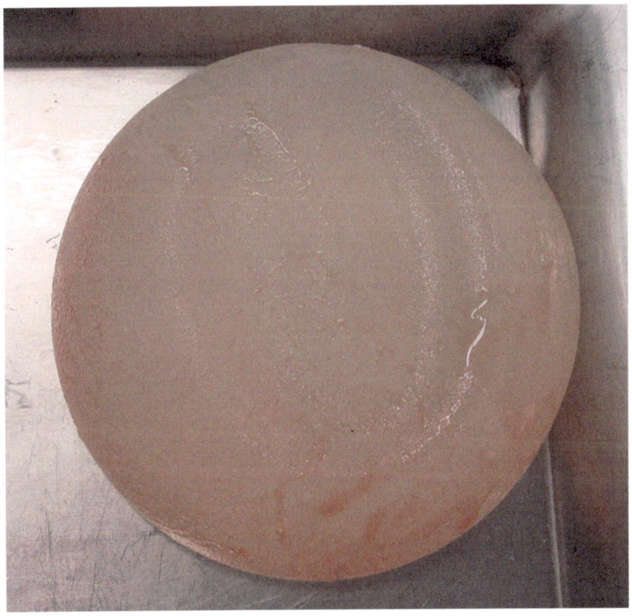

Fig. 6.110 A modern breast implant is shown following removal from the body. Removal of breast implants is not a requirement but has been undertaken here to demonstrate normality. Such implants can be re-sited during the autopsy

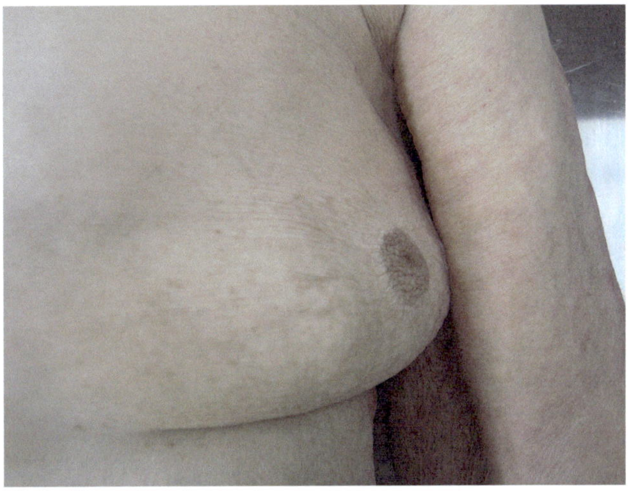

Fig. 6.111 The presence of breast cancer is often seen as an ill-defined lump (here, medial to the in-drawn nipple) on naked eye examination

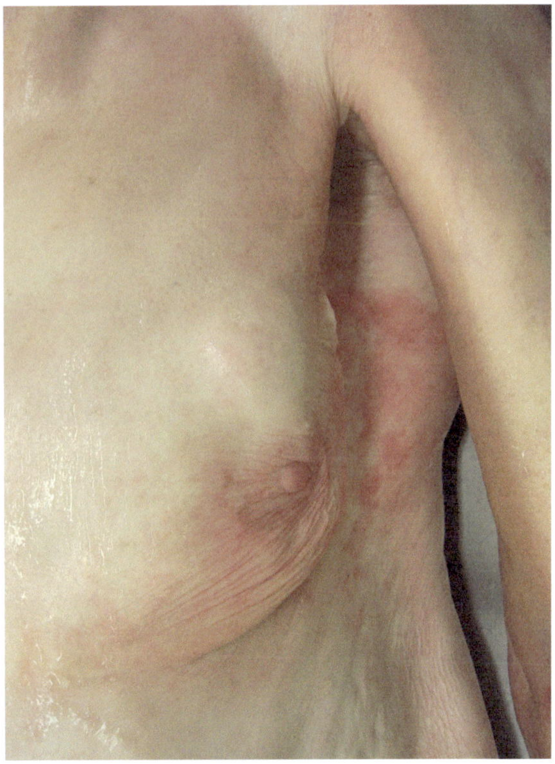

Fig. 6.112 Another case of breast cancer is seen from the external aspect. There is a tumour above the nipple

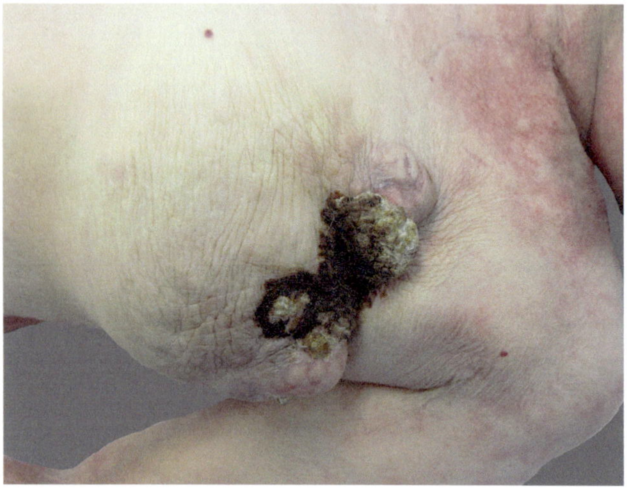

Fig. 6.113 Advanced breast cancer is seen here as a fungating tumour surrounded by subcutaneous nodules with overlying skin changes. This appearance of advanced disease is uncommon in modern healthcare settings. However, occasionally patients present late with such disease

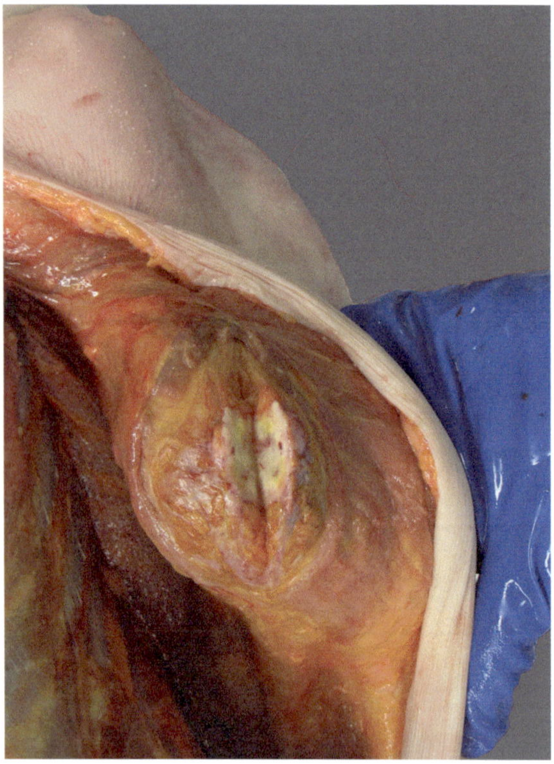

Fig. 6.114 Primary breast cancer is seen with a fatty and scirrhous cut surface, sliced from the inner aspect

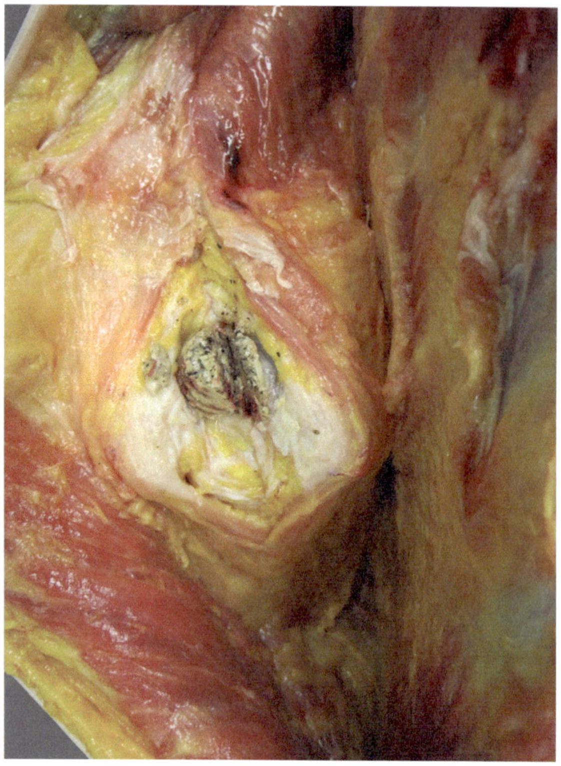

Fig. 6.115 The breast cancer here has been treated with radiotherapy. Note the enhanced sclerosis, zone of old haemorrhage and necrosis centrally

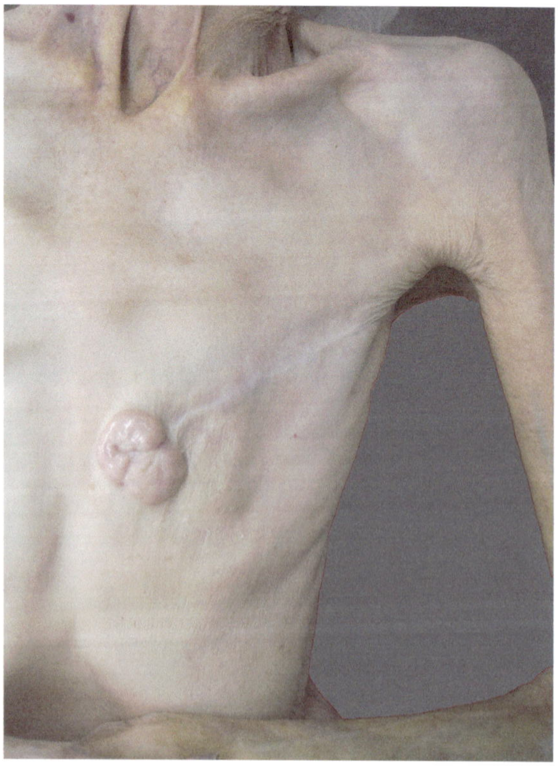

Fig. 6.116 This previous mastectomy site is noted to have recurrent tumour at the medial end. This may suggest disseminated disease elsewhere in the body. Due diligence to consider metastatic sites is recommended

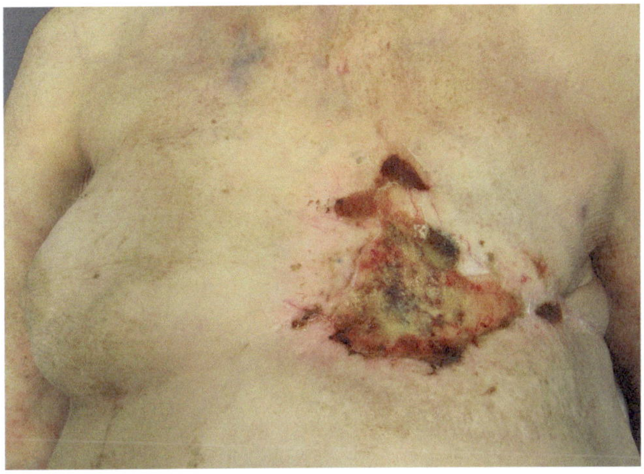

Fig. 6.117 Recurrent breast cancer can be widespread on the chest and destructive in nature. This previous mastectomy site showed extensive skin infiltration by tumour that ran into the local musculature, deeper parenchyma and indeed the bone. Widespread distant metastases were also present

can be associated with sepsis, particularly in the early post-operative period. Natural tissue breast infections are rare, but tumours should always be sought initially by internal and external palpation. Slicing the breast from the internal aspect (i.e. after the chest has had the skin/soft tissues dissected free from the rib cage) will allow detailed review of the breast parenchyma. One should ideally not cut into the skin overlying the breast for cosmetic and reconstructive reasons. Benign tumours (e.g. fibroadenomas) are occasionally found, but malignancy is a not uncommon reality in the autopsy room. Malignant tumours of the breast may be pertinent to the cause of death, although disseminated disease is usually the pathology of significance.

Suggested Reading

Amin MB, Tickoo SK. Diagnostic pathology: genitourinary. 2nd ed. Philadelphia, PA: Elsevier; 2016.

Burton JL, Rutty G. The hospital autopsy. 3rd ed. Hodder Arnold; 2010. p. 115–58, 203–15.

Connolly AJ, Finkbeiner WE, Ursell PC, Davis RL, editors. Autopsy pathology: a manual and atlas. 3rd ed. Philadelphia, PA: Elsevier; 2016.

Cooke RA, Stewart B. Renal system; male genital system; breast and female genital system. In: Colour atlas of anatomical pathology. 3rd ed. Edinburgh: Churchill Livingstone; 2004. p. 131–44, 145–52, 153–82.

Curran RC, Jones EL. Kidneys and bladder; male generative system; female generative system including breast. In: Gross pathology. A color atlas. Harvey Millar HM + M Publishers; 1974. p. 91–101, 102–6, 107–18.

Goldblum JR, Lamps LW, McKenney JK, Myers JL. Genitourinary pathology, female reproductive system, breast. In: Rosai and Ackerman's surgical pathology. 11th ed. Edinburgh: Elsevier; 2017. p. 936–1529.

Kumar V, Abbas AK, Aster JC, Deyrup AT, Das A. Kidney, male genital system and lower urinary tract, female genital system and breast. In: Robbins & Kumar basic pathology. 11th ed. Elsevier; 2022. p. 449–82, 582–635.

Ludwig J. Handbook of autopsy practice. 3rd ed. Ottawa: Humana Press; 2002.

7 Lymphoreticular Tissues: Lymph Node, Spleen, Thymus, Bone and Marrow

S. Kim Suvarna and Abigail K. Sharp

Introduction

The tissues of the lymphoreticular system are often examined almost incidentally as one performs an autopsy. These tissues are rarely the primary focus of the disease, unless considering the bony tissues and fractures. Yet this widespread group of tissues is responsible for many aspects of haematological and immune function, so it is not uncommon to see minor pathology of relevance during the post-mortem examination.

The lymph nodes commonly vary in size and shape when one considers the various types of autopsy cases. Localised or generalised lymphadenopathy may point towards systemic infections, autoimmune conditions, or neoplasia. Some histology sampling of such nodes is recommended, but one also should not forget to consider reserving some tissue for microbiology testing. Correlation against clinical data is always important.

The spleen, found adjacent to the stomach and left kidney, is easy to identify. In most autopsies it will be of normal shape and configuration, but cystic change, nodularity, or gross enlargement may point to either local or systemic disorders. Softening of the tissues may point towards sepsis.

The thymus atrophies, in relative terms, as one ages. Whilst relatively easy to identify in infancy and early childhood, the thymus is more difficult to appreciate as the amount of mediastinal fat increases. Indeed, most autopsy practitioners say they cannot find the thymus in the elderly. It is often relatively easy to define at the superior boundary of the pericardial sac, however, even in the elderly. The thymus is rarely of significance unless a tumour is present.

Unless there are fractures, the bone and marrow are rarely pursued during the autopsy examination. The presence of osteoporosis is common with increasing age and may be a significant factor in terms of fractures and local complications. Histology may be relevant, but bone invariably needs fixation and decalcification.

Lymph Nodes and Related Tissues

The tonsils (Figs. 7.1, 7.2, and 7.3) form a ring of lymphoid tissue located in the soft tissues of the posterior oropharynx. They are principally abnormal in infections or involvement by lymphoma or head and neck squamous carcinomas.

Lymph nodes (Figs. 7.4, 7.5, 7.6, 7.7, 7.8, 7.9, 7.10, 7.11, 7.12, and 7.13) are often found to be variably enlarged at autopsy. In most cases, this reflects terminal septic conditions, principally in the chest. Reactive nodal hyperplasia and infections are a common reality of autopsy practice. For this reason, some lymph node tissue sampling (histology and microbiology) may be of assistance when faced with diffuse lymphadenopathy.

In the elderly, it is not uncommon to find low-grade, unsuspected chronic lymphocytic leukaemia or lymphocytic lymphoma. Metastatic carcinoma (sometimes unsuspected) requires both macroscopic assessment of abnormal tissue in the lymph nodes and histological confirmation. The primary site should be sought.

Rarely, atypical infections, autoimmune disease, and other infiltrates may present as nodal enlargement—highlighting the need for histology and for microbiology to exclude sepsis.

S. Kim Suvarna was deceased at the time of publication.

S. K. Suvarna (Deceased) · A. K. Sharp (✉)
Department of Histopathology, Sheffield Teaching Hospitals NHS Foundation Trust, Sheffield, UK
e-mail: abigail.sharp@nhs.net

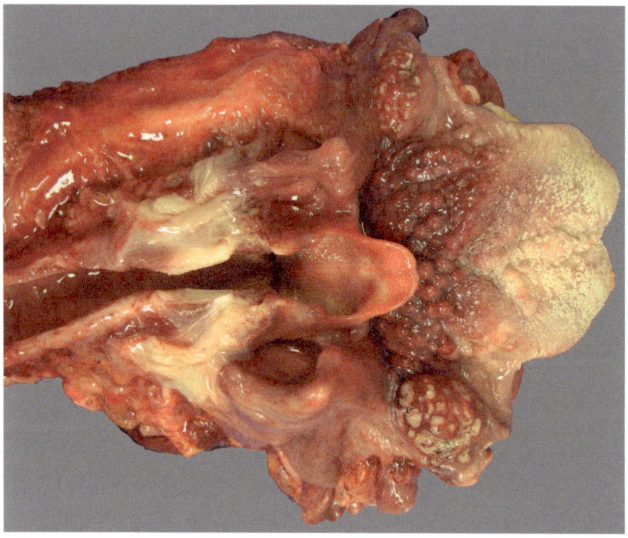

Fig. 7.1 Tonsillitis is a rare pathology in the autopsy room. Most cases reflect sepsis, as shown here with pus on the tonsil surface, but lymphomas must be considered

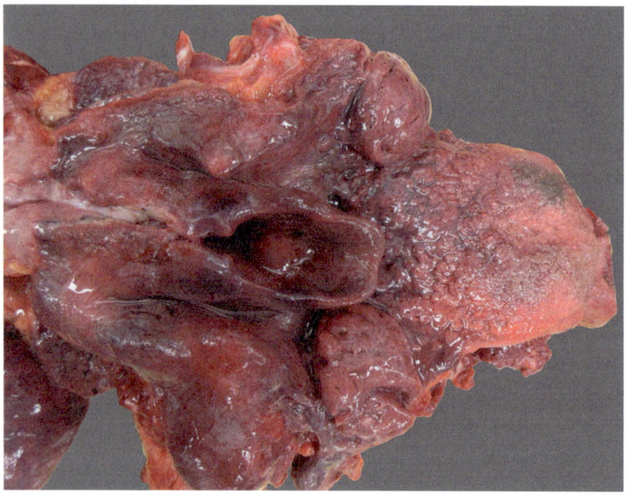

Fig. 7.2 The upper larynx and oropharynx are seen here with congestion and autolytic change. The tonsils are markedly enlarged and show pits present, without pus. This was a case of group A streptococcal infection with tonsillitis. There is widespread autolysis of tissues very early on following death of the individual. Note, there is no encroachment of the laryngeal airway but the systemic sepsis from the tonsilitis was sufficient to explain this person's death

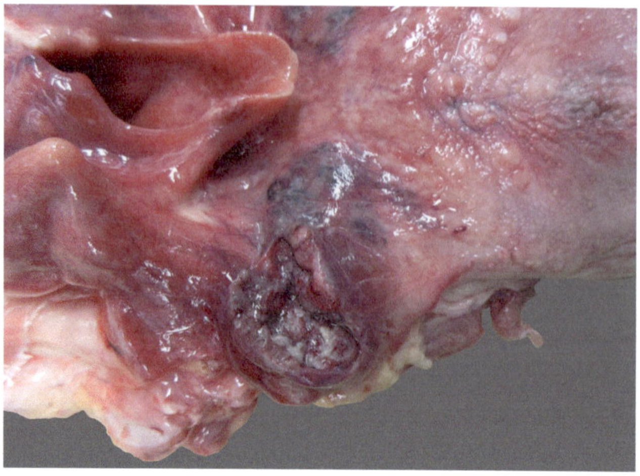

Fig. 7.3 Carcinoma of the tonsil is seen here with an ulcerated tumour on the right side of the oropharynx. The two most common lesions at this site include squamous carcinoma and lymphoma

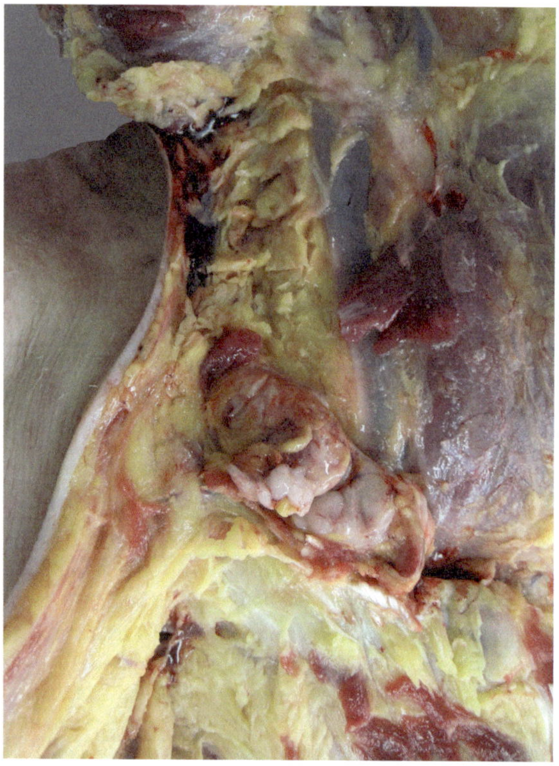

Fig. 7.4 Lymphadenopathy in the neck requires histology. It can reflect not only sepsis (*e.g.*, mycobacterial infections) but also thoracic, cranial, or distal metastatic neoplasia and primary lymphomas

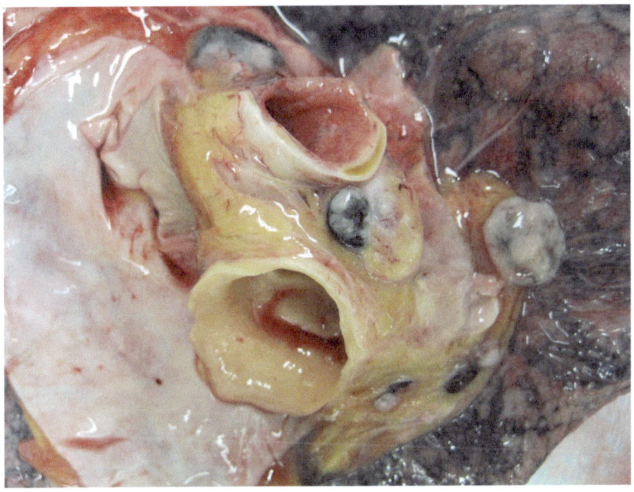

Fig. 7.5 Lymphadenopathy within the neck may represent thoracic disease or head and neck cancers. Some enlarged and partly necrotic nodes containing tumour are seen at the base of the neck structures immediately adjacent to the trachea

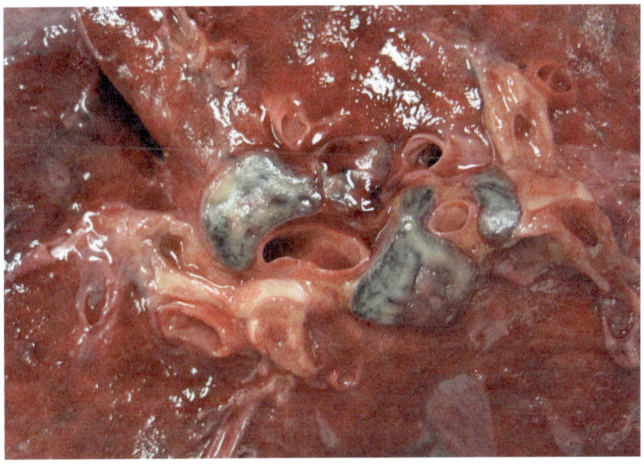

Fig. 7.6 The lymph nodes within the chest are often pigmented owing to inhaled particulates. Consequently, lymph nodes are often grey and black in colour. Variegation of the nodes, as seen in this image, does not automatically imply pathology, but any large nodes should be sampled for histology

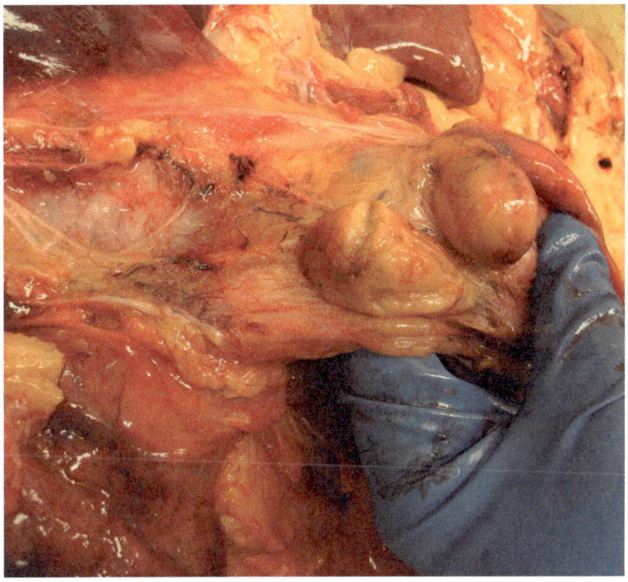

Fig. 7.7 Even single enlarged nodes in the body merit histology to consider the possibility of neoplasia and/or inflammatory conditions

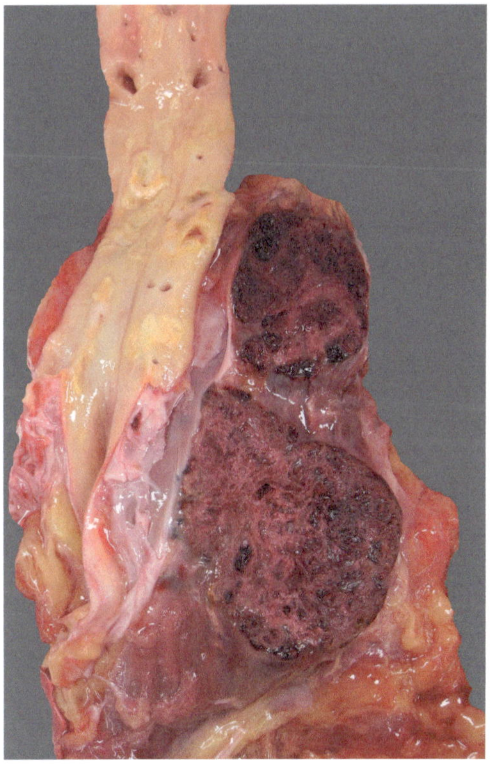

Fig. 7.8 Mediastinal nodal involvement often can occur with metastases. This case of choriocarcinoma was noted to widely infiltrate the soft tissues around the aorta and to compress local lung and cardiac tissues. Note the haemorrhagic and fleshy quality, akin to placental tissue

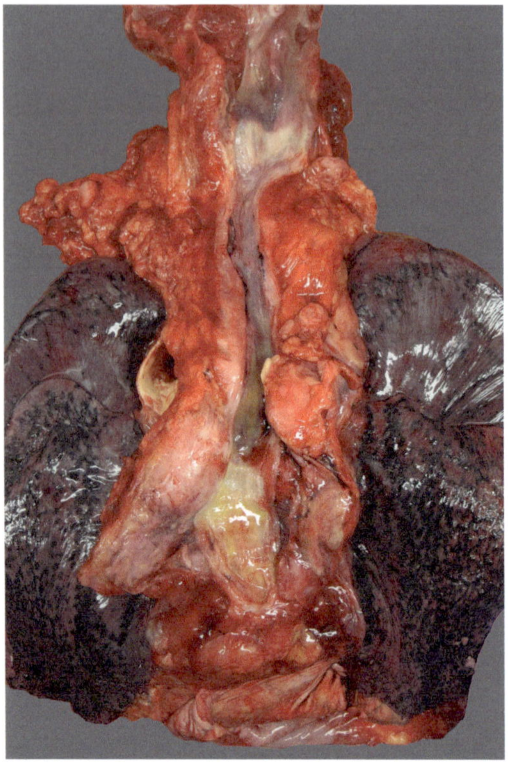

Fig. 7.9 Multiple-site thoracic lymphadenopathy may be a feature of inflammatory conditions (*e.g.*, sarcoid or mycobacterial infection), apart from lymphomas. The final interpretation requires histology and microbiology

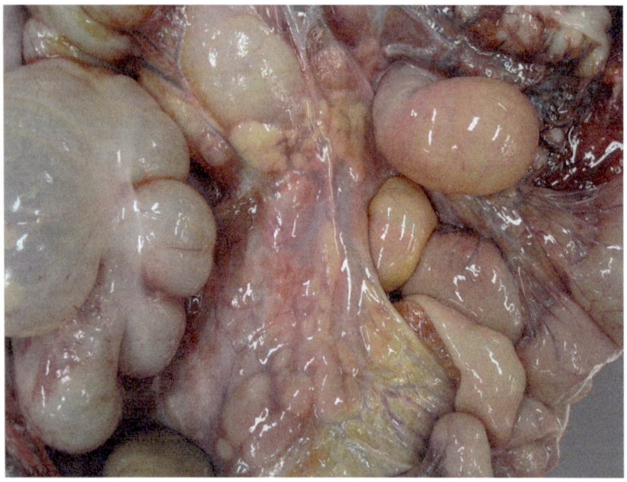

Fig. 7.10 If there is relative paucity of fat, then lymphadenopathy is relatively easy to identify. The lymph nodes in this view of the mesentery appear to be of variable size and clustered within the mesentery support tissues. Palpation of the mesentery should take place during resection of the bowel tissues at evisceration, to avoid missing adenopathy in individuals with adipose-rich mesentery

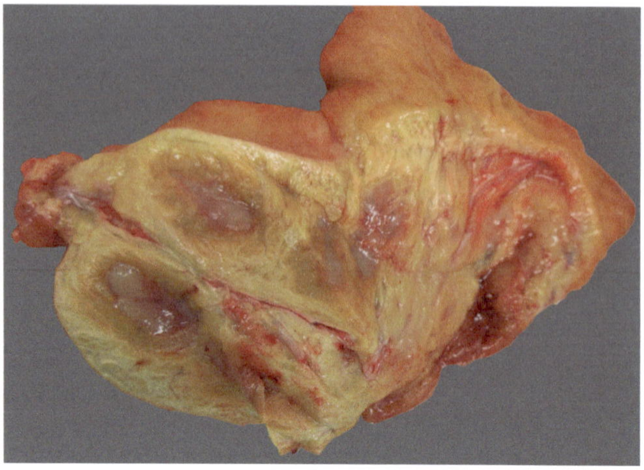

Fig. 7.11 This is fatty mesenteric tissue with some lymph nodes embedded within. These are probably reactive lymph nodes as they have no firm hard boundary and do not appear particularly enlarged. The driving force for reactive changes is often unclear at autopsy. A history of lymphoma or suspicion of lymphoma may prompt histological analysis of nodes with such an appearance

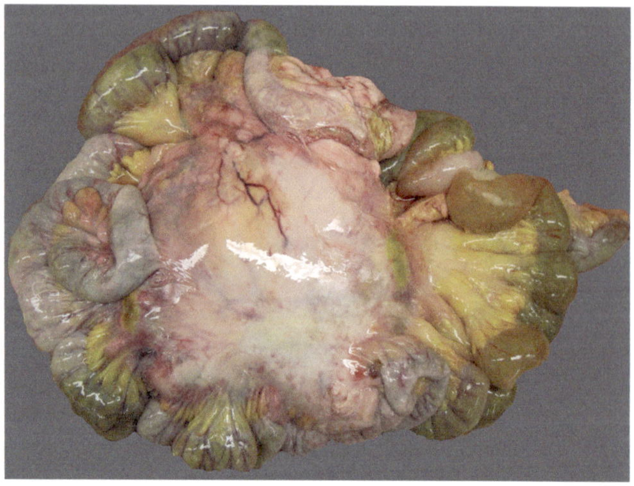

Fig. 7.12 Lymphadenopathy can be seen within the abdomen with enlarged nodes, occasionally merging into one large tumour mass, in the mesentery. Such cases often reflect lymphomatous neoplasia

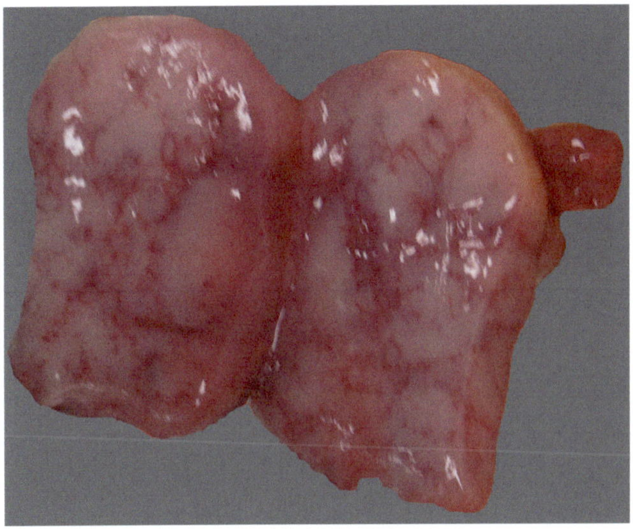

Fig. 7.13 The cut section of an enlarged node gives a clue as to the pathology. Carcinomas are often fibrous or sclerotic, whereas soft, fleshy nodes (such as this) often point towards lymphomatous disease. Rapid assessment can be undertaken by frozen section or imprint cytology, even at autopsy

Spleen

The spleen (Figs. 7.14, 7.15, 7.16, 7.17, 7.18, 7.19, 7.20, 7.21, 7.22, 7.23, and 7.24) normally weighs 100–150 g. It generally shows little relevance to the autopsy; that is, it is usually of normal weight, shape, and form. It may be enlarged, however, from background processes (*e.g.*, autoimmune conditions or cirrhosis). In these circumstances, the cut surface parenchyma usually is still unremarkable.

In terminal septicemia or bacteremia, the splenic tissues often appear soft and semifluid on section. If sepsis is suspected, the outer surface of the spleen should be sterilized by the application of alcohol and/or formalin, given that a hot metal to sear the surface is generally not a commonplace tool in the modern autopsy room.

The splenic tissues also can be involved by tumours. These commonly comprise lymphomas although metastatic carcinomas and angiomatous processes are also well recognised.

Splenic trauma is of particular importance. Any capsular tear or deficit should be recorded in terms of position and size, with an assessment of blood volume lost locally.

Gross enlargement should raise the suspicion of atypical infections such as malaria or leishmaniasis.

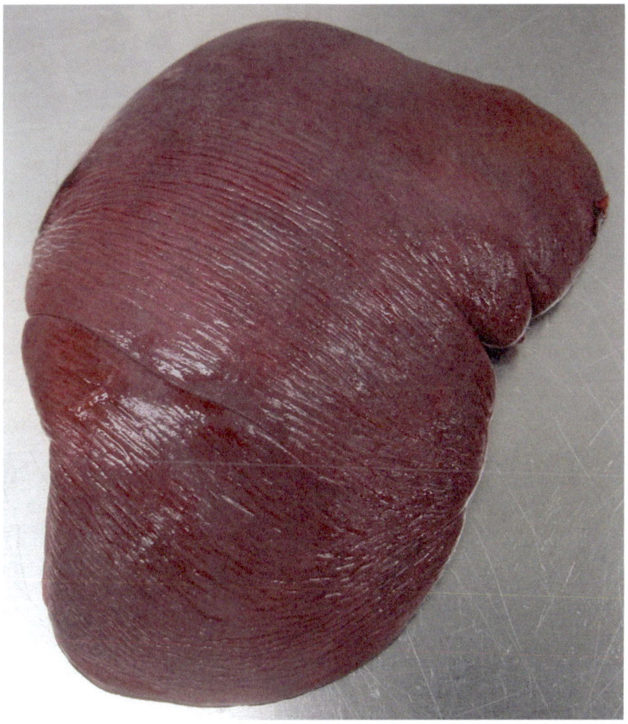

Fig. 7.14 The normal spleen (100–150 g) shows a characteristic slightly wrinkled capsular surface and abuts the tail of the pancreas. It lies adjacent to the stomach and under the rib cage

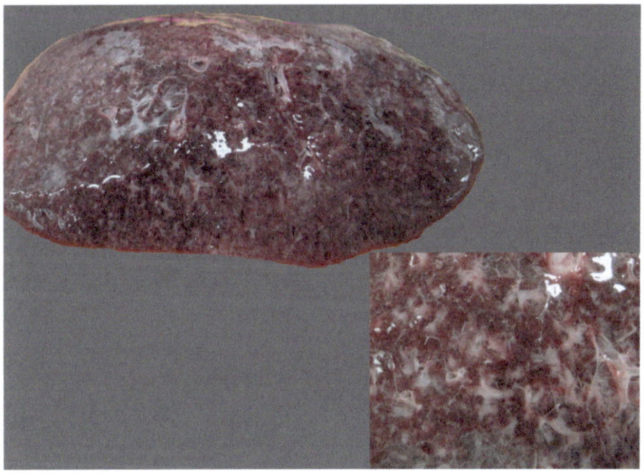

Fig. 7.15 The cut surface of the spleen shows a characteristic mottled architecture with different coloured elements. These are described as white pulp and red pulp, with the white elements representing periarterial lymphoid sheaths and connective tissues, which are active in immune states. The red pulp tissues are sinusoids in which effete circulating blood cells are removed along with other extraneous matter. The *low right inset* shows a high magnification of the spleen

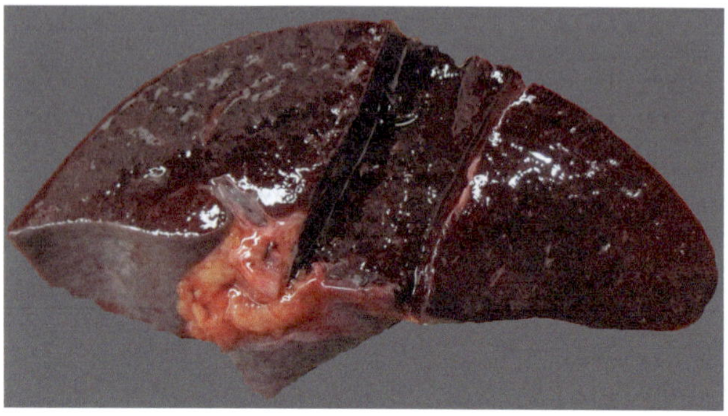

Fig. 7.16 When considering tissues to be sampled for genetic studies, the high density of lymphoid elements within the spleen favours this organ as a common source of DNA. It is recommended that a 1 to 2 cm cubed portion of tissue be removed from the spleen (as indicated in this post-sampling image) and placed in a sterile container. The DNA can be extracted immediately, or the sample may be frozen for subsequent DNA analysis

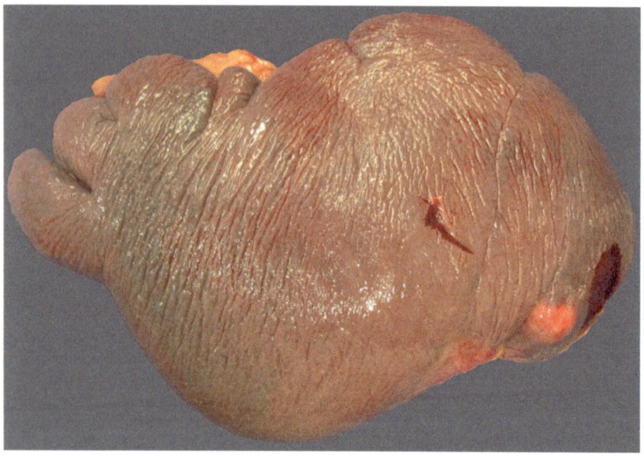

Fig. 7.17 Small tears of the spleen capsule often occur during evisceration and handling. These artefacts should not be construed as significant unless local bleeding is apparent, in which case they reflect ante-mortem problems

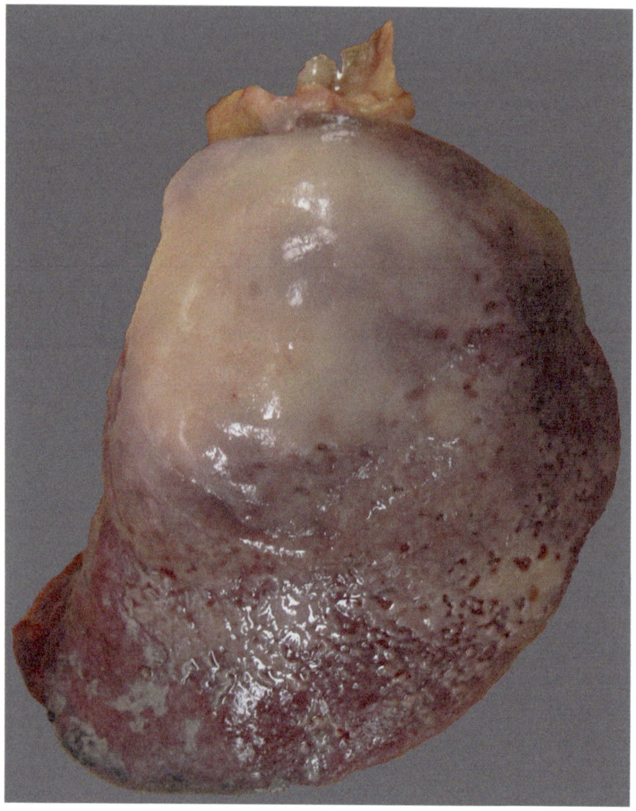

Fig. 7.18 A common feature of splenic tissues is a surface fibrinous exudate (generally described as 'sugar-icing') that is organized focally or entirely around the spleen tissues. It is of no pathological consequence

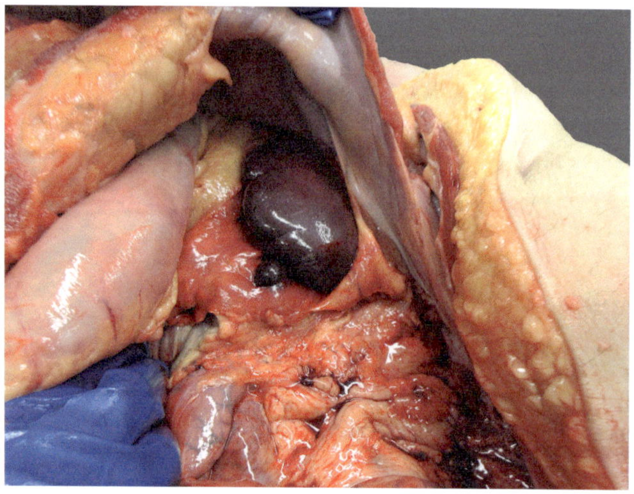

Fig. 7.19 A rounded splenunculus is seen adjacent to the normal spleen in the upper left quadrant of the abdomen. The spleen often has a small focus of similar spleen tissue adjacent. The splenunculus can vary in size and has exactly the same morphology and function as normal spleen tissues

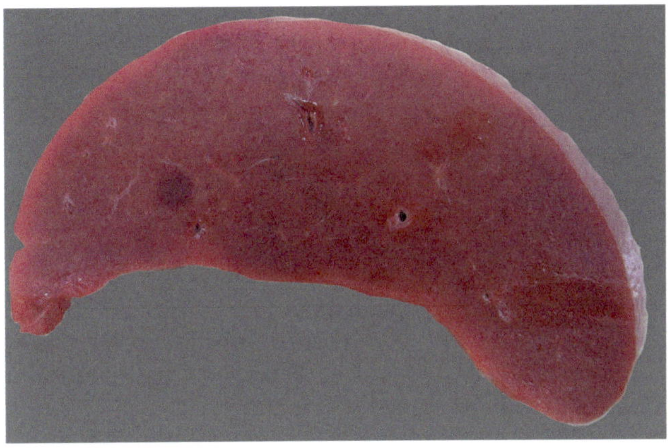

Fig. 7.20 This is lardaceous spleen showing firm enlarged splenic tissues with a rather colloid-like matrix. Histologically, this tissue comprised more than 50% amyloid parenchyma with only residual splenic elements being seen

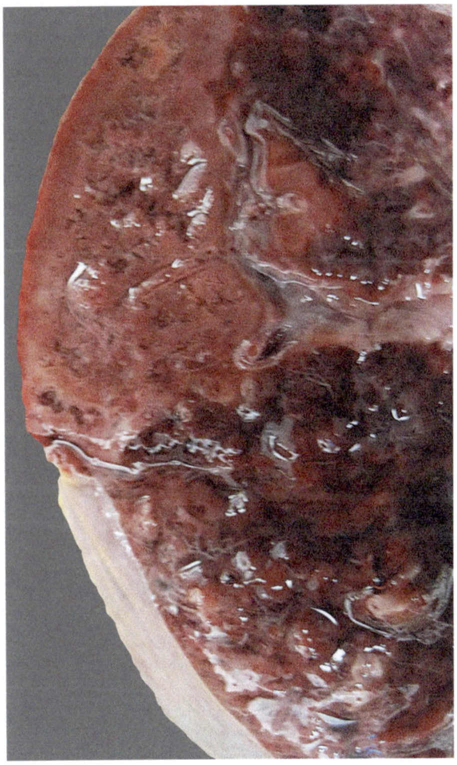

Fig. 7.21 This close-up of the edge of a spleen shows a wedge-shaped splenic infarct, representing an embolus from a case of infective endocarditis

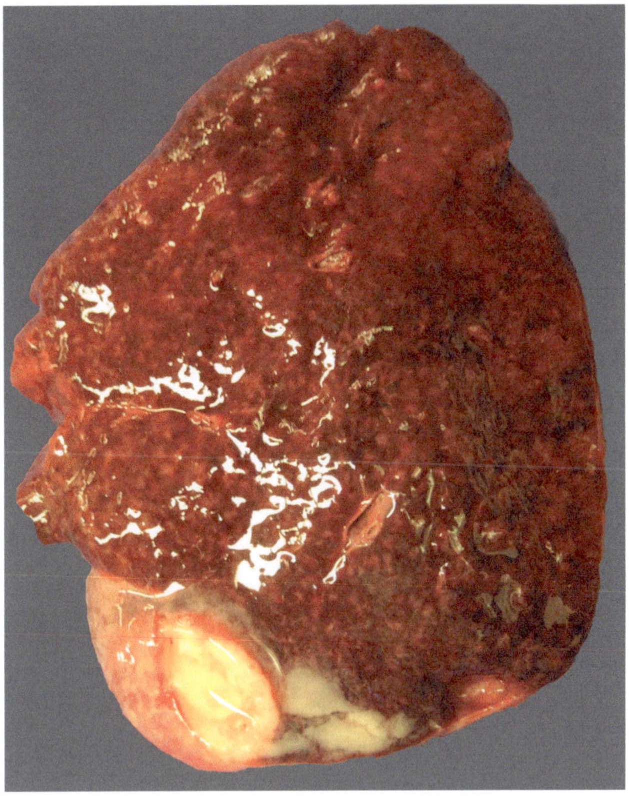

Fig. 7.22 Splenic tissues can be involved by neoplasia. The commonest are tumours of the haemopoietic system (leukaemia or lymphoma), although metastatic lung cancer (as in this case) also can be found in splenic tissues

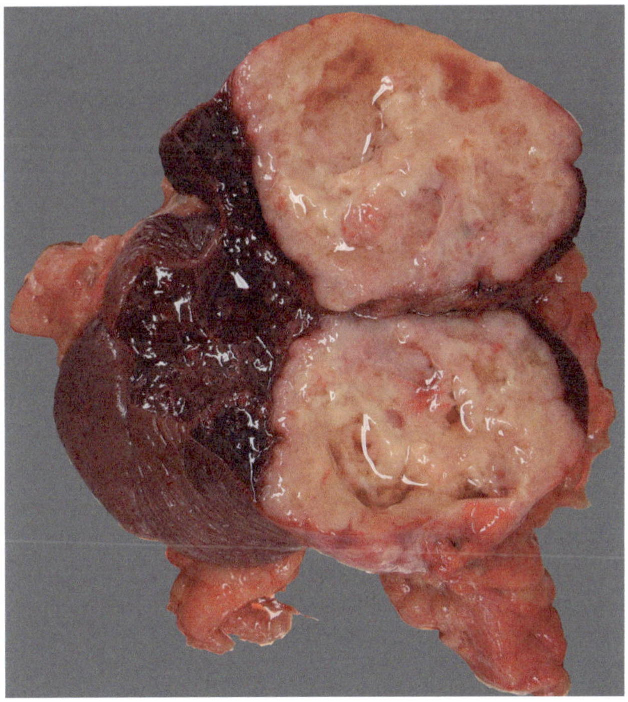

Fig. 7.23 Metastatic tumour is seen within the spleen shown here. Unusually, in this case this is an example of mesothelioma

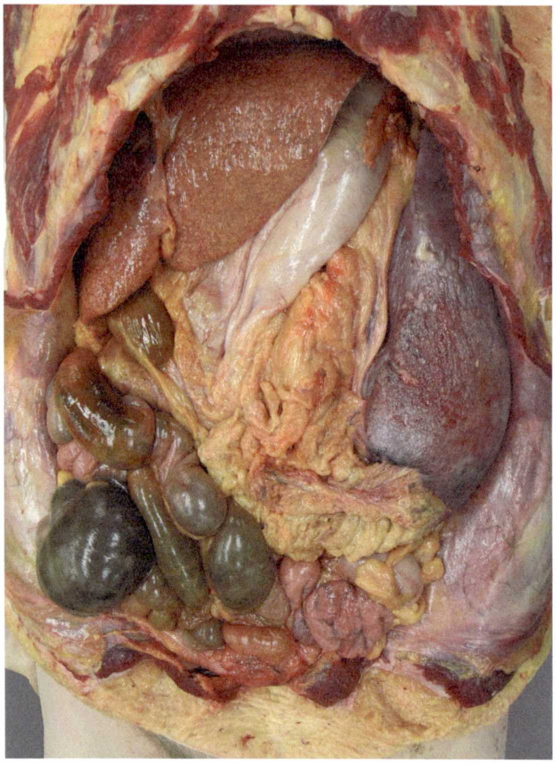

Fig. 7.24 Gross splenic enlargement may be an unsuspected finding at autopsy. In this case, the splenic enlargement was due to chronic lymphocytic leukaemia. One should always be aware of the possibility of other malignant infiltrates, and one should also consider leishmaniasis in those coming from abroad

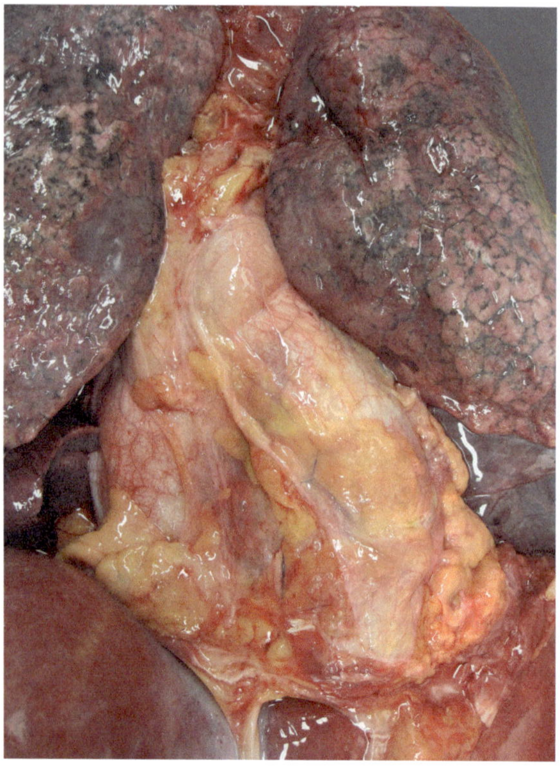

Fig. 7.25 The position of the normal thymus may be seen centrally and high within the mediastinum of this 20-year-old man. There is a clear 'bulge' where the tissue lies

Thymus

The thymus (Figs. 7.25, 7.26, 7.27, 7.28, 7.29, 7.30, 7.31, 7.32, 7.33, and 7.34) is normally found at the superior/anterior aspect of the pericardial sac, immediately behind the sternal tissues. Its size can be quite variable, but generally it is about 40 mm in cross-section. The weight varies depending on the amount of fatty tissue and the diligence with which one dissects normal fatty tissue away from the thymic parenchyma.

It is fair to state that the thymus is rarely involved in pathology of importance at autopsy. Mild prominence of fatty thymic tissues in the adult is often nonspecific macroscopically. Nevertheless, basic examination of the thymic tissues should occur at the time of opening the pericardial sac, in order to exclude localised neoplasia, cystic change, or indeed hyperplastic phenomena. If these are present, then histological interpretation is advised.

Thymic pathology in rare cases tends to occur in autoimmune disorders and also can occur in generalised inflammatory conditions. In such cases, histology is recommended for assessment. Likewise, thymic tissues can be enlarged by infiltration of the parenchyma by lymphoma. Rare tumours include carcinoid, germ cell, and thymic epithelial neoplasia. All possible neoplastic processes require histological assessment.

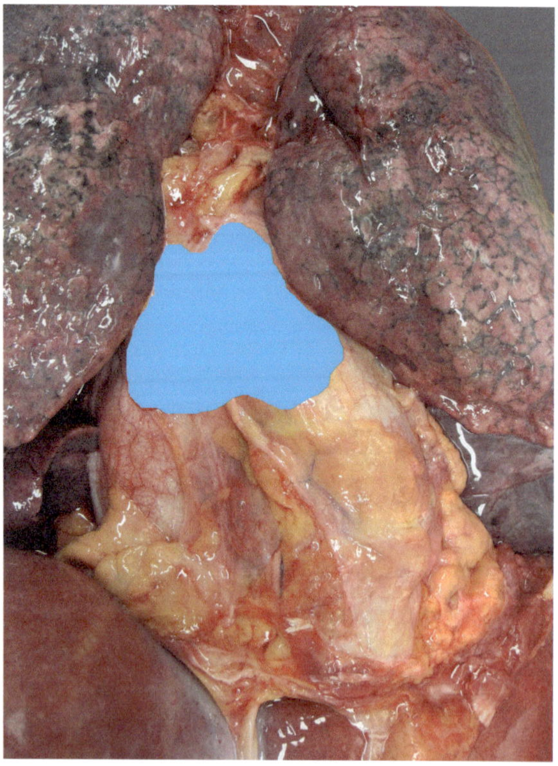

Fig. 7.26 The same view as Fig. 7.25 is shown with the position and shape of the thymus marked in blue

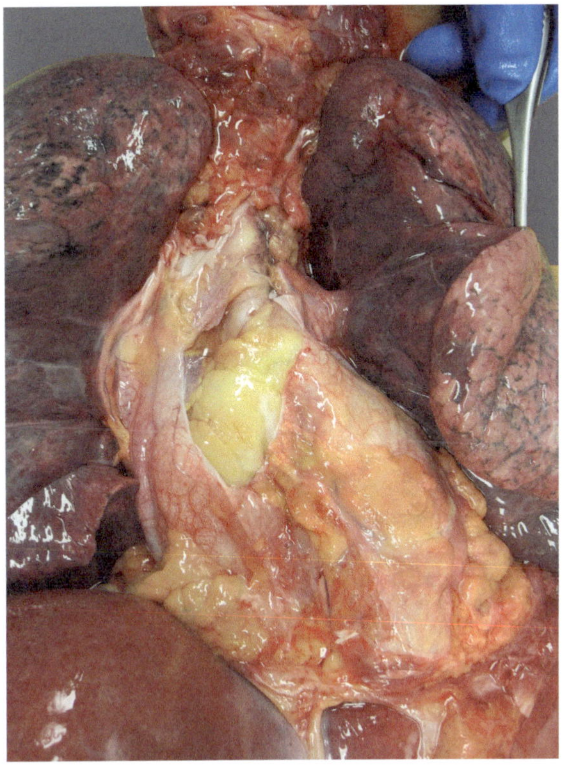

Fig. 7.27 The upper mediastinal tissue is shown with the thymus now resected

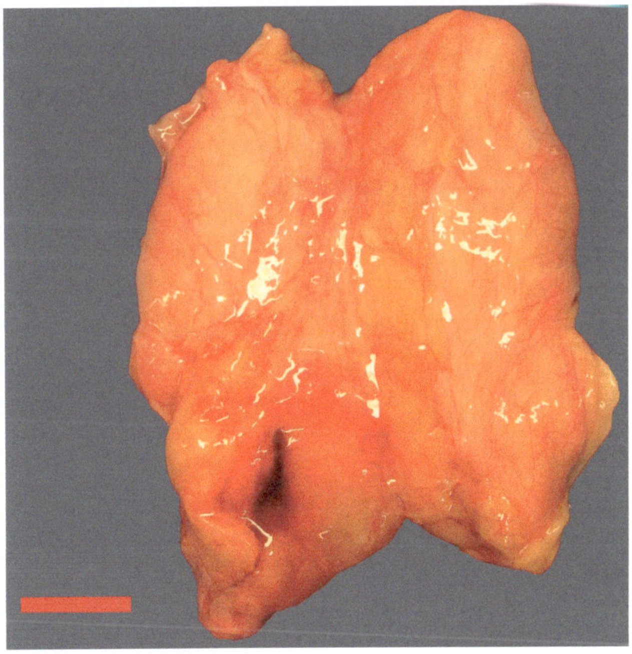

Fig. 7.28 The resected thymus is seen from the anterior aspect

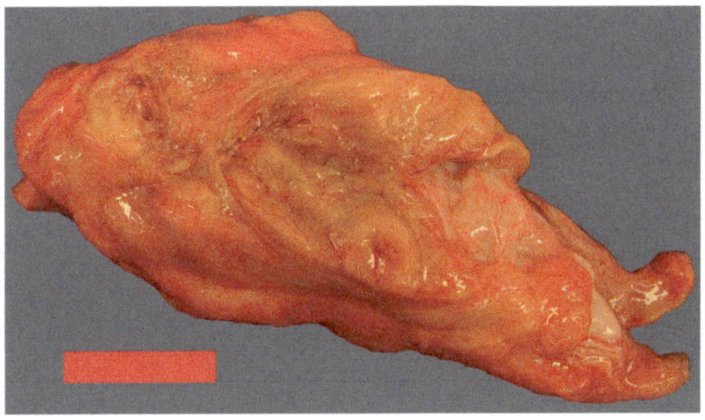

Fig. 7.29 The thymic cut surface is displayed

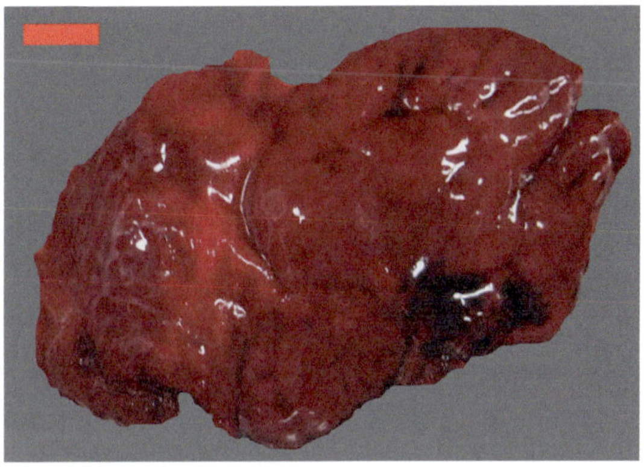

Fig. 7.30 The thymus of a teenager often appears more congested and has less fat than that of an elderly person. The appearance does not automatically imply disease, but softening of the tissue may point towards inflammatory or septic processes

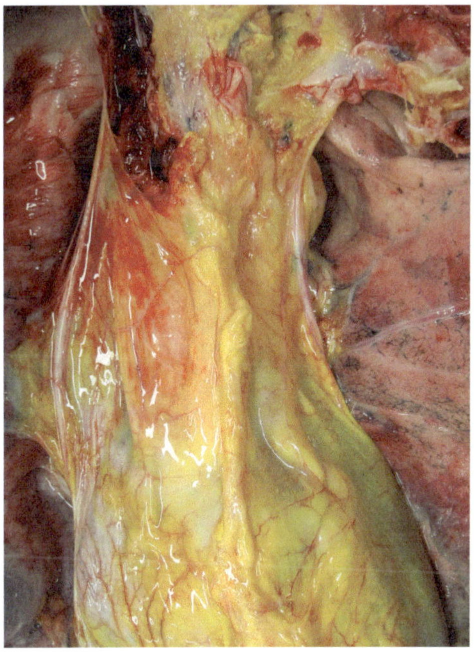

Fig. 7.31 The atrophic thymus in the elderly is more difficult to identify within the mediastinal soft tissues. This image shows fatty tissue over the front of the heart and upper mediastinum without a clearly defined thymus being evident. Nevertheless, if one sections in the central part of the tissue, atrophic elements of thymic tissue will be identified. There is some haemorrhage towards the upper right side of the mediastinum in this case, in keeping with placement of an intravenous central line

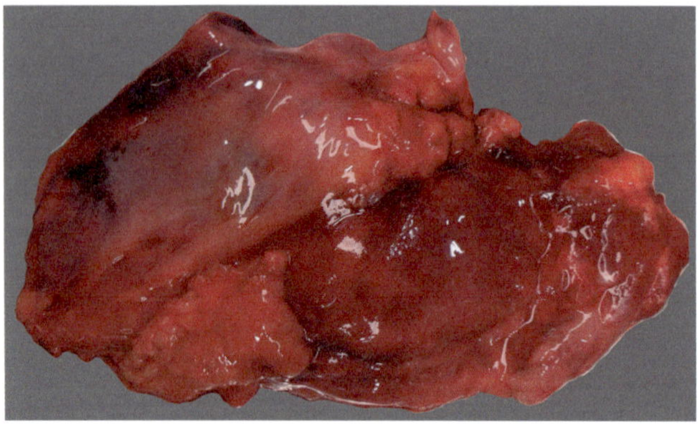

Fig. 7.32 This is a large thymus, which histologically showed only hyperplastic phenomena. No neoplasia was identified

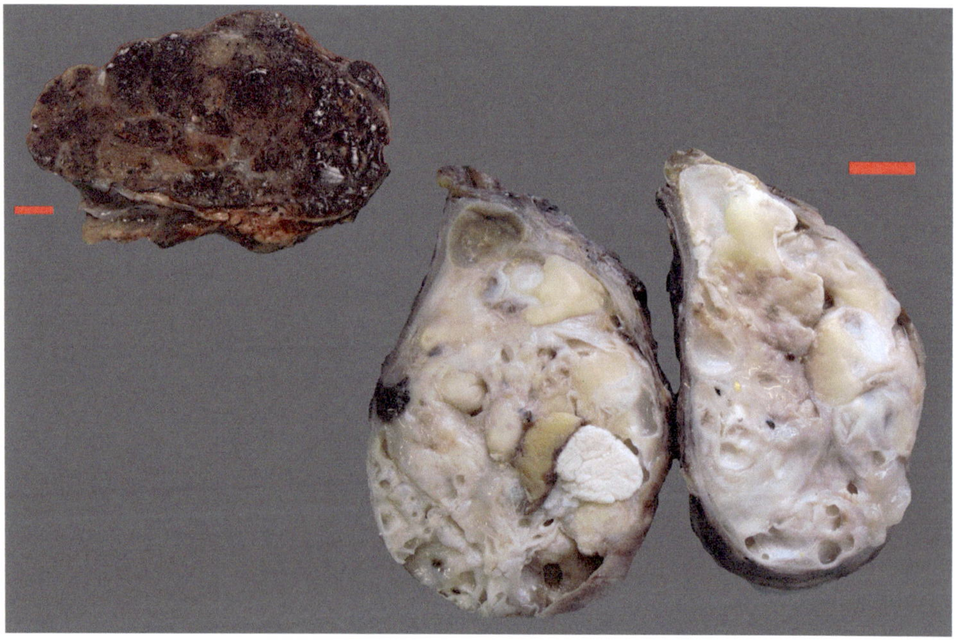

Fig. 7.33 *Upper left*. This multicystic and focally haemorrhagic mass within the upper mediastinum comprised retrosternal thyroid tissue of benign format. Increasing heterotopic thyroid tissue enlargement can cause pressure on local structures, much as thymic and other neoplasia can in this site. *Lower right*. Another cystic thymic mass is seen in this surgical sample. This case had cysts with different epithelia, muscle, and cartilage. The features were those of a mature teratoma with no malignant features

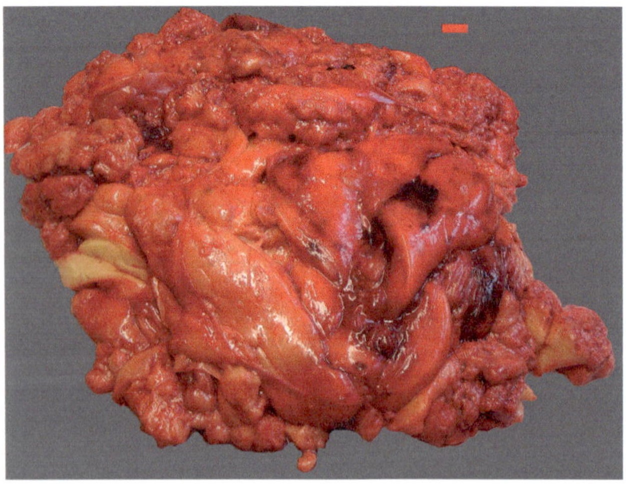

Fig. 7.34 This large, fatty mass was surgically resected from the anterior mediastinum of an elderly individual. Histologically it was a liposarcoma. Soft tissue neoplasia in the mediastinum is rare, but it is important to understand that not all anterior mediastinal tumours are thymomas or lymphomas

Bone and Marrow

The bone and cartilage tissues (Figs. 7.35, 7.36, 7.37, 7.38, 7.39, 7.40, 7.41, 7.42, 7.43, 7.44, 7.45, 7.46, 7.47, 7.48, 7.49, 7.50, 7.51, 7.52, 7.53, 7.54, 7.55, 7.56, 7.57, 7.58, 7.59, 7.60, 7.61, 7.62, and 7.63) are rarely the focus of an autopsy, but if so, it is likely that the commonest task is to consider primary

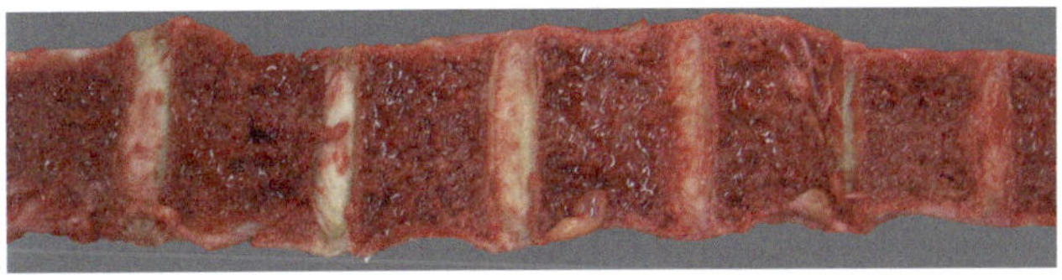

Fig. 7.35 In an autopsy case, the normal vertebral bone must be seen both as the external tissue architecture (see Chap. 3) and the internal structure, which is more important. Here the normal bone cortex is seen with red medullary tissues. There is no fracture or tumour

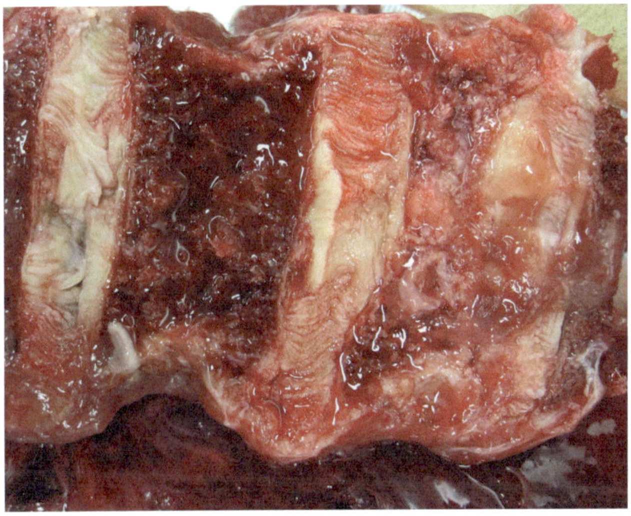

Fig. 7.36 Examination of the cut surface of the bony tissues from the spine may show variable areas of distal distortion and bony collapse, often due to osteoporosis. The beige/grey tissue present around the site of fracture and collapse of one vertebral body—chronic features of osteoporotic fractures—may also point to the possibility of metastatic tumour at this site. Histology will be required to confirm the nature of the fracture

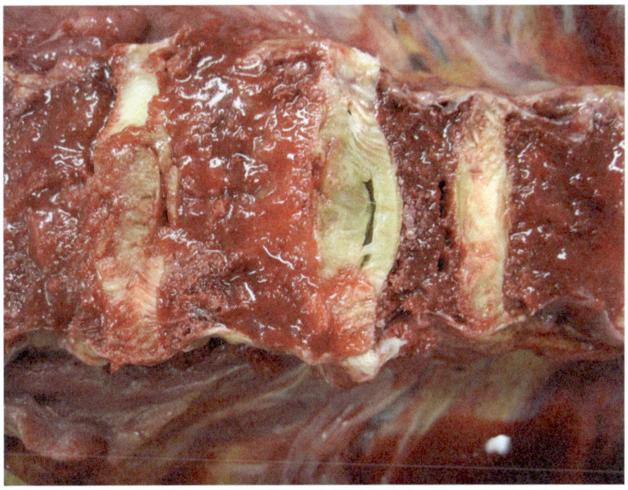

Fig. 7.37 Osteoporosis is characteristically associated with multiple fractures and collapse of the vertebral column bones. The different sizes of the vertebral bodies seen in longitudinal sections assists in confirming this interpretation. Palpation of the cut surface of relatively normal vertebral bodies should allow assessment of osteoporosis. In these cases, the thumb can be easily pressed into the bone tissue surface, a maneuver that is not possible in the bones of the young, where a normal bone framework exists

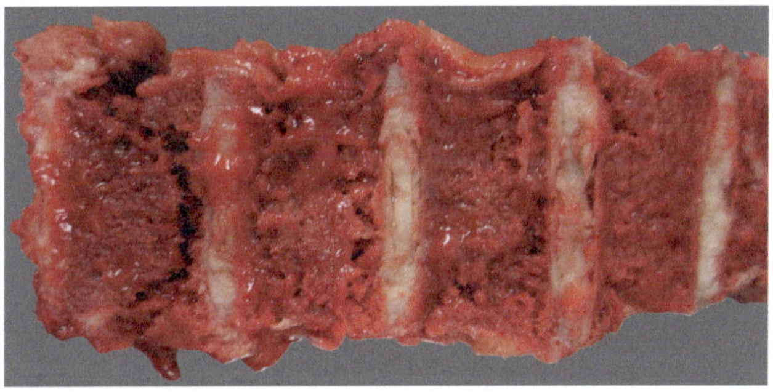

Fig. 7.38 Another example of osteoporotic bone tissue is seen. In this case, the kyphotic realities of the patient's spine show a degree of distraction and separation of the bony tissues once laid flat. The bone itself is under a normal alignment architecture although there is some suggestion of collapse of the vertebral bodies overall

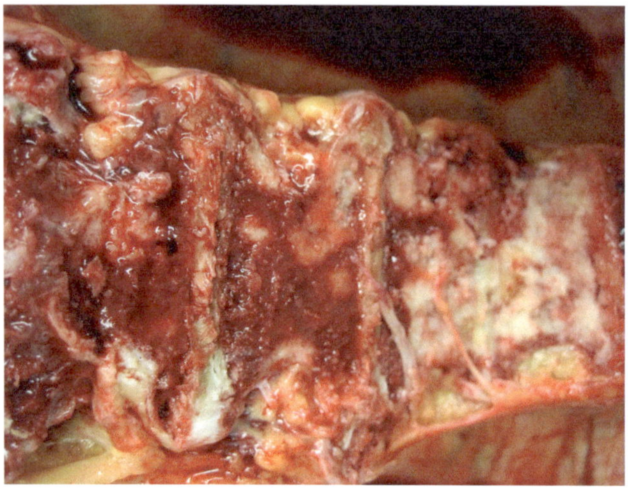

Fig. 7.39 This longitudinal section through the vertebral bodies shows multiple foci of tumour (disseminated lung cancer) involving the vertebral bony tissues

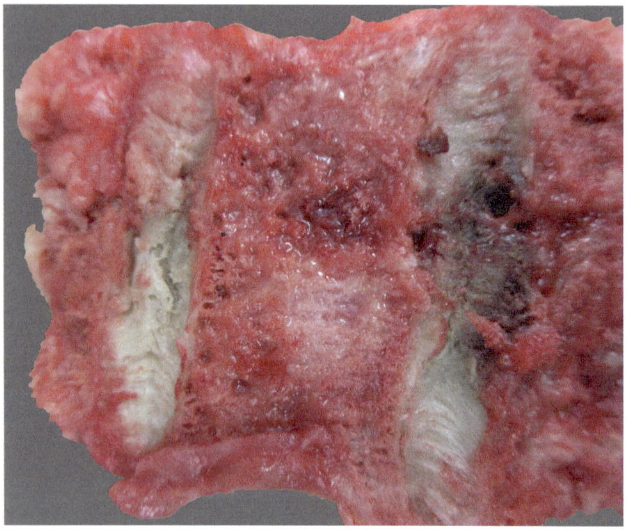

Fig. 7.40 A single focus of grey/cream tumour is seen within one of the vertebral bodies focally. This was a case of metastatic breast cancer in the somewhat osteoporotic bony tissues of the spine

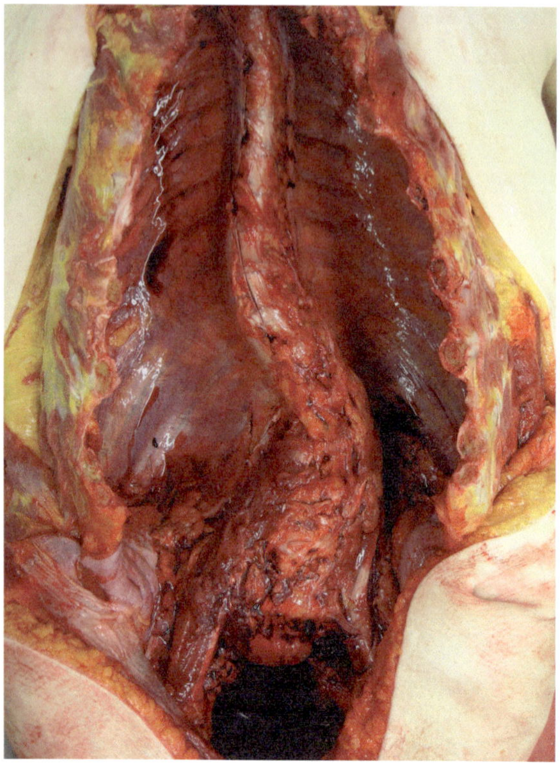

Fig. 7.41 Severe kyphoscoliosis should always be recorded. It has significant bearing upon thoracic function and may be pertinent to the cause of death

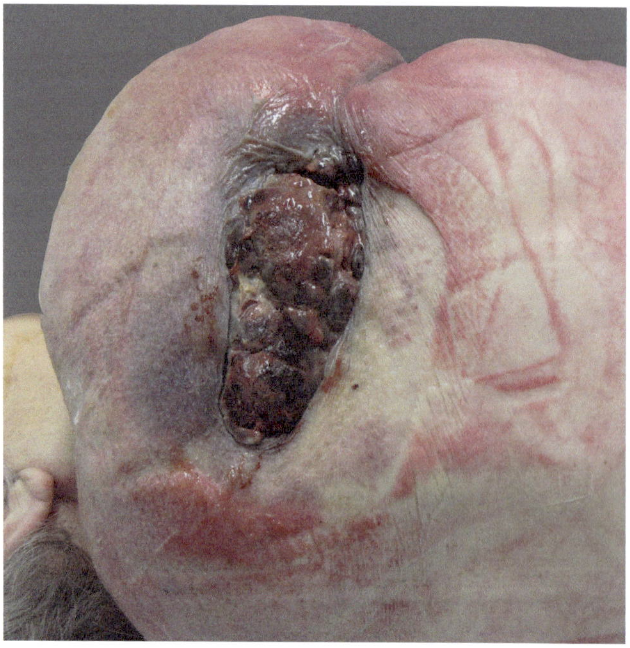

Fig. 7.42 This is a close up view of an unusual primary bone tumour eroding through the soft tissues onto the skin surface. This scapular-based giant cell tumour of the bone is seen to have thinned and eroded the skin surface with local congestion. It is not overtly infected although there is congestion around the site of the tumour encroachment. The tumour itself shows an unusual brown discolouration

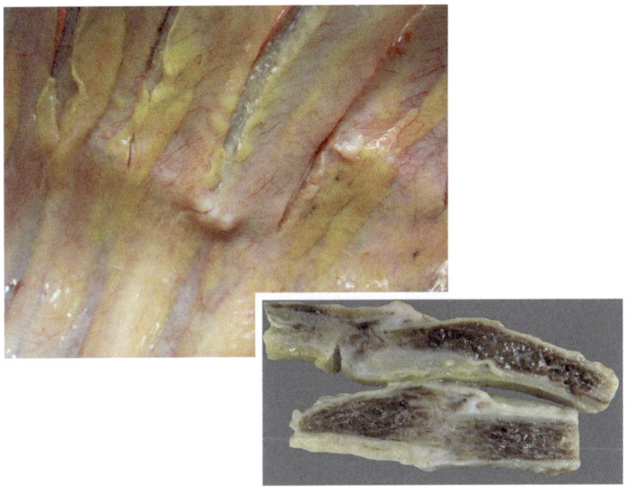

Fig. 7.43 Fractures of the ribs are common. In this case, there is a multi-step deformity of the inner aspect of the chest wall, with focal reparative cartilaginous tissue being seen clearly on the pleural aspect. This patient had suffered rib fractures some 6 weeks before death, with poor alignment of the broken ends of the bone. The lower right image shows the bone tissues from the rib fractures on either side of the fracture site. In this case, fixation and then decalcification has allowed longitudinal slicing through the bone tissues to demonstrate the poorly aligned fusion of the bone tissues and some pseudoarthrosis

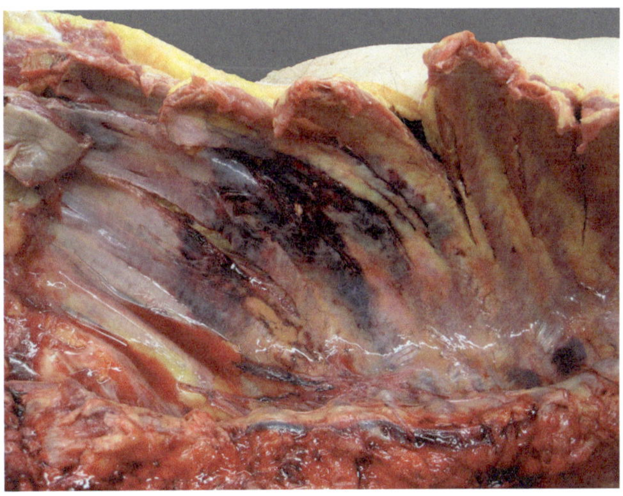

Fig. 7.44 Significant injuries to the chest often incur rib fractures with local haemorrhage. In such cases, one of the most important techniques is slicing between the ribs to allow the fracture sites to be explored and to define the amount of blood lost

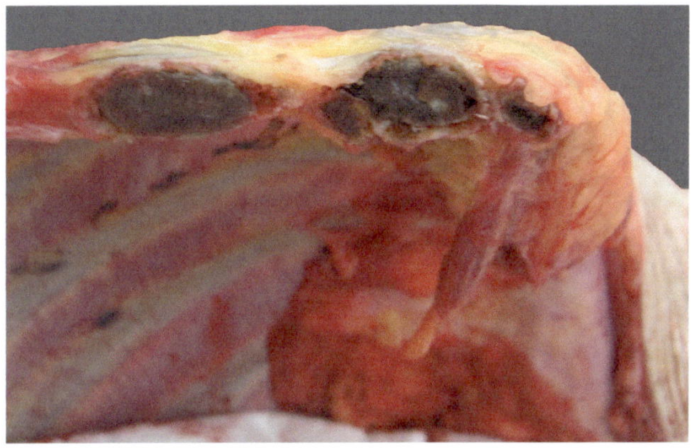

Fig. 7.45 Examination of the bone and cartilage tissues occasionally shows unusual phenomena. This is a case of ochronosis/alkaptonuria) with brown/black discolouration of the sternal and other cartilage surfaces

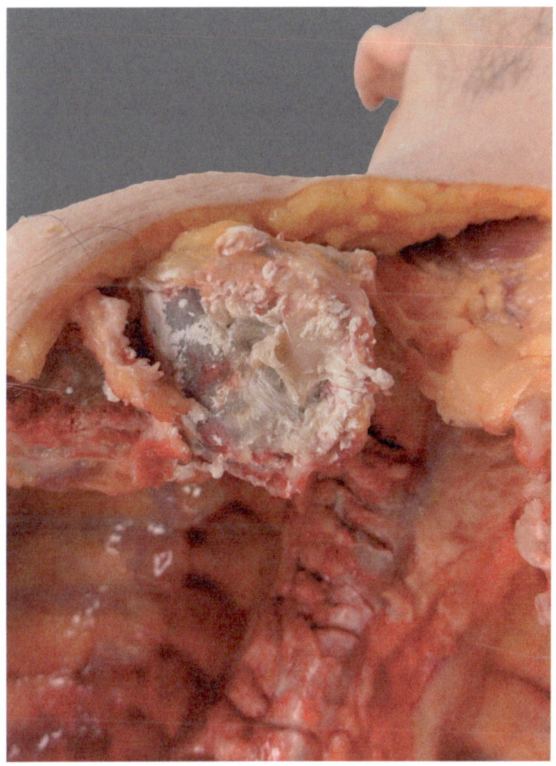

Fig. 7.46 This is the sternoclavicular junction which has been opened by knife, allowing separation of the clavicular and manubrial junction. There is granular white matrix present around the joint which is in keeping with pyrophosphate arthropathy

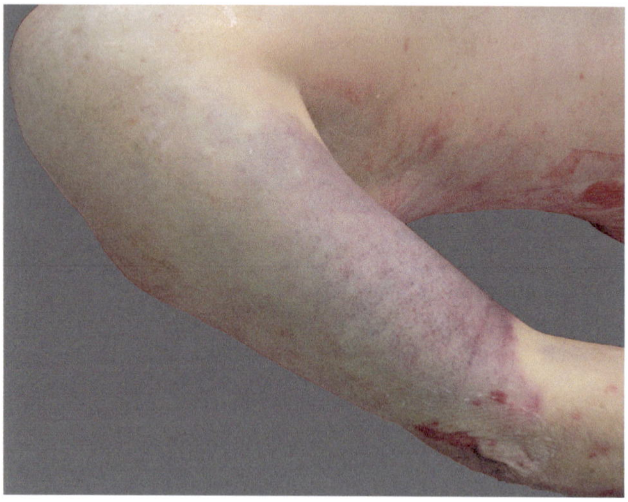

Fig. 7.47 Some bone fractures are suggested by the presence of significant haemorrhage around the site of fracture. In this case, a subcondylar fracture of the humerus was present and had been noted on ante-mortem radiology. The pronounced haemorrhage in the soft tissues of the upper arm points towards significant bone trauma. In such cases, it could be argued that dissection of the fracture site does not advance case analysis

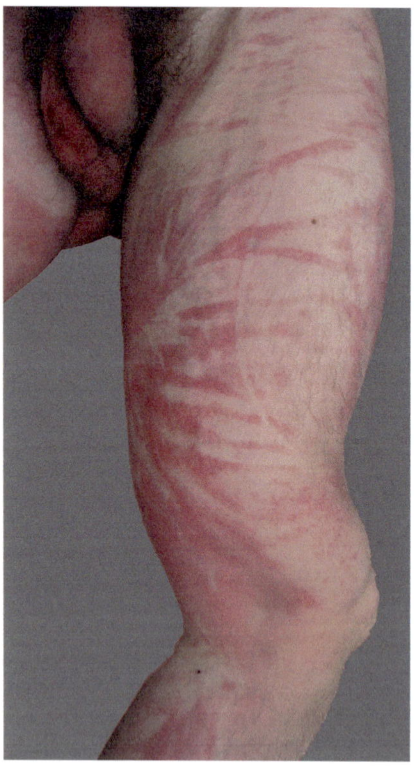

Fig. 7.48 It is not necessary to incise joints or limbs if bony fractures are clearly evident. The gross distortion of this left thigh points towards a severe acute fracture—in this case related to a road traffic collision. Ante-mortem radiology, if available, may augment understanding of any bone fractures, and post-mortem CT scans (see Chap. 13) are also valuable

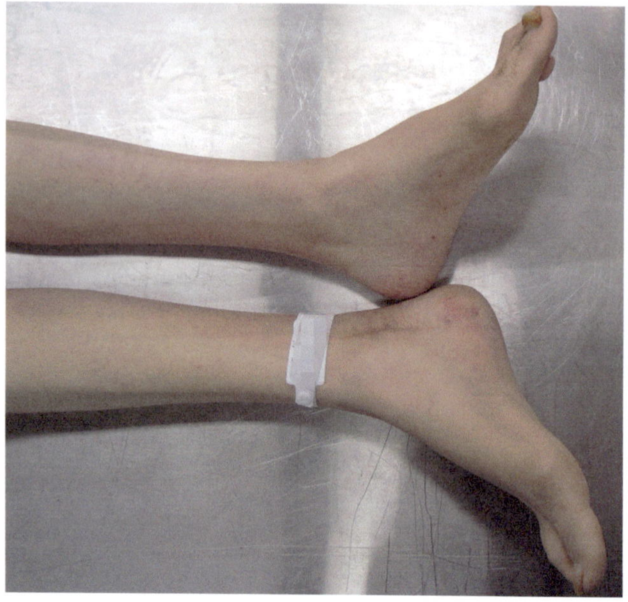

Fig. 7.49 Fractures often can be easily interpreted externally. In this case, the external rotation and shortening of the left leg points toward hip fracture

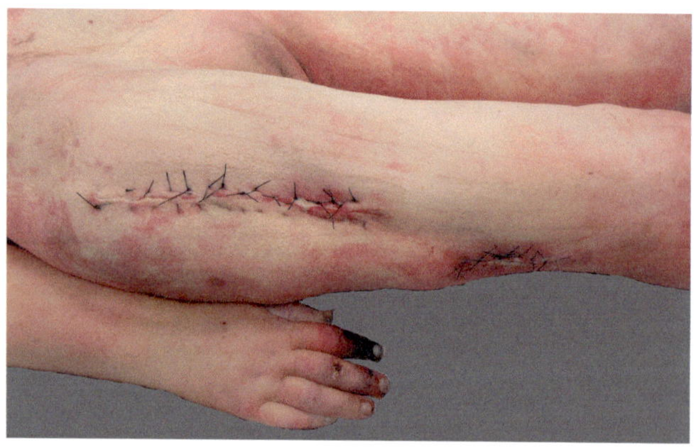

Fig. 7.50 This person has died from complications of sepsis following hip/femur surgery. In this operation an intra-femoral nail was inserted along the length of the femur, explaining the two different sutures on the lateral aspect of the knee and more anteriorly. The sutures are correctly positioned, but with some features of possible pus and reddening at one or two points, suggesting sepsis. The distal digital gangrene present in some of the fingers is in keeping with the septic event

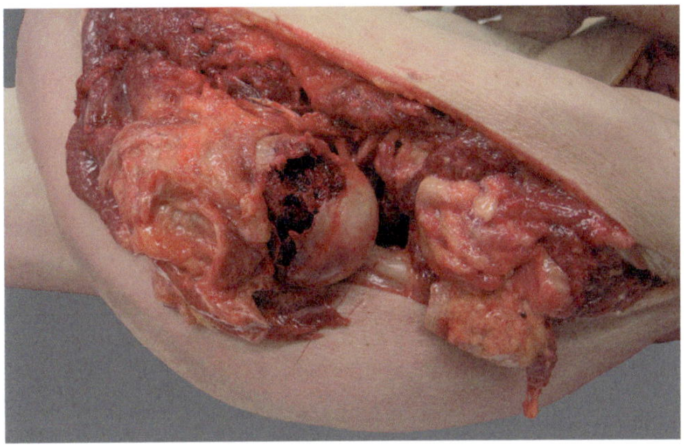

Fig. 7.51 Demonstration of hip fractures, particularly those involving the neck of the femur, can be complicated. A wide incision has been made over the left hip lateral aspect, with the thigh folded toward the right side. Dissection down onto the articular tissues should allow the hip joint to be 'popped out'. Any fracture should be easily discernible, and samples may be taken if required. Photography is all that is needed for documentation in most cases

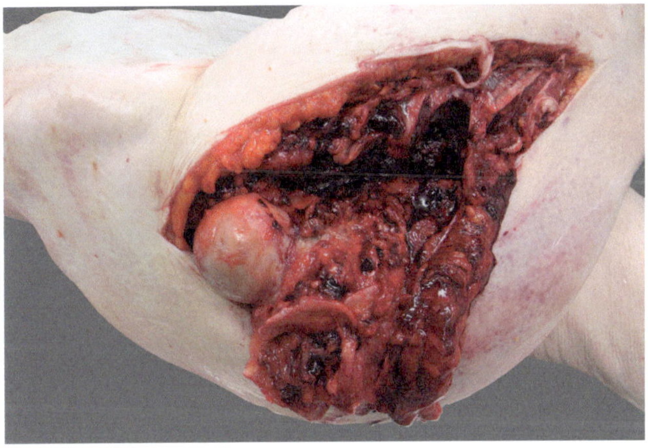

Fig. 7.52 The site of a hip fracture has been opened and explored, allowing one to confirm the degree and nature of the fracture along with tissue sampling to exclude malignancy. Note that it is not required to take the entire femur out in such cases unless there is some other issue present with the bone. This limited "popping-out" of the upper femoral head allows good inspection of the femoral parenchyma with ease and a cosmetically good closure subsequently

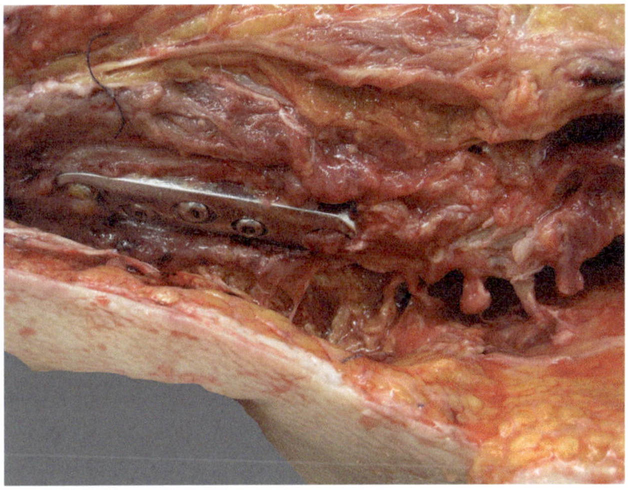

Fig. 7.53 Bony tissues with fractures often are repaired with metal devices being left in situ. These are rarely of consequence later, but there is the potential for sepsis, so some examination of the tissues may be required. In this case, repair of the femur with a screw and plate was undertaken with good effect. There is no sepsis in the local soft tissues

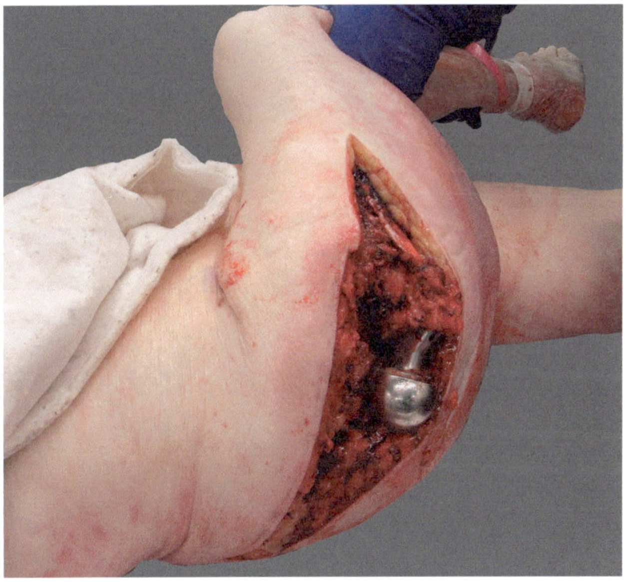

Fig. 7.54 A femoral neck and head repair is seen in this view. Opening the hip joint across the area of previous surgery and then putting the leg into marked adduction with rotation of the knee laterally allows the head of the prosthesis to pop out so that it can be inspected for correct alignment and absence of infection

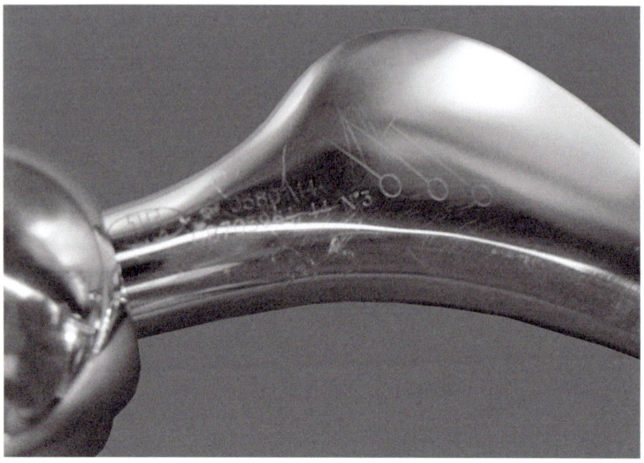

Fig. 7.55 Confirmation of the identity of a deceased individual, especially if significantly decomposed, may be assisted by checking the registry numbers of prosthetic devices such as hip implants

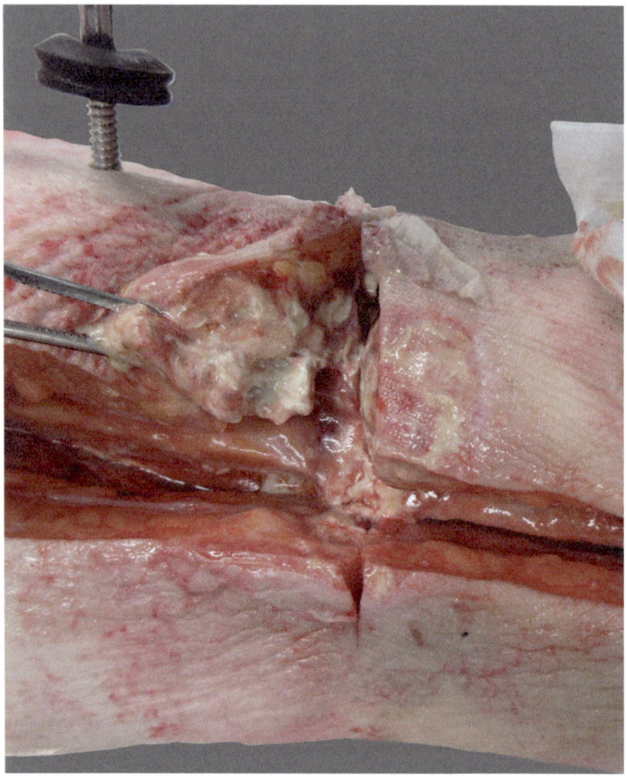

Fig. 7.56 This individual was known to have a focus of TB osteomyelitis at the site of previous bone fracture. The infection persisted despite treatment and the tissue has been opened focally to allow histopathology sampling and microbiological cultures of the areas of concern. It is not required to explant the entire bone in order to proceed with appropriate tissue sampling, but adequate exposure of the tissues and photography often suffices

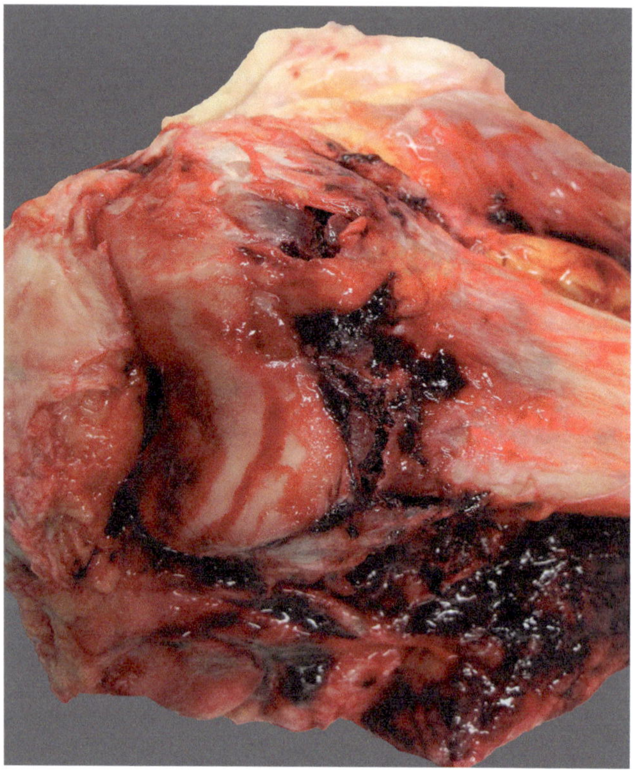

Fig. 7.57 The bony tissues of long bones are commonly involved by fractures, particularly in the elderly with a background of osteoporosis and falls. This fracture ran across the distal femur. It is notable that considerable haemorrhage was incurred around the fracture site, adding to the debility and pain experienced ante-mortem

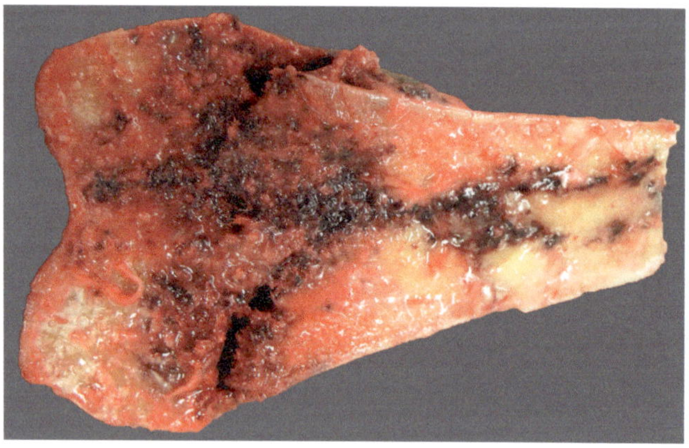

Fig. 7.58 The same fracture is now seen, having been partially excised with a cut running in a coronal plane along the long axis of the bone. This view clearly demonstrates the fracture site and local bony tissues. Performing this task allows targeted sampling, fixation, decalcification, and then appropriate block sampling

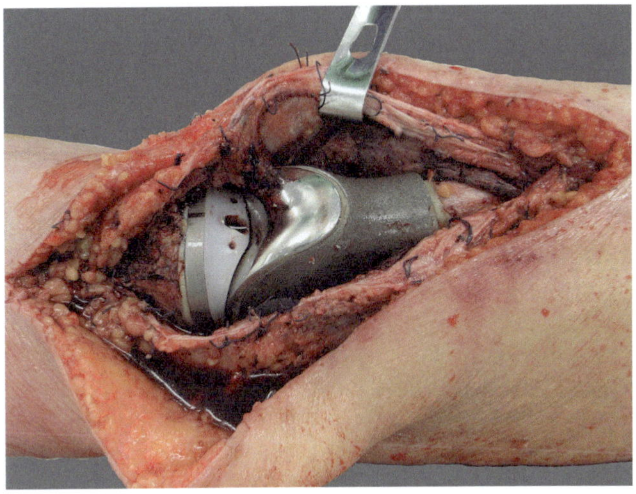

Fig. 7.59 This is a knee prosthetic replacement showing a variety of different features. Firstly, there is the bone of the femur seen towards the right side of the picture with the metal prosthesis immediately below it and with the burnished articular aspect seen as the shiny area. The plastic interface at the tibial insertion point is clearly evident with a metal collar below this. There is some light yellow matrix between the metal of the tibial and the femoral prosthesis, representing cement. The patella is seen with some arthritic change immediately adjacent to the retracting device towards the upper part of the image

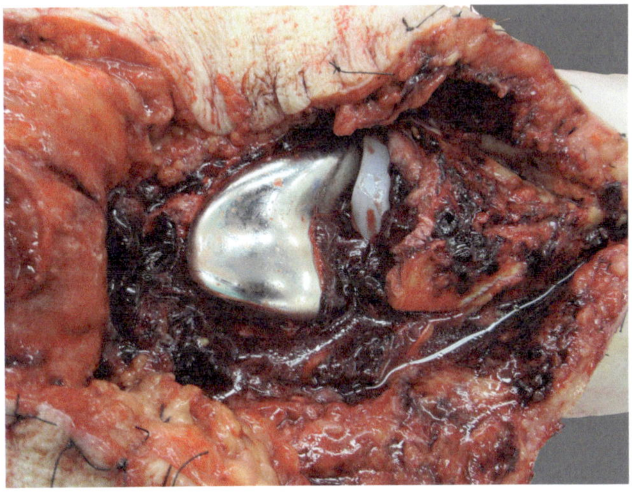

Fig. 7.60 This is another example of a knee replacement surgical procedure post-operatively. The patient died shortly after the surgical event and one can see here the metal plate from the upper knee/femur prosthesis together with a plastic spacer/interface tying into the tibial component. Sutures, blood and serosanguinous fluid are present, in keeping with the recent surgical realities of the operation

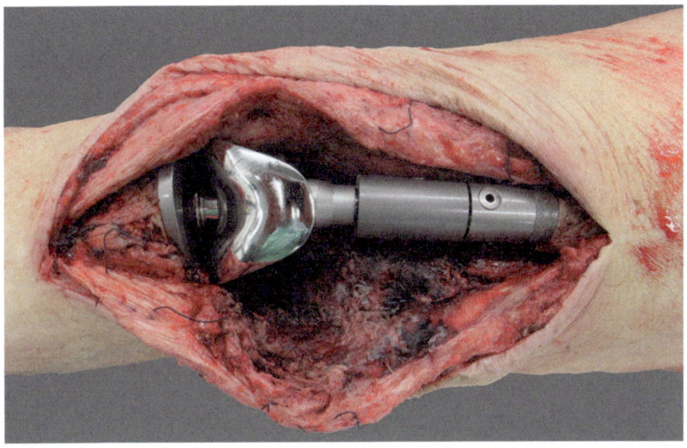

Fig. 7.61 This is a different type of knee replacement showing the femoral metal prosthesis with the moulded joint which is tied on to the end of the tibial plateau device. This patent has died following surgery, albeit several days subsequently, with congestion of the tissues but without overt local sepsis

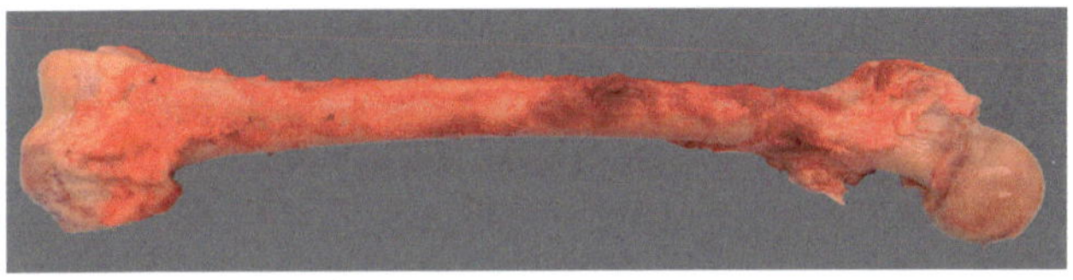

Fig. 7.62 This is an example of an adult femur which has been taken out for specialist study following the death of the individual. Note, that it has been cleaned of much of the fat and adherent tissues on the surface. Specialist samples can be taken from various points in the bone, with the bone being re-inserted later for reconstruction of the body

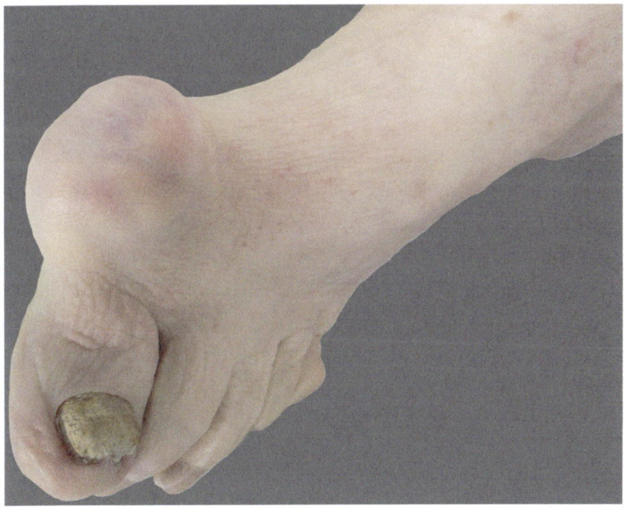

Fig. 7.63 An osteochondroma of the proximal medial phalanx of the left foot has produced a particularly marked deformity of the forefoot. A differential diagnosis would include a pronounced bunion, although ante-mortem investigations had confirmed the standard cartilaginous cap and collar-like assembly on radiology for this individual

or metastatic neoplasia. Metastatic neoplasia is more common, but primary tumorifactive leukemic and lymphomatous neoplasms also may present with pathological fractures.

Another prime area of pathology involving bone is the issue of trauma in the form of fractures with local haemorrhage (sometimes significant). In many cases, these may involve osteoporosis, although one should always be aware of possible metabolic bone disease. Ante-mortem radiology is often of benefit in assessing cases, and one may argue that it provides better data than a standard autopsy. Post-mortem radiology (see Chap. 13) is also making a significant impact in the arena of fractures. If skeletal evaluation is needed, then the sites, degree, number, and types of fracture should be recorded as a minimum.

Osteoporotic bones break easily, and all autopsies should assess for osteoporosis. The direct pressure of one's thumb into the cut surface of an osteoporotic individual's vertebral body will often indent the bone. This yields a simple assessment of bone volume since osteoporotic marrow is readily deformed. The alternative method is to use isolated ribs during initial dissection (slicing either side of rib tissues), with a subsequent attempt to break them by simple, direct finger pressure. In this test, osteoporotic bones break easily and yet can be realigned before body reconstruction.

Formal assessment of osteoporosis will require histology, in which decalcified tissues can be assessed in terms of bone volume (*i.e.*, the volume of ossified tissues over the total bone volume). In cases of metabolic bone disease, specialist techniques for assessment of bone mineralization may require consultation with specialist bone pathology services before one undertakes the autopsy.

Complications Adjacent to Fractures

The degree of blood loss in association with any fracture should be estimated, as it can be significant and pertinent to the cause of death. Such blood loss may occur from the bone fracture site itself. Multiple fractures will necessarily incur a greater degree of blood loss than small bone fractures. Local trauma to large arteries and veins may also complicate even small fractures. Any preexisting anticoagulation will further aggravate matters.

The autopsy must consider aspects of medical and surgical interventions with bone fractures, particularly in the form of metallic and other prostheses.

Finally, one must remember that bony tissues can be involved by sepsis, mostly following surgery and involving prostheses.

Cervical Vertebral Tissues and Cord

The approach to the spinal cord (Figs. 7.64, 7.65, 7.66, 7.67, 7.68, 7.69, 7.70, 7.71, 7.72, 7.73, 7.74, 7.75, and 7.76) is particularly complex when dealing with cervical bone injuries. The close relationship of the skull and the complex bone and ligaments at the base of the skull means that the assessment of cervical spinal pathology is technically difficult. In addition, the standard incisions provide limited access to this site.

One approach to this issue is to remove en bloc the central base of the skull and the cervical bony structures. Thereafter, the back of the spinal canal is removed, allowing access to the spinal cord. Lastly, the vertebral body block is cut (with an oscillating saw) in a sagittal plane, allowing inspection of the bony tissues. This method allows significant inspection of the cervical bone and neurological tissues. The alternative is to rely upon radiological images from ante-mortem studies.

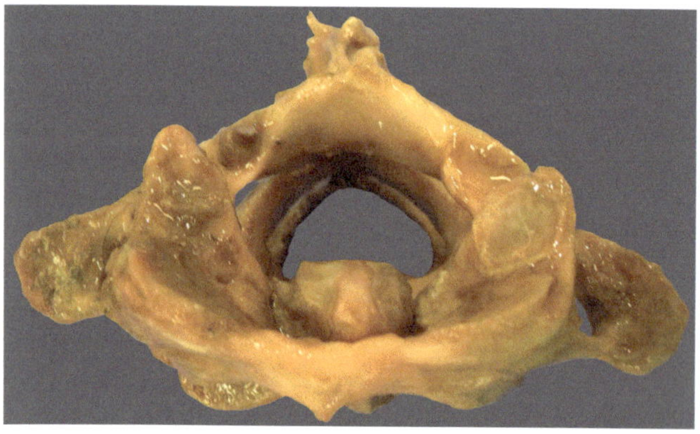

Fig. 7.64 This is a superior view of the C1, C2, and C3 vertebral bodies from the cranial aspect downwards. The decomposed body in this case allowed full appreciation of the close interaction of these vertebra, with preservation of the odontoid peg of C2 projecting immediately behind the anterior ring of the C1 vertebral tissue

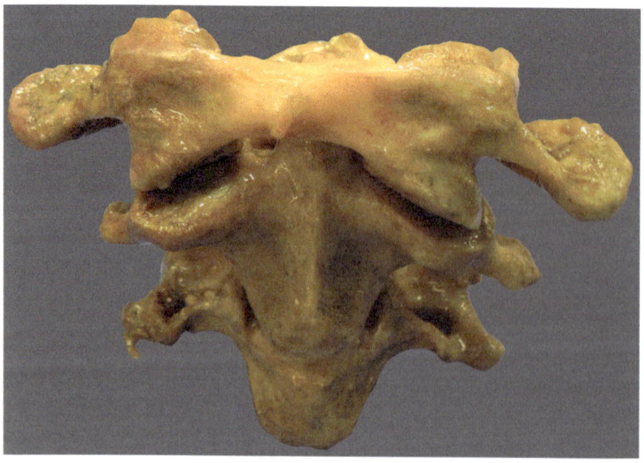

Fig. 7.65 The same tissue as in Fig. 7.64 is seen from the anterior perspective, highlighting the normal anatomy. This view allows certain pathologies such as spine trauma to be excluded, whether it is achieved by decomposition or by excarnation/defleshing (Chap. 12)

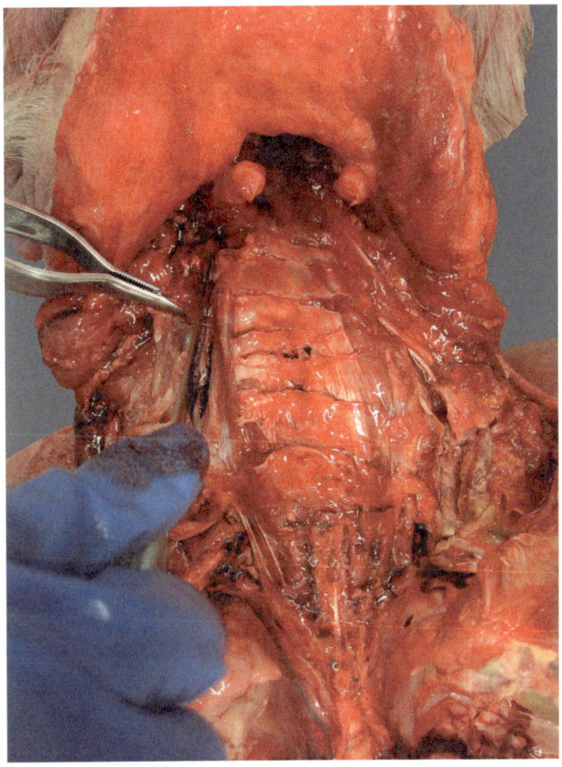

Fig. 7.66 Assessing the cervical spine in neck injuries is complicated. Good access to the neck is required, with cuts being made into the soft tissues on either side of the cervical bony tissues

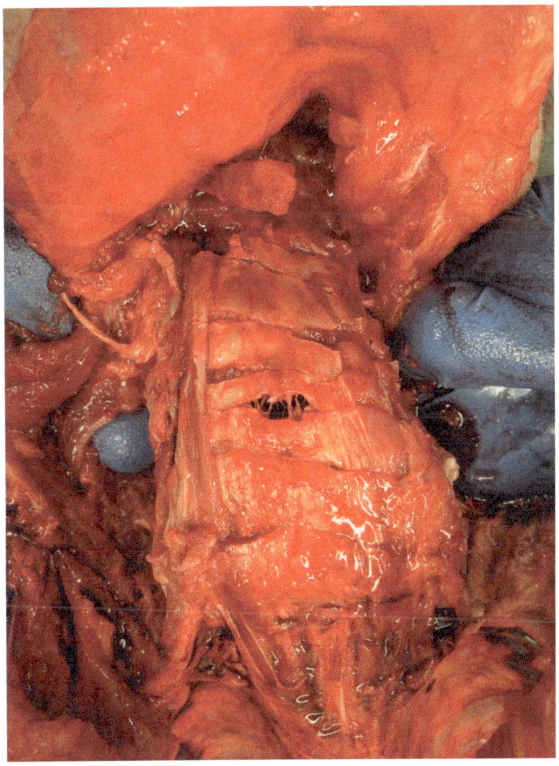

Fig. 7.67 The tissues are undermined on both sides so that the hand can be passed from one side to the other, confirming that the vertebral bony tissue block is now free of its local soft tissue attachments. At this point, the fracture dislocation site is seen centrally. This pathology was incurred during a fall

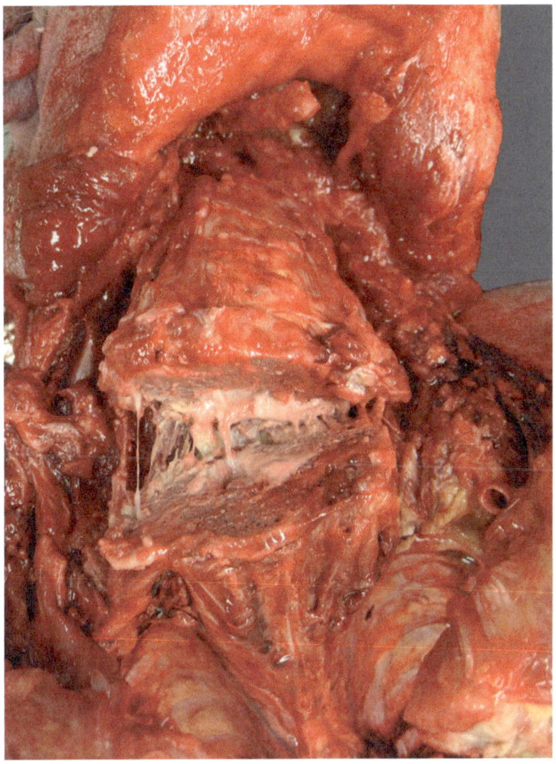

Fig. 7.68 The lower cervical bony tissues are now cut horizontally using a saw, at least 20 mm below the spinal cord area of significance

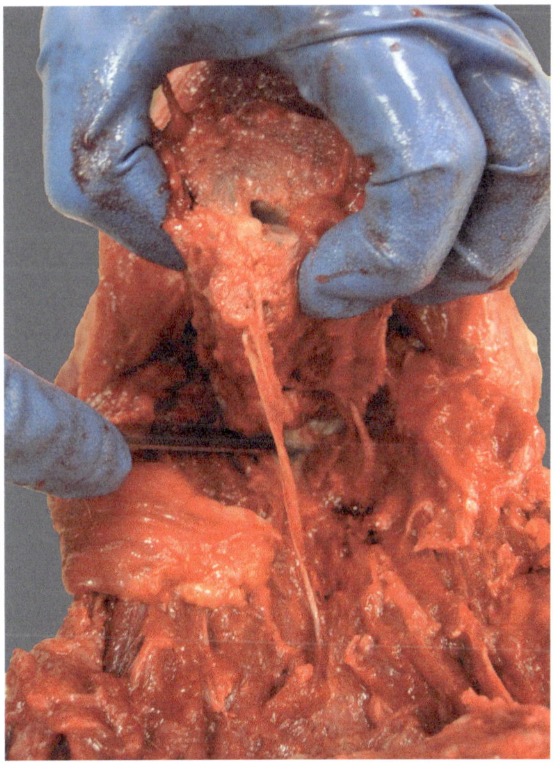

Fig. 7.69 The base of the spinal vertebral block may now be lifted gently upwards and away from the back of the soft tissues of the neck and skin. The spinal canal can be seen in relation to the vertebral bodies. Soft tissue dissection continues upwards towards the base of the skull

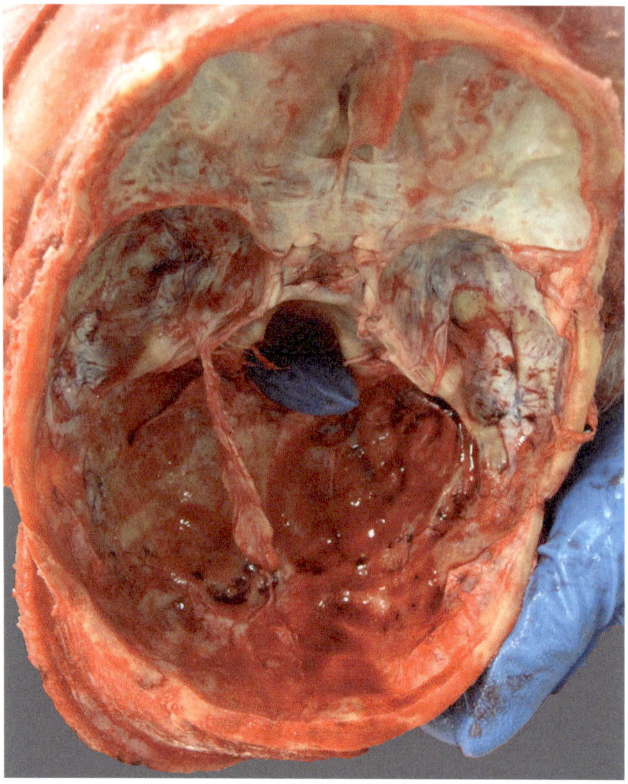

Fig. 7.70 A set of four cuts are made into the base of the skull around the front of the foramen magnum. There is no way to illustrate this dissection process, as the saw blocks the view, but the resultant hole is shown here. A finger has been passed into the defect to highlight the size of the hole required

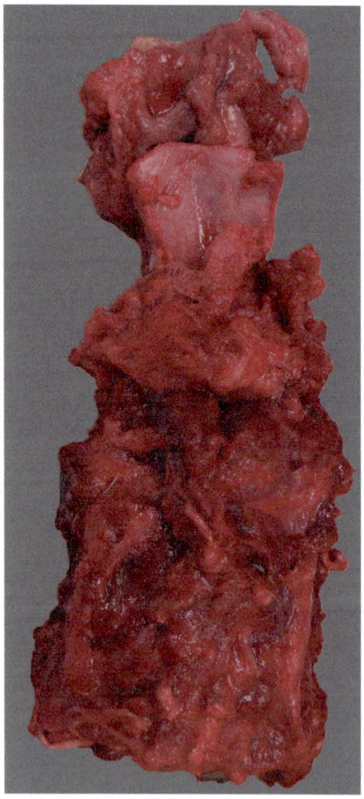

Fig. 7.71 The tissue block, incorporating soft tissues, basal skull, and vertebral bodies, is seen from the posterior aspect in this view

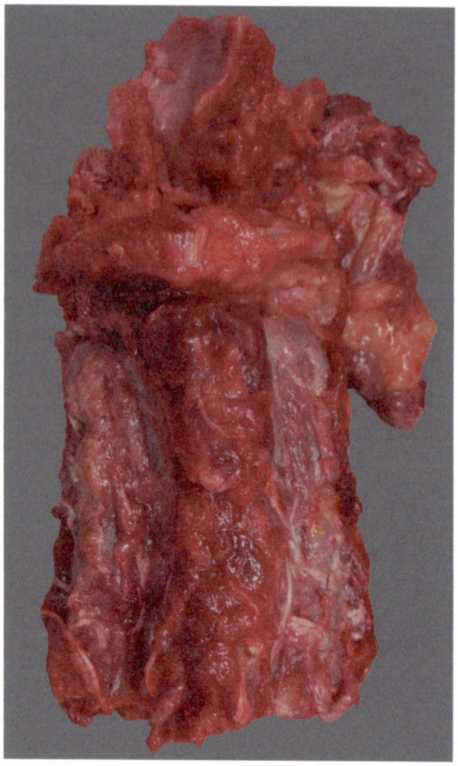

Fig. 7.72 Further dissection of the soft tissues adjacent to the skull base and the sides of the vertebral bodies continues, with this tissue now being removed. The tissue at the top end is the base of the skull

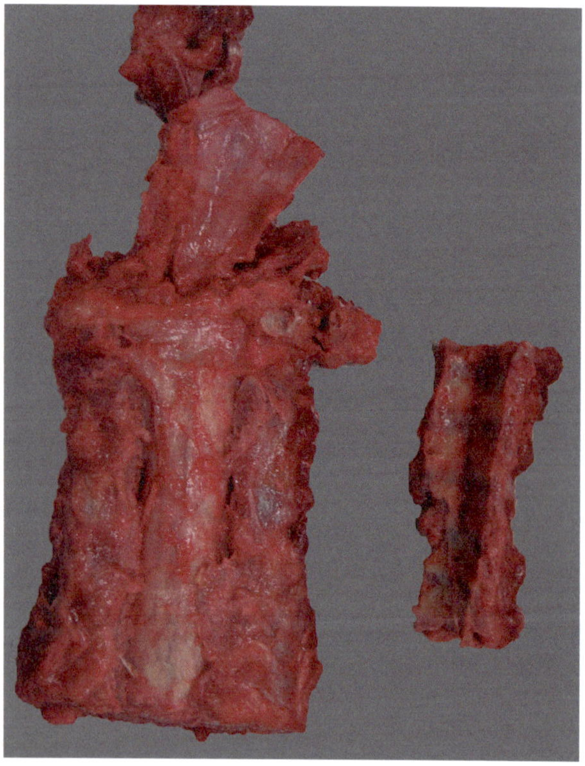

Fig. 7.73 The back of the spinal canal is exposed by cutting through the bony structures at the back. The spinal cord is seen in situ and the posterior aspect of the spinal canal has been turned around so that one can inspect this aspect of the spinal canal. Any areas of tumour, haemorrhage, or sepsis can be identified readily in this view

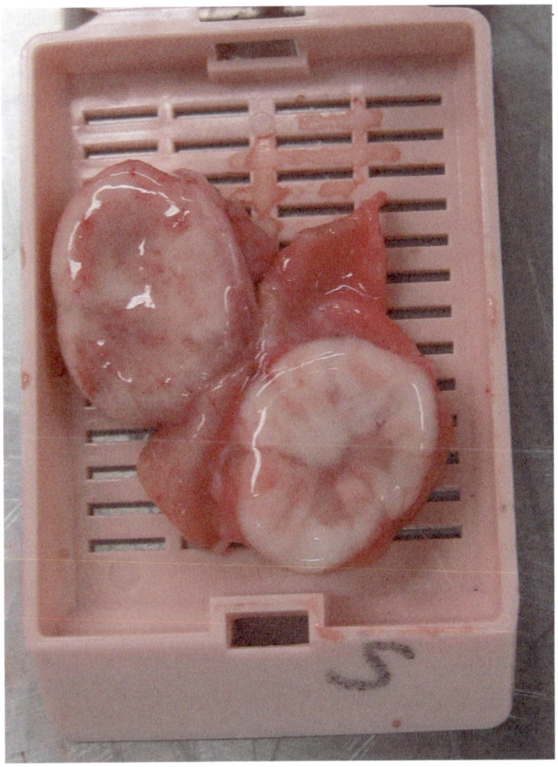

Fig. 7.74 The spinal cord is removed carefully and without significant traction. Ideally, this segment of spinal cord is left to fix and then sectioned for histology, but if histologically sampling is required immediately, then transverse sections of the spinal cord can be taken, using a fresh scalpel blade to ensure a sharp cut and minimal fresh damage to the soft tissues of the cord. Do not use an old blade!

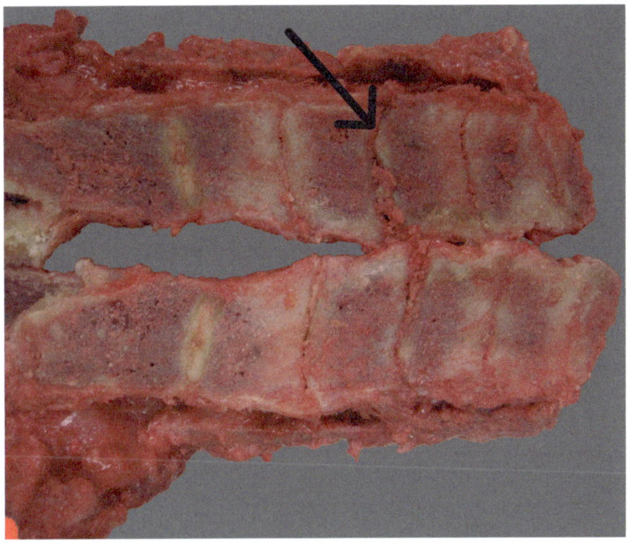

Fig. 7.75 The bony tissues have now been cut in a sagittal fashion, exposing the alignment of the cervical spine. It is noted that there is some separation at the disc interface (*arrow*) that was responsible for cervical injury. These samples can be reserved for fixation, decalcification, and then histological study if required, although photography alone is usually enough for any medicolegal purposes

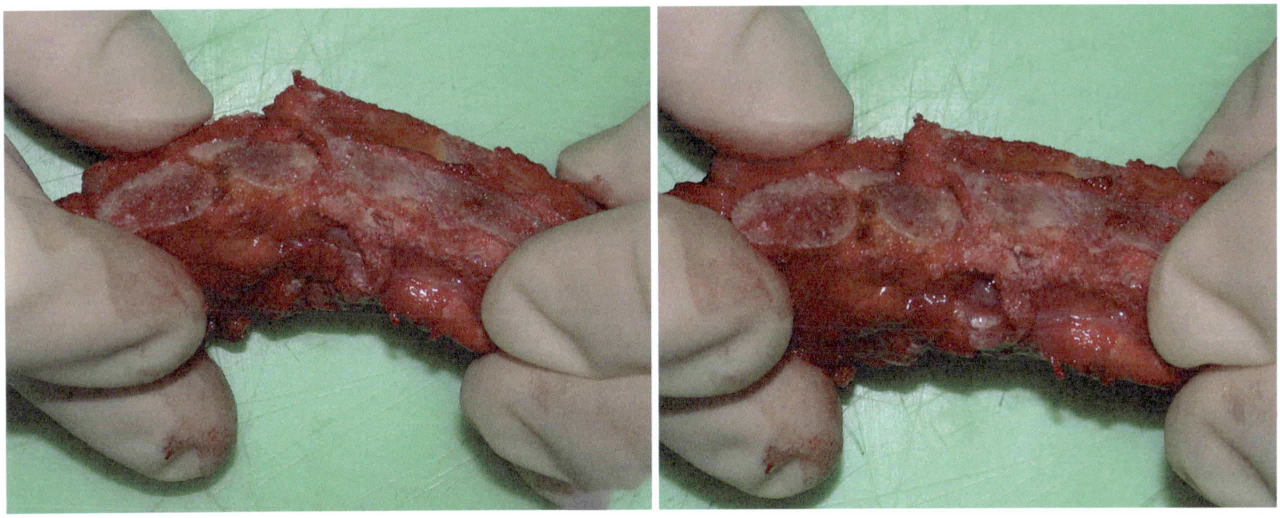

Fig. 7.76 These two images show another case. Here the cervical spine flexion and extension reveals clear separation of the vertebral bodies from each other during this maneuver. This patient had a high-level cervical cord injury associated with a fracture dislocation. Dissection of the vertebral tissues and examination of the different components allowed a full understanding of the injuries sustained

Suggested Reading

Burton JL, Rutty G. The hospital autopsy. 3rd ed. London: Hodder Arnold; 2010.

Connolly AJ, Finkbeiner WE, Ursell PC, Davis RL, (eds.). Autopsy pathology: a manual and atlas. 3rd ed. Philadelphia, PA: Elsevier; 2016.

Cooke RA, Stewart B. Lymph nodes and spleen. In: Colour atlas of anatomical pathology. 3rd ed. Edinburgh: Churchill Livingstone; 2004. p. 31–4.

Curran RC, Jones EL. Gross pathology: a colour atlas. Harvey Millar HM + M Publishers; 1974. p. 18–23.

Folpe AL, Inwards CY. Bone and soft tissue pathology. Philadelphia, PA: Elsevier—OHCE; 2013.

Goldblum JR, Lamps LW, McKenney JK, Myers JL. Hematopathology, bone and soft tissue pathology. In: Rosai and Ackerman's surgical pathology. 11th ed. Edinburgh: Elsevier; 2017. p. 1530–915.

Kumar V, Abbas AK, Aster JC, Deyrup AT, Das A. Hematopoietic and lymphoid systems, bones, joints and soft tissue tumors. In: Robbins & Kumar basic pathology. 11th ed. Elsevier; 2022. p. 345–399, 680–713.

Ludwig J. Handbook of autopsy practice. 3rd ed. Ottawa: Humana Press; 2002. p. 136–58, 262–76.

Medeiros LJ, Miranda RN. Diagnostic pathology: lymph nodes and extranodal lymphomas. 2nd ed. Philadelphia, PA: Elsevier—OHCE; 2018.

Endocrine Glands: Thyroid, Parathyroid and Adrenal

8

S. Kim Suvarna and Abigail K. Sharp

Introduction

The general autopsy often gives scant or cursory attention to the endocrine tissues. However, consideration of the possible impact of endocrine tissues to the individual's health, and death, should be made on all occasions.

This chapter covers the thyroid, parathyroid and adrenal glands. These endocrine tissues exist as separate glands. Nevertheless, it is also recognised that many other tissues are capable of secreting hormones and other circulating factors into the bloodstream, perhaps most notably the pancreas (covered in the gastrointestinal section). The pancreas is linked to diabetes and thereby cardiovascular disease, sepsis and metabolic issues, which are covered elsewhere in this book. The pituitary, intimately linked to the brain, is also covered later.

For the three glands under consideration, in most cases review of the clinical data before the autopsy and subsequent macroscopic glandular tissue assessment will suffice as the examination needed at autopsy. Thus, general dissection/slicing of the tissues in situ may well be enough to confirm normality. Nevertheless, if there is any concern that the endocrine tissues are of pathological quality, then the glands should be dissected free of the local structures, carefully checked in terms of architecture, weighed and sliced. Photography is often of value. Furthermore, some tissue may be submitted for histology.

The endocrine glands should be fully sampled in cases of unusual deaths and, in particular, all maternal or sudden unexpected deaths.

In all the following images, where present, the red bar marker is 10 mm.

S. Kim Suvarna was deceased at the time of publication.

S. K. Suvarna (Deceased) · A. K. Sharp (✉)
Department of Histopathology, Sheffield Teaching Hospitals NHS Foundation Trust, Sheffield, UK
e-mail: abigail.sharp@nhs.net

Thyroid

The thyroid gland (Figs. 8.1, 8.2, 8.3, 8.4, 8.5, 8.6, 8.7, 8.8, 8.9, 8.10, 8.11, 8.12, 8.13, 8.14, 8.15, 8.16, 8.17, 8.18, 8.19, 8.20, 8.21, 8.22, 8.23, 8.24, and 8.25) is not an uncommon site of pathology. In many cases, clues of thyroid disease are present externally in the form of macroscopic neck scarring and/or goiter.

The thyroid gland is situated immediately in front of the thyroid cartilage and upper trachea. It is a bi-lobed structure, with a weight of 20–40 g in health. Its size will reflect the individual, with some variation occurring during growth, health, pregnancy and systemic disease. It is

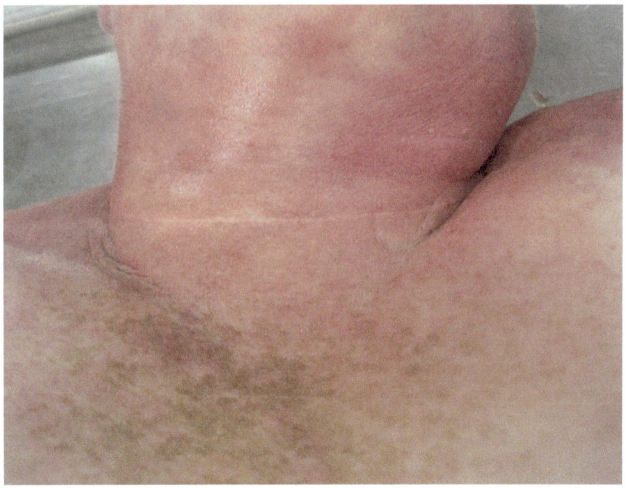

Fig. 8.1 External inspection of the neck of all cases should look for features of previous thyroid and/or parathyroid surgery. In this case, a well-healed transverse low cervical scar is seen

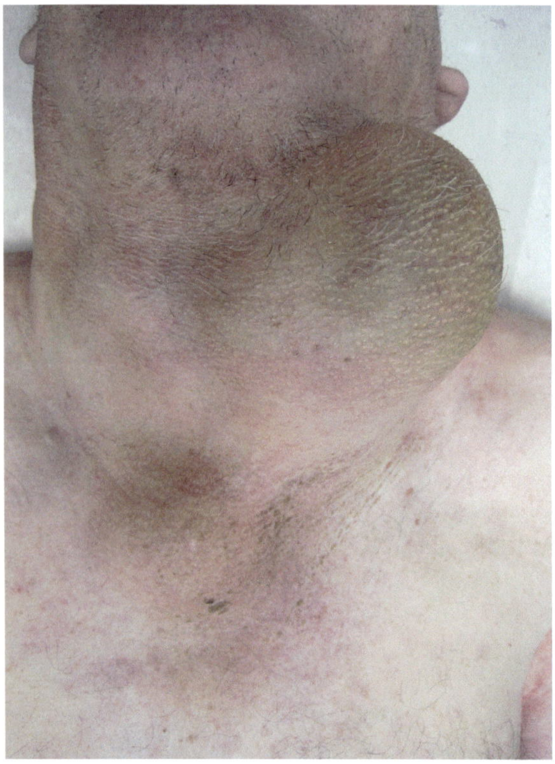

Fig. 8.2 The macroscopic features of thyroid enlargement may be obvious. The cervical tissues appear distorted by a rounded, firm mass, which appears most pronounced on the *left side*, though some palpable fullness and enlargement of the contralateral thyroid tissues was also evident

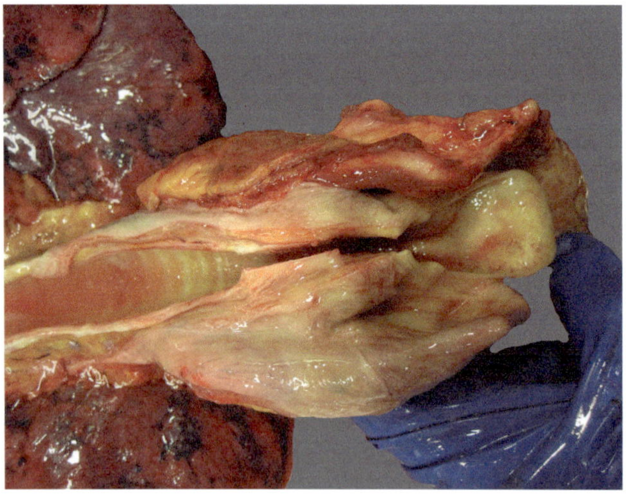

Fig. 8.3 The upper neck structures are seen from behind. The thyroid and parathyroid tissues are not immediately apparent, but rather are eased into view by careful dissection of the fascial planes, as discussed below

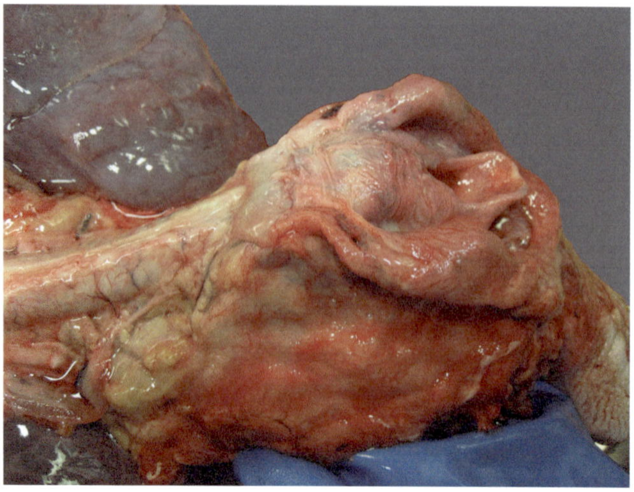

Fig. 8.4 The posterior view of the neck structures is viewed from the right side oblique perspective, with tension applied to the neck parenchyma, allowing the broad position of the thyroid and parathyroid glands to be defined

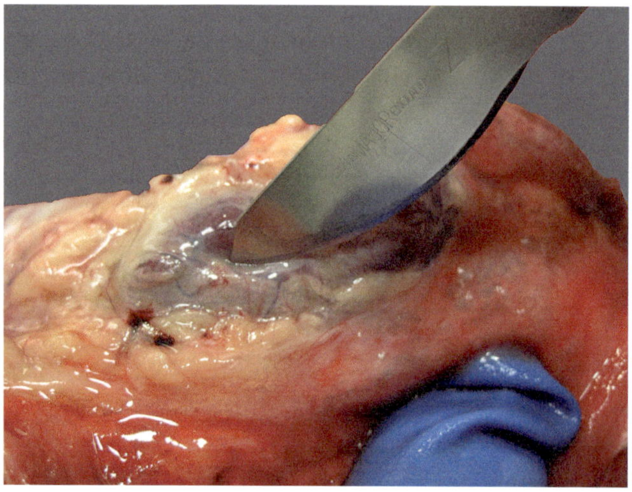

Fig. 8.5 The scalpel blade is run gently along the thyroid capsule to allow separation of the tissues at this fascial plane

surrounded by a thin capsule, often with the four parathyroid glands adjacent. Heterotopic thyroid tissue can also be found within the low neck or even the mediastinum. Furthermore, one may find both normal and neoplastic thyroid tissues in some ovarian neoplasia (struma ovarii).

The thyroid and parathyroid glands are best approached from a posterior perspective, rather than dissecting through the layers of the anterior strap muscles. By holding the neck structures in the cup of the hand, some grasping-style ten-

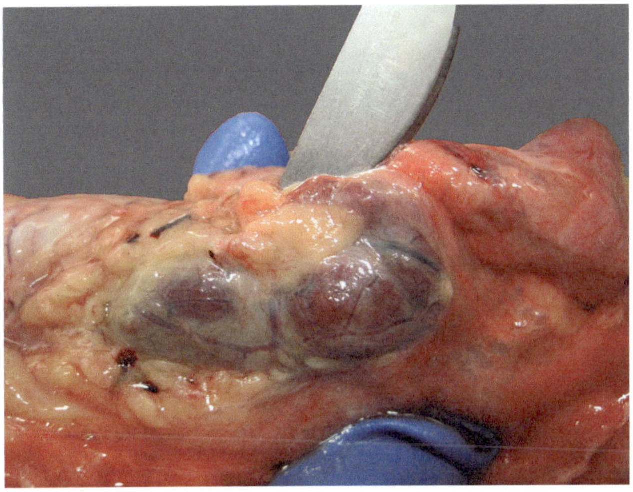

Fig. 8.6 The tension and gentle dissection allow the thyroid gland to emerge into view. The scalpel blade has been "stroked" gently across the lateral/posterior surface of the thyroid, allowing the gland, with slight nodularity, to be seen with local vasculature

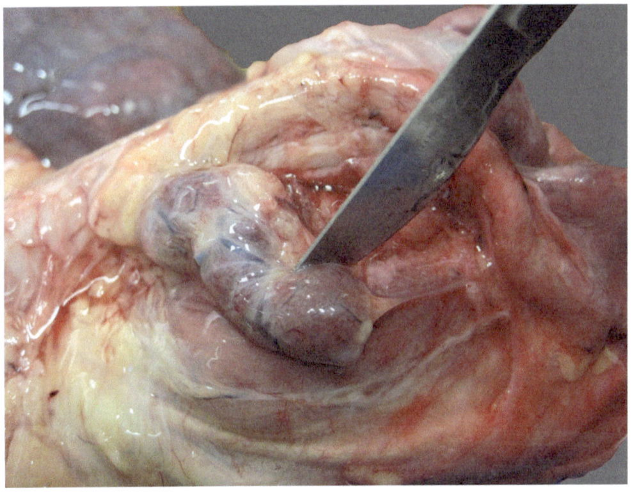

Fig. 8.7 The thyroid gland can now be gently pulled away from the central neck structures, and the gentle incision of fascia tissues continues across the posterior aspect of the gland. The thyroid is dissected free from the local trachea by running the scalpel blade gently between the thyroid capsule and airway tissues. One should be careful not to incise into the thyroid gland

sion can be applied on both sides of the neck tissue, around the trachea. This allows a broad appreciation of where the thyroid will be, with the likely positions of the parathyroids.

The thyroid gland, once dissected free, is slightly irregular in terms of external morphology, although nodularity (small amounts) is probably within the range of normality. The cut section of the gland shows a meaty red-brown architecture of an even quality.

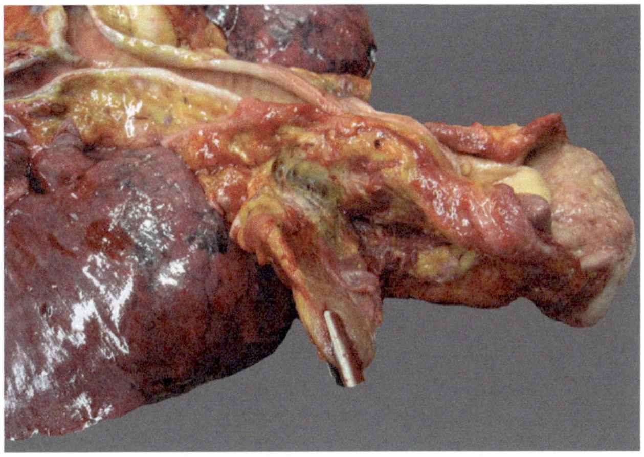

Fig. 8.8 The thyroid parenchyma has been dissected to reveal the smooth external lobar architecture. It is being pulled forwards by forceps to aid dissection

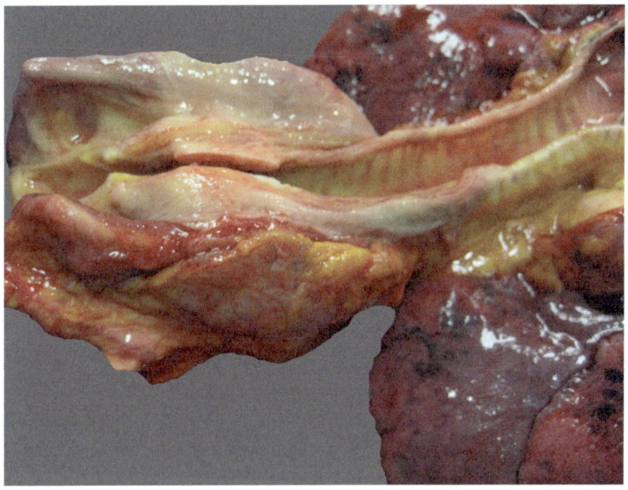

Fig. 8.9 The same process is completed on the other side, with one clearly visualizing the gland

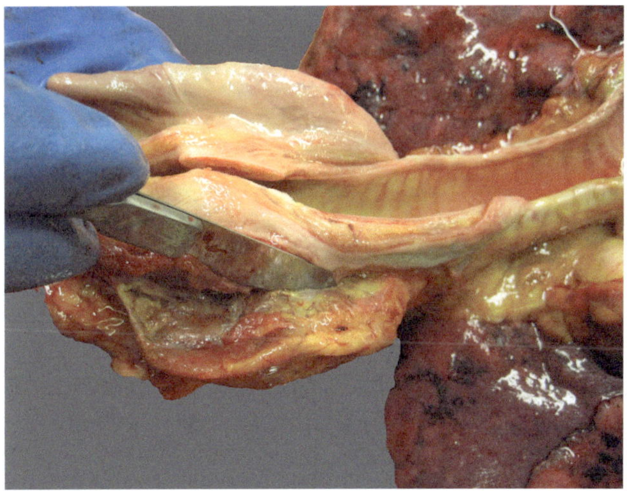

Fig. 8.10 The posterior aspect of the thyroid is exposed by very gentle stroking of the scalpel. It is emphasized that the blade should not have much pressure applied

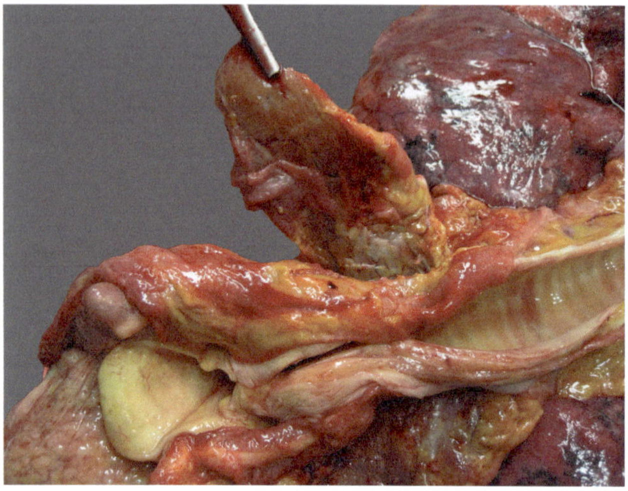

Fig. 8.11 The right side of the thyroid is now free

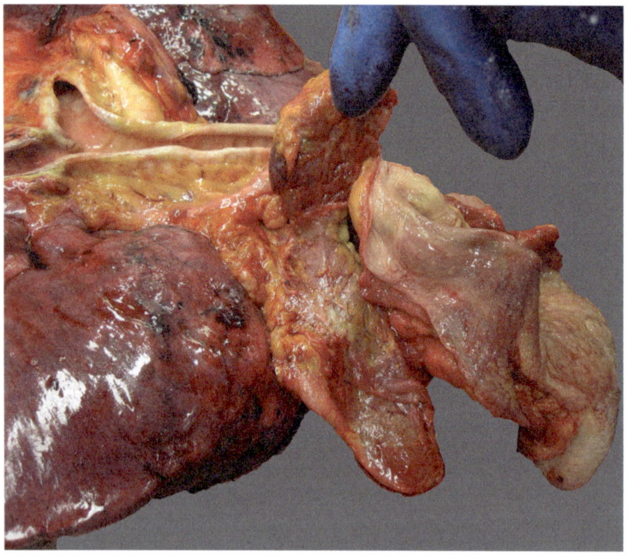

Fig. 8.12 The left side of the thyroid is similarly mobilized, and the dissection plane is extended onto the tracheal external surface. The left thyroid lobe may now be 'passed' to the right side, in front of the trachea. This allows the gland to be resected intact, and with minimal local soft tissues

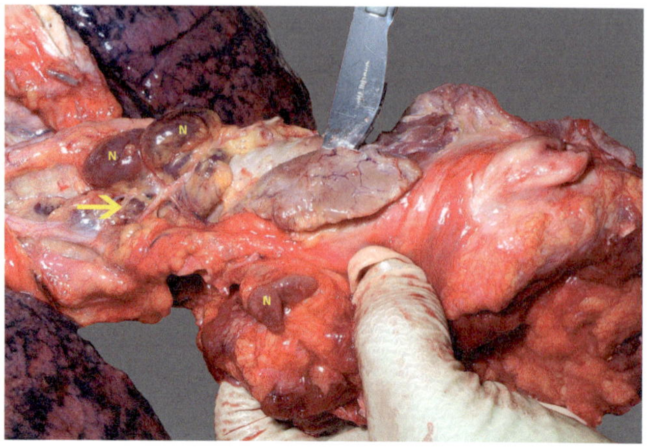

Fig. 8.13 Note the tension applied (by the hand grip) to the neck structures, to allow the thyroid to be gently mobilized. Below the thyroid and towards the lung interface are several rounded, mid-brown lymph nodes (N). These nodes should not be mistaken for parathyroid elements, although one possible parathyroid is noted (arrow)

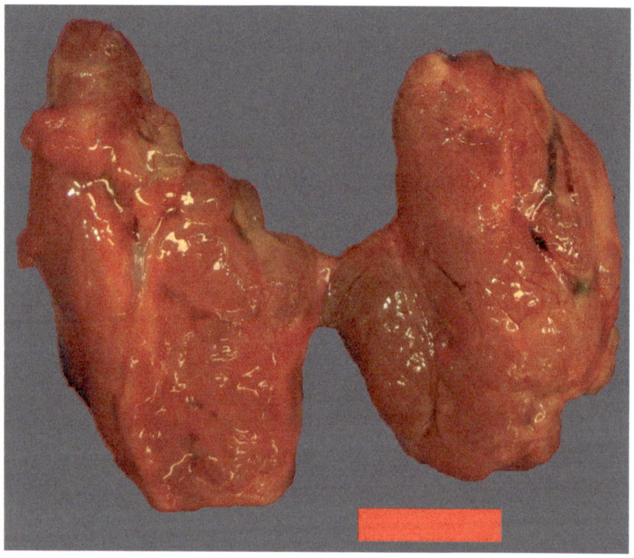

Fig. 8.14 The normal thyroid has a 'bow tie' architecture, with two large lobes and a small central isthmus

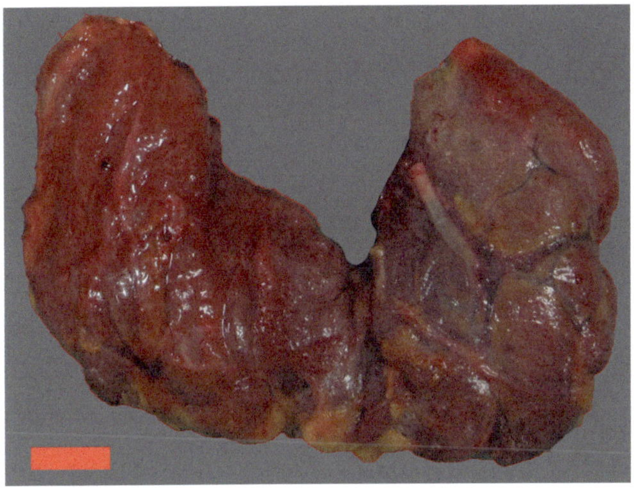

Fig. 8.15 An enlarged thyroid is seen with a very meaty architecture and some nodularity. This colloid goiter was clearly evident in the neck but was producing no direct pathological problem

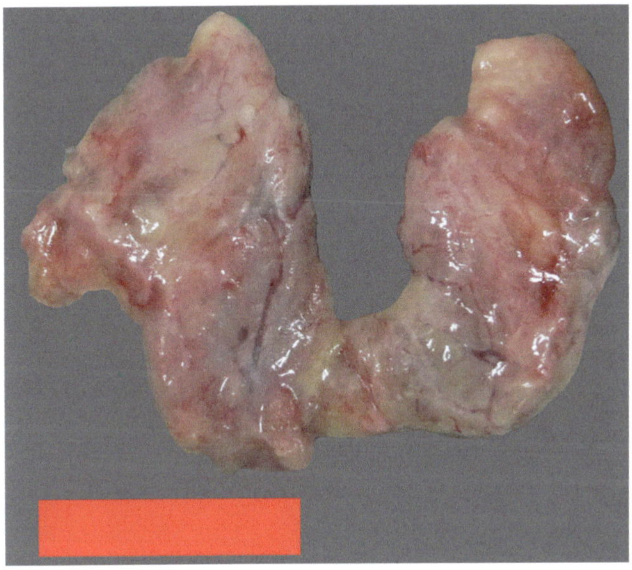

Fig. 8.16 The thyroid gland in many elderly individuals is subject to autoimmune destruction, with tissue atrophy and fibrosis. In this case of Hashimoto's/autoimmune thyroiditis, the gland is shrunken and fibrotic

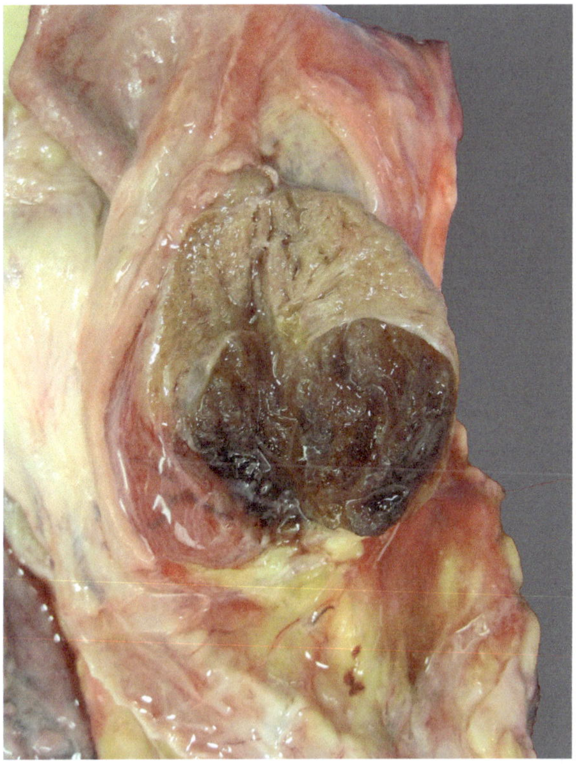

Fig. 8.17 This thyroid tissue has a brown, colloid nodule seen towards the lower end. The thyroid gland in this case has simply been incised along the long axis of the lobe to demonstrate the lesion, rather than undergoing complete resection and display

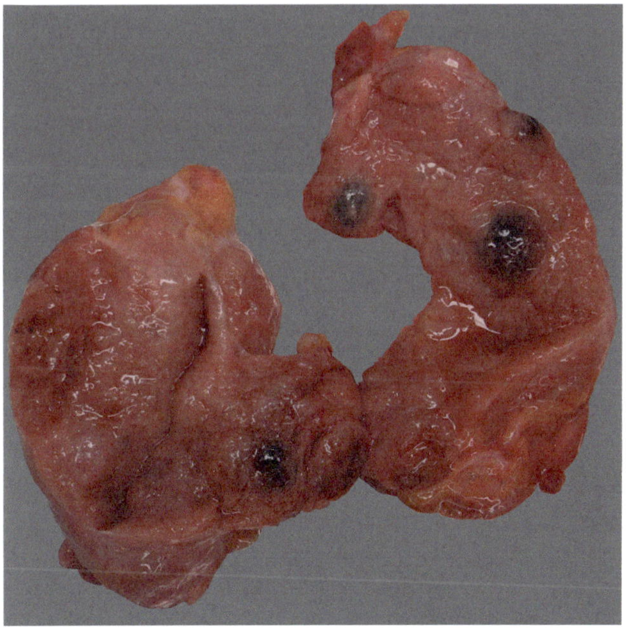

Fig. 8.18 Multiple small benign colloid cysts are seen in this thyroid tissue

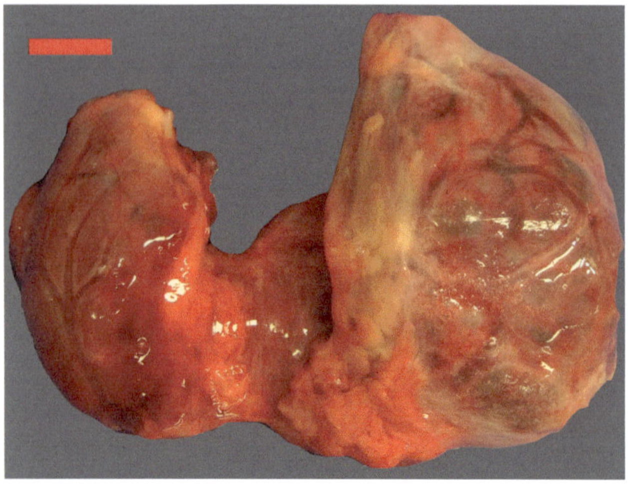

Fig. 8.19 Disproportion between the lobes of the thyroid is quite common and may produce localised goiter externally, as well as clearly defined overgrowth at autopsy. Such goiter may be associated with underproduction or overproduction of thyroid hormones, or indeed a euthyroid status

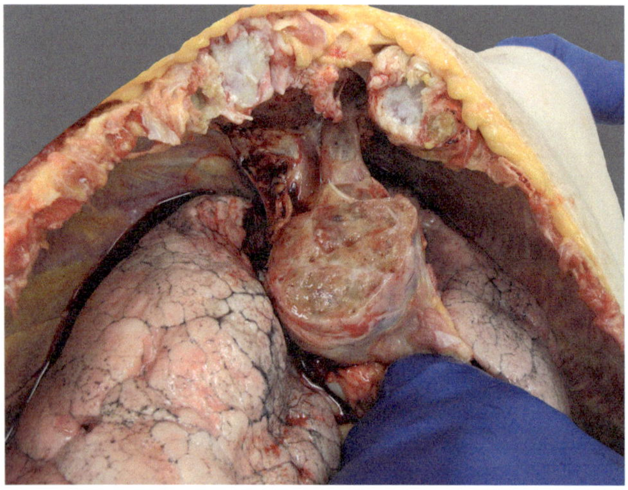

Fig. 8.20 This upper thoracic dissection shows a large colloid goiter which has been pulled downwards and forwards and away from the spinal column. It is partly obstructing the thoracic inlet but has not caused airway or vasculature compromise. Note the fibrosis and variegated architecture of the tissue, on section, with a smooth capsule externally. The total weight of this tissue was 87 g

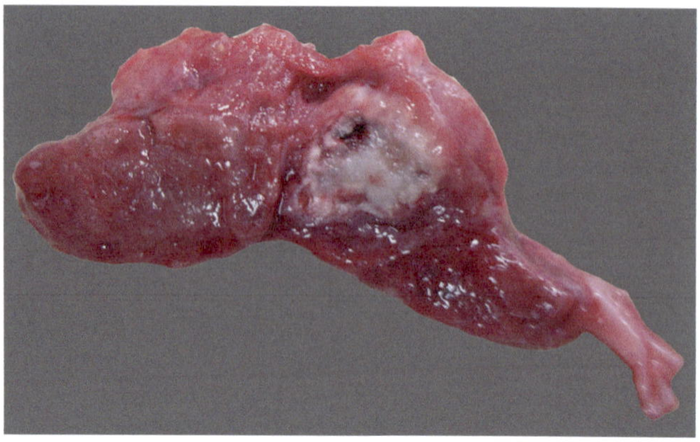

Fig. 8.21 This thyroid tissue shows an incidental, partly calcified, grey thyroid neoplasm. It has a gritty cut surface and histologically turned out to be a papillary thyroid cancer. Note that the lesion had not penetrated the thyroid capsule. Given the absence of tumour elsewhere in the body, this was deemed of no significance overall

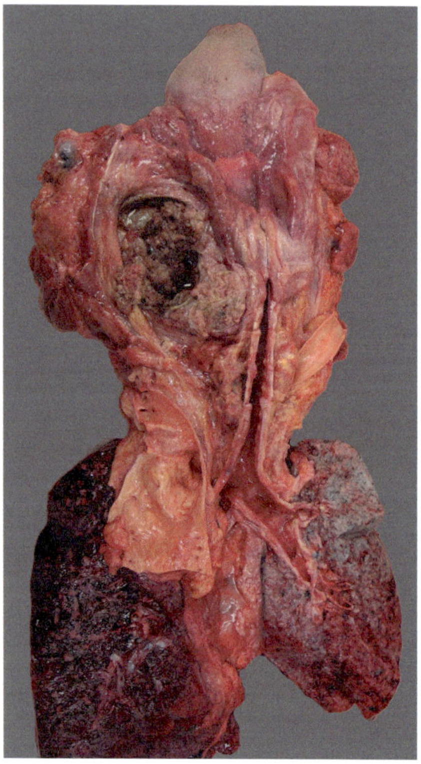

Fig. 8.22 This dissection shows the tongue superiorly, neck structures centrally, and lungs towards the base. There is distortion of the tracheal parenchyma by a partly necrotic thyroid tumor, particularly in the middle and upper cervical region

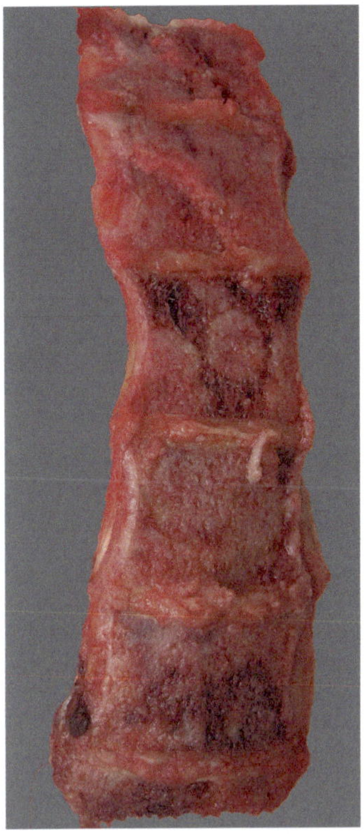

Fig. 8.23 Metastatic follicular carcinoma is seen in the vertebral tissue block

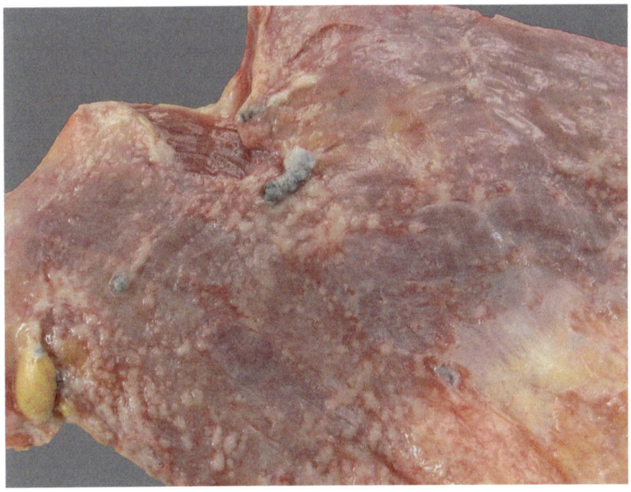

Fig. 8.24 Metastatic thyroid cancer can be seen in many sites, some being unusual. Here, follicular carcinoma deposits are seen on the superior aspect of the diaphragm. Immunohistochemistry can be applied to autopsy tissues and is of use in identifying thyroglobulin-positive neoplasia

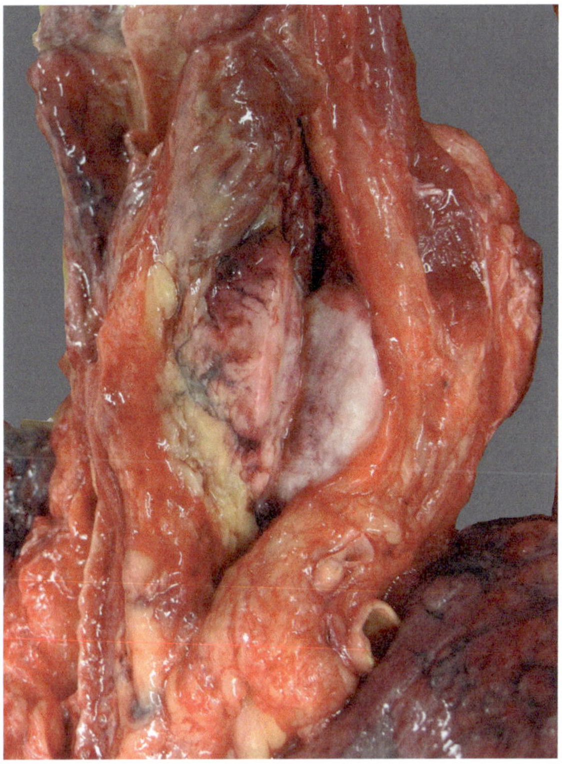

Fig. 8.25 The thyroid can be the site of metastasis, often in late-stage disseminated cancers. It can also be a primary site for lymphoma. This view shows lung cancer that has spread to the thyroid lobe, with widespread loss of the normal parenchyma

Parathyroids

The parathyroid glands (Figs. 8.26, 8.27, 8.28, 8.29, 8.30, 8.31, 8.32, 8.33, and 8.34) are often best examined and appreciated during thyroid dissection. There are usually four macroscopically identifiable glands, with an average weight in surgical biopsies of 20–40 mg. In almost all autopsy cases, the parathyroid glands are unremarkable, being small. They are often easily missed. Thus, many pathologists do not search for these small tissue elements, arguing that (unless the glands are obviously enlarged) they will likely be normal.

The majority of parathyroid pathology seen at autopsy will be found in cases of renal disease, with secondary hyperparathyroidism. This is manifest as generalized gland enlargement/hyperplasia, affecting all four glands to a roughly similar extent. In these cases, the glands are very easy to identify, potentially being up to 20 mm in diameter.

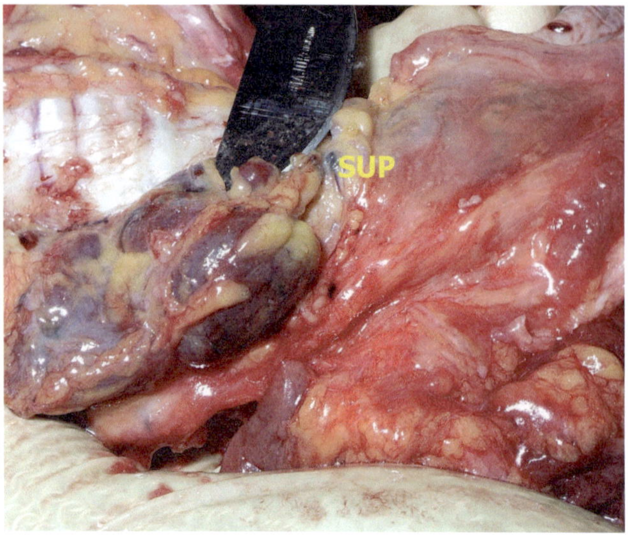

Fig. 8.26 As one dissects the posterior aspect of the thyroid gland, one should look closely for parathyroid elements. This close-up view shows that the thyroid parenchyma has been largely exposed and is being defined with tension applied to the neck structures. The right superior parathyroid gland (*SUP* here under the point of the scalpel) stands out from the thyroid capsule

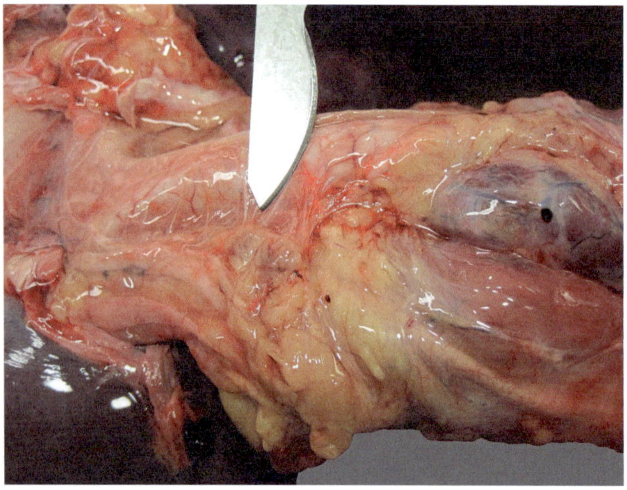

Fig. 8.27 Often the parathyroids are not easily identified, lying within fatty cervical soft tissue. If one is unsure as to the position of the glands, then it is advisable to fully resect the fatty tissues around the likely position. These tissues can then be fixed 'en masse' and later examined by histology

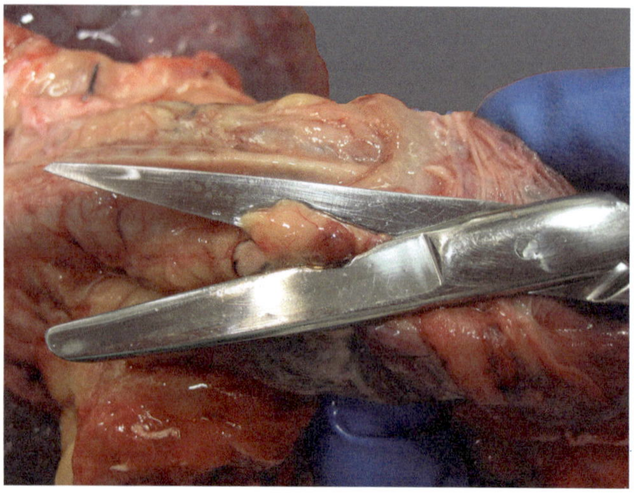

Fig. 8.28 In this case, scissors are used to lift and gently resect the parathyroid gland tissues. This is a particularly useful technique since the parathyroid glands stand out when the tissues of the neck are placed under tension

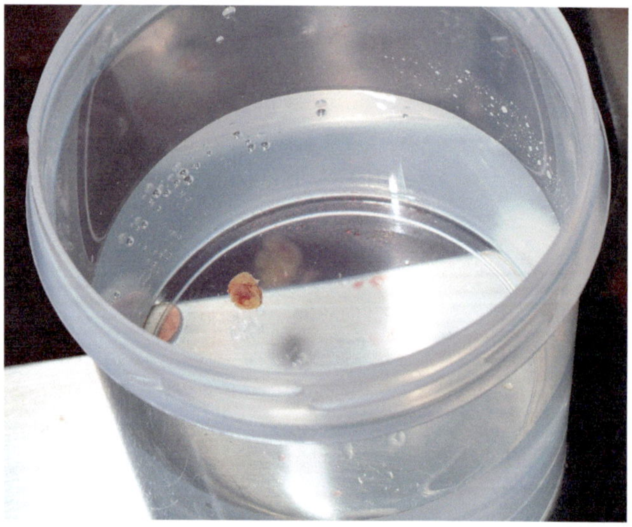

Fig. 8.29 Parathyroid glands tend to float when placed into formalin, contrasting with lymph nodes, which mostly sink. This crude technique is useful to confirm that one has captured all four glands

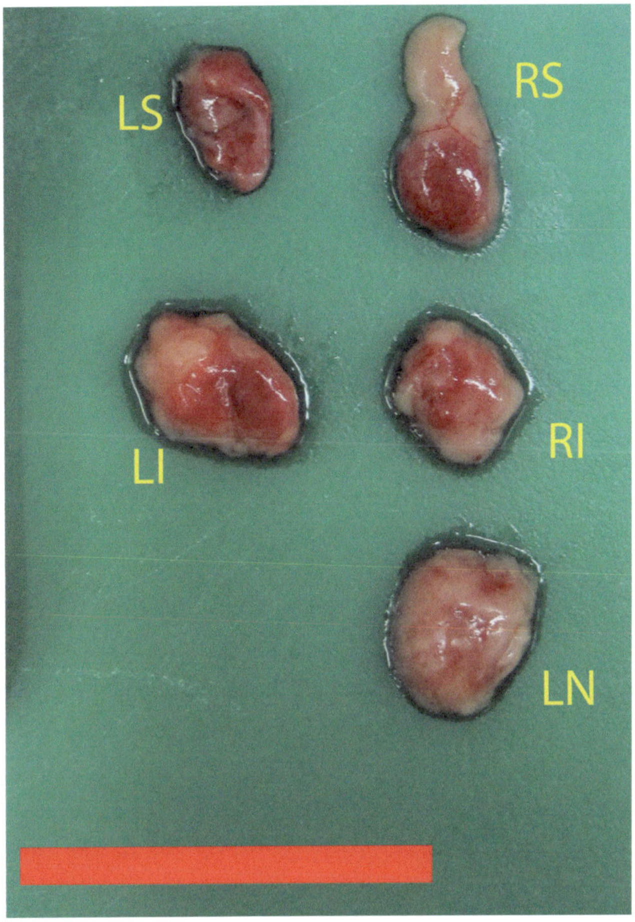

Fig. 8.30 This view of the four parathyroid glands (viewed from behind) serves to show the right superior (RS), right inferior (RI), left superior (LS) and left inferior (LI) glands. A local lymph node (LN) is included to emphasise how easy it is to mistake nodes and parathyroid tissues

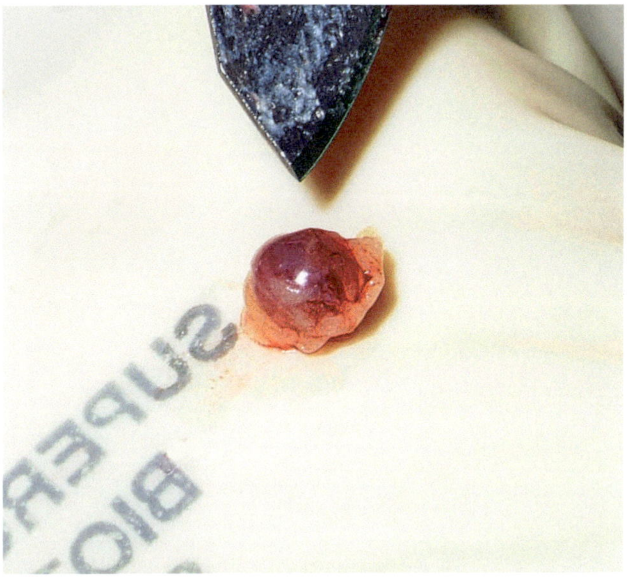

Fig. 8.31 Close-up of the parathyroid gland shows a fine vascular network around the gland tissue, which is closely attached to local fatty soft tissue and the back of the thyroid gland

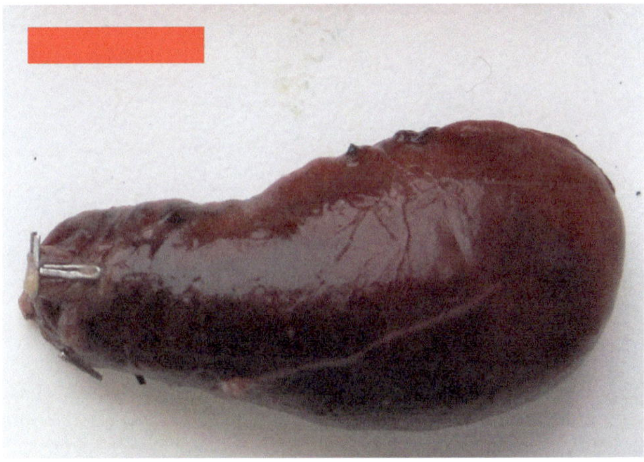

Fig. 8.32 A parathyroid adenoma (surgical case), showing considerable glandular enlargement. The other glands were normal in size

Fig. 8.33 On occasion, parathyroid resection would have been undertaken previously, usually as a consequence of chronic kidney disease. A small amount of residual parathyroid tissue is often implanted into the forearm, and this too may become hyperplastic. This surgically resected sample shows somewhat grey tissue with surrounding brown muscle (top left), with the histology (bottom right)

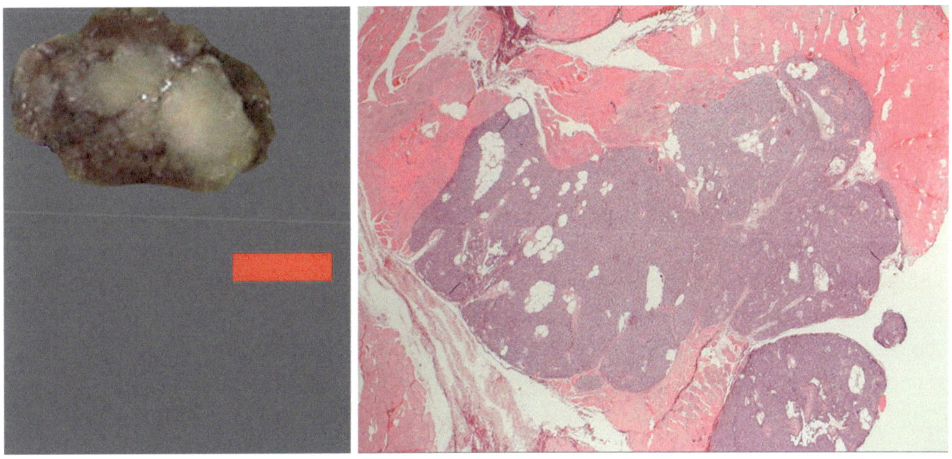

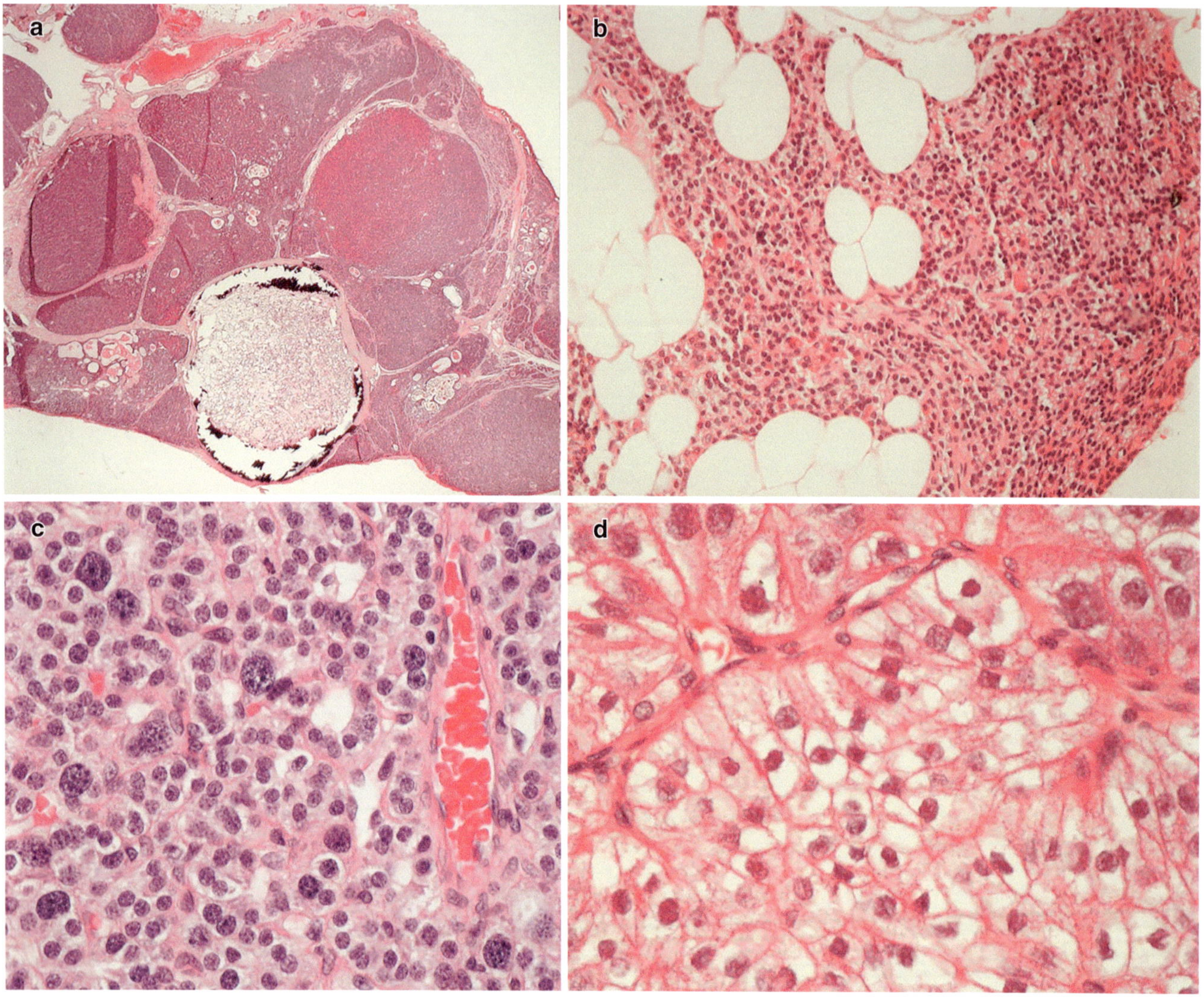

Fig. 8.34 Many aspects of parathyroid tissues are really appreciated only under the microscope. (**a**) Parathyroid hyperplasia can have a variable nodularity with some calcification. (**b**) Normal parathyroid tissues have chief and oxyphil cells mixed with fat. (**c**) Nuclear pleomorphism may be found in hyperplastic glands and does not signify malignancy. (**d**) Parathyroid carcinoma may appear relatively bland but often has pronounced clear cytoplasm

Contrastingly, it is rare to find complete absence of the parathyroid tissues, unless part of a syndrome (e.g. DiGeorge syndrome). Therefore, in most cases, the absence of parathyroid gland enlargement (together with no ante-mortem history of significance) may allow one to judge that the glands are within normal limits.

The parathyroids are best identified by means of careful dissection of the thyroid. This section demonstrates a posterior approach, grasping the anterior neck tissues firmly and applying tension towards the front of the cervical block. This allows the scalpel blade to gently scrape along the edge of the posterior thyroid. As one applies gentle sweeping movements with the scalpel blade, the parathyroids will begin to "pop" into view and often are clearly evident without any detailed dissection.

Firm incision into the soft tissues and thyroid is not recommended, as this will distort the thyroid parenchyma/capsule with the blood and fluid loss often obscuring the dissection plane.

If the glands cannot be identified, then the soft tissues (including fat, lymph nodes and possible parathyroid tissue) adjacent to the thyroid are resected en-bloc in order to guarantee capture of the parathyroids. It should also be remembered that the upper thymic tissue can contain some embryologically-derived parathyroid parenchyma. If it is important to understand all sites for parathyroid histology then these sites may need to be resected for histology examination.

Adrenals

The adrenal tissues (Figs. 8.35, 8.36, 8.37, 8.38, 8.39, 8.40, 8.41, 8.42, 8.43, 8.44, 8.45, 8.46, 8.47, 8.48, 8.49, 8.50, 8.51, and 8.52) have two significantly different endocrine functions. The outer cortex, appreciated histologically as three discrete layers, is the site of production of a variety of steroids. These have effects in terms of mineral metabolism, general health and sexual function. The inner medullary tissues are concerned with the production of adrenalin and noradrenalin, principally. The weight of the adrenals varies according to the body frame of the individual, but is generally 5–10 g, per gland.

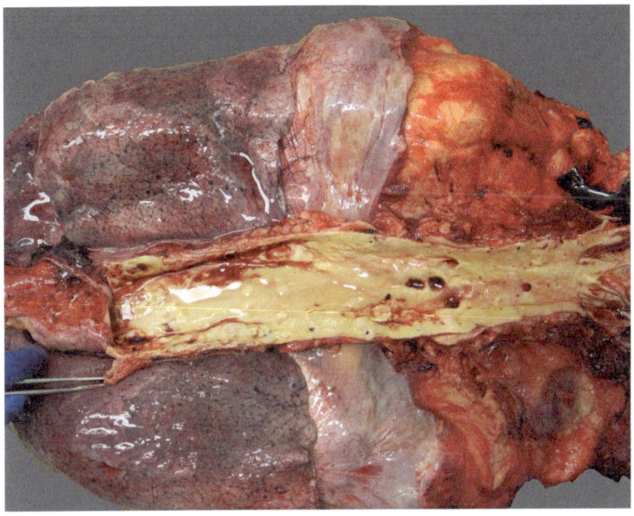

Fig. 8.35 The adrenal glands require a staged dissection for identification in most cases. The eviscerated retroperitoneal block (see Chap. 3) is seen from the back. The aorta has been opened in this initial dissection view, with the lungs being seen above the diaphragm (towards the left). The fatty retroperitoneal tissues are seen below the diaphragm. It is possible to palpate the kidney tissues and thereby derive a rough position for the adrenal glands which lie above and medial to the kidney upper poles. Removal of the diaphragms will often assist identification of the likely adrenal sites. However, in those with minimal fat, the adrenals are often clearly visible on direct inspection

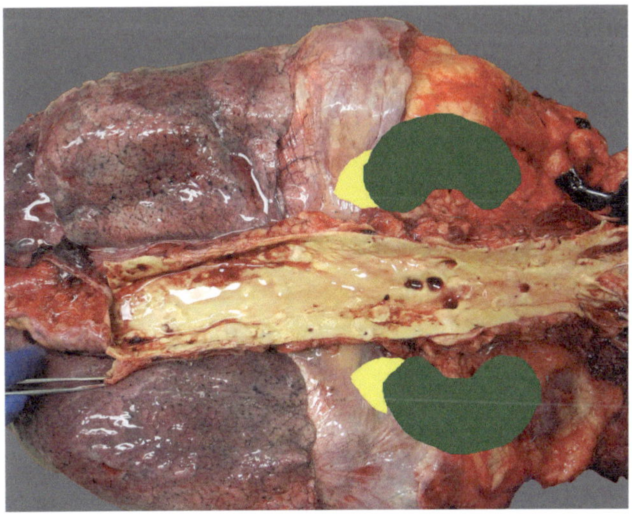

Fig. 8.36 The same thoracic/retroperitoneal block of tissue has overlaid two green kidney shapes to represent the positions of the renal parenchyma. The approximate position of the adrenals (yellow) is seen on the superior aspect of both kidneys. Awareness of this localization can assist the search for these glands

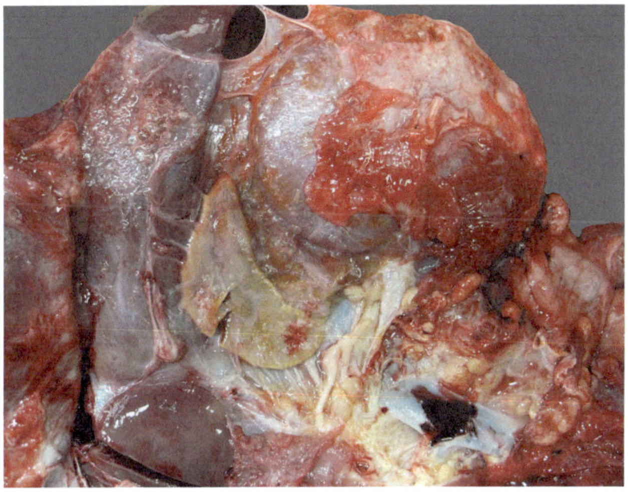

Fig. 8.37 The right side posterior retroperitoneum is seen from the back. The adrenal is positioned above and slightly medial to the kidney tissues. The relative paucity of fat in this case allows one to fully appreciate the shape and architecture of the adrenal in relation to the liver and kidney

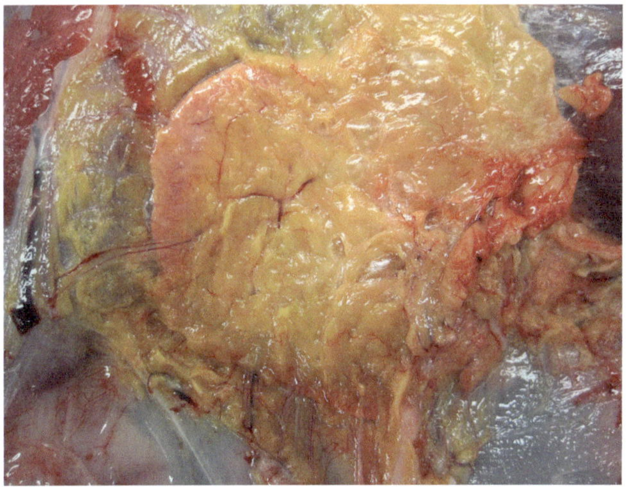

Fig. 8.38 The adrenal has been partly dissected free of the surrounding fat. There is a fine fibrous capsule around the cortex

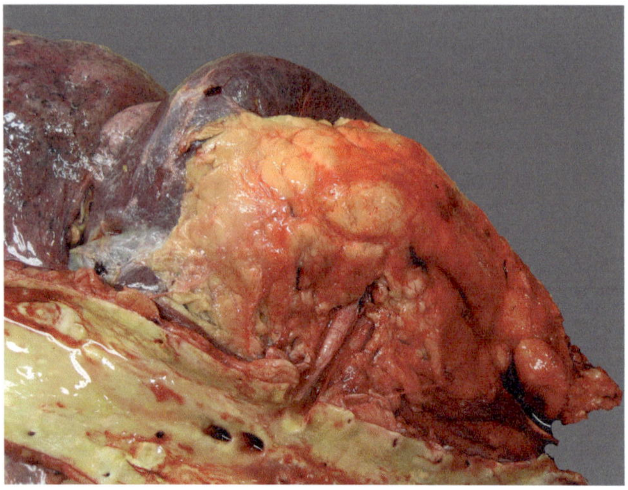

Fig. 8.39 The aortic tissues have been opened and the proximal renal artery is likewise open. The vague outline of the kidney can be identified, but the adrenal gland is not immediately apparent. One therefore has a choice as to whether one dissects directly into the fat in order to identify the gland, and then trace/dissect around the adrenal, or to resect the entire fatty tissue block that lies superior to the kidney, and then serially section this tissue

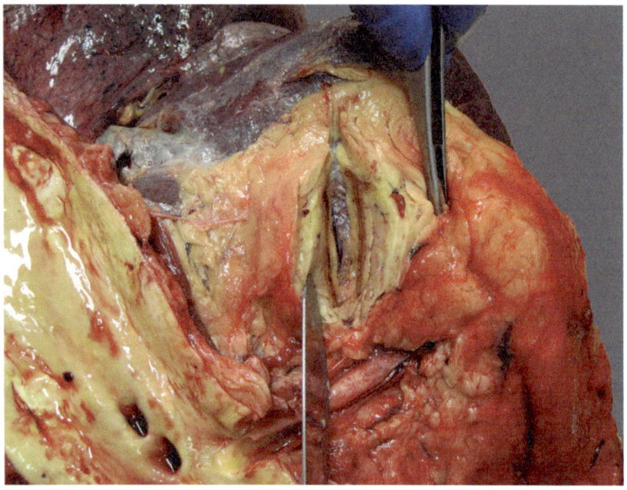

Fig. 8.40 When pronounced fat is obscuring the adrenal position, one may choose to identify the adrenal by making a single cut into the fat and then dissecting around the adrenal once it is found. Alternatively, one can proceed along the course of the adrenal artery to identify the gland tissue, although this is a more time-consuming technique

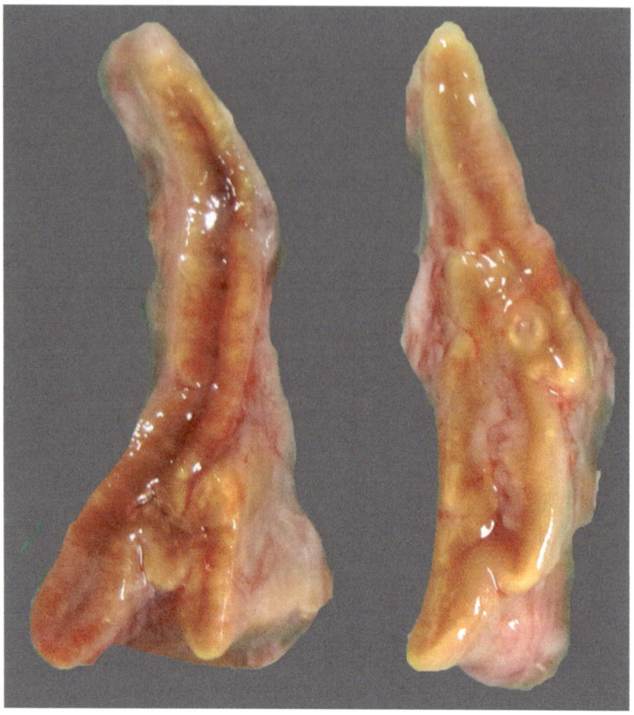

Fig. 8.41 The cut surface of the normal adrenal shows a yellow/orange cortex, reflecting the steroid production of the three zones or layers of the cortex. The medullary tissue is often a tan/brown color, although it may be difficult to define on occasion. It is noted that the adrenal has a somewhat lumpy, irregular quality on the external and internal cut surface, without defined nodularity or other focal pathology. In some areas the adrenal tissue is folded, potentially giving a false impression of cortical hyperplasia

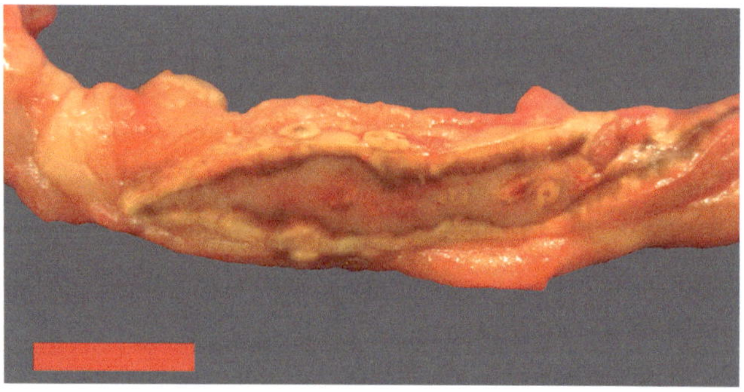

Fig. 8.42 This adrenal, with some peripheral fat, shows a relatively thin cortex in relation to the medullary parenchyma. Although one might interpret this as medullary hyperplasia, it is in fact cortical atrophy in an individual who was systemically stressed by several episodes of surgery over the 2 weeks prior to death. In this case, the depletion and thinning of the cortical tissues is a stress response. One can see similar changes in individuals given long-term exogenous corticosteroids, with secondary ACTH suppression and thereby cortical atrophy

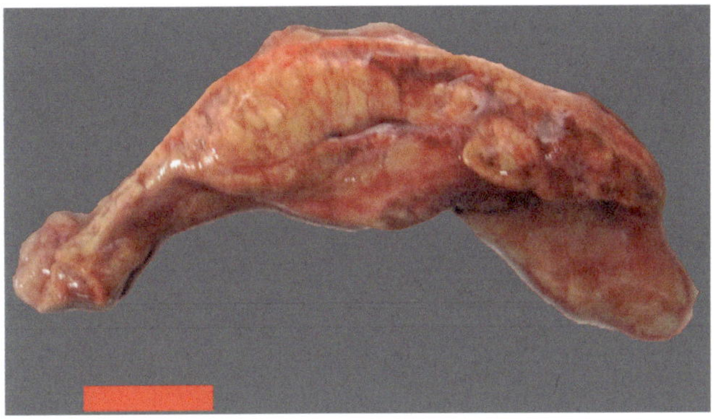

Fig. 8.43 This adrenal shows nodular hyperplasia of the cortex, with variable thickness of the cortical tissues. The hyperplasia is not uniform along the tissue length

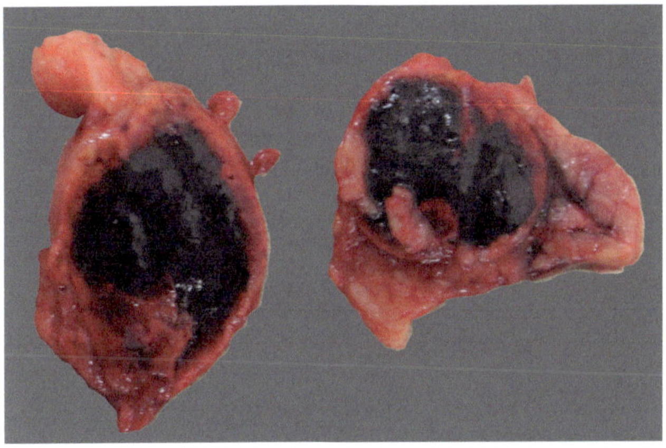

Fig. 8.44 This adrenal has been opened to reveal marked parenchymal haemorrhage, principally in the medullary parenchyma, in a case of disseminated sepsis. Such changes are common in cases of significant bacteraemia (e.g., meningococcal meningitis or group A streptococcal septicaemia)

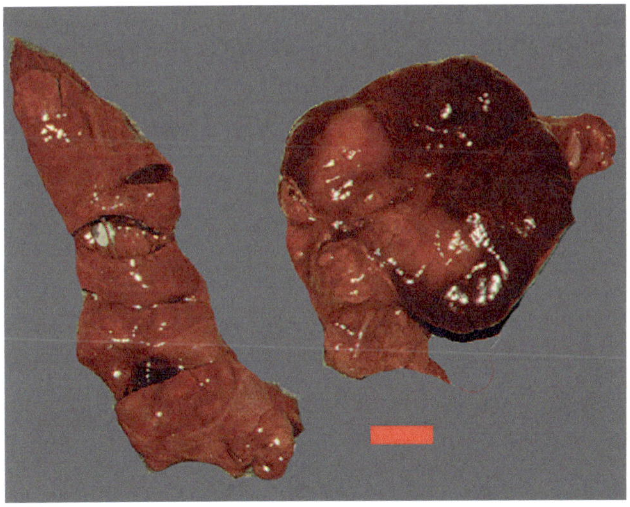

Fig. 8.45 An adrenal myelolipoma is seen in a case with associated sickle cell disease (HbSS). The adrenal on the left side is normal. The right-side adrenal had a soft, haemorrhagic tumour. Histological examination confirmed the presence of all three types of hematological elements, although there was pronounced hyperplasia of the erythron, in keeping with the sickle cell anaemia

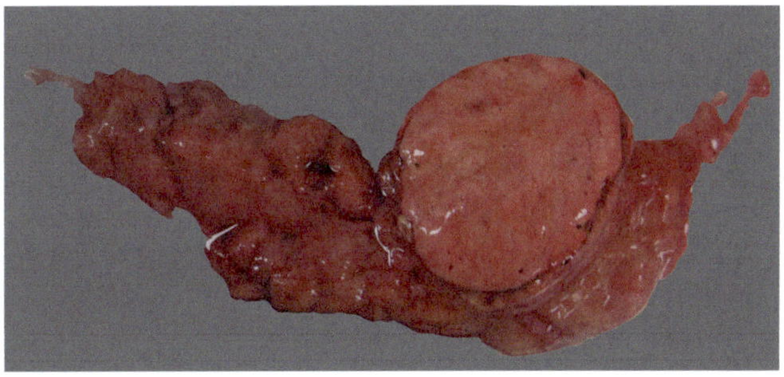

Fig. 8.46 A rounded yellow adrenal adenoma is seen on the right hand aspect of this adrenal gland. Such tumours may be found incidentally at autopsy. They may be functional (actively secreting hormones) or without endocrine secretion or effects

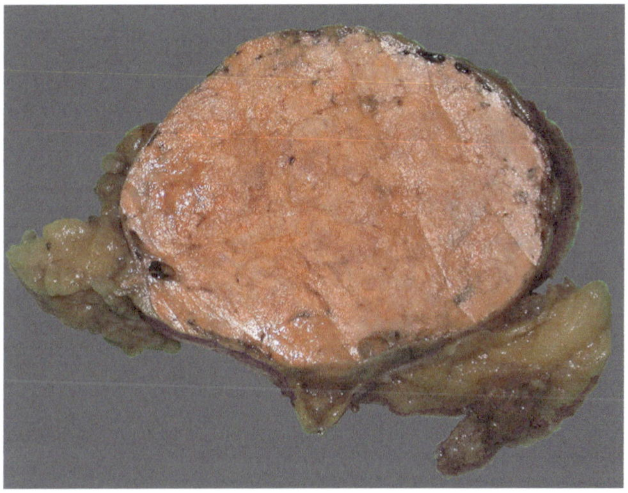

Fig. 8.47 An incidental rounded adrenal neoplasm, with no features of malignancy. This had no secretory activity and was an unexpected autopsy finding

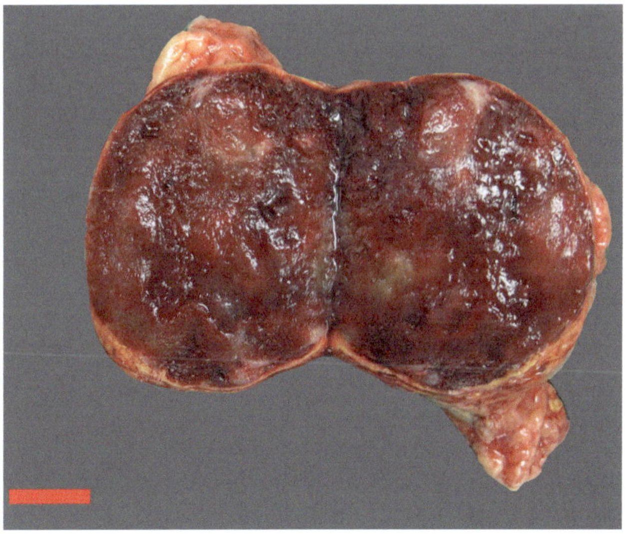

Fig. 8.48 An adrenal paraganglioma is present, with a thin rind of normal adrenal tissue stretched around the mid brown adrenal tumour. Such tumours may be functional with significant cardiovascular consequences, or they may be hormonally silent

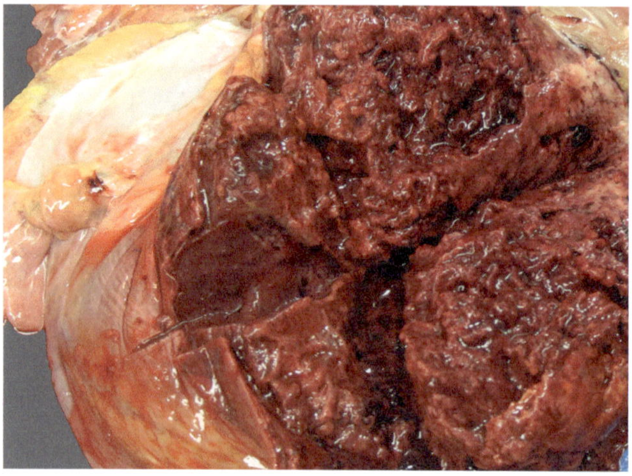

Fig. 8.49 The retroperitoneal tissues of this case have been partially dissected and exposed in a case of adrenal cortical carcinoma. The tumour had been treated by both radiotherapy and chemotherapy. Tissue necrosis has occurred because the tumour outgrew its own blood supply, and because of the oncological treatments, resulting in a large zone of haemorrhage and necrotic tissue. It is not easy to find viable tumour elements in necrotic tumors, and widespread sampling is recommended for histology

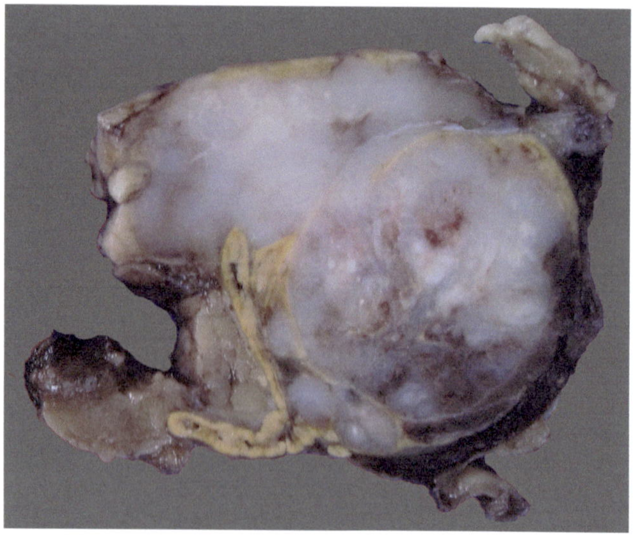

Fig. 8.51 This fixed adrenal tissue has been widely invaded by metastatic lung carcinoma, with expansion of the tumour into adjacent soft tissues. Residual adrenal tissue can be seen focally, but the carcinoma has widely infiltrated and disrupted the gland

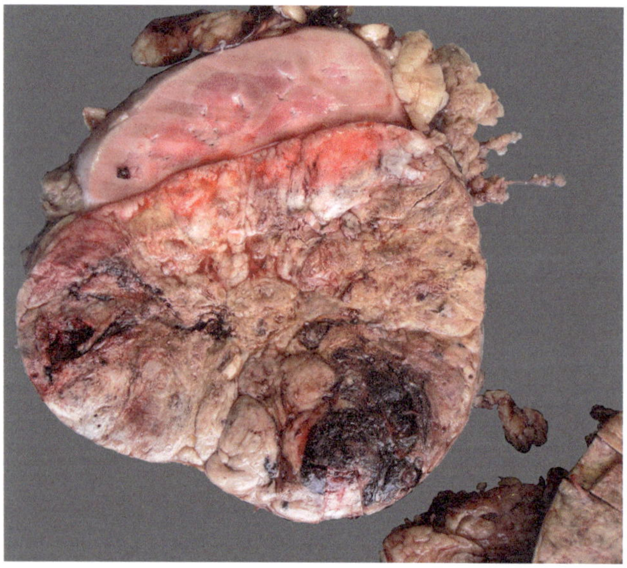

Fig. 8.50 An adrenal carcinoma (with partial necrosis and degeneration) is seen with focal haemorrhage. Normal kidney tissue is seen adjacent

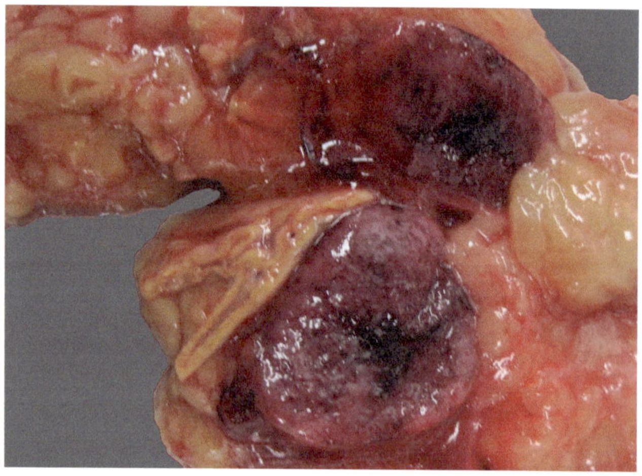

Fig. 8.52 This case of alleged adrenal tumor actually reflected lymphadenopathy adjacent to the adrenal rather than tumour within the parenchyma. Metastatic tumours to the para-aortic site can be mistaken for adrenal neoplasia (either primary or secondary), so histological sampling is often important

The adrenal gland tissues are sited close to the kidney superior pole/capsule. Very rarely, heterotopic rests may be seen in the para-ovarian/testis sites. The glands are often deep within a significant amount of retroperitoneal fat, hindering identification. Blind dissection or slicing into the fat at the likely gland site should allow one to inspect the tissues directly. This process is obviously easier if the glands are not deep in retroperitoneal fatty parenchyma. However, whether found by direct vision or by serial slices, the direct visualization of the parenchyma during the course of a routine autopsy is often all that is necessary to confirm normality.

This basic examination technique allows confirmation of the normal arrangement of cortical and medullary tissues and exclusion of nodularity, tumors, hemorrhage or necrosis. However, histology is of benefit in review of metabolic dysfunction, particularly if implicated in the cause of death (e.g. Cushing's disease and hypoadrenalism).

Suggested Reading

Connolly AJ, Finkbeiner WE, Ursell PC, Davis RL, editors. Autopsy pathology: a manual and atlas. 3rd ed. Philadelphia, PA: Elsevier; 2016.

Cooke RA, Stewart B. Endocrine system. In: Colour atlas of anatomical pathology. 3rd ed. Edinburgh: Churchill Livingstone; 2004. p. 183–204.

Curran RC, Jones EL. Endocrine organs. In: Gross pathology. A colour atlas. Harvey Millar HM + M Publishers; 1974. p. 70–5.

Goldblum JR, Lamps LW, McKenney JK, Myers JL. Thyroid gland, parathyroid gland, adrenal gland and other paraganglia. In: Rosai and Ackerman's surgical pathology. 11th ed. Edinburgh: Elsevier; 2017. p. 278–371, 1190–223.

Ludwig J. Autopsy practice. 3rd ed. Ottawa: Humana Press; 2002.

Maitra A. Endocrine system. In: Kumar V, Abbas AK, Aster JC, editors. Robbins basic pathology. 10th ed. Elsevier; 2021. p. 1065–132.

Newell-Price JDC, Gibb FW. Endocrinology. In: Penman ID, Ralston SH, Strachan MWJ, Hobson RP, editors. Davidson's principles and practice of medicine. 24th ed. Elsevier; 2018. p. 647–702.

Nosé V. Diagnostic pathology: endocrine. 3rd ed. Elsevier; 2022.

The Central Nervous System, with Pituitary, Eye and Ear

9

Stephen B. Wharton and Abigail K. Sharp

Introduction

Examination of the brain is an emotive issue for some relatives as it involves opening the head. Some pathologists and medicolegal authorities prefer to examine the brain only when examination of the organs within the torso has not yielded a definitive cause of death. It may be argued that this approach is seen as more acceptable (i.e., less disfiguring) by the relatives of the deceased. This view may have some merit if ante-mortem CT imaging of the head is available and there is no likelihood of new intracranial disease.

Nevertheless, ideally the brain should be examined in every autopsy. An argument against progressing to intracranial examination only because of time constraints (cited by some pathologists) cannot be used. The autopsy examination must be sufficient to allow the pathologist to determine the cause of death reliably.

Intracranial pathology may be linked with systemic effects that result in death or that contribute to the cause of death. For example, raised intracranial pressure due to an intracranial haemorrhage may result in systemic hypertension that precipitates rupture of an abdominal aortic aneurysm. Similarly, systemic disease and its treatment may have an effect on the central nervous system (CNS) with impact upon the cause of death. Examples include cerebral infarction following myocardial infarction, metastatic malignancy, and fat embolism following femoral fracture. Examination of the brain should not significantly add to the time taken to perform the post-mortem examination or reconstruct the body in a well-run mortuary.

The pathologist should be familiar with the techniques used to extract the brain, though in practise this procedure is normally performed by the anatomical pathology technician.

Examination of the pituitary gland, middle ears, eyes and spinal cord are not required in every post-mortem examination, but the techniques used to examine these structures are included in this chapter and the pathologist engaged in autopsy practise should be familiar with their use.

This chapter initially details the standard dissection process for the brain and then shows the various pathologies linked to this tissue. The final part of the chapter focuses on the less commonly assessed areas: the eye, ear and spinal cord.

The Brain

Extraction of the Brain

The brain may be extracted/eviscerated before or after evisceration of the organs within the torso. When there are concerns that death may be the result of pressure to the neck, the brain should be removed prior to opening the neck. This helps to decompress the vessels within the neck, reducing the risk of generating artefactual haemorrhages during dissection. Examination of the scalp, skull and meninges at the time of brain removal is an important part of the examination. Dural sinuses can be opened if there is suspicion of thrombosis and stripping of the dura allows more detailed

S. B. Wharton (✉)
Division of Neuroscience, School of Medicine and Population Health, University of Sheffield, Sheffield, UK

Department of Histopathology, Sheffield Teaching Hospitals NHS Foundation Trust, Sheffield, UK
e-mail: s.wharton@sheffield.ac.uk

A. K. Sharp
Department of Histopathology, Sheffield Teaching Hospitals NHS Foundation Trust, Sheffield, UK

S. K. Suvarna (represented by Grace Horne), A. K. Sharp (eds.), *Atlas of Adult Autopsy*,
https://doi.org/10.1007/978-3-031-72207-3_9

assessment of the skull base in cases where there may be a suspicion of fracture. Relationship of any haemorrhage to extradural, subdural or subarachnoid spaces should be noted at this stage of the examination.

Fixing the Brain for Neuropathological Examination

In cases where microscopic pathology of the brain is suspected (*e.g.*, dementia or demyelinating disease), the brain may be retained and fixed to allow subsequent transport and detailed examination by a neuropathologist. The brain is fixed in formalin, which should be changed after 3 days, and then every week thereafter for 3 weeks. A minimum of 3 weeks of fixation is needed before the brain is transported to a neuropathologist.

Dissection of the Brain

Examination of the fresh brain (Figs. 9.1, 9.2, 9.3, 9.4, 9.5, 9.6, 9.7, 9.8, 9.9, 9.10, 9.11, 9.12, 9.13, 9.14, 9.15, 9.16, 9.17, 9.18, 9.19, 9.20, 9.21, 9.22, and 9.23) is a relatively crude form of examination, allowing initial inspection of the external gross morphology, the meninges, circle of Willis, cranial nerves and the gyral and sulcal surfaces. It should also be sufficient, after sectioning, to allow review of the internal parenchyma for gross lesions, but more subtle and diffuse pathologies may be missed. Sampling of focal lesions for histology can be undertaken in the fresh brain. Whilst assessment of pathologies requiring microscopy, such as neurodegenerative diseases, is best performed in the fixed brain, it is possible to sample systematically for microscopic examination in the fresh brain. Although this approach is suboptimal with a risk that the assessment may be inadequate, this approach may provide useful diagnostic information in cases where consent does not permit retention, and the advice of a neuropathologist may be valuable to guide sampling.

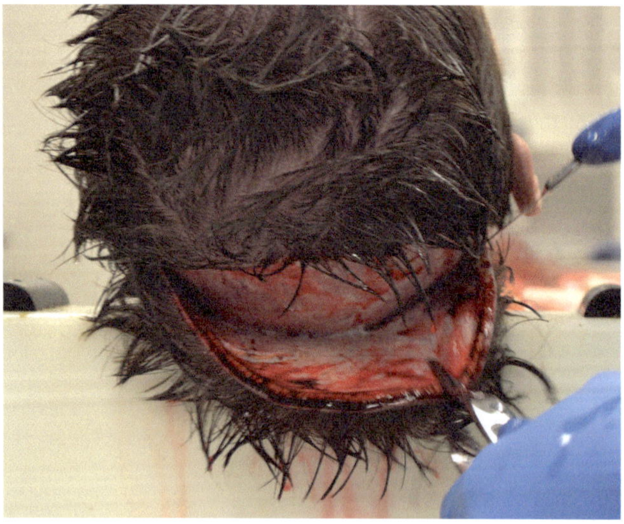

Fig. 9.1 The hair is parted and the scalp is incised over the occiput from ear to ear

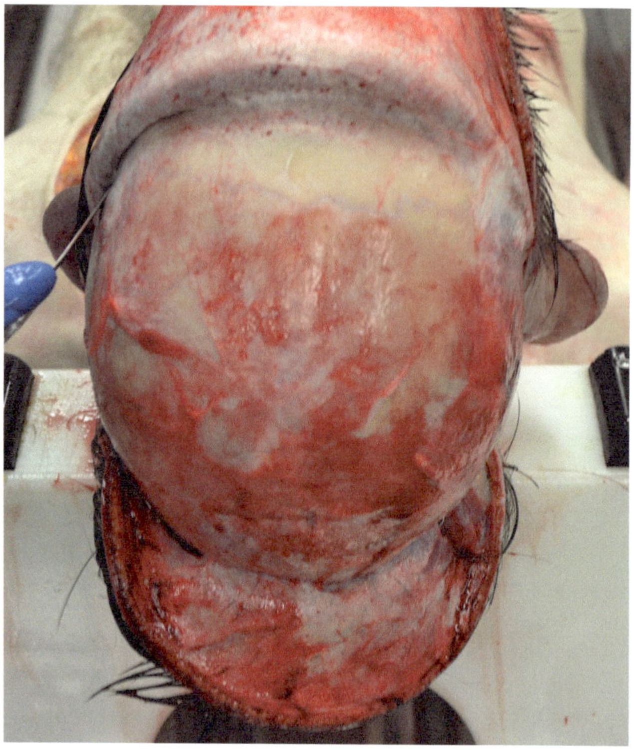

Fig. 9.2 The scalp is reflected

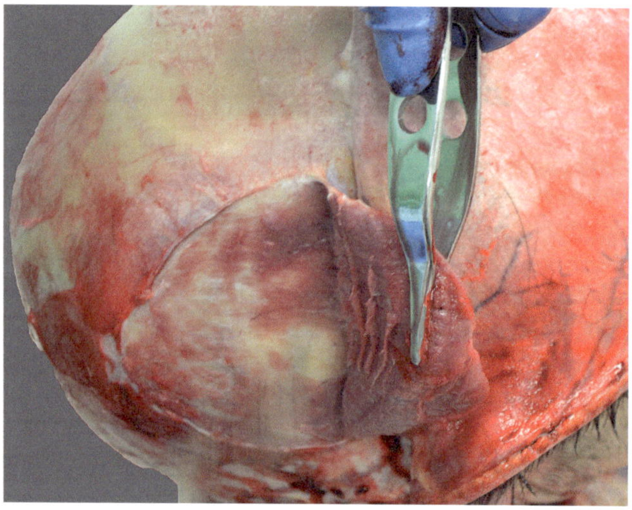

Fig. 9.3 The temporalis muscles are incised and reflected

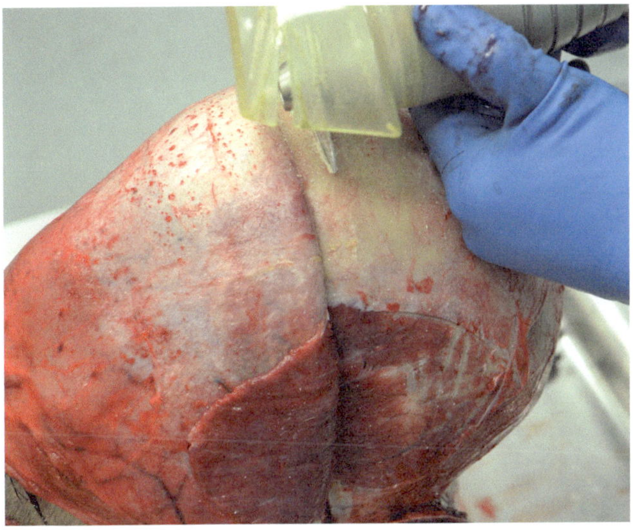

Fig. 9.4 Incising the skull is normally performed with a motorised saw with extractor unit

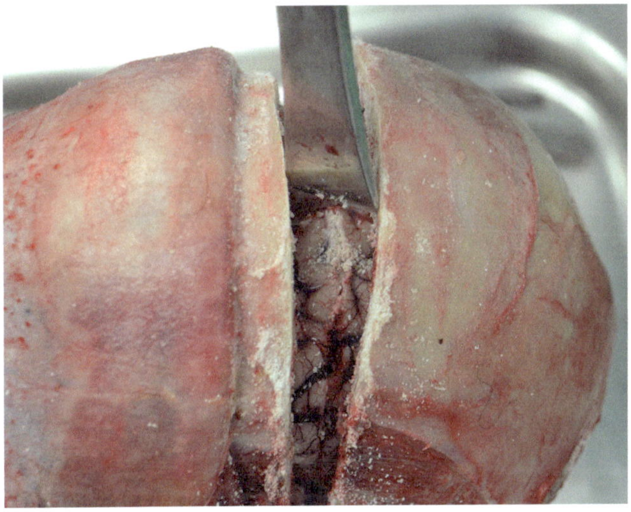

Fig. 9.5 The calvaria is separated from the skull base using a skull key

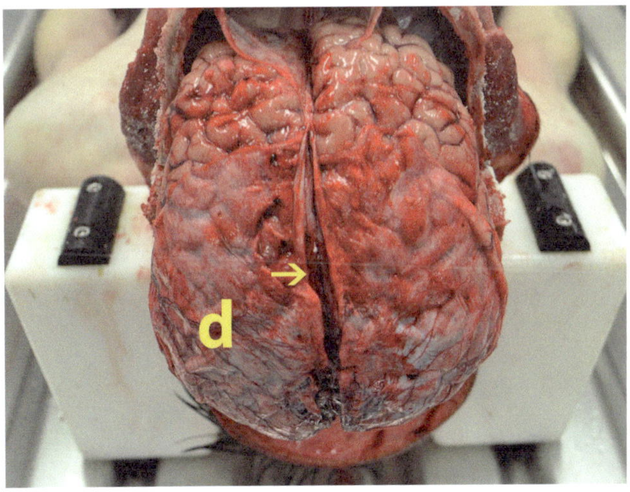

Fig. 9.6 The brain and dura are exposed by lifting off the skull cap. Some remaining dura (*d*) can be seen on the brain surface, and the superior sagittal sinus (*arrow*) has been opened

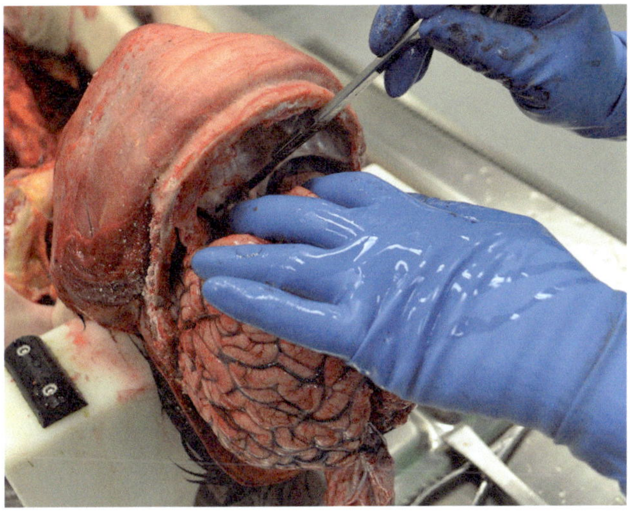

Fig. 9.7 Working from front to back under the brain, the cranial nerves and spinal cord are transected

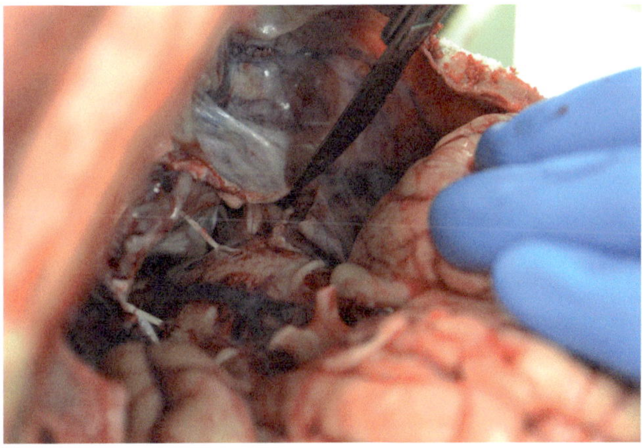

Fig. 9.8 The falx cerebri and tentorium cerebelli are incised

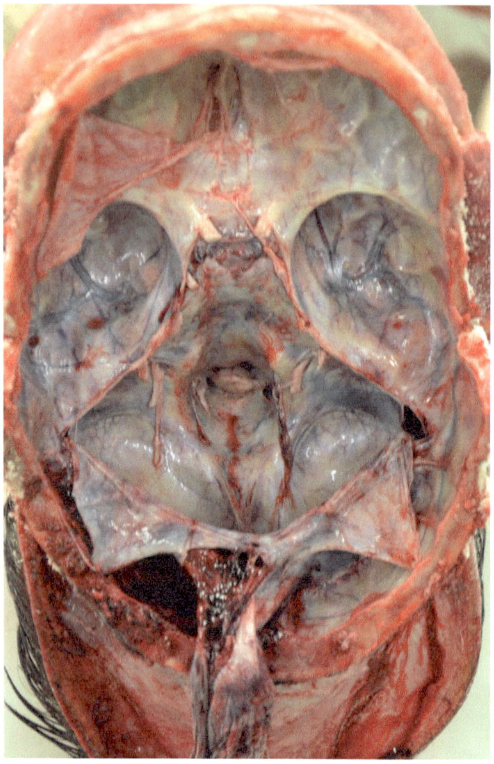

Fig. 9.9 The brain is lifted free from the head, exposing the lower cranial cavity boundary

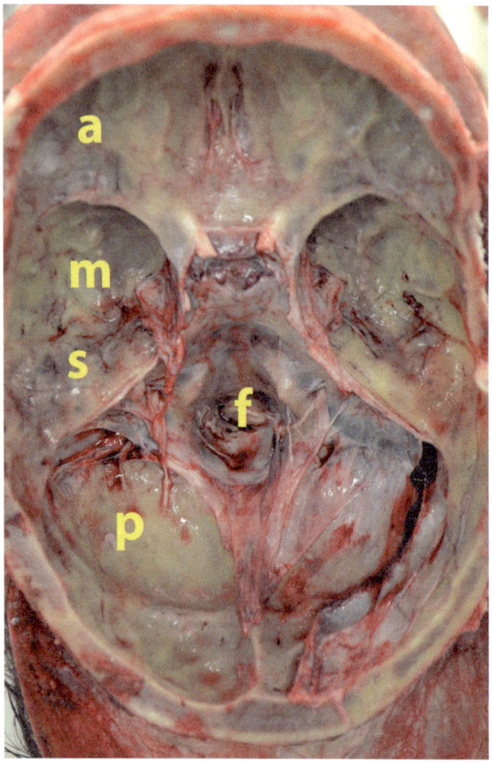

Fig. 9.10 The dura is stripped, exposing the skull base. One may identify the anterior fossa (*a*), middle fossa (*m*), posterior fossa (*p*), transected cord in the foramen magnum (*f*), and sphenoid bone tissue (*s*)

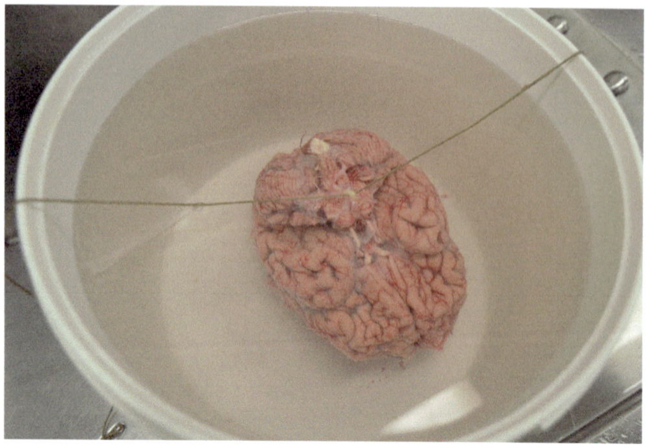

Fig. 9.11 The brain is suspended in a bucket of 10% neutral buffered formalin by a string that is passed beneath the basilar artery. The ends of the string are tied to the bucket handles, thus suspending the brain in the formalin

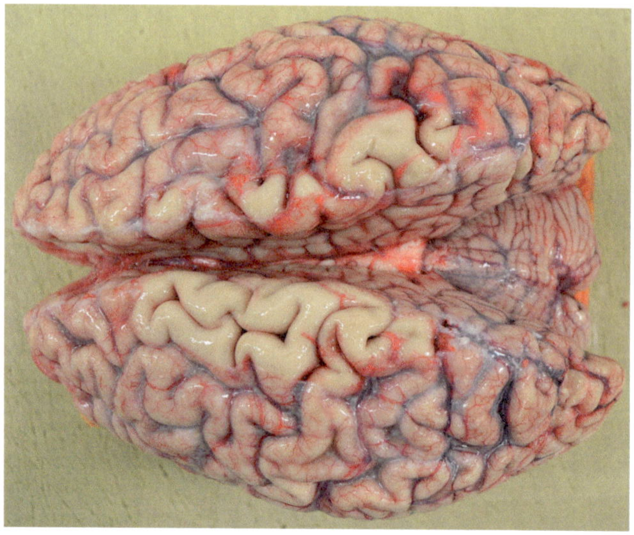

Fig. 9.12 The brain is inspected: superior surface

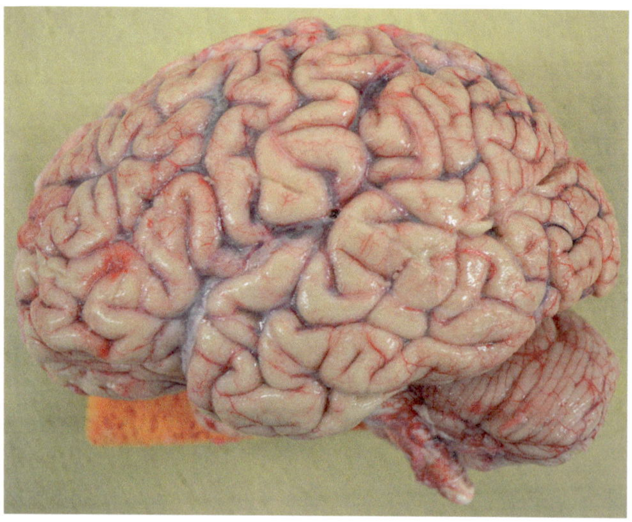

Fig. 9.13 The brain is inspected: lateral view, using a sponge to balance the brain on edge

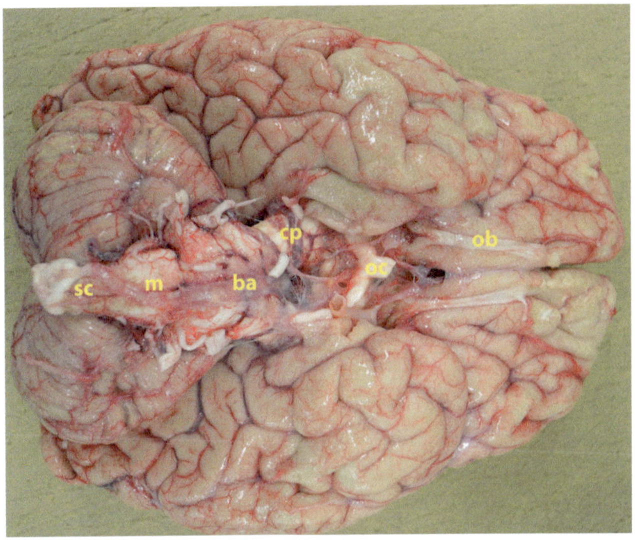

Fig. 9.14 The brain is inspected: basal view showing olfactory bulbs (*ob*), optic chiasm (*oc*), cerebral peduncle (*cp*), basilar artery (*ba*), medulla (*m*) and spinal cord (*sc*)

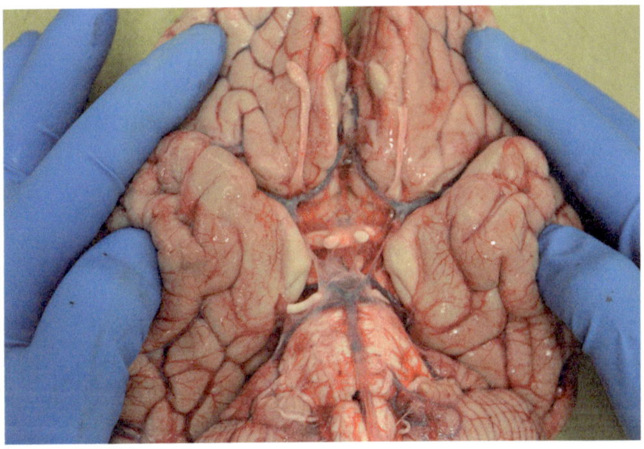

Fig. 9.15 The circle of Willis is inspected and may be dissected free for demonstration purposes. All of the branch points should be inspected for berry aneurysms, including the branching of the middle cerebral arteries in the Sylvian fissure

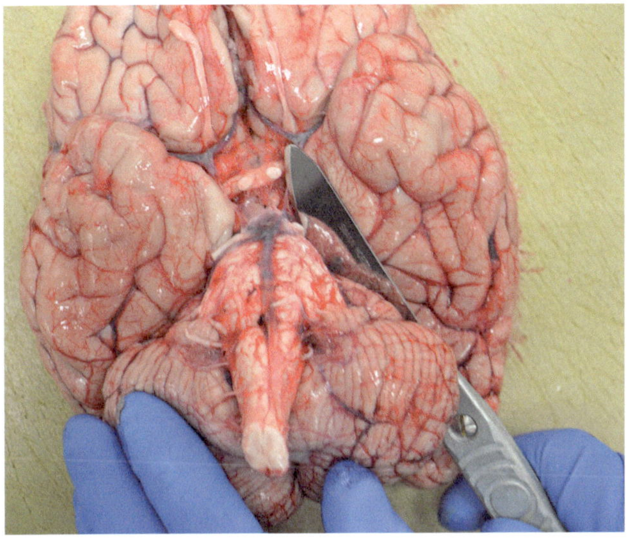

Fig. 9.16 The cerebellum and brainstem are removed by a cut through the upper midbrain, perpendicular to the long axis of the brainstem

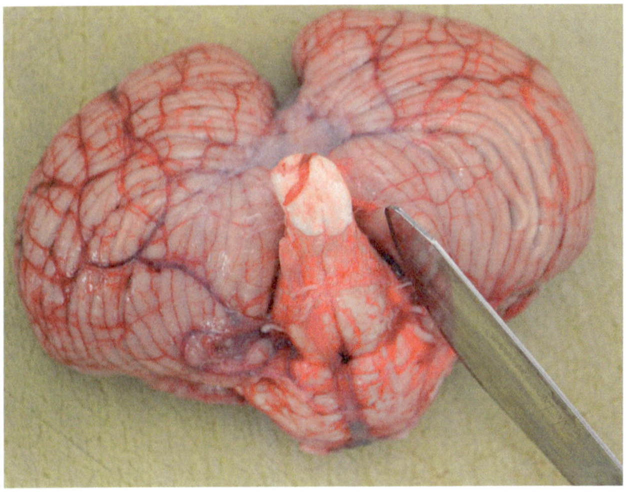

Fig. 9.17 The cerebellar peduncles are divided

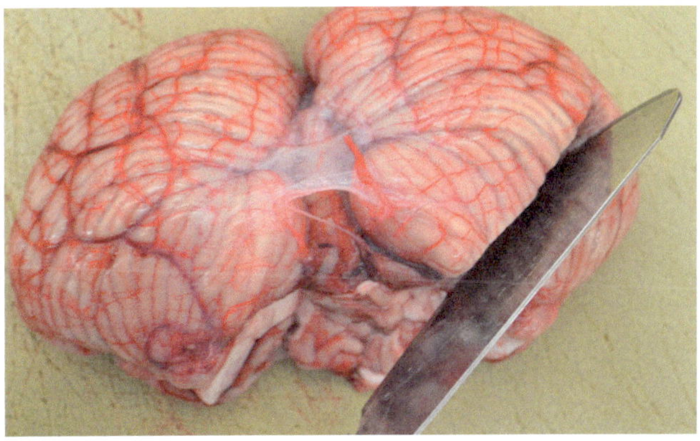

Fig. 9.18 The cerebellum is radially sliced (shown here). Alternatively, the cerebellum can be bisected in a horizontal fashion

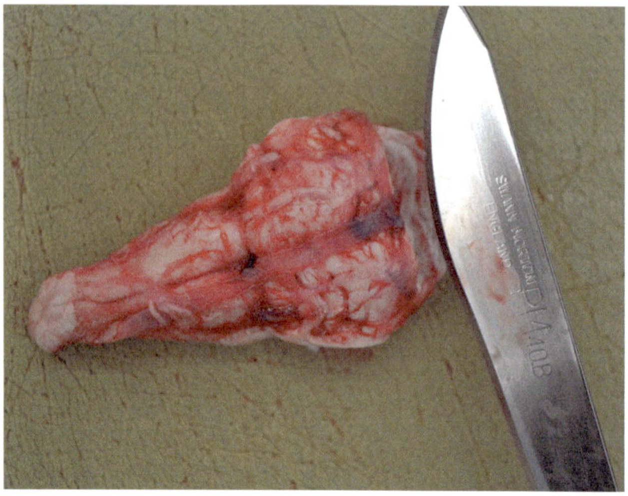

Fig. 9.19 The medulla and pons are sliced at 5 mm intervals

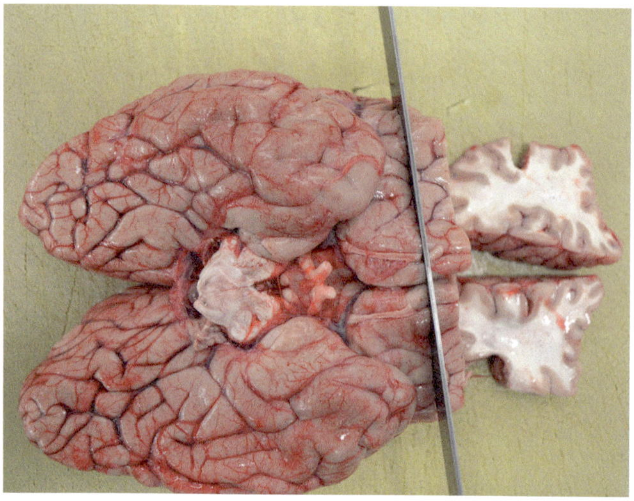

Fig. 9.20 The brain is coronally sliced at 1–2 cm intervals. For dissection of a fixed brain, the use of right-angled guide bars can guide slicing at even 1 cm intervals and thinner slices (0.5 cm) can be made if smaller lesions are sought

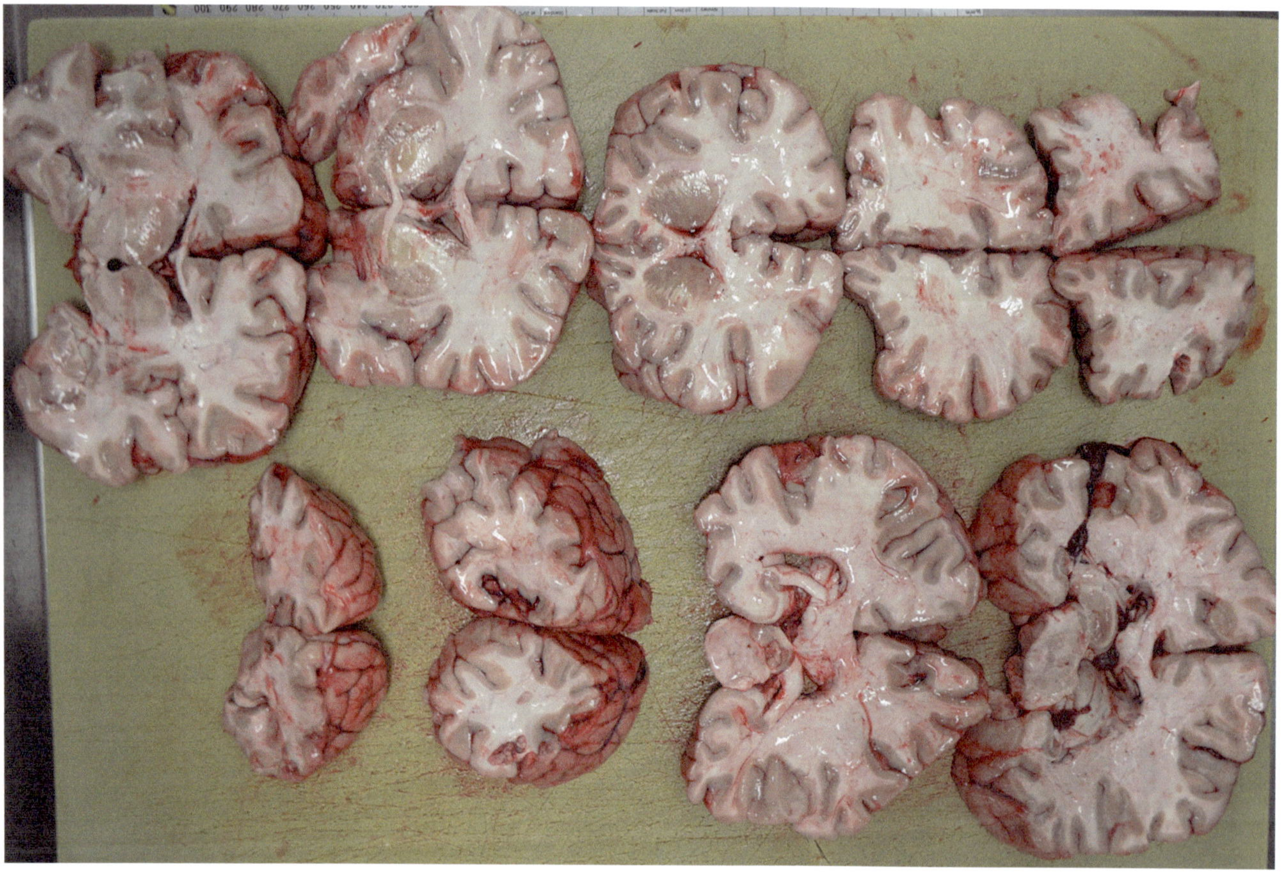

Fig. 9.21 The brain slices can be laid out for demonstration

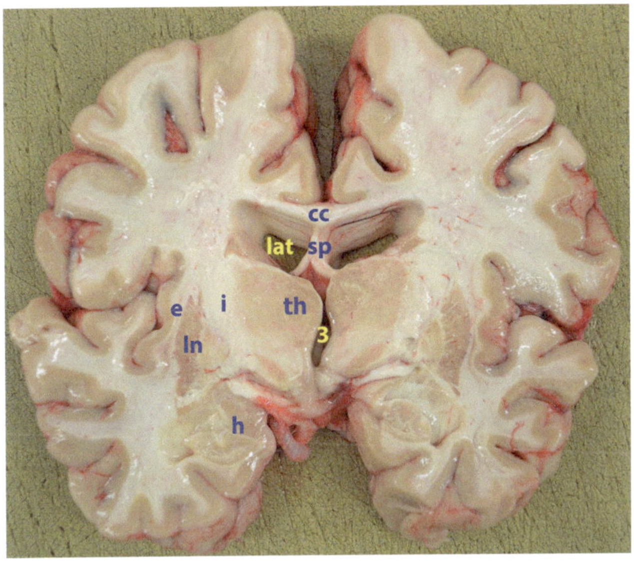

Fig. 9.22 Neuroanatomy visible in a coronal section close to the level of the mammillary bodies: corpus callosum (*cc*), septum pellucidum (*sp*), lateral ventricle (*lat*), thalamus (*th*), third ventricle (*3*), anterior hippocampus (*h*), lentiform nucleus (*ln*), external capsule (*e*), and internal capsule (*i*)

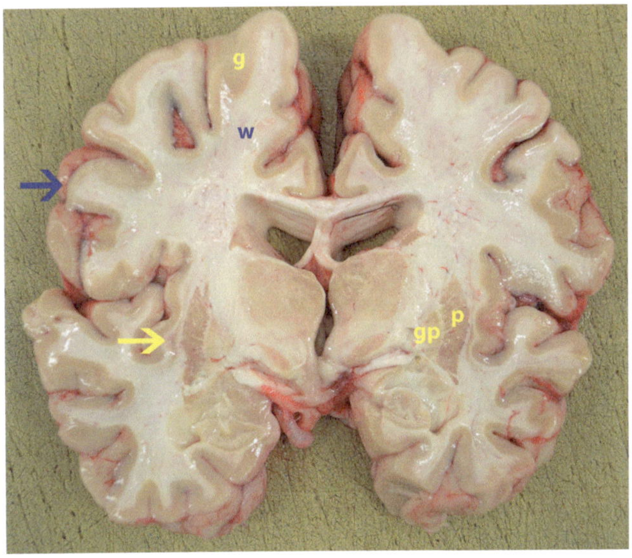

Fig. 9.23 Neuroanatomy visible in a coronal section close to the level of the mammillary bodies (same picture as Fig. 9.22): putamen (*p*), globus pallidus (*gp*), white matter (*w*), cortical grey matter (*g*), surface arachnoid/pia meninges (*blue arrow*), and claustrum (*yellow arrow*)

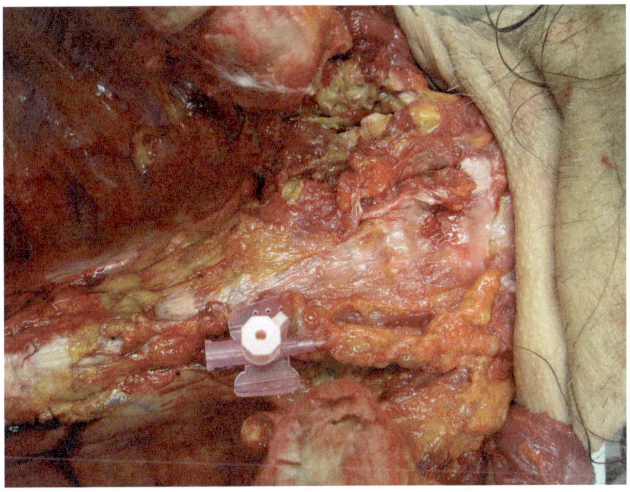

Fig. 9.24 Testing the basilar artery system can involve dissecting out the vertebral arteries from the foramina transversaria on both sides of the neck. Alternatively, one can cannulate and perfuse the vertebral artery at the start of the subclavian artery

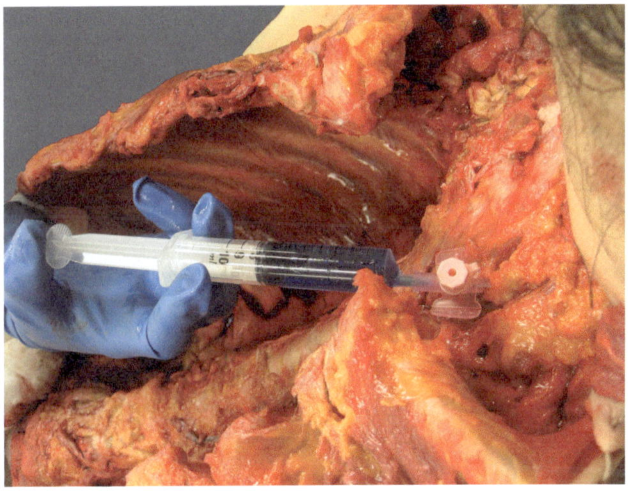

Fig. 9.25 The artery is instilled gently with water containing blue dye

Common Pathologies

Figures 9.24, 9.25, 9.26, 9.27, 9.28, 9.29, 9.30, 9.31, 9.32, 9.33, 9.34, 9.35, 9.36, 9.37, 9.38, 9.39, 9.40, 9.41, 9.42, 9.43, 9.44, 9.45, 9.46, 9.47, 9.48, 9.49, 9.50, 9.51, 9.52, 9.53, 9.54, 9.55, 9.56, 9.57, 9.58, 9.59, 9.60, 9.61, 9.62, 9.63, 9.64, 9.65, 9.66, 9.67, 9.68, 9.69, 9.70, 9.71, 9.72, 9.73, 9.74, 9.75, 9.76, 9.77,

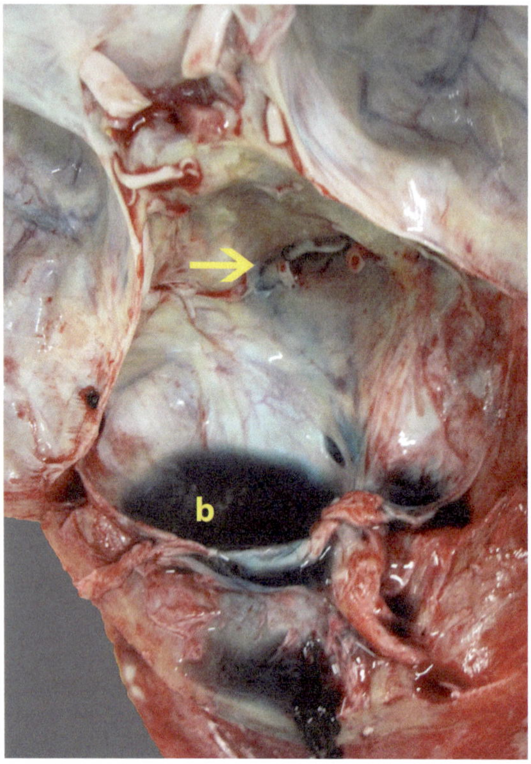

Fig. 9.26 This artery is patent and blue dye is seen emerging from the cut end of the vertebral artery (*arrow*) to pool as blue fluid (*b*) in the posterior fossa

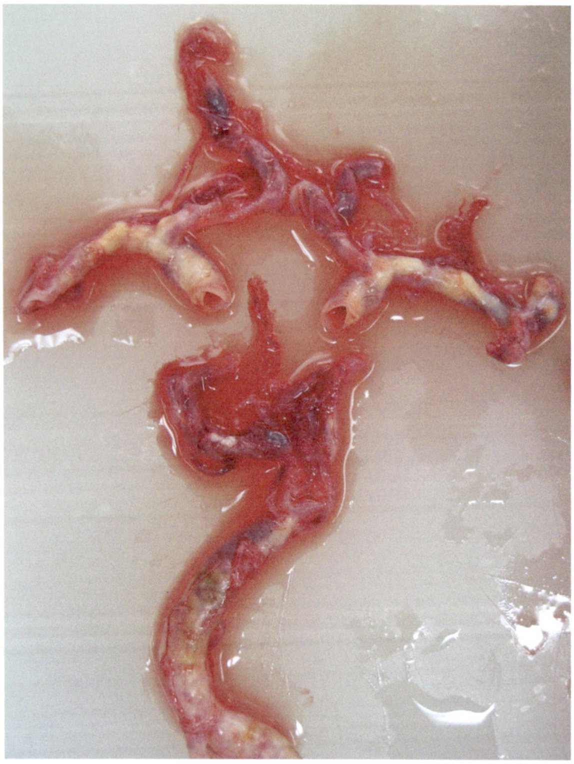

Fig. 9.27 The circle of Willis can be dissected from the base of the brain. Atheromatous disease can make the tissues both rigid and fragile, often making dissection difficult. Atheromatous disease is strongly associated with cerebrovascular ischaemia and cerebral infarction

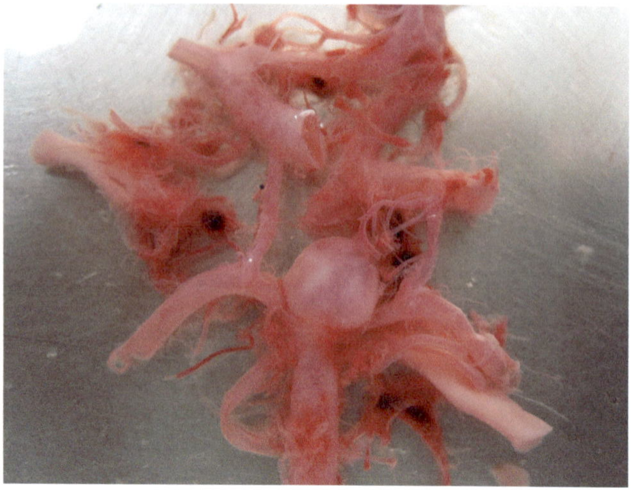

Fig. 9.28 The circle of Willis is a common site for aneurysmal change. This circle of Willis has been dissected and then floated in water to show the relative positions of the arteries, as well as a saccular aneurysm close to the origin of the posterior cerebellar artery

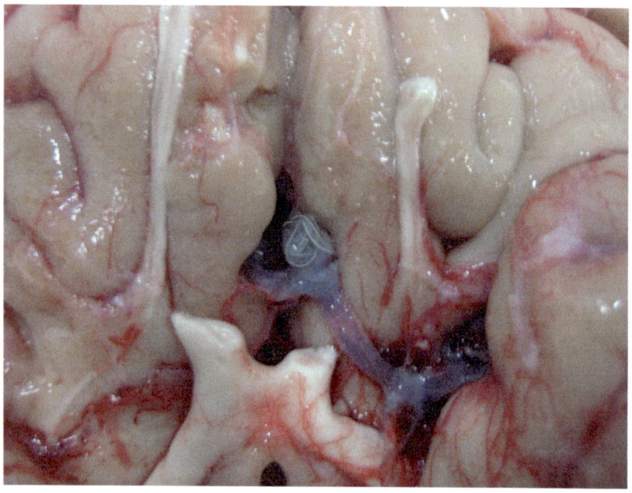

Fig. 9.29 This aneurysm has been treated by the placing of a metal coil within the dilated, aneurysmal artery. This process aims to induce local thrombosis and diminish the risk of any subsequent haemorrhage from the weakened artery site

9.78, 9.79, 9.80, 9.81, 9.82, 9.83, 9.84, 9.85, 9.86, 9.87, 9.88, 9.89, 9.90, 9.91, 9.92, 9.93, 9.94, 9.95, 9.96, 9.97, 9.98, 9.99, 9.100, 9.101, and 9.102 illustrate a variety of pathologies that may be identified. Trauma to the head may result in skull fractures or bleeding between the skull and dura (extradural haematoma) or between the dura and arachnoid layers (subdural haematoma). Berry aneurysms of the circle of Willis are common and rupture of such an aneurysm results in subarachnoid haemorrhage. Subarachnoid haemorrhage may also complicate a cerebral haemorrhage. Occlusion of the cerebral vasculature results in cerebral infarction. Benign tumours of the meninges (meningiomas) are common and are usually asymptomatic incidental autopsy findings. Tumours from many sites, particularly the lungs, may metastasise to the brain.

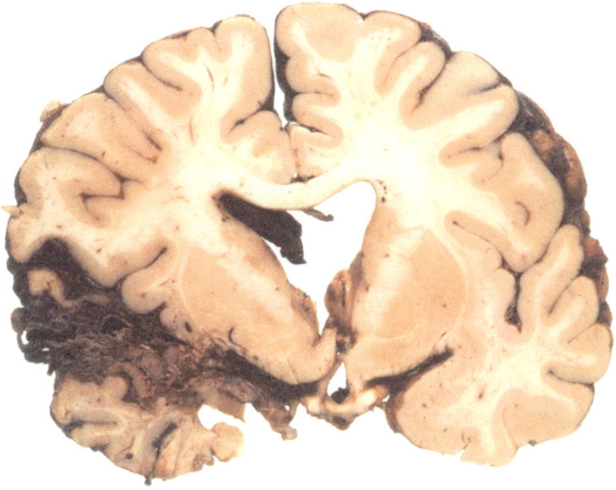

Fig. 9.30 A common vascular intracranial anomaly is the arteriovenous malformation (AVM). This characteristic appearance of a *sac of worms* is seen arising around the Sylvian fissure. Complications of AVMs include rupture and mass effect

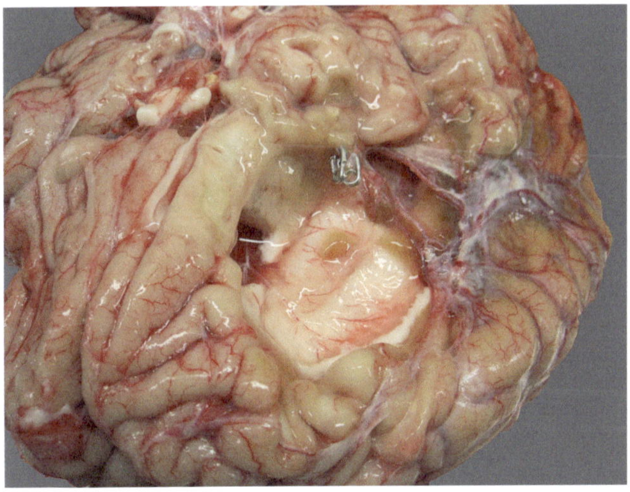

Fig. 9.31 Cerebral infarction (haemorrhagic or ischaemic) often undergoes liquefactive degeneration. The relationship to an aneurysmal vessel had been recognised earlier in this patient. A surgical clip had been placed to seal off the aneurysm in order to prevent haemorrhage

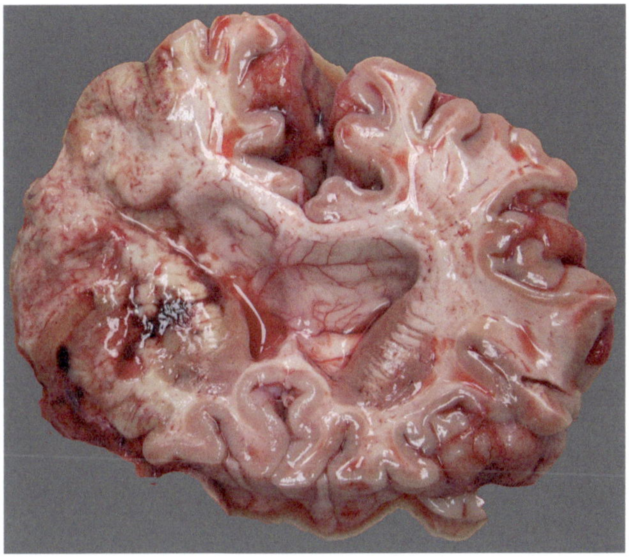

Fig. 9.32 Shown here is a middle cerebral artery infarction, with localised haemorrhage, some weeks after the initial event. Note the unilateral, wedge-shaped circumscribed change in the brain parenchyma, which was softer than the unaffected brain tissues

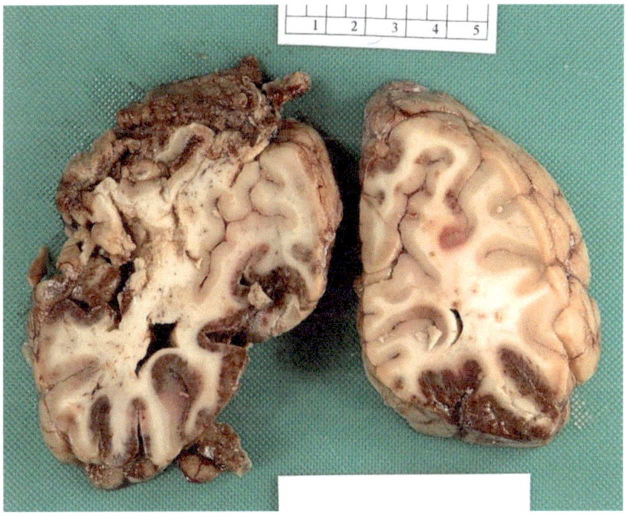

Fig. 9.33 Cerebral vasospasm due to stimulant illicit drug use can cause infarction. This is a case of amphetamine abuse. The extensive bilateral haemorrhagic infarction seen is in keeping with involvement of multiple cerebral vessels by vasoconstrictive effects caused by the substance misuse

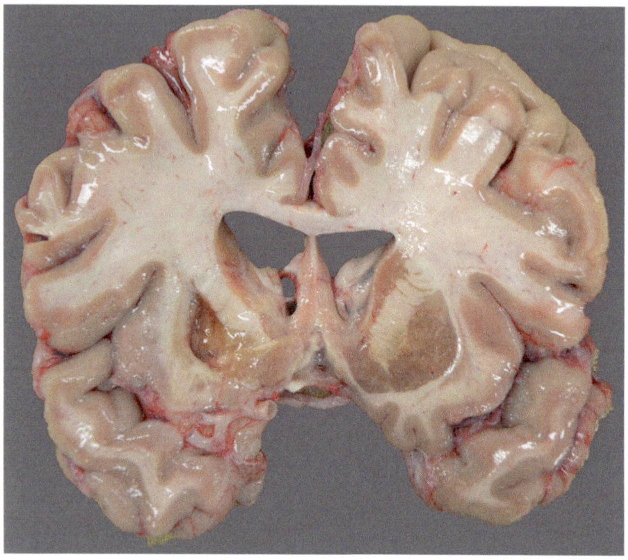

Fig. 9.34 A well-circumscribed area of cystic change and gliosis in the cerebral deep nuclei (basal ganglia) due to a vascular event. The yellow discolouration is from focal haemosiderin deposition and is suggestive of previous haemorrhage

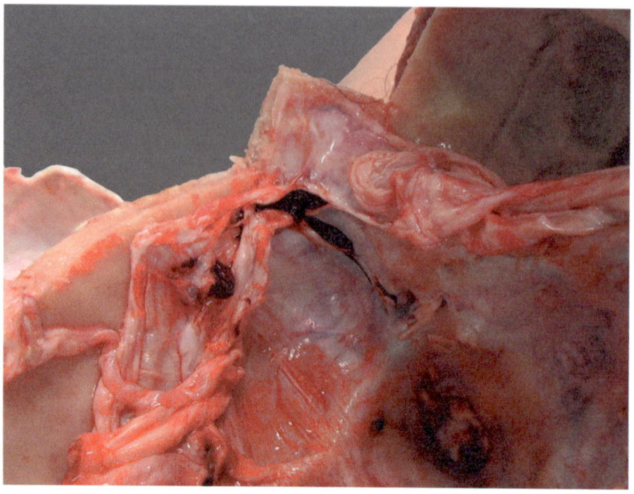

Fig. 9.36 This image shows the left base of the skull with the dura mater partially stripped. There is thrombosis of the transverse venous sinus, seen as blood clot emanating from the cut vessels. Causes of central venous sinus thrombosis (CVST) include thrombophilia disorders, malignancy and pregnancy, among others

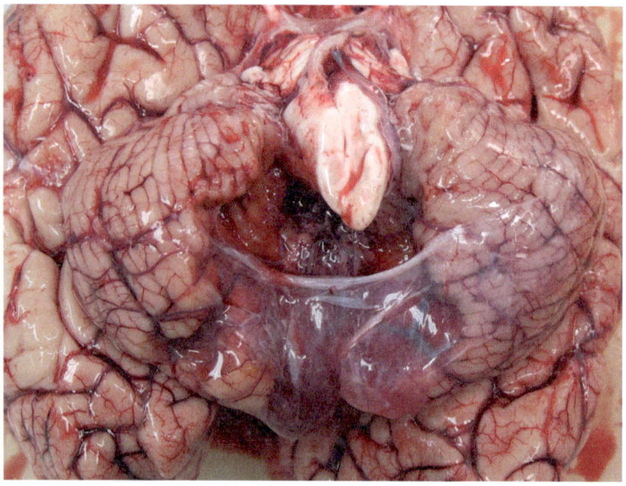

Fig. 9.35 Old cerebellar infarction is often seen as a cystic area, in this case involving the central inferior cerebellar aspect

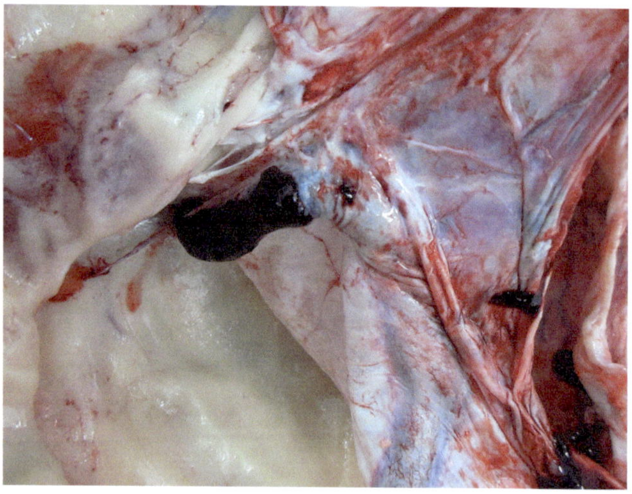

Fig. 9.37 Another example of central venous sinus thrombosis, with clot exiting the cerebral veins. This person died soon after vaccination against COVID-19. Death was due to cerebral haemorrhagic infarction because of the CVST

Neurosurgical interventions may be encountered at autopsy. Burr holes may be drilled into the skull to relieve raised intracranial pressure. These are typically located over the parietal bones and are 10–12 mm in diameter. When wider access to the brain is needed, a craniotomy is used. Intracranial pressure monitors are commonly used to monitor patients who have undergone neurosurgery.

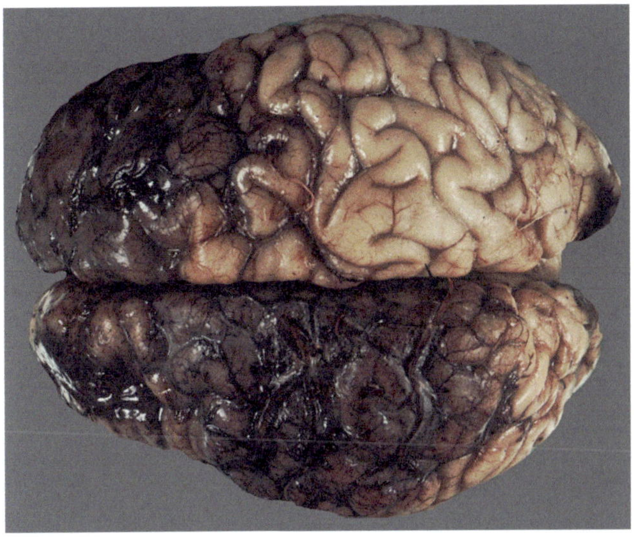

Fig. 9.38 Thrombosis of the sagittal sinus produces bilateral congestion and venous infarction of local draining brain tissues. The degree of thrombotic change is clearly evident in the draining radicals that run on the surface of the cerebral hemispheres (*Courtesy of* Professor Paul G. Ince, Sheffield, UK)

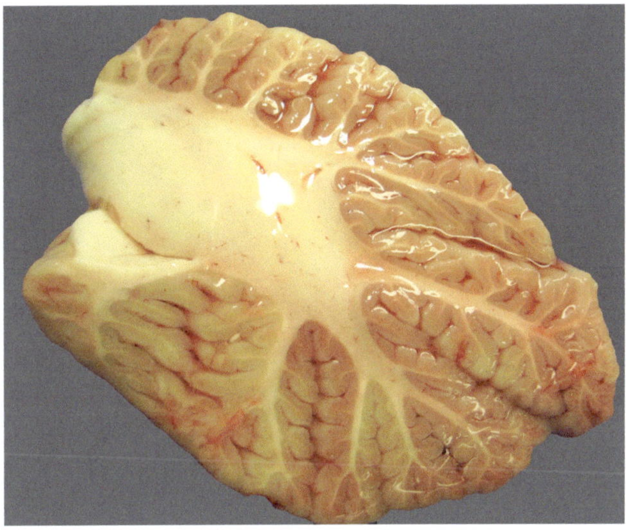

Fig. 9.40 Hypoxic brain injury can cause localised swelling due to ischaemic damage. Very early changes are seen as swollen brain parenchyma, which is evident in this view of the cerebellum, where the inferior and posterior pole of the tissues appear more prominent, firm and closely opposed than that of the superior surface

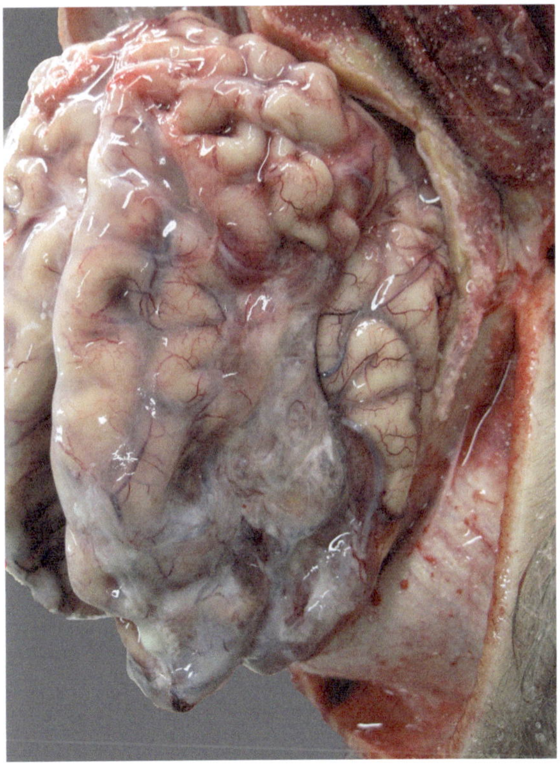

Fig. 9.39 Significant brain injury can occur at birth. This adult had experienced significant hypoxic-ischaemic injury in the immediate perinatal period, resulting in gross tissue loss from the right cerebral hemisphere, and to a lesser degree the left. Significant neurological deficit was present throughout life, involving higher intellect functions as well as motor and sensory skills

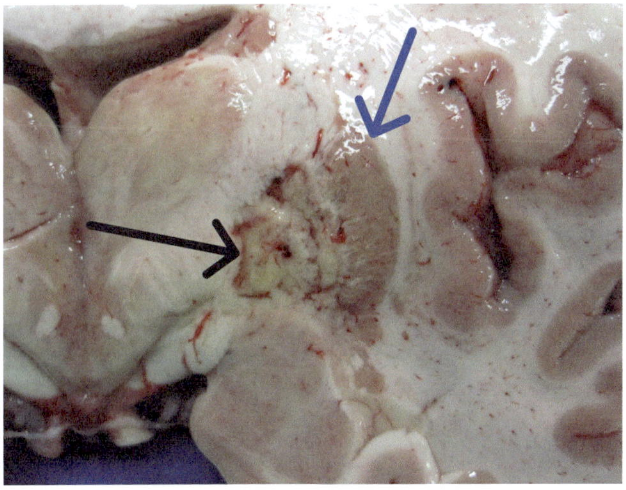

Fig. 9.41 Hypoxic brain damage can occur in relation to multiple aetiological factors. The globus pallidus (*black arrow*) is necrotic and the putamen (*blue arrow*) is relatively unaffected. There is also some swelling of the tissues. Bilateral pallidal necrosis is a particular feature of carbon monoxide poisoning, although the appearance may be seen in other hypoxic conditions

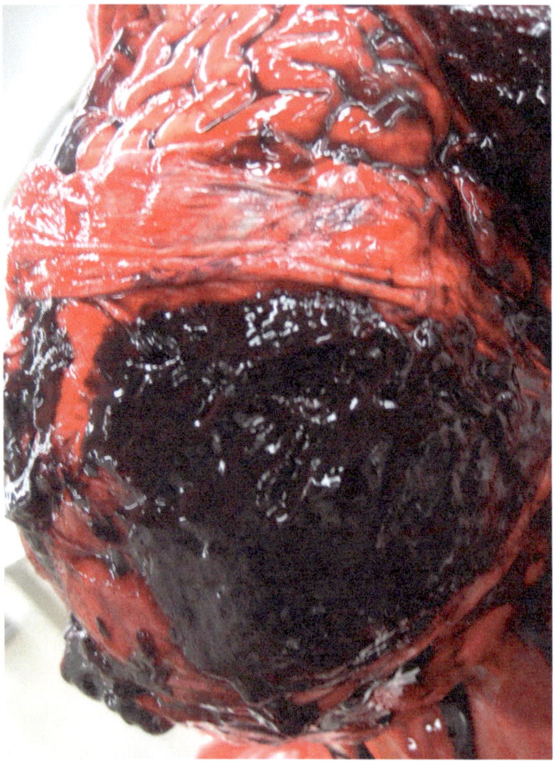

Fig. 9.42 An extradural haemorrhage is seen, with blood that has accumulated above the dura and below the skull vault. This type of haemorrhage commonly follows significant head trauma tearing the middle meningeal artery

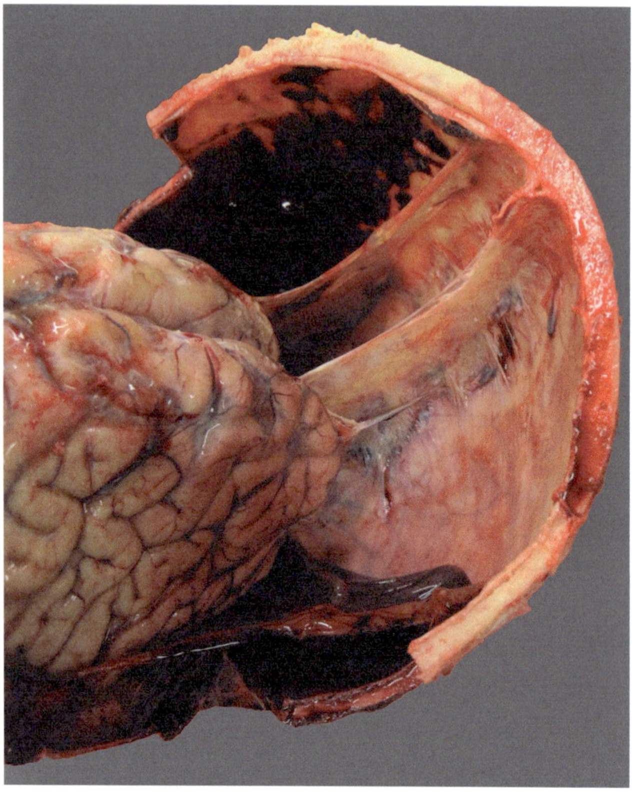

Fig. 9.44 Subdural bleeding is seen under the right side dura as one removes the skull cap. One should try to estimate the volume of blood that has accumulated

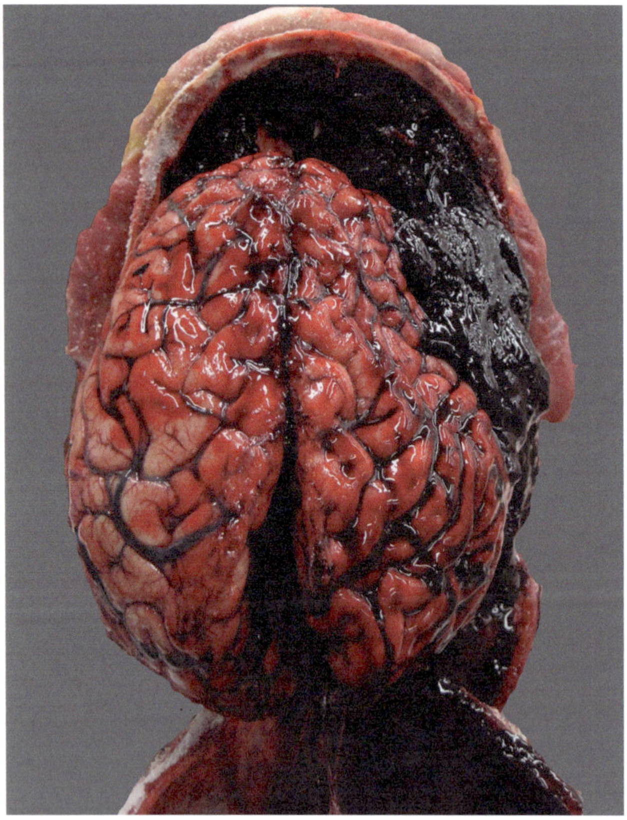

Fig. 9.43 Subdural haemorrhage, also typically traumatic in origin, can be associated with significant mass effect, with compression of the local brain

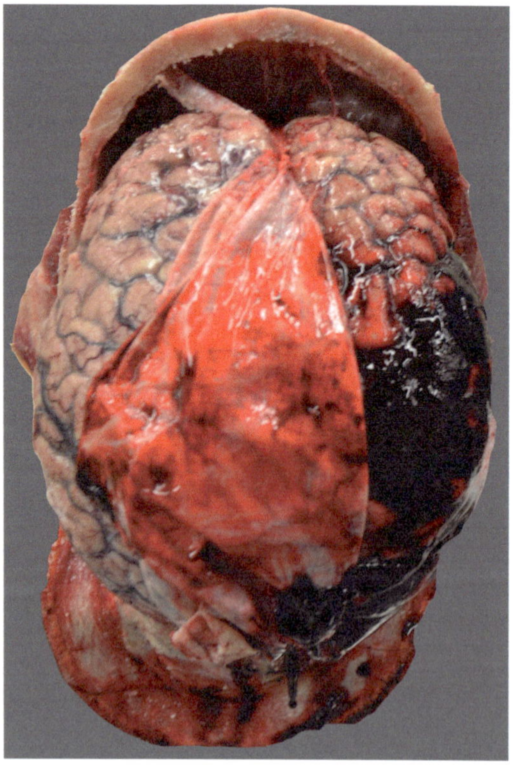

Fig. 9.45 Subdural haemorrhage is seen on the right side with the dura reflected

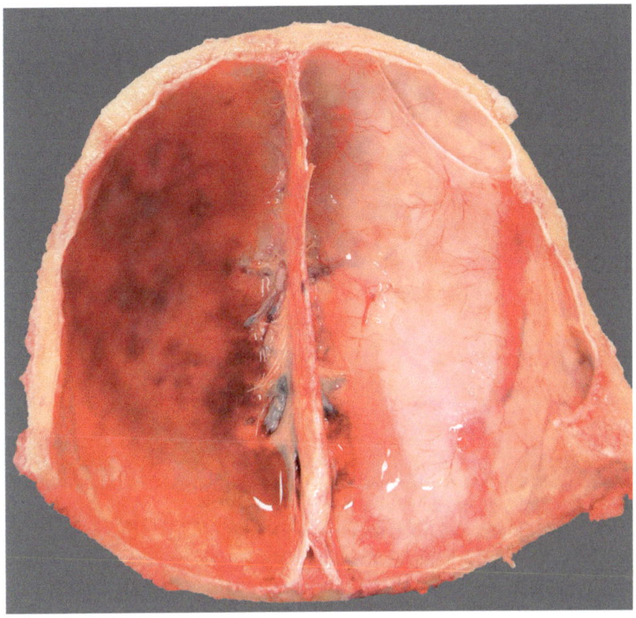

Fig. 9.46 In this image of the skull vault, unilateral subacute subdural haemorrhage is adherent to the dura. Although removal of the brain may be performed by technical mortuary staff, the removed skull cap should always be examined by the pathologist, as should the cranial vault

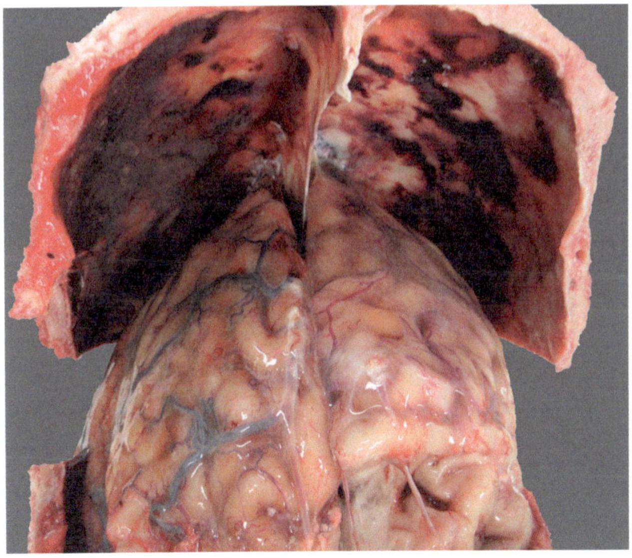

Fig. 9.47 Subdural haemorrhage may be present bilaterally, as shown here. This appearance is not uncommon in elderly patients or people with alcoholism who may be prone to low-impact falls, causing small haemorrhages. The dura remains adherent to the undersurface of the calvaria in this case

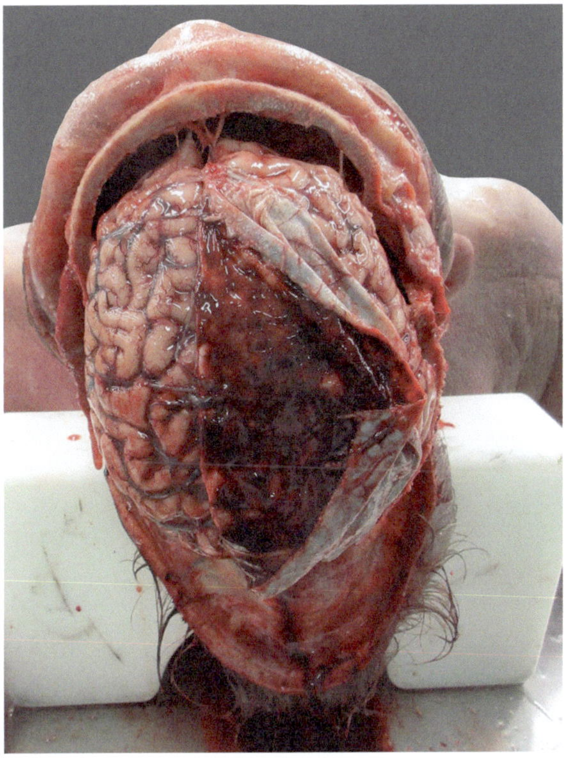

Fig. 9.48 The left side dura here shows features of recent bleeding and some yellow discolouration indicating older haemorrhage. These findings are of acute on chronic subdural haemorrhage. Such situations are not uncommon in elderly patients with cerebral atrophy who are prone to bleeding from the bridging veins between the brain and cranium following even minor trauma

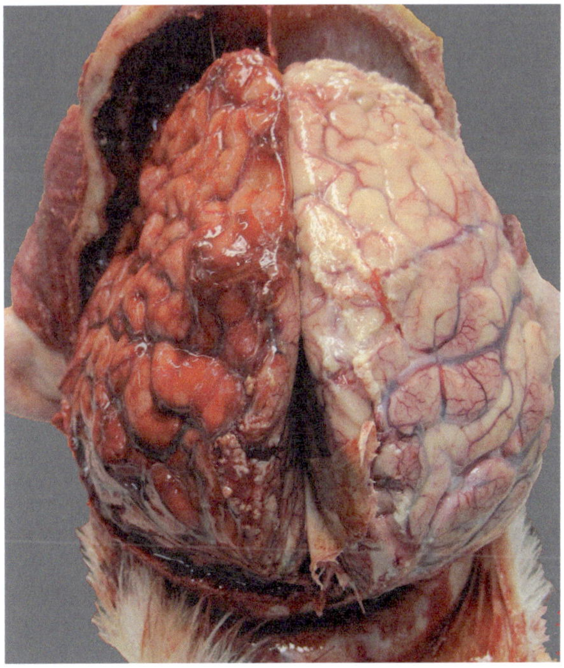

Fig. 9.49 Old subdural haemorrhage is often associated with some flattening of the cerebral surface. Here, there is flattening of the left sided cerebral tissue outer surface, with yellow discolouration of the meninges

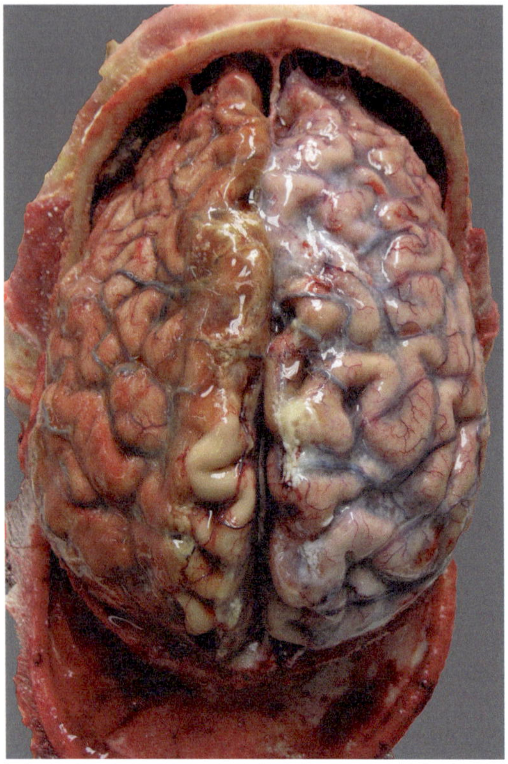

Fig. 9.50 Chronic subdural haemorrhage is seen with blood-stained discolouration of the outer brain tissues and with a hint of yellow discolouration

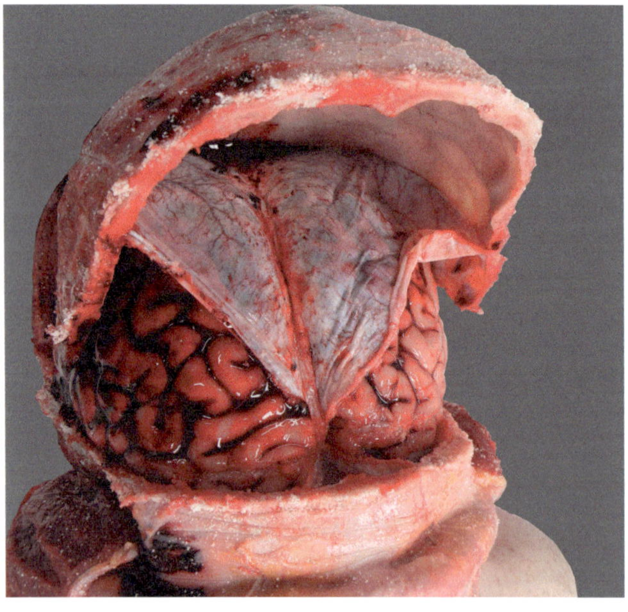

Fig. 9.51 Here is an example of a subarachnoid haemorrhage, seen immediately on opening the cranium and lifting the dura. The deep soft tissue bruise of the left lower scalp provides a clue towards a traumatic cause of this intracranial bleed

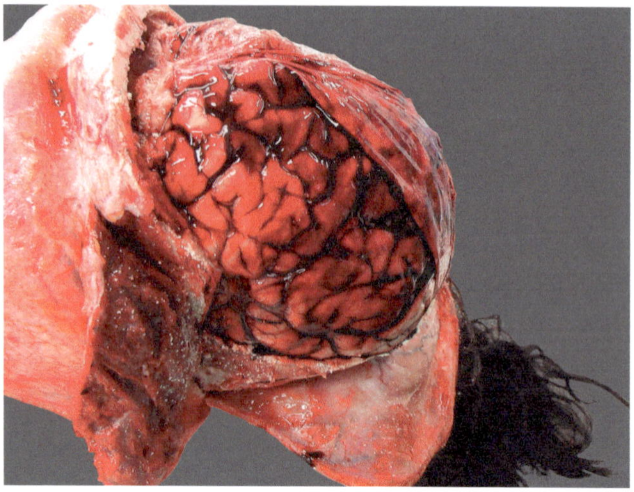

Fig. 9.52 In this subarachnoid haemorrhage, blood can be seen filling the sulci and held beneath the shiny surface of the arachnoid mater. Causes of subarachnoid haemorrhages include aneurysm rupture, trauma, arteriovenous malformation rupture, cocaine use and arterial dissection

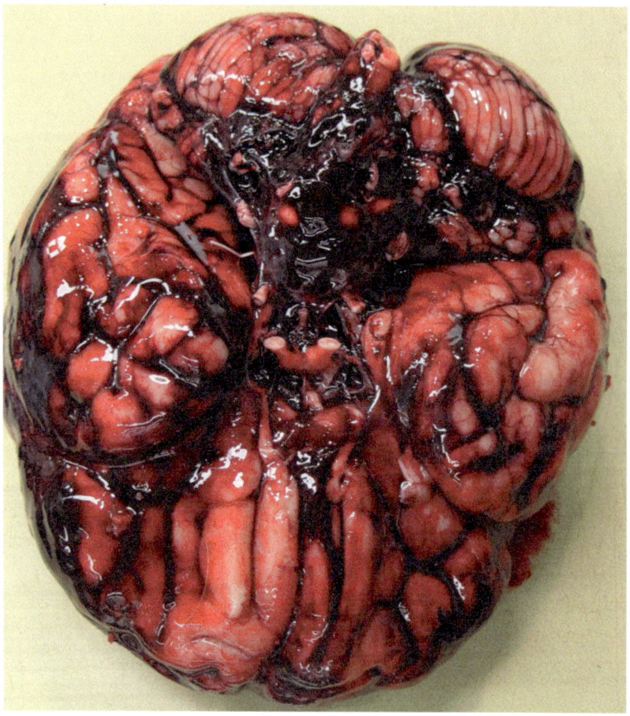

Fig. 9.53 Significant subarachnoid haemorrhage is seen in a case of a ruptured circle of Willis aneurysm. The heavy contamination of blood around the undersurface of the brain makes identification of the bleeding point difficult. If the brain is to be fixed, it is important to carefully wash or dissect away the blood in its fresh state to look for an aneurysm. This is because blood hardened by fixation is difficult to remove without destroying adjacent structures such as the vessels

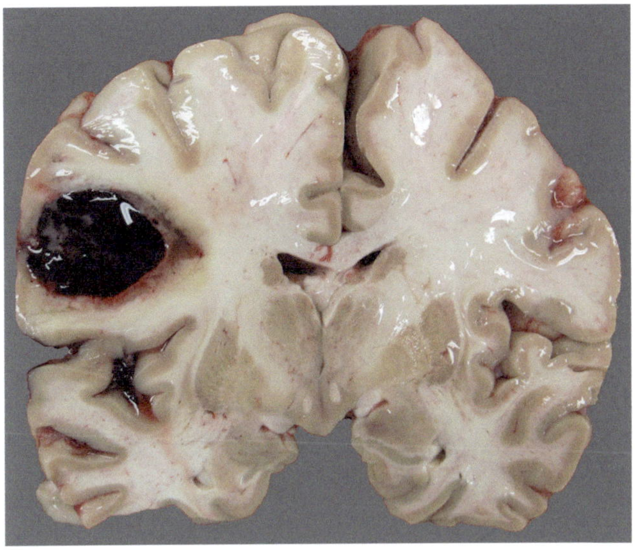

Fig. 9.54 Examination of brain tissues following haemorrhage may be fraught with difficulty in that the brain parenchyma is soft and distorted. Some would say that radiological investigation of such events is superior to transverse slicing of the fresh brain. If significant study of the brain parenchyma is required, then the tissues ideally must be fixed for about 6 weeks, and then sliced. However, despite all these limitations, slicing the brain in a fresh state and taking photographs can still provide significant information for clinical teams. This image shows a large spontaneous cerebral bleed with some midline (mild left to right) shift. This haemorrhage is lobar in distribution. Histology is of importance in cases of lobar haematoma to define the cause of haemorrhage, such as cerebral amyloid angiopathy, tumour or vascular malformation

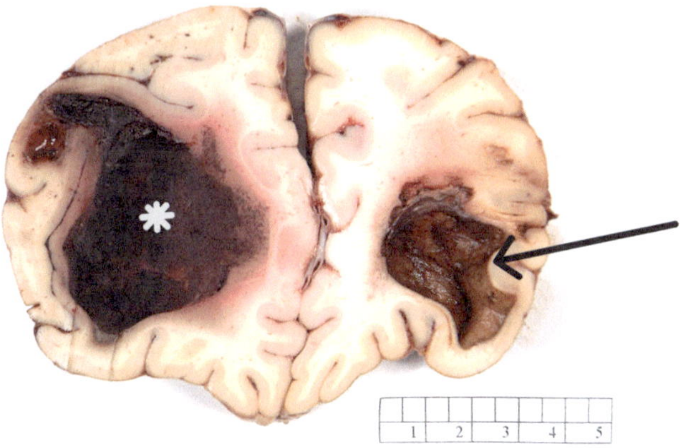

Fig. 9.55 This example shows an old lobar haemorrhage (*arrow*) and a recent lobar haemorrhage (*asterisk*) due to cerebral amyloid angiopathy. This pattern of multiple lesions often happens in this disease

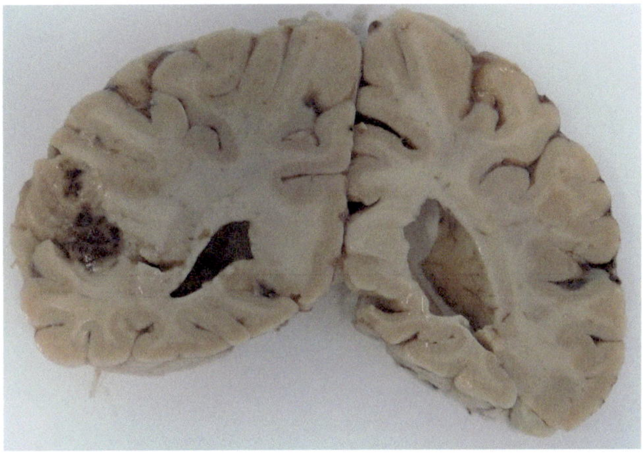

Fig. 9.56 An acute haemorrhagic stroke affecting the middle cerebral artery has caused focal destruction of the cerebral tissue. It can be seen that the texture of the affected brain is altered, appearing softer and more friable, with haemorrhagic change into the tissue architecture (as opposed to a solid mass of blood in a haematoma)

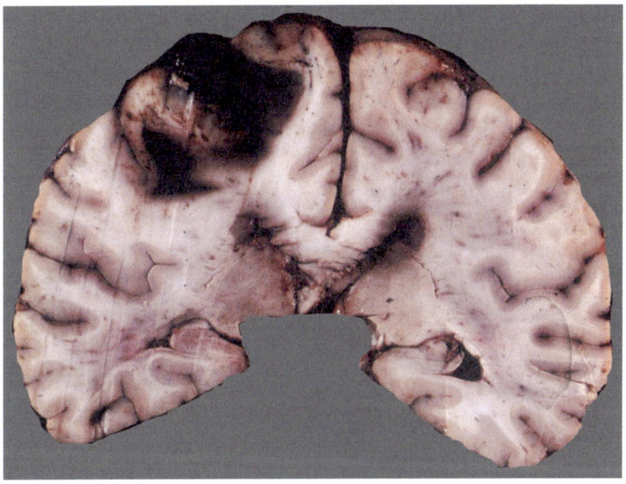

Fig. 9.57 This view of a brain shows significant cerebral microvascular haemorrhages as well as a large cerebral bleed, in a case of eclampsia (*Courtesy of* Professor Paul G. Ince, Sheffield, UK)

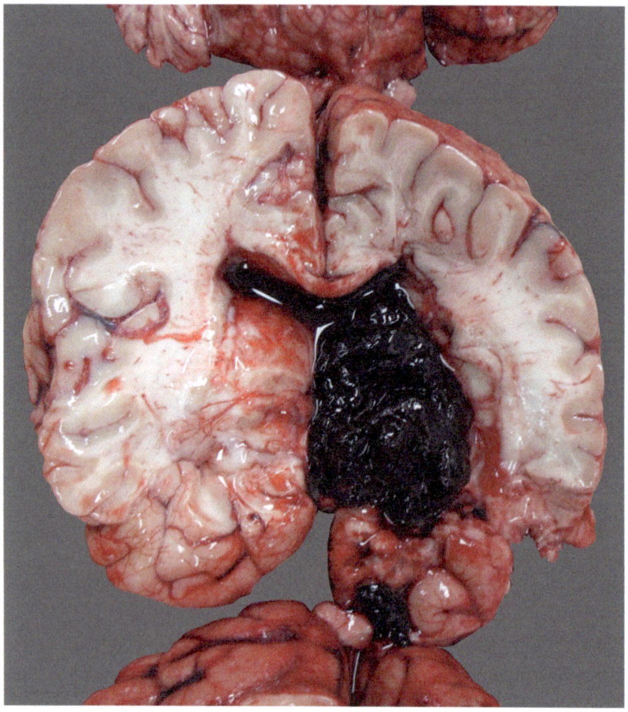

Fig. 9.58 A parenchymal bleed in the deep brain structures. The haemorrhage has destroyed much of the ipsilateral thalamus and basal ganglia. The central ganglionic location of this bleed is most in keeping with a hypertensive aetiology

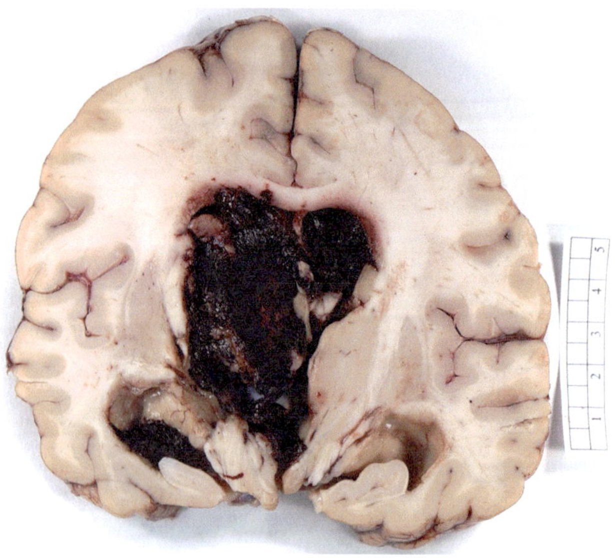

Fig. 9.59 A fresh thalamic haemorrhage is seen with extension into the ventricles in this fixed specimen. Death was from sudden raised intracranial pressure from the extension into the ventricle in this hypertensive ganglionic bleed

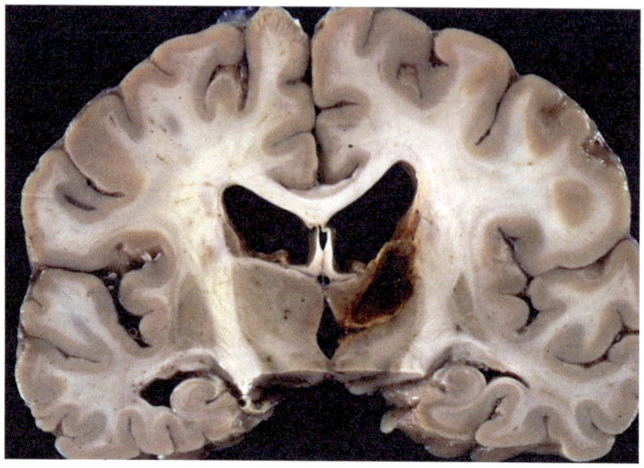

Fig. 9.60 Another example of an older hypertensive haemorrhage in the basal ganglia in a fixed specimen. The affected area contains altered blood and is undergoing cystic degeneration, with a circumscribed border. The yellow/brown discolouration of haemosiderin is present. These features point to this haemorrhage having occurred sometime before death, with a subsequent period of survival

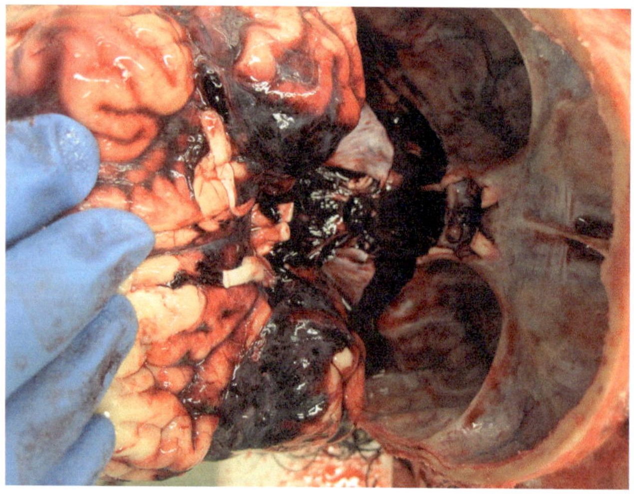

Fig. 9.61 Significant bleeding around the brainstem has been identified during brain tissue removal. Such changes can occur in relation to fractures of the skull base or subarachnoid haemorrhages due to aneurysms or vertebral artery transections

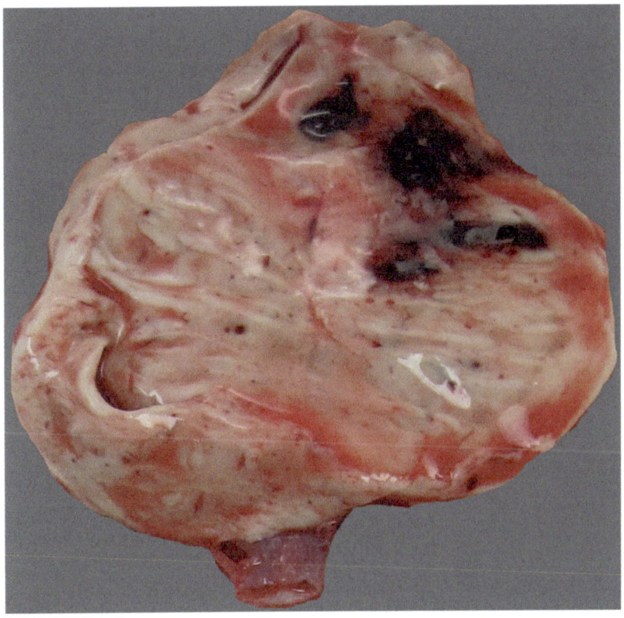

Fig. 9.62 Haemorrhages in the brainstem, midbrain and pons can occur in situations of raised intracranial pressure. These 'Duret' haemorrhages are a secondary consequence of the raised intracranial pressure and shearing of the brainstem tissues and blood vessels, rather than primary pathology

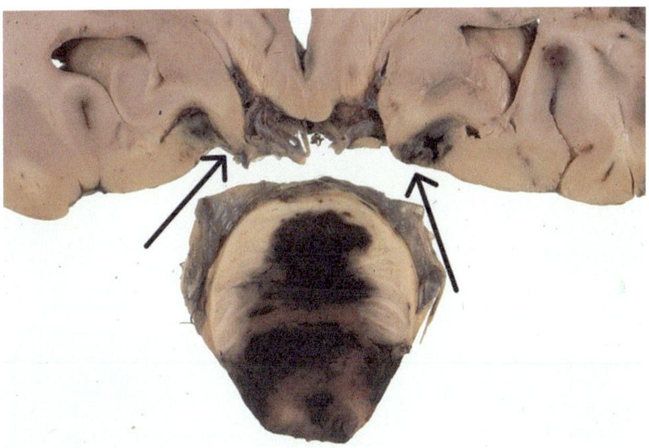

Fig. 9.63 Another example of Duret haemorrhage, seen in the midline of the pons. At the top of the image is the inferior surface of the brain showing bilateral uncal herniation (*arrows*) caused by raised intracranial pressure in this case due to a head injury

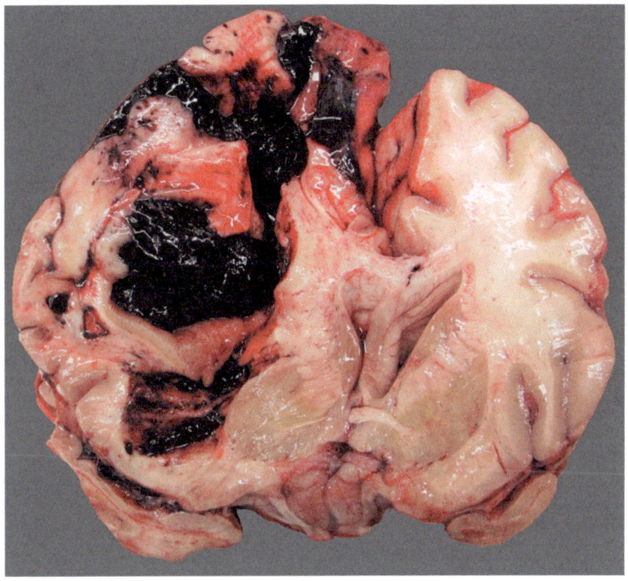

Fig. 9.64 Fresh cerebral haemorrhage can often be associated with massive brain disruption. Death occurs promptly due to the effects of raised intracranial pressure in these cases

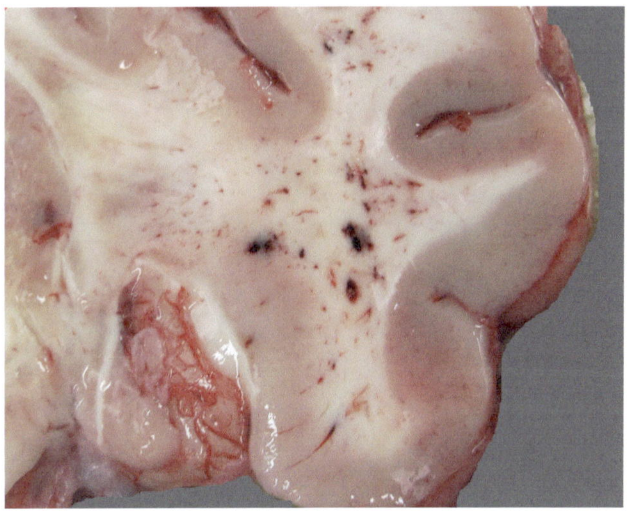

Fig. 9.65 Cerebral trauma can produce significant vascular injury, usually reflecting shearing effects. Bleeding occurs diffusely across the brain tissues and is often rapidly fatal. Such vascular lesions often reflect diffuse axonal injury, which should be sought microscopically

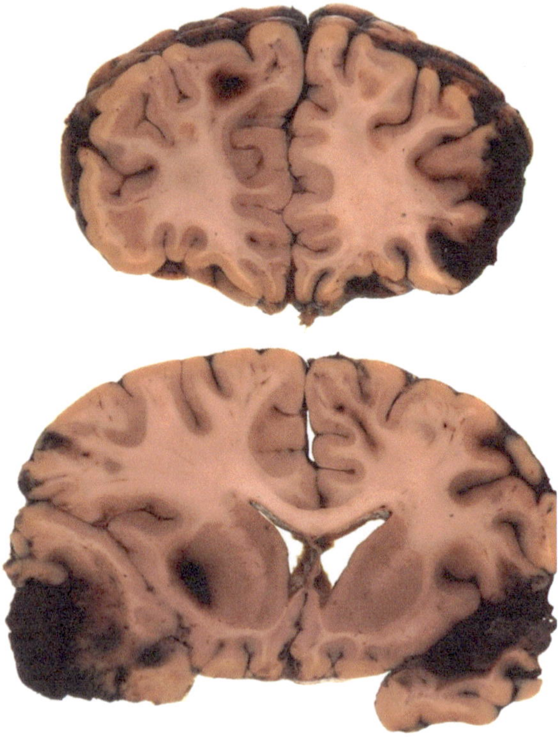

Fig. 9.66 Another pattern of injury seen in traumatic brain injury is that of contusional haemorrhage, seen here in a typical distribution affecting the inferior frontal and temporal areas bilaterally. Contusions represent bruising of the brain, with damage to small vessels and neural tissue. The mechanisms for brain contusion formation are discussed in Chap. 12—The Forensic Autopsy

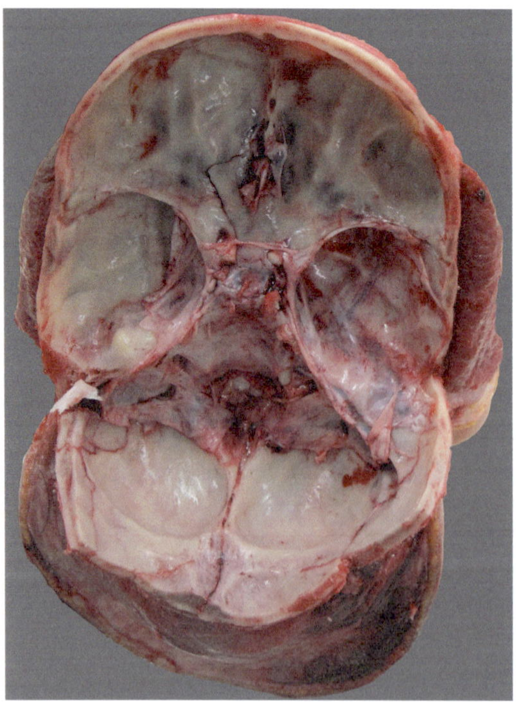

Fig. 9.67 This complex skull fracture involves multiple bones of the skull and the skull base. It is often easiest to appreciate skull fractures by flexing and extending the skull tissues to demonstrate separation planes. Often, a picture is most valuable in these cases, rather than having to laboriously document the length and angle of every single fracture line

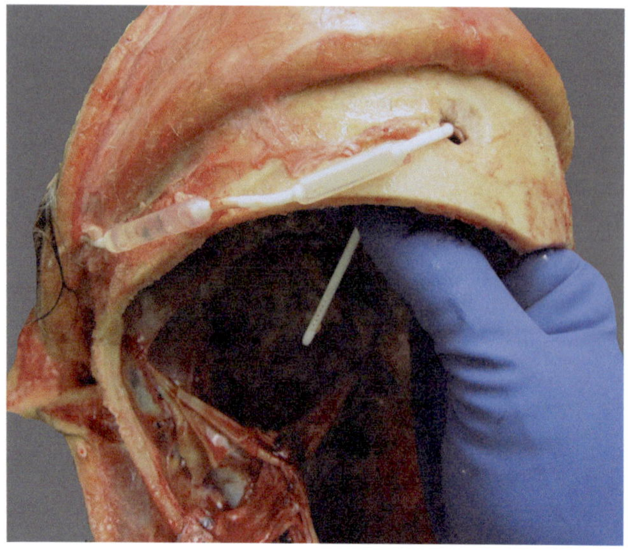

Fig. 9.68 The entry point of a ventriculoperitoneal shunt is illustrated. The catheter running into the cerebral ventricles has been left intact so that the depth of penetration can be demonstrated

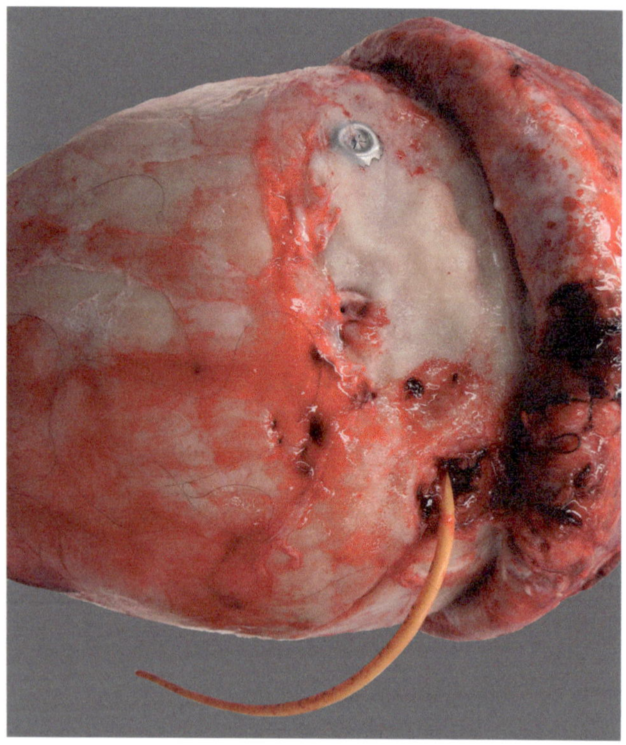

Fig. 9.69 Soft tissue bruising of the scalp is shown, in keeping with recent intervention to insert a ventriculoperitoneal shunt (*yellow tube*). An anchoring screw with fibrous overgrowth can be seen, indicating that previous neurosurgery has occurred

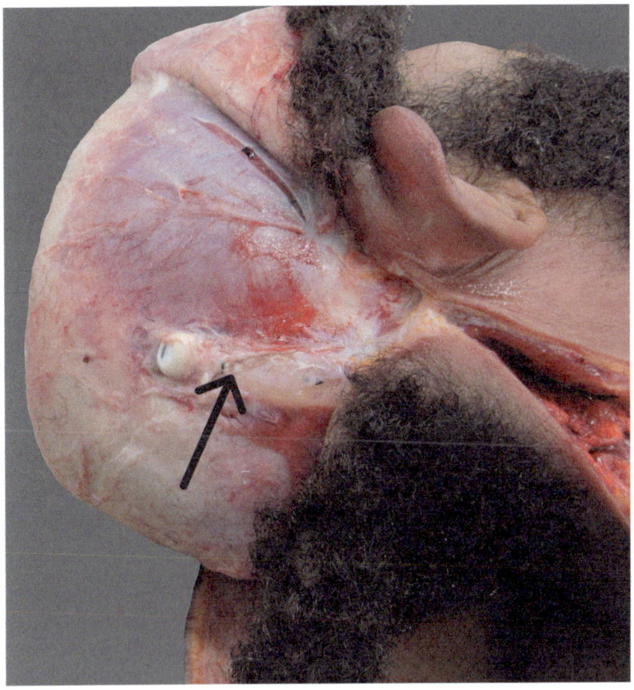

Fig. 9.70 Another example of a ventriculoperitoneal shunt is shown here, towards its origin. Cerebrospinal fluid is drained into the abdomen (See also Figs. 11.13 and 11.14), reducing the effects of hydrocephalus

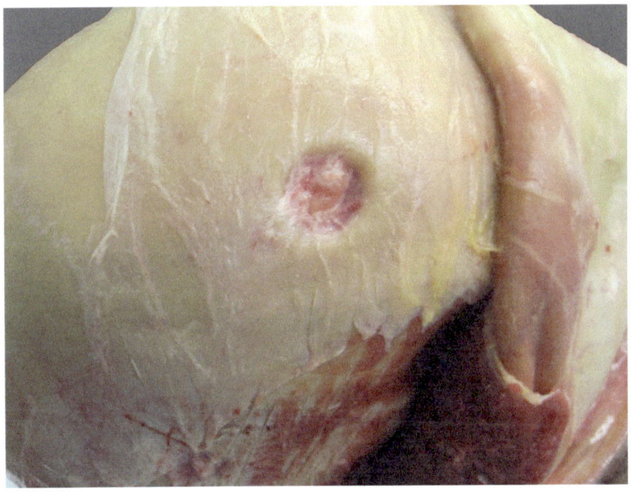

Fig. 9.71 A burr hole is present from previous drainage of a subdural collection

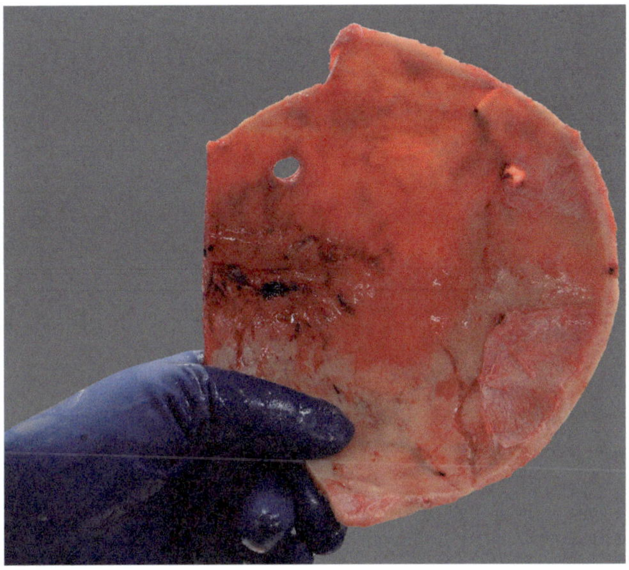

Fig. 9.72 The removed calvaria shows a rounded hole, in keeping with prior burr hole formation during neurosurgical interventions

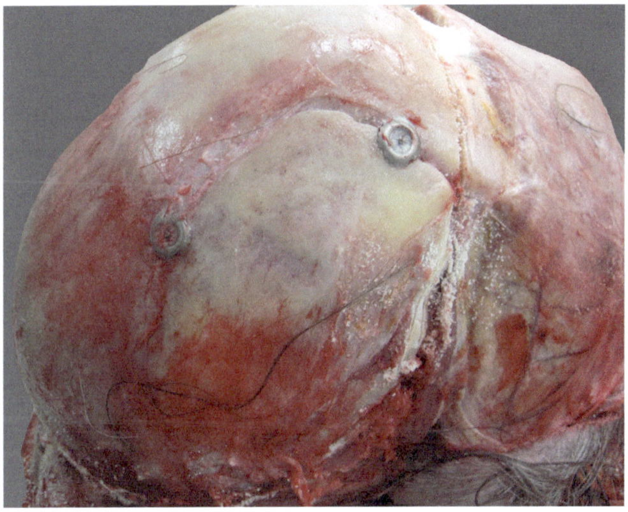

Fig. 9.73 Previous cranial surgery is seen, with a bone flap and several anchoring screws. The space between the edges of the bony tissues has been filled by fibrous tissue

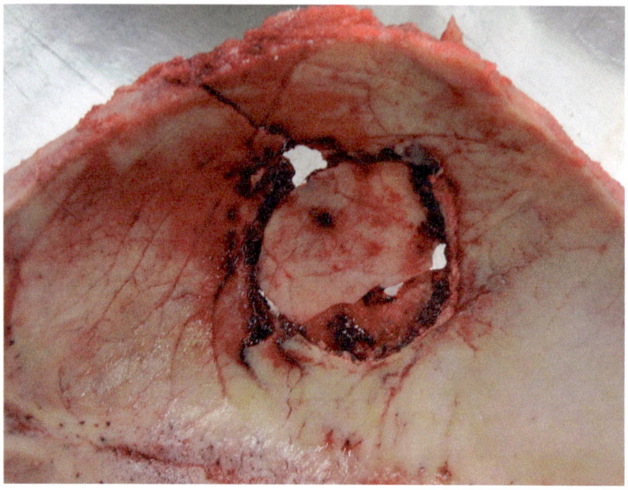

Fig. 9.74 This repair of an acute fracture of the skull involved fixing it in position with screws. The inner aspect has no metal projecting into the cranial cavity

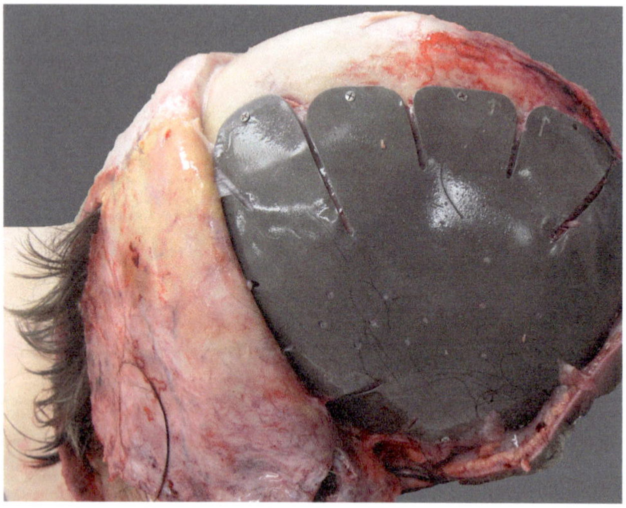

Fig. 9.75 When cerebral tissues have had a significant pathological insult, it may be necessary to remove quite large areas of skull bony tissue to avoid raised intracranial pressure and death when the brain inevitably swells with cerebral oedema. In this case there was cerebral trauma and skull fracture with secondary infection. The integrity of the cranial vault is reestablished by using a metal plate. The individual metal leaflets are folded directly onto the cranial vault and screwed into place

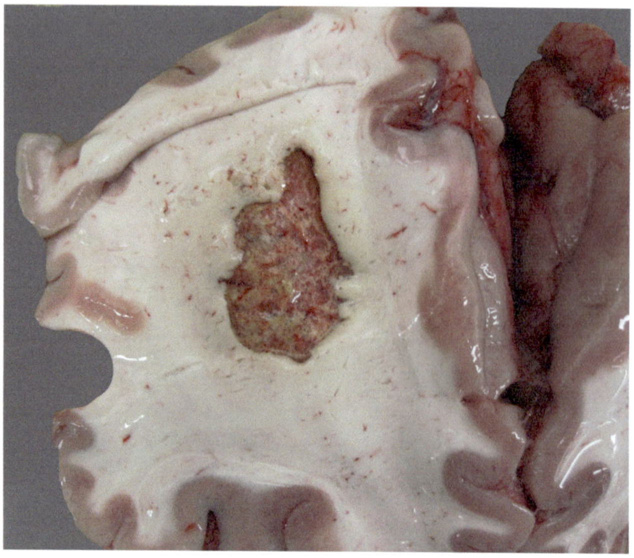

Fig. 9.76 A central nervous system abscess is seen in a case of an intravenous drug user. Surprisingly, there were no ante-mortem symptoms and the individual died as result of an overdose

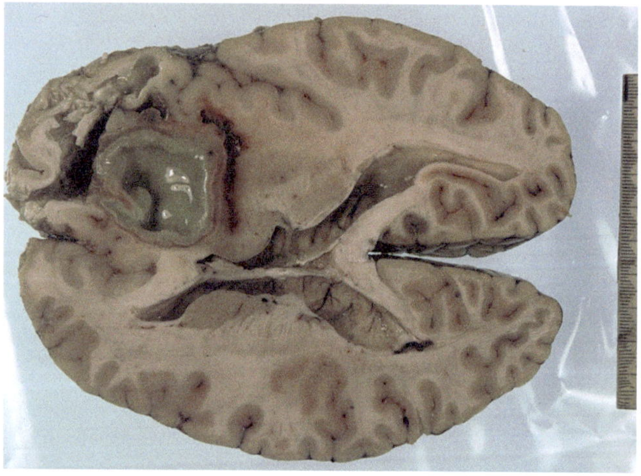

Fig. 9.77 This axial section of brain shows another example of a bacterial cerebral abscess with central liquefied necrosis/pus. Note the rim of affected brain tissue surrounding the abscess with softening and oedema of the tissue and some mass effect

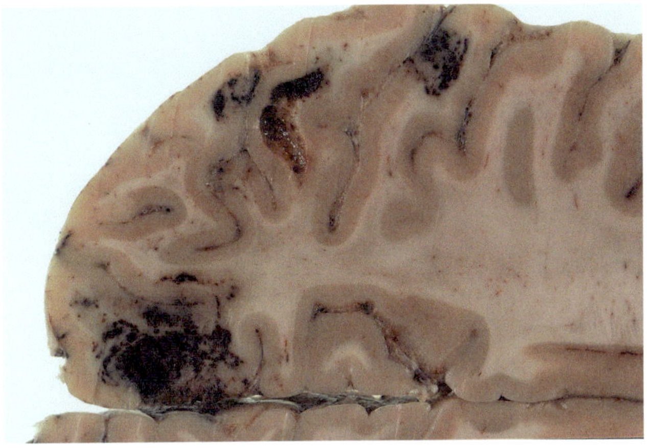

Fig. 9.78 There are multiple sites of cerebral haemorrhagic infarction in this case of subacute bacterial endocarditis. Septic emboli from vegetations on the mitral valve have travelled to the small intracranial vessels via the arterial circulation. In such cases of showering emboli, it is likely that there will be infarcts in other organs, such as the kidneys, spleen and bowel

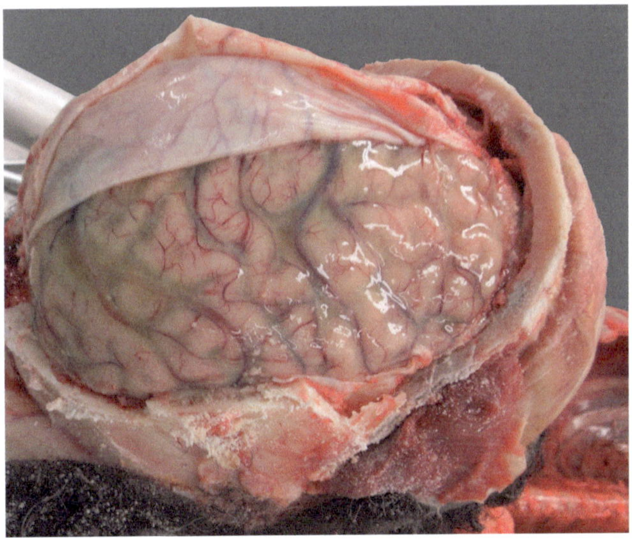

Fig. 9.79 Here is the appearance of bacterial meningitis, seen as yellow discolouration of the leptomeninges, indicating infection at this site. Microbiological swabs should be taken as soon as possible after opening the intracranial cavity to avoid contamination

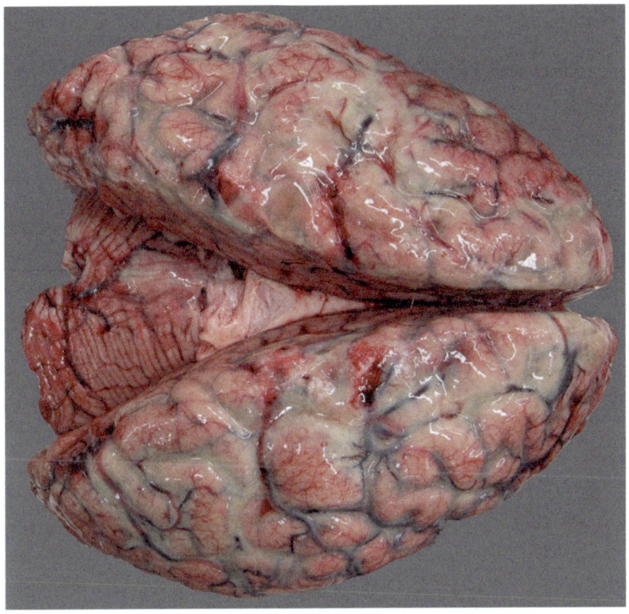

Fig. 9.80 Purulent meningitis is shown in this case of a young adult student. This is a relatively rare, but well recognised, cause of sudden death. Material should always be sent to microbiology for typing of the organism, and notification of local authorities is often required. Contact tracing may be relevant

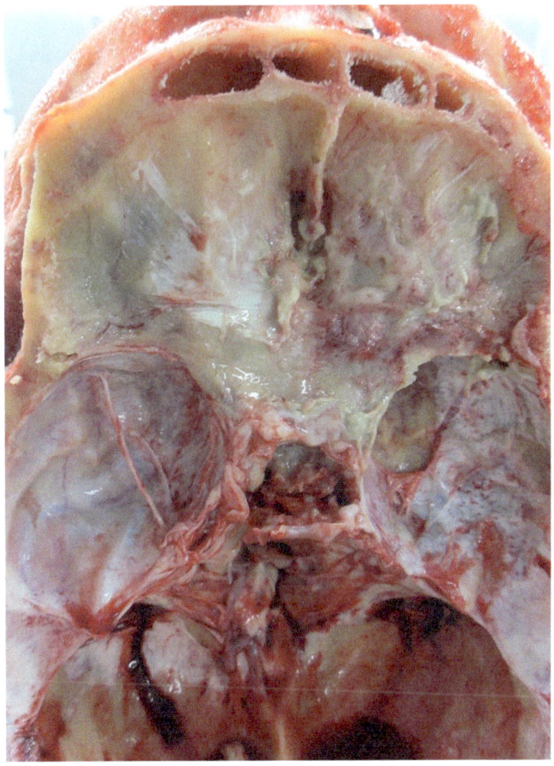

Fig. 9.81 The anterior cranial fossa of this skull base is covered in yellow/green pus. This is a rare case of meningitis originating from sinusitis

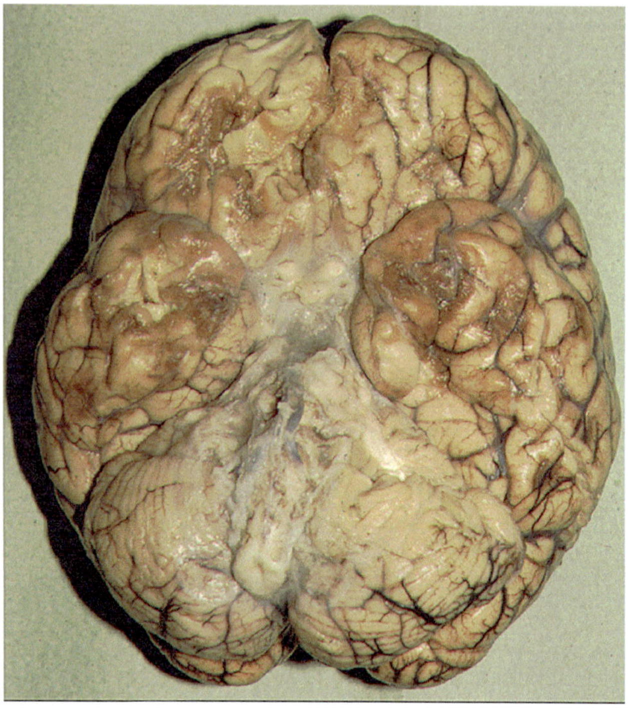

Fig. 9.82 *Mycobacterium avium-intracellulare* meningitis in an individual with HIV infection

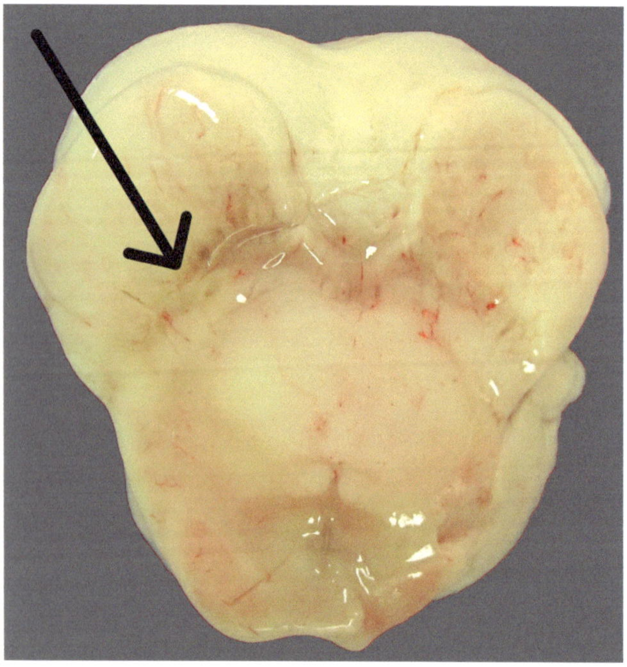

Fig. 9.83 A section through the midbrain (lower) shows significant loss of pigmentation at the site of the substantia nigra (*arrow*) in a case of idiopathic Parkinson's disease. Identification of this process in relation to falls, accidents and natural disease (chest infections) is of value as there is a strong link between the neurological impairment and secondary pathologies such as subdural haemorrhage

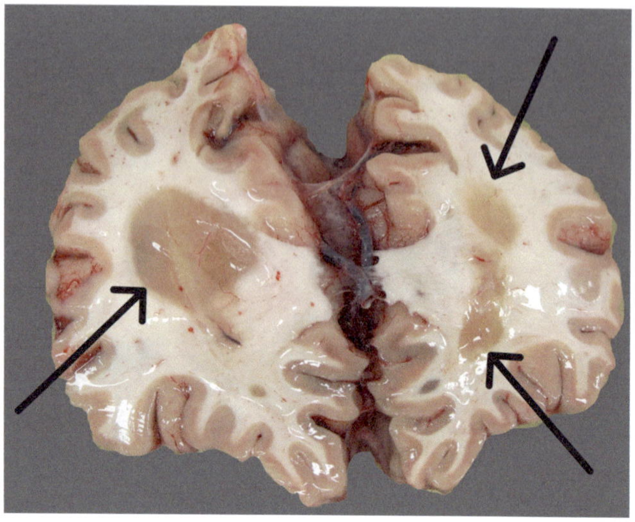

Fig. 9.84 Multiple sclerosis is normally recognised clinically before death. Several plaques (*arrows*) are evident in the deep white matter in the coronal section through the frontal lobes, mapping to the antemortem symptoms experienced

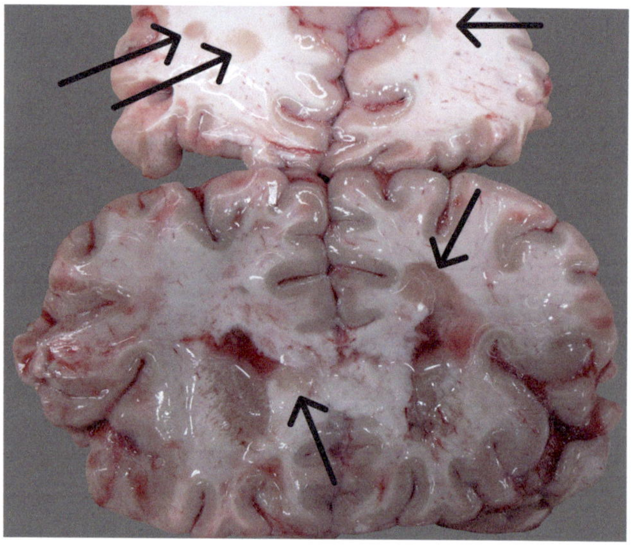

Fig. 9.85 Another example of the plaques (*arrows*) seen in multiple sclerosis is shown here in the frontal white matter

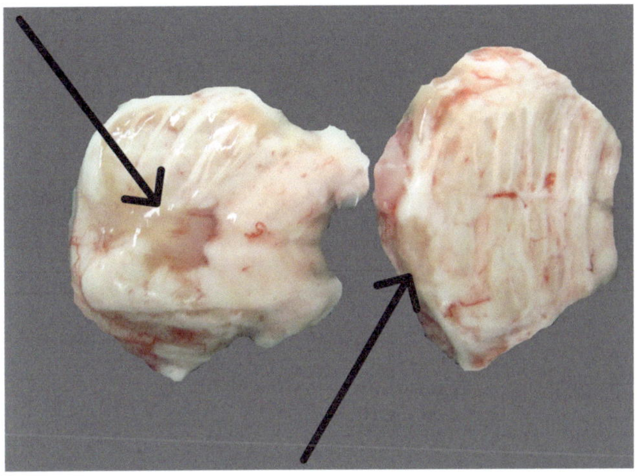

Fig. 9.86 Multiple sclerosis can affect the brainstem, cerebellum and spinal cord as well as cerebral tissues (*arrows*)

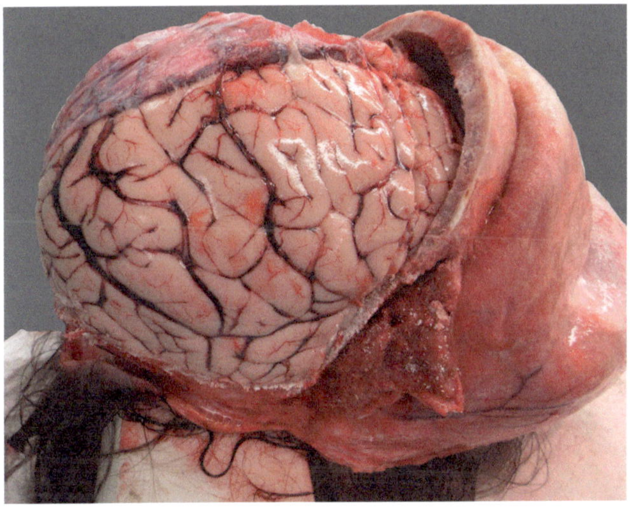

Fig. 9.87 In this image, the surface of the brain appears flattened, with loss of the gyri and sulci of normal brain. This is an example of cerebral oedema. This is a non-specific finding, which can be caused by trauma, tumours, ischaemia or obstructing hydrocephalus, among other pathologies. Raised intracranial pressure from cerebral oedema may result in death

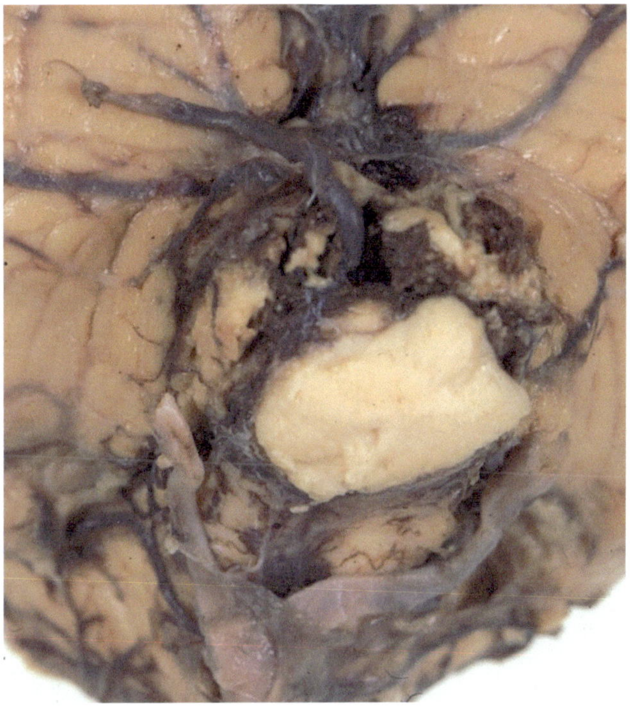

Fig. 9.88 Tonsillar herniation (*coning*) is due to raised intracranial pressure of any cause. The inferior parts of the cerebellum, the cerebellar tonsils, are pushed into the foramen magnum. This results in haemorrhagic necrosis of the tonsils and compression of the medulla

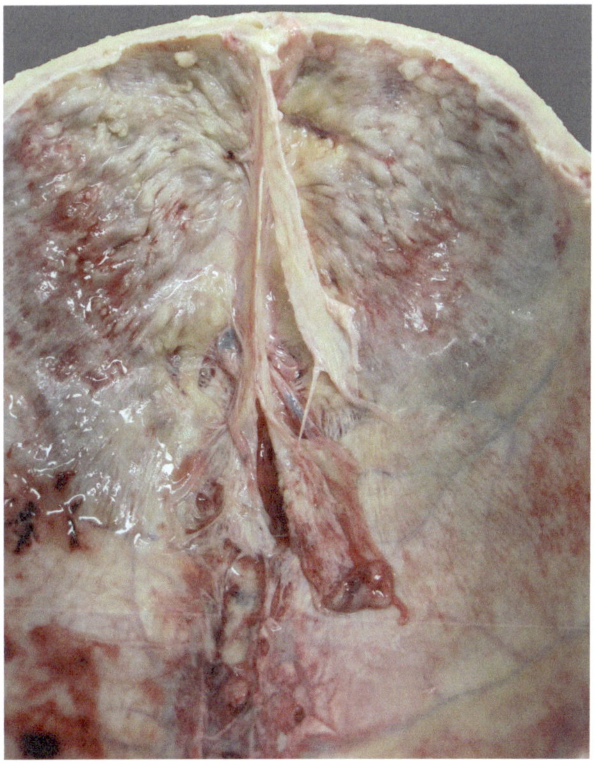

Fig. 9.89 Hyperostosis frontalis interna is a benign condition of the cranial vault involving overgrowth of the bony tissues

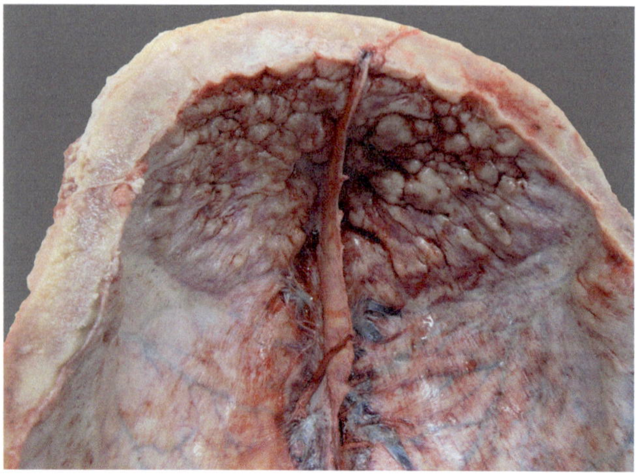

Fig. 9.90 Another example of hyperostosis frontalis is shown here

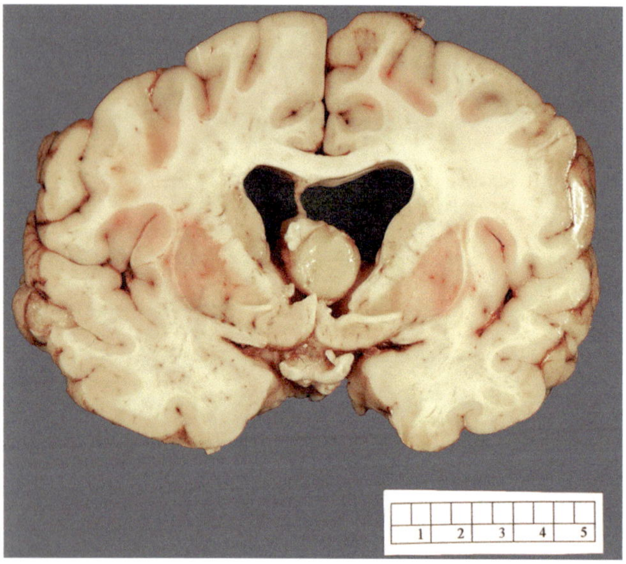

Fig. 9.91 A colloid cyst of the third ventricle. This type of benign tumour is a cause of sudden death

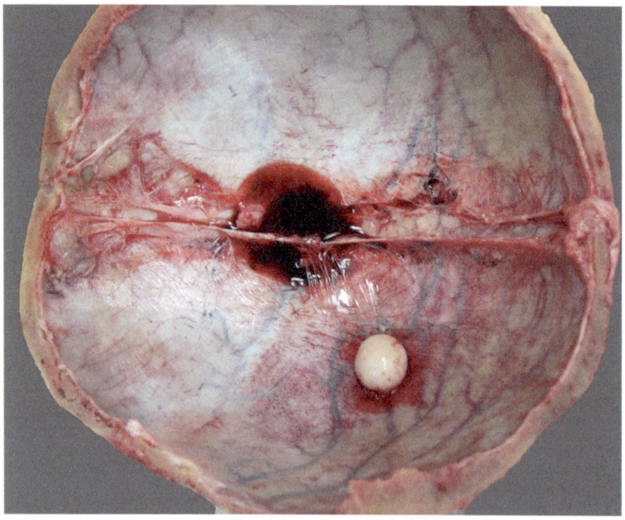

Fig. 9.92 This meningioma was an incidental finding at autopsy

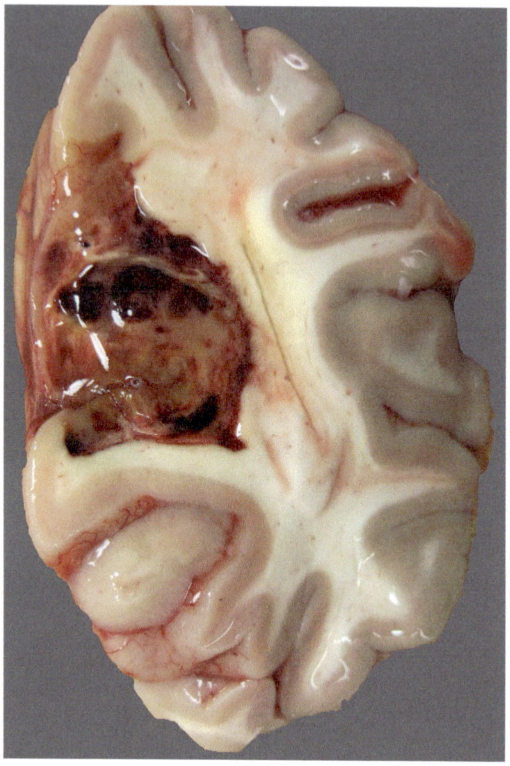

Fig. 9.93 Primary brain neoplasia is an uncommon finding at autopsy, although it does explain sudden death on occasion. This case shows a high-grade glioma with significant brain destruction and necrosis

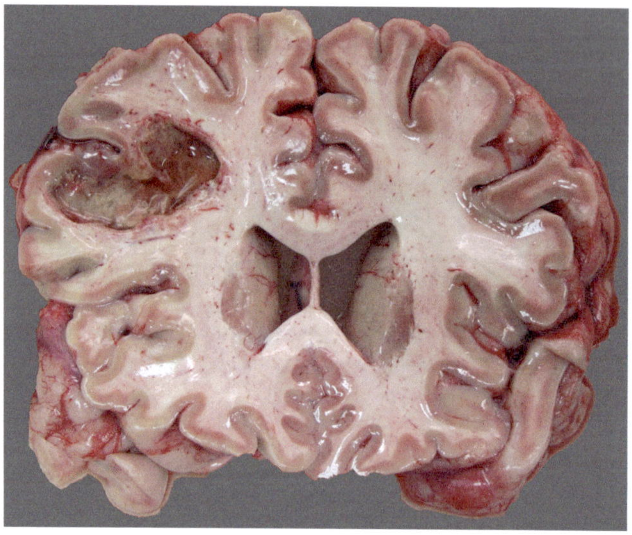

Fig. 9.94 Gliomas are often identified before death and treated. The pronounced cystic degeneration and necrosis points to significant tumour destruction by means of external beam radiotherapy

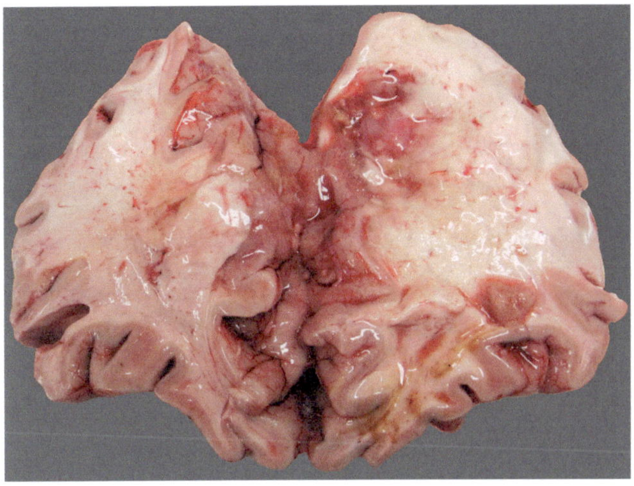

Fig. 9.95 The brain tissues are widely softened, distorted and friable in this case of advanced, high-grade oligodendroglioma

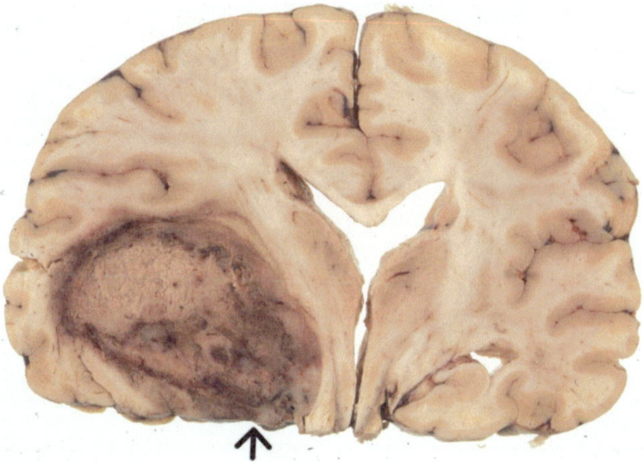

Fig. 9.96 This case of glioblastoma has caused mass effect. There is left to right asymmetry due to midline shift and a raised ipsilateral Sylvian fissure. The tumour is circumscribed with a variegated appearance. The yellow areas in the tumour represent necrosis. It has effaced much of the temporal lobe and adjacent deep cerebral nuclei. Tumour also infiltrates the uncus, which is notched (*arrow*) due to herniation (a lateral tentorial hernia) leading to death

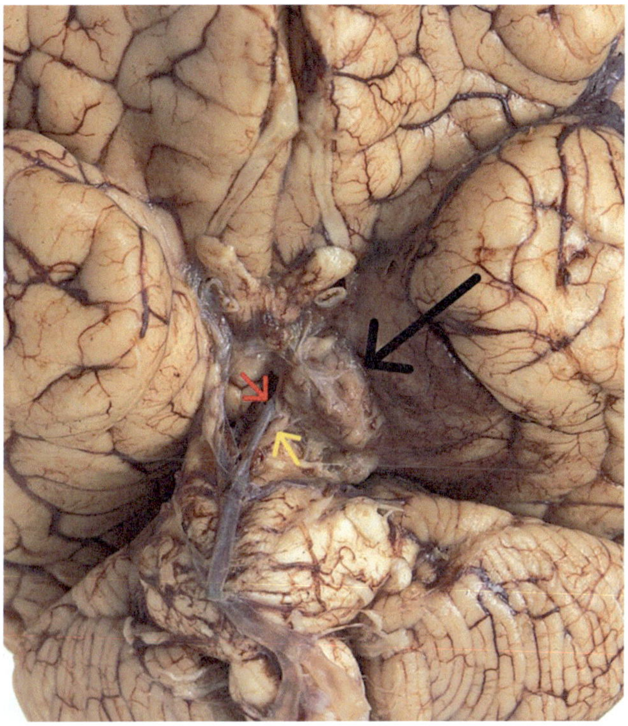

Fig. 9.97 This is the base of the brain in the case of glioblastoma shown in Fig. 9.96. Mass effect from the tumour has caused uncal herniation (*black arrow*). Also seen here are compression of the posterior cerebral artery (*red arrow*) and oculomotor nerve (*yellow arrow*)

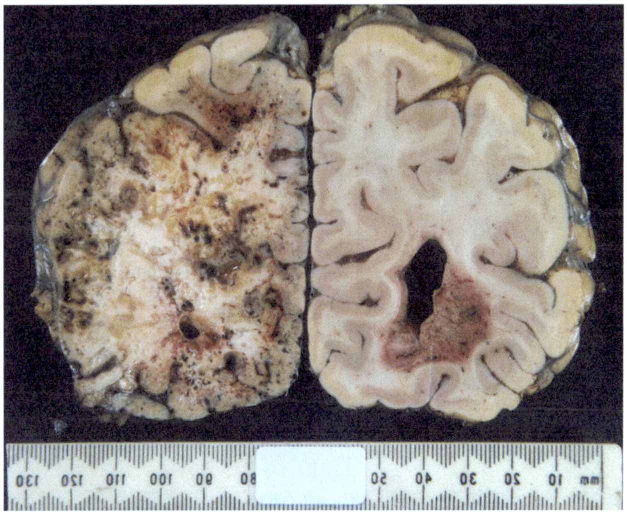

Fig. 9.98 Widespread cerebral involvement by glioblastoma is seen with a significantly necrotic and haemorrhagic tumour, affecting both cerebral hemispheres. (*Courtesy of* Professor Paul G. Ince, Sheffield, UK)

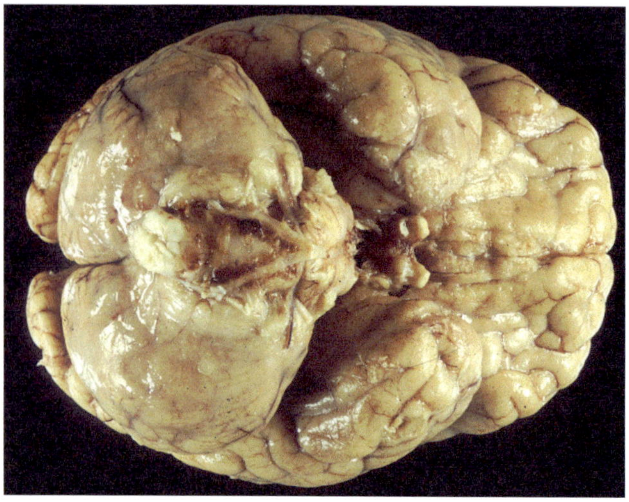

Fig. 9.99 Diffuse meningeal spread of tumour is relatively rare, but it is a recognised cause of progressive cognitive decline and thereby the death of the individual (*Courtesy of* Professor Paul G. Ince, Sheffield, UK)

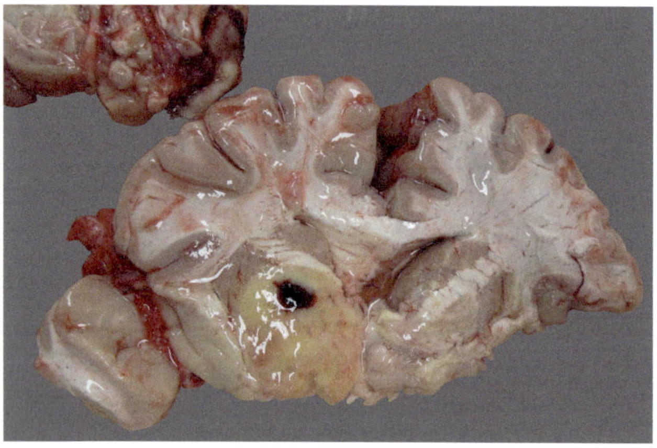

Fig. 9.100 In this case of primary central nervous system lymphoma, the yellow tumour can be seen replacing the deep cerebral nuclei, with a focus of haemorrhage

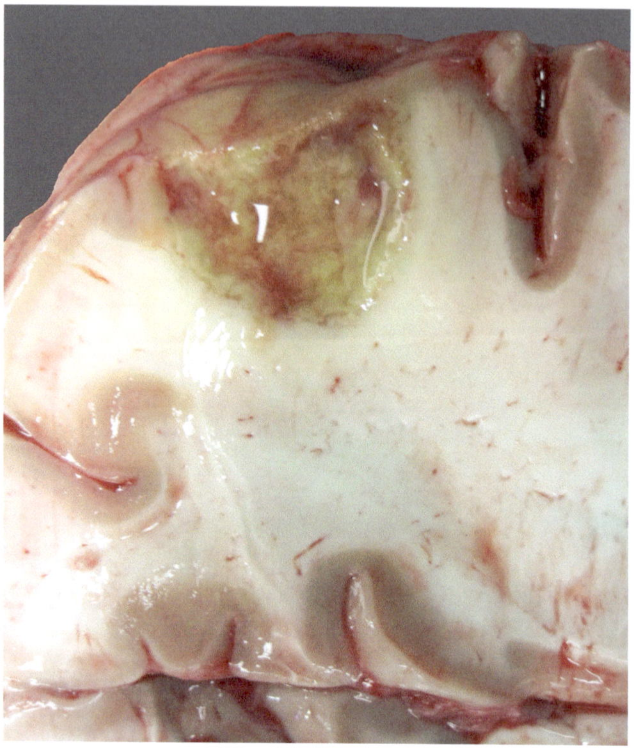

Fig. 9.101 Metastatic neoplasia involving the brain often appears as relatively well-defined lesions. This case shows a largely necrotic, cystic focus of metastatic lung cancer involving the outer grey cortical ribbon

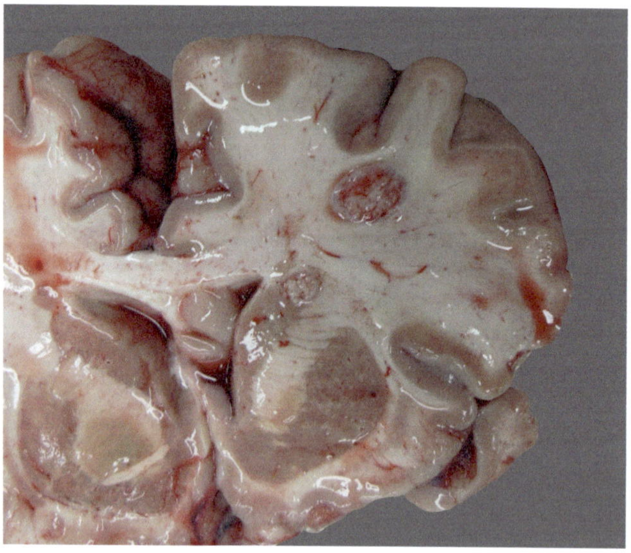

Fig. 9.102 The brain parenchyma contains multiple rounded lesions in keeping with metastatic disease from an extracranial primary malignancy, such as the lung

The Pituitary

The pituitary gland (Figs. 9.103, 9.104, 9.105, 9.106, 9.107, 9.108, 9.109, 9.110, 9.111, 9.112, 9.113, 9.114, 9.115, and 9.116) is removed once the brain has been eviscerated and the dura stripped from the base of the skull. It sits in the sella turcica at the skull base, adjacent to the optic chiasm. Pituitary dissection is rarely an issue, given that the gland is removed whole after knocking the posterior clinoid processes backwards with the skull key. The pituitary is then 'scooped' out by running the scalpel blade around the sella boundary and gently extracting the gland with toothed forceps.

At autopsy, the pituitary gland is about 10 mm in diameter and generally weighs about 1 g. It comprises two main parts, termed *anterior* and *posterior*. There may be a small, macroscopically indiscernible embryological remnant (*pars intermedia*) between the two lobes.

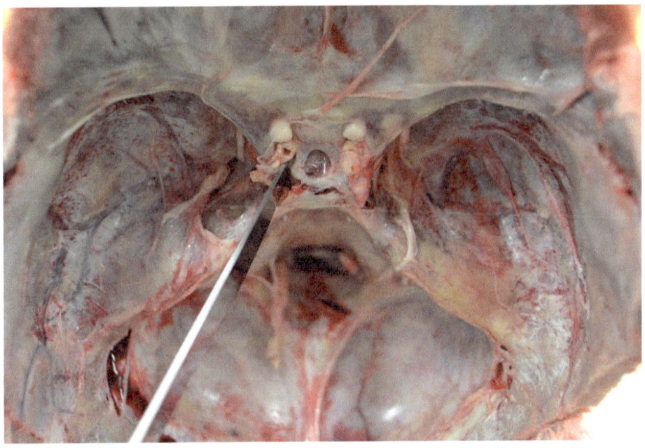

Fig. 9.103 Cuts are made around the sella turcica

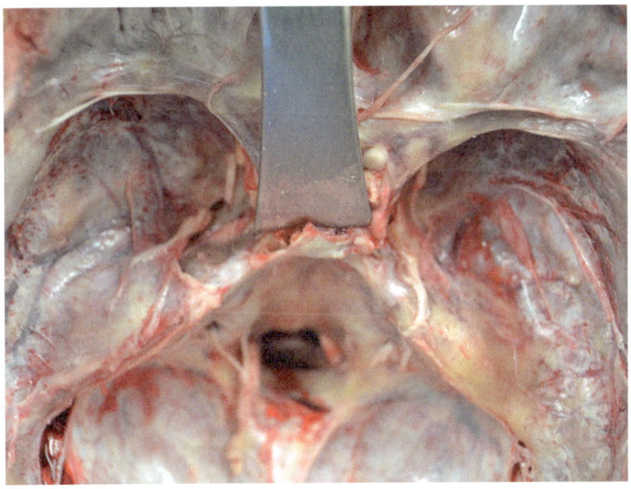

Fig. 9.104 The posterior part of the clinoid processes are wedged backwards by the skull key

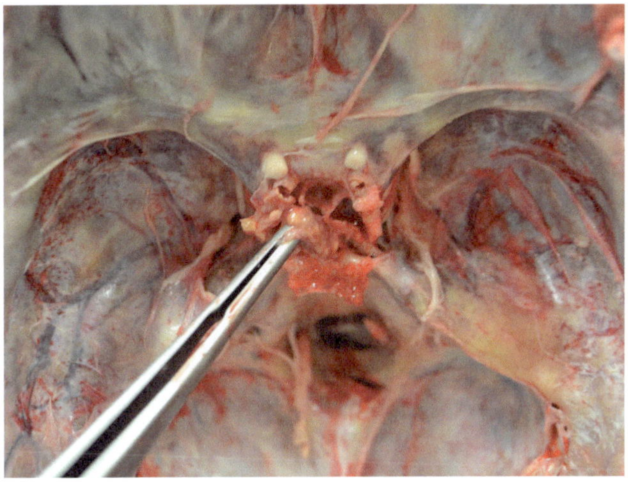

Fig. 9.105 The pituitary is gently dissected and lifted out

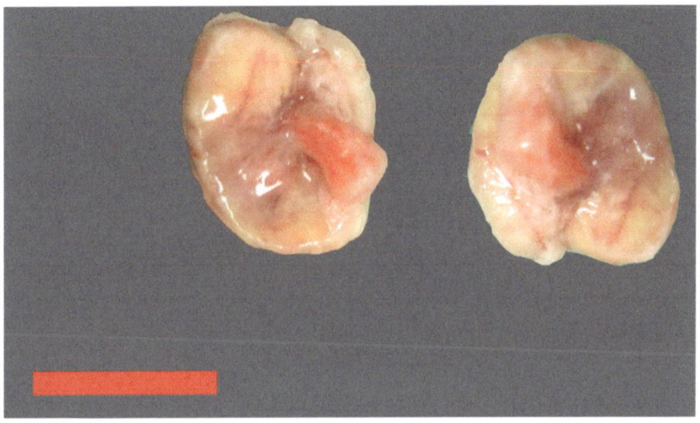

Fig. 9.106 This normal pituitary is seen from the superior (*left*) and inferior (*right*) aspects. The stalk is present, entering the pituitary from the superior aspect

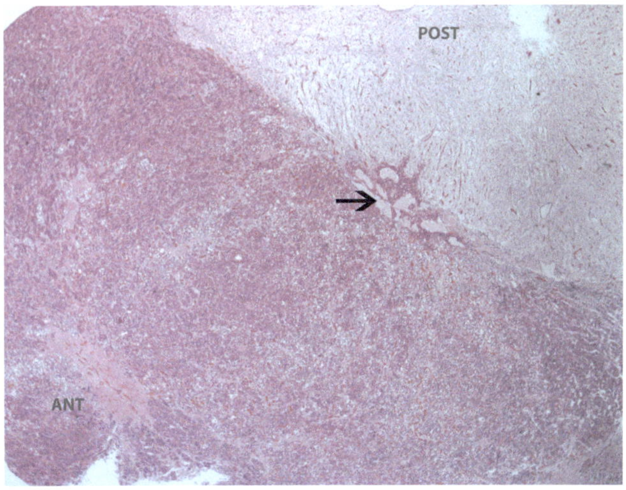

Fig. 9.107 Histology of the pituitary demonstrates the anterior lobe (*ANT*) with closely packed polygonal cells and the neuronal elements of the posterior lobe (*POST*). The two parts are clearly separate entities, with the partly cystic pars intermedia (*arrow*)

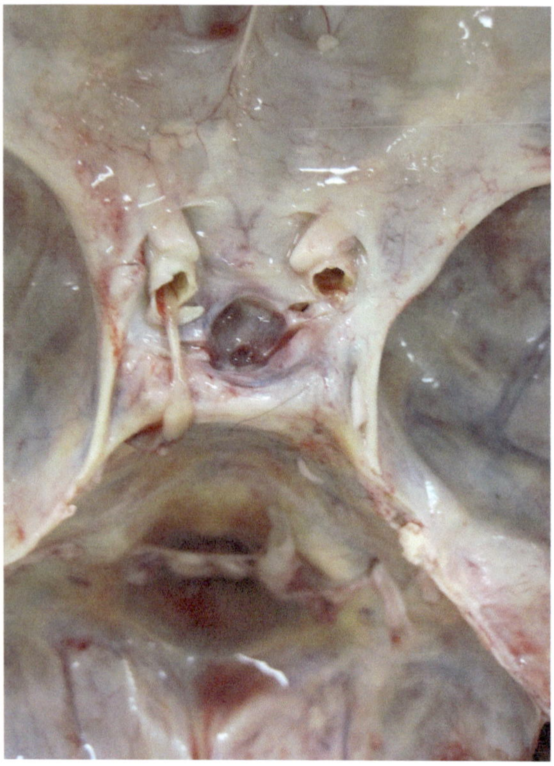

Fig. 9.108 An empty sella can be found in autopsy studies in cases with no antemortem irregularity of hormone production, visual fields or symptoms. There is often a thin rind of gland parenchyma around the base of the sella, which is still producing adequate levels of hormones

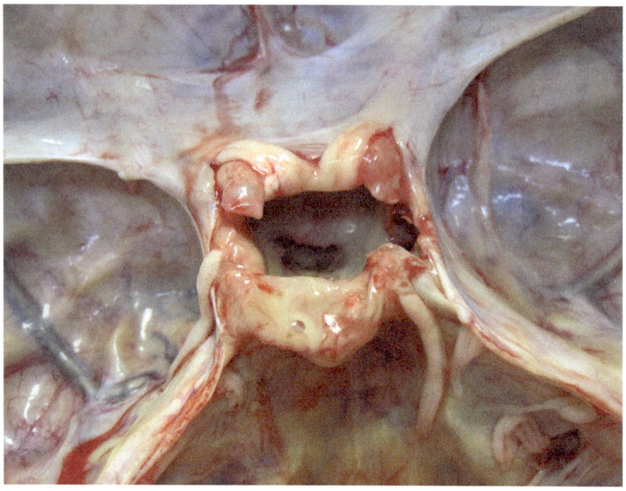

Fig. 9.109 This pituitary site has been subject to previous surgery with dissolution of the adenomatous parenchyma. A hole at the base indicates the point of entry of the surgical procedure via a transsphenoidal approach

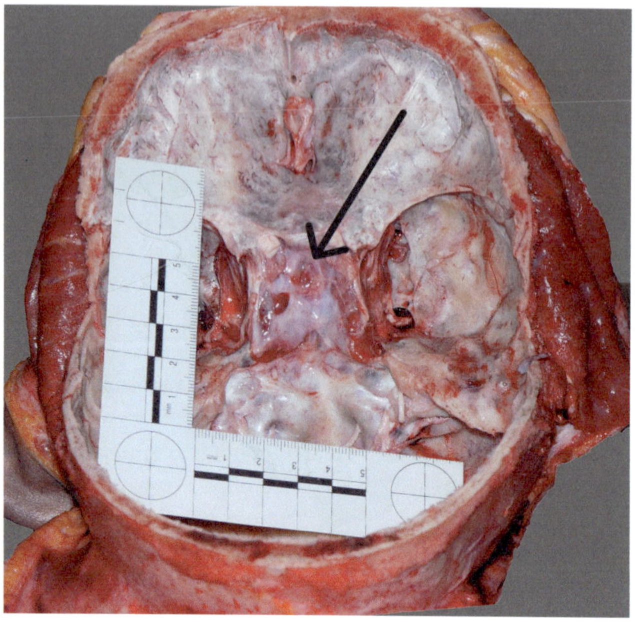

Fig. 9.110 A pituitary neuroendocrine tumour (pituitary adenoma) is seen in situ, expanding and distorting the local sella tissues and bulging upwards focally in a diffuse fashion

Histologically, the anterior lobe contains polygonal endocrine cells with varying histology colour (chromophobe, acidophil, basophil) in sections stained with haematoxylin and eosin. The cells have a rich vascular supply locally and secrete hormones directly into the bloodstream. The hormones secreted include follicle-stimulating hormone, prolactin, luteinizing hormone, thyroid stimulating hormone, growth hormone and adrenocorticotrophic hormone.

The posterior lobe may secrete oxytocin and anti-diuretic hormone. It is a direct extension of the brain parenchyma. The hormones enter the blood stream from the ends of the nerves that extend from the local brain tissues.

The bulk of pituitary pathology at autopsy reflects adenomatous neoplasia and the effects of therapy. Other tumours and inflammatory conditions rarely may have a detrimental effect on pituitary status, so histology is often valuable.

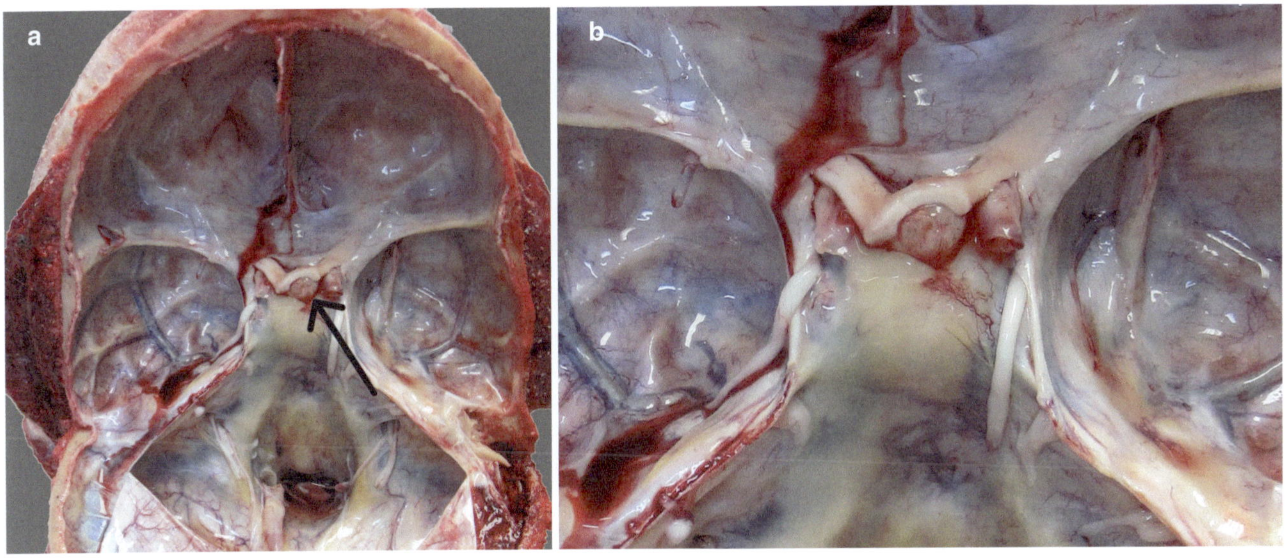

Fig. 9.111 (**a** and **b**) This pituitary neuroendocrine tumour, seen as cream-colored tissue, is expanding the sella and bulging upwards. The higher power image shows the pituitary tumour pressing on and stretching the crossing fibres of the optic chiasm, the clinicopathological correlate of bitemporal hemianopia

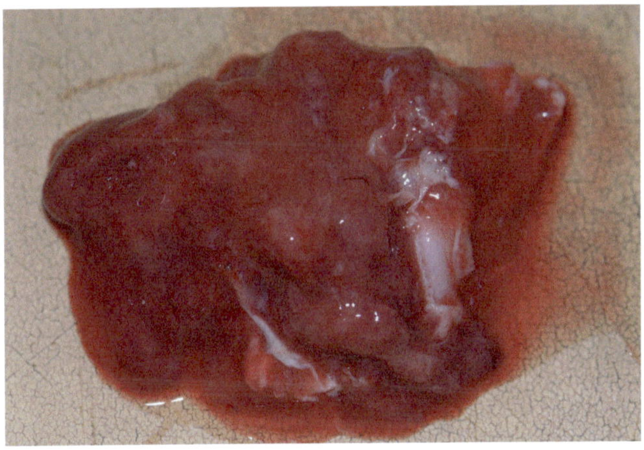

Fig. 9.112 A close up view of a pituitary adenoma which had a very soft and focally liquefied quality, indicating partial necrosis. This individual had been treated for his adenomatous tumour, but clearly much of the lesion was viable. This tumour weighed 8 g and measured up to 3 cm, both expanding the sella and protruding upwards towards the optic chiasm

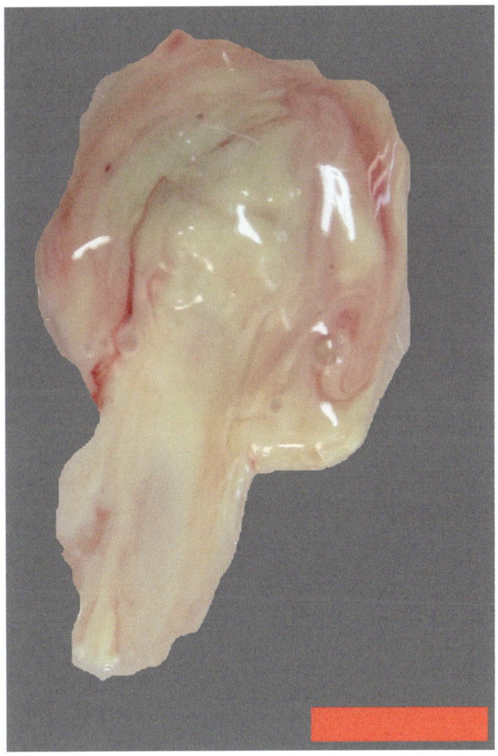

Fig. 9.113 The liquefied pituitary fossa contents are seen in a case of adenomatous disease. The antemortem oncological treatment has caused significant degeneration of the pituitary neoplasm. Histology is often unrewarding, but it can be undertaken in order to assess the therapeutic effectiveness (i.e., the tumour cell kill fraction)

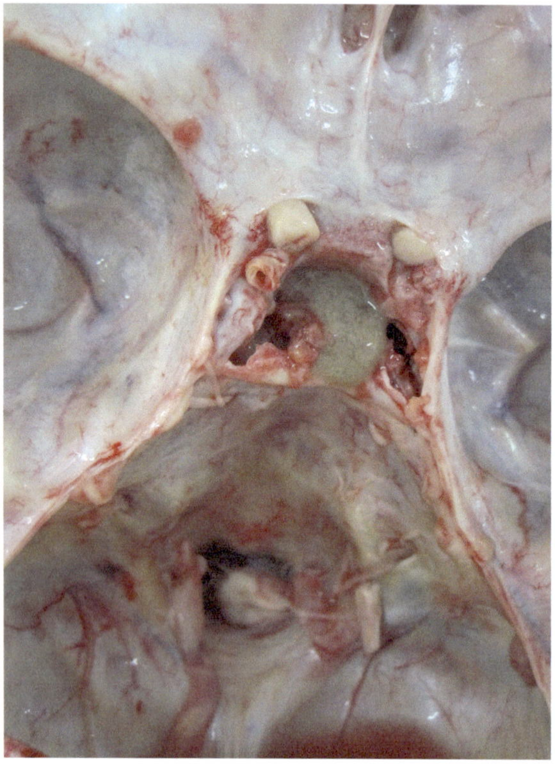

Fig. 9.114 The skull base shows the sella turcica to contain partially liquefied grey/yellow tissue, in a case of treated pituitary adenoma. These cases are difficult to define macroscopically. Histology may be the only way to truly appreciate any residual tissue elements

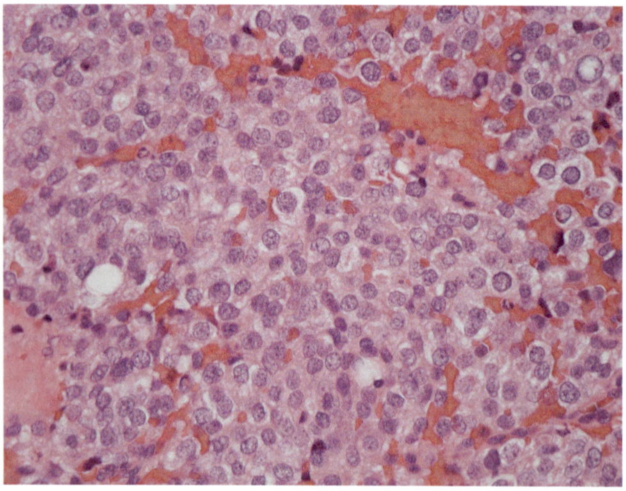

Fig. 9.115 Histological examination of a viable pituitary neuroendocrine tumour/adenoma shows closely packed polygonal cells of a classically neuroendocrine quality set within a vascular stroma. Histological assessment of these cases involves immunohistochemistry for adenohypophyseal hormones and for pituitary transcription factors to define the lineage

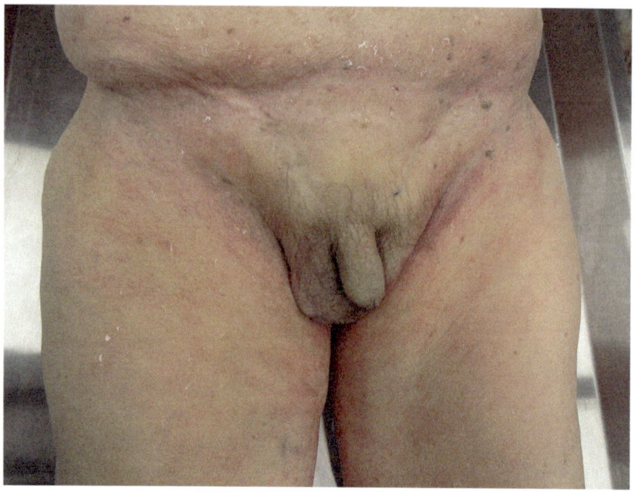

Fig. 9.116 This patient had previous hormone-secreting pituitary adenomatous disease which was treated by surgery and ultimately radiotherapy. There has been consequential genital and gonadal atrophy. Incidental hernia scars are noted

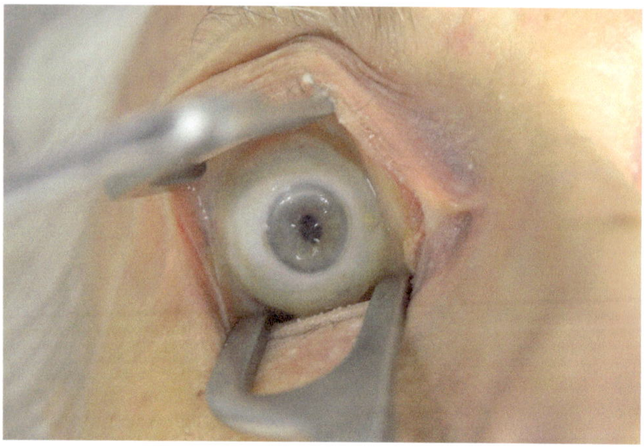

Fig. 9.117 The eye is removed in stages. One begins by retracting the eyelids

The Eye

On rare occasions, it may be necessary to remove one or both eyes for detailed examination by an ophthalmic pathologist, or to explore and sample the orbit (Figs. 9.117, 9.118, 9.119, 9.120, and 9.121). For example, examination may be necessary if there is concern regarding possible ocular or orbital tumours or an acute disease that may have affected visual acuity, contributing to death.

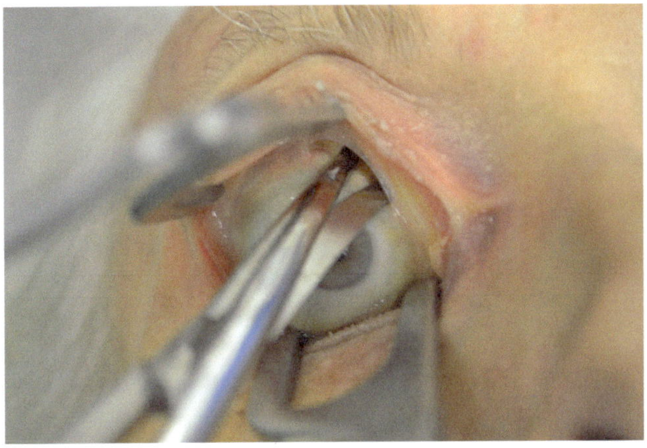

Fig. 9.118 The conjunctiva is incised and the muscles are cut, followed by the optic nerve

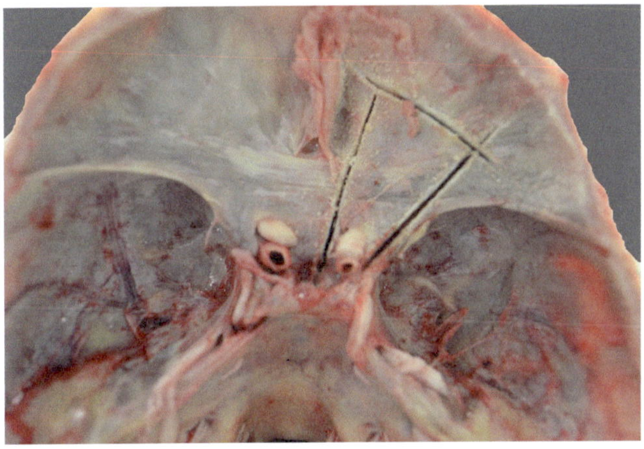

Fig. 9.119 Using the oscillating saw, three cuts are made in the floor of the anterior cranial fossa

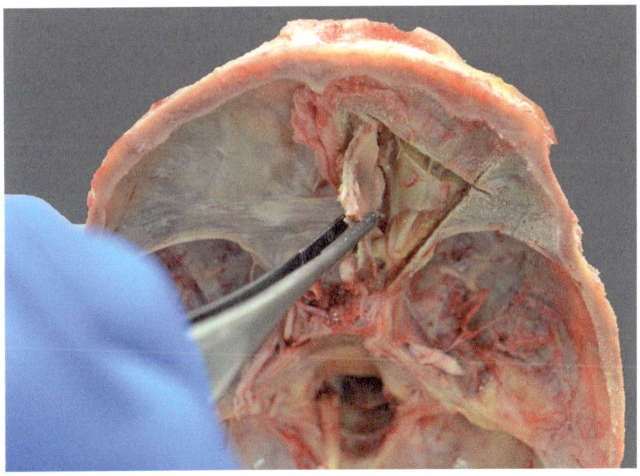

Fig. 9.120 The bone segment is removed

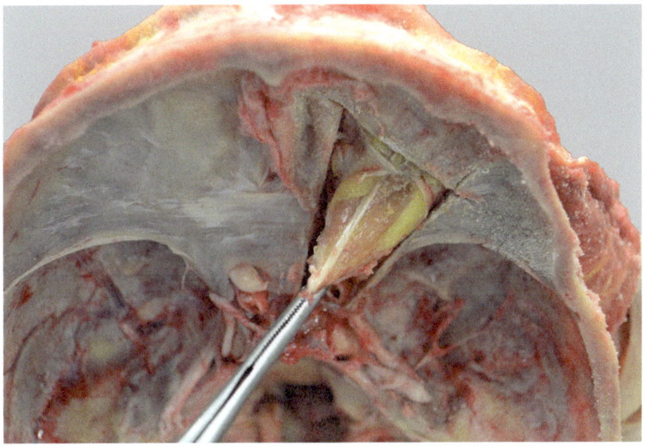

Fig. 9.121 The eye connections can be removed from the superior approach using curved scissors

The anterior approach is appropriate in cases where examination of the orbital structures, other than the eye, is not required.

The posterior approach is preferred in cases where there are concerns that the deceased may have had an ocular tumour. This approach allows the globe to be removed in continuity with the other orbital contents, allowing staging of such tumours. The conjunctiva is first incised, as per the anterior approach.

To achieve an adequate cosmetic result on reconstruction, great care must be taken not to damage the eyelids or eyelashes when removing the eyes. Following the removal of the eye, the orbit must be reconstructed. The back of the orbit is packed with wet cotton wool, and dry cotton wool is then placed in front. An eye shield is placed over the top of the cotton wool and the eyelid is then closed. Methyl methacrylate glue may be used to hold the eyelid in place, but care must be taken not to allow the glue to come into contact with the external surface of the eyelids.

The Middle Ear

The middle ear (Figs. 9.122 and 9.123) should be examined in cases of sepsis of unknown source, and in some cases of meningitis, to look for a source of infection. The middle ear cavities can be swabbed for microbiological examination (see Chap. 10).

The middle ears are exposed once the brain has been eviscerated and the dura stripped from the base of the skull. No specific reconstruction is required beyond that used to reconstruct the skull following evisceration of the brain.

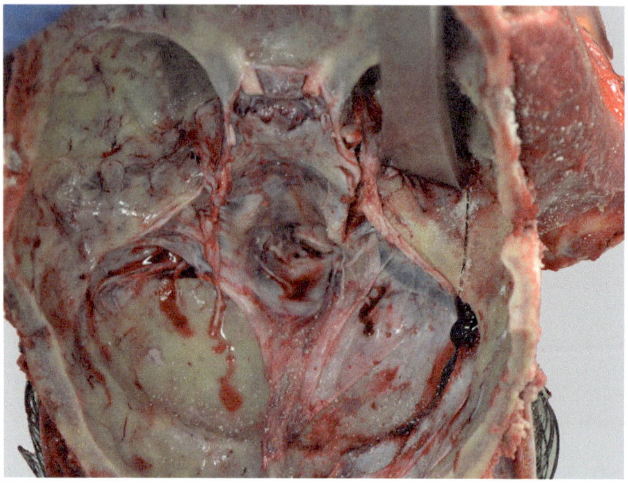

Fig. 9.122 The ear is approached by cutting into the sphenoid. Two parallel cuts are made. The bone segment is levered out with the skull key or osteotome

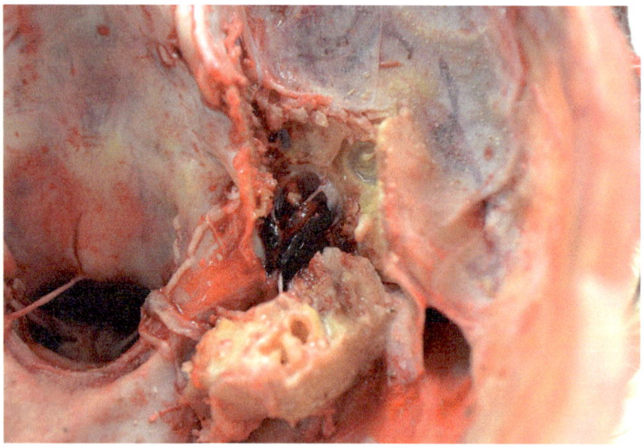

Fig. 9.123 The inner ear is exposed

The Spinal Cord

The spinal cord (Figs. 9.124, 9.125, 9.126, 9.127, 9.128, 9.129, and 9.130) may require examination in cases where trauma, tumour, inflammatory diseases or degenerative diseases are suspected. Care must be taken when handling the cord to keep it as straight as possible. Angulation of the cord may produce artefacts that make histopathological interpretation difficult.

On very rare occasions, it may be necessary to remove the cord in continuity with the brain. This is best done by using the anterior approach for removal of the cord, as the body is then in the correct position for removal of the brain.

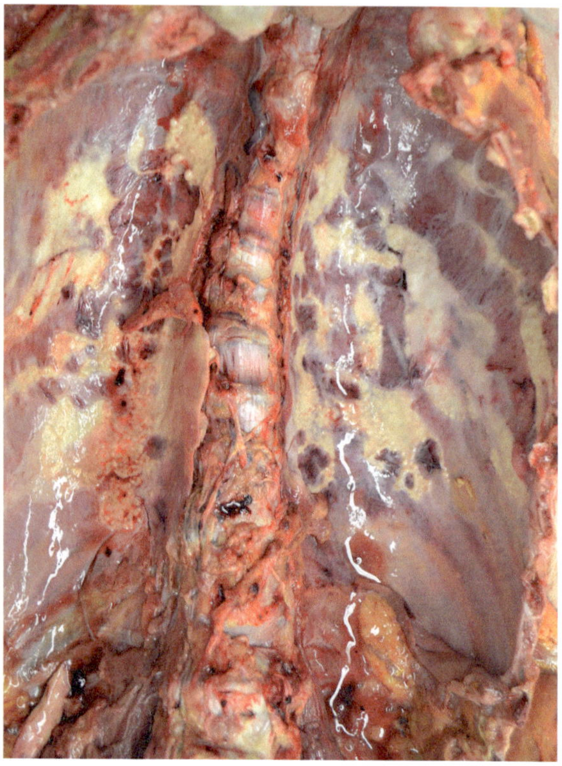

Fig. 9.124 The examination and removal of the spinal cord is a complex task. Here, one starts by having the thoracic and lumbar vertebral bone exposed. The muscle and other soft tissues are removed on either side

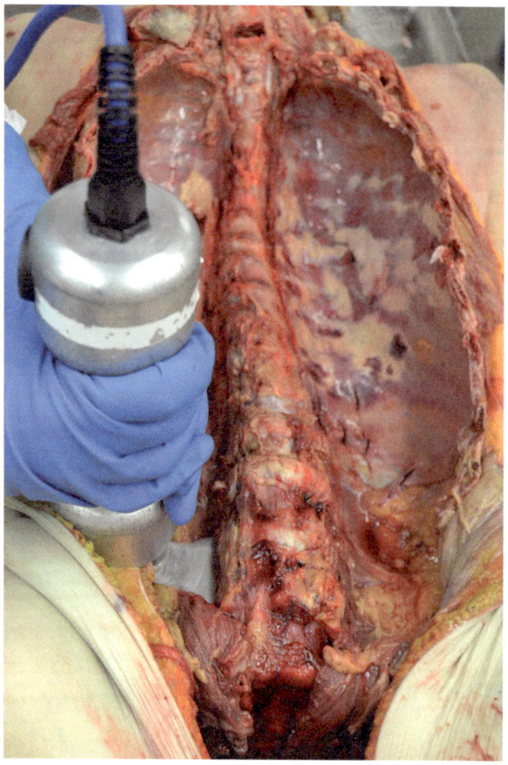

Fig. 9.125 The lateral bone boundaries of the spinal canal are cut with the oscillating saw. Each vertebral body must be cut. The lower end (L5/S1 disc) is transected by a long knife

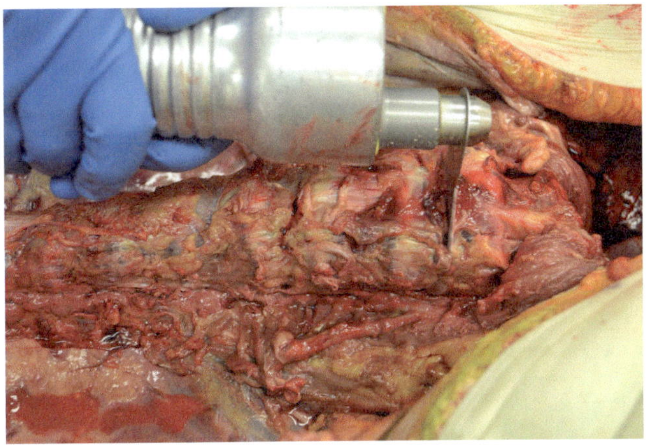

Fig. 9.126 Alternatively, one can use the saw to cut across the bone transversely. This cut, or that made at the disc, will be below the distal end of the cord

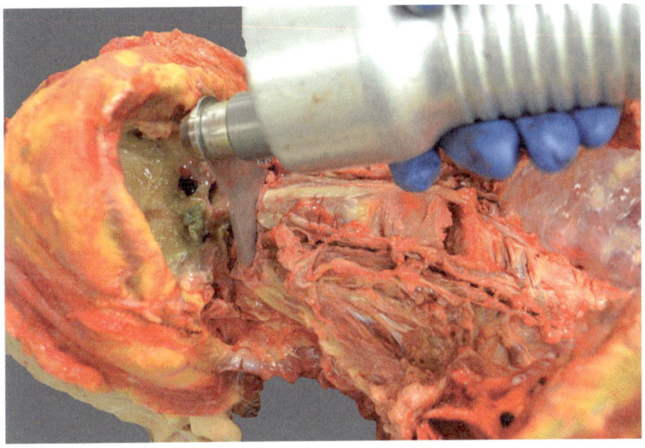

Fig. 9.127 The upper end of the cord is accessed by a high cervical vertebral bone cut

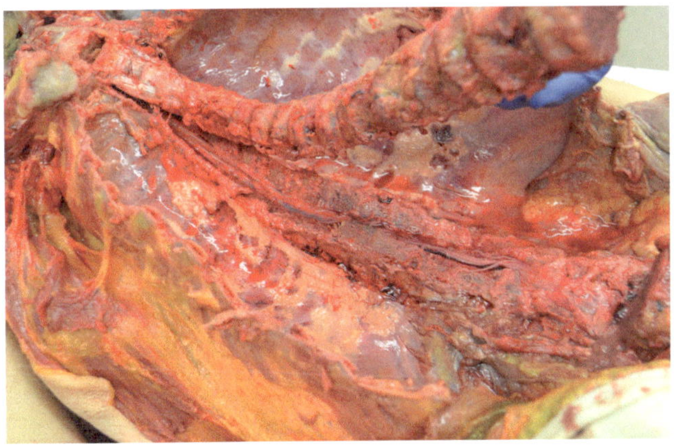

Fig. 9.128 The vertebral bodies are levered upwards, gently exposing the spinal cord in the spinal canal

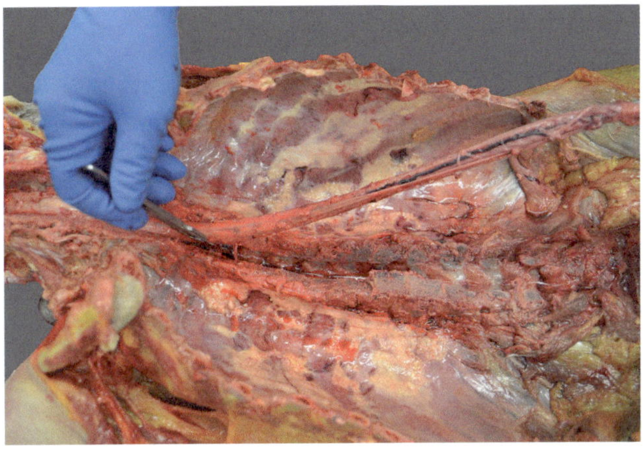

Fig. 9.129 The side branches of the spinal nerves are sequentially cut, allowing the cord to be removed gently

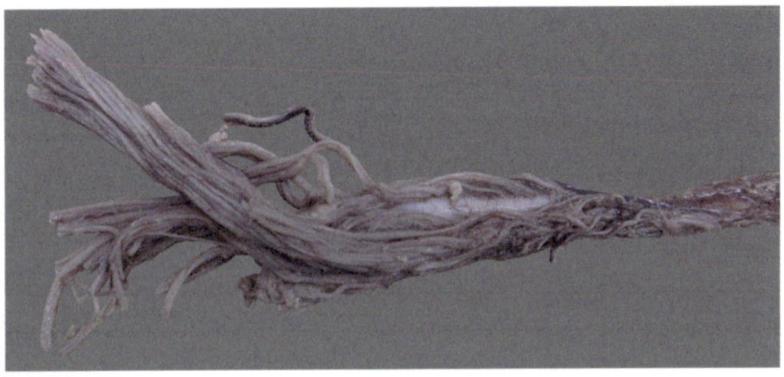

Fig. 9.130 When removed, the spinal cord is extremely fragile and susceptible to artefactual damage. Fixation prior to sectioning is beneficial in most cases. Where avoidance of artifact is important, the cord can be fixed suspended in a tube. The distal spinal cord section, the cauda equina, is shown here

Exposing and Removing the Spinal Cord—Anterior Approach

Most often, the spinal cord is removed using an anterior approach once the organs of the neck, thorax and abdomen have been eviscerated. This approach allows the spinal cord to be removed in continuity with its associated ganglia.

Exposing and Removing the Spinal Cord—Posterior Approach

When the spinal cord is to be examined without its associated ganglia, it may be removed via a posterior approach. This approach is easier than the anterior approach, as the angle of the saw cuts is uniform in all regions of the spine, but it requires the body to be placed into a prone position and it generates a further skin incision. See also Chap. 7, cervical vertebrae dissection Figs. 7.64 to 7.76.

Reconstructing the Head

It is not practicable to attempt to replace the brain in the cranial cavity because of its soft consistency and the risk of later leakage. When the examination of the brain and skull is complete, the brain is returned to the body with the organs from the torso.

The head is normally reconstructed by an experienced anatomical pathology technician, who will ensure good cosmesis. However, the pathologist should be familiar with the process. The cranial cavity is first packed with cotton wool, and the calvaria is replaced. The calvaria can be secured in place using methyl methacrylate glue. The temporalis muscles are returned to their anatomical positions and the scalp is then replaced over the calvaria. The scalp incision is sutured closed.

The authors would like to acknowledge the significant contributions of Professor Julian Burton and Professor S. Kim Suvarna for provision of the images and text in this chapter from this book's first edition.

Suggested Reading

Burton JL, Rutty G. The hospital autopsy. 3rd ed. London: Hodder Arnold; 2010. p. 136–58, 262–76.

Connolly AJ, Finkbeiner WE, Ursell PC, Davis RL, editors. Autopsy pathology: a manual and atlas. 3rd ed. Philadelphia: Elsevier; 2016.

Cooke RA, Stewart B. Nervous system. In: Colour atlas of anatomical pathology. 3rd ed. Edinburgh: Churchill Livingstone; 2004. p. 229–82.

Curran RC, Jones EL. Central nervous system and eye. In: Curran RC, Jones EL, editors. Gross pathology: a colour atlas. Aylesbury: HM + M Publishers; 1974. p. 76–90.

Gray F, Duyckaerts C, De Girolami U, editors. Escourolle and Poirier's manual of basic neuropathology. 6th ed. Oxford Academic; 2018.

Love S. Post mortem sampling of the brain and other tissues in neurodegenerative disease. Histopathology. 2004;44(4):309–17.

Love S, Perry A, Ironside J, Budka H. Greenfield's neuropathology. 9th ed. CRC Press; 2015.

Ludwig J. Autopsy practice. 3rd ed. Ottawa: Humana Press; 2002.

Standard and Special Tests

10

Julian L. Burton and Abigail K. Sharp

Introduction

In many autopsies, the cause of death can be determined by macroscopic examination alone, or with macroscopic and histopathological examination of the major organs. Frequently, however, further investigations are needed to determine or refine the cause of death.

This chapter illustrates the methods used to collect samples for toxicology, microbiology, virology, immunology, and histology. It should be noted that the technique shown to collect blood for toxicological analysis is also largely appropriate for the collection of blood for virology and/or immunological investigation, although an aseptic technique is more appropriate for microbiology samples. The initial set of images deals with toxicology samples, with microbiology samples following.

Consideration should be given to the potential collection of these samples prior to the start of every autopsy. Once the organs have been eviscerated, the opportunity to collect these samples is frequently limited, or even lost.

When samples are submitted for analysis, it is imperative that they be placed into the appropriate containers and correctly labelled with patient identifier information (ideally name, date of birth/death, and unique numerical coding). The samples should be accompanied by adequate clinical and case history details.

Toxicology samples should be accompanied by details that include the circumstances surrounding the death, the nature of any prescribed medication or suspected illicit drugs, and the nature and site of collection of the samples.

Samples submitted for bacteriological or virological examination should likewise be accompanied by details of the clinical history, the deceased's address (for contact tracing purposes), any antimicrobial therapies given in life, and the post-mortem interval.

Autopsy microbiology poses its own special challenges of interpretation. It should be remembered that organisms detected may be due to post-mortem colonisation of the body (usually originating from the intestines), and that a test may be negative because there is no infection (true negative) or because the infecting organism has died in the interval between death and autopsy. Sampling error also may yield false negative results.

All samples obtained should be submitted to the appropriate laboratory as soon as possible. If immediate transportation is not possible, they should be stored at 4 °C.

Toxicology

The collection of samples for toxicology should be considered in every autopsy. Samples are best collected before or during full evisceration, or potentially as the autopsy starts. Where possible, both plain and preserved samples should be collected and placed into the appropriate specimen containers. Tissue samples should be placed dry into a sterile container that has never contained formalin or another product.

Vitreous Humour

Vitreous humour may be collected for both clinical chemistry and toxicological analysis by direct aspiration of the eye contents using a syringe and needle (Figs. 10.1, 10.2, 10.3, 10.4, and 10.5). An unpreserved sample is required for sodium ion, urea, and creatinine quantification. A preserved sample is required for glucose, alcohol, cocaine, and 6-monoacetylmorphine

J. L. Burton (✉)
Medical Education, Division of Clinical Medicine, School of Medicine and Population Health, The University of Sheffield, Sheffield, UK
e-mail: j.l.burton@sheffield.ac.uk

A. K. Sharp
Histopathology Department, Sheffield Teaching Hospitals NHS Foundation Trust, Sheffield, UK

S. K. Suvarna (represented by Grace Horne), A. K. Sharp (eds.), *Atlas of Adult Autopsy*,
https://doi.org/10.1007/978-3-031-72207-3_10

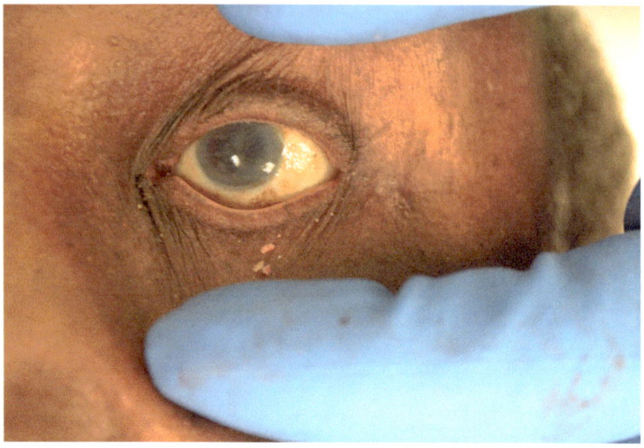

Fig. 10.1 The eyelids are retracted

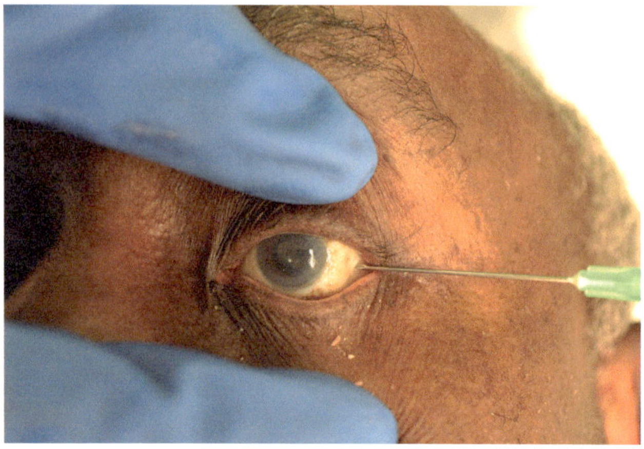

Fig. 10.2 Using a 19G needle attached to a 10 mL syringe, puncture the sclera as distally and laterally as possible. The needle should be angled inwards at 30–45°

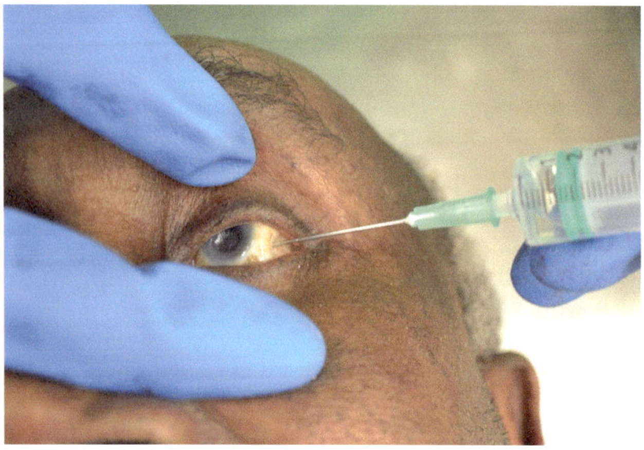

Fig. 10.3 Aspirate 2–3 mL of vitreous humour

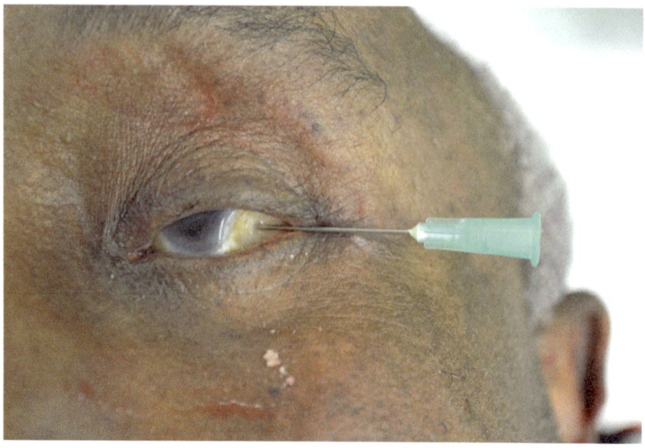

Fig. 10.4 Remove the syringe from the needle, leaving the needle in situ

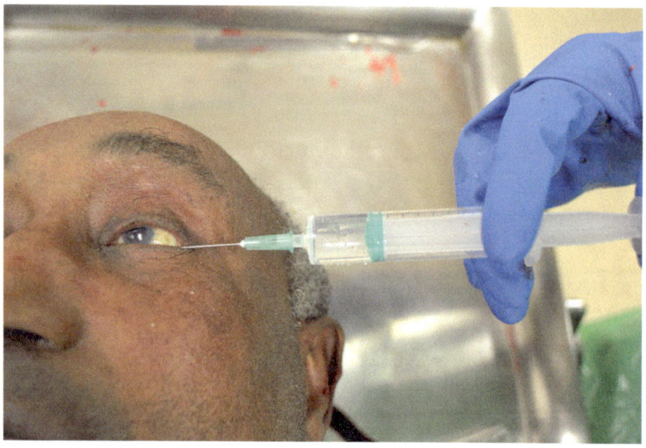

Fig. 10.5 Reinflate the globe using 2–3 mL of water, and then remove the needle

quantification. The structure and shape of the eye should be reconstituted by instilling water afterwards.

Blood

Blood for toxicological analysis (ideally 10–20 mL) should be obtained either by needle puncture of the femoral vein prior to evisceration (Figs. 10.6, 10.7, and 10.8) or from the common iliac vein on opening the body, prior to evisceration of the internal organs. It is not common practice to sample blood from the abdominal or thoracic tissues, to prevent issues with post-mortem redistribution of drugs or toxins. On rare occasions, when little peripheral blood is available, the venous sinuses in the cranial cavity may be accessed directly with syringe aspiration of their contents.

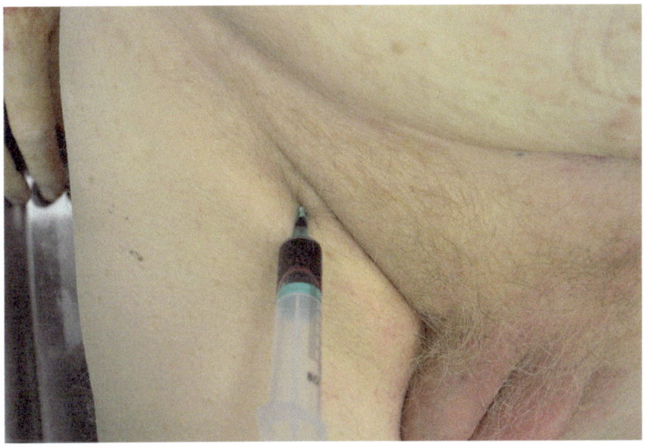

Fig. 10.6 Blood for toxicology can be aspirated from the femoral vein, which lies medial to the midpoint of the inguinal ligament

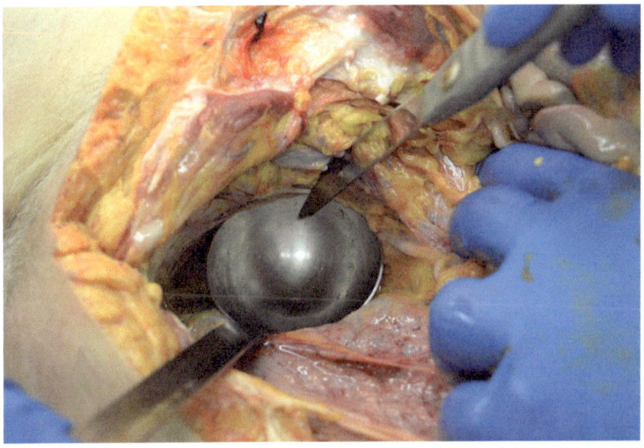

Fig. 10.7 On opening the abdomen, use blunt dissection to free the pelvic organs from the pelvic side walls. Place a specimen container or clean ladle into the pelvis, below the common iliac vein

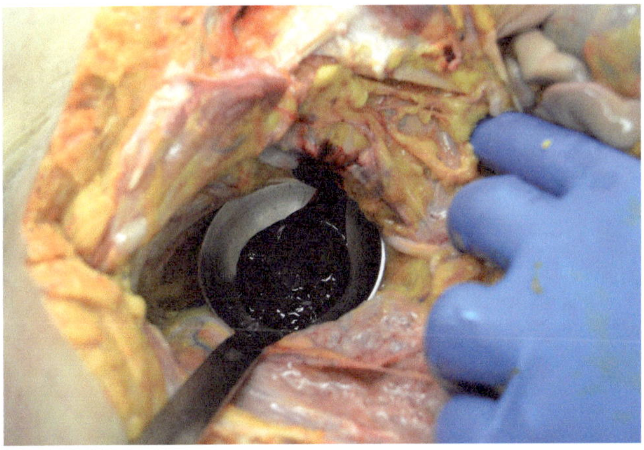

Fig. 10.8 Incise the iliac vein using a knife. Blood usually flows freely into the specimen container or ladle. If necessary, gently massage the inner thigh, from knee to groin, to express blood

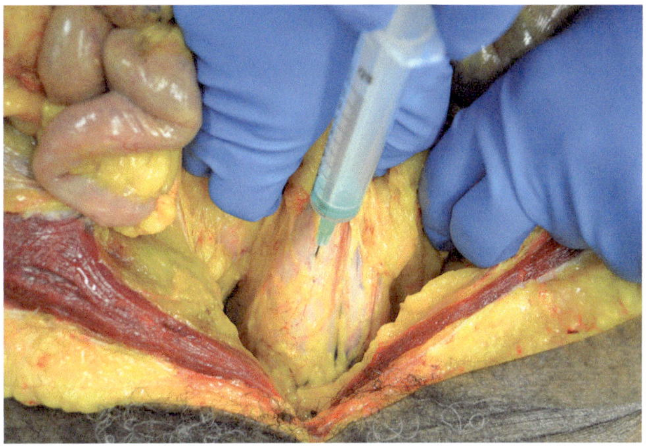

Fig. 10.9 Urine for toxicology is best obtained using a needle and syringe, on opening the abdomen. Take care not to contaminate the sample with blood. Insert the needle through the dome of the bladder

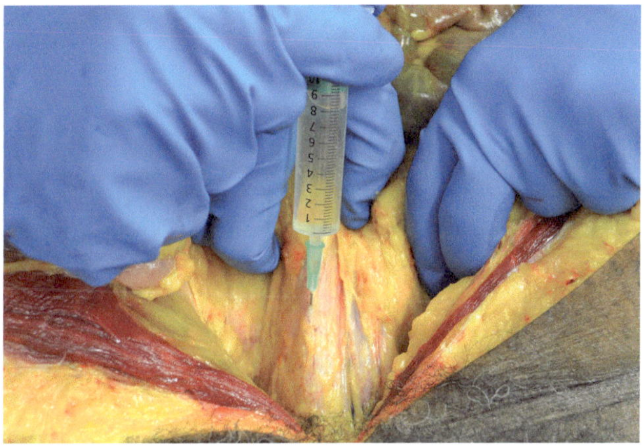

Fig. 10.10 Aspirate 10 mL of urine and place it into the appropriate specimen containers

Urine

Urine is most easily obtained immediately after the peritoneal cavity has been opened, using a needle and syringe (Figs. 10.9 and 10.10). If the volume of urine within the bladder is small, a sample may be obtained by incising the dome of the bladder to visualise the sample to be collected.

Gastric Contents

It is useful to collect a sample of gastric contents if there is suspicion that the deceased may have ingested a toxin or drug overdose. The entire contents should be extracted (Figs. 10.11, 10.12, and 10.13). The total volume of the stomach contents should be noted and a representative sample (generally 20 mL) should be submitted for analysis. The total volume of the

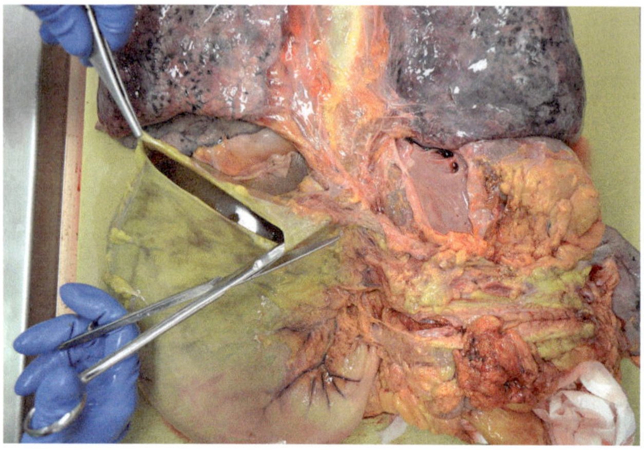

Fig. 10.11 A 10 cm incision is made into the gastric fundus using scissors, taking care not to contaminate the gastric contents with blood

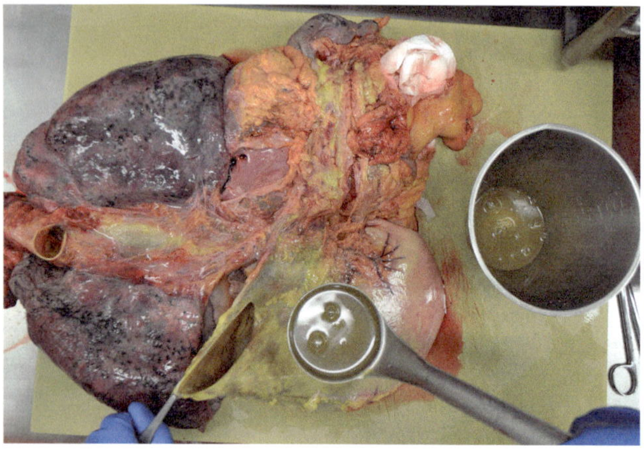

Fig. 10.12 The gastric contents are removed into a clean, dry measuring jug using a clean, dry ladle

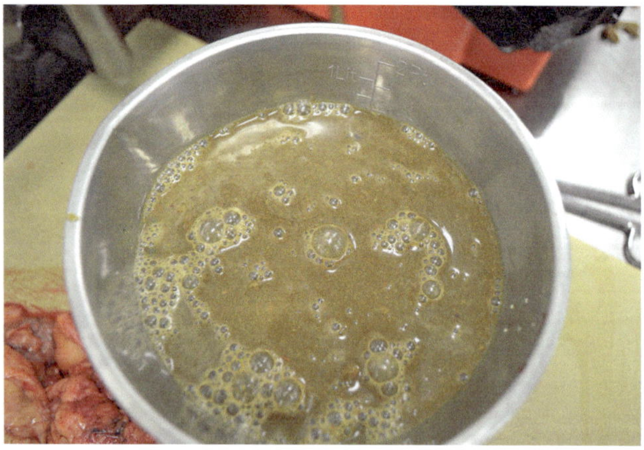

Fig. 10.13 Record the volume of the gastric contents, noting the presence or absence of any tablet residues. Reserve a sample for toxicology, but the entire volume may not be required

stomach contents should be recorded. Close attention to the contents is advised, looking for solid or partly brokendown tablet residues. If there is concern that death may be due to anaphylaxis, the stomach contents should be photographed.

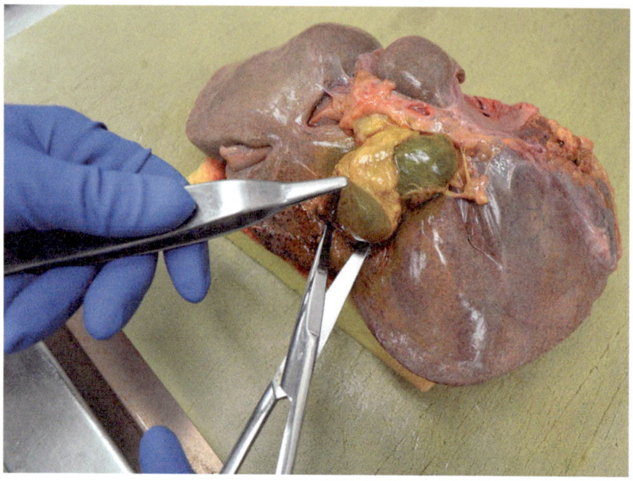

Fig. 10.14 Carefully dissect the intact gallbladder free of the gallbladder bed. Alternatively, take the sample by syringe aspiration of the gallbladder at the start of the examination, after opening the abdomen

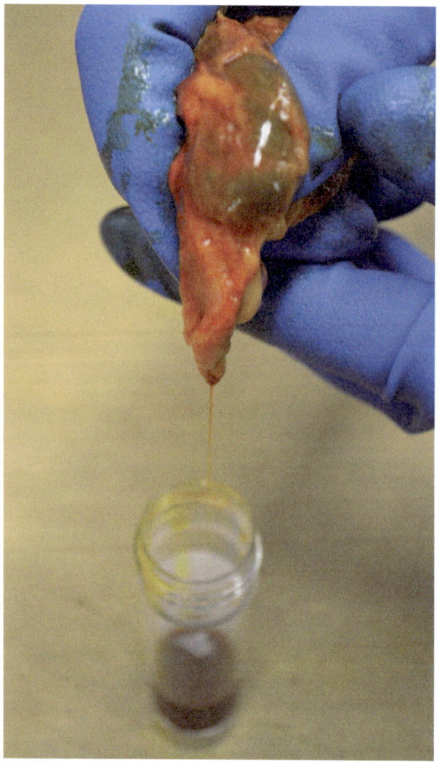

Fig. 10.15 Invert the gallbladder over an appropriate specimen container and squeeze gently, taking care not to contaminate the sample with blood

Bile

When it is not possible to obtain samples of blood or urine, a sample of bile may be collected and submitted for toxicological analysis (Figs. 10.14 and 10.15). The range of drugs that can be tested may be more limited than with blood.

Liver

If no fluid samples can be obtained from the body, a sample (generally 2–3 cm^3) of the right lobe of the liver can be submitted for toxicological analysis (Figs. 10.16 and 10.17). A sample of psoas muscle is also acceptable, either in place of liver or as an additional specimen.

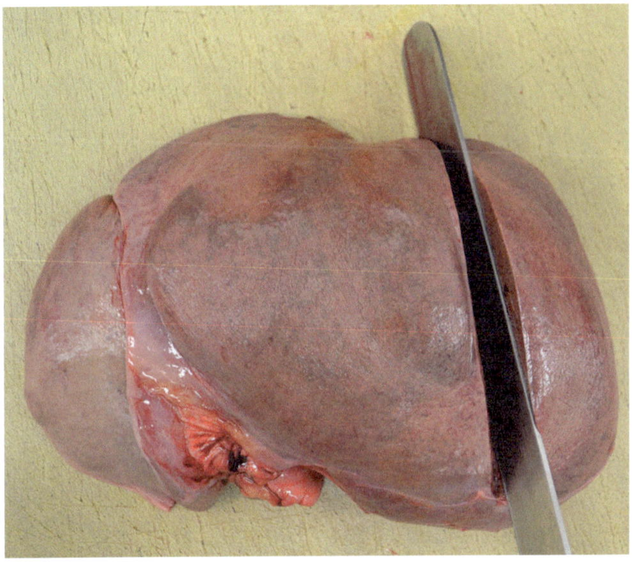

Fig. 10.16 Having dissected the liver free of its attachments, make a parasagittal slice through the middle of the right lobe, using a clean, dry knife

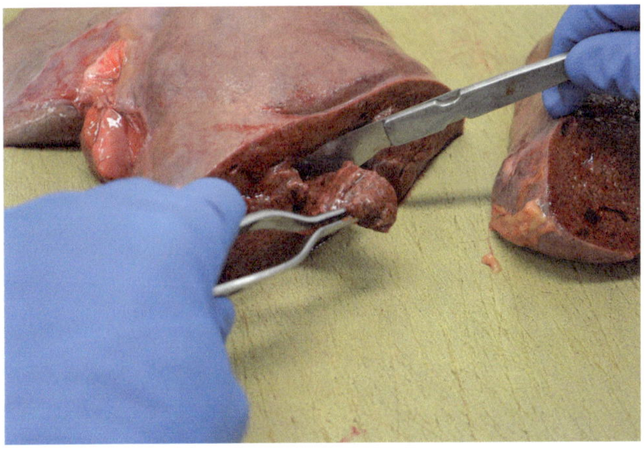

Fig. 10.17 Use a clean, dry scalpel to excise a portion of liver from deep within the right lobe of the liver

Microbiology and Virology

In cases where infection is suspected, samples should be collected for microbiology. When collecting transdermal samples, the skin should be cleaned with alcohol, povidone-iodine solution, or chlorhexidine and allowed to dry. If these are not available, then formalin-soaked tissue may be used.

Sterile instruments must be used, and needles should not be changed.

Specimens must be placed into empty, sterile universal containers that have never contained formalin or other products. When tissue is collected, it may be placed into a sterile container containing sterile 0.9% saline to prevent it from drying out. Samples should be stored at 4 °C if they cannot be immediately transported to the laboratory. Modern virological investigations examine for the presence of viral DNA/RNA rather than viral culture, and viral transport medium is generally no longer required.

Blood

Blood for microbiological culture should be collected prior to opening the body. It is best collected from a site remote from the intestines. The jugular or subclavian veins are often ideal sites (Figs. 10.18 and 10.19).

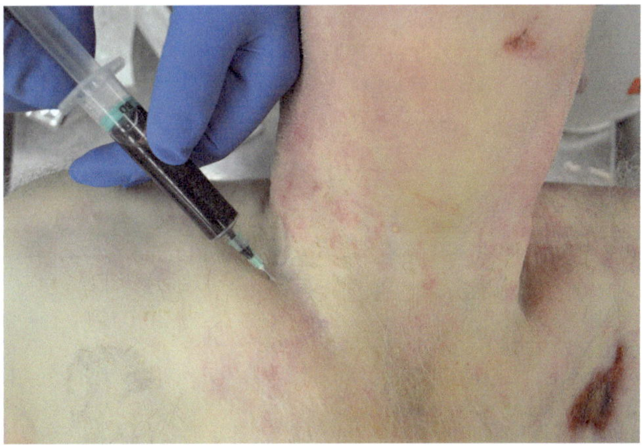

Fig. 10.18 Taking blood for microbiology starts with cleaning the skin of the anterior neck using alcohol, chlorhexidine, or povidone-iodine solution, and allowing it to dry. Using a green needle attached to a 10 or 20 mL syringe, insert the needle above the junction of the inner and middle thirds of the clavicle. Angle the needle at 80° from the vertical, and aim towards the contralateral sternoclavicular joint. Gradually advance the needle while gently aspirating on the syringe. Aspirate 10–20 mL of blood

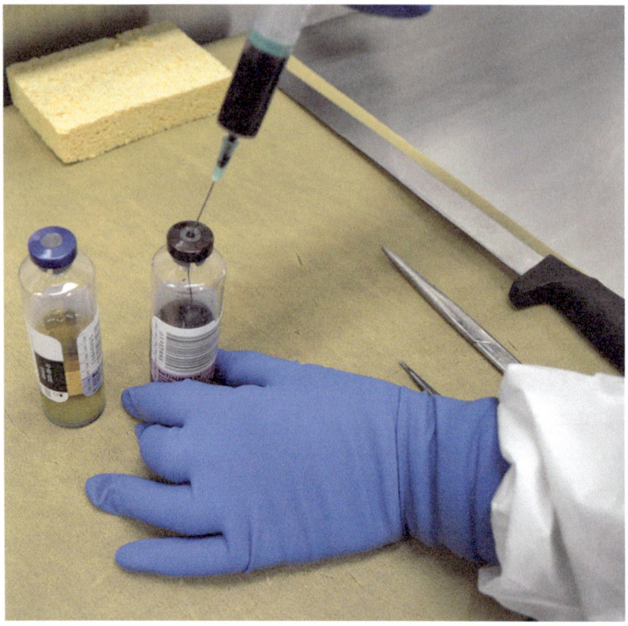

Fig. 10.19 Withdraw the needle, and inject directly into blood culture bottles. *Do not change the needle*

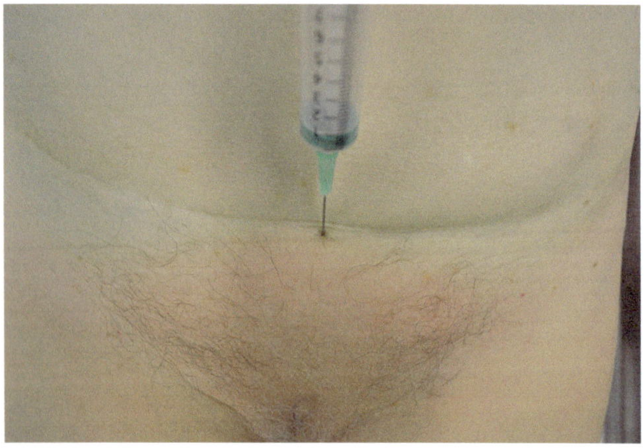

Fig. 10.20 Microbiology assessment of urine may be approached using a green needle attached to a 10 mL syringe. Insert the needle above the symphysis pubis

Urine

Urine for microbiological examination is best obtained from the bladder prior to opening the body (Figs. 10.20, 10.21, 10.22, and 10.23). If this is not possible, the method described for the collection of urine for toxicology can be used. If there is no urine within the bladder, the bladder mucosa can be swabbed. It is emphasised that urine present within catheter bags is not appropriate for microbiology.

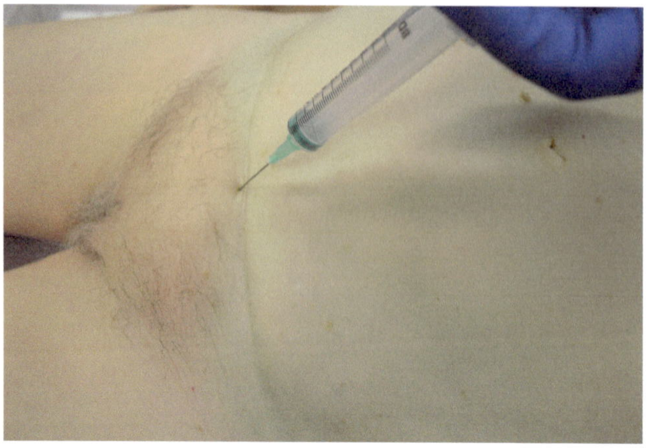

Fig. 10.21 Angle the needle inferiorly, at an angle of 45°

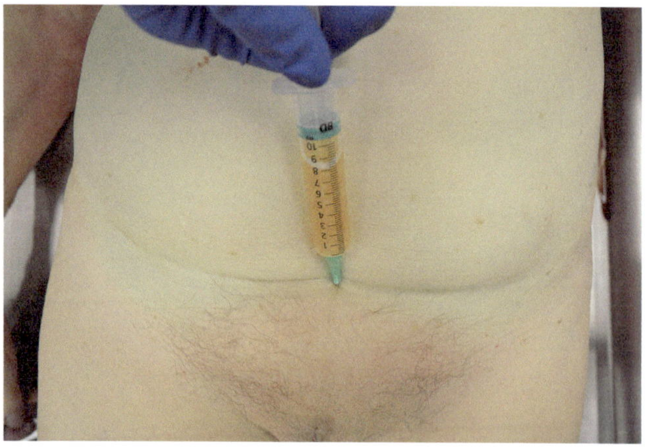

Fig. 10.22 Gradually advance the needle, while gently aspirating on the syringe. Aspirate 10 mL of urine

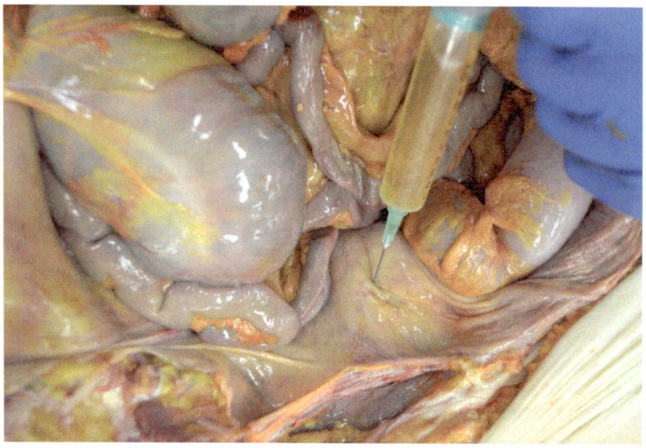

Fig. 10.23 Alternatively, use a needle and syringe to aspirate urine via the dome of the bladder immediately on opening the peritoneal cavity

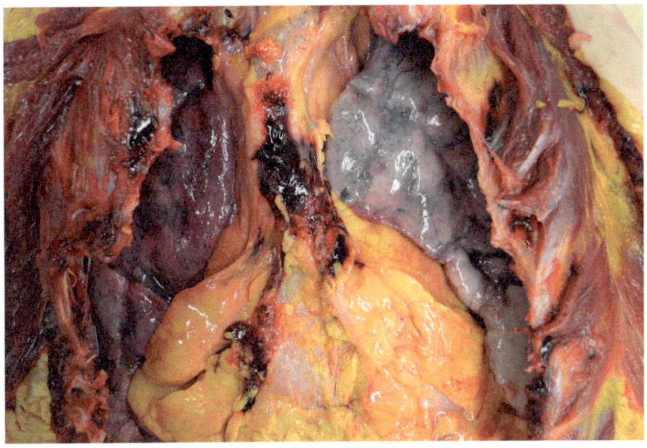

Fig. 10.24 One may sample lung for microbiology. This sampling is accomplished by opening the chest cavity as normal, taking care not to handle the lungs directly

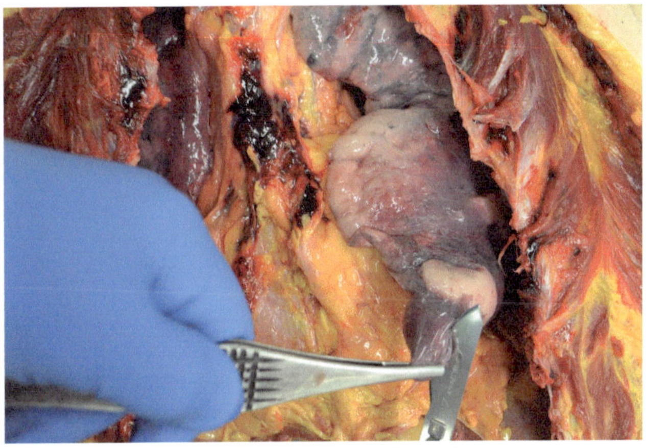

Fig. 10.25 Using a sterile scalpel blade and forceps, remove a cube of lung (1–2 cm^3) from the lower lobe or area of interest

Lung

Lung tissue should be collected for standard microbiology (bacterial) studies and/or virology when either pneumonia or viral pneumonitis are suspected from the history (Figs. 10.24 and 10.25). One should not overlook possible fungal infections. A sample for histology should also be reserved for cross comparison.

Cerebrospinal Fluid

When meningitis or encephalitis is suspected, samples of cerebrospinal fluid (CSF) should be collected for microbiology and virology. Samples can be easily obtained from the cisterna magna by direct aspiration (Figs. 10.26, 10.27, 10.28, and 10.29). Swabs and samples of brain tissue also can be collected, and a pharyngeal swab for microbiology should also be collected.

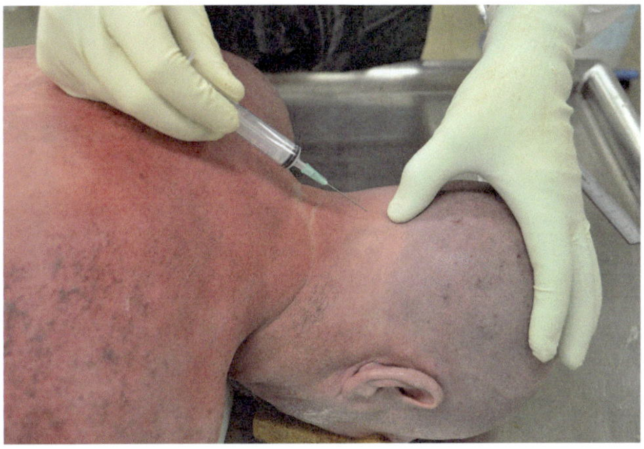

Fig. 10.26 Cerebrospinal fluid (CSF) sampling involves access via the back of the neck. Lay the body prone, with a block under the chest to flex the neck. Palpate the atlanto-occipital membrane in the midline. This will be the site of needle insertion

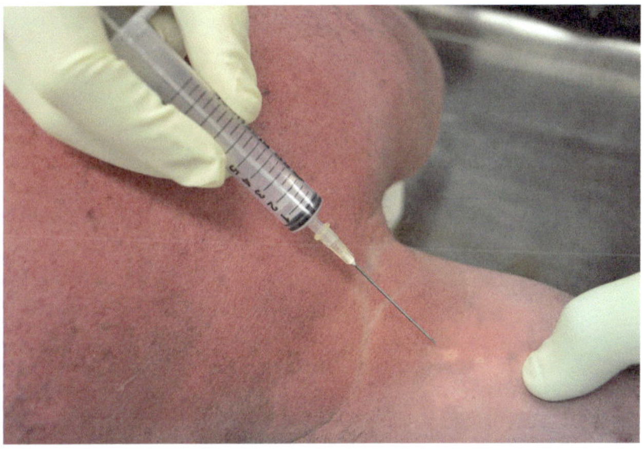

Fig. 10.27 Use a wide-bore needle attached to a 5 or 10 mL syringe

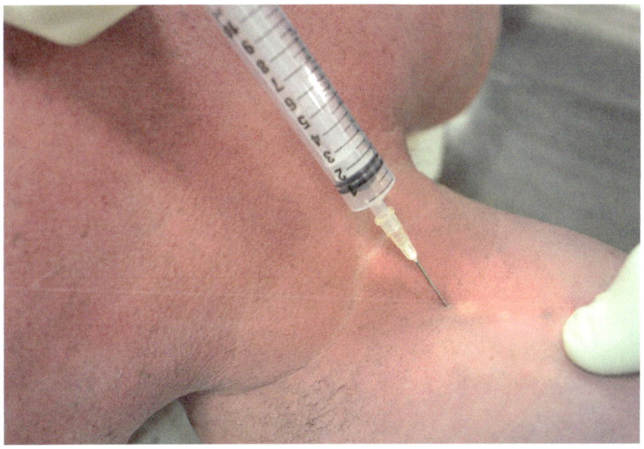

Fig. 10.28 Slowly advance the needle, aiming towards the bridge of the nose

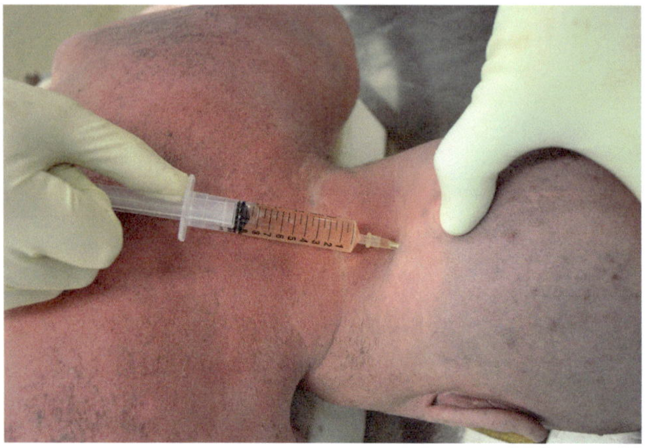

Fig. 10.29 At a depth of approximately 20 mm, you will feel the needle "give" and will be able to aspirate between 2 and 10 mL of CSF

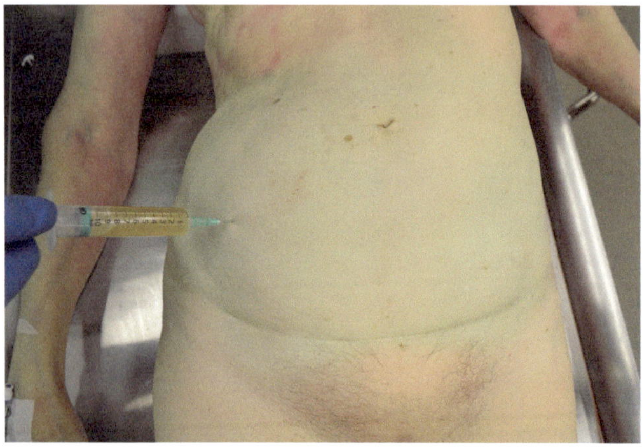

Fig. 10.30 To sample ascites, use a green needle attached to a syringe. Insert the needle in the mid-clavicular line, aiming for the spine, and aspirate 10 mL of ascites

Ascites

Patients with cirrhosis of the liver may develop spontaneous bacterial peritonitis. Collecting a sample of ascites for microbiological examination helps to confirm the diagnosis and is best done before the body is opened (Fig. 10.30).

Spleen

If blood cultures are desirable but unobtainable, a sample of spleen can be collected for microbiological culture as soon as the peritoneal cavity has been opened (Figs. 10.31 and 10.32).

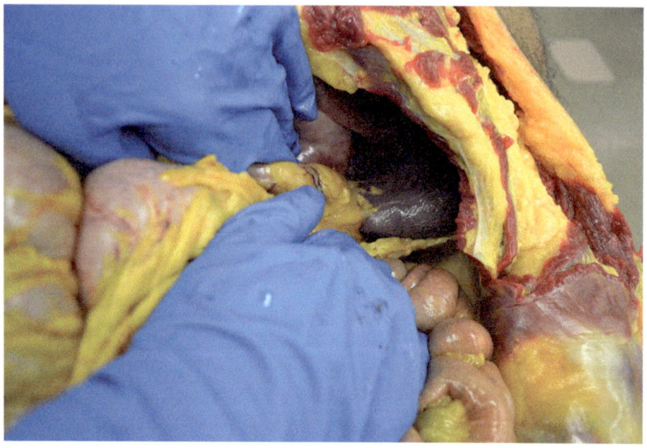

Fig. 10.31 To collect a sample of spleen for microbiological culture, have an assistant retract the intestines towards the right iliac fossa, taking care not to touch the spleen

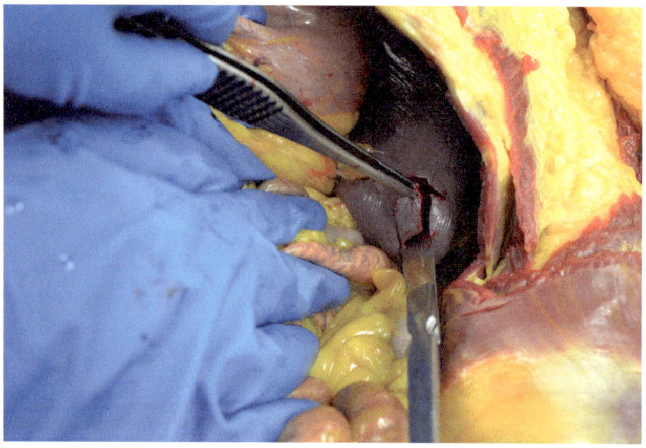

Fig. 10.32 Using a sterile scalpel blade and forceps, remove a 1–2 cm^3 cube of spleen

Bile

When biliary sepsis is suspected, a sample of bile may be collected for culture. This is best done on opening the peritoneal cavity, prior to evisceration of the internal organs (Fig. 10.33).

Faeces

If gastroenteritis (including viral causes) or pseudomembranous colitis is suspected, sample of faeces can be collected during evisceration or organ dissection for stool culture (Fig. 10.34).

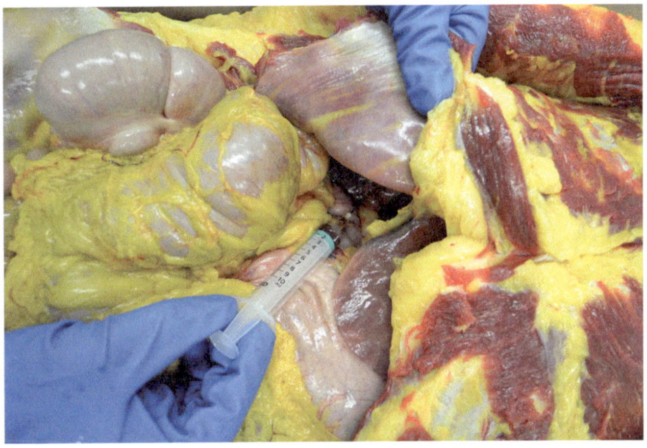

Fig. 10.33 To collect a sample of bile for microbiological culture, use a white needle attached to a 10 mL syringe to puncture the gallbladder fundus and aspirate up to 10 mL of bile

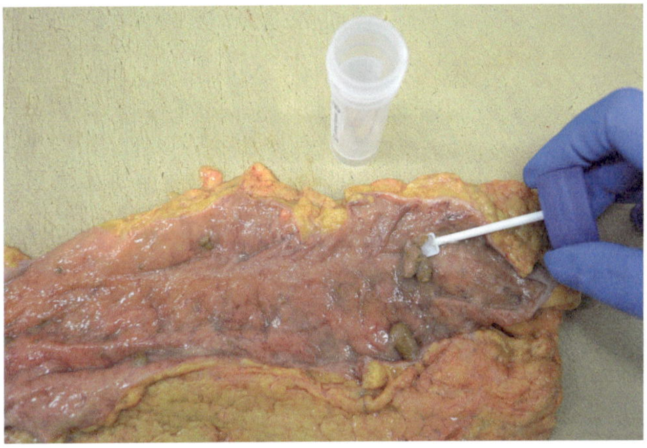

Fig. 10.34 A sample of faeces can also be collected by opening the sigmoid colon after evisceration

DNA Sampling

Any tissue with nucleated cell content will have DNA available for extraction and testing, but the best source will be tissue with a high cell nuclear content, generally taken to be spleen. A sample of spleen is generally advocated for DNA testing purposes. The sample is taken in a similar manner to that employed for microbiology. The sample may have the DNA extracted soon after sampling for storage, or the spleen sample may be frozen for later DNA extraction and assessment.

Histopathology Sampling

If the cause of death is not evident from macroscopic examination, or if there is concern about diseases that can be accurately identified only using microscopic examination, samples of tissues should be collected for histology.

Samples of the major organs and other tissues of interest are collected using a knife and are placed directly into appropriately labelled cassettes. The tissue samples should be approximately 2 mm thick. Soft tissues may need more than 24 h of fixation. Heavily calcified tissues require fixation and decalcification prior to histology sampling. Samples of similar density, or those that require similar staining techniques (for example, liver and kidney) may be placed into the same cassette for efficiency.

Suggested Reading

Burton JL, Rutty G. The hospital autopsy. 3rd ed. London: Hodder Arnold; 2010.

Connolly AJ, Finkbeiner WE, Ursell PC, Davis RL, editors. Autopsy pathology: a manual and atlas. 3rd ed. Philadelphia: Elsevier; 2016.

Saukko P, Knight B. Knight's forensic pathology. 4th ed. Boca Raton: CRC Press; 2016.

11 Devices: Foreign Items Encountered During the Autopsy

S. Kim Suvarna and Abigail K. Sharp

Introduction

Modern medicine has developed a variety of lines, tubes, joints and electronic instruments to be implanted during life. These devices (for want of a better word) are many in type and varied in design. They have symptomatic, reconstructive and therapeutic functionality.

Among the devices often seen at autopsy are cardiac valves, pacemakers and joint replacements. Many bodies arrive in the mortuary without full notes. One may be perplexed to find an unexpected or unusual item during the examination, for which the function is not immediately apparent. Whilst not all-encompassing, this chapter aims to demonstrate a substantial range of items that many be found, with some basic data about their functionality.

External Devices

Modern medicine provides a range of different devices that are used to assist monitoring and treatment of patients in the surgical and medical setting. Many, such as the pulse oximeter and ECG electrodes, are temporary and are removed before the patient is transferred to the mortuary after death. Nevertheless, general advice to those looking after the deceased is that any device or item that could have an effect upon the body is generally left in situ following death. If the body is not subject to autopsy examination, then the devices may be removed before funeral preparations.

For those cases requiring autopsy, the presence of any device which may have bearing upon the cause of death require the device to be considered as part of the post-mortem examination process. By the nature of this topic, there is some overlap with the material covered in Chap. 2.

Personal devices attached to the body are common (Figs. 11.1, 11.2, 11.3, and 11.4). Such devices include hearing aids and false eyes. Some may indicate significant underlying disease (e.g., surgery for ocular neoplasia). Other items include piercings (commonly in the ear, but perhaps almost anywhere). The site, type and number of piercings should be noted. Although they are not usually matters to be considered at autopsy, skin-related sepsis may be pertinent. Unusual devices that have been placed in position by the deceased may also be relevant to the cause of death.

The presence of drug patches should be noted, with the name of the drug and dose being recorded. It follows that the provision of therapy will often point to the terminal realities of the deceased.

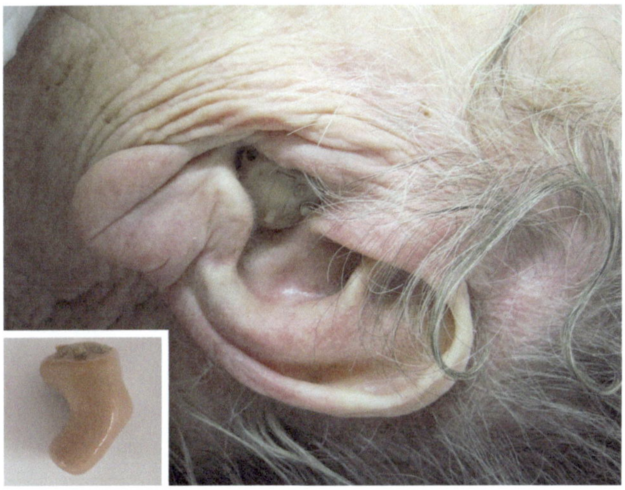

Fig. 11.1 A hearing aid, seen in situ and outside the ear canal (*inset*)

S. Kim Suvarna was deceased at the time of publication.

S. K. Suvarna (Deceased) · A. K. Sharp (✉)
Department of Histopathology, Sheffield Teaching Hospitals NHS Foundation Trust, Sheffield, UK
e-mail: abigail.sharp@nhs.net

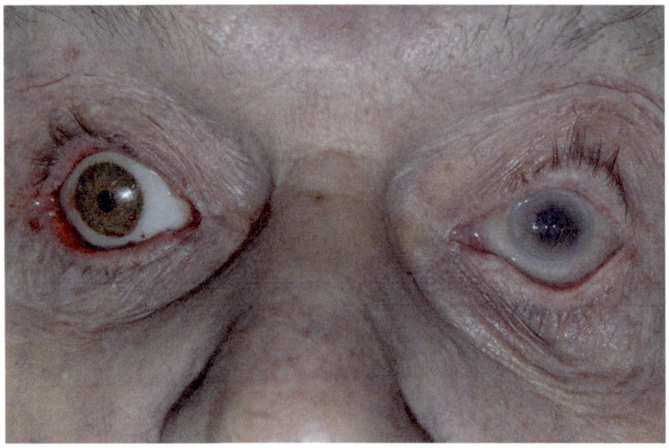

Fig. 11.2 A glass eye (*right side*) is an unusual finding in autopsy. Often, it is marked by appearing normal, compared with a post-mortem eye (*left side*)

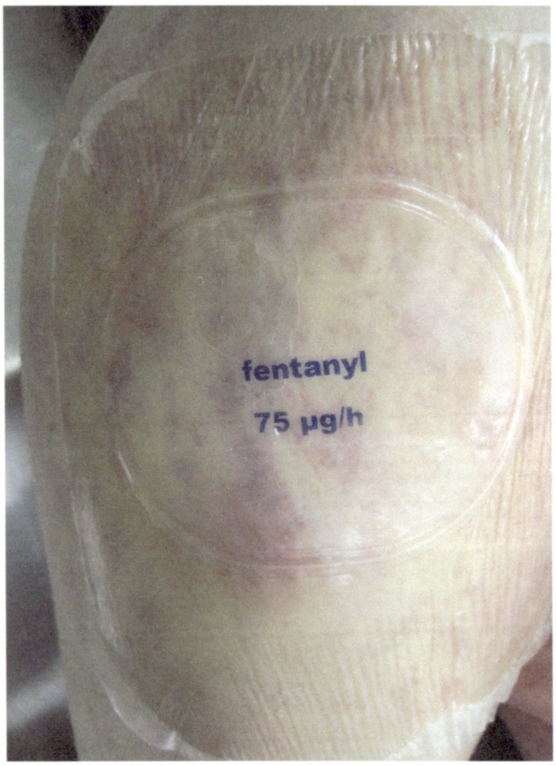

Fig. 11.3 A drug-delivery patch, on which the drug, the dose and the delivery rate are clearly marked

Examples of devices include a variety of lines that access the internal aspects of the body, including intravenous, intraarterial, intraosseous, subcutaneous, intrathecal, percutaneous, and intraabdominal lines (Figs. 11.5, 11.6, 11.7, 11.8, 11.9, 11.10, 11.11, 11.12, 11.13, 11.14, 11.15, and 11.16). It must be understood that these all

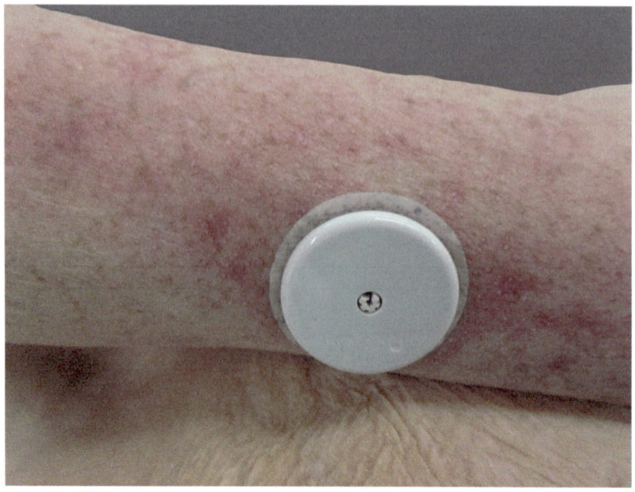

Fig. 11.4 This is a continuous glucose monitoring device, commonly placed on the upper arm. It is an increasingly common finding at autopsy examination of patients with diabetes. Note that there is a thin needle on the underside of these discs. Some of these devices can communicate with insulin pumps to create a closed-loop system of glucose monitoring and insulin delivery

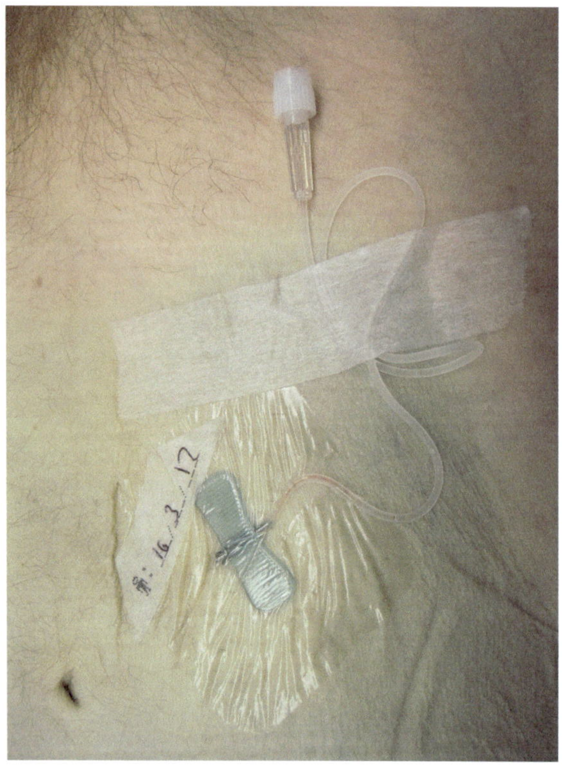

Fig. 11.5 A butterfly needle is present on the abdomen. This simple subcutaneous drug delivery device is useful for instilling small volumes of drugs, particularly in the palliative care setting. There is a date written on the dressing, indicating when it was positioned

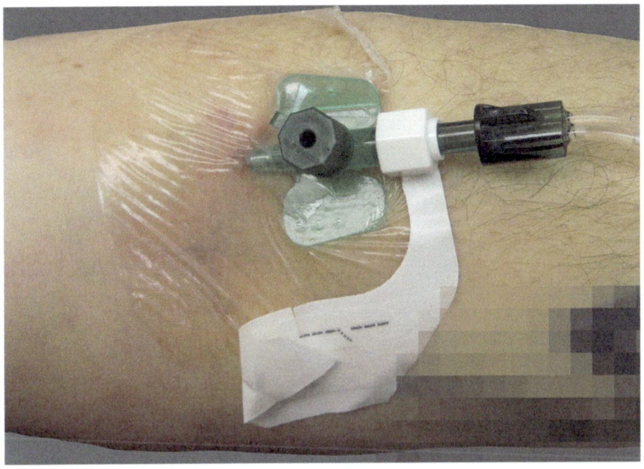

Fig. 11.6 Many types of intravenous line exist. This one is covered with a clear dressing to assist early identification of skin inflammation or sepsis

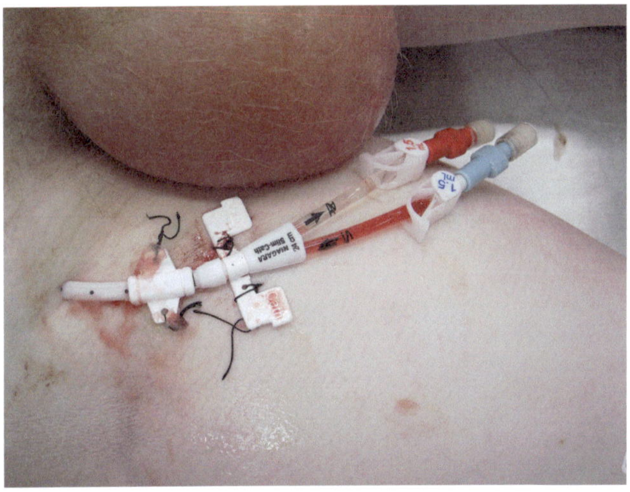

Fig. 11.7 Various external-sited vascular lines can be seen around the torso. This groin red and blue coded line with twin arms is characteristic of a haemodialysis line, mapping to the connections for a dialysis unit. Pronounced scrotal edema is noted adjacent to it

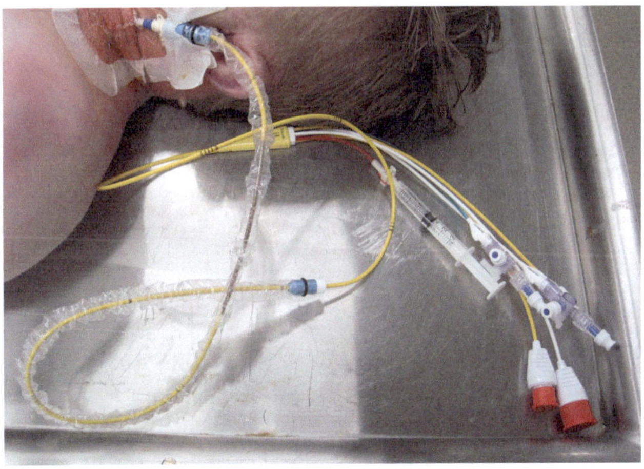

Fig. 11.8 A multiple-channel pulmonary artery catheter is present on the left side of the neck. This device allows monitoring of central pressures as well as the instillation of a range of different drugs or fluids

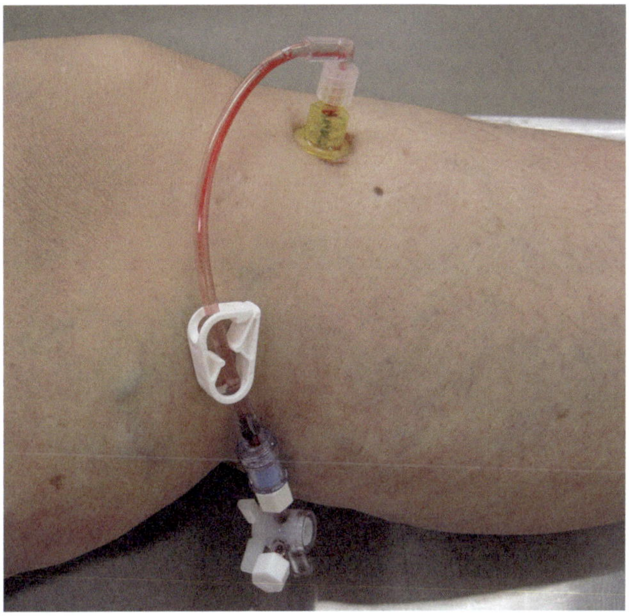

Fig. 11.9 An intraosseous vascular line to secure rapid access to the circulatory system is seen in a patient with 'vascular shut-down'. This type of line is increasingly used in emergency settings

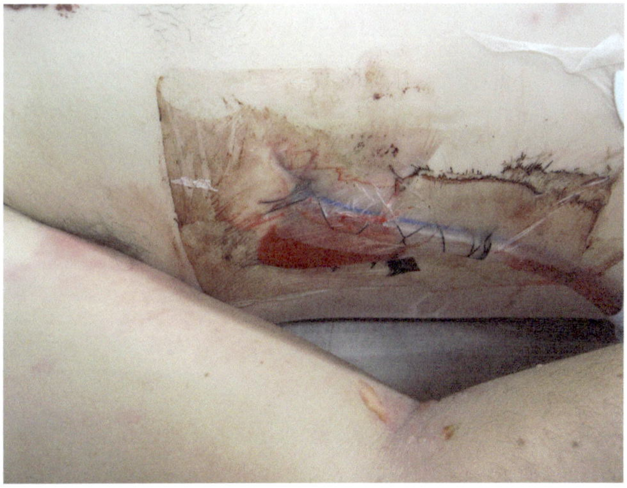

Fig. 11.10 A chest drain is seen in situ. It is secured by suture and covered in a clear dressing

provide a portal through the skin barrier directly into the body and may be the source of sepsis. On occasion, the lines may interact adversely with underlying structures, causing pathology in their own right, such as significant haemorrhage from arterial puncture in a patient on anticoagulation medication. Internal lines must be traced to the point of interaction. Thus, intravenous and intraarterial lines may need to be cut flush with the skin and pushed slightly inwards to allow the autopsy incision to then consider whether the lines have been placed correctly.

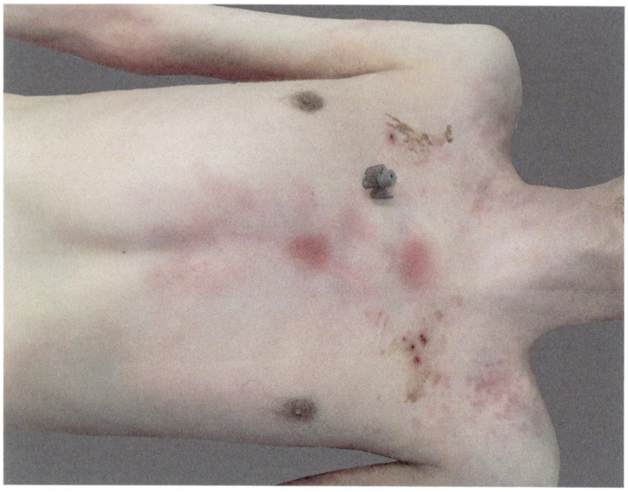

Fig. 11.11 This image of a young male's chest shows a grey, large bore cannula inserted in the right side anterior chest wall to attempt decompression of a suspected tension pneumothorax. Multiple needle puncture wounds on the left side and another puncture wound on the right represent other attempts at this procedure

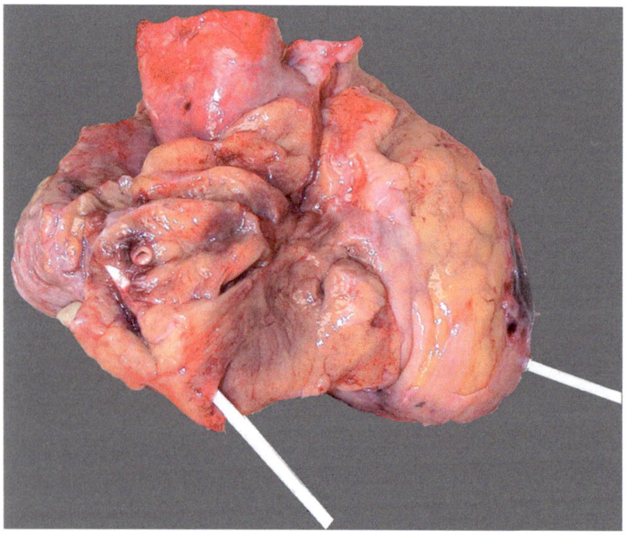

Fig. 11.12 This heart demonstrates two attempts to drain a pericardial fluid collection. Both lines penetrated the cardiac tissues and caused death. The role of photography is clearly evident as it demonstrates the cause of death and can be used as evidence in court, if needed

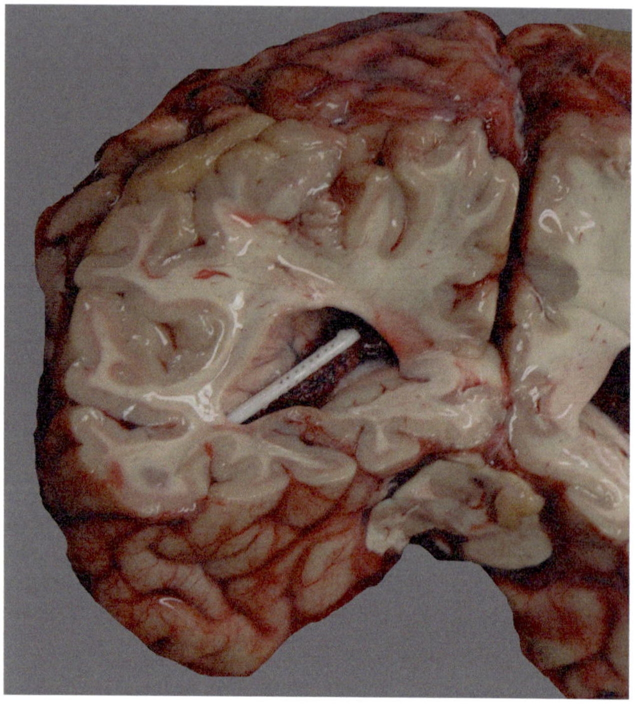

Fig. 11.13 The tip of a cerebrospinal fluid (CSF) drainage tube, inserted because of hydrocephalus, is present in the lateral ventricle. This tube ran into the scalp soft tissues, and then downwards alongside the body to end in the peritoneal cavity

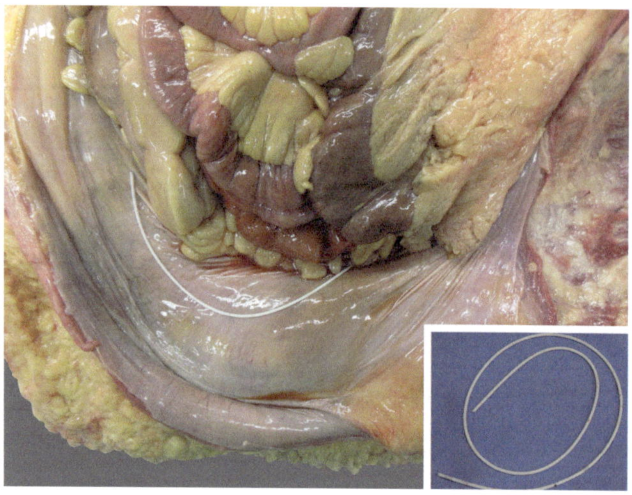

Fig. 11.14 The CSF drain tube is seen entering the abdomen. The drain fluid is discharged into the peritoneal cavity. The *inset* shows the coiled tube after extraction, with a total length of 85 cm in this case

Some knowledge of the types of lines is required, if one is to understand the pathophysiology of the patient prior to death. In this regard, one should be familiar with long lines that monitor central pressures, and those which provide portals for multiple drug access (e.g., Swan-Ganz catheter etc.). Haemodialysis and intraarterial lines should be identified and understood in terms of their basic function. Haemodialysis lines, for instance, remove blood for filtration/dialysis and then return it to the circulation.

Drainage lines and tubes are generally placed into cavities and are often connected to bags and other drainage devices. The amount and type of fluid in the drain collection point should be considered because significant fluid collections, particularly those with blood, may be relevant to the cause of death. It is important not to just pull such tubes out at the

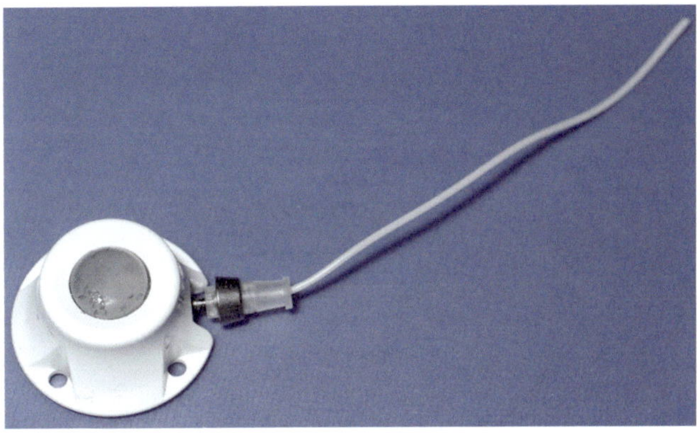

Fig. 11.15 Some drugs are introduced into the intrathecal space by means of a drug-eluting reservoir sitting immediately below the skin, with the drug delivery point running from the unit towards the site desired. The injection-site hub unit and part of the tube are seen

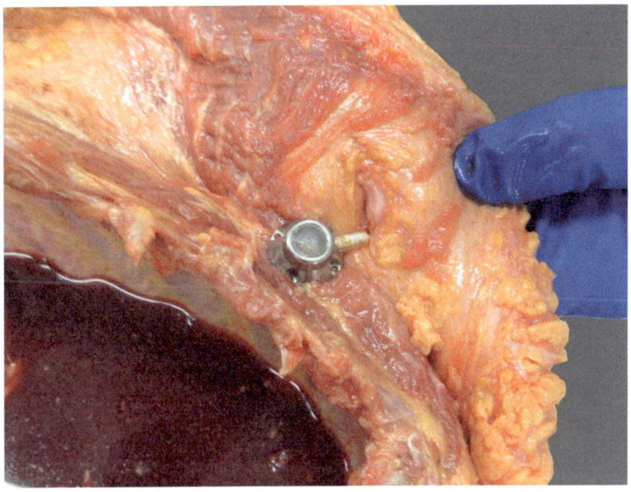

Fig. 11.16 This is an implanted drug delivery port, also called a porta-cath, used for long term drug delivery. It is seen in the soft tissues of the chest

start of the autopsy. Any tubes and lines that penetrate into cavities below the skin surface, such as chest or surgical drains, also need to be checked in terms of their pathway.

Surgical operation closure is often an easily identified external feature, particularly if the surgery was performed shortly before death (Figs. 11.17, 11.18, 11.19, and 11.20). Many surgical incisions are closed in layers with different types of suture. These can be prone to infection. External skin closure, the final layer, is usually made via surgical suture, or on occasion, metal staple. These external closures are often removed after the skin has begun to heal, with deeper tissue

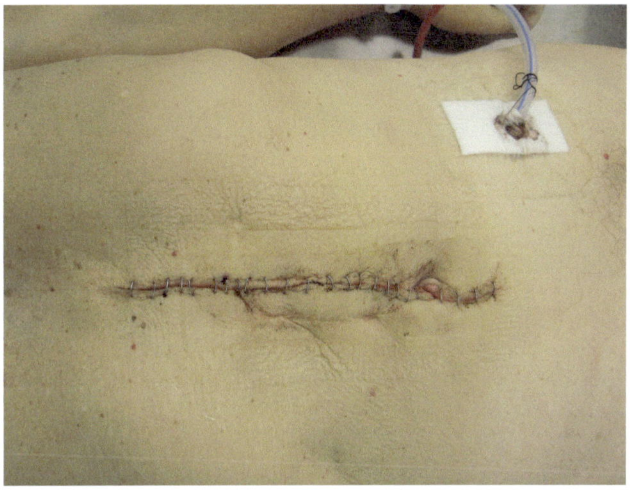

Fig. 11.17 A stapled surgery closure is seen with a local peritoneal drain tube. Knowledge of the surgical procedure is advised before starting the examination in order to secure the best analysis of the case

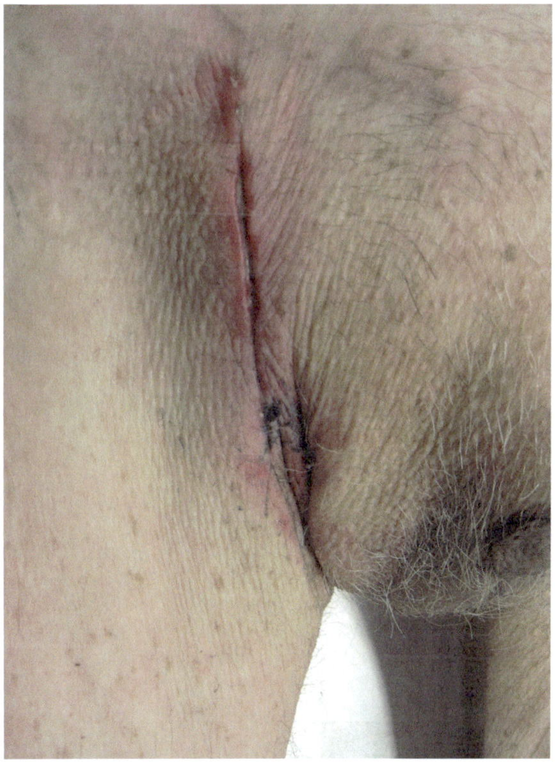

Fig. 11.18 Grafted tissues may become infected via sepsis extending from or towards the skin surface. Close inspection of any surgery site is recommended with swabs/tissue sampling if infection is suspected. The erythema here represented local infection of this wound following surgery

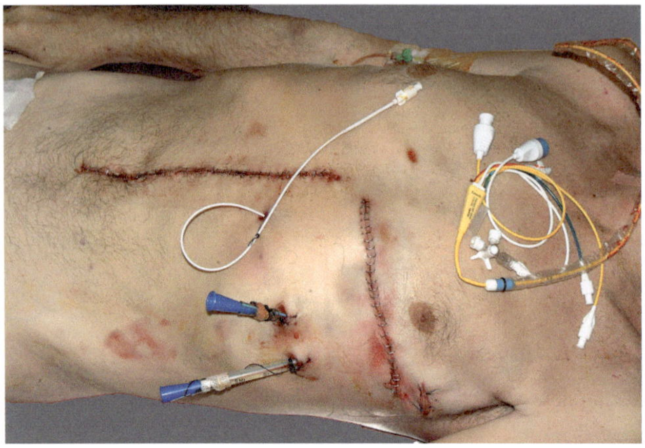

Fig. 11.19 Investigating the death of an individual with complicated medical problems and recent surgery often is seen externally as "a complicated area". Two drainage tubes are present immediately below the left costal boundary, which were positioned within the left pleural space. A pericardial drain site is present, entering under the xiphisternum. A multiple channel pulmonary artery catheter was present on the right side of the neck, the end of which has been curled round onto the front of the chest. Freshly sutured and stapled wounds are present in the midline of the abdomen and the left lateral chest, and a freshly sutured chest drain point is seen in the lateral midline of the left chest

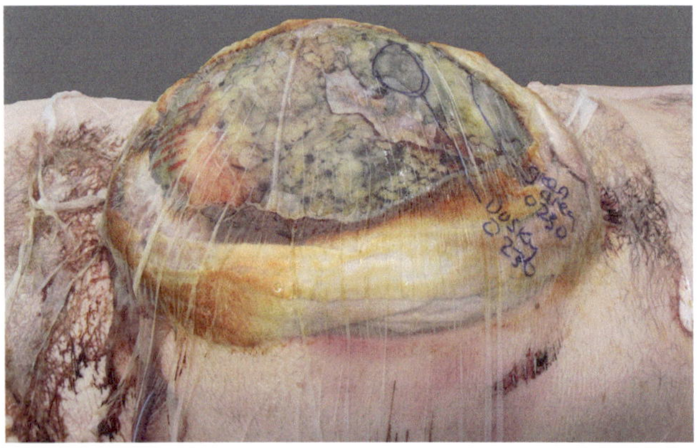

Fig. 11.20 This abdomen has been left open because the abdominal content is grossly distended and any attempt to close would cause tissue necrosis (akin to compartment syndrome). Several gauze packs are also present within the abdomen. Critically compromised tissues may recover with this approach, with later abdominal closure. Note the plastic dressing and comments written onto the surface. This may assist monitoring of sepsis or peri-ischaemic phenomena

sutures being left in situ. On occasion, closure is not possible and the wound is left open, either to allow the pathology to subside or to permit secondary closure by scarring. In this regard, the absence of a device for closure is potentially a pathology in its own right or indicator of other issues.

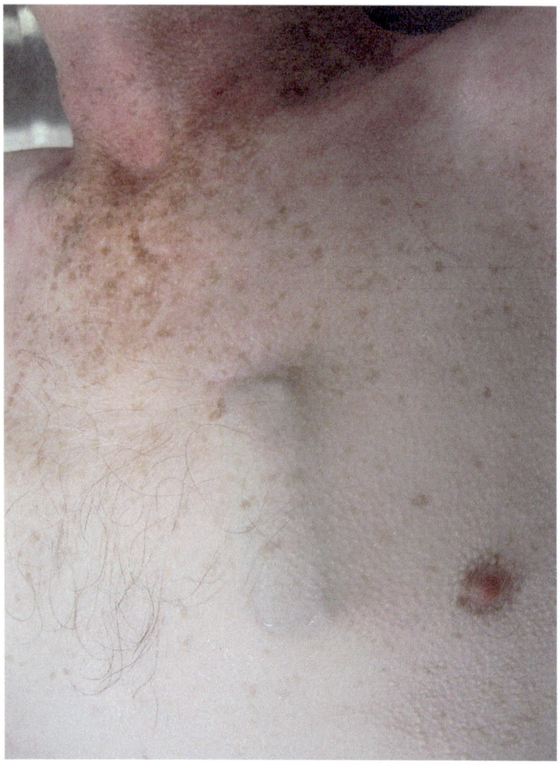

Fig. 11.21 A Reveal® electronic sensor unit (Medtronic) is seen below the skin surface. This is an internal cardiac monitor that can have data remotely downloaded about the cardiac cycle

Electronic Devices

A variety of electronic devices are available (Figs. 11.21, 11.22, 11.23, 11.24, 11.25, 11.26, 11.27, 11.28, 11.29, 11.30, 11.31, 11.32, and 11.33). Pacemakers are covered principally in Chap. 4, but some examples are given in this chapter, including devices used for monitoring of cardiac rhythms. Dissection of the entire unit should be considered before the autopsy starts if there is a suspicion of pacemaker malfunction.

Other pacemaker-like devices are occasionally found within the body. These include stimulator devices for the treatment of Parkinson's disease and vagal stimulators in cases of persistent epilepsy.

There are also devices with muscle stimulatory function, such as those assisting diaphragm function. These are usually activated by external electrical generators. Aural cranial nerve stimulators and other similar items act on nerve tissues around the spine. Often, review of the clinical record and interaction with the relatives or caregivers will assist in the identification and understanding of these devices.

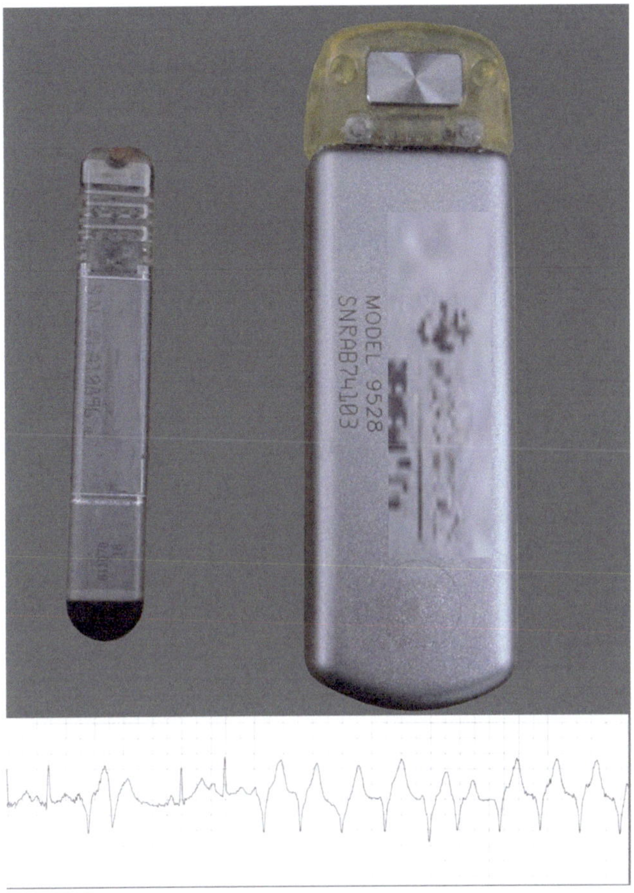

Fig. 11.22 The Reveal® ECG monitoring device, once removed, comprises a single, sealed box capable of assessing cardiac rhythm and later having that data downloaded. Two examples are shown here. In the ECG recording, a device has captured a ventricular tachycardia arrest

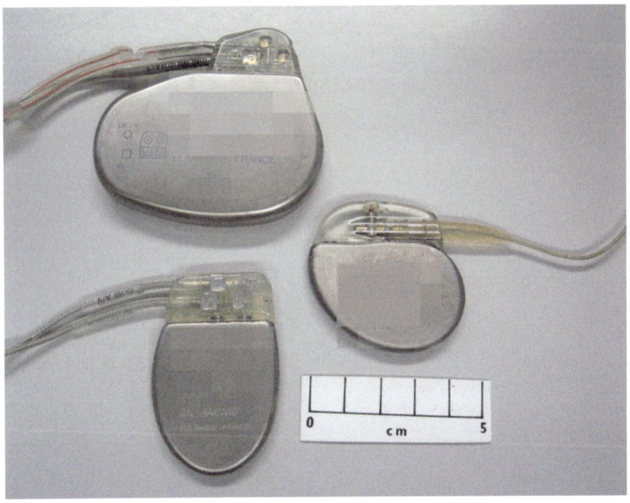

Fig. 11.23 A range of cardiac pacemakers is seen. The modern variety have a smooth external case, with manufacturer's data and serial numbers. Leads emerge from one point on the device and pass onwards to the heart. At autopsy, most cases have the generator unit (box) cut free from the wires to allow easy extraction. In cases where the device may have not worked adequately, the entire unit with wires and electrodes needs to be retrieved intact and sent for specialized analysis

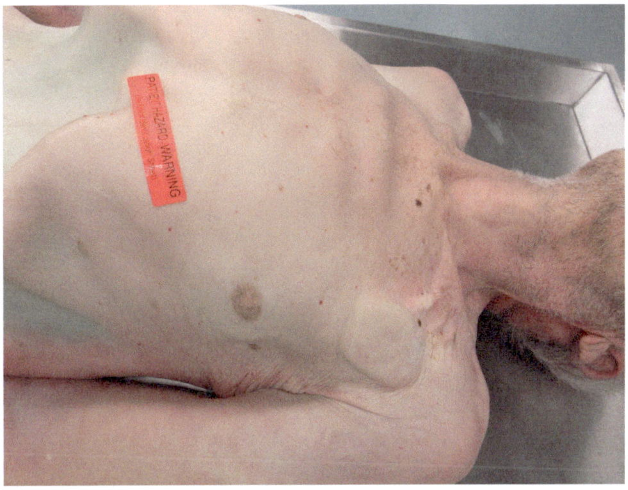

Fig. 11.24 The left upper chest soft tissues show a typical plateaued prominence due to an implanted pacemaker device. In this case, it was an implantable cardioverter defibrillator. These devices can deliver electrical shocks, warranting the warning label due to the small risk posed to staff in the mortuary. The device should be inactivated prior to attempting its removal

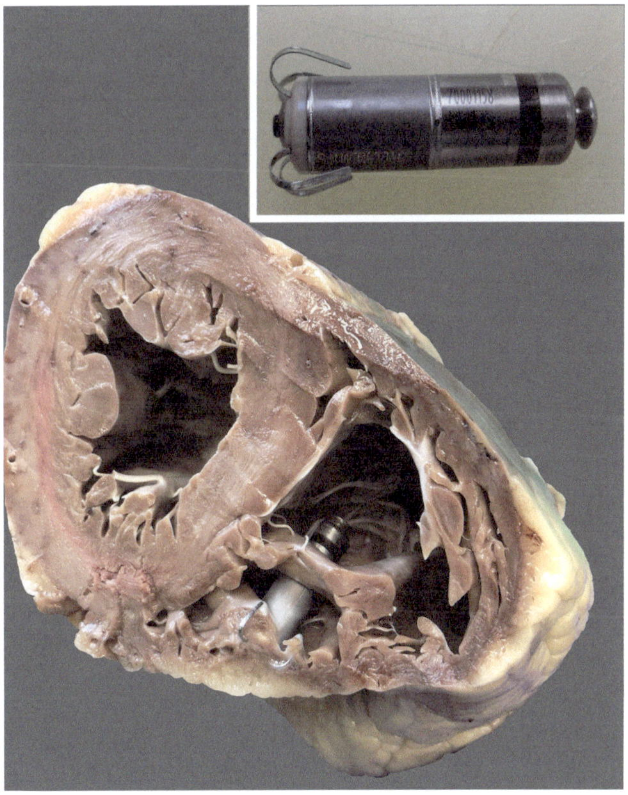

Fig. 11.25 A lesser seen pacemaker is the intracardiac permanent pacemaker, shown here in situ and once extracted (*inset*). It is a self-contained device and there is no separate subcutaneous pocket to house the generator. It usually resides in the right ventricle, where it is introduced by catheter and secured in place

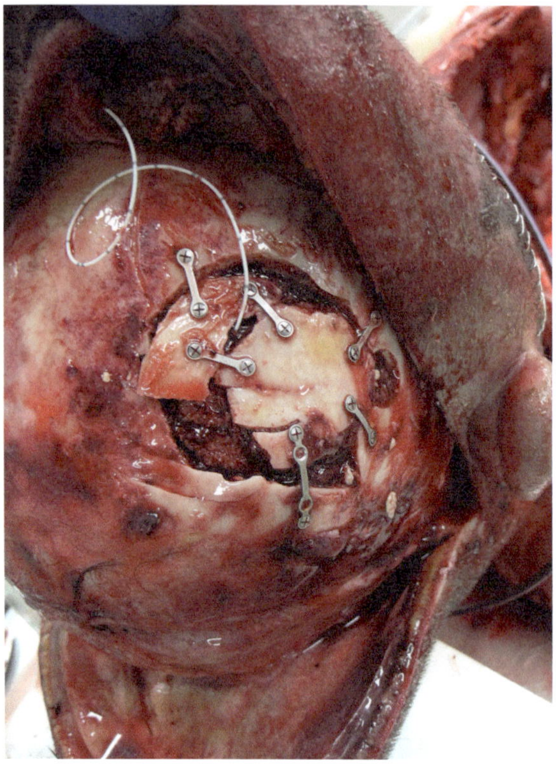

Fig. 11.26 A complex and depressed skull fracture has been closed with original skull bone, anchored by metal struts. A central nervous system pressure transducer is entering the intracranial tissues through part of the defect left after surgery

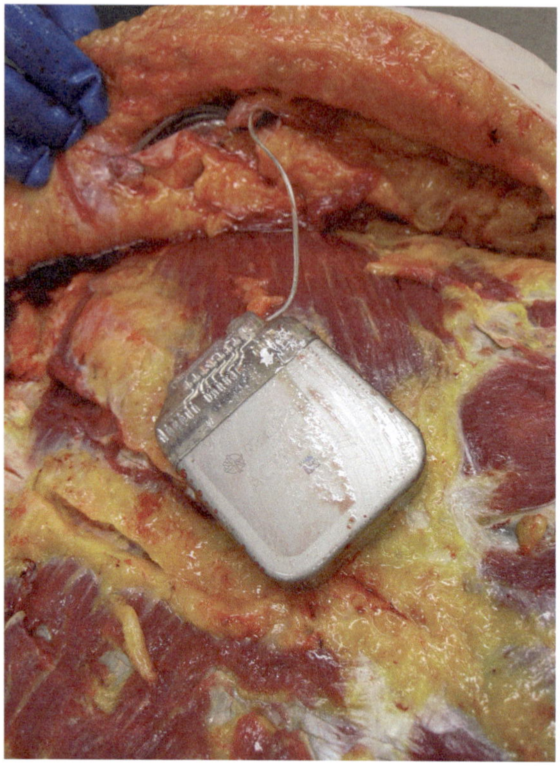

Fig. 11.28 The stimulator unit for Parkinson's disease was situated in a subcutaneous pocket, akin to a pacemaker. However, the electrical lead ran towards the brain tissue rather than into the mediastinal/vascular compartment. This was the same patient as Fig. 11.27

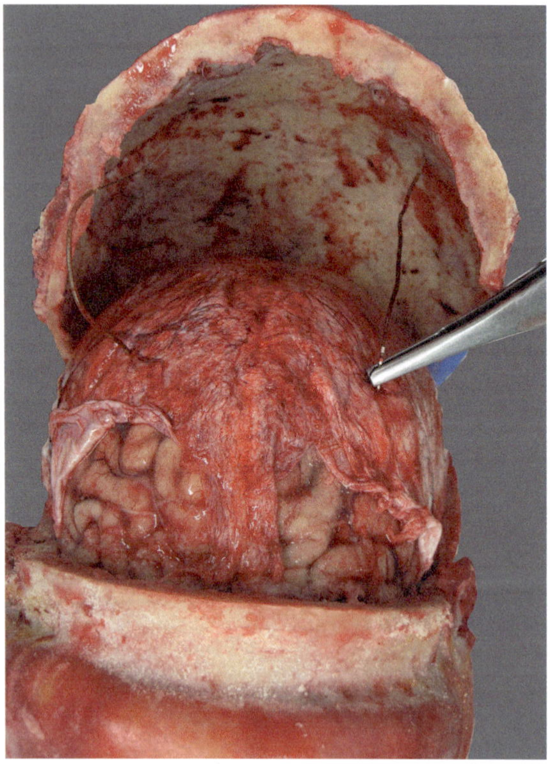

Fig. 11.27 Two thin wires are present running through the skull and into the brain tissues. This patient had significant Parkinson's disease and had direct electrical stimulation of relevant nerve nuclei and pathways to control symptoms

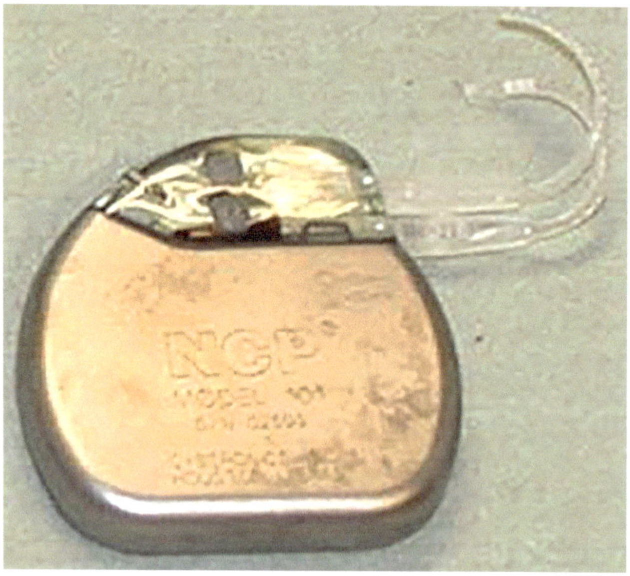

Fig. 11.29 A vagal nerve stimulator can be used in cases of epilepsy. This device, with the wires progressing towards the base of the skull, should not be confused with a cardiac pacemaker

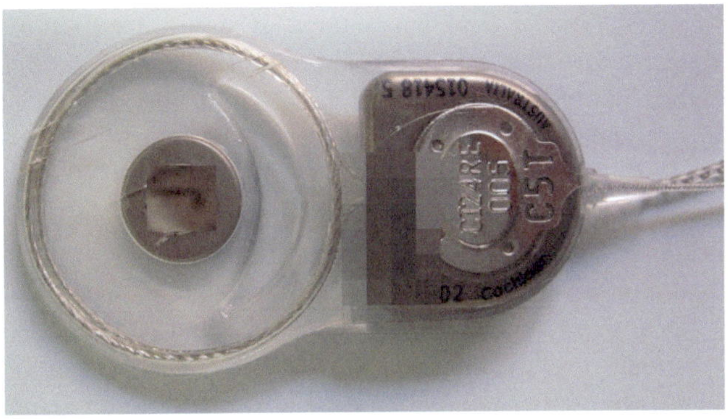

Fig. 11.30 An aural nerve stimulator is present in the soft tissues around the neck. This is an unusual device to find within the body. It often requires review of the clinical notes or information from medical practitioners to confirm its nature

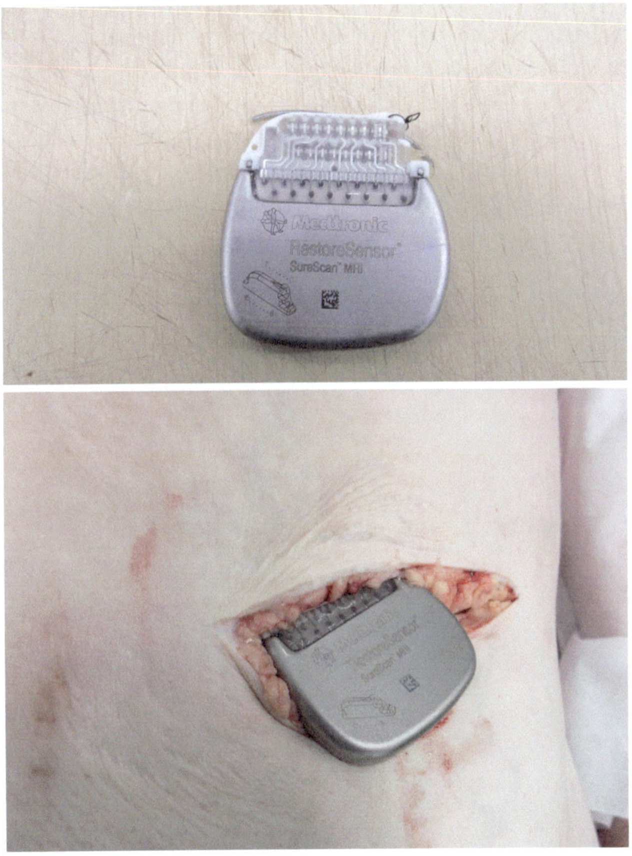

Fig. 11.31 A device which may be mistaken for a pacemaker is shown here, typically implanted in the chest, abdomen or buttocks. This is a spinal cord neurostimulation device and the electrodes would have been placed in the epidural space. It may be used in cases of chronic pain

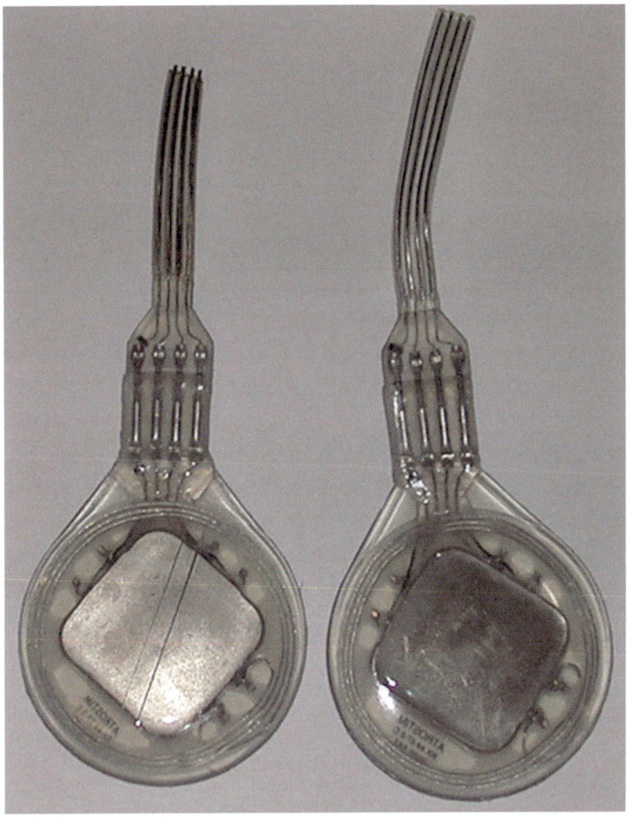

Fig. 11.32 These electrical transducers with wires running to the low chest served to stimulate the diaphragms. An external electrical stimulator device produced electrical activity in these receivers

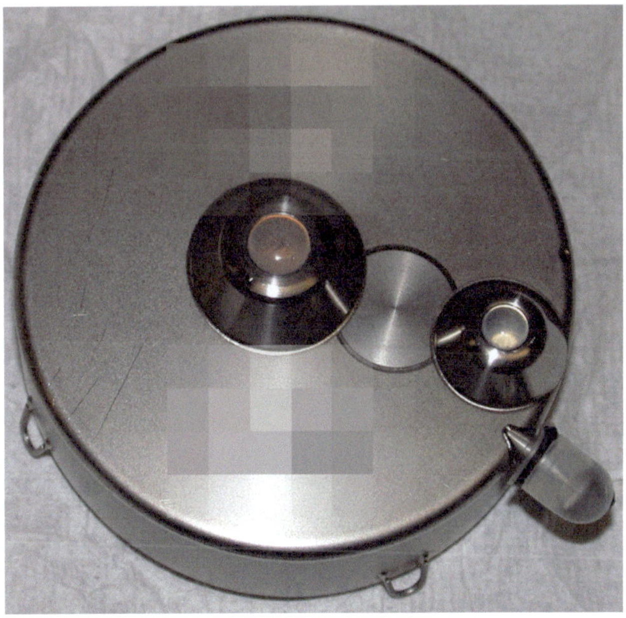

Fig. 11.33 A baclofen pump/drug-delivery device is seen with a drug installation portal towards the front and a central metallic body. This device is occasionally seen in spinal injury patients who have significant pelvic floor muscle/sphincter problems

Structural Cardiovascular Devices

Intracardiac devices are complex and multiple (Figs. 11.34, 11.35, 11.36, 11.37, 11.38, 11.39, 11.40, 11.41, 11.42, 11.43, 11.44, 11.45, 11.46, 11.47, 11.48, 11.49, 11.50, and 11.51). Cardiac valves, as discussed and illustrated in Chap. 4, with some examples provided here, are now frequently encountered in the autopsy room. Less commonly, one may find devices related to septal defects. These congenital and acquired holes through septal tissues can be closed by means of devices delivered by intravascular access. Such devices placed across the septal defect will permit thrombosis around the metal device, closure of the defect and ultimately reendothelialisation. These devices have a potential risk of infective endocarditis, although this is rare.

In the immediate postoperative setting, coronary bypass surgery and valve placement need to be considered from the point of view of clips and sutures. If significant haemorrhage occurs at the time of surgery, then pledget sutures (fabric-buttressed sutures) can be placed to assist surgical closure and procoagulant matrix (e.g., Surgicel®) can be employed.

Vascular stents are increasingly common, both within the coronary system and in the arterial and venous circuits. Issues to consider at autopsy are the presence and degree of internal thrombosis, any issues with regard to infection and the effectiveness of the device. Many such devices are placed internally by means of an endovascular approach, although open surgery is occasionally employed. Sepsis is an important issue with stents, and any infection at the skin surface can potentially spread to the internal vascular device, with significant consequences.

Some intravascular devices (inferior vena cava filters) are designed to capture embolic fragments of clot. If these are present, then commentary with regard to the amount of clot and effectiveness of the device should be made.

Another vascular device, often used in the intensive care setting, is the intra-aortic balloon pump. If present, its position should be confirmed, although it will invariably be deflated at the time of autopsy examination.

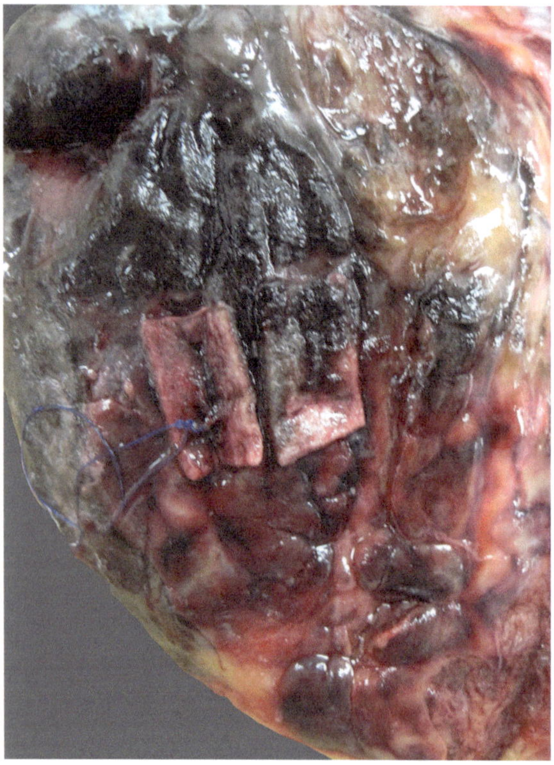

Fig. 11.34 Pledgets (cloth-buttressed sutures) are used to try and seal bleeding points on friable cardiac tissues

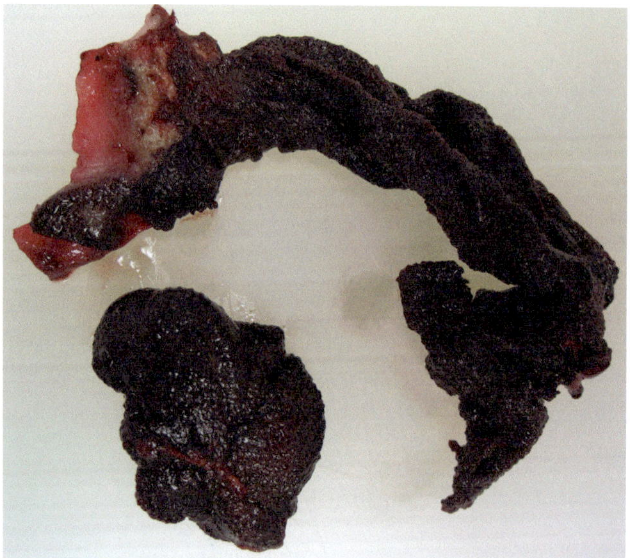

Fig. 11.35 Surgicel® matrix is occasionally used in cardiac surgery cases to enhance coagulation around the heart. It is invariably heavily blood stained and has a rather granular quality

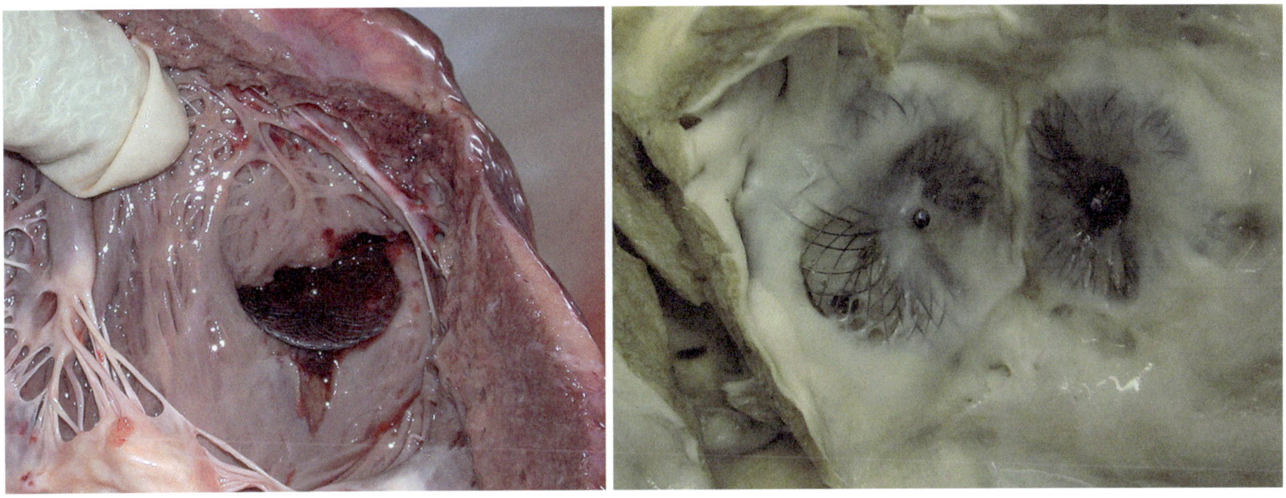

Fig. 11.36 The left shows a septal closure device which was deployed into an area of infarction-related ventricular septal defect. The device could not be deployed adequately and the individual died. The metal device is seen in an atypical position, preventing deployment. The right side image shows two septal closure devices that have served their purpose in closing the defects. With time, local fibrosis and re-endothelialisation occur; no sepsis is seen

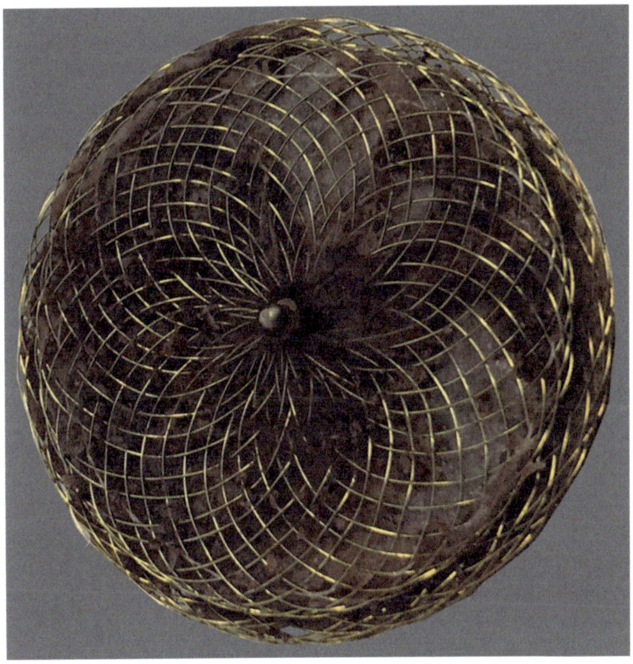

Fig. 11.37 Shown here is a similar septal occluder device, used to plug the hole in an atrial septal defect, having been removed from the tissues. This type of device is introduced by a minimally invasive approach via percutaneous catheter

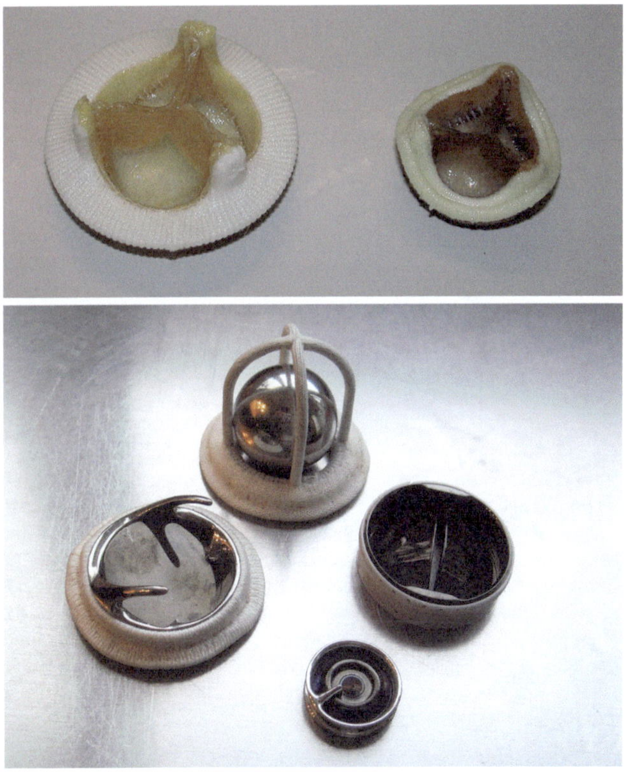

Fig. 11.38 Prosthetic cardiac valves are broadly of two main types: tissue and metal disc varieties. The types currently favoured are natural (tissue) trileaflet valves and twin metal leaflet devices

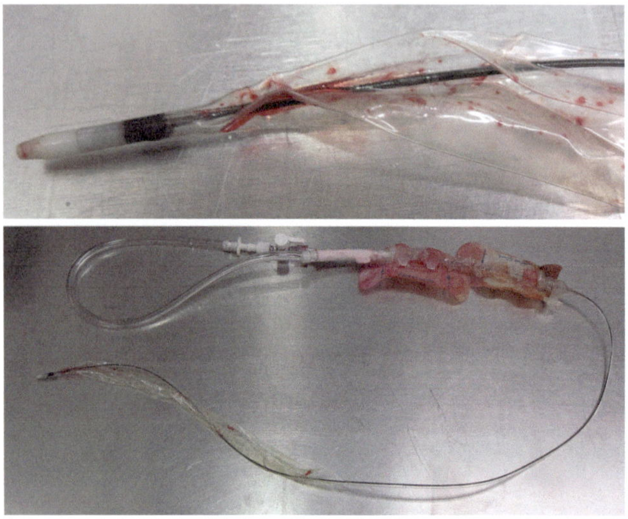

Fig. 11.39 An aortic balloon pump is can be used to help maintain systemic blood pressure to vital structures in cases of acute cardiac failure. It normally lies within the aorta and will invariably be in the collapsed state at autopsy

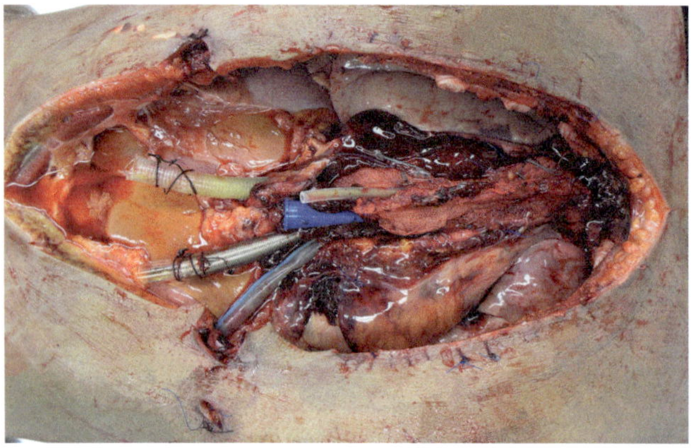

Fig. 11.40 This image shows the complicated appearance of a torso following attempted extracorporeal membrane oxygenation (ECMO) which was abandoned due to complications. Photographic imaging in such cases is strongly recommended to document the findings of the staged dissection. ECMO is a technique used when the circulation needs to be redirected from the heart and lungs, generally as a temporary measure to rest these vital organs. Precise knowledge of the attempted procedure is necessary to interpret the post mortem findings correctly because there are multiple types of ECMO involving different vessels. The cut, sutured ends of the tubes can be seen caudally, kept in situ for the internal examination

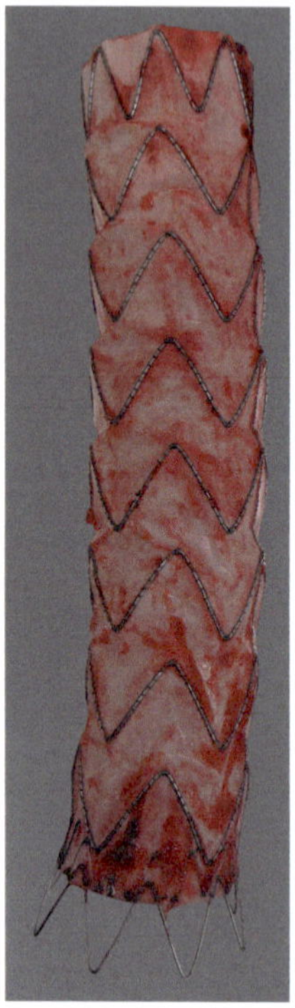

Fig. 11.41 Treatment for aneurysms can sometimes be done with minimally invasive endovascular aneurysm repair (EVAR). This image shows one type of single-lumened repair device which may be found in such cases

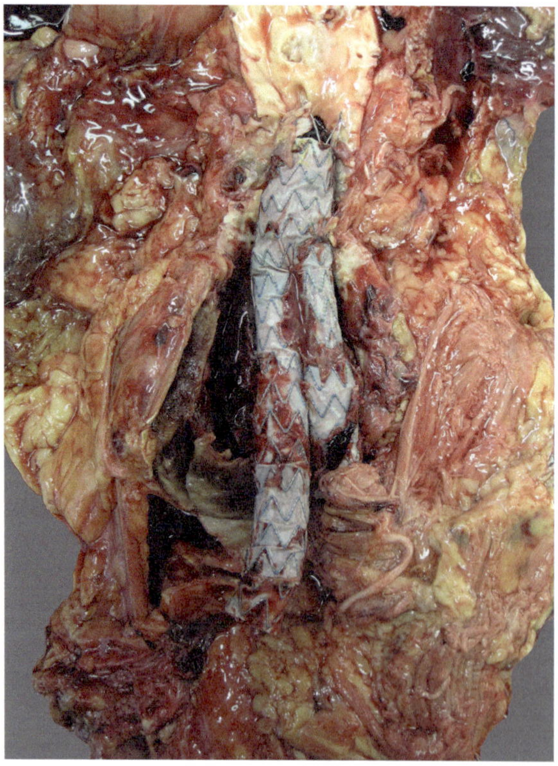

Fig. 11.42 The endoluminal trouser graft was used with good effect in an area of aneurysm and atheromatous disease of the lower aorta. The local aneurysmal changes and thrombus are seen compartmentalized, away from the lumen of the low aortic graft

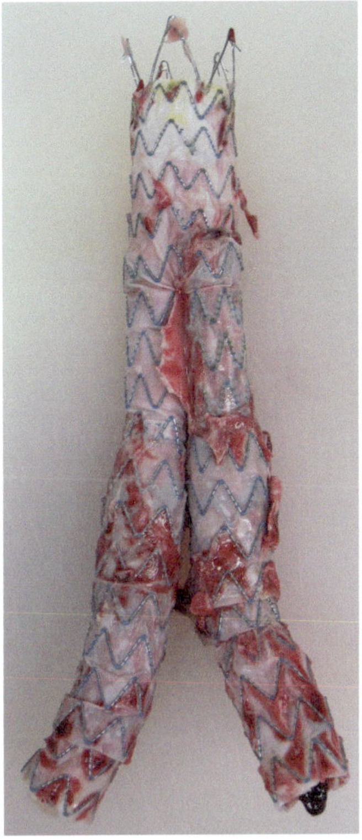

Fig. 11.43 The same graft repair from Fig. 11.42 is seen, having been freed from the local tissues to allow confirmation of lumen patency and absence of sepsis

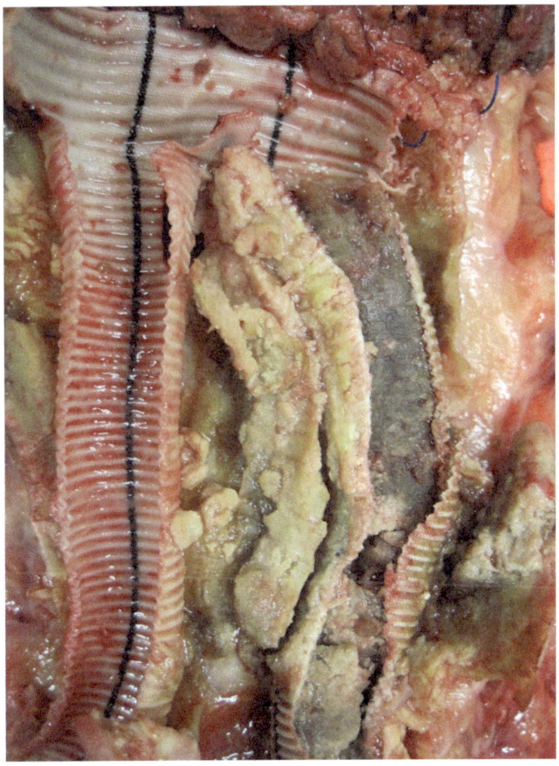

Fig. 11.44 An open operative trouser graft repair, using Dacron®, has been successful on one side of the tissues, but the luminal aspect of the other limb shows abundant grey thrombotic material, indicating complete occlusion of the graft

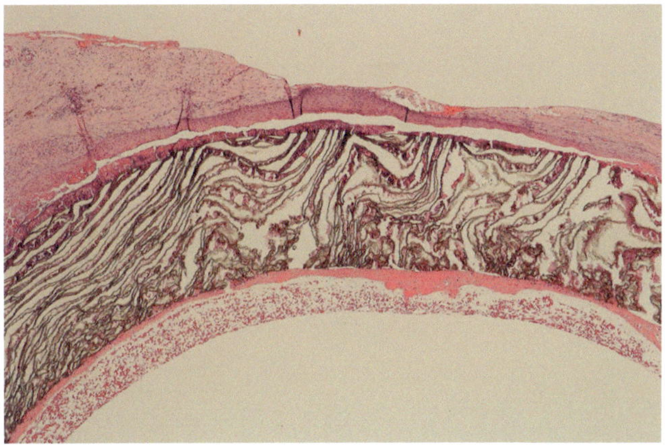

Fig. 11.45 Another material used for vascular conduits is polytetrafluoroethylene (PTFE) which appears as a featureless white-grey plastic. Histologically it has a characteristic quality. It can cause local fibrosis, calcification, and occasionally local squamous epithelial metaplasia. It can be used to assist the creation of an arteriovenous fistula for haemodialysis

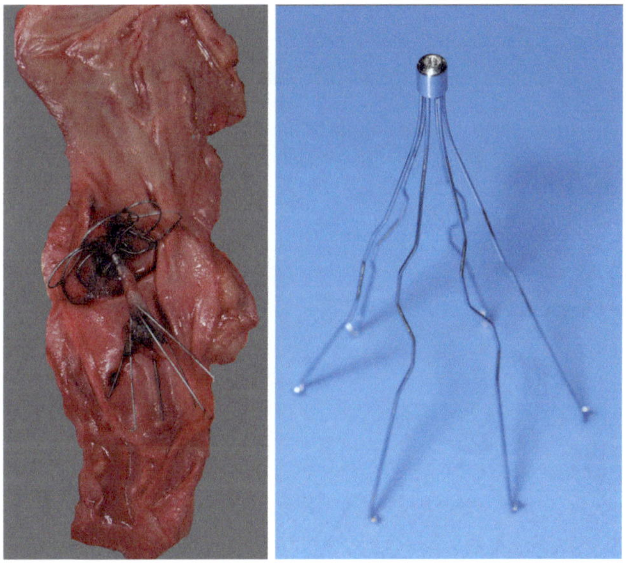

Fig. 11.46 The venous system is occasionally used as a site for placement of endovascular cages to prevent venous embolization from leg to lung. The inferior vena cava (IVC) is a common site for a cage filter, which is aimed at preventing such thromboembolic events, particularly in patients with issues of anticoagulation control. Here, the device is seen with a small amount of thrombus captured. An explanted filter is seen on the right side

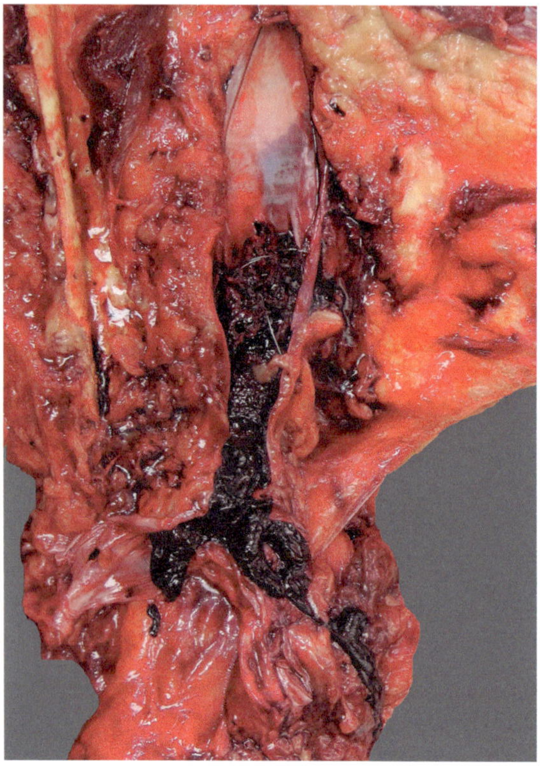

Fig. 11.47 This case demonstrates the value of the IVC filter, having captured many embolic fragments of thrombus

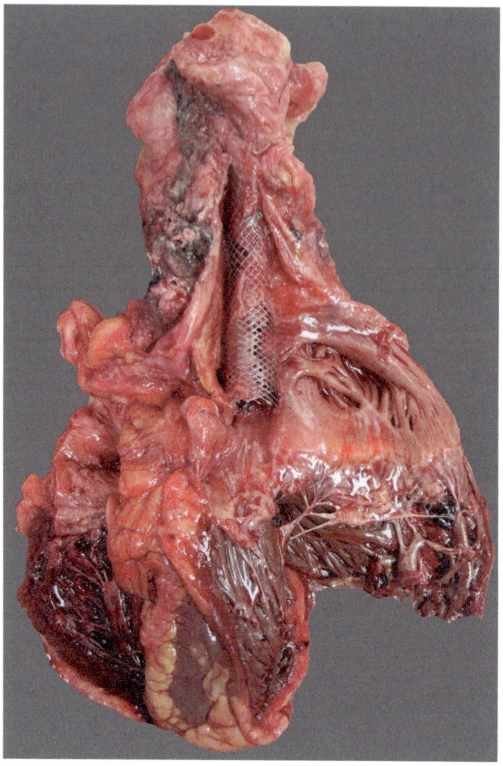

Fig. 11.49 Another case of SVC stenting is seen, with the metallic cage protecting the lumen of the SVC as it runs towards the right atrium

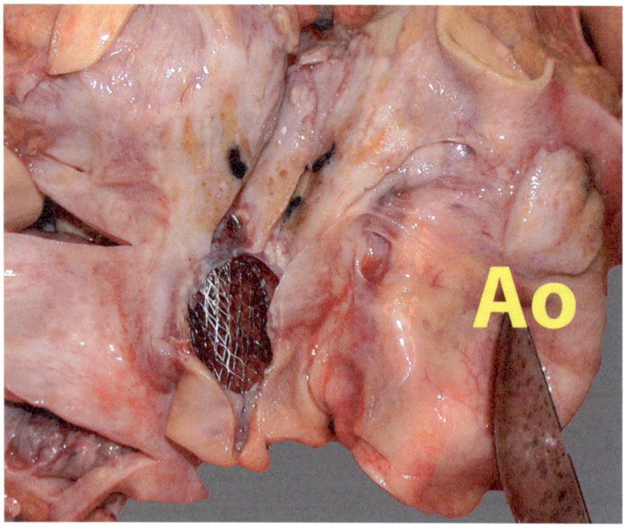

Fig. 11.48 A superior vena cava (SVC) stent is often used to hold open the SVC when there is significant compressive tumour locally. This view shows the dense sclerotic thoracic tumour around the SVC, adjacent to the aorta (*Ao*)

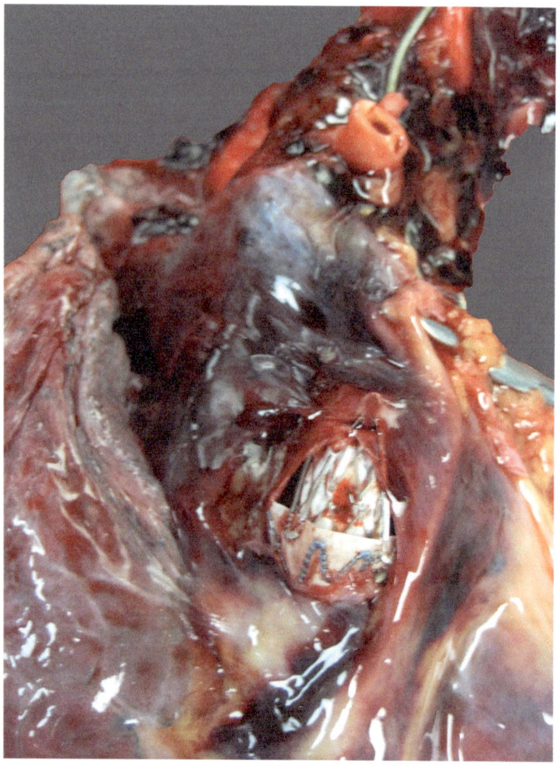

Fig. 11.50 Longstanding pacemaker leads can become adherent to the SVC. An attempt to remove these leads may very rarely result in SVC tearing, causing massive right-side haemothorax. An emergency endovascular approach, attempting to seal the hole, was undertaken, without success. The endovascular device is seen directly at the site of the large tear/defect

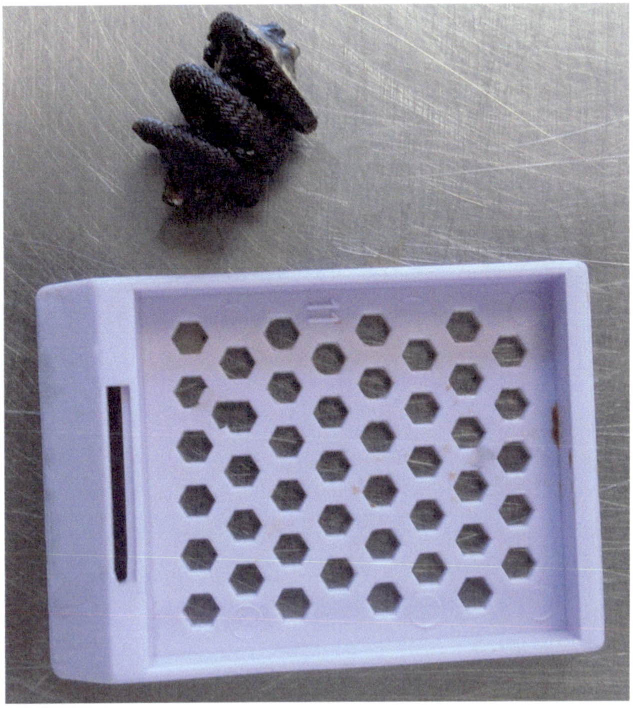

Fig. 11.51 This is an endovascular prothrombotic plug device used in peripheral vessels requiring embolization. Indications prompting use of this device may include aneurysms, arteriovenous malformations and following vascular trauma

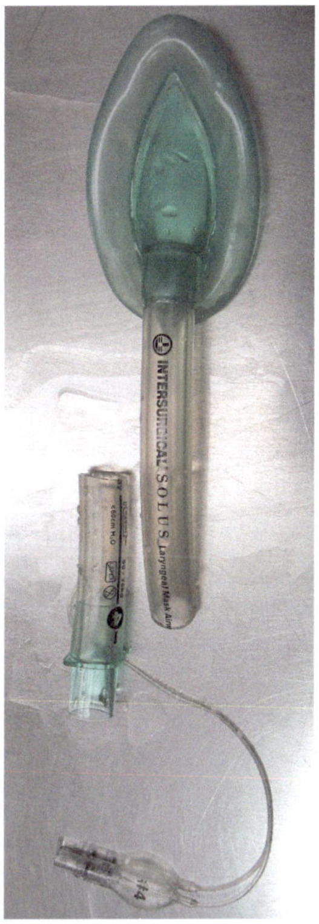

Fig. 11.52 A laryngeal mask airway has been used in this individual rather than an endotracheal tube. To facilitate its extraction and analysis in situ, the outer end of the tube has been cut, allowing the airway end to be left in situ for inspection at the time when the neck tissues are mobilized

Respiratory System

In the respiratory system, endotracheal tubes are regularly seen. It is important to verify that the tube has been positioned in the larynx and trachea, rather than misplaced into the oesophagus (see Fig. 4.160). On occasion, laryngeal masks may be found as an alternative and simpler method of ventilating the unconscious patient. Unusual devices that may be found, particularly in the context of previously treated laryngeal cancer, include valves within the oesophagus or trachea to assist phonation. Figures 11.52 and 11.53 illustrate some of these devices.

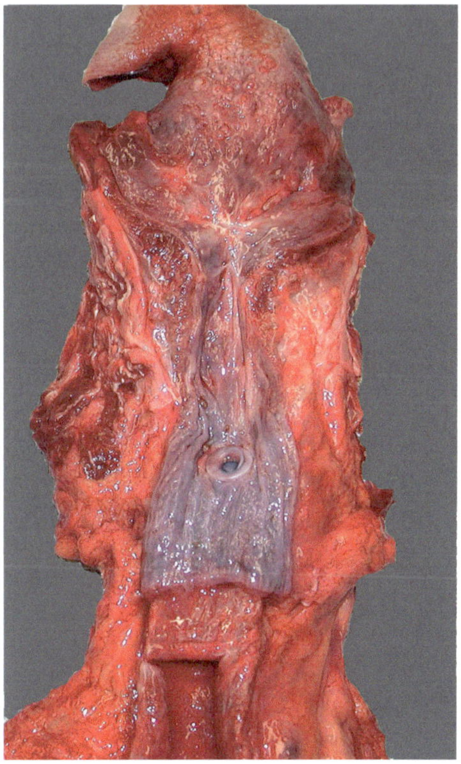

Fig. 11.53 A valve is present at the upper end of the oesophagus, linked to the trachea, to allow some phonation in those who have had laryngeal cancer treatments or surgery

Gastrointestinal Devices

Gastrointestinal devices are principally of two main types; stents and feeding tubes (Figs. 11.54, 11.55, 11.56, 11.57, and 11.58). Stents are applied across inflammatory or neoplastic strictures. The most common sites include the oesophagus and colon, although the biliary system and other parts of the bowel may be treated similarly. Feeding tubes usually interact with upper gastrointestinal tissues (e.g., percutaneous endoscopic gastrostomy (PEG) tube). On occasion, some unusual devices may be encountered, such as an external flatus tube.

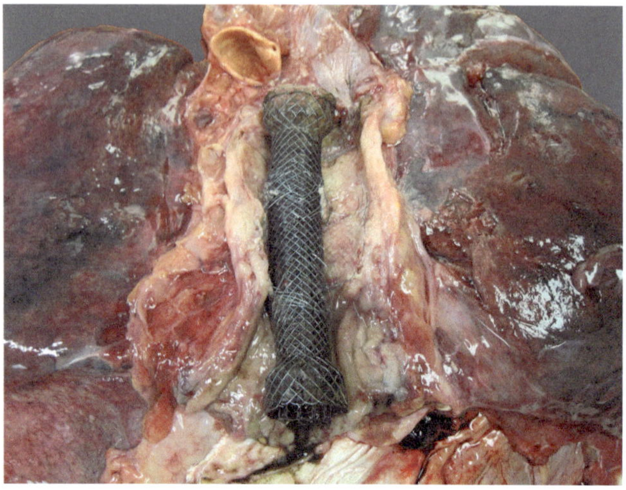

Fig. 11.54 The oesophagus is commonly stented in cases of malignant narrowing or inflammatory strictures. Several interlocking metal stent devices have been inserted to allow oesophageal lumen patency. Whilst tumour can grow into the lumen itself, it is often not a significant problem as further endoscopic treatments can be used and it is also degraded by food materials passed along the oesophageal lumen. Such stents can cause oesophageal rupture (and thereby mediastinitis) at the time of placement. It is important to look for infections and involvement of local structures when considering large stents

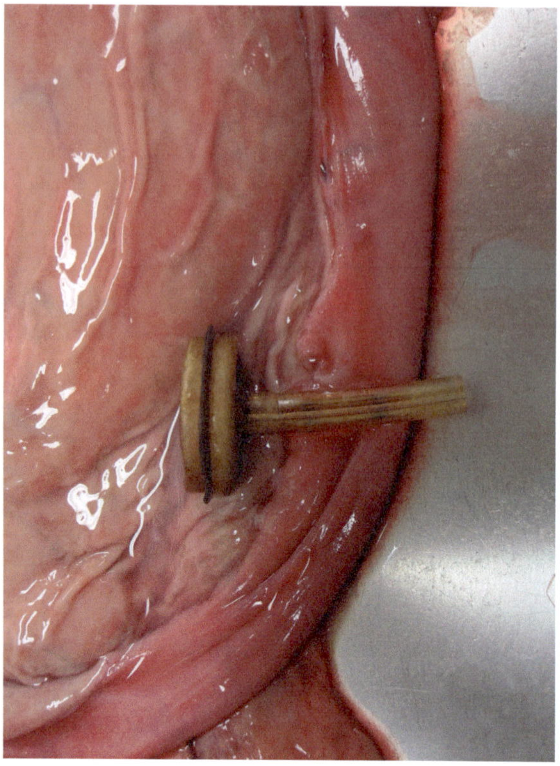

Fig. 11.55 Percutaneous endoscopic gastrostomy (PEG) tube feeding is a common procedure in patients unable to take fluids and foods by oral means. Whether placed using endoscopic support or directly through the abdominal wall, the feeding tube is passed directly into the stomach. A similar process can be used for the proximal small bowel. The cushioned, soft, disclike end prevents the unit from being pulled backwards out of the bowel site and allows direct instillation of fluids, foods and drugs at an appropriate rate into the bowel tissues. An autopsy with a PEG tube in situ requires consideration of the tube's entry point to the abdominal tissues as well as the point where the tube interacts with the bowel

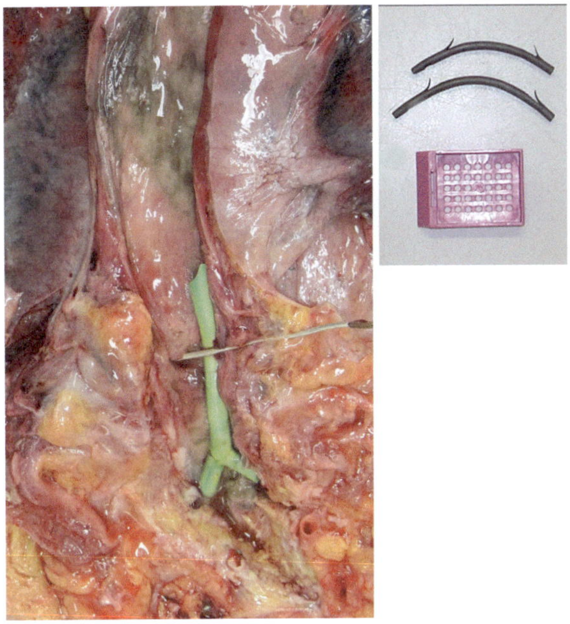

Fig. 11.56 Plastic-type tubes are often employed in allowing materials to flow along bowel or related structures. On the left, a green T tube allows oesophageal content to flow towards the anastomosed small bowel (following oesophagogastrectomy). Suture line dehiscence is noted, with a probe being passed through the defect. On the right, two plastic stents from a case of biliary obstruction due to cholangiocarcinoma are seen. Note the flanges to prevent stent slippage. These stents are normally placed by endoscopic routes

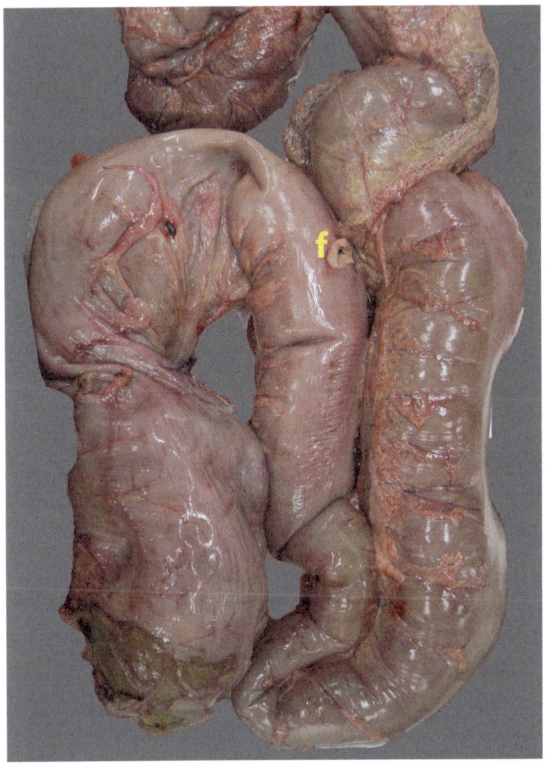

Fig. 11.57 Although stomas can be placed directly into the upper bowel tissues for feeding purposes, one occasionally can find a flatus stoma (*f*) sited in the colon to prevent excessive gas production and thereby a risk of colon volvulus. A PEG-like flatus decompression tube was present in this loaded colon

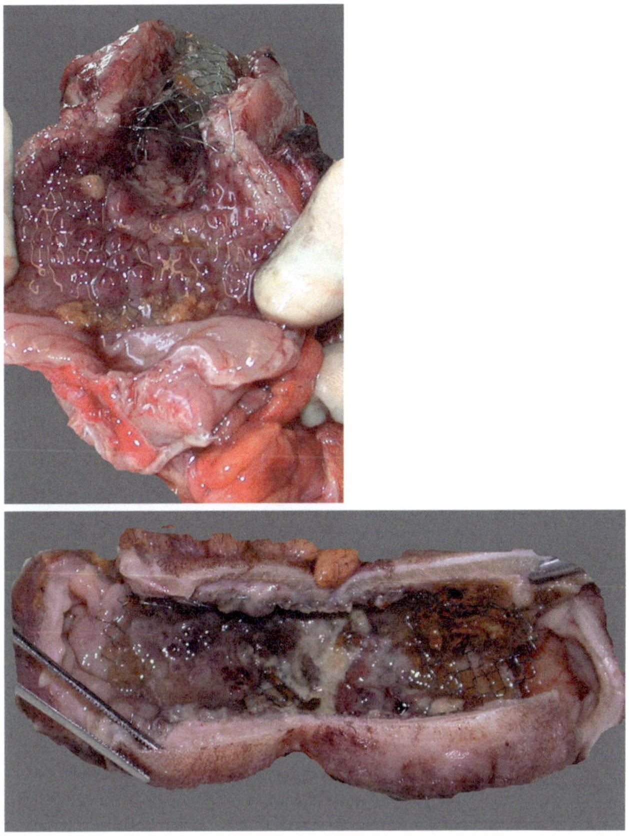

Fig. 11.58 Strictures at the site of inoperable rectal cancers often may be treated by means of stents. These metal cages will hold open the lumen of the bowel tissues and prevent intestinal obstruction. They do not treat the tumour itself. These devices are for palliation only. The stent may suffer failure because of tumour ingrowth into the lumen, and necrotic or infected material around the tumour may involve the metal stent frame itself and thereby local tissues. Two views of such devices are seen with the stents in situ

The Genitourinary System

The urinary catheter is a common finding at autopsy. Some degree of bladder reddening is a consequence of inflating the tip of the urinary catheter, causing bladder surface irritation. Exclusion of sepsis around the catheter is important, but it is difficult to confirm because the urothelium is often shed early, mimicking urinary septic change (see Chap. 6). However, if frank pus is seen, then a swab of the material may be pertinent. Other urinary devices found at autopsy include urostomies to the skin, pigtail catheters running between the kidney and bladder, and occasionally intraprostate metal devices (Figs. 11.59, 11.60, and 11.61).

Devices may also be encountered in the genital tract (Figs. 11.62, 11.63, 11.64, 11.65, 11.66, and 11.67). Many are commonly used in the female genital tract, including ring pessaries or other pessaries, intrauterine contraceptive devices and uterine (Fallopian) tube clips. In the male, penile implants are rarely encountered.

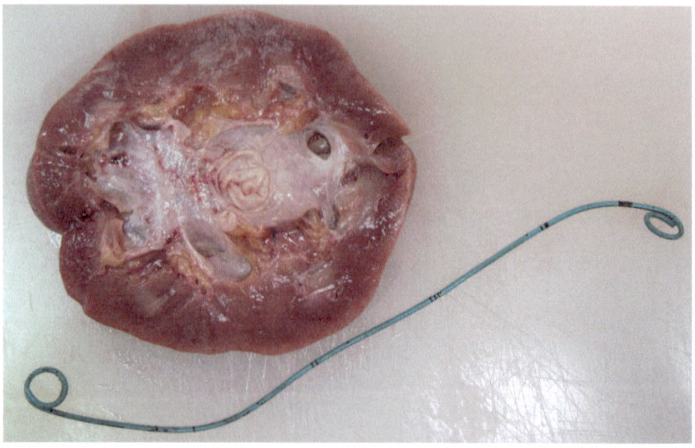

Fig. 11.59 A pigtail catheter is used to drain urine from an obstructed kidney. One end of the pigtail will be present in the renal pelvis, with the other end in the bladder. *Pigtail* refers to the coiled nature of the distal end of the drainage tube

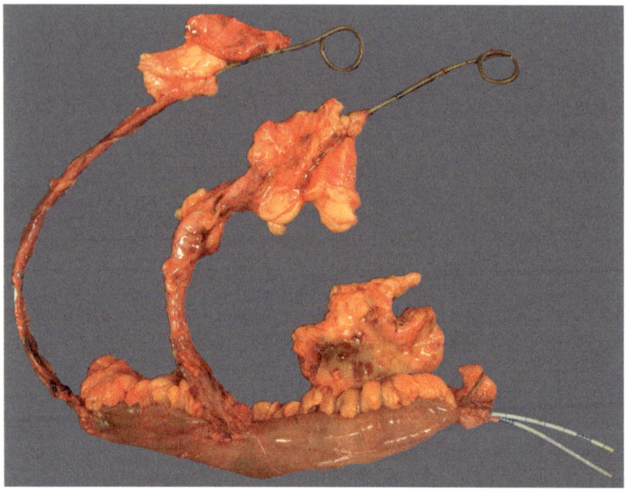

Fig. 11.60 A dissected urinary ileal conduit has been assisted in terms of drainage by inserting two tubes that ran into the renal pelves. Such tubes normally accompany ileal conduit surgery, as a method of initially assisting the kidney urine outflow and thereby recovery

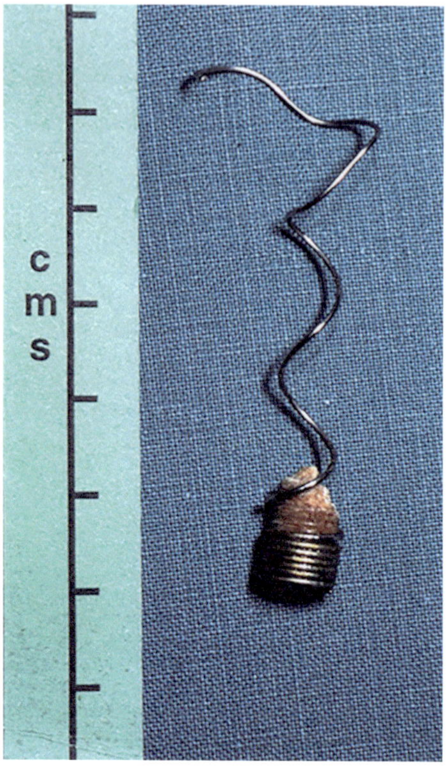

Fig. 11.61 Some urinary stents are placed at sites of strictures in the prostate and bladder outlet. These can become encrusted with bladder stone material and thereby obstruct the urine outflow. This stent has been partially pulled apart in order to reveal the obstructing calculus material

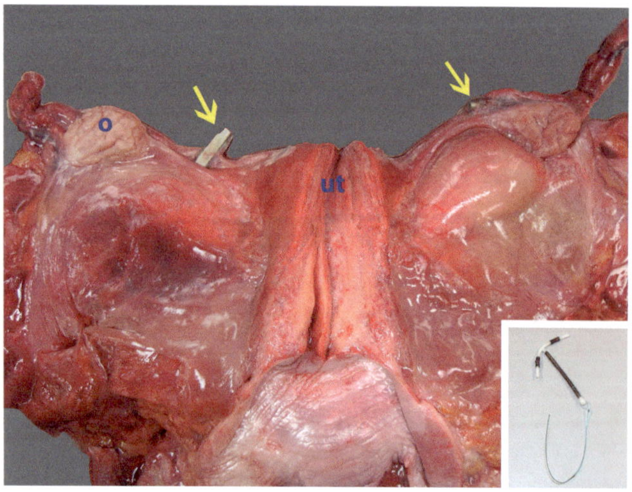

Fig. 11.62 This view of the uterine tissue (*ut*) shows sterilization clips (*arrows*) on the tubes leading to the ovary (*o*). The inset shows an intrauterine contraceptive device

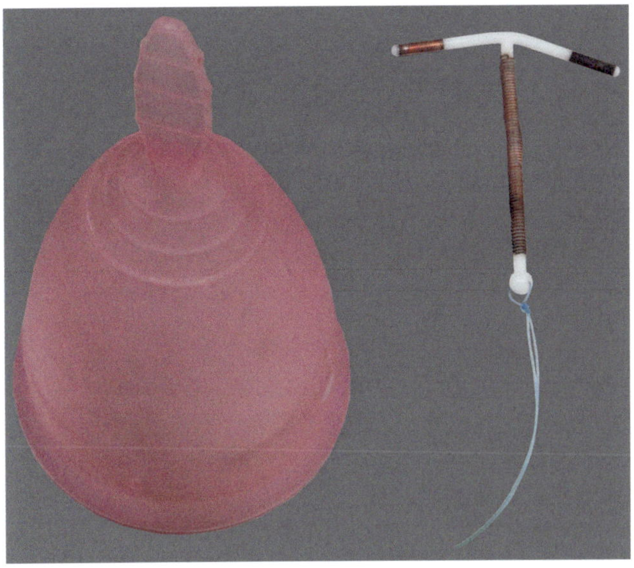

Fig. 11.63 This image shows two contraceptive devices which may be found in the female genital tract. On the left is a menstrual cup and on the right is an intrauterine contraceptive device

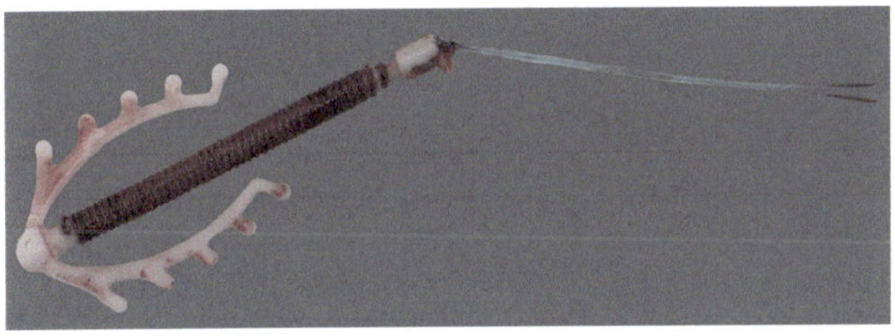

Fig. 11.64 Another example of an intrauterine contraceptive device is shown here

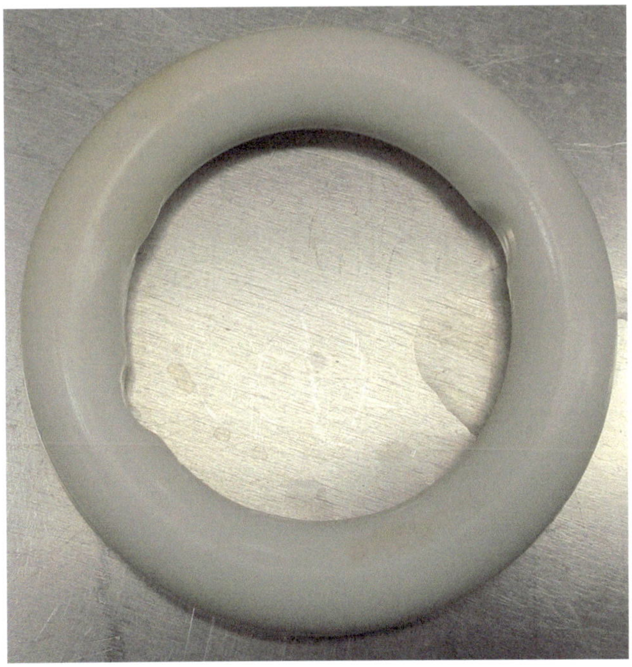

Fig. 11.65 Here is a ring pessary used to support the pelvic floor muscles in cases of vaginal prolapse or stress incontinence

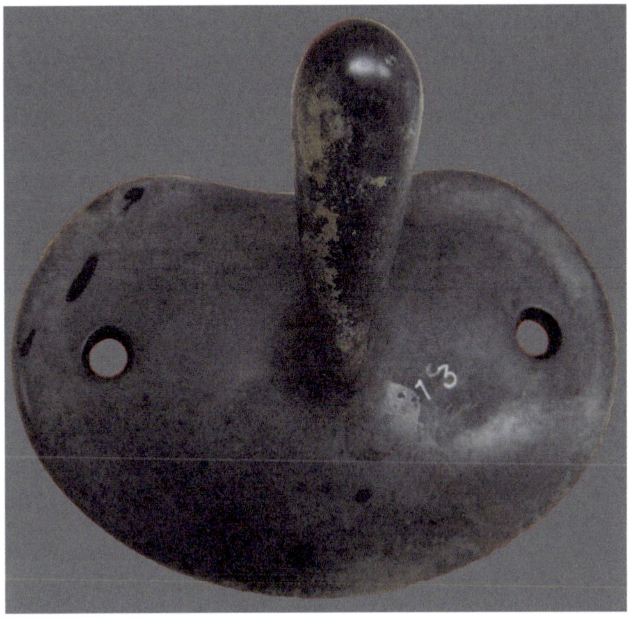

Fig. 11.66 A vaginal pessary. Not all are ring shaped

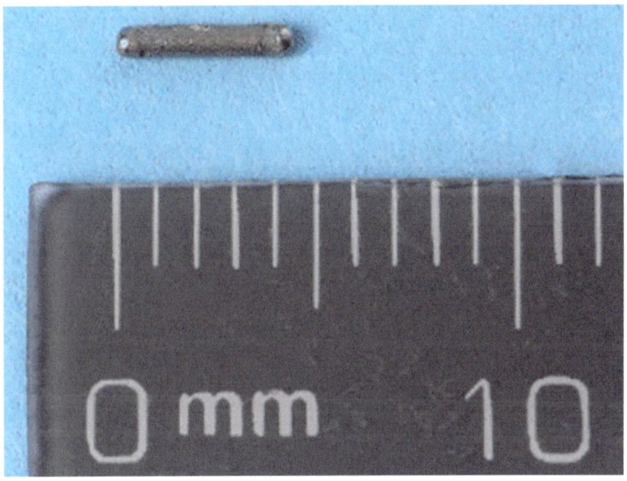

Fig. 11.67 Radioactive beads (and other radioactive implants) such as the one shown here are a potential hazard for those performing autopsies. They often appear innocuous but one should have a high index of suspicion, even if not declared beforehand, if present in an area of tumour. Reproduced with permission from Start RD, Tindale W, Singleton M, Conway M and Richardson C. Radioactive prostatic implants: a potential autopsy hazard. 2007. Histopathology; 51: 246–248

Hazardous materials, applied as beads or a needle, delivering radiation to the local tissues may be found in some tumours. This therapy often focuses on breast and prostate tumours, but conceivably radioactive devices may be encountered anywhere. Care with handling these items is mandatory and disposal of radioactive materials will always be governed by strict regulations.

Supports for Soft Tissues and Bones

Many devices are used to support structures (Figs. 11.68, 11.69, 11.70, 11.71, 11.72, and 11.73), such as mesh for abdominal hernias, bone prostheses and metal plates for cra-

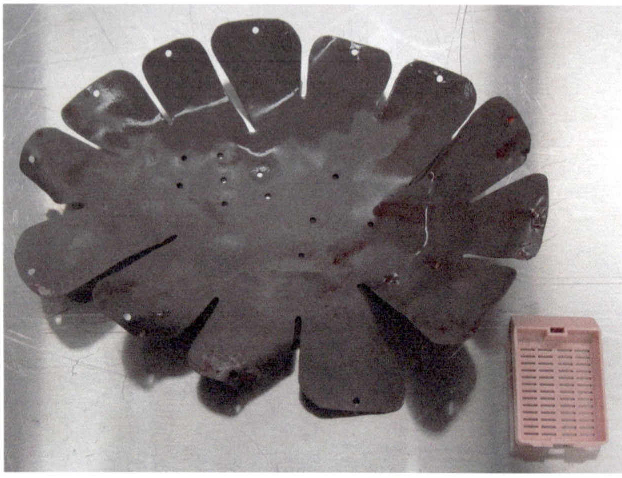

Fig. 11.68 A large skull fracture and bone defect can be treated with a metal plate to protect the brain. This metal plate device is bent to fit the patient's outer cranial vault and fixed in position by small screws at the edge. Here it has been dissected free (see also Chap. 9, Fig. 9.75)

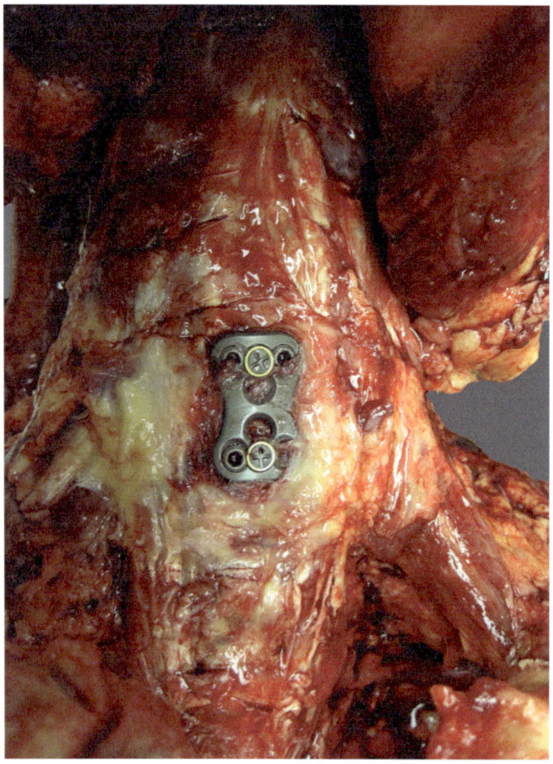

Fig. 11.69 Features of spinal stabilization may be evident when the body is open and the cervical, thoracic and abdominal tissues have been removed. This metal device had been positioned many years beforehand to stabilize a fracture/dislocation of the spine. In cases of recently completed surgery, it is important to check for local sepsis

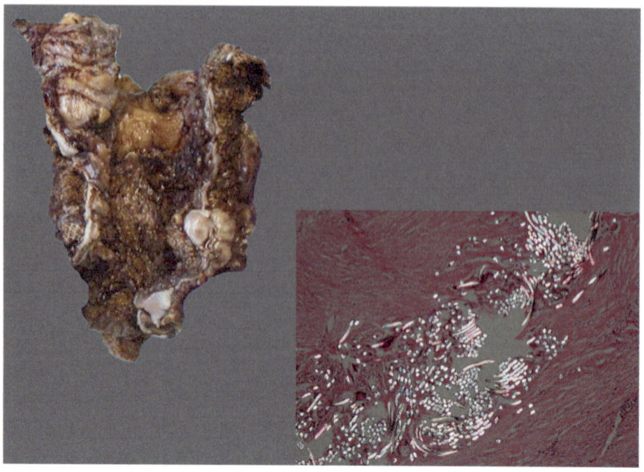

Fig. 11.70 Laparoscopic hernia surgery with synthetic mesh devices is increasingly common. This left side image shows a case involving chronic sepsis and extensive fibrosis into the local tissues. Samples for microbiology should be sent. The histology (*inset*) shows the mesh highlighted (in a non-septic case) with polarized light

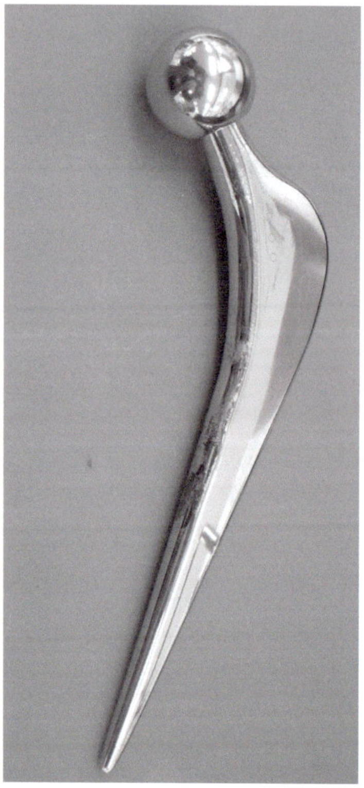

Fig. 11.71 A variety of metal joint replacements exist, as exemplified by this hip prosthesis. This type of device is commonly found in autopsy cases following acute fractures or elective replacement surgery. If the bone alignment is good and there is no antemortem issue, then complete explantation is not needed. However, if there is any issue of sepsis or mechanical failure, then prosthesis examination is advised

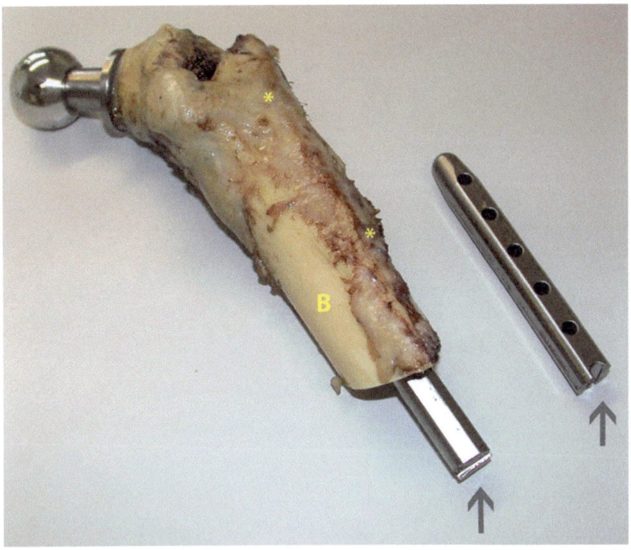

Fig. 11.72 This complicated hip fracture needed a metal prosthesis and reinforcement with allograft bone and cement (*asterisk*). Whilst this procedure was a success with regard to allowing incorporation into native bone (*B*), the metal device failed, with fracture of the metal stem adjacent to a drilled hole (*arrows*)

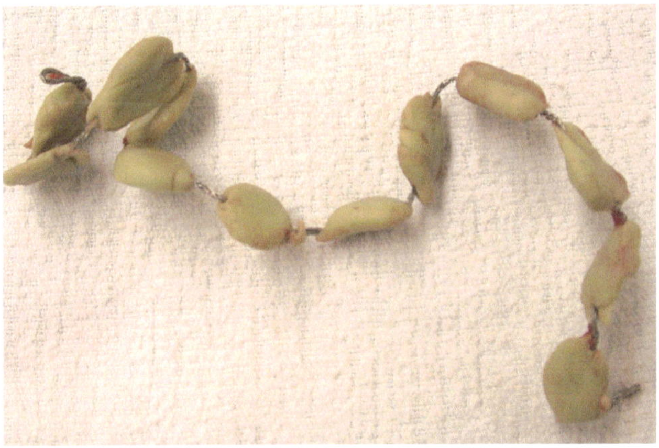

Fig. 11.73 Antibiotic beads are an uncommon therapy. These drug-loaded beads elute antimicrobial therapy directly into a cavity or other site that may have poor vascularity

niotomy wounds. In all autopsies where such devices are present, their position must be recorded and sepsis must be considered. In most cases, if there is no overt pathology, then the device does not need to be removed. However, one should be able to extract metal devices and bony tissue or soft tissue support devices en bloc if there is an issue with regard to the alignment of the repair or consideration of neoplasia or sepsis. Clearly, if the device has failed, then photography and radiology may be of assistance. Review by the manufacturer may also be helpful.

Suggested Reading

Burton JL, Rutty G. The hospital autopsy. 3rd ed. London: Hodder Arnold; 2010.

Burton J, Saunders S, Hamilton S. Atlas adult autopsy pathology. Boca Raton: CRC Press; 2015.

Connolly AJ, Finkbeiner WE, Ursell PC, Davis RL, editors. Autopsy pathology: a manual and atlas. 3rd ed. Philadelphia: Elsevier; 2016.

Singleton M, Start RD, Tindale W, Richardson C, Conway M. The radioactive autopsy: safe working practices. Histopathology. 2007;51:289–304.

The Forensic Autopsy

12

Philip D. Lumb

Introduction

Not all cases coming to autopsy examination reflect deaths that are natural. Some have medicolegal considerations regarding, for example, nursing care, medical negligence, violent deaths, industrial accidents, suicide, homicide, and so on. The investigating police officers may require urgent examination of a deceased individual to determine if a crime has been committed, so that they can manage and progress their investigation. For those undertaking any autopsy examination, whether anatomical technician or pathologist, a degree of dutiful suspicion should always exist but not at the expense of objective, unbiased analysis. This rigor in the investigative process is essential to uphold the integrity of the autopsy findings, which may have significant legal and societal implications. This careful scrutiny must continue throughout the entire examination, and one should always be prepared to consider stopping the case if any suspicious features are found, to refer the case to a forensic pathologist.

In simple terms, the forensic autopsy covers the same ground as a standard autopsy, but it goes into greater detail in terms of analysing the pathology, recording the injuries (if present), retaining samples (e.g., evidence and other tests), and liaising with the police and other relevant parties. To this end, performing the autopsy with other personnel (police, scene of crime officer, photographer, etc.) is required. The principles of forensic pathology mandate a meticulous and impartial approach, ensuring that conclusions are drawn solely from the medical and scientific evidence presented by the body.

The examination often must go beyond the routine incisions, extending the dissection around various parts of the body. Assessment of the deceased in situ at the site of discovery can also provide valuable information.

P. D. Lumb (✉)
Department of Forensic Pathology, Medicolegal Centre,
Sheffield, UK

Scenes

Investigation of a scene or scenes can form an important part of the forensic pathologist's investigation into a death but also often impacts, at an early stage, upon how the police may manage the case. Critical roles for the pathologist include an early indication into the manner and mechanism of death, estimation of time of death, the identification of any weapons and the preservation and collection of fragile evidence for further scientific investigation. On arrival at the scene of a death, the forensic pathologist should elicit from the Senior Investigating Police Officer the history of events and determine, from the Crime Scene Manager, the stage of the scene investigation—can the body be approached; has fragile evidence been recovered; has the body been photographed? The requirements of the pathologist should be documented as part of the overall forensic strategy for the scene visit and agreed between police, pathologist and crime scene investigators. Urgent attendance of the pathologist to a scene is not usually necessary. However, in some circumstances, such as when the deceased rests in a public place, urgent DNA profiling is needed or when a body temperature may be critical (e.g., a case of excited delirium), it may be of value for the pathologist to attend as soon as practicable. Assessment and removal of deceased persons at the scene may lead to leakage of bodily fluids and may require considerable disturbance of the scene about the deceased, so it may be of value to permit other experts (e.g., a biologist) to attend first to recover fragile evidence (e.g., blood spatter patterns). Collection of evidence from the body at a scene prevents it becoming contaminated or destroyed during transportation to the mortuary. If the scene permits, then samples such as fingernail scrapings, head hair combings, anogenital swabs, oronasal swabs and skin swabs can be taken in situ. All samples taken by the pathologist should be carefully documented.

S. K. Suvarna (represented by Grace Horne), A. K. Sharp (eds.), *Atlas of Adult Autopsy*,
https://doi.org/10.1007/978-3-031-72207-3_12

The Forensic Autopsy Specialist Dissections

The Neck

Detailed examination of the neck should take place in a "dry" bloodless field in order to prevent artefacts such as the Prinsloo-Gordon lesion. Decompression of the neck should be made by initially removing the brain, draining the head of blood. A wide superficial "V" incision should then be extended from the region of the upper chest, along the lateral aspect of the neck, and behind both ears. The angle of the "V" is just below the top of the sternum centrally. The chest and abdomen should then be opened in the usual manner (including removal of the sternum) with a clamp placed across the trachea just above the carina. The trachea and associated soft tissues are divided above the clamp and the thoracic pluck is separated from the neck structures. This isolates the neck structures, permitting effective drainage. The skin of the neck, between the "V" incisions, should then be reflected over the chin. The initial reflection should keep the platysma muscle intact for inspection and the under surface of the skin should also be reviewed for hidden bruising. Each of the strap muscles are sequentially dissected, layer-by-layer, and photographed. Each muscle can also be individually incised to examine for subtle internal bruises. For completeness, the posterior triangles of the neck also should be exposed, and the fold of skin over the occiput also can be dissected inferiorly to reveal the posterior musculature at the back of the neck. Once the musculature has been inspected, the other neck structures can be readily exposed and carefully dissected away from the spinal column. The laryngeal inlet and any obstruction process are readily visualized at this point, using this technique.

The Face

Standard forensic autopsies usually involve dissection of the subcutaneous tissues of the face. The "V" neck incision fully exposes the neck structures and is then extended behind both external auditory meatuses and over the mental process of the chin. The buccal surfaces are exposed and the incision can be extended to the orbits, which also allows access to the orbital contents. This dissection allows assessment of deep facial bruising and fracturing. The lips also can be examined in detail. The dissections can be extended over much of the nose to expose fracturing to the nasal bones and cartilages, although some residual tissue is kept here, to ensure that the facial tissues remain attached to the face. Reconstruction is relatively straightforward; in the hands of a skilled technician, the individual's appearance will not be altered, even for identification purposes.

Posterior Skin Flay, Including Upper Limbs

Dissection of the back can reveal very extensive injuries that are not visible on the skin surface but which may cause or contribute to death. Such injuries include large hematomas causing exsanguination, or pulping of the subcutaneous fat, producing fat embolism. The dissections also permit assessment of the path of, for example, stab wounds, and in particular their relationship to the spinal column. The scapulae can also be fully inspected at this stage. The deceased should be positioned face down on the dissection table with a mortuary block underneath the upper chest to facilitate dissection. It may also be pertinent to position a cloth or sponge underneath the face at this time to prevent any artefactual damage. A cruciate incision should be made and extended down the back. Extension can also be made down the arms to reveal deep bruising, such as that which may be caused by restraint or gripping. The dorsum of the neck can also be exposed to assess the posterior ligamentous attachments, spinous processes, and laminae of the cervical vertebrae. Each muscle layer should be sequentially revealed to expose hidden injury.

The Lips

Following deep dissection of the face, the inner aspects of the lips are exposed. Some incisions can be made to assess for deep lip bruising. Deep lip bruising may be encountered in blunt force assaults, although subtle bruising seen in smothering cases may also be exposed by using this technique. Detailed imaging of the lips can also be made at this stage.

The Orbit

Following dissection of the face, it is then possible to extend the dissection to expose the tissues and bony walls of the orbit. This is particularly useful when investigating the cause of periorbital hematomas. These "blowout" fractures of the floor of the orbit suggest direct force to the ocular globe, such as from a punch. Indeed, it is important to remember that, rarely, oculocardiac reflexes can be the cause of death. Care must be taken during the orbital dissection to prevent artefactual fractures to the thin walls of the orbit. The lateral orbital margin is exposed and blunt dissection is made posteriorly into soft tissues of the orbit using snub-nosed scissors. Freeing this tissue should expose the optic nerve, which is then cut with scissors. Gentle retraction on the soft tissues surrounding the globe, and further blunt dissection posteriorly and medially, free the globe from the orbit. Note that the globe remains attached to the inner aspect of the eyelids by the conjunctivae, allowing simple reconstruction of the face afterwards.

The Vertebral Arteries

The extracranial and intracranial portions of the vertebral arteries may become damaged with blows causing rotation of the head upon the spinal column, leading to basal subarachnoid haemorrhage (see also below). Careful dissection of the extracranial vertebral arteries is mandatory in such cases, as dissection and stretch-related changes may be identified. The vertebral artery canal is deroofed with small bone clippers (tailor-made equipment is also available), and the arteries are carefully removed. It is recognized that accessing the upper extracranial vertebral artery (between C1 and the dural insertion) is difficult and is best done by exposing the area with the deceased lying face downwards. Alternatively, the entire cervical spinal column can be removed in continuity with a rectangle of bone surrounding the foramen magnum. The specimen may then be fixed and decalcified, permitting serial sectioning of the entire specimen for histological assessment. In some centres, this is the preferred method of examination of the extracranial vertebral arteries.

Anterior Skin Flay

Subcutaneous dissection of the front of the chest and abdomen can reveal subtle bruising that may not be visible externally. It is important to remember that not all blunt force trauma to the front of the abdomen may cause local skin injury despite catastrophic internal organ damage.

Forearm and Hand Flay

The incision lines should be extended from the base of the proximal phalanx of the little finger, ulnar aspect, along the ulnar aspect of the forearm towards the elbow. A second incision can then be extended from the metacarpophalangeal joint of the thumb and up the radial aspect of the forearm. A third transverse incision then should join the outer forearm incisions, and the skin can be dissected back from the forearm over the metacarpophalangeal joints of the knuckles, facilitating the assessment of subtle deep bruising and hidden needle puncture marks. The knuckles can be assessed for offensive injuries (e.g., punching). Reconstruction preserves much of the skin of the hand and is thus more satisfactory for relatives of the deceased than the more traditional hand incisions along the length of each finger/knuckle.

Anogenital Block (Female)

A marker should be placed at the anal verge in the 12 o'clock position, so that the location of injuries can later be identified after dissection. Internally, the bladder, uterus, and rectum should be freed from the pelvic wall by blunt dissection. An incision to form an ellipse of skin is then made around the pudenda to include the anus and vulva. The subcutaneous tissues are then carefully dissected and deepened into the pelvic outlet, to free up the entire block. The pubic symphysis can be divided with a saw to facilitate this dissection although this is not always necessary. Following removal, the anus, rectum, vulva, and vagina are easy to access for detailed inspection and photographic documentation of injuries.

Excarnation/Defleshing

Decomposition of the corpse can hamper careful inspection of the skeleton for features that may be relevant to the identity of the deceased or the cause of death (such as subtle bony incisions from stab wounds). After general tissue examination and preservation of samples for additional tests (e.g., toxicology, DNA), bone cleansing may be used. This specialist technique is simple and effective. Different methods are available, but they generally involve the incubation of partially defleshed tissue in a bath of proteolytic enzymes (commonly encountered in biological washing powders). During the process, it is imperative to check upon progress each day as prolonged immersion can cause the bone to become friable and damaged.

Sharp Force Trauma

Sharp force injuries can be generally categorized into incised wounds and stab wounds. Puncture wounds often are also included in this group and can be defined as shallow penetration of the tip of an implement. Sharp force injuries can be differentiated from lacerations by examination of the wound edges, which are cleanly divided and without tissue bridges. Hairs crossing over the wound also may be divided neatly. Unlike with lacerations, abrasions at the edge of the wound are relatively uncommon, unless severe force has been used (for example, the hilt of a weapon had been driven into the skin).

The Stab Wound

A stab wound can be defined as a sharp force injury that has a wound tract that is deeper than the width of the injury at the skin surface. Stab wounds are usually caused by bladed weapons such as knives, which are thrust into the tissues.

The following information should be gathered about each stab wound: location in terms of height from the heel and distance from the midline on the torso (or other fixed point on the body); length; shape of the ends of the wound, direction of the track; tissues penetrated; and depth of the track. These features can help identify the weapon used.

Stab wounds that are orientated across Langer's lines (tension lines in the skin and subcuticular tissues) can gape open and become shortened, misrepresenting the width of the blade. In this situation, gentle tension should be applied to reform the wound. Sharp or pointed wound ends indicate that it is likely that there has been contact with the forged cutting edge of the blade, whereas a squared or blunt end indicates contact with the unforged spine of the blade.

Stabbing Injuries: Force

The force used to cause a stab wound should be assessed. Many pathologists use a scale of mild, moderate, and severe force. Mild force usually implies slow movement of the weapon; deeply penetrating wounds caused by mild force are usually seen only when the individual is restrained and unable to fend off the weapon as it is relatively slowly inserted into the tissues. By contrast, severe force has been used when thick, bony buttresses such as the sternum, the full thickness of a rib, or the calvarium are penetrated. Moderate force lies somewhere between, with the blade moving quickly enough to overcome the evasive actions of the deceased but not necessarily having the force to penetrate through thick bone. When assessing the force used to describe a deeply penetrating stab wound without bony injury (or with minor bony injury), the term "at least moderate force" is used in the autopsy report. Whilst moderate force may have been used to cause such deep injuries, severe force cannot be excluded; it just so happens that the stab wound has not struck bone that might serve as a marker of force. Hilt marks (or more rarely, fingernail marks) alongside the stab wound suggest that the weapon has been driven in deeply with severe force.

Defence Injuries

The discovery of incised wounds or stab wounds to the hands or ulnar aspects of the upper limbs raises the possibility of sharp force defence injuries and that the individual has been attacked by an assailant. During the course of an assault with a sharp weapon, the hands and forearms are often instinctively raised to protect the torso and head from injury. The bladed weapon may even have been grasped in the hand and, upon removal, incised injuries can be seen across the palm or palmar aspects of the fingers, not uncommonly in the interphalangeal skin creases. The weapon also may be drawn through the web of skin between the index finger and thumb, causing deep incision. Similarly, as the individual fends off a sharp force attack with the upper limbs, the back of the hands and often the ulnar aspect of the forearm are presented to the oncoming weapon, causing incised wounds to be inflicted at these sites.

Self-Inflicted Fatal Stab and Incised Wounds

It is critical to consider whether sharp force injuries might have been self-inflicted during an episode of self-harm, as opposed to being inflicted by an assailant. One should be mindful of the circumstances surrounding the death, but assumptions must not be made on the history alone. Fatal self-inflicted stab wounds are not uncommon, being more frequently encountered in males. The individual is more likely to lift their clothing to inflict the fatal injury, and the weapon may remain in the deceased's body or may be close by. Occasionally, because stab wounds do not necessarily cause immediate collapse and death, the weapon may even be tidied away. Some stab wounds can permit a period of purposeful activity, and the individual may even be capable of quite vigorous activity until overwhelmed by blood loss or other tissue damage.

Self-inflicted injuries must be in a location accessible to the deceased's own hand; fatal stab wounds or incised wounds are most frequently encountered in the torso or neck (usually incisions here). The fatal injury is often accompanied by tentative wounds or hesitation marks—shallow stab wounds or puncture wounds caused by the tip of a knife, presumably testing out the pain to be expected prior to the fatal blow. Self-inflicted stab wounds usually do not penetrate through thick, bony buttresses such as the sternum, and penetration of such bones should elevate the suspicion of the forensic pathologist that assault has taken place. Incised wounds to the upper limb can injure the main vessels (e.g., radial or ulnar arteries), leading to severe and fatal haemorrhage.

A word of caution is necessary at this point regarding post-mortem incised and stab wounds. Although the accompanying injuries may suggest that the wound is self-inflicted, it would never be entirely possible for the forensic pathologist, when considering the pathological findings alone, to entirely exclude third-party intervention with regard to the fatal injury. Indeed, old self-harm scars may not necessarily indicate that a single stab wound to the chest is self-inflicted.

Blunt Force Trauma and Friction Injury

Blunt force trauma is caused by blunt, non-sharp, impacts to the skin tissue. Two characteristic injuries occur: the bruise and the laceration.

The bruise appears as an area of discolouration upon the skin, sometimes accompanied by tissue swelling. The bruise is caused by bleeding from crushed and ruptured vessels in the tissues. Not all bruises are visible from external inspection of the body, and deep body dissections are required to reveal them (see above). The age of bruises can be broadly gauged by colour and their histological appearances, although forensic pathologists often encounter clearly old bruises retaining their blue colour and showing little or no inflammation upon histological inspection. Haemorrhage from basal skull fractures and other deep injuries can emerge upon the skin surface to mimic localized injuries (for example, a "black eye" caused by a basal skull fracture).

Lacerations are skin splits caused by blunt force. They can be rather irregular, with an associated abrasion rim. Invariably, a degree of bruising accompanies lacerations. Lacerations occurring over bony ridges, such as the orbit, can split in a rather linear fashion making differentiation from incised wounds sometimes difficult. The use of a bright light source and magnification (e.g., surgical loupes or magnifying glass) should still reveal helpful, albeit subtle, features such as deep tissue bridges within the injury to assist in its characterisation.

Friction injuries occur when a rough surface rubs across the skin surface, leading to the development of abrasion. Abrasion typically involves only the epidermis, although bleeding may ensue from the injury if the papillary dermis (or deeper) becomes involved.

Patterned Bruise

Patterned bruising may be critical in identifying a weapon or offending footwear. The pathologist is required to carefully document and measure the pattern and ensure that it is appropriately recorded photographically, with standardised scale. Patterns may be modified or lost due to the interposition of clothing or the healing process.

Tramline Bruises

Tramline bruises are characteristic of impacts from cylindrical objects, such as bats and poles. The tramline comprises two outer linear bruises, separated by an area of sparing. As the cylindrical object impacts, the area of most skin deforming occurs at the edges of the impacting object, tearing blood vessels and leading to the development of bruising. Centrally, the skin is depressed inwards rather than deformed, with less vascular injury. Broader weapons cause broader tramlines, although it is important to be cautious about estimating the width of a potential weapon from the width of the tramline bruise alone.

Lacerations

Lacerations occur in areas where the skin is relatively tightly applied to the underlying soft tissues, such as in the scalp. The blunt force applied is sufficient to split the skin and underlying tissues. Linear lacerations caused by blunt linear implements may have thin rims of abrasion along the wound margin. In addition, within the depths of the wound there are tissue bridges, rather than the neat division encountered with incised wounds. Falls onto surfaces such as pavement or roadway often cause a central complex laceration surrounded by patchy abrasion ("gravel rash"). Bruising and swelling are often more marked with blunt force trauma than with a sharp force wound.

Bite Marks

Curved bruises and earlobe injuries (particularly if part of the ear is missing) should always raise the consideration that an injury has been caused by teeth (human or other). A forensic odontologist should be consulted for specialist advice and interpretation. Dissection of a bite mark may alter its shape and size, so ideally the odontologist should be asked for advice prior to dissection. Swabbing of the marks for possible DNA is also required, potentially assisting future identification of the perpetrator.

Grip Marks

Ovoid bruises on the inner aspects of the upper limbs or thighs suggest tight gripping. Such injuries on the upper arms are often caused during the resuscitation procedure, usually by attempts to move the collapsed individual into a favourable position for chest compressions. Multiple grip marks to the upper limbs are often encountered in those individuals who repeatedly fall over, such as those with alcohol dependency syndrome, with acquaintances helping them to their feet. Bruising may be more prominent in these cases due to the presence of liver disease.

Bruising on the thighs, particularly the inner aspects, may indicate forced ante-mortem sexual activity.

Abrasion Injuries

Many of these injuries will be familiar to all, such as common knee abrasions or grazes caused by collapse or falls to the ground. Facial abrasions, centred on the nose, philtrum, central lips, chin and over the bony prominences may indicate sudden collapse. Rather parchmented and bloodless abrasions might suggest that the injury was sustained as the circulation collapsed. Linear abrasions to the back and buttocks are commonly encountered as a consequence of a collapse onto the edge of an object such as a step edge. Large abrasions with multiple linear lines of brushing are typically encountered in road traffic collisions, produced as the individual skids across the roadway or pavement.

Abrasion Scrolls

The direction that the friction force was applied to the skin can be determined by the observation of abrasion scrolls. Scrolls of skin (and sometimes large skin flaps) are raised, with the base of the scroll (or flap) showing the direction of travel.

Deaths on the Highway

Deaths on the highway should be considered from the perspective of what the person was doing when death occurred. Realities to be considered differ for driver versus pedestrian deaths, cyclist versus motor vehicle, and passenger/driver injuries. Persons injured as pedestrians need a different approach.

For the sake of simplicity, this section assumes the vehicle is a car, although one must accept that different injuries will follow collisions involving motorcycles, lorries, coaches, and other vehicles. In this regard, close interaction with traffic police, forensic collision reconstruction experts, and civil highway engineers may be needed.

Pedestrian Injuries: Primary, Secondary, and Tertiary Impacts

Impacts with pedestrians can be classified into primary, secondary, and tertiary impacts. The primary impact is the point of first contact of the oncoming vehicle with the pedestrian and should be identified, if possible.

Primary impacts caused by the vehicle bumper on the lower limbs often appear as horizontal bruises, and the distance from the heel should be measured. This information can assist the forensic collision reconstruction experts in their assessment of the case; low bumper marks could indicate braking of the oncoming vehicle. Radiographs or CT scans of fractured lower limbs, assessing the shape of the injury, can also identify the direction in which the collision occurred. Horizontal or wedge-shaped fractures to the tibia are typical of primary impacts, with the base of the wedge to the point being in the same direction as the travel of the vehicle.

Secondary collisions often involve the head striking an upper part of the vehicle, such as the window screen or vehicle frame. The secondary injury is often fatal. Tertiary impacts are caused by contact with the roadway and include large abrasions or fractures. Long bone fractures from these impacts are often spiral in nature, rather than transverse.

Pedestrian Injuries: Patterned Injuries

Patterned injuries discovered upon the body of a "hit and run" victim can be critical in the identification or exclusion of a suspect vehicle. Grills and other patterned parts of the vehicle may leave imprinted bruises. Careful, scaled photography can assist the investigating officers in comparing the injury to a suspect vehicle. If possible, the injuries can also be traced upon paper, to allow rapid comparison of a suspect vehicle to the injury in the field.

Vehicle Occupants

Critical to many investigations is identification of the driver of the vehicle at the time of the fatal collision. Often, this is straightforward, with the driver remaining strapped in the driver's seat, but the collision may alter the position of deceased individuals in the vehicle or may project individuals out of the vehicle.

The pathologist can help the investigating officers determine who was driving the vehicle at the time of a fatal collision. Transmitted forces through the foot pedals can leave impressions on footwear, which can be recovered at autopsy for the officers. Examination of the chest may identify specific features of the steering wheel, if it has been in contact with the deceased. However, one caveat should be considered: mechanical resuscitators used by some emergency services can leave rounded or curved bruises upon the chest, which may be mistaken for steering wheel injuries.

The position of a seat belt mark also can assist in determining who was sitting where in the vehicle. Classic seat belt marks or abrasions are uncommonly encountered, as clothing often protects the skin. More commonly encountered are broad but linear abrasions at the base of the neck, caused as the upper part of the seat belt tightens against exposed skin. Horizontal marks across the abdomen, caused by the lap belt, may also indicate the use of a seat belt. These abdominal injuries sometimes are not evident externally, but subcutaneous dissection can reveal a band of linear laceration in the lower abdominal soft tissues.

Road Traffic Collision with Natural Disease

For both pedestrian versus vehicle collisions and fatal vehicle collisions, natural disease is often relevant. For example, pedestrians may collapse in front of a vehicle as a result of epilepsy or syncope from coronary artery atheroma. Alternatively, one may find an acute natural pathology affecting the driver of a vehicle. All such disease data must be evaluated alongside the forensic injuries.

Consideration of the senses can be difficult to assess as a pathologist. The best information with regard to an individual's vision or hearing comes from ante-mortem clinical data or statements of witnesses (such as family). It may be appropriate under some circumstances to remove the eyes for formal ophthalmological assessment. Recovery of items such as contact lenses may also help investigators inquire into why a collision occurred.

Pressure to the Neck

When pressure to the neck is applied with sufficient force and over a sufficient time, compression of the structures within the neck may lead to a cardiac arrest and death. The mechanisms of death include airway obstruction, vascular compression and possibly stimulation of abnormal nerve reflexes. The airway running through the neck (the trachea) may become compressed and, depending on the direction of force, the soft tissues of the neck may be pushed upwards, closing the air passages at the back of the mouth. Two of the main arteries that supply blood to the brain, the carotid arteries, may also become compressed, depriving the brain of its main blood supply (and therefore oxygen). Also within the neck are receptors which monitor the blood pressure. When compressed abnormally, the heart rate can fall and may even stop. This is sometimes referred to as "vagal inhibition" although the evidence for its significance in such deaths is inconclusive. The time taken for pressure to the neck to lead to these deleterious effects, culminating in cardiac arrest, depends upon the severity of the pressure, location/direction of pressure and consistency of pressure.

Commonly encountered causes of fatal pressure to the neck include manual strangulation, ligature strangulation and a number of other means (e.g., headlocks, garrotting, ligature self-strangulation). Pressure to the neck may be accompanied by the asphyxial signs.

Signs of Asphyxia (Petechiae and Congestion)

Petechiae are small, pin-prick sized haemorrhages visible upon the skin and on the inner aspects of the eyelids, which appear like a fine rash. They are commonly encountered in cases of death by asphyxia. The precise mechanism by which they develop is not known, although they are likely related to vascular over-pressure, which may involve aspects of hypoxia on small blood vessels and continued arterial supply of blood to the head during asphyxia, whilst venous return may be impaired. Petechiae are not exclusive to asphyxial deaths. They may be encountered in other circumstances, including natural deaths. Hypostasis may also mimic the development of petechiae in the face, particularly if the deceased assumed a "face down" posture, although in the author's experience, hypostatic petechiae tend to be coarser than the finer true asphyxial petechiae.

Congestion, causing a purple discolouration to the head, often accompanies other asphyxial signs such as petechiae, nose bleeds, and facial oedema. Indeed, congestion is responsible for artefactual haemorrhages in the neck, such as the Prinsloo-Gordon lesion, and decompression of this congestion is required when assessing deaths caused by pressure to the neck.

Pressure to the Neck: Internal Injuries

Ligatures or hand grips (manual strangulation) are capable of causing fractures to the hyoid bone and larynx. Younger individuals may be less susceptible to such fractures, as these joints and cartilages are often flexible and not ossified. Bruising often accompanies these injuries. Occasionally, the cricoid cartilage may also be fractured. To assist, histological assessment should be made. A lack of an inflammatory infiltrate indicates death soon after the injuries were inflicted (i.e., death was caused by the pressure to the neck), whereas a well-established inflammatory infiltrate may indicate a period of survival, and death by another mechanism.

Hanging

Hanging is death caused by exerting pressure upon the neck, usually using the weight of the body through a ligature tethered to a suspension point. This is quite unlike judicial hanging, which causes death by cervical spinal column disruption following precipitation of the individual from a height with a ligature about the neck. Self-suspension with a ligature usually causes unconsciousness very rapidly, with death ensuing within a few minutes. Respiratory movements, whilst suspended by the neck, along with decorticate/decerebrate posturing during the hanging process, can occasionally cause additional injuries over the bony prominences of the face. One must be aware of these minor injuries, as they do not necessarily indicate third-party participation or additional suspicious circumstances. For death to occur, full suspension of the body is not necessary; partial suspension with the feet or knees touching the floor can exert enough pressure to bring about death.

Several critical features should be assessed at autopsy. Firstly, the ligature mark must be compared to the ligature that is believed to have been used to cause death. Any mismatch in the patterns must be highlighted to the investigating officers. Secondly, the point of suspension should be sought; it is often characterized by the ligature marks on either side of the neck rising towards a single point. Horizontal or encircling ligature marks are more suspicious of ligature strangulation. Thirdly, other suspicious marks to the neck (or elsewhere) need to be assessed to exclude other modes of pressure to the neck or additional injuries used to subdue a victim.

Manual Strangulation

Manual strangulation can be defined as pressure to the neck exerted by a third party by use of the hand or hands. Manual strangulation is often characterized by multifocal areas of irregular abrasion and ovoid bruising to the neck—injuries that occur during a dynamic struggle between two individuals. Curved abrasions may also be identified, caused by the fingernails of either the perpetrator or victim attempting to remove the gripping hands. Objects such as clothing or necklaces may be pushed into the skin, simulating the application of a ligature. Examination of the internal neck structures often identifies widespread, multifocal bruising to the strap muscles, mirroring the external findings. The larynx, cricoid, and/or hyoid may be fractured, but there may be no injury in younger individuals because the cartilages are flexible and mainly cartilaginous.

Ligature Strangulation

Ligature strangulation can be defined as pressure to the neck exerted by a third party by use of a ligature. Ligature strangulation is usually characterized by the presence of a ligature mark upon the neck. Such ligature marks may not necessarily be particularly well defined. Some marks are characterized by linear bruises only, and broad ligatures may not leave any ligature mark. Ligature marks caused during ligature strangulation do not have suspension points such as those encountered in hanging, and the marks tend to be horizontal as they cross the sides of the neck. Signs of a struggle may also be present, with fingernail marks about the ligature mark. Documentation of the injuries must capture any patterning within the ligature mark, and it is often of value to measure the circumference of the neck. These records may assist in determining the nature of the ligature.

Choking

Exposure of the neck by a wide "V" incision (see above) permits careful access to the oropharynx, preventing items from becoming dislodged, which may occur with single neck low incisions that require removal of the tongue from low in the neck. Choking should be suspected particularly in cases where an individual has died suddenly whilst eating a meal, particularly if they have any disorder that may alter the ability to swallow, such as degenerative neurological conditions.

Traumatic Asphyxia

When the chest becomes compressed and it is no longer possible to ventilate the lungs owing to failure of the chest to expand and contract, the situation is best termed traumatic asphyxia. Traumatic asphyxia can be encountered in a number of situations, including motor vehicle accidents, industrial accidents, and crowd crushes or stampedes. Although the exact mechanisms are debated in the medical literature, the back pressure in the venous system and continued cardiac output may account for the intense congestion of the head, neck, and upper limbs; intense petechiae of the face; and scleral haemorrhage. Examination of the chest can identify accompanying external injuries and rib fractures, although little injury may be present in the young because of relative chest flexibility.

Postural/Positional Asphyxia

These terms describe asphyxial deaths caused when the body adopts such a posture or is placed in such a position that ventilatory movements become compromised. If the individual cannot escape from the situation, then fatal postural or positional asphyxia may take place. Flexion of the lower limbs and abdomen can displace the abdomen viscera upwards, making downward movement of the chest difficult. This can be further compromised by flexion of the upper chest and neck. Support of the body weight by extension of the upper limbs away from the chest wall, with elevation above the shoulders, can also prevent normal expansion of the chest, leading to positional asphyxia.

Intoxication with alcohol or drugs is a risk factor for postural or positional asphyxia, as the individual may be rendered incapable of escape. Natural disease, particularly if affecting muscle power (such as motor neuron disease, muscular dystrophy, or multiple sclerosis) also can increase the possibility of accidental postural asphyxia, although practically any condition than can cause a person to fall into unconsciousness might lead to death by this mechanism. Diagnosis of fatal postural/positional asphyxia cannot be made without assessing the scene. Post-mortem examination reveals typical features of asphyxia, with congestion and petechiae often extending onto the chest. Hypostatic pallor can also assist in the assessment of the position of the deceased.

Electrocution

Sudden death in the workplace (or elsewhere, for that matter) without obvious explanation should raise the suspicion of possible electrocution, as the autopsy findings can be minimal. The mechanism of death is usually disturbance of cardiac rhythm, although extensive burns may also sometimes be a feature.

Electrocution burns can be subtle and easily overlooked. They can appear as small blisters or focal areas of carbonization and occasionally can appear similar to abrasions. Histological assessment of electrical burns reveals characteristic features: the epidermis is focally denuded, and nuclear streaming is identified at the edge of the burn. Deep to the burn site, the dermal collagen is often hypereosinophilic. Embedded metallic particles may also be identified.

Fire Deaths

Fires may kill from the effects of direct thermal injury, but fatalities more commonly result from smoke inhalation. Fires often occur in accidental settings, although fire investigations (which may take considerable time) may later indicate arson. Fires may also be set in order to hide evidence of a homicide. The autopsy needs to establish whether the individual died prior to the fire or during the fire, and if the person died during the fire, the autopsy must attempt to discover why the individual did not escape from the heat and/or smoke.

Vital Signs

The presence of soot below the level of the vocal cords indicates active inhalation of smoke. It indicates that the individual was alive whilst the fire was producing smoke. Individuals who are deceased prior to commencement of the production of smoke have airways free of soot, although soot may percolate into the mouth, onto the tongue and pharynx.

External examination may reveal the typical cherry pink discolouration of the skin caused by carboxyhaemoglobin (the combination of carbon monoxide with haemoglobin, which displaces oxygen). The internal tissues and blood also show this similar discolouration.

Carboxyhaemoglobin saturations of 50% and above may prove fatal in healthy adults. In individuals with other conditions, such as ischaemic heart disease, lower carboxyhaemoglobin saturations may lead to death.

For those surviving a blaze for a period of time, when medical assistance is rendered, fatalities will necessarily have modulation of their injuries. In these cases, case note/record assessment will be important, as well as consideration of the physiological effects of the treated injuries (e.g., sepsis on a large zone of burn injury, or respiratory distress syndrome from exposure to smoke or fumes).

Artefacts of Fire: Heat Haematoma

Some caution is needed in looking at bodies retrieved from fires. Artefacts of heat may mimic intracranial haemorrhage, skin lacerations, or bony fractures. One artefact of concern is the heat hematoma. These are usually associated with carbonization and loss of the scalp over the head. The heated blood from the venous sinuses of the dura leaks into the extradural space, where it coagulates and occasionally may form a substantial hematoma. These are not to be confused with true extradural hematomas, which are invariably caused by skull fractures.

Artefacts of Fire: Heat Lacerations

Heated skin, particularly when carbonized, can shrivel and split, thereby mimicking injury. Under most circumstances, these can be distinguished from true injuries by a lack of haemorrhage into the underlying subcutaneous fatty tissues.

Post-Mortem Phenomena on the Boundary of Natural and Non-Natural Death

A complicated group of post-mortem changes confuse many pathologists. One needs to be aware of these issues, first to identify when a non-natural death has occurred and second, to avoid mistakenly raising alarm over a case.

Post-Mortem Injuries

Post-mortem injuries may be sustained when the body is moved to the mortuary from the scene of the death. Many are unintentional. These injuries may be inflicted by the pathologist or technician during the autopsy. Resuscitation also may be a cause of peri-mortem injury.

Rarely, an assailant may inflict additional injury on a body as part of the assault/mutilation after death has occurred. In general terms, post-mortem injuries show no vital reaction, no bleeding, or no swelling. Decomposition increases the risk of accidental skin tears, but medical conditions (e.g., steroid medication causing thin skin) also may increase the risk of injury.

Hypostasis

Hypostasis (or post-mortem lividity) is the discolouration of the skin caused by gravitational pooling of blood after death. Relatives who view the body after death can sometimes confuse hypostasis with true injury—a question sometimes raised at inquest.

After several hours, hypostasis becomes fixed or partially fixed within the tissues. Thus, it can be used to determine whether a body has been moved from one position to another after death. Hypostasis also can be identified within the internal organs and must be distinguished from naturally occurring disease processes. In the heart, posterior hypostasis can even be mistaken for myocardial infarction.

Skin Slippage and Depigmentation

Skin slippage and depigmentation is a particular problem often encountered in bodies recovered from water, when the identity is not known. Of course, it is useful in identifying an individual to know the person's ethnic origin and skin colour, but maceration and slippage of the skin due to decomposition can lead to loss of the pigmented layer, exposing the underlying dermis and making identification of the deceased more difficult.

Post-Mortem Animal Predation

Individuals may die in a sealed environment with their pets. The pets, when starving, will resort to feeding on the corpse. The post-mortem injuries can be widespread and may mimic true injury. Rodents, other vermin, insects, and crustaceans also can inflict a variety of post-mortem injuries if they have access to the body.

Hypothermia

Hypothermia is typically associated with exposure to very low ambient temperature, although it can be encountered in environments where the temperature may be as high as 12 °C. Disease processes or intoxicants that interfere with homeothermic mechanisms (e.g., hypothyroidism or acute alcohol intoxication) can increase the risk of developing hypothermia.

The diagnosis of hypothermia requires careful consideration of the circumstances of death. Of course, the individual needs to be in a cold environment. Although not fully understood, unusual behaviours can develop in the hypothermic individual. Paradoxically, before death, the affected individual may remove items of clothing, and the individual may be discovered semi-naked or naked. This situation can be of concern to investigating officers, particularly with females, as it raises the possibility of sexual assault.

Confusion often also ensues in cases of hypothermia, and a scene may show signs of great disturbance or chaos, again mimicking the scene of an assault. The hypothermic individual also may be found in an enclosed space (sometimes referred to as the "hide and die" syndrome or "terminal burrowing". Presumably this behaviour is an attempt to escape from the cold.

Hypothermia may produce reddish discolouration over the main joints and sometimes over the nose and cheeks. When exposure to cold has been prolonged, the extremities occasionally may show blistering or tissue necrosis (frost nip and frost bite).

Multiple gastric erosions (Wischnewski spots/ulcers) are also characteristic of hypothermia deaths. Microscopically, the ulcers usually involve only the mucosa. A heavy polymorph infiltrate is also characteristic of these ulcers. Pancreatitis sometimes is also encountered.

Drowning

The post-mortem features indicating that death was caused by drowning are often minimal. Froth (caused by the mixture of water, mucus, and surfactant) may be present in the airways. In addition, silt or other material may also become deeply inhaled or swallowed. Occasionally, large quantities of extruded foam may be seen at the nose and nostrils.

The lungs typically are hyperinflated and feel crepitant. Other features, such as middle ear haemorrhage and maceration of the limbs, are nonspecific and only indicate immersion in water, rather than specifically death by drowning.

Microscopic inspection of the lungs may show emphysema aquosum. This irregular expansion of the alveolar spaces is not specific for drowning. Specialist tests, such as assessment of bone marrow, liver, and splenic diatoms can sometimes assist in the diagnosis of drowning. The pathologist should also consider why an individual has drowned. Why were they incapable of saving themselves? The answer to such questions may lie in an assessment of the circumstances (such as fast-flowing rivers and strong currents), although it also is paramount to assess natural disease and toxicology in these cases.

Firearms

Firearms injuries can generally be categorized into those caused by rifled weapons and those caused by shotguns firing pellet cartridges. Rifled weapons fire bullets, and the rifling of the spiral-grooved gun barrel causes the bullet to spin and remain in stable flight. Shotguns usually fire a bolus of small projectiles (shot), housed in a cartridge. Both the pellets, cartridge, propellant, and expelled gases are capable of causing injuries from shotgun discharges.

Standard assessment of firearm injuries includes description of the number of missiles fired, direction of the shot, internal injury, and range of fire. Prior to post-mortem assessment, full body radiographs should be undertaken to identify the number of retained missiles. A ballistics expert should also be consulted prior to the external examination, so that the correct samples can be retrieved for later forensic assessment in the laboratory.

If the gunshot wound is believed to have been self-inflicted, it is important to assess the hands for minor injury or soot staining, which may be caused when the weapon discharges. Swabbing for gunshot residue using specially designed kits (to reduced artefactual contamination) may be important to perform on such cases. Measurements of the limbs should also be recorded, to ensure that the individual is capable of pulling the trigger of a weapon.

Rifled Weapon: Entry Wounds

A typical entry wound comprises a central defect surrounded by a rim of abrasion, which is caused as the bullet passes through the epidermis. At the abrasion rim, oils from the missile may be wiped off, which may be of forensic significance. The shape of the entry hole and width of the surrounding abrasion rim should be carefully noted, as this can indicate the direction that the missile passed into the skin. A wider abrasion rim on one side of an oval gunshot entry, with under-shelving of the wound opposite, indicates that the strike was angled towards the skin towards the abraded end.

Rifled Weapon: Exit Wounds

Exit wounds are often rather ragged and are sometimes accompanied by additional lacerations caused by bone being driven into the skin. A typical exit wound has no abrasion rim. However, if the skin is resting against a firm object when the missile exits, the edges of the wound can become crushed, leading to the formation of abrasion. This shored-up exit wound, because of the abrasion, can sometimes be confused with an entry wound.

Bone Injury

When it is unclear from the external examination of the skin whether a gunshot wound is an entry or an exit wound, bone injury may be able to assist. Skull bone comprises an inner and outer table. A smaller hole is formed in the table that the missile first penetrates, and a larger hole is formed in the second table passed through. Thus, with an entry wound, the inner table has a larger defect than the outer table, and with an exit wound the reverse is true: the outer table has the larger defect. If multiple entry wounds are present in the skull, causing radiating skull fractures, it is possible to determine the order that each missile was fired using Puppe's rule, wherein a new fracture will terminate when it comes to a pre-existing fracture. This means that the pattern of interlocking fractures may be seen as a sequence of successive injuries, allowing the first and later events to be defined.

Shotgun Entry Wound

Contact shotgun wounds can be devastating, and it may be difficult to identify the precise location of discharge. Soot staining can assist in determining the location of the weapon discharge, and careful reconstruction of the edges of lacerations can re-form the entry hole. Contact wounds may also show a distinct muzzle mark: as the gases from the discharge enter the skin, the skin is forced back against the metal of the muzzle to form a well-defined rim of abrasion. Double-barreled shotguns can leave two muzzle marks, one with a ragged central hole from the discharge.

Upon exiting the barrel of a shotgun, the pellet mass begins to spread out. With increasing range, the shape of the shotgun entry wounds changes. Scalloping of the wounds edges and separate entry holes caused by individual pellets are observed with increasing range. The presence of any of these features must raise the suspicion that the discharge was made by a third party, rather than being a self-inflicted wound.

Blunt Force Head Injury

Blunt force head injury is a very common mode of death in forensic practice. Detailed external examination of the face and scalp can assist in determining the implement used to cause injury. Indeed, the head hair should be shaved off to reveal subtle injuries, so that they may be documented photographically. The under surface of the scalp and face should be inspected for deep bruising not otherwise visible externally. The calvarium should be inspected for fractures. Removal of the temporalis muscles and aponeurosis (which can be rubbed off with a blade or abrasive pad) should be undertaken to expose subtle hairline fractures. Similarly, it also may be necessary to strip muscle from the bones of the face to reveal fractures.

The calvarium should be opened carefully, so as not to damage the underlying dura mater. The cranial contents can then be inspected for extradural haemorrhage, before the dura is incised. Observation of the subdural space can then be made for bleeding. At this stage, the frontal lobes can be gently lifted in order to visualize the base of the brain, enabling assessment for basal subarachnoid haemorrhage. Once satisfied, the brain can be removed in the standard way. The dura at the base of the brain can then be stripped to expose the base of the skull, permitting inspection of the basal skull bone.

Extradural Haematoma

Extradural haemorrhage (the collection of blood is known as a haematoma) is the accumulation of blood between the under surface of the inner cranial bone and the external surface of the dura mater. Invariably it is associated with skull fracture, as the fracture lines damage underlying calvarial arteries. The middle meningeal arteries are particularly vulnerable, as they are covered by the relatively thin squamous part of the temporal bone. As with subdural haemorrhage, individuals with extradural haemorrhage may be characterized by a variable period of lucidity before later collapse.

Subdural Haematoma

Subdural haematomas accumulate beneath the dura mater, above the surface of the brain. When force is transmitted through the cranial cavity, the brain tissue can deform to an extent. The bridging veins, which are tethered to the dura mater, stretch as the brain tissue deforms, and can then shear. The sheared vessels result in bleeding, causing subdural haematoma formation. In individuals with cerebral atrophy, the bridging veins become slightly stretched and are more vulnerable to shearing, so less force may be necessary to cause subdural bleeding. Subdural haematomas are almost invariably caused by trauma. Very rarely, ruptured cerebral aneurysms can force jets of haemorrhage through the brain tissue to erupt into the subdural space, mimicking injury. Similarly, other natural intracranial haemorrhages can enter the subdural space, but they are usually readily distinguished from true trauma.

Cerebral Contusions, Coup and Contre-Coup

Cerebral contusions, bruises to the brain surface, are often accompanied by superficial laceration. Direct blows with a blunt weapon may cause contusion to the brain directly beneath the impact site—a "coup" lesion contusion. Conversely, falls onto a hard, unyielding surface, such as the pavement or tarmac, cause contusion on the opposite side of the brain. Typically, unprotected falls onto the back of the head cause abrasion about the occiput with skull fracturing radiating forwards towards the foramen magnum. Subdural haemorrhage is invariably present, but the characteristic finding is of contre-coup contusions over the poles of the frontal and temporal lobes and contusion in the region of the olfactory bulbs. Another common finding that accompanies contre-coup head injuries is fractures to the supraorbital plates. The precise mechanism by which the supraorbital fractures develop is poorly understood, although radiated force or changes in the intracranial pressure may be responsible. They are of forensic significance, and bleeding from these fractures may spread to the periorbital tissues, mimicking a "black eye" caused by a blow such as a punch.

Traumatic Basal Subarachnoid Haemorrhage

When there is a forceful angular rotation of the skull upon the spinal column, the vertebral arteries may traumatically rupture, causing fatal basal traumatic subarachnoid haemorrhage. The rupture may be caused by direct shearing forces placed on the arteries at the junction, although a water hammer effect may also cause rupturing. Typically, deep dissection of the facial tissues reveals injury in the region of one of the angles of the jaw. Dissection of the extracranial vertebral arteries is detailed above, and the intracranial portion of the vertebral arteries should also be carefully examined. Removal of the cerebral hemispheres above the tentorium gives much easier access to the intracranial portions and basilar artery, facilitating easy removal. In addition, sampling of other arteries elsewhere in the body is valuable, to exclude a vasculopathy. Histological assessment of the entire vertebral arteries should be made to exclude a natural cause for the haemorrhage. Trauma is characterized histologically by areas of nuclear lysis, focal dissection, and fibrin plugs.

Late Complications of Head Injury

Late complications of head injury can lead to death a considerable time after the injuries were originally sustained. Complications include posttraumatic epilepsy, bacterial meningitis, and bronchopneumonia from reduced mobility. In every case where epilepsy is believed to be the cause of death, the medical records should be carefully inspected, even traced back for years, to ensure that head injury was not the cause of the seizure activity.

Bacterial meningitis can complicate head injuries in which skull fractures traverse the airway, middle ears, or frontal sinuses. This complication of head injury usually occurs relatively early (days or weeks) following infliction of the head injury. Bronchopneumonia can be a terminal feature of head injury that can develop many months or years after the incident. In order to consider whether the pneumonia was caused by the head injury, a clinical review must be made to ensure that the head injury was the cause of immobility or gastric content aspiration, rather than another disease process acting independently.

Skull Fractures

Broadly, skull fractures can be classed as linear (simple or complex) or depressed. Higher-energy impacts can cause severe basal skull fractures, such as the "hinge" fracture or the "ring" fracture. Linear injuries can be encountered from practically any form of blunt force trauma applied to the skull, but depressed skull fractures always raise the possibility that a blunt weapon has been used, and caution should be employed upon their discovery.

Skull fractures also may be hidden beneath the dura mater, so this should be carefully stripped away from the calvarium to expose the underling bone. Occasionally, fractures may also develop away from the impact site, commonly within the thin supraorbital plates. The precise mechanism is not fully understood, but this phenomenon is likely the result of transmitted forces or rapid changes in intracranial pressure caused by the initial impact. The form and length of skull fractures should be documented. Where possible, it is also of value to document the thickness of the skull in the region of the fracture. Puppe's rule may be relevant in these cases.

Forensic Radiology

Forensic pathologists have used radiology as an investigative tool since the inception of forensic pathology as a specialty. Plain radiographs were commonly used to identify metallic fragments within the body, including bullets and knife tips amongst other foreign objects. Other uses, which are still pertinent today, include the radiological study of foetal/infant/childhood skeletons for the identification of a separate existence, gestational age, skeletal dysplasia and skeletal injury. In recent years, there has been increasing use of post mortem computed tomography (PMCT) in forensic pathology as an adjunct to the traditional post mortem examination. The additional information provided by the PMCT can be particularly helpful in elucidating all the pathological features, pre-planning the approach to an autopsy and also potentially limiting some dissections. One particular use of PMCT in forensic pathology is assisting a court in understanding the nature of the pathology without necessarily having to present the decision makers (judge, jury) with confronting images of injuries. Furthermore, it is also possible to three-dimensionally reconstruct and print out some injuries (particularly bone fractures) to assist the courts. More recently, forensic pathology has also enjoyed the use of MicroCT scanning. Detailed three-dimensional images are now possible of smaller structures, such as the adult larynx, to identify the location of fractures. This can help focus pathological sampling and three-dimensional reconstruction can be used in the court room.

Figures 12.1, 12.2, 12.3, 12.4, 12.5, 12.6, 12.7, 12.8, 12.9, 12.10, 12.11, 12.12, 12.13, 12.14, 12.15, 12.16, 12.17, 12.18, 12.19, 12.20, 12.21, 12.22, 12.23, 12.24, 12.25, 12.26, 12.27, 12.28, 12.29, 12.30, 12.31, 12.32, 12.33, 12.34, 12.35, 12.36, 12.37, 12.38, 12.39, 12.40, 12.41, 12.42, 12.43, 12.44, 12.45, 12.46, 12.47, 12.48, 12.49, 12.50, 12.51, 12.52, 12.53, 12.54, 12.55, 12.56, 12.57, 12.58, 12.59, 12.60, 12.61, 12.62, 12.63, 12.64, 12.65, 12.66, 12.67, 12.68, 12.69, 12.70, 12.71, 12.72, 12.73, 12.74, 12.75, 12.76, 12.77, 12.78, 12.79, 12.80, 12.81, 12.82, 12.83, 12.84, 12.85, 12.86, 12.87, 12.88, 12.89, 12.90, 12.91, 12.92, 12.93, 12.94, 12.95, 12.96, 12.97, 12.98, 12.99, 12.100, 12.101, 12.102, 12.103, and 12.104 illustrate the points made in this chapter.

The author acknowledges Greater Manchester Police for their permission to use some of the materials in this chapter.

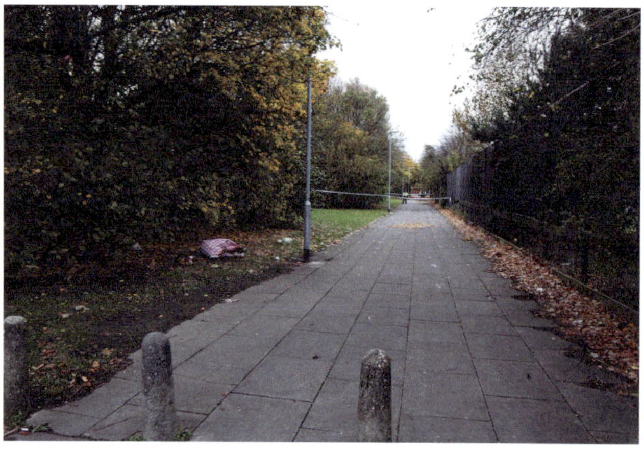

Fig. 12.1 A typical scene greeting a forensic pathologist. Protected by a police guard and cordoned off by taping, the outdoor nature of this incident in a public place warranted an urgent visit by the pathologist with a view to restoring the scene to public access

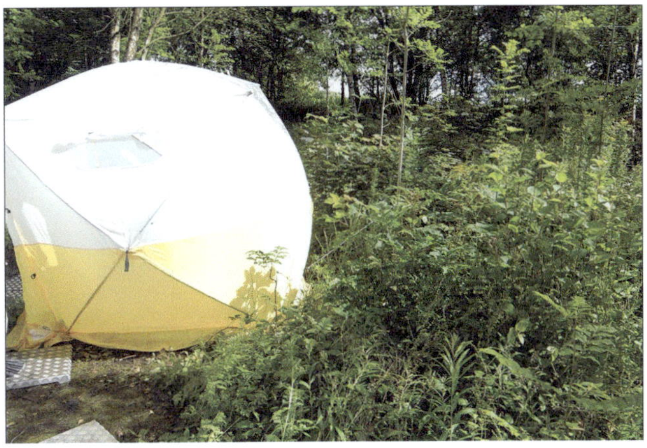

Fig. 12.2 Scene tents are often employed in outside scenes. In addition to providing privacy for the deceased from public gaze, the scene tent protects the body from exposure to the elements, ensuring critical evidence is recovered

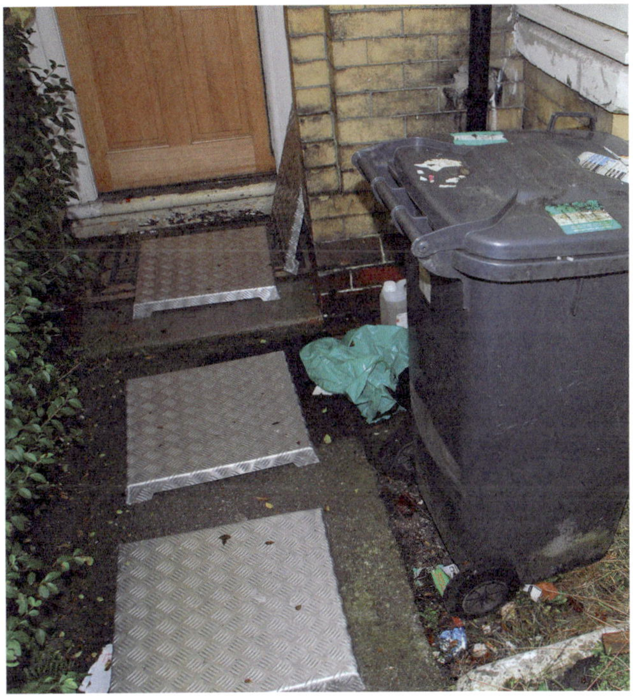

Fig. 12.3 Stepping plates show the pathologist the predetermined pathway into the scene, whilst protecting evidence, such as footprints in blood, from becoming damaged

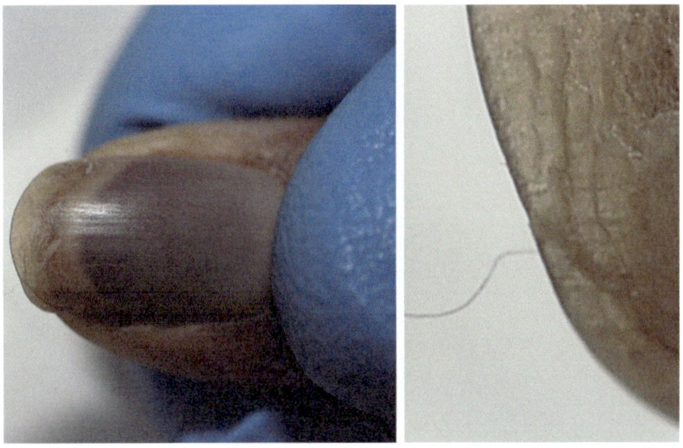

Fig. 12.4 Here is an example of subtle but critical evidence identified by the forensic pathologist under a fingernail at the scene of a death. Without sampling at the scene, this fibre would have been lost in transportation

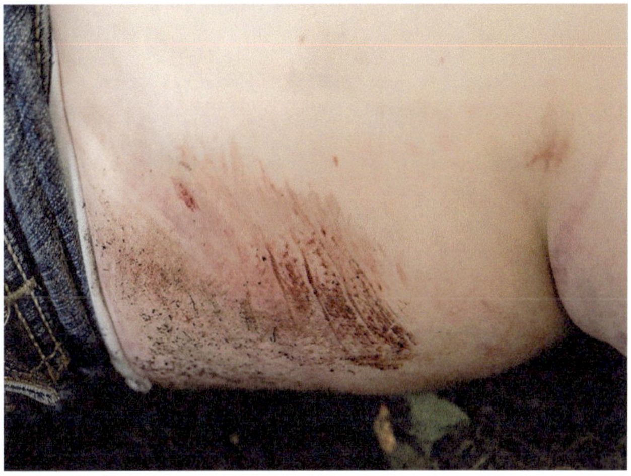

Fig. 12.5 A patterned stain in blood on the deceased's torso is shown here. The forensic pathologist identified this mark which was then photographically documented in the scene. The mark smeared off during transportation to the mortuary

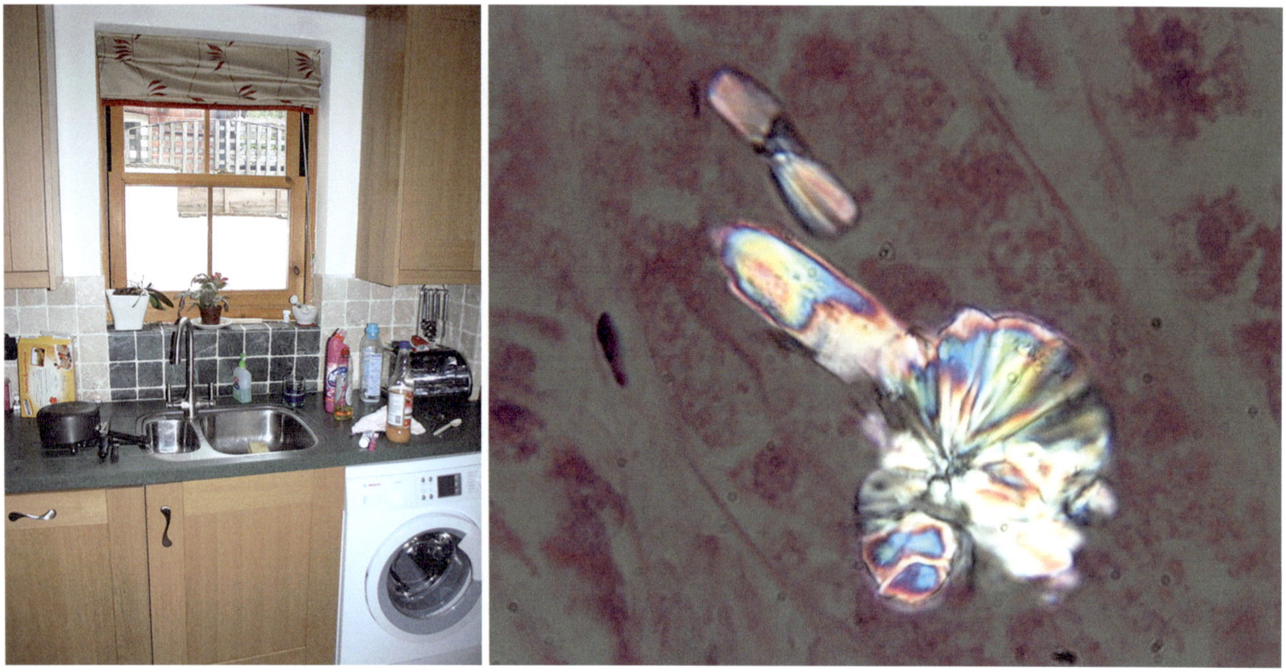

Fig. 12.6 This case involved a female, aged 36 years, in a relationship involving alleged domestic violence. Careful inspection of the scene helped expedite the case management, with the cause of death (ethylene glycol toxicity) confirmed histologically in the form of calcium oxalate crystals in the kidney

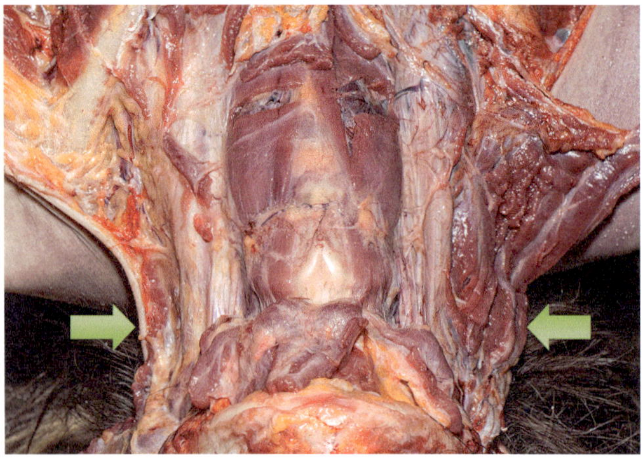

Fig. 12.7 The neck is shown exposed. Each individual muscle can be stripped back and inspected both externally and internally. The scalene muscles (*arrows*) can also be dissected

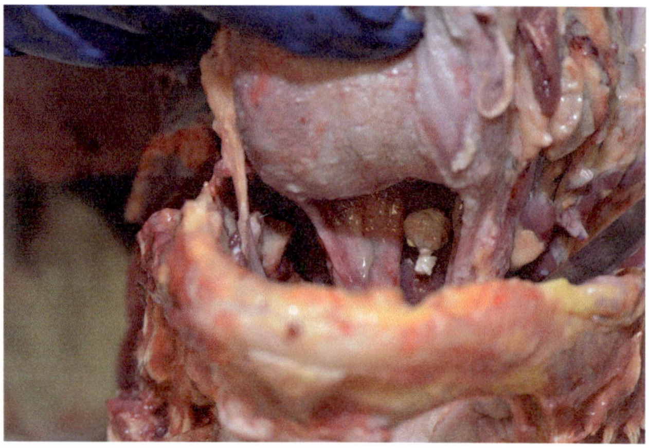

Fig. 12.8 An advantage of the "V" neck incision is that the contents of the nasopharynx can be exposed with minimal disturbance, allowing inspection of the contents. Here a drug wrap was occluding the upper airway

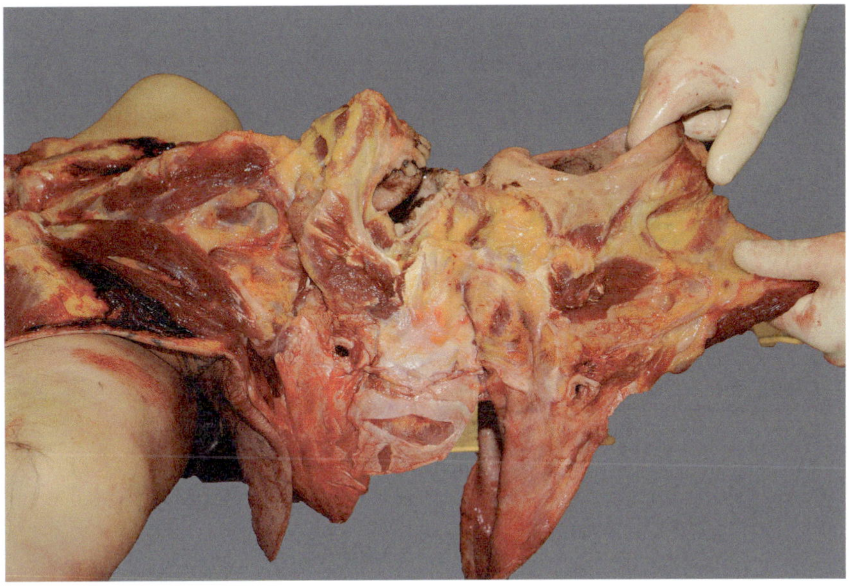

Fig. 12.9 The exposed facial tissues can be readily inspected for deep bruising and fractures

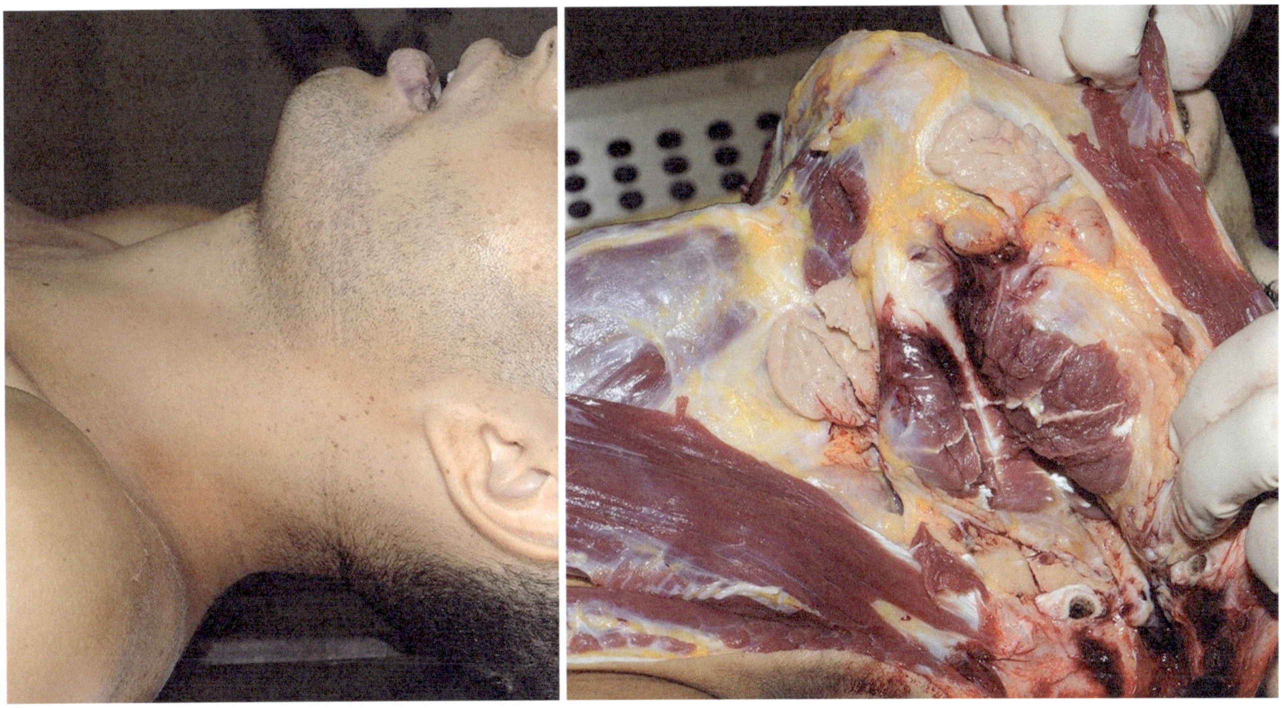

Fig. 12.10 A case of death from a subdural haematoma following an alleged blow. No external injury was visible but subcutaneous facial dissection revealed a bruise to the mandible

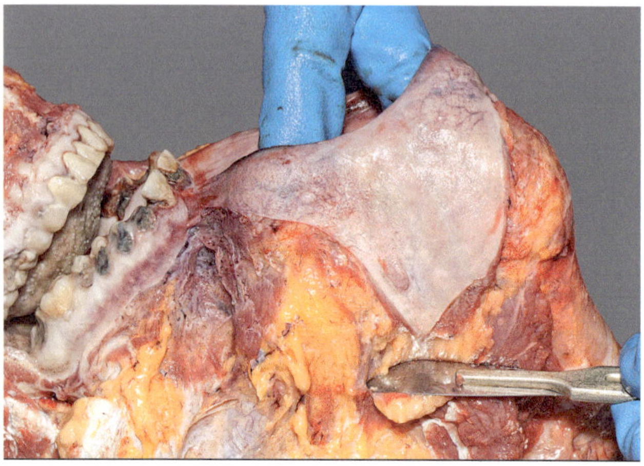

Fig. 12.11 The lips are carefully incised to expose subtle deep bruising. This is a case of smothering

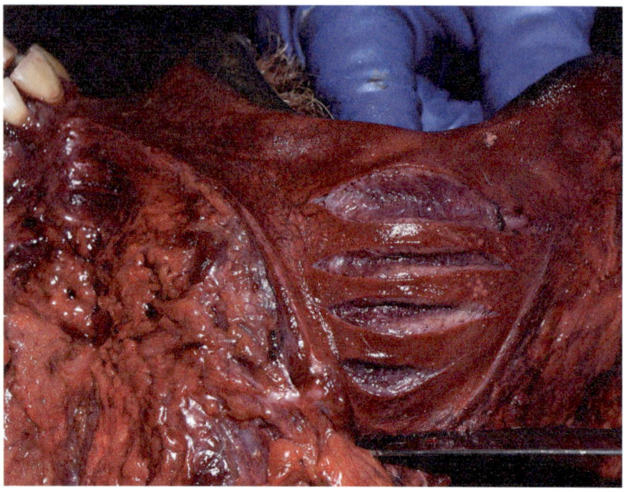

Fig. 12.12 In a lip dissection, superficial incisions are made to expose the underlying submucosa to reveal hidden bruising

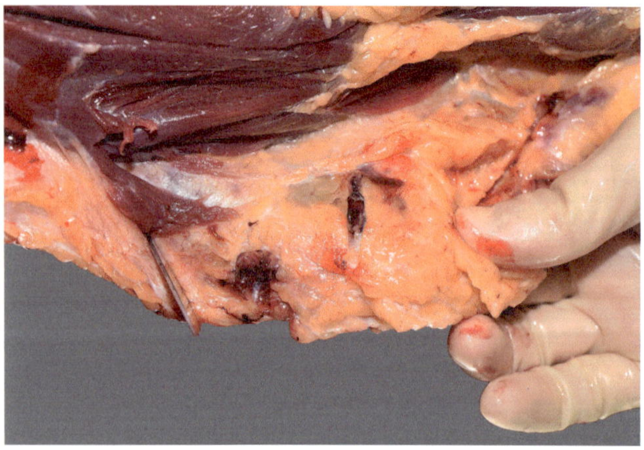

Fig. 12.13 The superficial fatty and deep subcutaneous tissues are carefully examined for hidden bruises

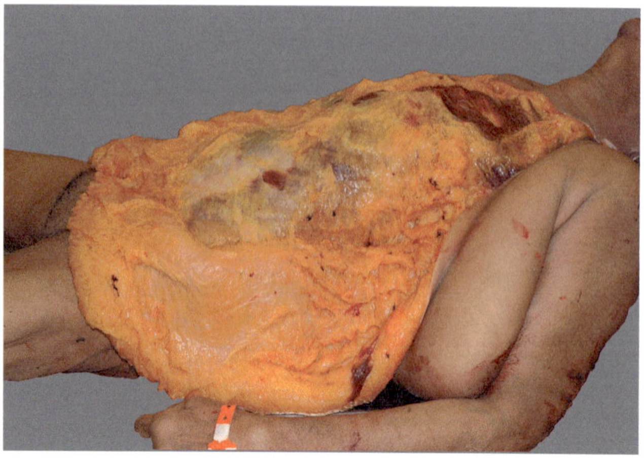

Fig. 12.14 The abdominal subcutis has been extensively dissected to look for deep bruising

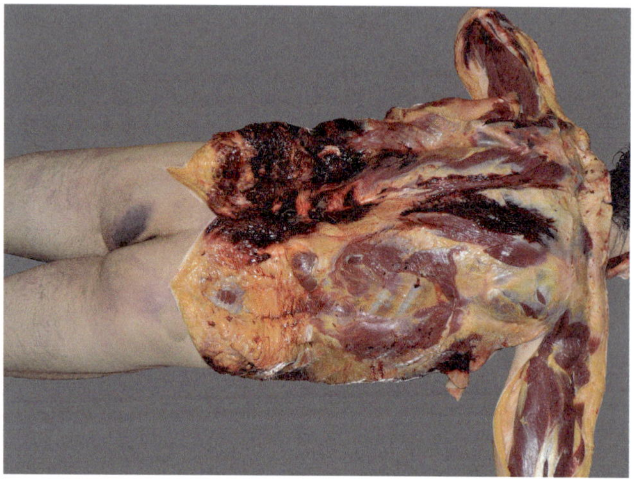

Fig. 12.15 Here is an example of subcutaneous dissection of the back revealing large bruises, not visible externally

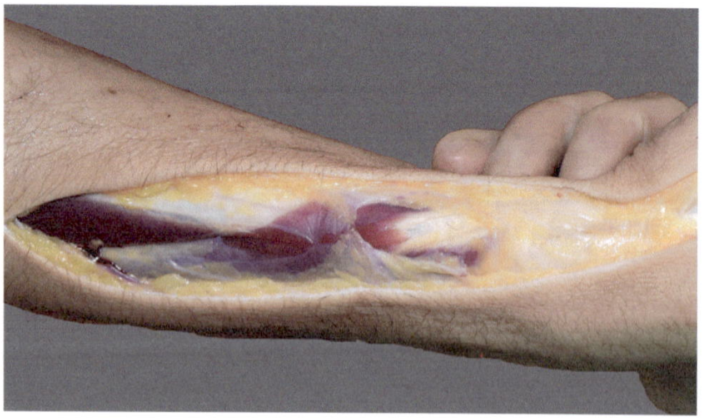

Fig. 12.16 Subcutaneous forearm dissection. Stage 1

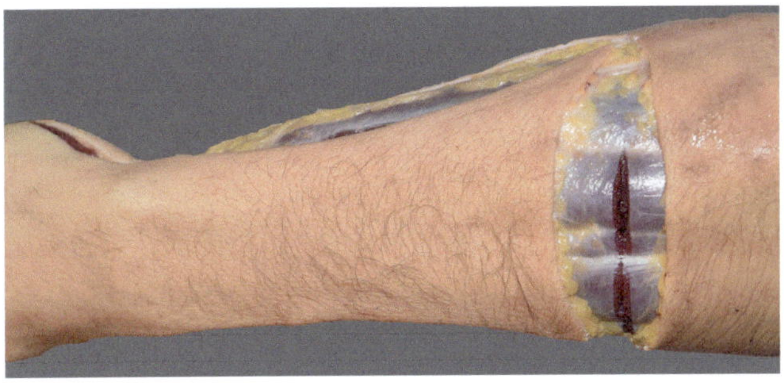

Fig. 12.17 Subcutaneous forearm dissection. Stage 2

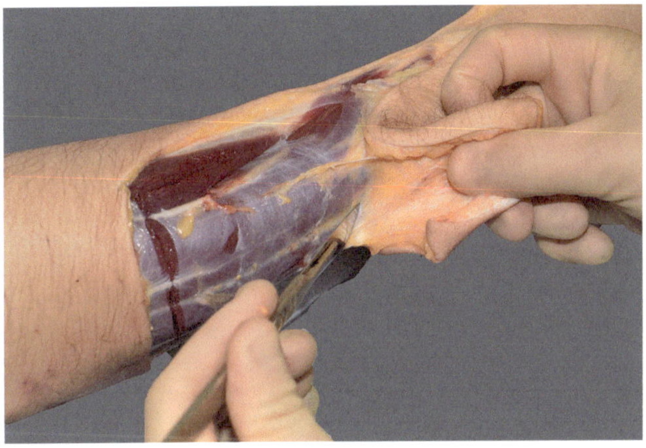

Fig. 12.18 Subcutaneous forearm dissection. Stage 3

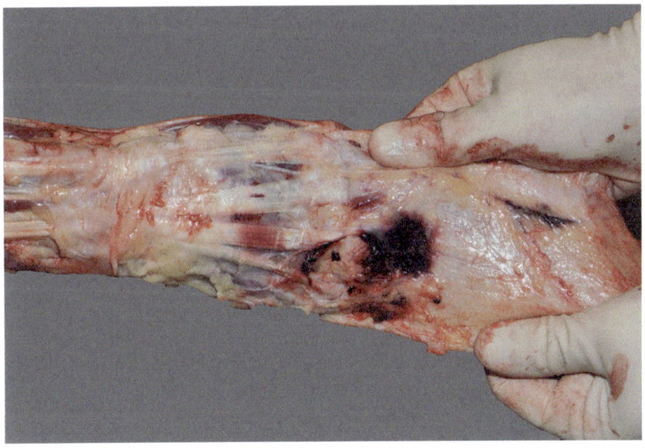

Fig. 12.19 Subcutaneous forearm dissection. Stage 4. The superficial incisions form the flap, which is dissected distally

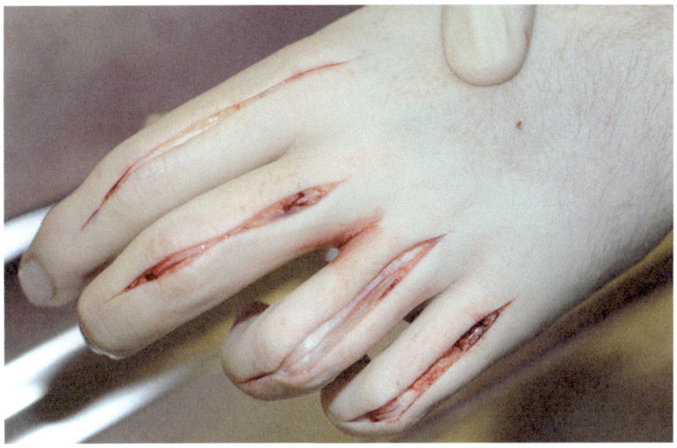

Fig. 12.20 The traditional method of inspection for knuckle bruising involves longitudinal incisions to the fingers. Although effective at identifying injury, such incisions can be distressing for the family during viewings

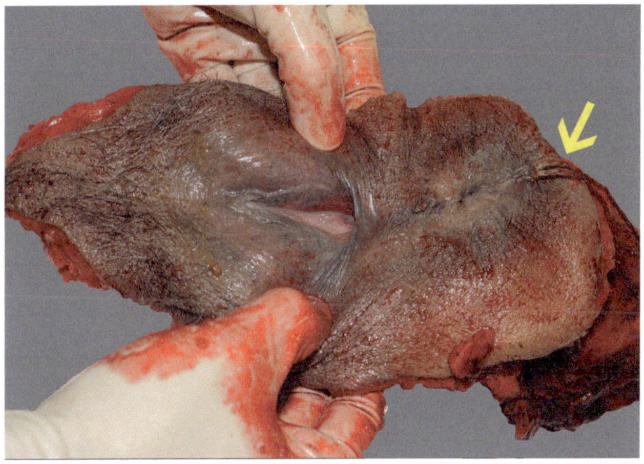

Fig. 12.21 An anogenital block is shown fully excised, permitting ready assessment and access for imaging. A marker is placed (*arrow*) for orientation

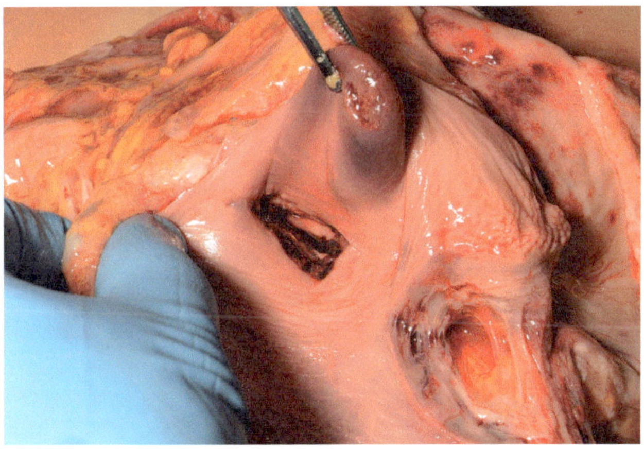

Fig. 12.22 The anogenital block in a female permits access to the intact genital tract, allowing careful inspection in the absence of autopsy artefacts. Here, a laceration to the posterior vaginal fornix is evident, an area often disrupted by standard dissection techniques

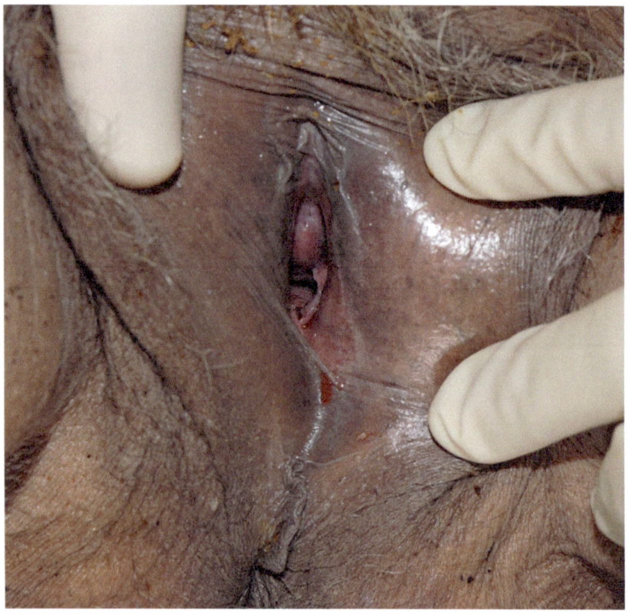

Fig. 12.23 Traditional inspection of the vulva, particularly with atrophic skin, can often induce injury artefact in areas such as the posterior labial commissure, as seen here

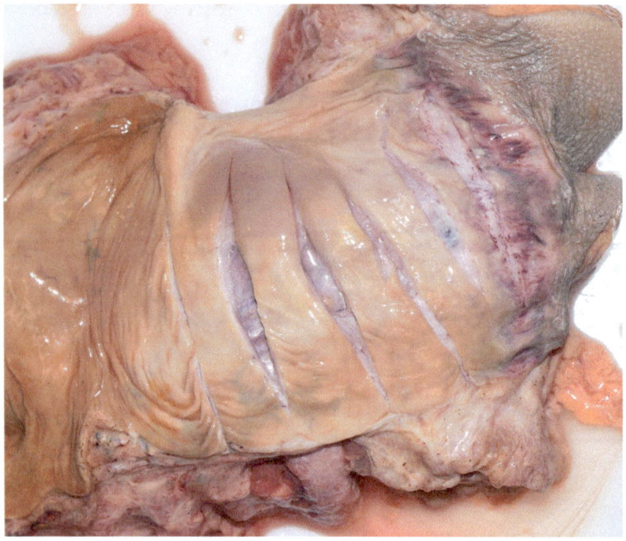

Fig. 12.24 Anogenital block dissection permits inspection of the anal skin, anal canal, rectal mucosa and, with incision as seen here, the rectal submucosa. Similar inspection can be made of the vagina

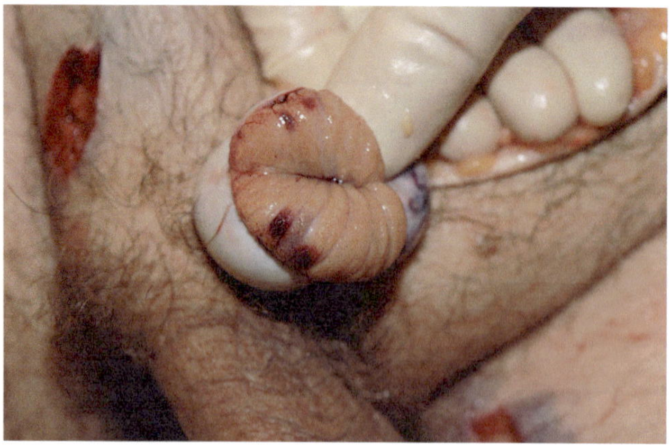

Fig. 12.25 Inspection of testes, accessed via the pelvic brim with blunt dissection into the scrotum, can reveal hidden injuries. Here parenchymal bruising to the testes is evident following a kick

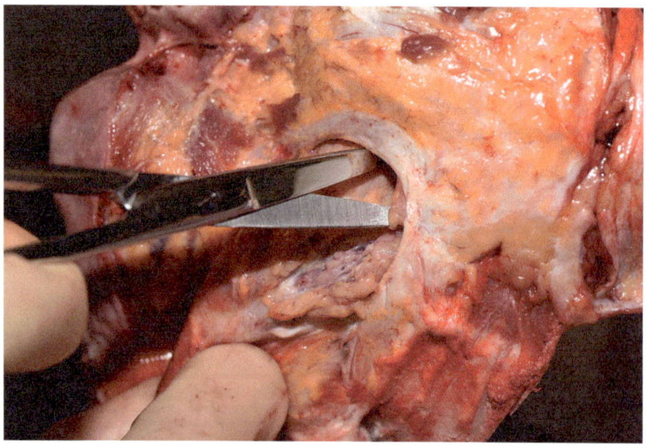

Fig. 12.26 Orbital dissection (1). Blunt dissection of the lateral wall tissues of the orbit is made

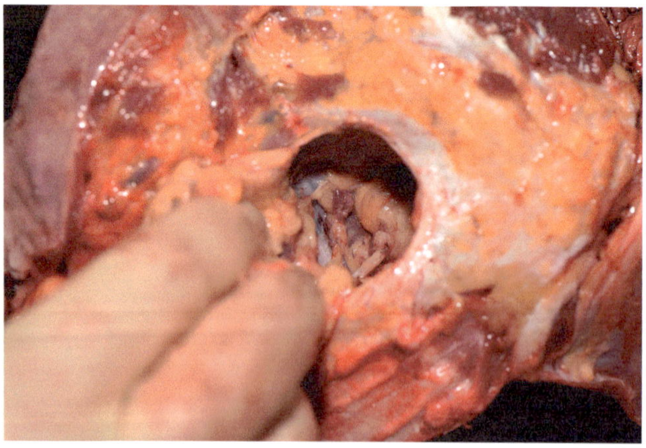

Fig. 12.27 Orbital dissection (2). The eye is removed after the optic nerve is cut

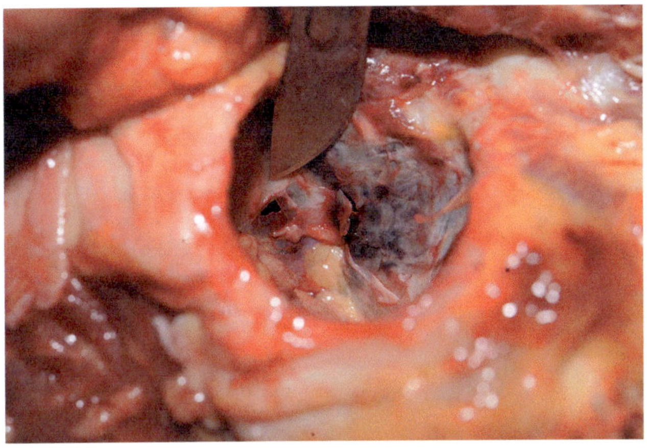

Fig. 12.28 The globe has been removed from the orbit to expose fractures of the medial orbital wall. Care should be taken when removing the globe, so not to introduce damage to the thin ethmoid bones. In this case, the fracturing was complex and associated with haemorrhage, the vital reaction reassuring of true injury

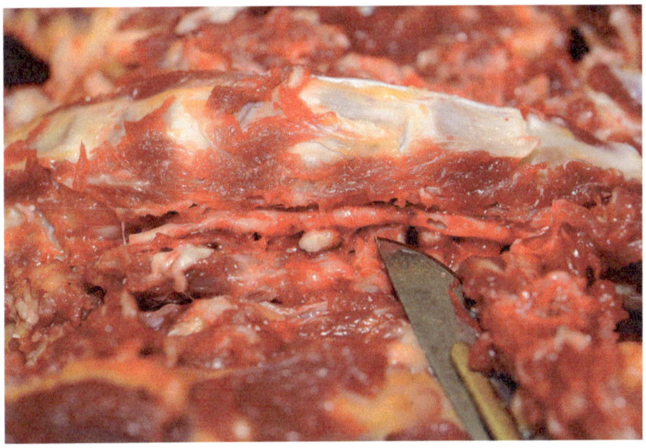

Fig. 12.29 Deroofing the vertebral canal with bone clippers will expose the vertebral canal and artery

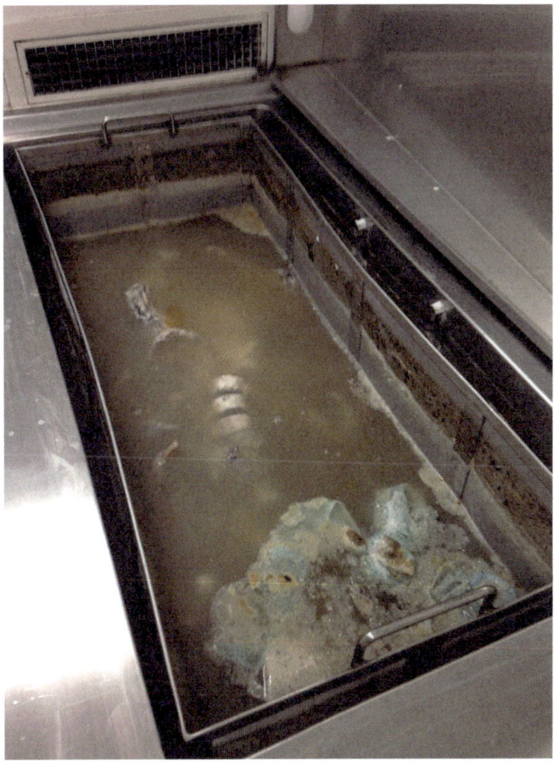

Fig. 12.30 Excarnation or defleshing. Partial defleshing is done using dissection initially. The partially defleshed bones are placed in a bath with biological washing powder at about 37 °C for a week

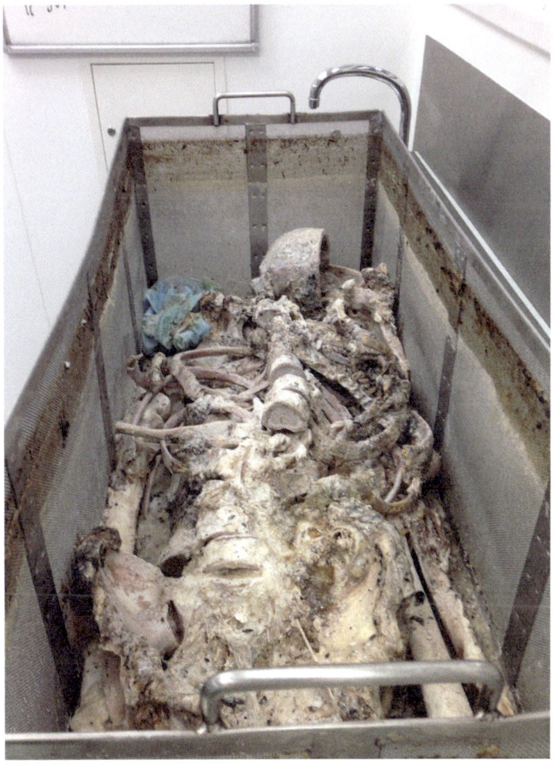

Fig. 12.31 Following drainage of the fluid, the skeleton remains with some adherent soft tissues

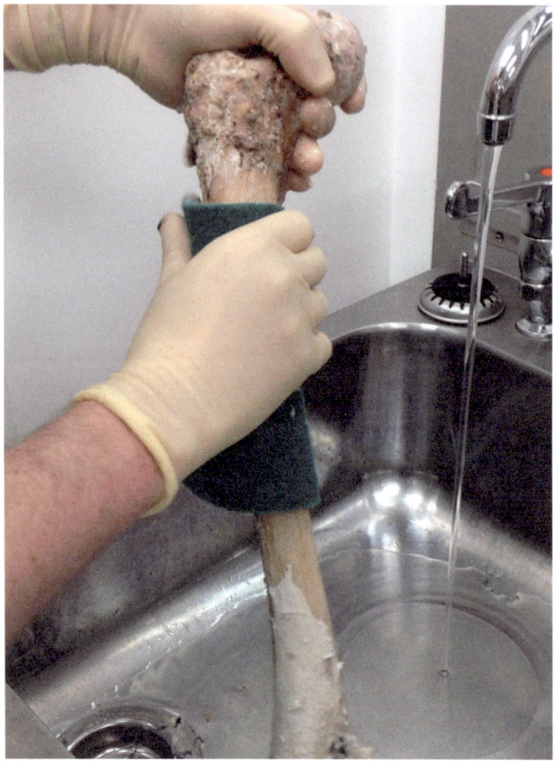

Fig. 12.32 The tissue had loosened enough for simple removal with an abrasive pad

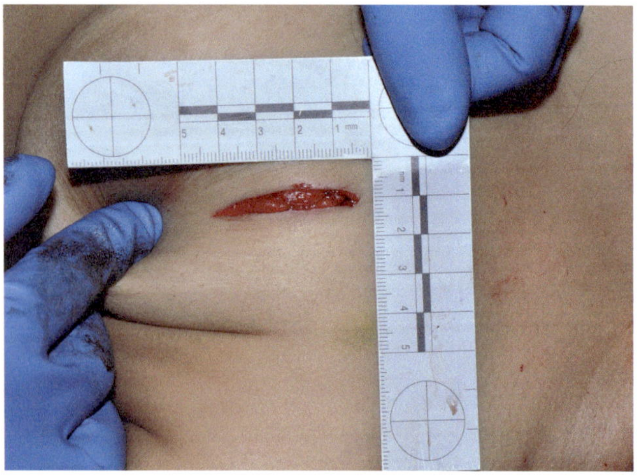

Fig. 12.33 Stab wound. Note the slight tension applied to reflect the true length of the injury. The shape of this injury indicates the passage of a single-edged weapon

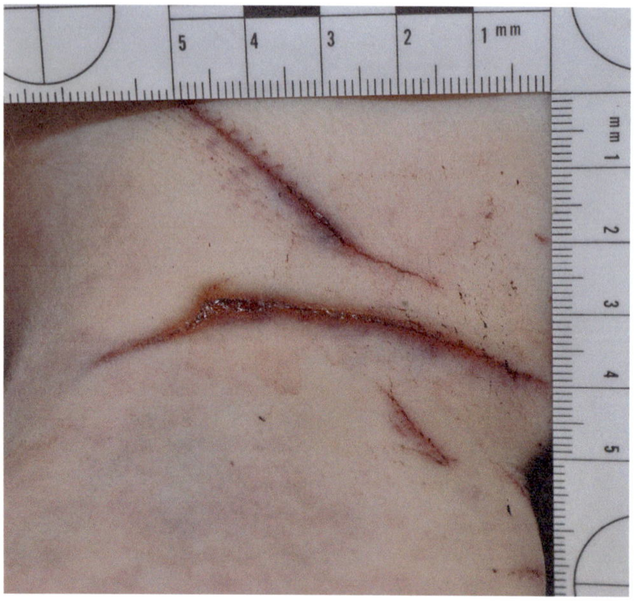

Fig. 12.34 Brushing of the sharp implement across the skin in this case of a fatal stabbing revealed a pattern suggestive of the use of a serrated weapon

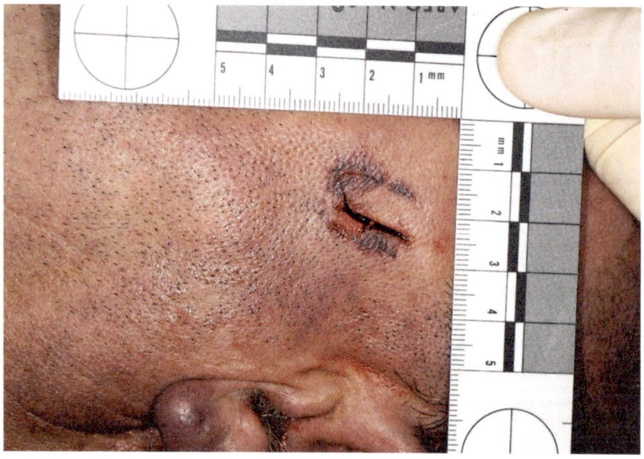

Fig. 12.35 This stab wound penetrated the calvarium, indicating the use of severe force. The curved injury is the assailant's fingernail penetrating the skin, also implying that severe force was used

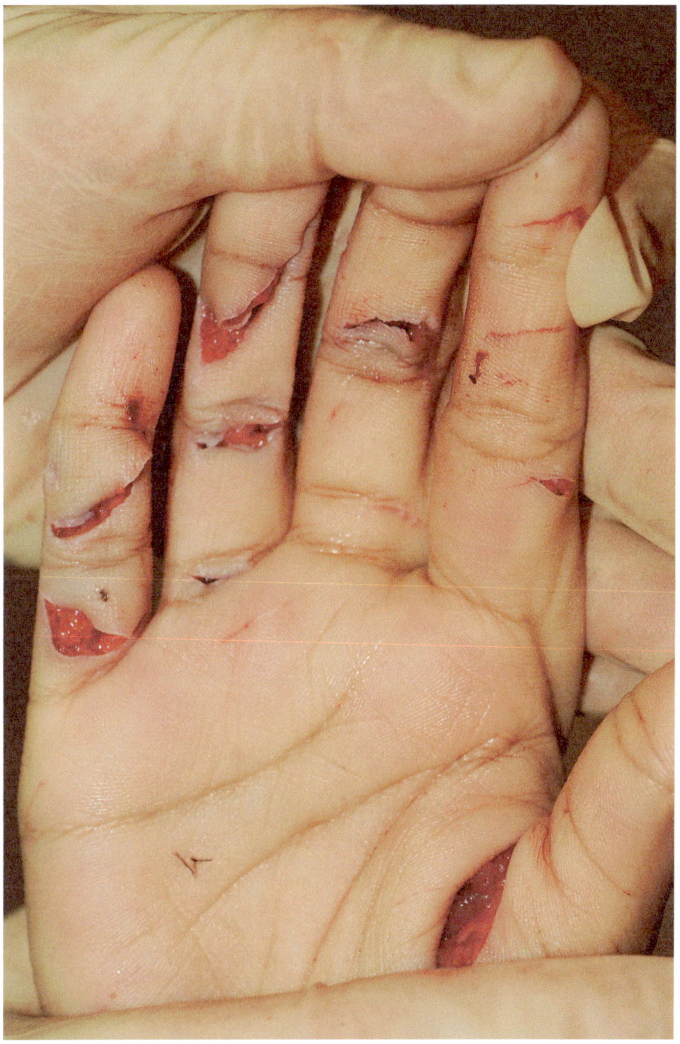

Fig. 12.36 Injuries to the palm caused by grasping a knife—defence injuries

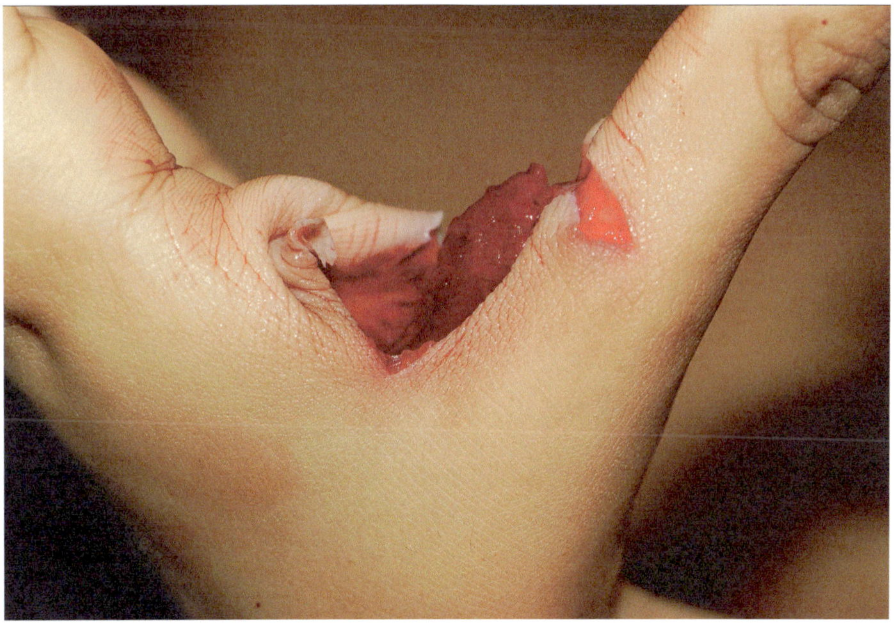

Fig. 12.37 A typical defence injury comprising an incision between the index finger and thumb

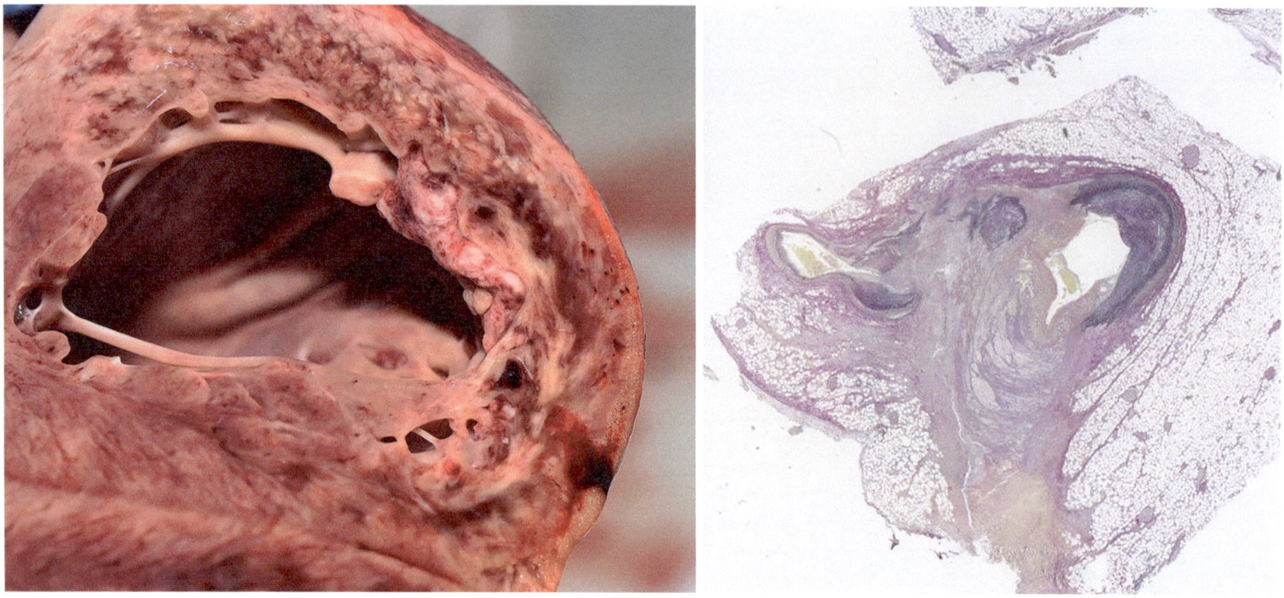

Fig. 12.38 Shown here is a late complication of a stab wound. The initial acute complications of this stab wound involving the left anterior descending coronary artery were survived. Death came 2 weeks later due to myocardial infarction from the injury (seen macroscopically on the left side image). The histological image on the right shows marked disruption of the usual coronary artery architecture at the site of injury

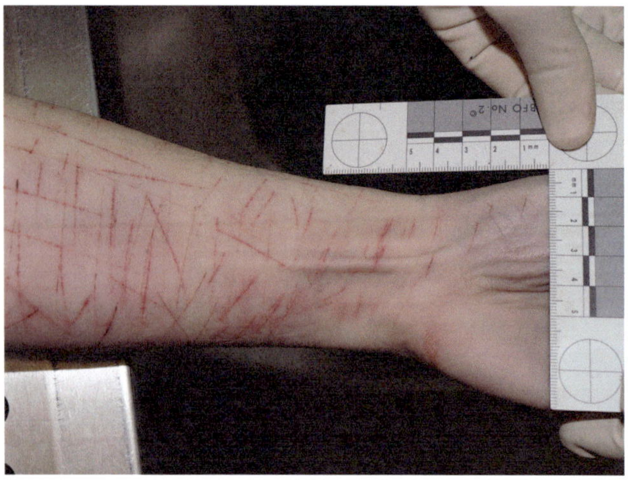

Fig. 12.39 Parallel, superficial and horizontal linear incised wounds, typical of self-inflicted wounds

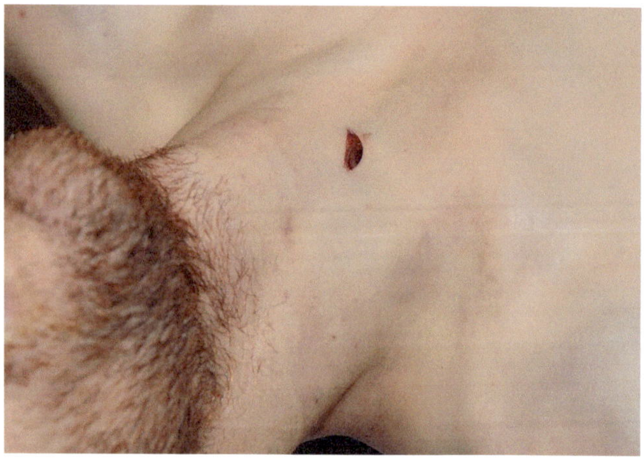

Fig. 12.40 This image is from the same case as Fig. 12.39. The single fatal stab wound is identified in the lower neck. Despite the presence of self-harm injuries, inspection of CCTV footage revealed this was homicidal. The single stab wound to the chest is a difficult entity to interpret

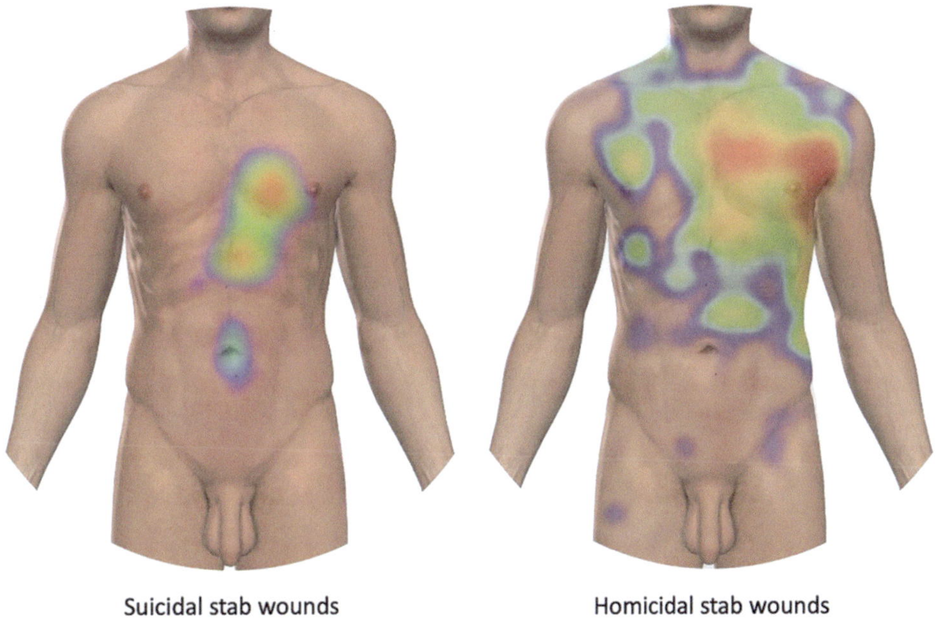

Fig. 12.41 Distribution of fatal self-harm chest stab wounds and homicidal stab wounds (author's own data; red most frequent, to blue, least frequent). Fatal incised wounds are not considered in this diagram

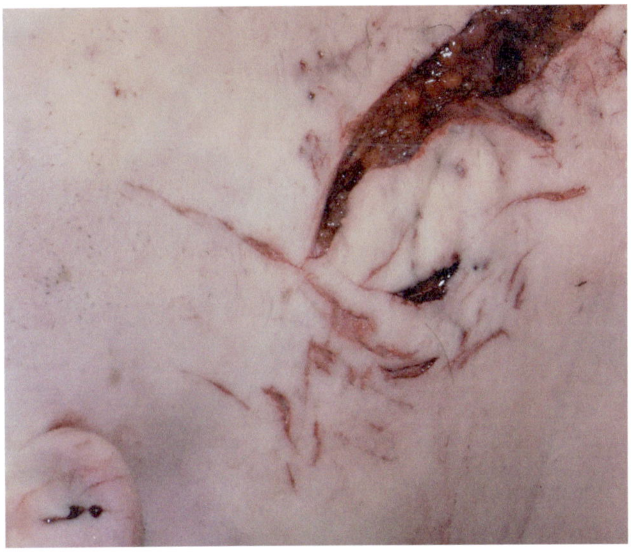

Fig. 12.42 A case of fatal glass injury wherein a beer glass was thrust into the neck. Note the complex pattern of incision. One shard had penetrated the carotid artery leading to death at the scene

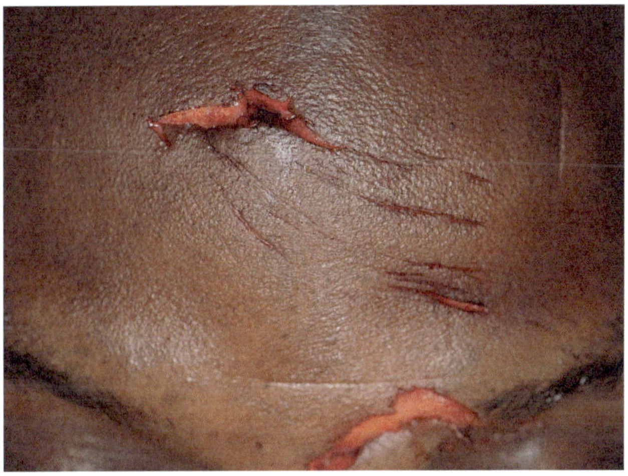

Fig. 12.43 A fatal assault due to a glass bottle smashed upon the forehead causing sweeping complex incised wounds

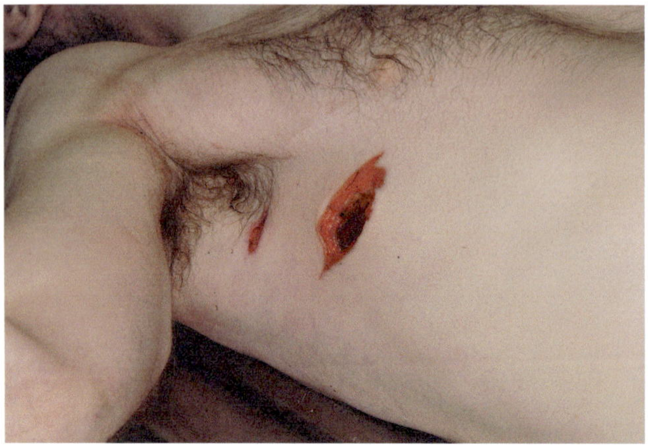

Fig. 12.44 It is imperative to have the emergency medical notes available at the time of an autopsy. As seen here, medical intervention can mimic injury. The superior injury is true stab wound and the inferior injury is from thoracostomy during resuscitation attempts

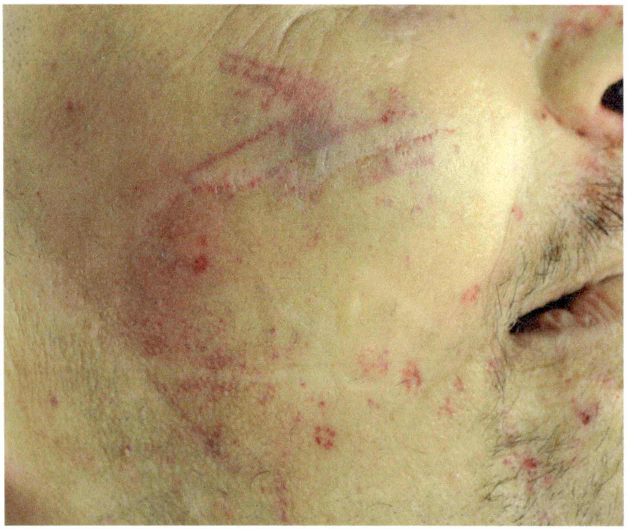

Fig. 12.45 A footwear mark on the face with red intradermal bruising

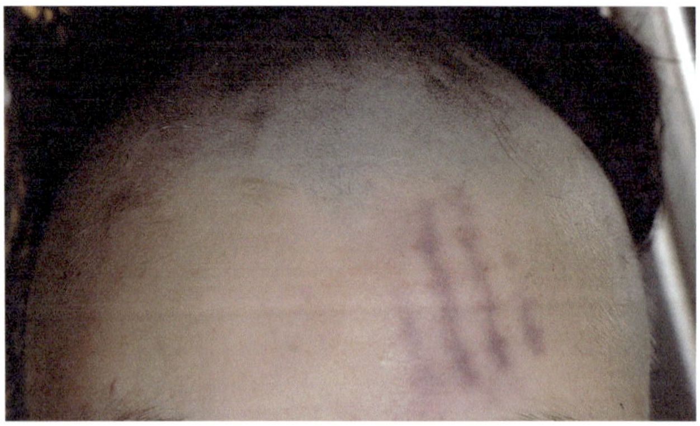

Fig. 12.46 A footwear mark on the forehead. Note the head hair has been shaved by the pathologist. This can reveal hidden injuries, as in this case

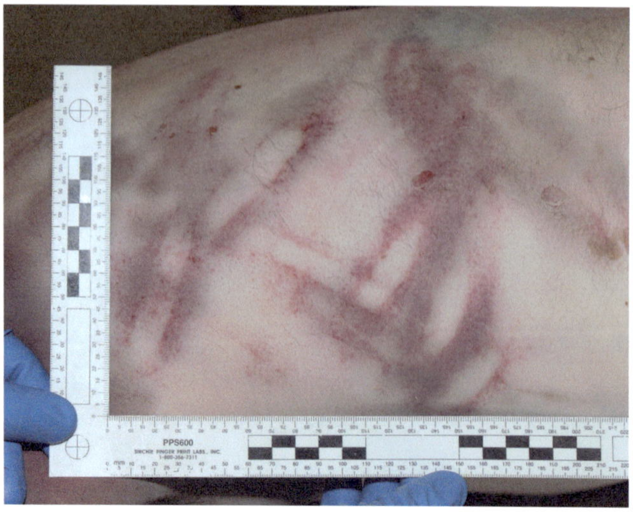

Fig. 12.47 Tramline bruise caused by repeated strikes from a baseball bat

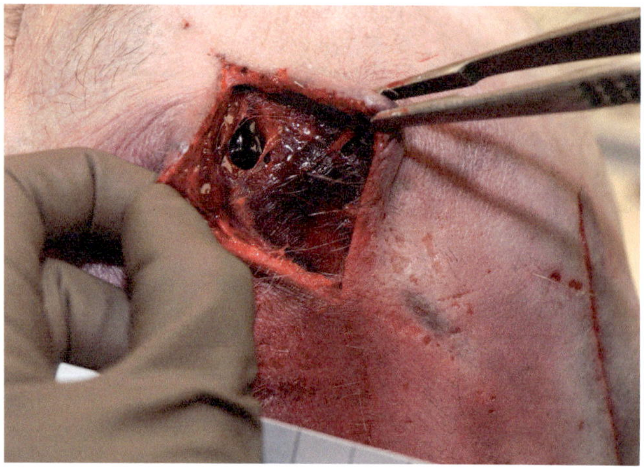

Fig. 12.48 Linear laceration mimicking an incised wound. Tissue bridges are evident deep within the injury, indicating the use of blunt force

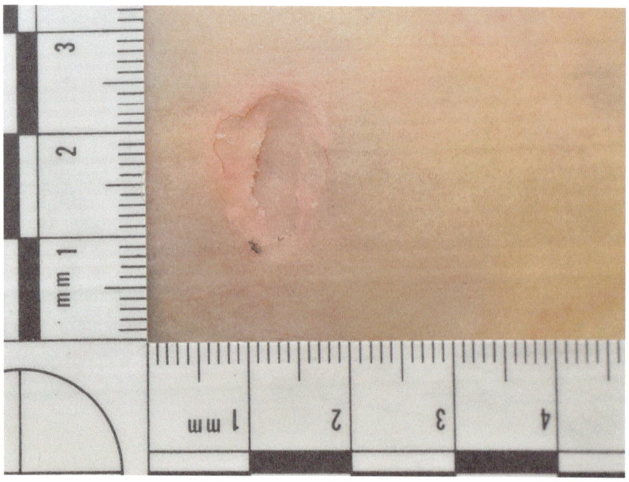

Fig. 12.49 Depressed skull fracture underneath a curved laceration: a typical hammer blow

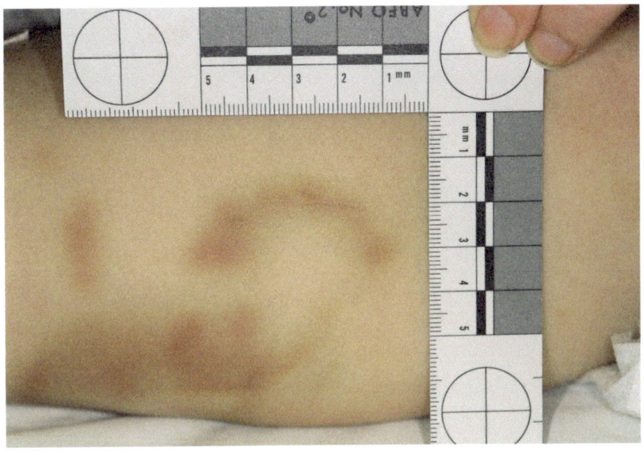

Fig. 12.50 This is a curve of bruising. An odontologist confirmed that this was a bite mark caused by an adult

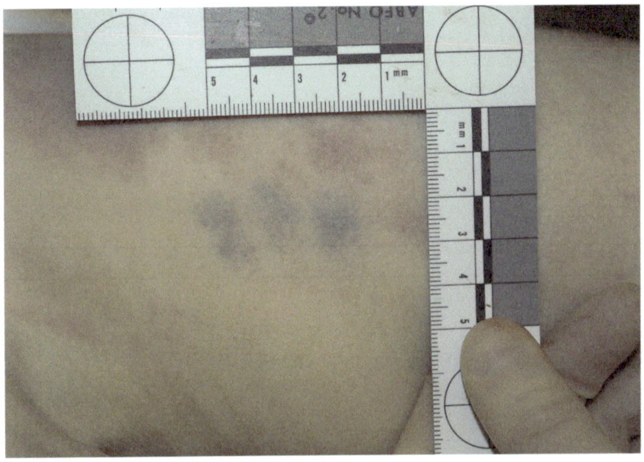

Fig. 12.51 Grip mark on the inner thigh in a suspicious death

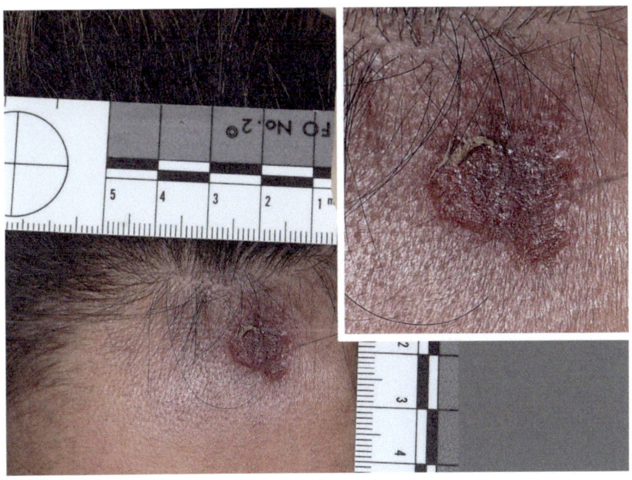

Fig. 12.52 An abrasion scroll is seen at the upper edge of the injury. The individual was dragged by the heels. High magnification (inset) shows the scroll towards the edge

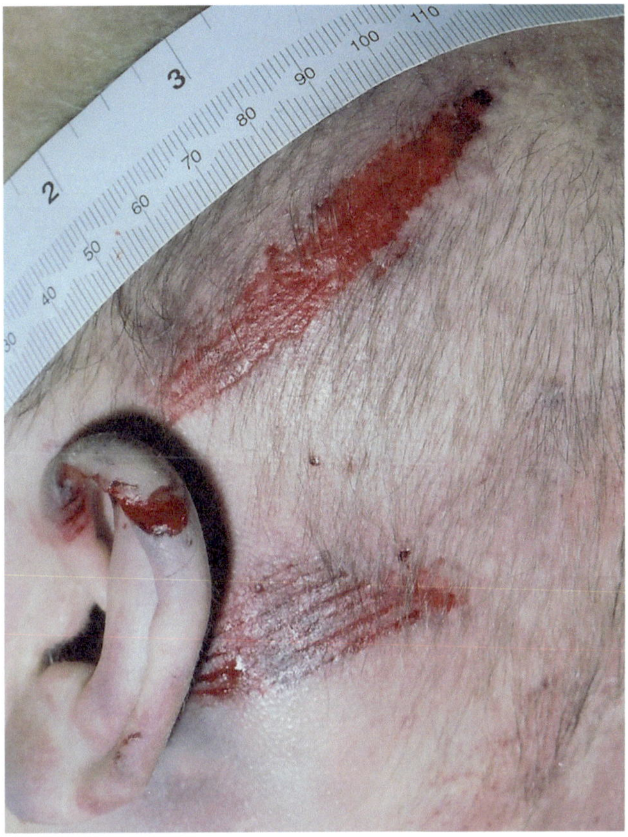

Fig. 12.53 Striped patterning within a bruise-abrasion is seen here. This is a pattern often associated with an impact from weathered wood. In this case, a fence plank was used

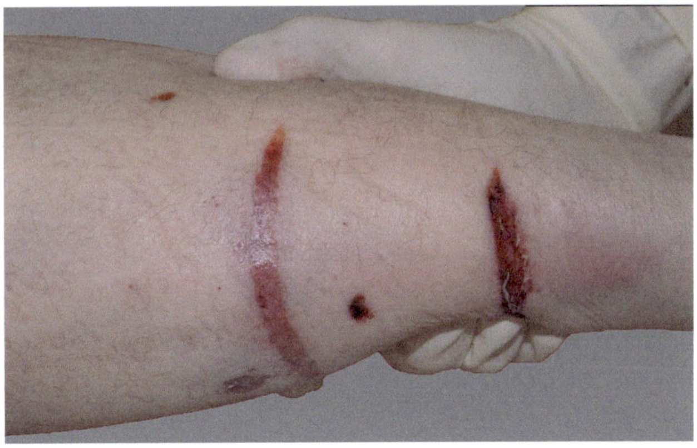

Fig. 12.54 Primary impact of a vehicle striking a pedestrian: linear bumper strike injuries

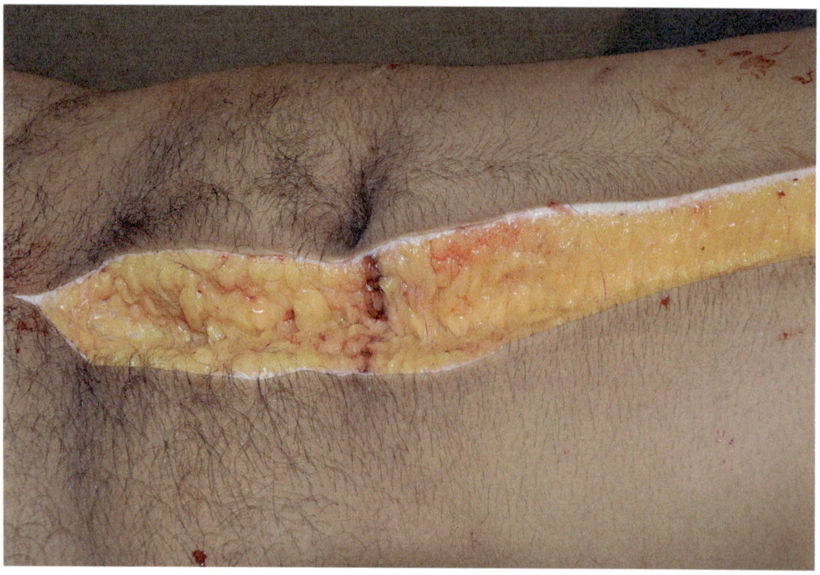

Fig. 12.55 Horizontal panniculus injury caused by a seatbelt

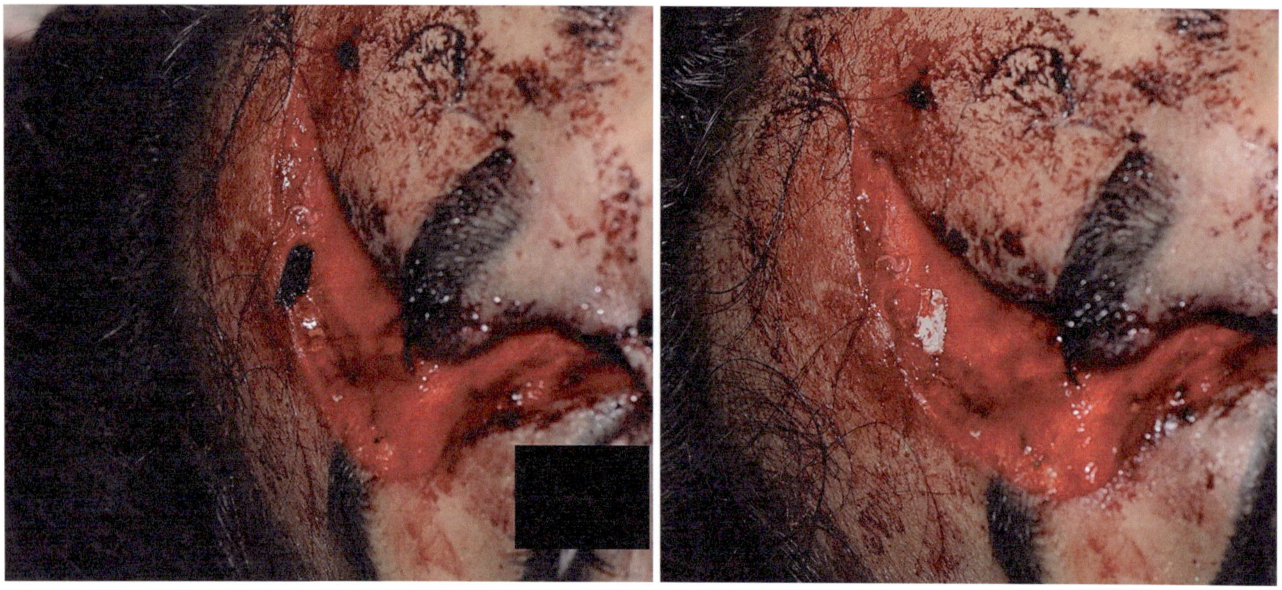

Fig. 12.56 These images show a critical finding within an injury in a "failure to stop" fatal pedestrian collision case. Vehicle paint (black and white) is contained within an injury. Inspection of the body prior to cleaning is important as such findings can easily be lost

Fig. 12.57 Shown here are multiple facial incised wounds in a pedestrian whose head penetrated the windscreen of a motor vehicle

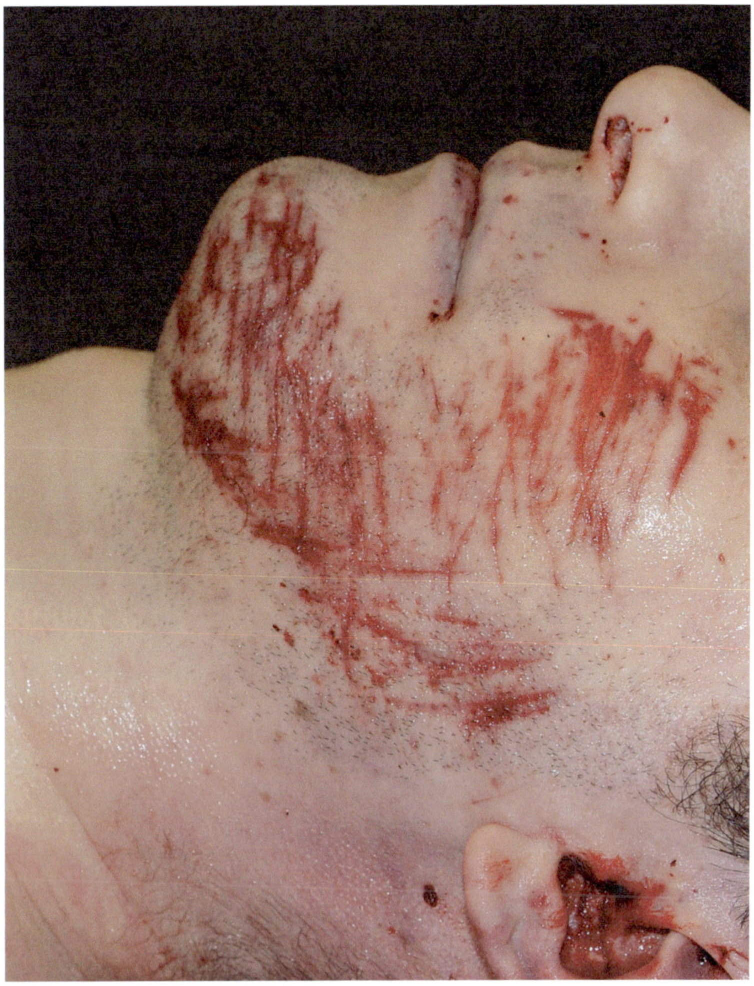

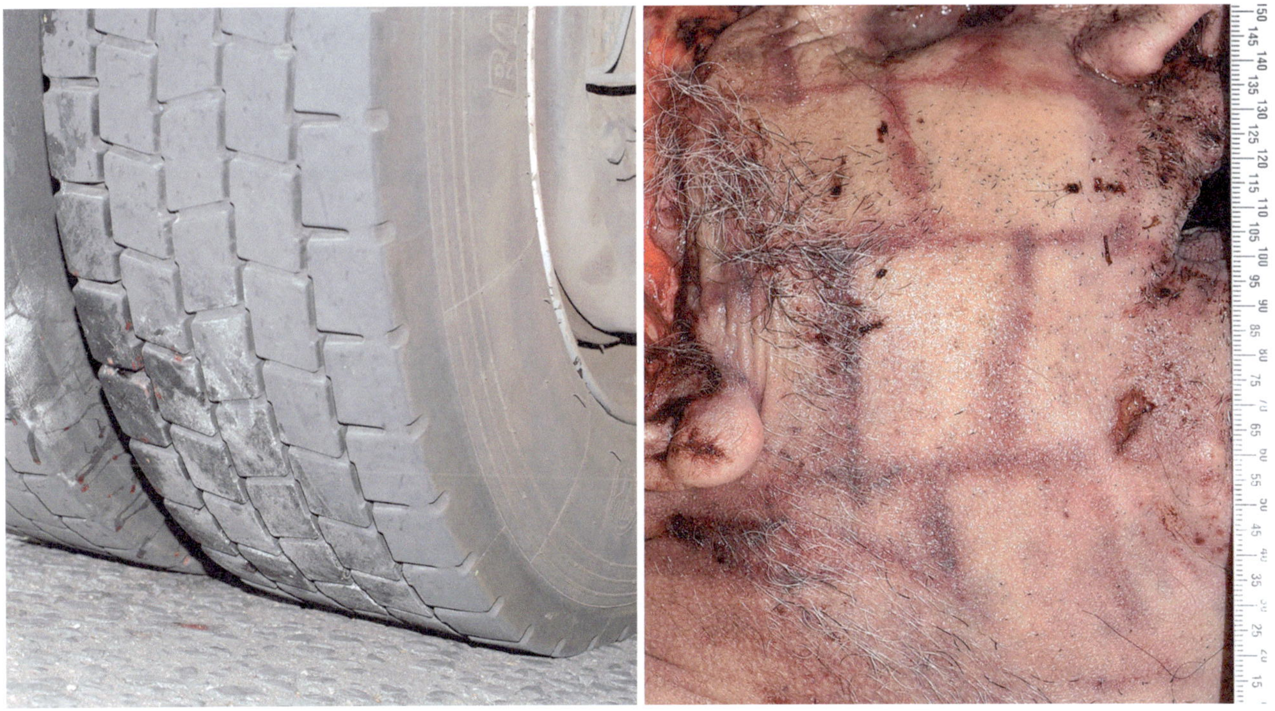

Fig. 12.58 Pattern matching injuries in road traffic collisions can assist in the identification of offending vehicles; the injury to the pedestrian's face in this case mirrored that of the suspect vehicle

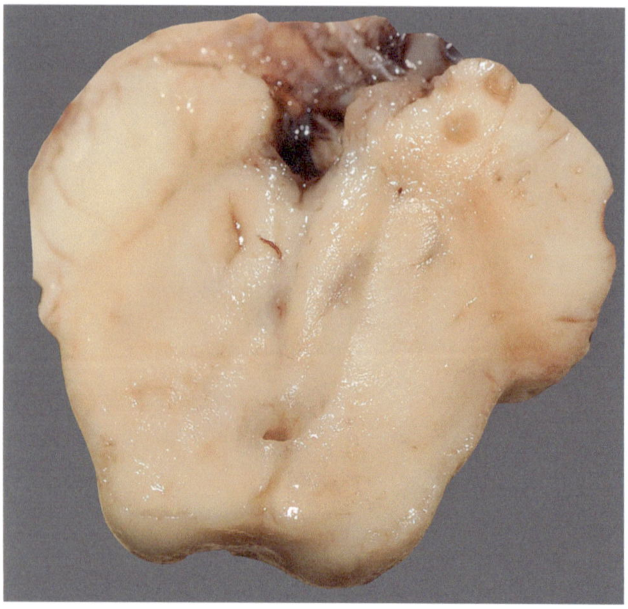

Fig. 12.59 Pale substantia nigra in a case of Parkinson's disease . The deceased had a festinant gait, which caused this pedestrian to walk unexpectedly into the roadway

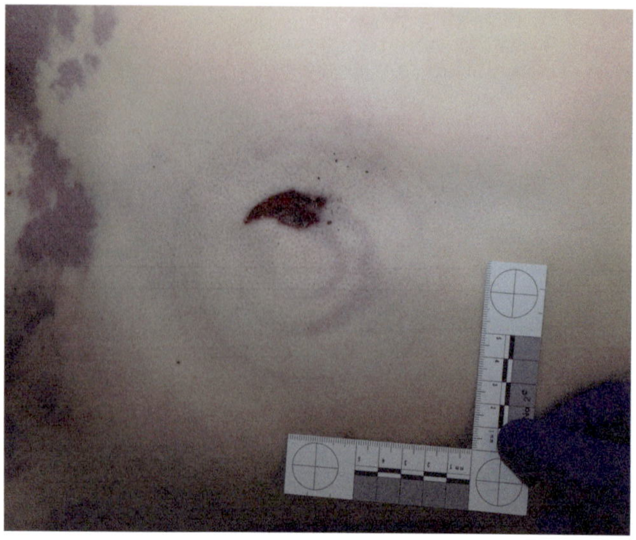

Fig. 12.61 An automated chest compression delivery system mark following a road traffic collision. This may be mistaken by those unfamiliar as steering wheel injuries

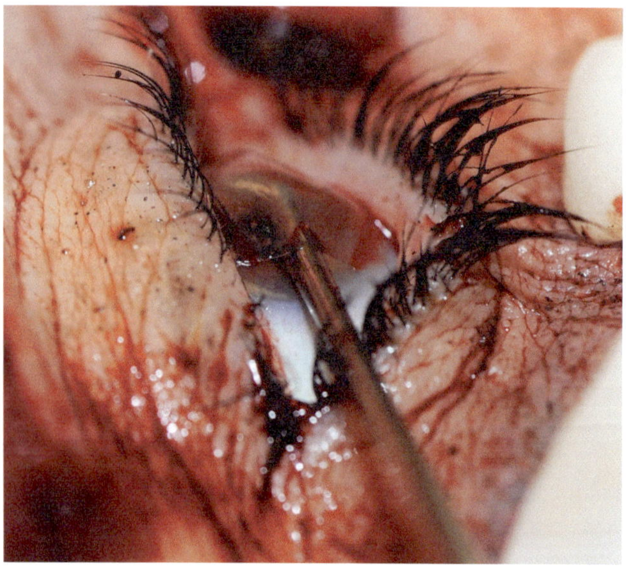

Fig. 12.60 Removal of the contact lenses for expert assessment. This individual crashed his car shortly after visiting the optician

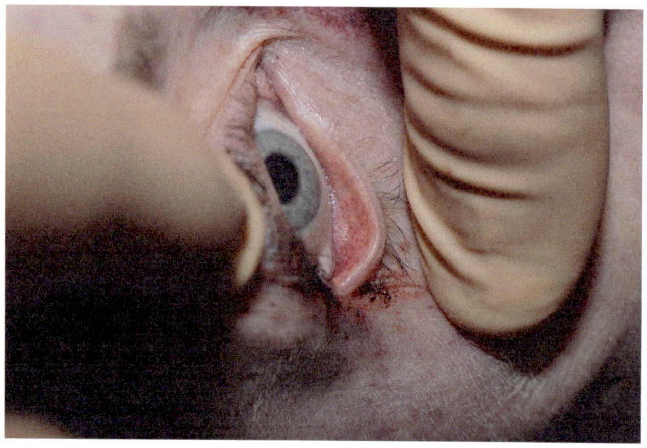

Fig. 12.62 Conjunctival petechiae in a case of strangulation

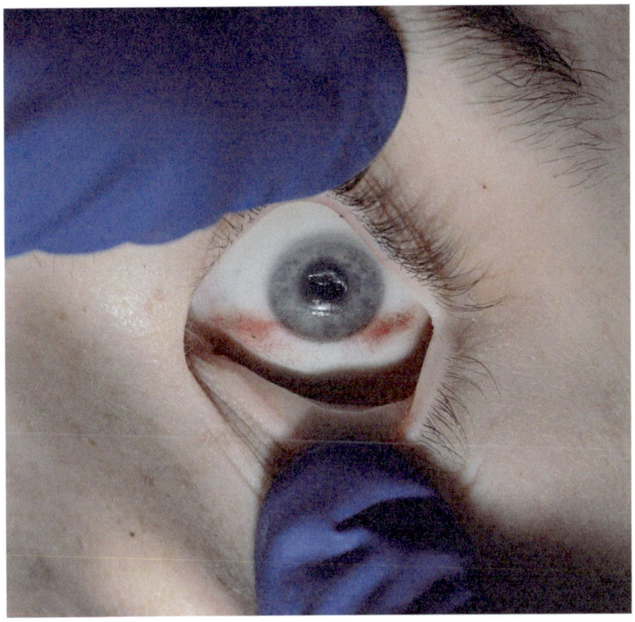

Fig. 12.63 This post mortem artefact, tache noir (early), can be mistaken for an asphyxial change

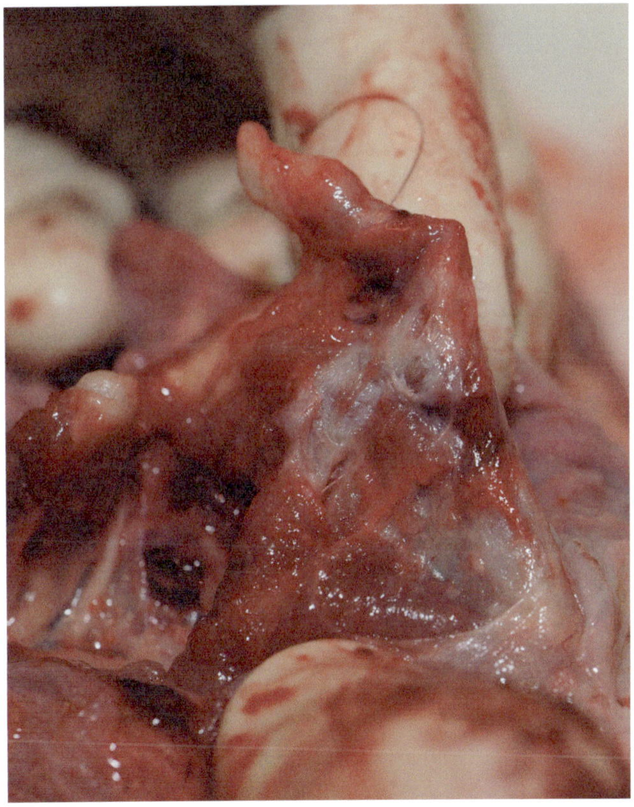

Fig. 12.64 Fracture to the larynx (laryngeal horn) in a case of manual strangulation

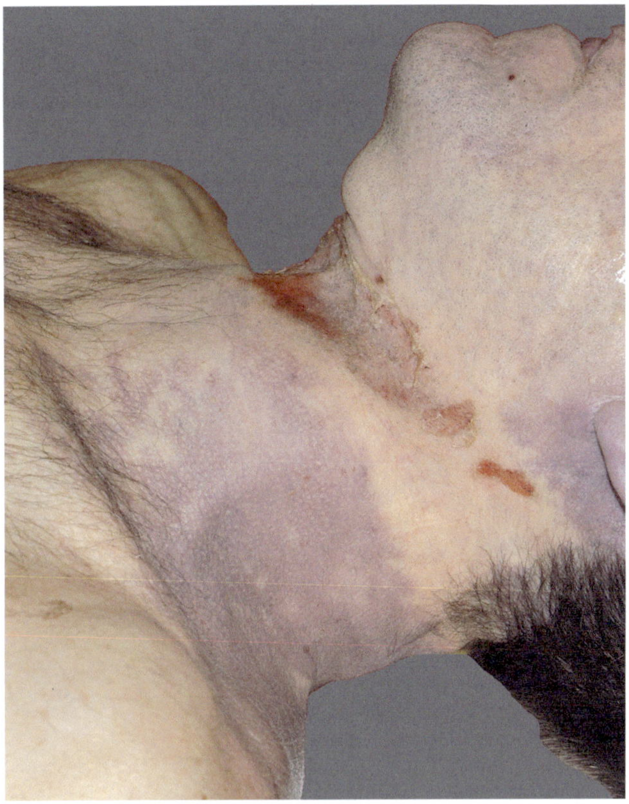

Fig. 12.65 A typical ligature mark with suspension point in a hanging death

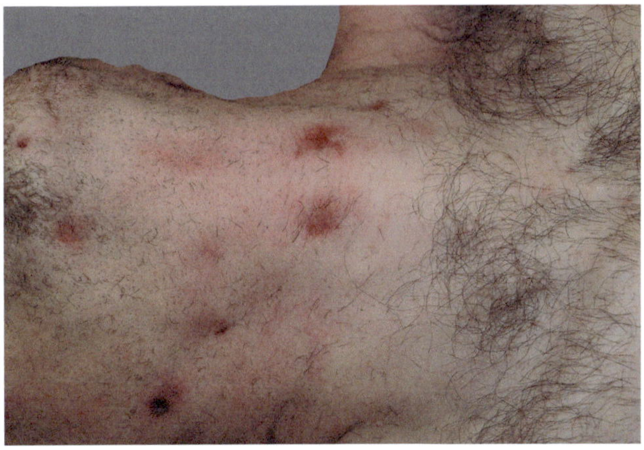

Fig. 12.66 Manual strangulation: multiple foci of bruising and abrasion over the neck, with fingernail marks

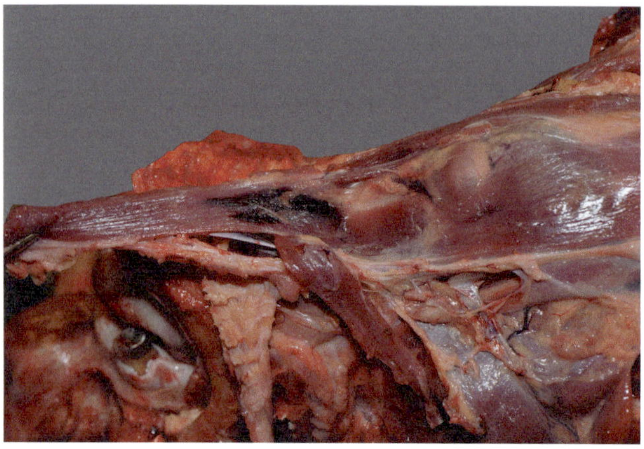

Fig. 12.67 Manual strangulation: multiple foci of bruising in the deep soft tissues and muscle

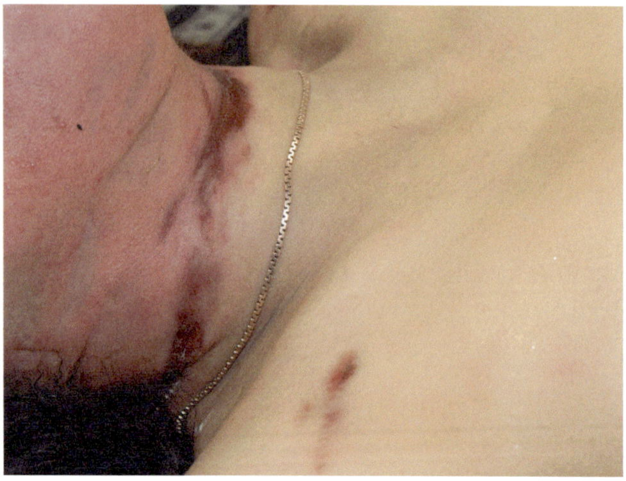

Fig. 12.68 Ligature strangulation of the neck. Note the congestion rising above the ligature mark

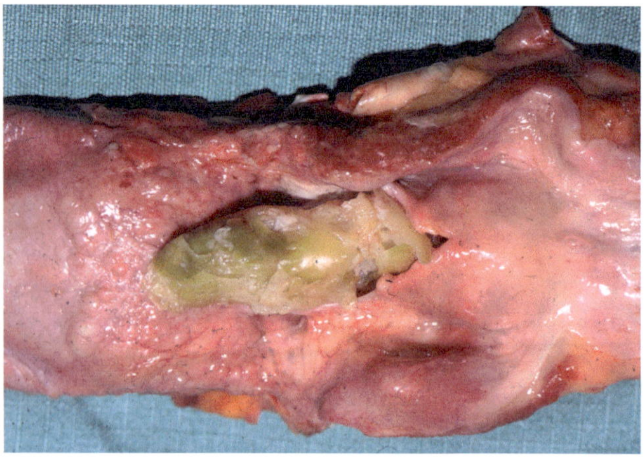

Fig. 12.69 Choking in an elderly individual who had swallowing difficulties due to cerebrovascular accident. A bolus of food is lodged in the laryngeal inlet, blocking the airway

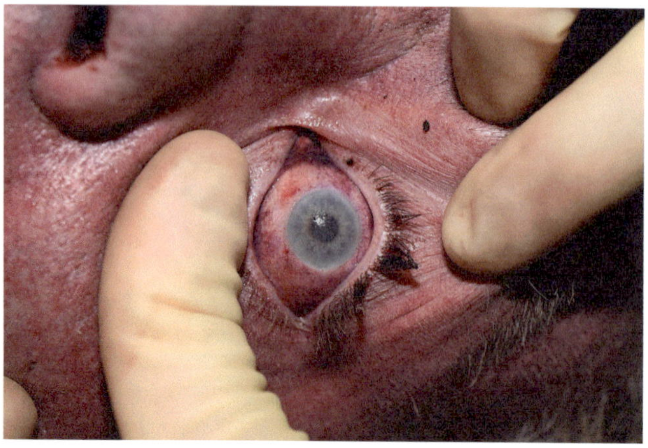

Fig. 12.70 Scleral haemorrhage, florid petechial haemorrhages, and intense facial congestion in a case of traumatic asphyxia

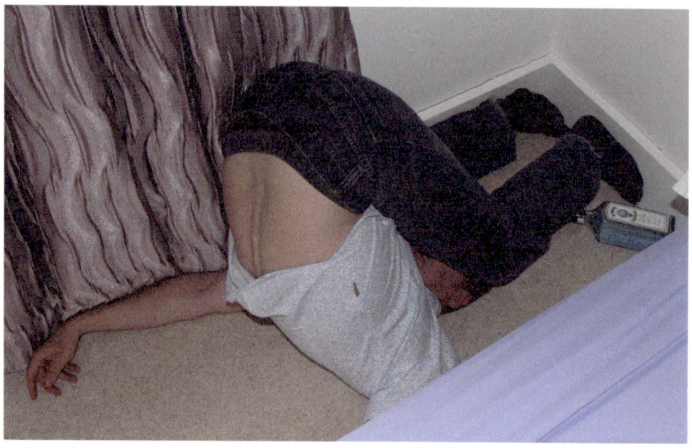

Fig. 12.71 Postural asphyxia. This heavily intoxicated man became trapped between the wall and a bed, resulting in airway occlusion and respiratory muscle inefficiency. Note that the bed has been pulled to the side to assist photography

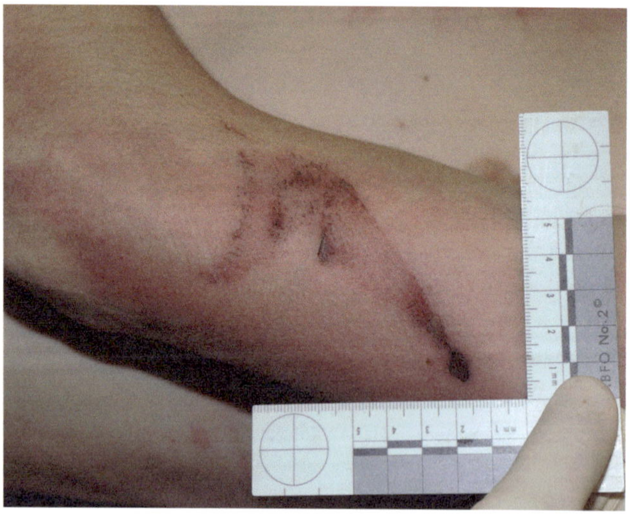

Fig. 12.72 An electric burn on the skin mimicking an abrasion. Close inspection revealed carbonization

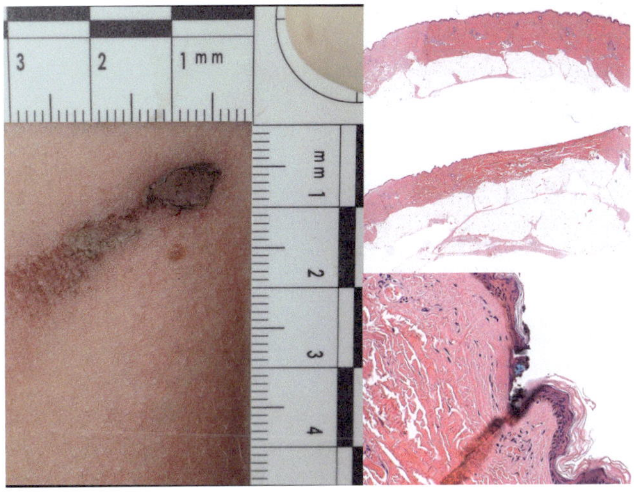

Fig. 12.73 Shown here is an example of electrical burn macroscopy with histology. Typically, the nuclei at the edges of the lesion show streaming artefact. The dermis is hypereosinophilic. Embedded copper from the electric cabling with which the deceased came into contact is seen in this example

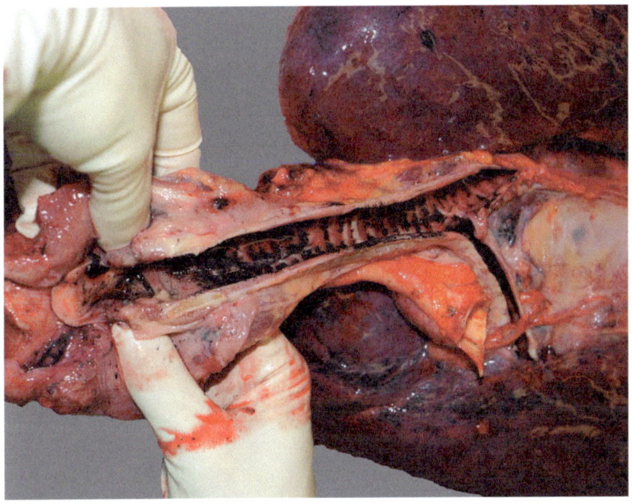

Fig. 12.74 Soot below the level of the vocal cords, in the trachea, indicating active inhalation of smoke

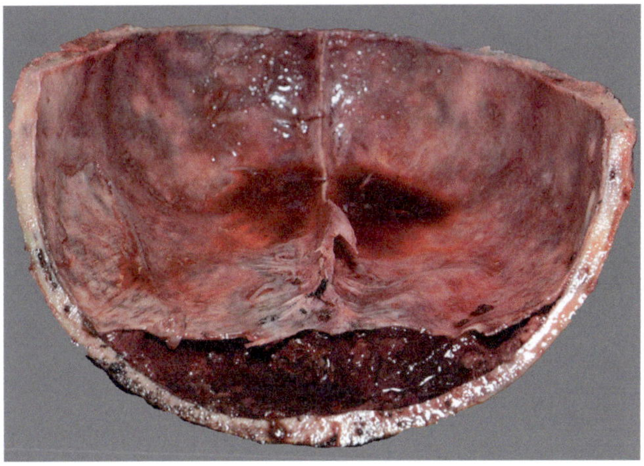

Fig. 12.75 Heat haematoma: the overlying skull and scalp are carbonized. The skull often shows superficial fracturing above (a patina effect)

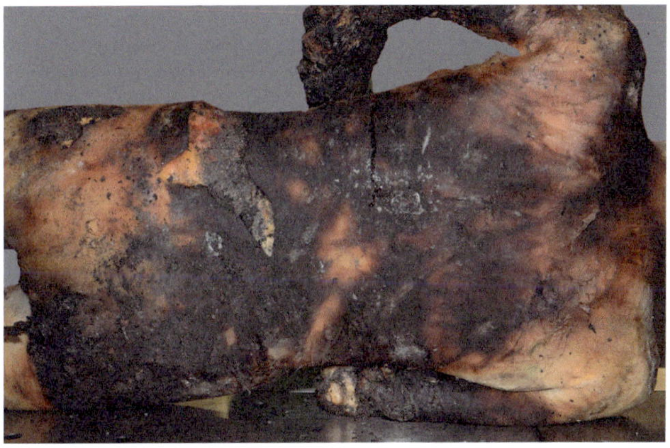

Fig. 12.76 Heat skin splits. These can be confused with true laceration, but the underlying fat shows no haemorrhage

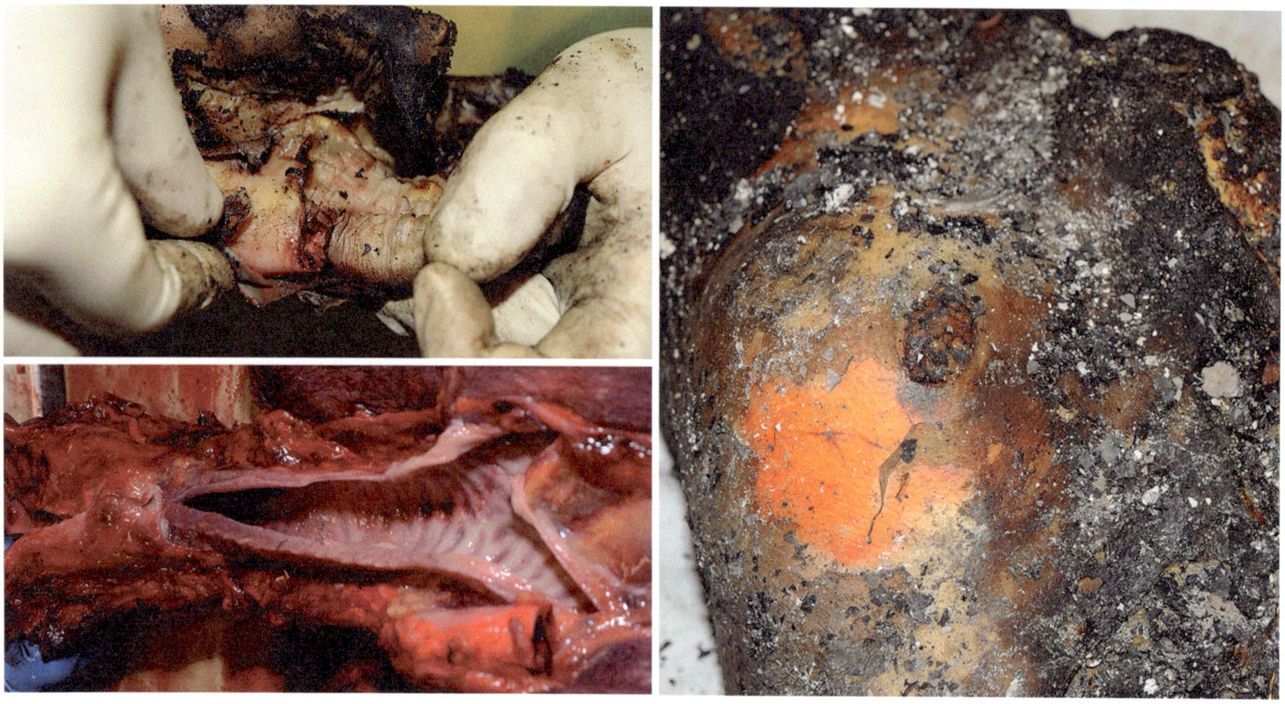

Fig. 12.77 Beware fire deaths. It is not uncommon that an attempt to cover a crime is made by burning the body. Here, stab wounds can just be made out. Soot has not extended down the airway, indicating death occurred prior to the fire

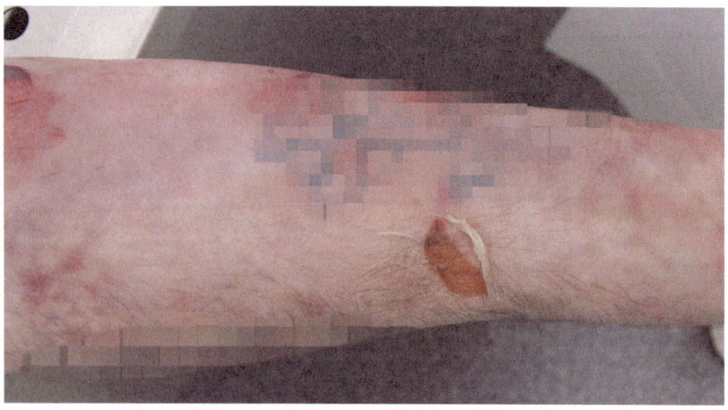

Fig. 12.78 Post mortem skin laceration without any associated bleeding or tissue haemorrhage

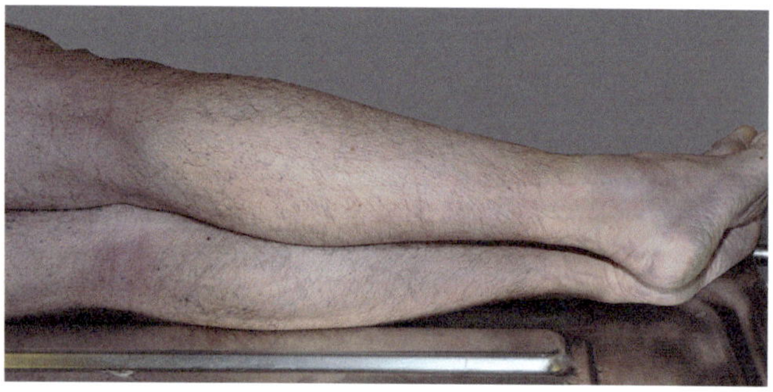

Fig. 12.80 Hypostasis in the soles of the feet in a case of partial suspension hanging. Hypostasis has also moved to the front of the shin, sparing the calves, reflecting the deceased's position after death

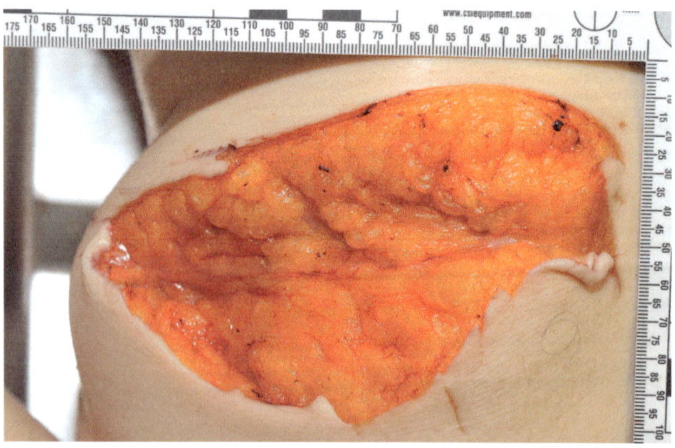

Fig. 12.79 Here is an example of post mortem sharp force mutilation of a breast. Note the complete absence of haemorrhage

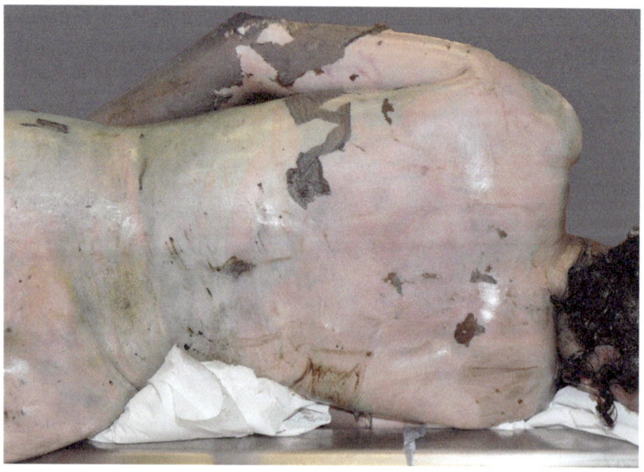

Fig. 12.81 Loss of the epidermis in a dark-skinned individual, exposing the underlying white dermis. When the loss is extensive, the ethnicity of the individual can be misinterpreted

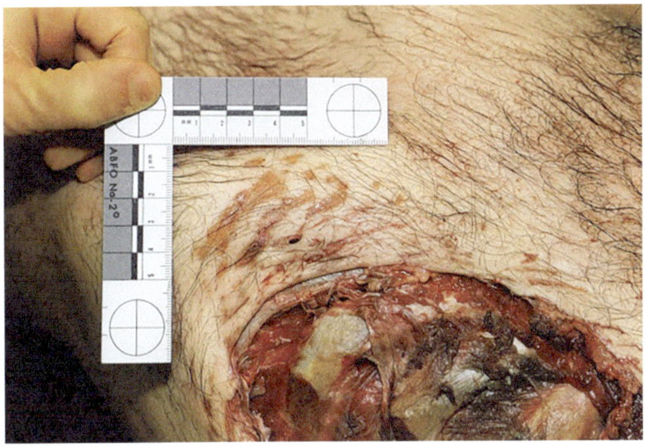

Fig. 12.82 Post-mortem decapitation by a pet dog left for approximately 10 days, locked in a residence without food

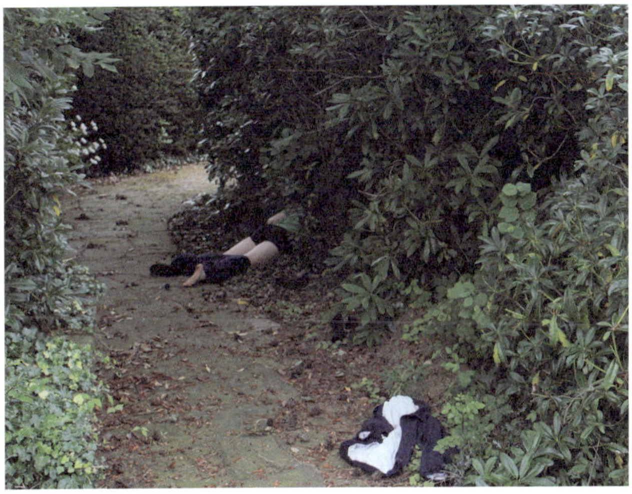

Fig. 12.83 An example of a hypothermic death is shown here. The previous evening, this individual was intoxicated and never arrived home. Clothing is partially removed, and he has tried to enter a bush. The blood alcohol concentration was more than 280 mg/dL

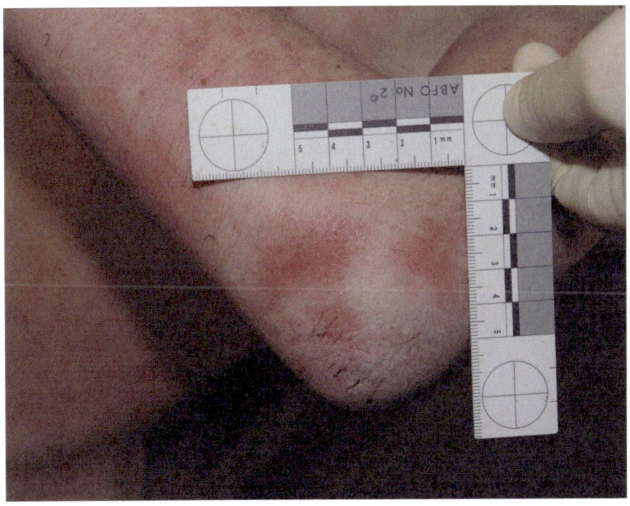

Fig. 12.84 Reddish discolouration of the joint in an individual who died of hypothermia

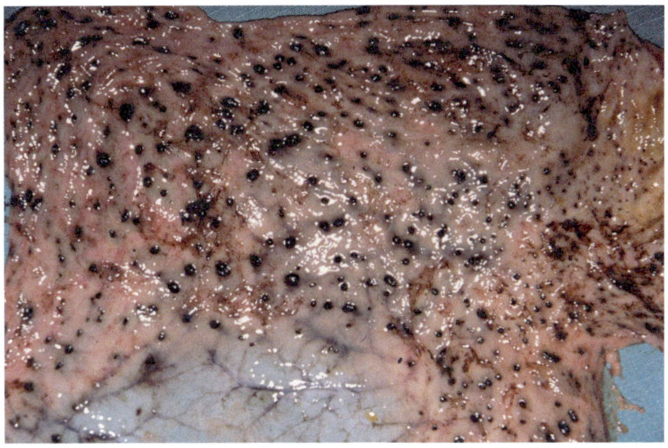

Fig. 12.85 Gastric ulcerations in a case of hypothermia

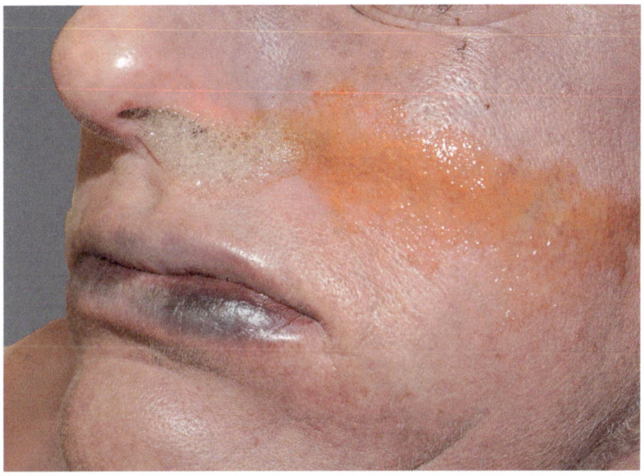

Fig. 12.86 Foam exuding from the nostrils of a drowned individual

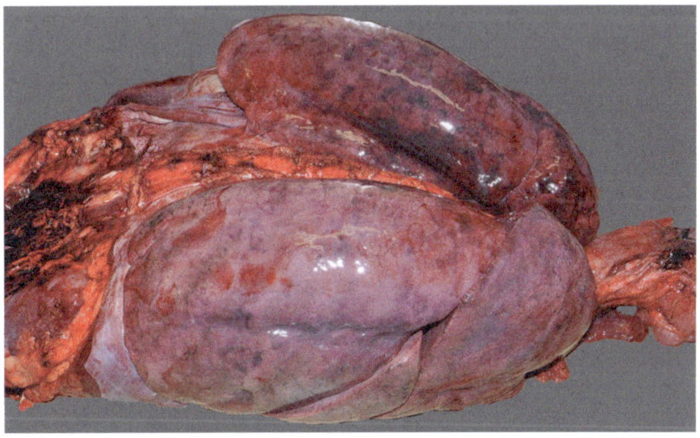

Fig. 12.87 Hyperinflated lungs in a case of drowning

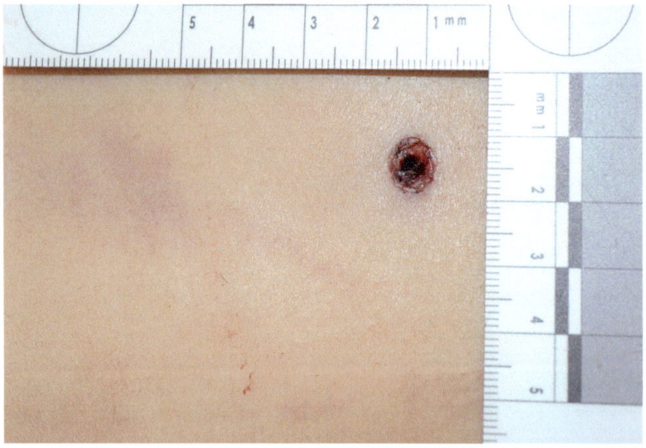

Fig. 12.88 Gunshot entry wound with typical abrasion rim

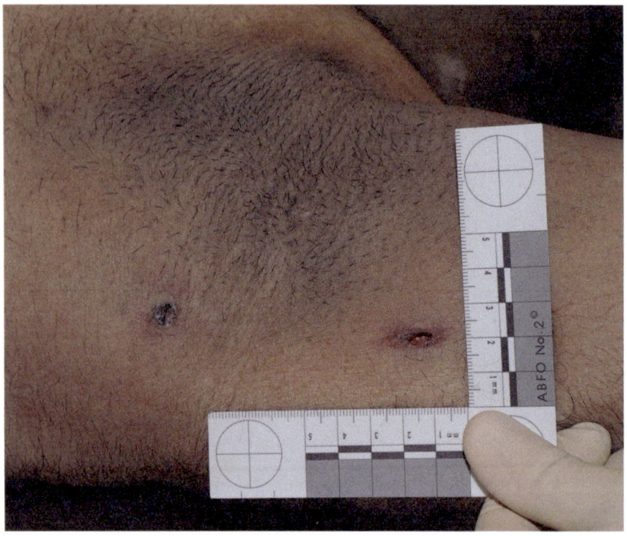

Fig. 12.89 A shored up exit wound on the inner arm, showing abrasion around the exit wound. This exit wound was shored up against a jacket that was being worn on the chest (a second entry wound is visible on the chest)

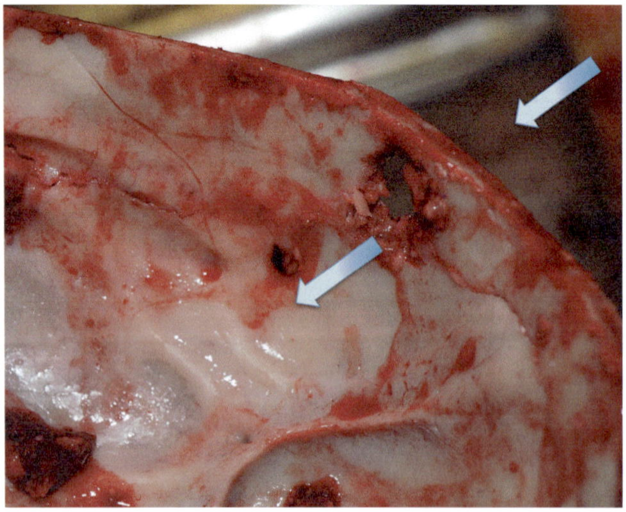

Fig. 12.90 A gunshot wound through the skull is shown here. Collapse of the inner table confirmed the impression that the external injury was an entry wound

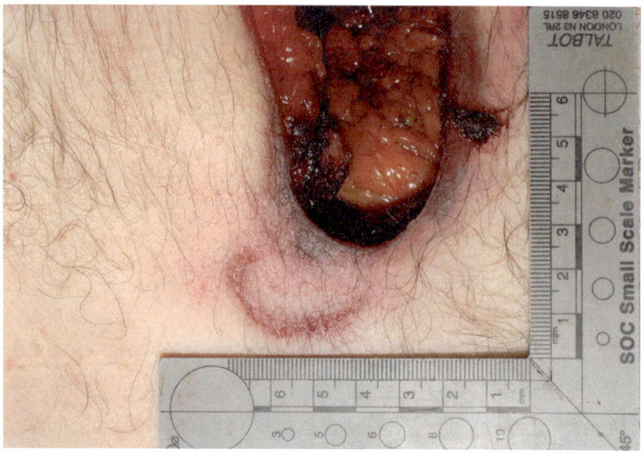

Fig. 12.91 Contact gunshot wound from a double-barreled (side-by-side) shotgun. One barrel has discharged, and the expansion of the gases has compressed the skin against the non-discharged barrel to produce an abrasion ring

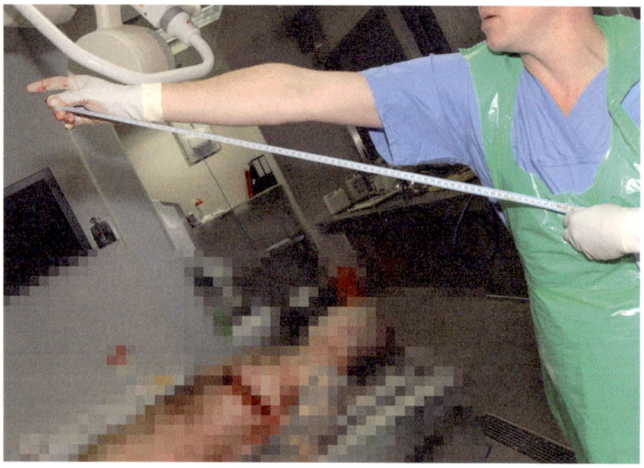

Fig. 12.92 Coincidentally, the pathologist's upper limbs were the same length as the deceased's. Using a tape measure, it was possible to demonstrate that the deceased was capable of reaching the weapon trigger to discharge the shotgun into his chest

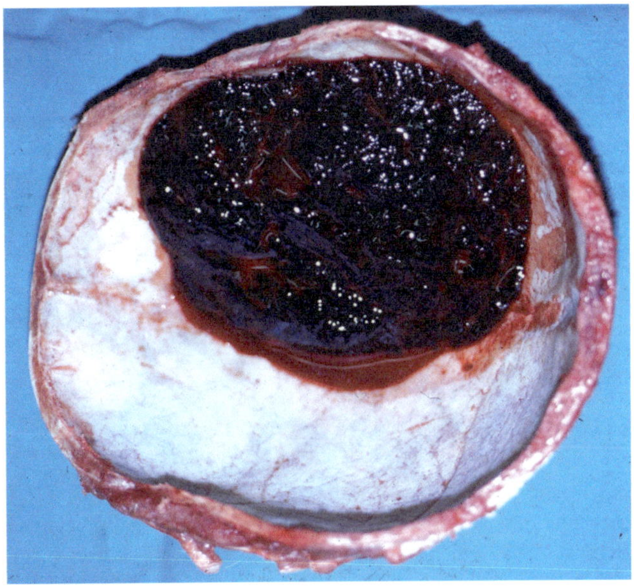

Fig. 12.93 Extradural haematoma: skull fracture following an assault

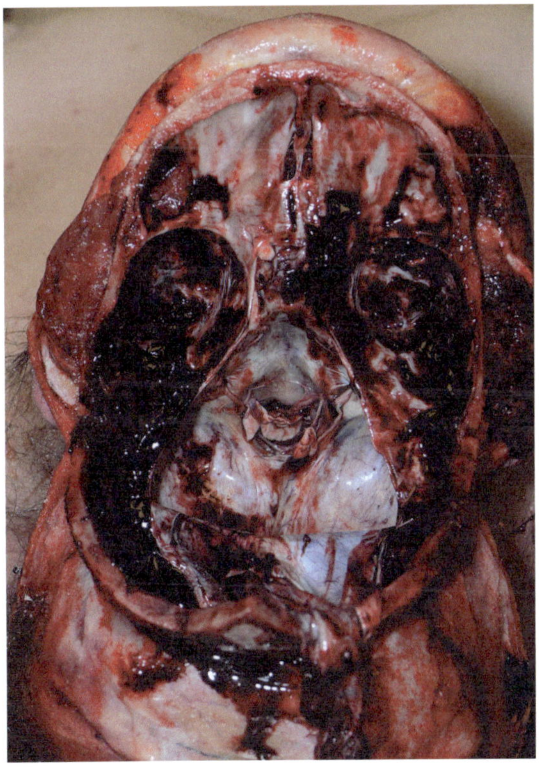

Fig. 12.94 Subdural haematoma shown within the cranial fossae

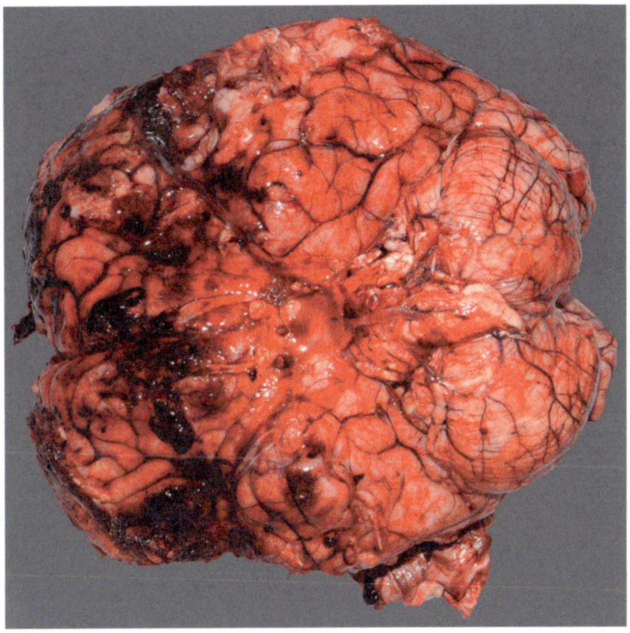

Fig. 12.95 Contre-coup pattern of brain injury following a fall onto the back of the head

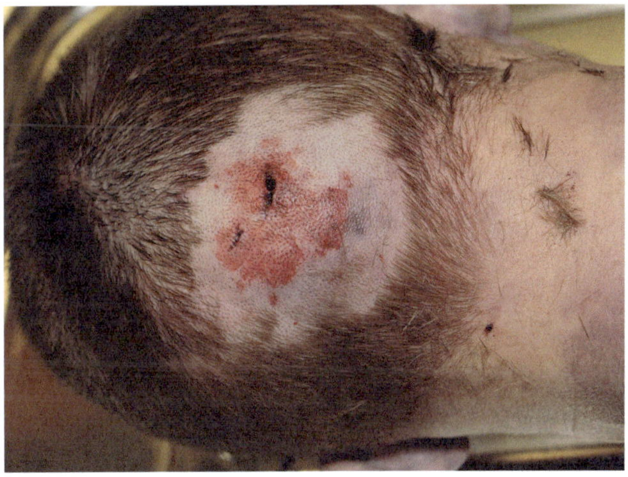

Fig. 12.96 Typical laceration and abrasion ("gravel rash") injuries to the back of the head following a fall precipitated by a blow to the face are seen here. Death was caused by a contre-coup head injury

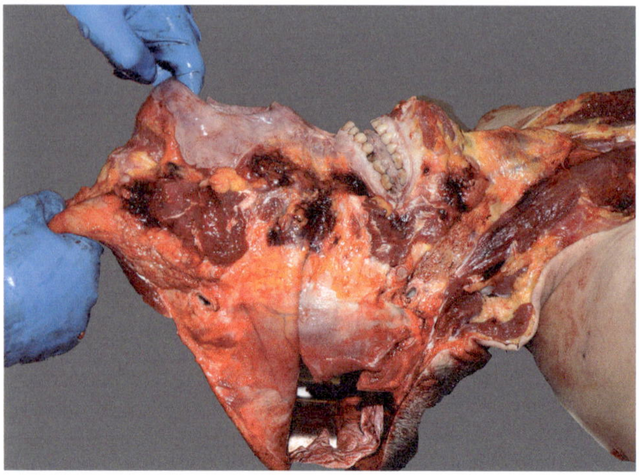

Fig. 12.97 An example of traumatic basal subarachnoid haemorrhage. Deep dissection of the face revealed a bruise at the angle of the right side of the jaw from a single punch delivered in a brawl

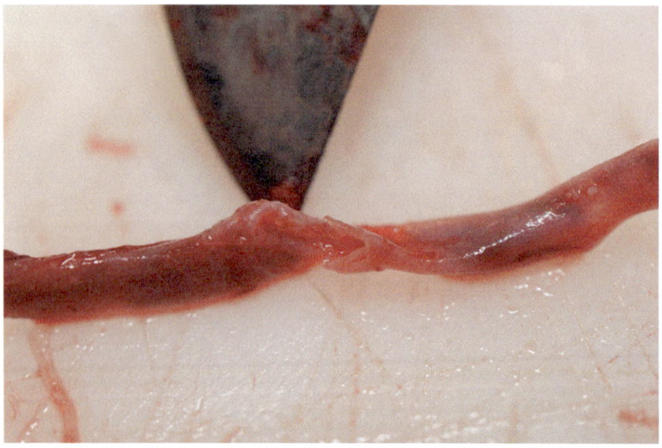

Fig. 12.98 A close up image of an ipsilateral traumatic rupture to a vertebral artery caused by a blow close to the angle of the mandible, causing fatal basal subarachnoid haemorrhage. The rupture should be inspected microscopically to exclude natural disease and confirm traumatic changes to the artery, including anuclear regions of the media and loss of staining of the vascular smooth muscle

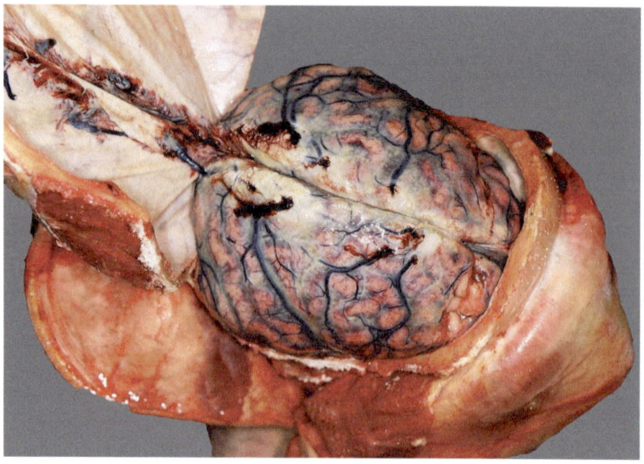

Fig. 12.99 Post-traumatic meningitis (1). This individual died several days after sustaining a skull fracture following a push forwards onto the floor. The meningeal membranes are thickened and inflamed

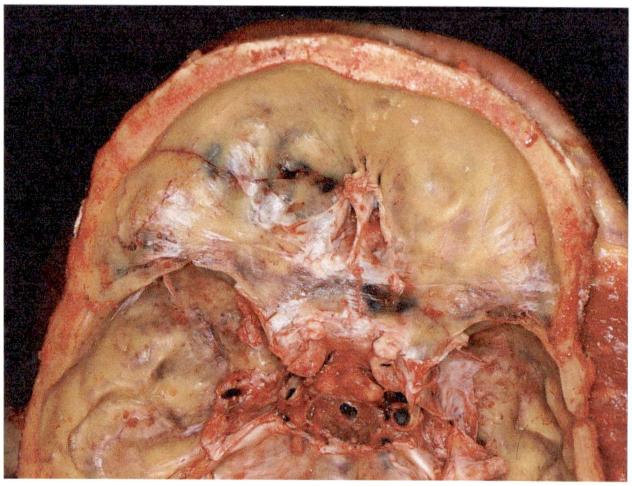

Fig. 12.100 Post-traumatic meningitis (2). The fracture crossed the cribriform plate, presumably admitting bacteria (streptococcus) into the normally sterile environment of the skull cavity

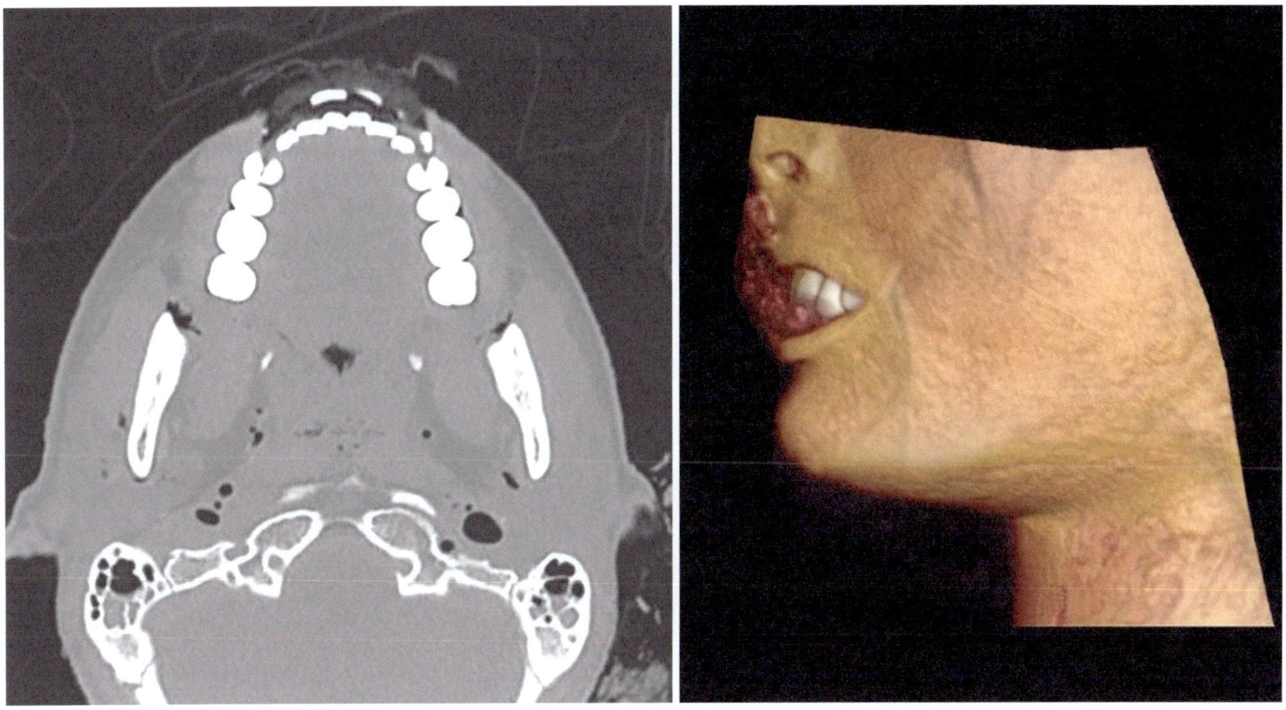

Fig. 12.101 This is a case of a 23-year-old male who was bound and gagged. The injury images were too severe to show to the jury, so PMCT cross-sectional images and volume rendering were used to demonstrate part of a sock gripped between the teeth

Fig. 12.102 Three-dimensional reconstruction from a PMCT scan clearly demonstrates a machete injury to the left forehead. Additional 3D rendering software has been used here to enhance the lighting effects

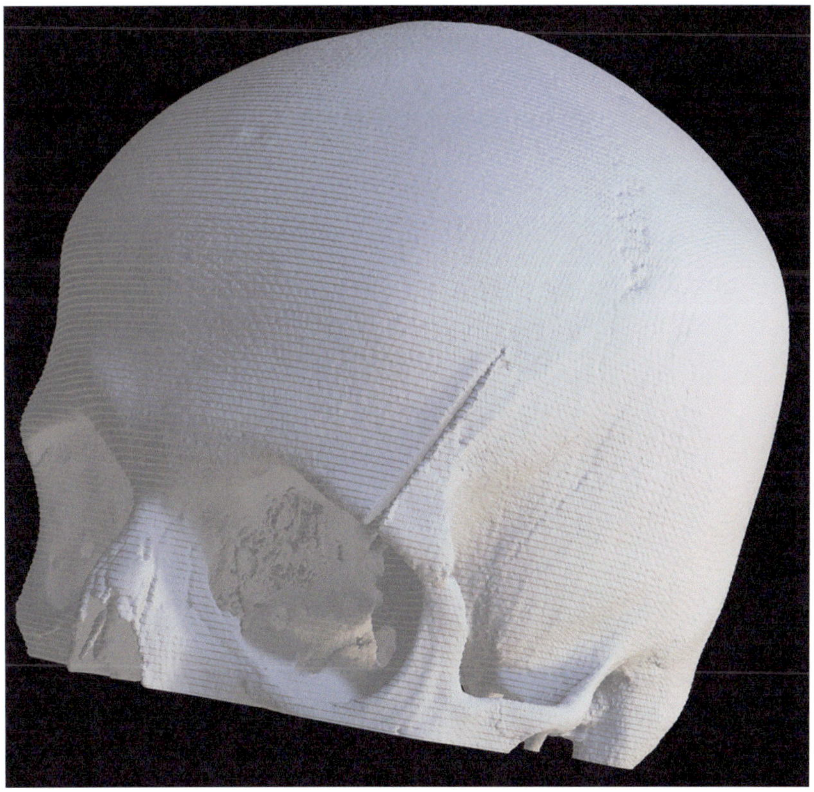

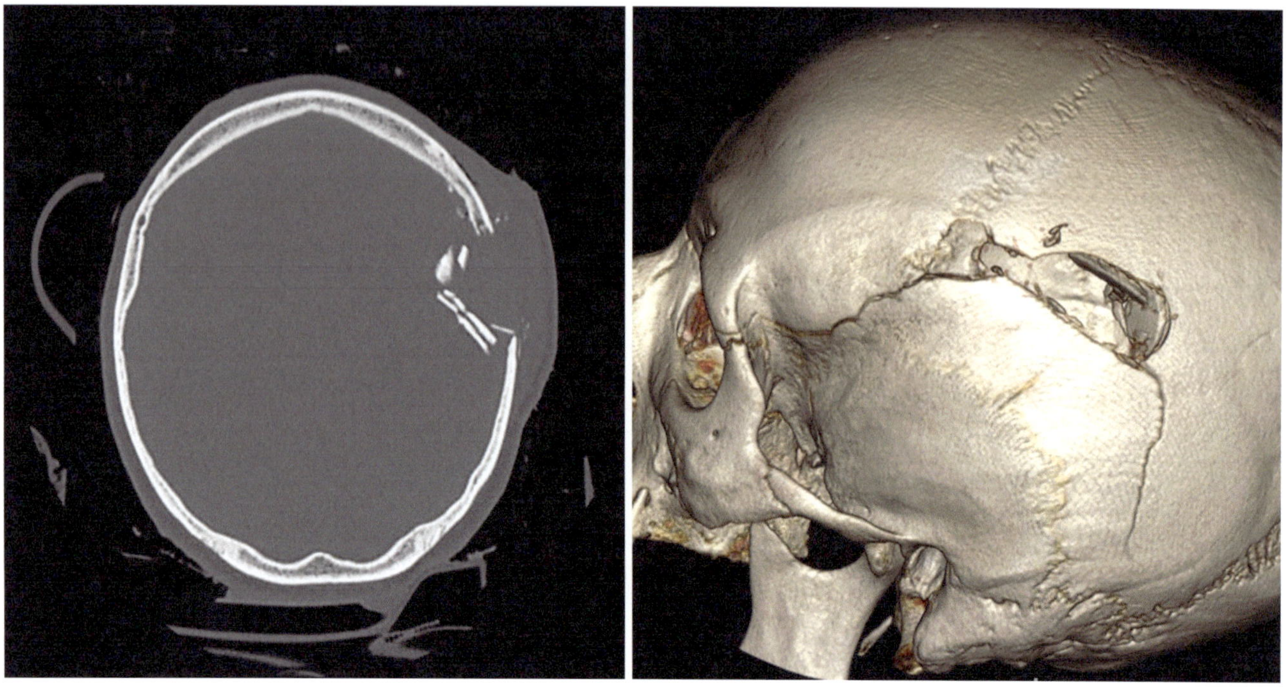

Fig. 12.103 A 35-year-old male was assaulted in his house with a golf club. The digital reconstruction from the cross-sectional data revealed the nature of the injury to the court

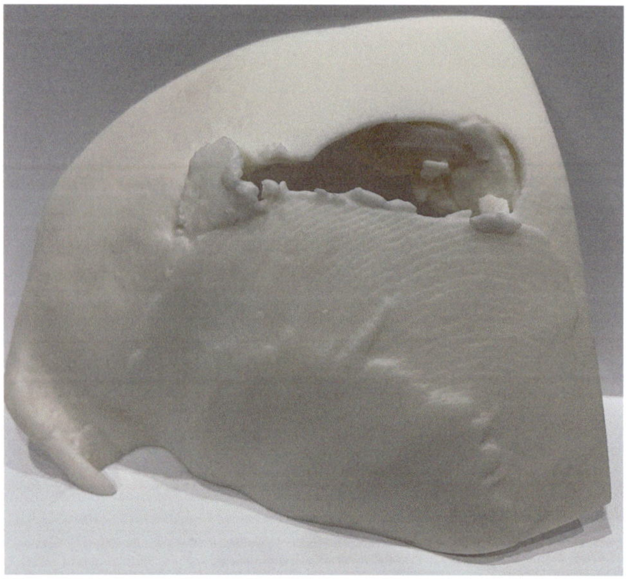

Fig. 12.104 Here is a plastic three-dimensional print of the injury seen in Fig. 12.103, which was passed around the jury

Suggested Reading

Burke MP. Forensic medical investigation of motor vehicle incidents. Boca Raton: CRC Press Taylor & Francis Group; 2007.

DiMaio VJM, Molina DK. DiMaio's forensic pathology. 3rd ed. Boca Raton: CRC Press; 2021.

Mason JK, Purdue BN. The pathology of trauma. 3rd ed. London: Arnold Publishing; 2000.

Pollanen MS, Deck JH, Blenkinsop B. Injury of the tunica media in fatal rupture of the vertebral artery. Am J Forensic Med Pathol. 1996;17(3):197–201.

Saukko P, Knight B, editors. Knight's forensic pathology. 4th ed. Boca Raton: CRC Press; 2015.

Sauvageau A, Geberth V. Autoerotic deaths, practical forensic and investigative perspectives. CRC Press; 2013.

Thali MJ, Viner BG, Brogdon BG. Brogdon's forensic radiology. 2nd ed. CRC Press; 2011.

Vanezis P. The pathology of sharp force trauma. CRC Press; 2021.

13 The Radiological Autopsy

Ian S. D. Roberts and Zoë C. Traill

Introduction

Post-mortem imaging is widely used to supplement dissection in the forensic investigation of traumatic deaths. Post-mortem computerised tomography (PMCT) is particularly effective for the identification of fractures, internal haemorrhage, and foreign bodies. Unlike dissection, it is non-destructive and produces a permanent record of the findings for review by pathologists or other parties. The imaging findings can be demonstrated in court in order to facilitate understanding of the injuries incurred.

Increasingly, post-mortem imaging is being used as an alternative, rather than merely a supplement, to traditional autopsy. Such autopsies are described as 'virtual autopsies' or digital autopsies. They are now the primary method of death investigation in some countries [1]. As an example, in England and Wales, a large number of autopsies are carried out; in 2022, 36% of all deaths were reported to a Coroner, and post-mortem examinations were ordered in 43% of these cases [2]. However, only a minority of Coroners use a digital autopsy approach; of 90,191 post-mortem examinations ordered by Coroners only 8564 used less-invasive techniques such as PMCT. In contrast, there is a low invasive autopsy rate (2%) in Japan, and post-mortem imaging is widely used both as an alternative to an invasive autopsy and as a screening tool to determine whether invasive autopsy is necessary in the case of a death of unknown cause. Indeed, 89% of large hospitals in Japan perform post-mortem imaging, with 20,000 post-mortem CT scans reported each year [3].

I. S. D. Roberts (✉)
Department of Cellular Pathology, Oxford University Hospitals Foundation Trust, John Radcliffe Hospital, Oxford, UK
e-mail: ian.roberts@ouh.nhs.uk

Z. C. Traill
Department of Radiology, Oxford University Hospitals Foundation Trust, Churchill Hospital, Oxford, UK
e-mail: zoe.traill@ouh.nhs.uk

The emergence of the digital autopsy has also been driven by religious and cultural objections to invasive autopsy. The accuracy of early digital autopsy services was questionable, because they lacked a strong evidence base and appropriate governance [4, 5]. However, research in recent years has defined the accuracy of the various imaging techniques, identified their strengths and weaknesses, and optimised imaging protocols [6]. The development of angiographic techniques has improved the diagnostic accuracy of imaging, particularly in the assessment of coronary heart disease [7–9].

Imaging can be combined with (minimally) invasive techniques. Of particular value, for example, are aspiration of fluids for toxicology in suspected drug-related deaths [10] and needle biopsy of tumours or solid organs in order to obtain a precise histological diagnosis [11, 12]. If an invasive autopsy is necessary, the imaging findings can be used to direct and/or limit dissection. A knowledge and understanding of the applications of post-mortem imaging is essential if it is to be used appropriately.

Decision Making During the Digital Autopsy

In this section we discuss the decisions that a pathologist should make at each stage of the autopsy process. This relates to the coronial system in the UK but can be applied widely. The primary function of the UK Coroner (who has a legal rather than medical role) is to identify and investigate unnatural deaths. The Coroner's pathologist is tasked with (1) identifying the cause of death in cases of sudden death of unknown cause in order to identify unnatural deaths, and (2) collecting information that will inform the Coroner's investigation into unnatural deaths.

Although PMCT is less accurate than traditional invasive autopsy in identifying and distinguishing the pathologies that result in many natural deaths, such as inflammatory and infective diseases, it may be superior to dissection in identi-

S. K. Suvarna (represented by Grace Horne), A. K. Sharp (eds.), *Atlas of Adult Autopsy*,
https://doi.org/10.1007/978-3-031-72207-3_13

Full body CT + external examination → issue report & cause of death

↓ no definitive cause of death

CT coronary angiography → issue report & cause of death

↓ no definitive cause of death

Conventional autopsy, limited according to imaging findings

Other minimally invasive investigations performed as indicated – aspiration of fluids for toxicology and biochemistry, biopsy of tumours identified at imaging.

Fig. 13.1 A protocol for the use of post-mortem imaging to avoid traditional medicolegal autopsy, and to guide and limit dissection in those cases in which an invasive element to the examination is required

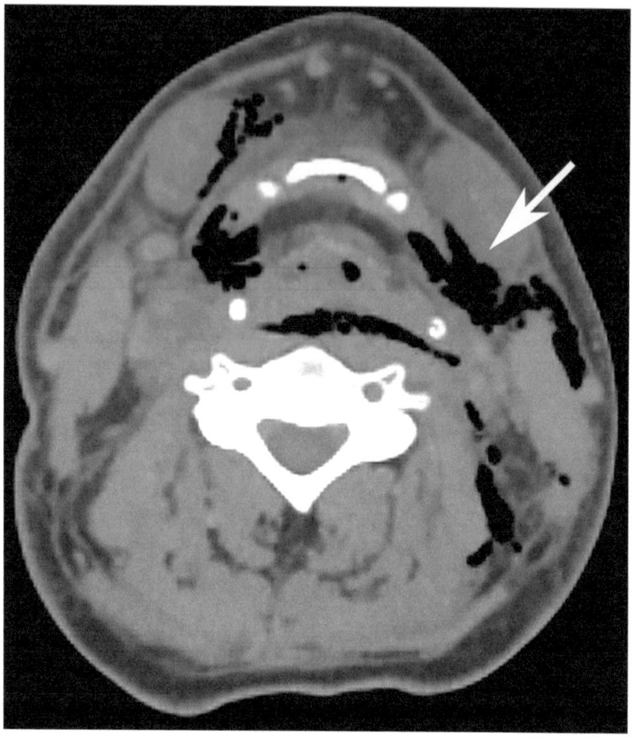

Fig. 13.2 Necrotising fasciitis of the neck following dental infection. An axial CT image showing soft tissue gas tracking down the neck (arrow)

fying unnatural deaths, such as those resulting from unsuspected injuries, which is the primary function of the Coroner's autopsy. This is illustrated below in the section on trauma. Knowledge of the strengths and limitations of PMCT, in addition to careful correlation of the imaging findings with the clinical history and circumstances of the death, is essential if correct decisions are to be made.

The digital autopsy protocol used by the authors is illustrated in Fig. 13.1. It is a staged process, with the aim of limiting the invasive component of the autopsy. Sequentially, the following set of questions must be answered:

Is This Case Suitable for a Digital Autopsy Approach?

The majority of sudden adult deaths, both natural and unnatural, can be diagnosed with PMCT when combined with angiographic techniques [13]. PMCT is more accurate than traditional autopsy in the identification of certain injuries, such as fractures and pneumothorax, which might be missed on dissection.

Relative contraindications to the digital autopsy are deaths suspected to be due to metabolic disorders or sepsis, or deaths in hospital following extensive investigation in life, including imaging. Nevertheless, even in such cases, post-mortem imaging might be used to answer specific questions and enable a limited invasive procedure to be performed. Certain infections can be diagnosed on PMCT, including pneumonia, abscesses and soft tissue infections that result in gas production, such as necrotising fasciitis (Fig. 13.2).

Which Imaging Techniques Are Required? Is Angiography Indicated?

In general, CT is more accurate than MRI in the diagnosis of sudden adult death [6]. The converse is true for the investigation of fetal and infant deaths. If initial non-contrast CT identifies a definitive cause of death, then no further procedure is required. Conditions that can be diagnosed with certainty on CT alone include ruptured abdominal aortic aneurysm, haemopericardium due to ruptured myocardial infarct, or massive intracerebral haemorrhage.

In the absence of a definitive cause of death on non-contrast CT, the addition of coronary angiography may well identify coronary artery occlusion and early myocardial infarcts. In general, such angiography is more accurate than dissection in the assessment of coronary stenosis.

Following Imaging, Is an Invasive Procedure Necessary to Determine the Cause of Death?

Approximately three quarters of sudden adult deaths can be diagnosed with CT, supplemented by coronary angiography. In the remaining quarter of cases, other investigations or invasive procedures are required for one of the following reasons:

- The cause of death is unascertained on imaging. Examples include septic, metabolic, and drug-related deaths. Pulmonary embolism cannot be diagnosed on unenhanced PMCT, as it cannot distinguish between post mortem clot and ante mortem thrombus.

- An abnormality detected on imaging requires further investigation. Examples include pneumoperitoneum, suggesting a perforated viscus, or pulmonary lesions in which the differential diagnosis is between malignancy and infection. However, a Coroner may take a view that the cause of death has been found and no further investigations are needed.
- There is a discrepancy between the clinical history, the circumstances of the death, and the imaging findings. An example of such a case would be a history of severe abdominal pain or "coffee ground" vomit prior to sudden collapse, in which imaging demonstrates severe coronary heart disease but does not fully explain the abdominal symptoms.

Can Invasive Autopsy Be Limited?

It is rare for a full invasive autopsy to be required following digital autopsy. In general, opening the cranial cavity is considered unnecessary if no abnormality is detected on CT. Imaging is used to direct the invasive procedure. In the case of pneumoperitoneum, it is often necessary to explore only the abdominal cavity in order to identify the cause of perforation. In the case of a suspected pulmonary embolus, minimally invasive examination of the main pulmonary arteries might be the only procedure required to confirm the diagnosis.

Are Additional Investigations Required, Such as Aspiration of Fluids for Toxicology?

Toxicology is normally performed in suspected drug-related deaths and in many traumatic deaths. Needle biopsy of tumours detected on CT can be performed if a definitive histological diagnosis is required. These investigations can be performed with minimal intervention to the body.

Digital Autopsy Services

Both the UK Royal Colleges of Pathologists and Radiologists recommend that the pathologist should be at the centre of the decision-making process; they should include the radiology findings together with their external ± internal examination findings and cause of death in their report to the Coroner. It is recommended that a radiologist who is appropriately trained in post mortem imaging should report the PMCT [14]. Good communication between the radiologist and pathologist is critical to a well-functioning digital autopsy service.

In the authors' practice, both radiologist and pathologist are together in the CT unit during the scanning process. The pathologist carries out an external examination and performs angiography if necessary. Both radiologist and pathologist view the imaging together and discuss the significance of the radiology findings in the context of the circumstances of the death. Decisions on the need for angiography, or any other invasive procedure, are made on the basis of this discussion. The radiologist completes an imaging proforma and the pathologist includes the radiology findings in their autopsy report to the Coroner.

In contrast, for most digital autopsy services, neither the pathologist nor radiologist are present at the time of imaging. The radiologist reports the images remotely, sending an electronic report to the pathologist who then makes decisions on the basis of this report, carrying out an invasive procedure when indicated. In this type of service, it is essential that the radiologist is available if the pathologist needs to discuss the imaging findings, particularly when PMCT identifies a potential rather than definitive cause of death or makes a new diagnosis.

Issues Around Decomposition

Post-mortem changes such as free air and fluid collections and decomposition cause particular difficulties in radiological diagnosis. Post-mortem accumulation of gas in the abdominal cavity may be mistakenly attributed to a perforated viscus (Figs. 13.3, 13.4, and 13.5). In advanced decomposition, post-mortem imaging must be interpreted with particular care. This is illustrated in Fig. 13.6, in which post-

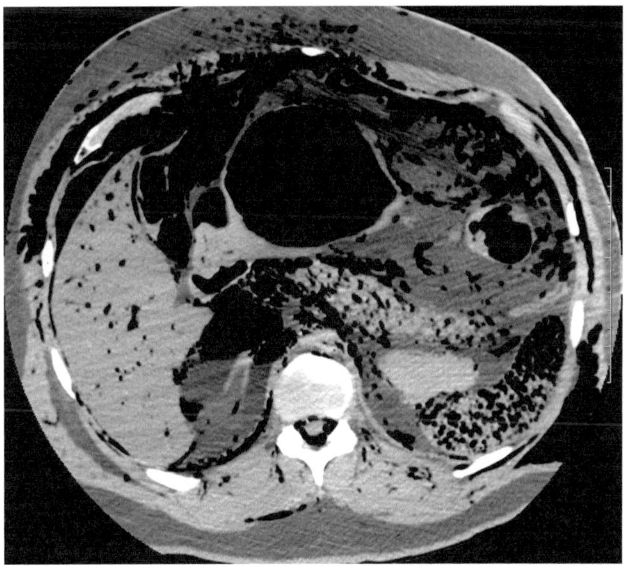

Fig. 13.3 Post-mortem decomposition. An axial CT image showing widespread gas, particularly in hepatic vessels, spleen, and pancreas

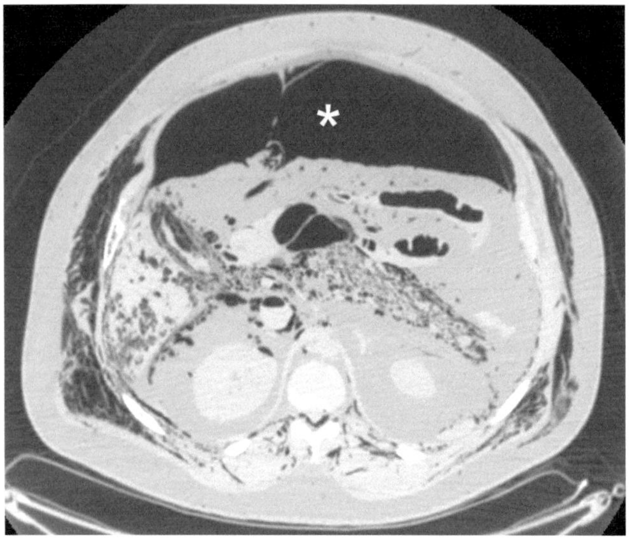

Fig. 13.4 Post-mortem decomposition. An axial CT image showing pneumoperitoneum (star) and extensive soft tissue gas

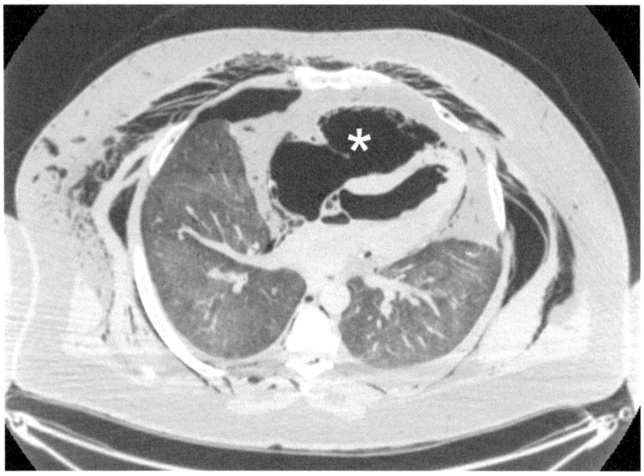

Fig. 13.5 Post-mortem decomposition. An axial CT image showing gas in the cardiac chambers (star)

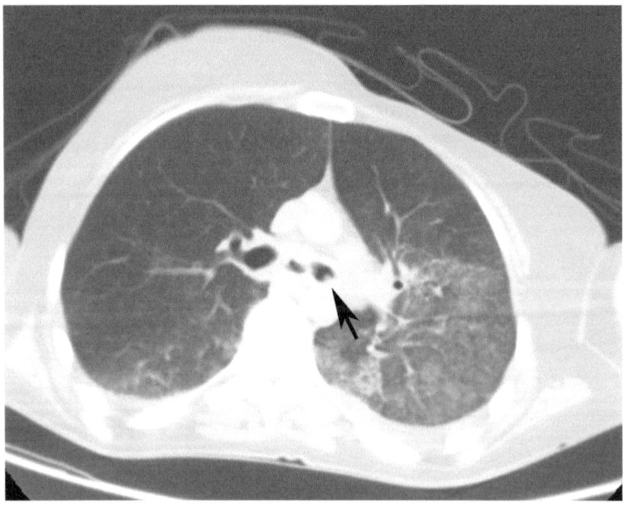

Fig. 13.6 Maggots in a bronchus (arrow), which may result in a misdiagnosis of bronchial obstruction as the cause of death

mortem CT of a decomposed body suggested bronchial obstruction as the probable cause of death. Subsequent autopsy demonstrated that the soft tissue mass noted in the airways on CT was in fact maggots crawling down the airways from the mouth. However, in advanced decomposition, PMCT can be a valuable adjunct to autopsy, enabling the demonstration of skeletal injuries that might be obscured by the decomposing soft tissues.

Trauma

PMCT is sensitive for the detection of fractures and is often superior to dissection in documenting skeletal injuries. In some cases, it is clear that PMCT is superior to dissection in identifying unnatural deaths. In a large series of digital autopsies, PMCT detected evidence of trauma that was missed at standard autopsy, such as femoral neck fracture (Fig. 13.7), and pneumothorax (Fig. 13.8) [12].

A scenario frequently encountered by the Coroner's pathologist is death of an elderly individual following a collapse/fall in which standard autopsy demonstrates significant coronary artery stenosis, without acute pathology or injuries. Death is then attributed to ischaemic heart disease with the assumption that myocardial ischaemia triggered a fatal ventricular arrhythmia. In the authors' digital autopsy service, several such cases have been encountered in which PMCT

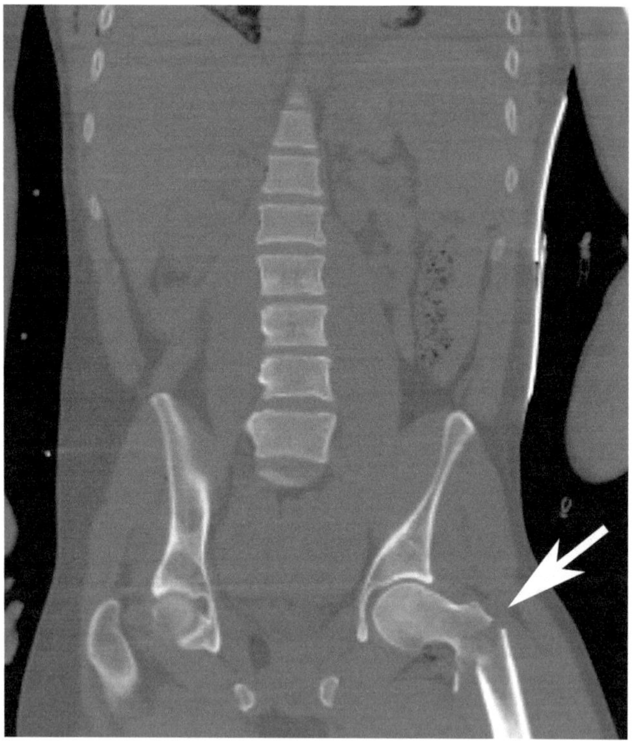

Fig. 13.7 Femoral fracture. A coronal CT image showing an intertrochanteric fracture of the left femur (arrow)

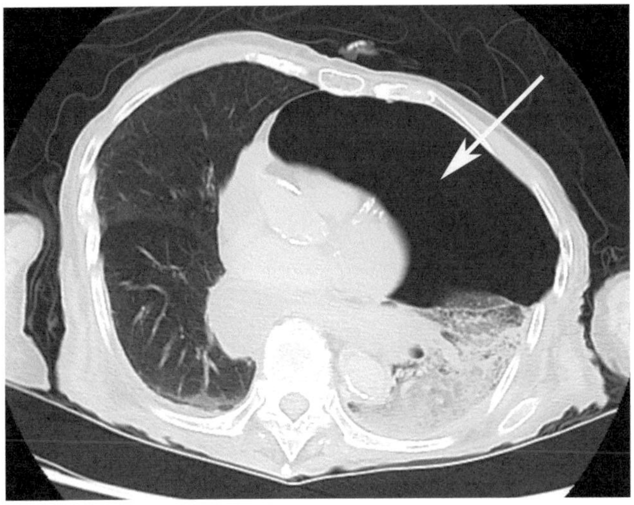

Fig. 13.8 Pneumothorax. An axial CT image demonstrating a left sided tension pneumothorax (arrow) with mediastinal shift to the right

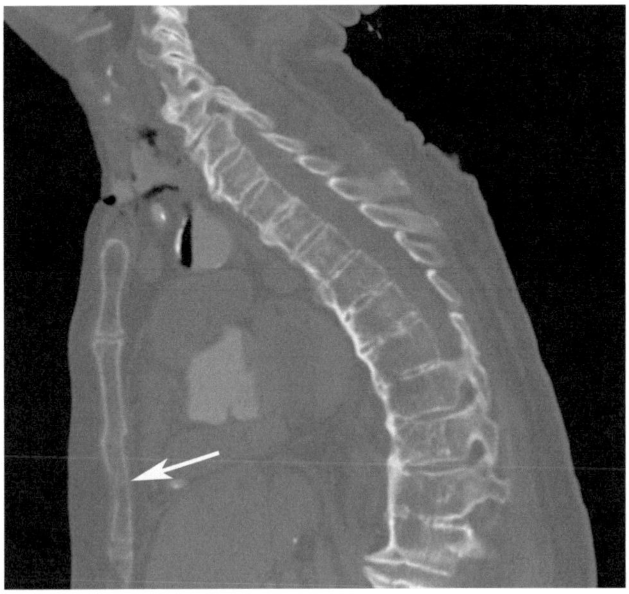

Fig. 13.10 Sternal fracture. A sagittal reformatted CT image showing a fracture of the sternal body (arrow) secondary to attempted cardiopulmonary resuscitation

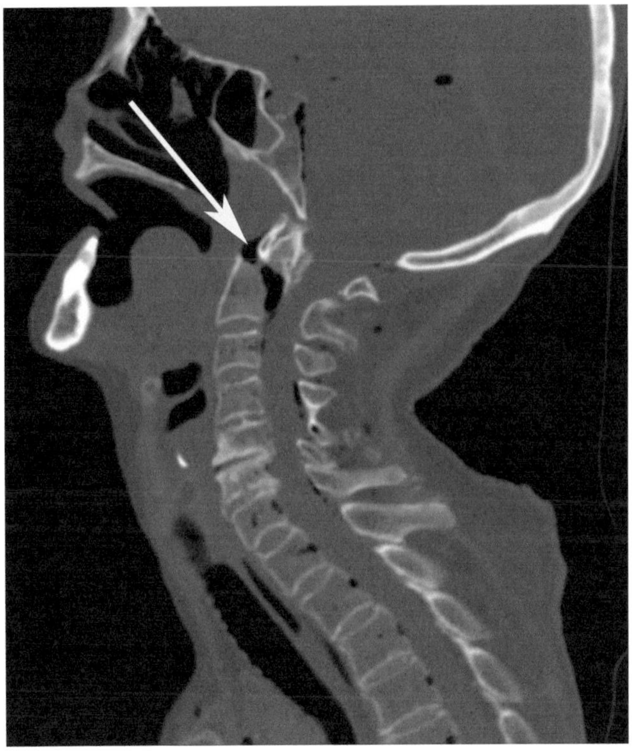

Fig. 13.9 C2 fracture. A sagittal reformatted CT image demonstrating a displaced fracture of the odontoid process of C2 (arrow)

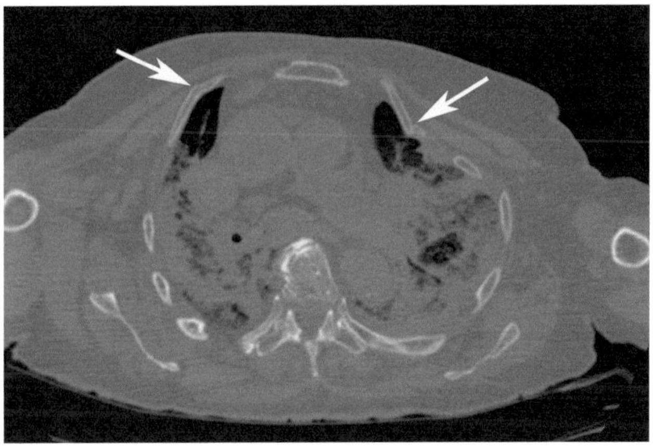

Fig. 13.11 Rib fractures. An axial CT image showing bilateral anterior rib fractures (arrows) secondary to attempted cardiopulmonary resuscitation

revealed a displaced C1/C2 fracture with spinal cord injury (Fig. 13.9) indicating that death resulted from trauma rather than natural causes. Such cervical spine fractures are frequently missed on standard autopsy.

The commonest injuries to be encountered on PMCT are anterior rib and sternal fractures secondary to attempted cardiopulmonary resuscitation (Figs. 13.10 and 13.11). The investigation of choice for the detection of metallic objects such as shot and pellets from gunshot wounds is PMCT (Figs. 13.12 and 13.13).

PMCT is superior to dissection in the assessment of head injuries that involve skull fractures (Figs. 13.14 and 13.15). In deaths resulting from major trauma, such as road traffic collisions, CT typically identifies many injuries that are missed on dissection; spinal, pelvic and limb fractures in particular (Figs. 13.16 and 13.17). Furthermore, three-dimensional reconstruction images provide additional information about how an injury was sustained and are valuable in explaining pathology to the public for illustration in court, as illustrated in these figures.

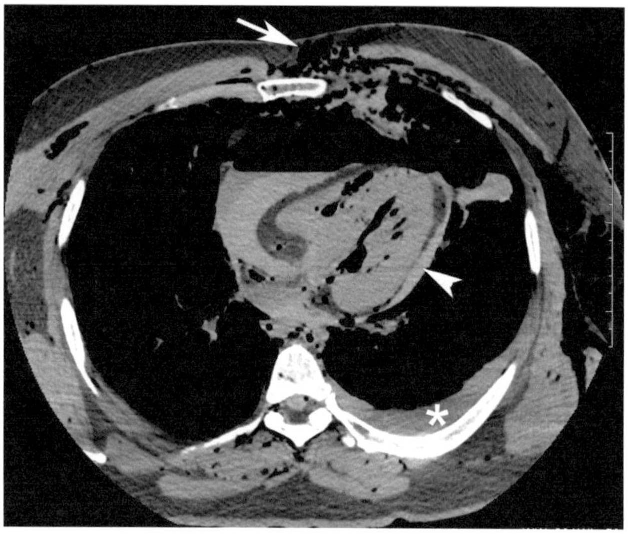

Fig. 13.12 Gunshot wound to the chest. An axial CT image showing the entry wound (arrow) with haemopericardium (arrowhead), and haemothorax (star)

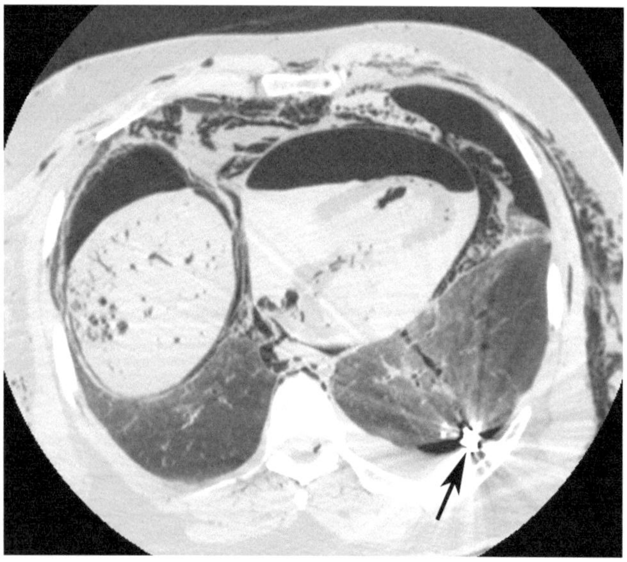

Fig. 13.13 Gunshot wound to chest (same patient as Fig. 13.12). An axial CT image showing pellets in the left hemithorax (arrow)

Demonstration of internal collections of blood secondary to trauma can be achieved by PMCT with considerable sensitivity (Fig. 13.18) and the use of angiographic techniques can demonstrate the precise source of haemorrhage (Fig. 13.19).

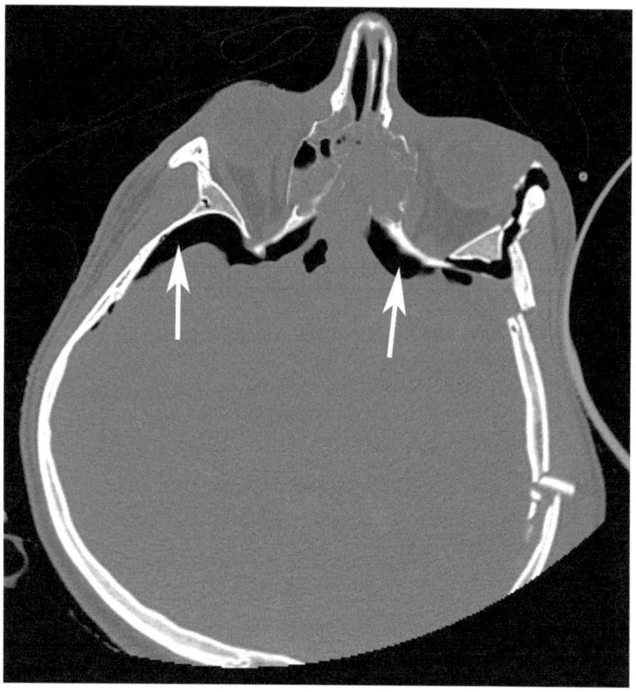

Fig. 13.14 Head injury. An axial CT image on bone windows showing multiple skull fractures and intracranial air (arrows)

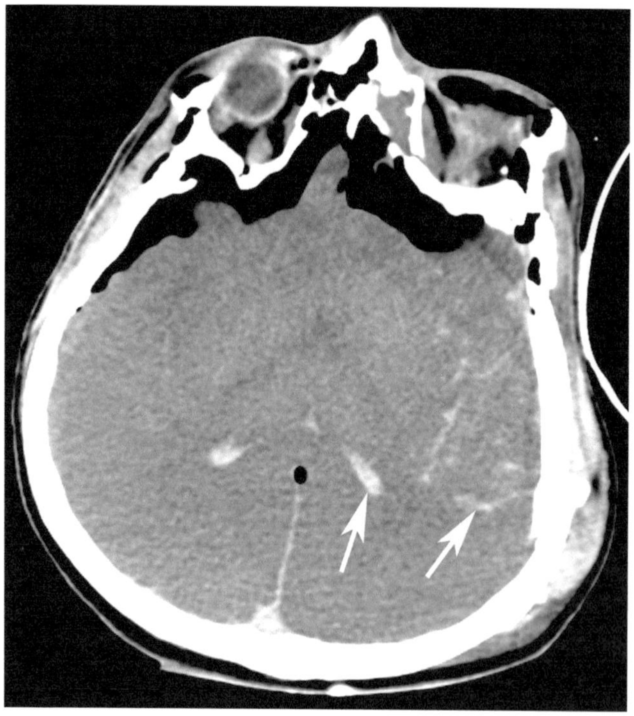

Fig. 13.15 Head injury (same patient as in Fig. 13.14). An axial CT image on soft tissue windows showing subarachnoid and intraventricular haemorrhage (arrows)

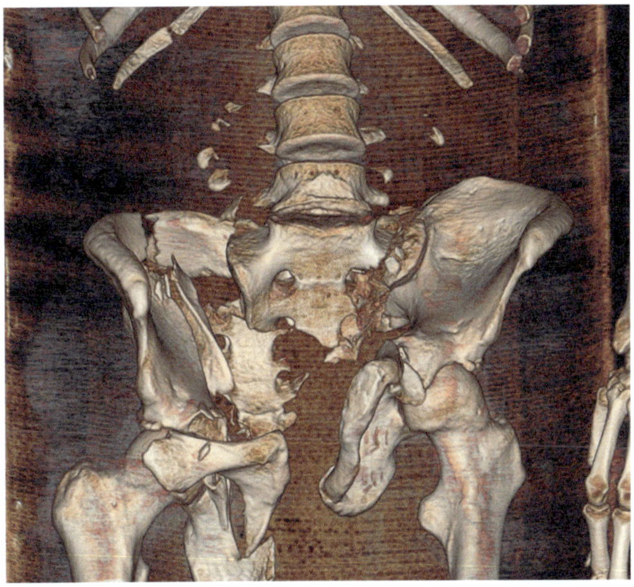

Fig. 13.16 Spinal and pelvic fractures. A 3D volume-rendered image showing multiple transverse process fractures and comminuted fractures of the pelvis and sacrum

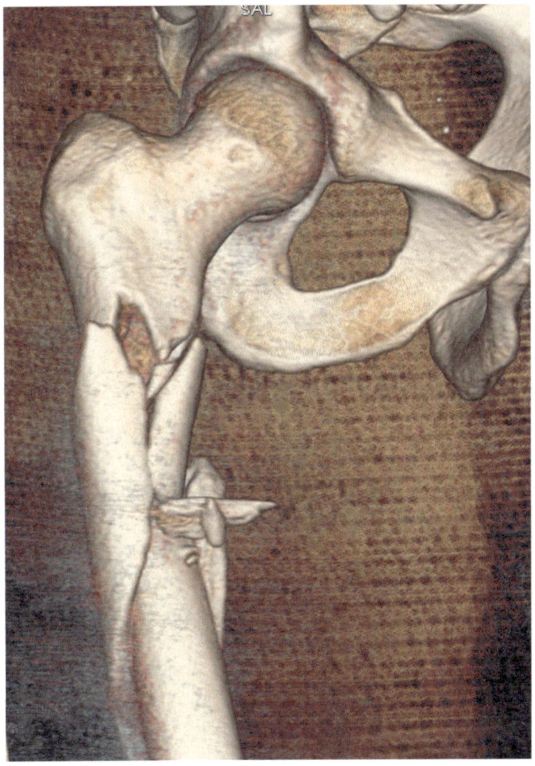

Fig. 13.17 Femoral fracture. A 3D volume-rendered image showing a comminuted fracture of the proximal right femoral shaft

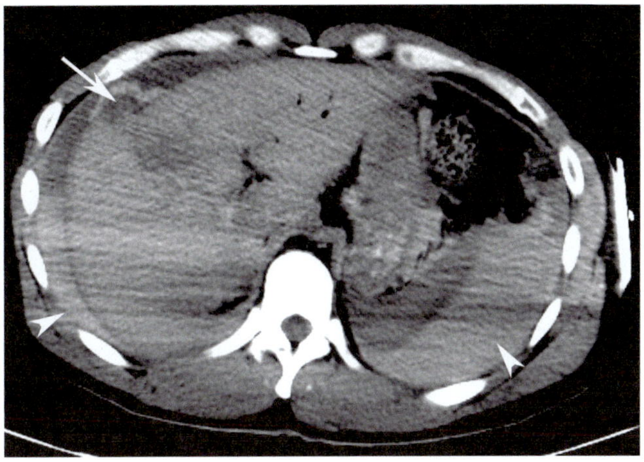

Fig. 13.18 Blunt injury to abdomen. An axial CT image showing a deep laceration of the liver (arrow) with intraperitoneal haemorrhage (arrowheads)

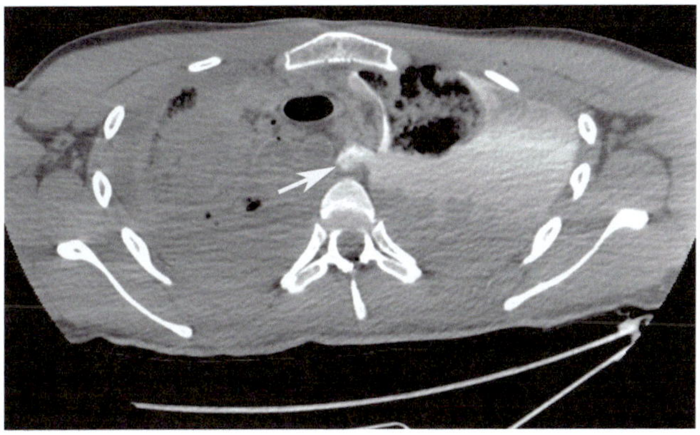

Fig. 13.19 Rupture of descending thoracic aorta secondary to deceleration injury suffered in a road traffic collision. An axial CT image showing contrast in the aorta (arrow) leaking through the tear in the wall and into the mediastinum and left chest cavity

Head

PMCT is sensitive in the detection of intracranial haemorrhage, cerebral infarction, and intracranial tumours (Figs. 13.20, 13.21, 13.22, and 13.23). MRI provides superior detail of most cerebral abnormalities but CT is extremely sensitive in the diagnosis of acute subarachnoid haemorrhage. In a large validation series of post-mortem imaging, the only significant intracranial pathology missed on CT and MRI was meningitis [6].

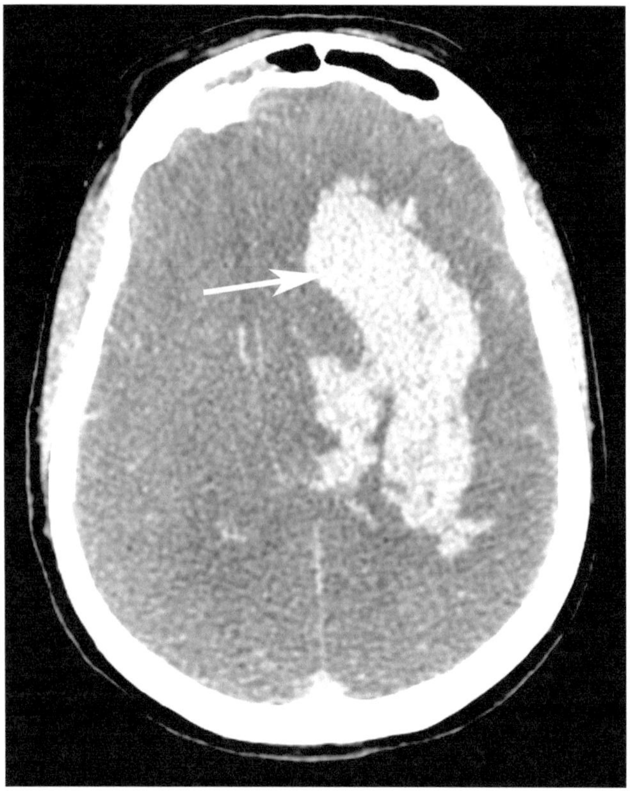

Fig. 13.20 Intracerebral haemorrhage. An axial CT image showing haemorrhage into the left cerebral hemisphere (arrow)

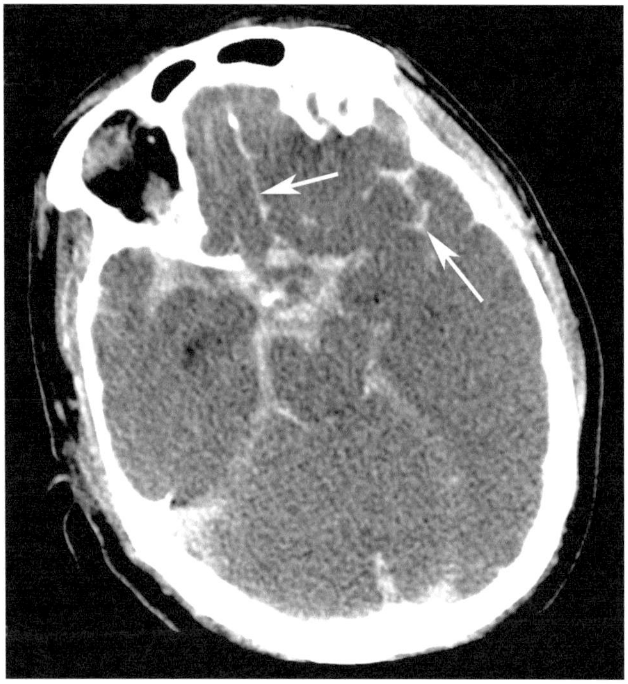

Fig. 13.21 Subarachnoid haemorrhage. An axial CT image showing extensive subarachnoid blood (arrows)

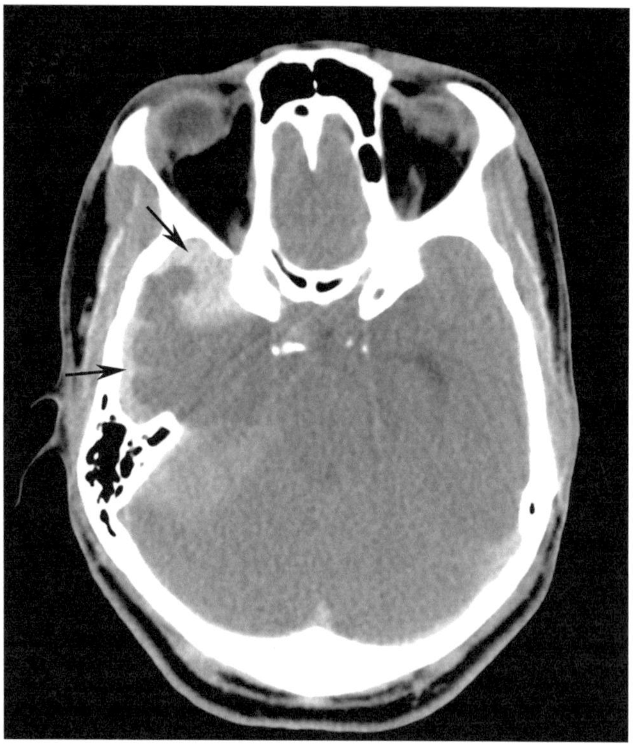

Fig. 13.22 Subdural haemorrhage. An axial CT image showing a subdural haematoma in the right middle cranial fossa (arrow)

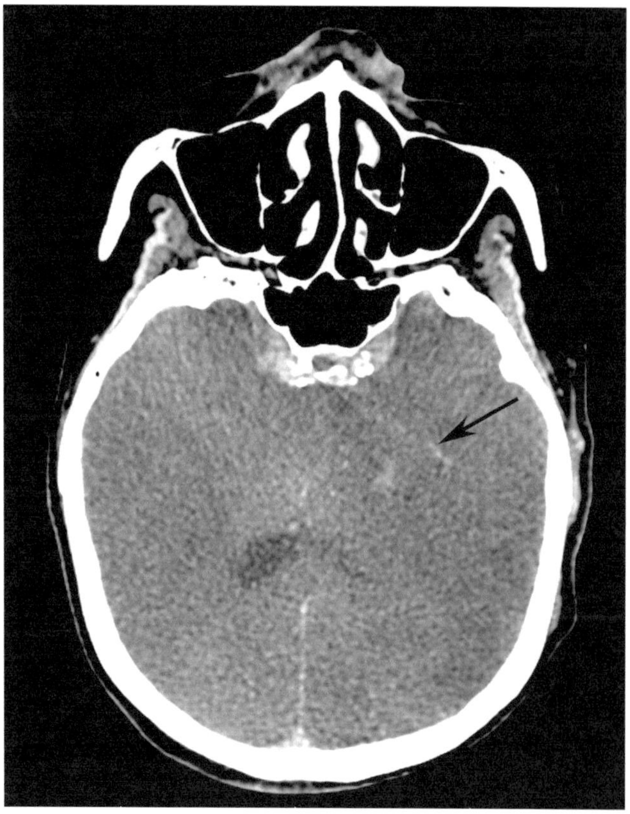

Fig. 13.23 Cerebral infarct. An axial CT image showing extensive cerebral infarction (more marked on the left) with predominant low density but with some small, high-density parenchymal haemorrhages (arrow)

Lungs

The lungs almost invariably appear abnormal on post-mortem imaging. A very common finding is the presence of ground-glass attenuation (a hazy increase in opacification with preservation of bronchial and vascular margins) in a dependent position, usually with a straight, horizontal anterior border, due to post-mortem hypostasis (Fig. 13.24).

Perihilar consolidation and/or ground-glass opacification, frequently with interlobular septal thickening, usually indicates pulmonary oedema (Fig. 13.25). Whilst this might be secondary to left ventricular failure and fluid retention in life, it is also commonly present as a consequence of attempted cardiopulmonary resuscitation.

Consolidation (a homogeneous increase in pulmonary parenchymal attenuation that obscures the margins of vessels and airway walls) is commonly due to pneumonia (Fig. 13.26). CT can demonstrate cavitating lung lesions such as those seen in tuberculosis (Fig. 13.27) and is sensitive for the detection of pulmonary fibrosis (Fig. 13.28).

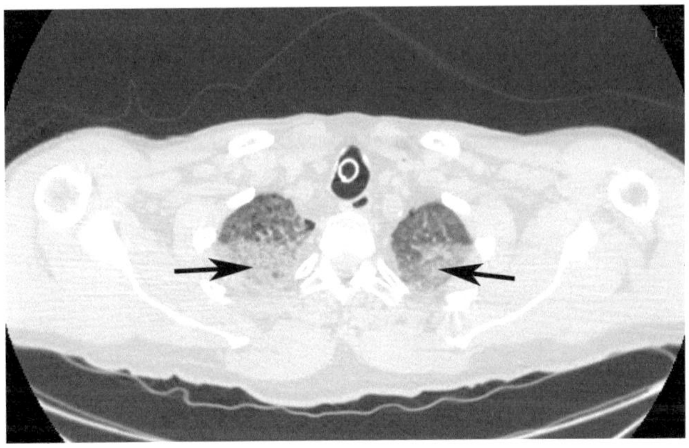

Fig. 13.24 Post-mortem hypostasis. Dependent ground-glass attenuation is seen at the lung apices (arrows), secondary to post-mortem hypostasis

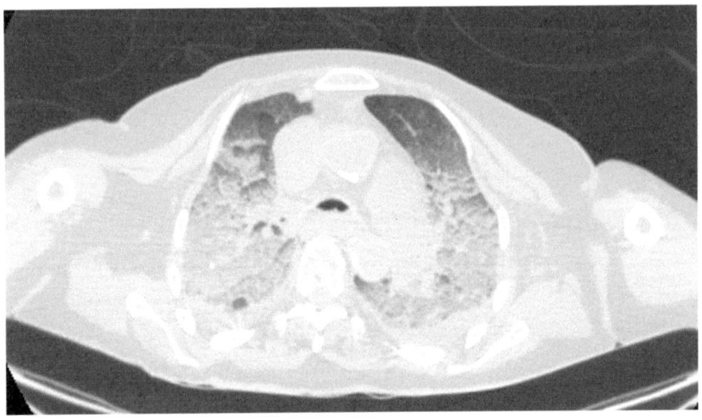

Fig. 13.25 Pulmonary oedema. An axial CT image showing perihilar ground-glass attenuation and interlobular septal thickening secondary to pulmonary oedema

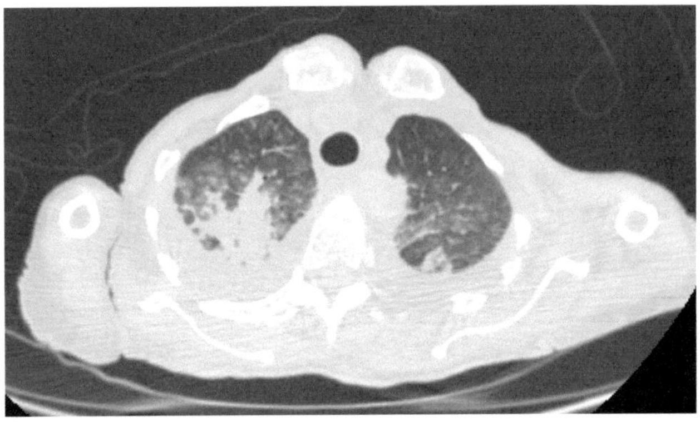

Fig. 13.26 Consolidation. An axial CT image showing bilateral upper lobe consolidation and pleural effusions

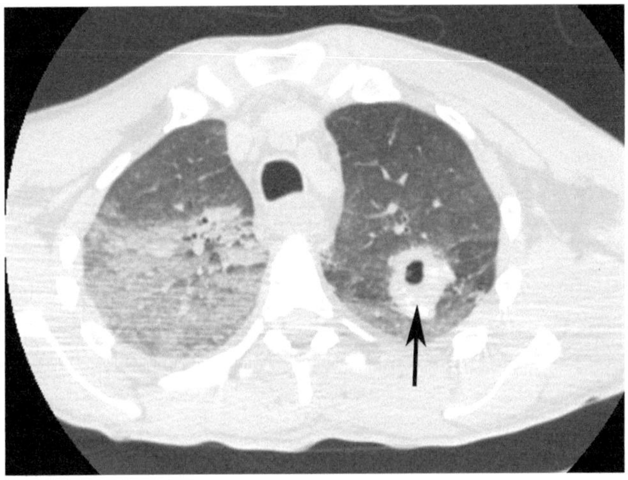

Fig. 13.27 Pulmonary tuberculosis. An axial CT image showing a cavitating mass (arrow) in the left upper lobe secondary to tuberculosis

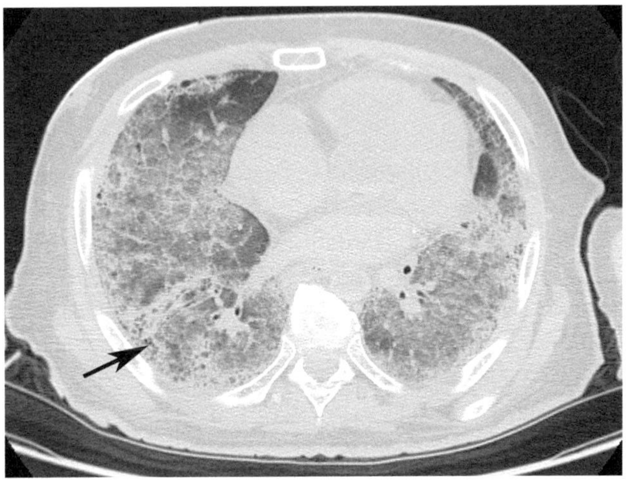

Fig. 13.28 Pulmonary fibrosis. An axial CT image showing honeycombing (arrow) with diffuse ground-glass attenuation and interlobular septal thickening

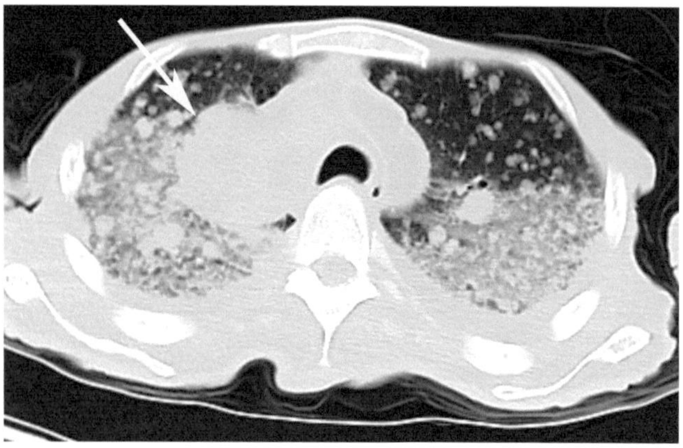

Fig. 13.29 Primary lung tumour and pulmonary metastases. An axial CT image demonstrating a right upper lobe mass (arrow), mediastinal lymphadenopathy and multiple lung metastases. There is also bilateral, dependent ground-glass attenuation due to hypostasis

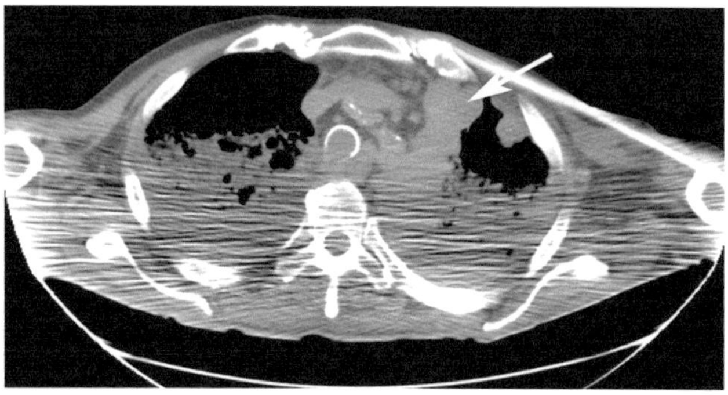

Fig. 13.30 Pleural mesothelioma. An axial CT image showing pleural based tumour in the left hemithorax (arrow). Artefact from the arms obscures views of the posterior hemithoraces

Primary lung tumours (Fig. 13.29), pulmonary metastases (also seen in Fig. 13.29) and pleural tumours (Fig. 13.30) may all be detected on PMCT.

Heart

Coronary calcification is very commonly demonstrated on PMCT (Fig. 13.31), but this finding does not necessarily equate to high-grade arterial stenosis or occlusion. Indeed, cases of patent calcified vessels are frequent, as are occluded noncalcified arteries. However, studies of living patients have demonstrated that extensive coronary calcification (Agatston score, a measure of calcification, of >400) is associated with >90% probability of at least one severe coronary stenosis. Therefore, in the presence of a supportive clinical history (such as chest pain followed by documented cardiac arrest) and absence of other findings on PMCT, an Agatston score of >400 is usually sufficient to attribute death to coronary heart disease. Recent myocardial infarcts cannot be seen on unenhanced PMCT, although myocardial thinning or calcification may be indicative of an old infarct (Fig. 13.32).

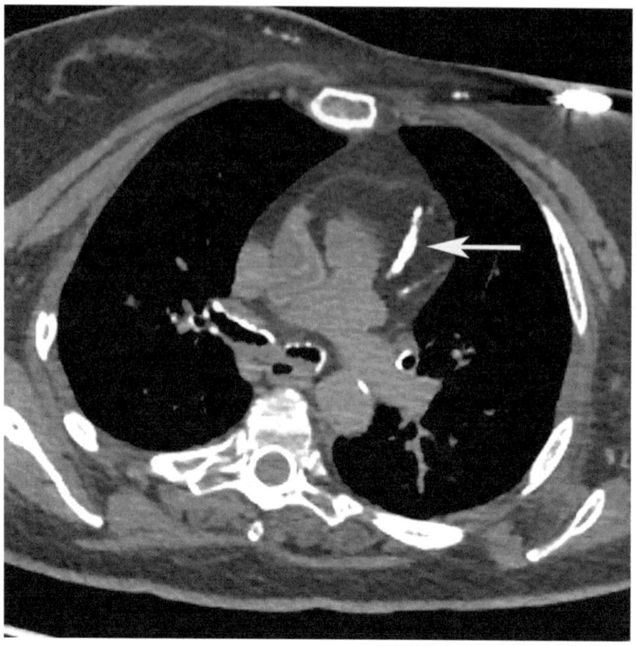

Fig. 13.31 Coronary artery calcification. An axial CT image showing a heavily calcified left anterior descending coronary artery (arrow)

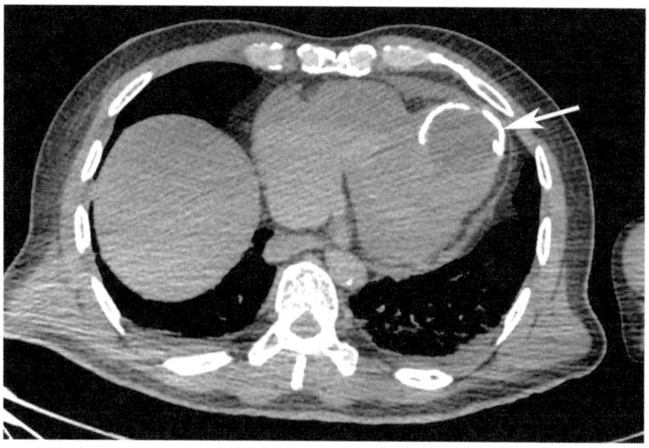

Fig. 13.32 Left ventricular aneurysm. An axial CT image showing a calcified aneurysm (arrow) secondary to previous myocardial infarction

Visualisation of coronary artery lesions is not possible on post-mortem MRI, although myocardial abnormalities indicative of infarction may be identified [15, 16]. In addition, MRI may reveal myocardial abnormalities in cases with normal-appearing myocardium on macroscopic and histological examination. These abnormalities correlate with severe coronary stenosis, suggesting that MRI may be able to demonstrate early ischaemic lesions, which are not detected at macroscopic autopsy.

Haemopericardium can be easily demonstrated on PMCT (Fig. 13.33), but without using angiographic techniques, it is not always possible to distinguish between the two commonest causes, ruptured myocardial infarction and aortic dissection. However, detection of a displaced, calcified intimal flap may allow the diagnosis of an aortic dissection (Fig. 13.34).

In the absence of haemopericardium or severe coronary calcification on PMCT, coronary angiography is required when there is a suspicion of sudden cardiac death. Targeted coronary angiography by cannulation of the left common carotid artery with a Foley catheter and ballooning of the ascending aorta [15], provides detailed visualisation of coronary arteries and is superior to dissection in the evaluation of coronary stenosis (Fig. 13.35). Angiography can also reveal areas of non-perfused myocardium indicative of recent myocardial infarction (Fig. 13.36).

Angiography can also be used to demonstrate congenital abnormalities of the heart, such as ventricular septal defects (Fig. 13.37) and anomalous coronary anatomy (Fig. 13.38).

The diagnosis of cardiomyopathies requires an invasive examination of the heart with histology. However, PMCT can identify cardiac abnormalities that are indicative of a cardiomyopathy, thus directing and limiting dissection to the heart. Figure 13.39 illustrates marked left ventricular hypertrophy in a 42-year-old man who suffered a cardiac

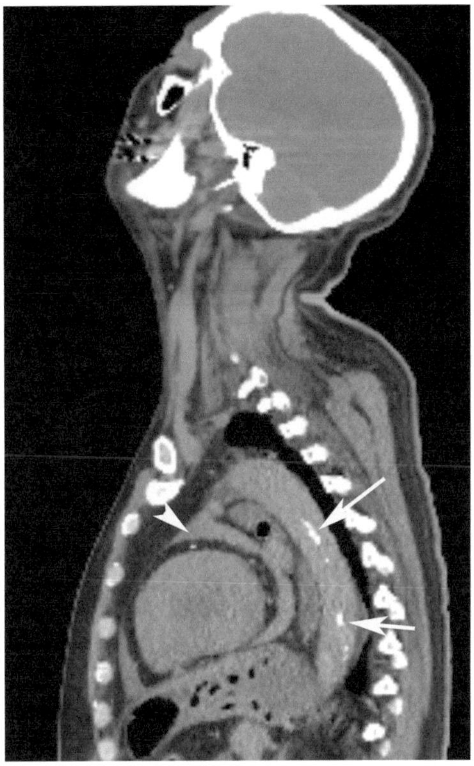

Fig. 13.34 Aortic dissection. A sagittal reformatted image demonstrating a haemopericardium (arrowhead) secondary to a ruptured aortic dissection, as evidenced by displacement of a calcified intimal flap (arrows)

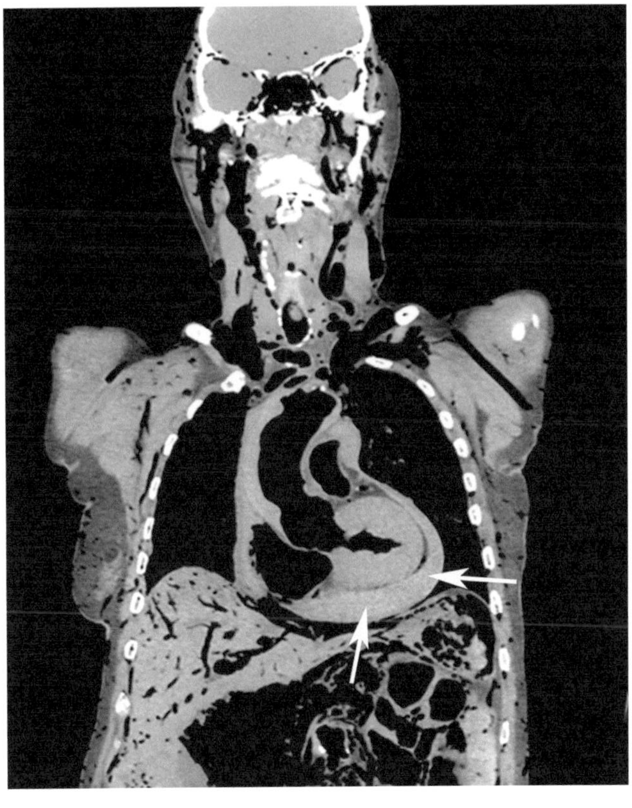

Fig. 13.33 Haemopericardium. A coronal CT image showing haemopericardium (arrows) secondary to a ruptured myocardial infarct

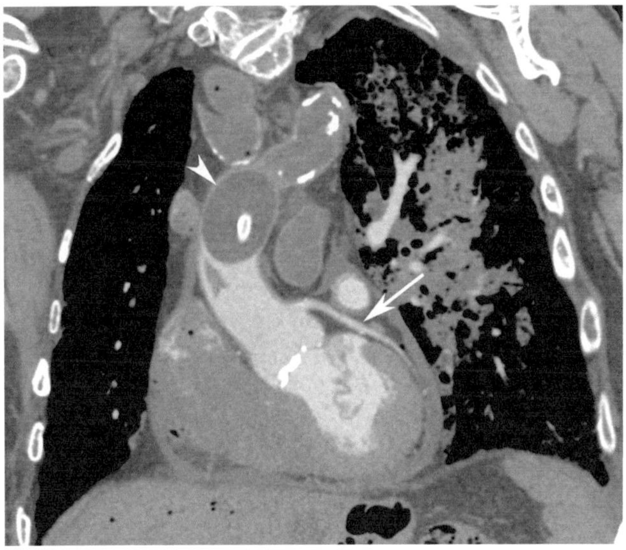

Fig. 13.35 Coronary angiography. An oblique sagittal reformatted image showing the catheter balloon within the ascending aorta (arrowhead), calcification in the aortic valve cusps, and contrast within the left circumflex coronary artery (arrow)

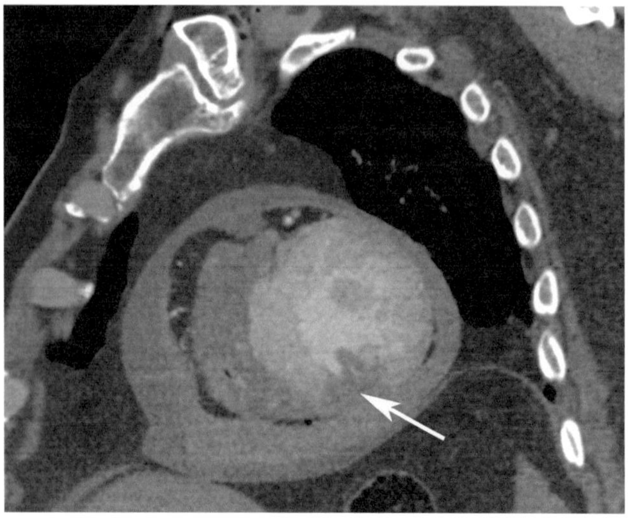

Fig. 13.36 Coronary angiography showing a perfusion defect in the inferior wall of the left ventricle (arrow) with haemopericardium secondary to a ruptured myocardial infarct

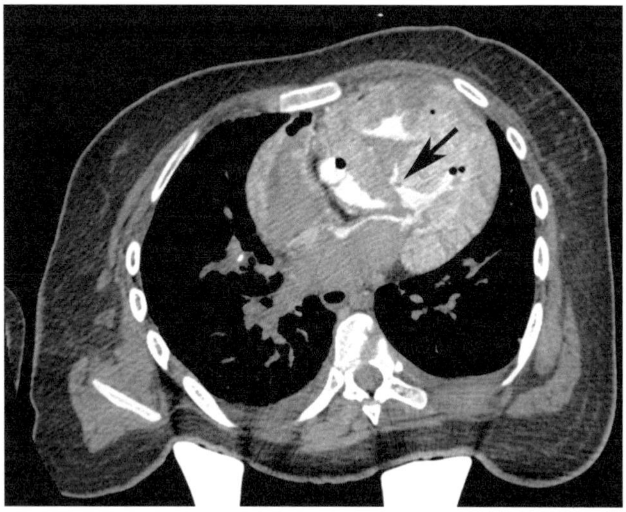

Fig. 13.37 Ventricular septal defect demonstrated on angiography. An axial CT image showing contrast passing from the cavity of the left ventricle into the right ventricle through a ventricular septal defect (arrow)

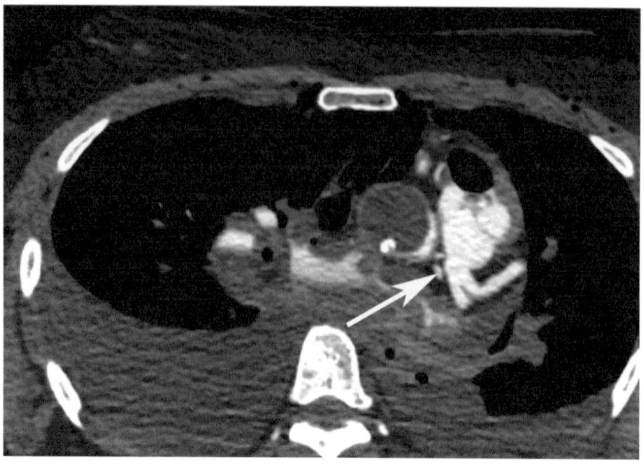

Fig. 13.38 Anomalous coronary anatomy demonstrated on angiography. An axial CT image showing anomalous origin of the left coronary artery from the pulmonary artery (arrow)

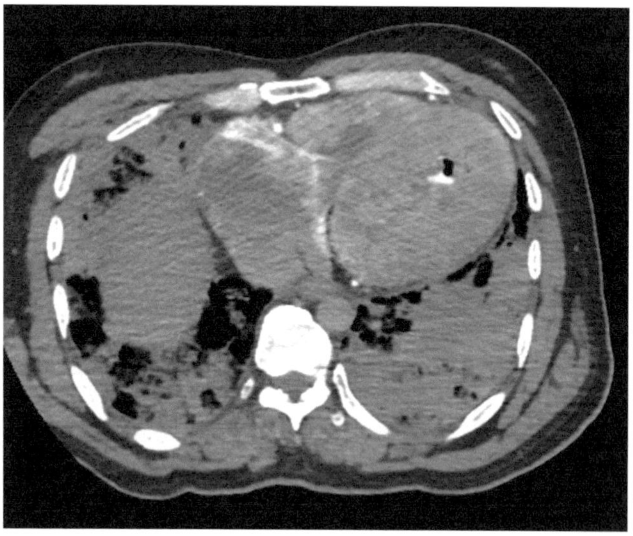

Fig. 13.39 Hypertrophic cardiomyopathy. An axial CT image following coronary angiography showing marked left ventricular hypertrophy

arrest. Coronary angiography demonstrated patent coronary arteries. Subsequent dissection was limited to the heart, removed through a 10 cm incision over the sternum. The heart weighed 609 g with a septal thickness of 30 mm. A diagnosis of hypertrophic cardiomyopathy was confirmed on histology.

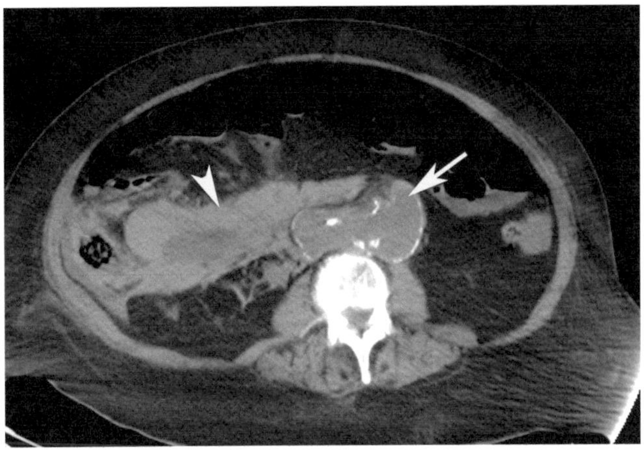

Fig. 13.40 Ruptured abdominal aortic aneurysm. An axial CT image showing a calcified aortic aneurysm (arrow) with retroperitoneal haemorrhage (arrowhead) secondary to rupture

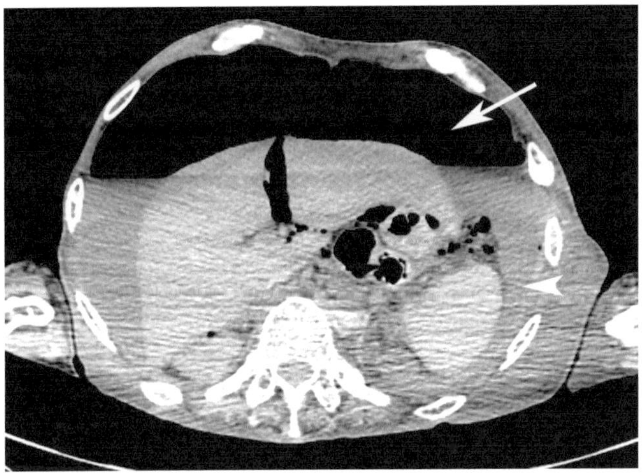

Fig. 13.41 Perforated duodenal ulcer. An axial CT image showing pneumoperitoneum (arrow) and free intraperitoneal fluid (arrowhead)

Abdomen

Post-mortem imaging is sensitive in the detection of tumours and other mass lesions. MRI is generally superior to CT in identifying tumours in solid organs. For example, hepatic metastases frequently are not visible using CT alone. Both techniques easily detect intra-abdominal haemorrhage such as ruptured abdominal aortic aneurysm (Fig. 13.40). PMCT is sensitive for the diagnosis of pneumoperitoneum secondary to a perforated viscus (Fig. 13.41), but it is usually impossible to identify the precise site of perforation. Abdominal wall and inguinal hernias are clearly visible on PMCT (Figs. 13.42 and 13.43).

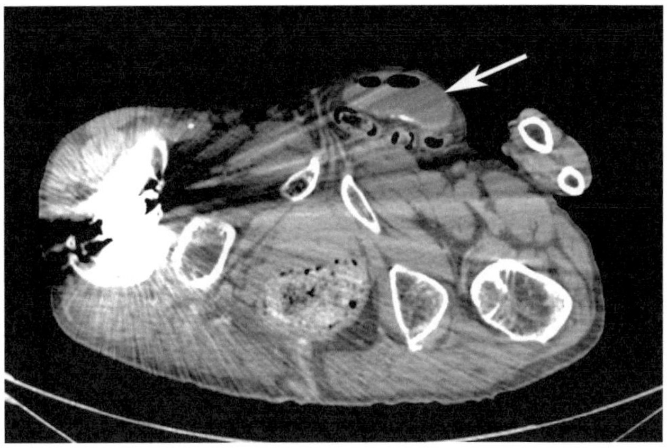

Fig. 13.42 Strangulated inguinal hernia. An axial CT image showing a left inguinal hernia (arrow)

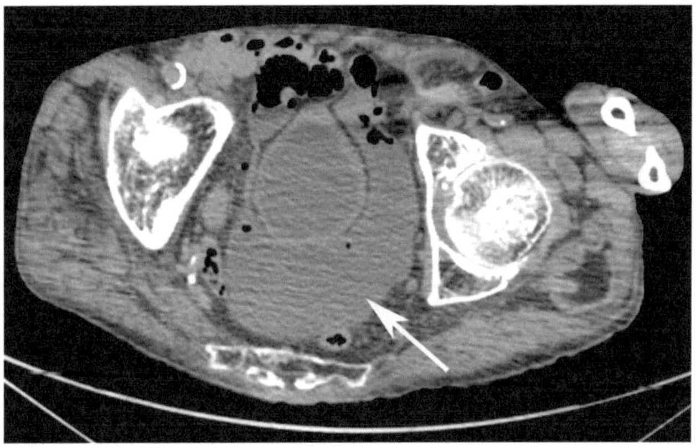

Fig. 13.43 Fluid in the pelvis (arrow) secondary to peritonitis related to the strangulated inguinal hernia (same patient as Fig. 13.42)

References

1. Norberti N, Tonelli P, Giaconi C, et al. State of the art in post-mortem computed tomography: a review of current literature. Virchows Arch. 2019;475:139–50.
2. Ministry of Justice. Coroners' statistics 2022: England and Wales. Available from: https://www.gov.uk/government/statistics/coroners-statistics-2022/coroners-statistics-2022-england-and-wales
3. Okuda T, Shiotani S, Sakamoto N, Kobayashi T. Background and current status of postmortem imaging in Japan: short history of "Autopsy imaging (Ai)". Forensic Sci Int. 2013;225:3–8.
4. Bisset RAL, Thomas NB, Turnbull IW, Lee S. Postmortem examinations using magnetic resonance imaging: four year review of a working service. BMJ. 2002;324:1423–4.
5. Roberts IS, Benbow EW, Bisset R, et al. Accuracy of magnetic resonance imaging in determining cause of sudden death in

adults: comparison with conventional autopsy. Histopathology. 2003;42:424–30.
6. Roberts ISD, Benamore RE, Benbow EW, et al. Could post-mortem imaging be an alternative to autopsy in the diagnosis of adult deaths? A validation study. Lancet. 2012;379:136–42.
7. Roberts ISD, Benamore RE, Peebles C, Roobottom C, Traill ZC. Diagnosis of coronary artery disease using minimally invasive autopsy: evaluation of a novel method of post-mortem coronary CT angiography. Clin Radiol. 2011;66:645–50.
8. Rutty GN, Morgan B, Robinson C, et al. Diagnostic accuracy of post-mortem CT with targeted coronary angiography versus autopsy for coroner-requested post-mortem investigations: a prospective, masked, comparison study. Lancet. 2017;390:145–54.
9. Grabherr S, Gygax E, Sollberger B, et al. Two-step postmortem angiography with a modified heart-lung machine: preliminary results. AJR Am J Roentgenol. 2008;190:345–51.
10. Fryer EP, Traill ZC, Benamore RE, Roberts ISD. High risk medico-legal autopsies: is a full postmortem examination necessary? J Clin Pathol. 2013;66:1–7.
11. Weustink AC, Hunink MGM, van Dijke CF, Renken NS, Krestin GP, Oosterhuis JW. Minimally invasive autopsy: an alternative to conventional autopsy? Radiology. 2009;50:897–904.
12. Bolliger SA, Filograna L, Spendlove D, Thali MJ, Dirnhofer S, Ross S. Postmortem imaging-guided biopsy as an adjuvant to minimally invasive autopsy with CT and postmortem angiography: a feasibility study. AJR Am J Roentgenol. 2010;195:1051–6.
13. Roberts ISD, Traill ZC. Minimally invasive autopsy employing postmortem CT and targeted coronary angiography: evaluation of its application to a routine Coronial service. Histopathology. 2014;64:211–7.
14. The Royal College of Pathologists and The Royal College of Radiologists. Guidelines for post-mortem cross-sectional imaging in adults for non-forensic deaths. 2021. https://www.rcpath.org/static/666dbf95-de06-44ad-89c3b4e5f1ceab79/G182-Guidelines-for-post-mortem-cross-sectional-imaging.pdf
15. Jackowski C, Schwendener N, Grabherr S, Persson A. Post-mortem cardiac 3-T magnetic resonance imaging: visualization of sudden cardiac death? J Am Coll Cardiol. 2013;62:617–29.
16. Michaud K, Genet P, Sabatasso S, Grabherr S. Postmortem imaging as a complementary tool for the investigation of cardiac death. Forensic Sci Res. 2019;4:211–22.

Suggested Reading

Shenton A, Kralt P, Suvarna SK. Post mortem CT for non-suspicious adult deaths. Springer; 2021.

14 Histology of the Autopsy

Esther Youd

Introduction

Histology is a valuable part of the autopsy examination. The wise autopsy pathologist will utilise microscopic examination as part of many autopsies.

Histology can be a useful tool to confirm macroscopic features, or to date the findings, for example in acute myocardial infarction, thromboembolism or subdural haemorrhage.

There are features of macroscopically identifiable pathology which can be refined and defined using histology, for example tumour types, or the cause of aortic dissection.

There are some diagnoses which can only be made using histology, for example myocarditis, encephalitis or the inheritable cardiomyopathies.

In an apparently negative autopsy macroscopically, microscopic examination of the organs may reveal a surprise diagnosis such as pyelonephritis, pancreatitis or cardiac amyloidosis.

Regular sampling of the major organs for histology will allow the pathologist to become familiar with the artefacts conferred by the post mortem period and the range of normal features encountered, in order to be able to recognise and define pathology and better understand the pathophysiological processes which led to death.

This chapter illustrates autopsy histology arranged by organ systems, covering normal appearances, autopsy artefacts and common and uncommon organ pathology.

Autopsy Artefacts

Within a few hours of death, the body will undergo deterioration. This will inevitably be seen in autopsy tissues to some degree. Cell nuclei die and cell membranes disintegrate. Enzyme activity breaks down cells and tissues. Bacterial activity then takes over.

The range of changes seen will vary with the length of time since the person died and the organ or tissue the pathologist is observing. For example, the gastrointestinal mucosa is rapidly affected by autolysis and loss of the epithelium is a common artefact of the post mortem period. This makes assessment of mucosal changes in the gastrointestinal tract challenging. Similarly, the pancreas contains a host of autoenzymes which, without the usual protective measures in life, cause rapid autolysis of the pancreas.

After several days, weeks or months histological features may be entirely uninterpretable in any or all organs. However, some pathological features, for example fibrosis in the heart, do persist even in the setting of advanced autolysis and therefore histology from a decomposed body can still be instructive.

Figures 14.1, 14.2, 14.3, 14.4, 14.5, and 14.6 show some of the artefacts seen in autopsy histology.

E. Youd (✉)
Forensic Medicine and Science, University of Glasgow, Glasgow, UK
e-mail: esther.youd@glasgow.ac.uk

S. K. Suvarna (represented by Grace Horne), A. K. Sharp (eds.), *Atlas of Adult Autopsy*,
https://doi.org/10.1007/978-3-031-72207-3_14

Autopsy Artefacts

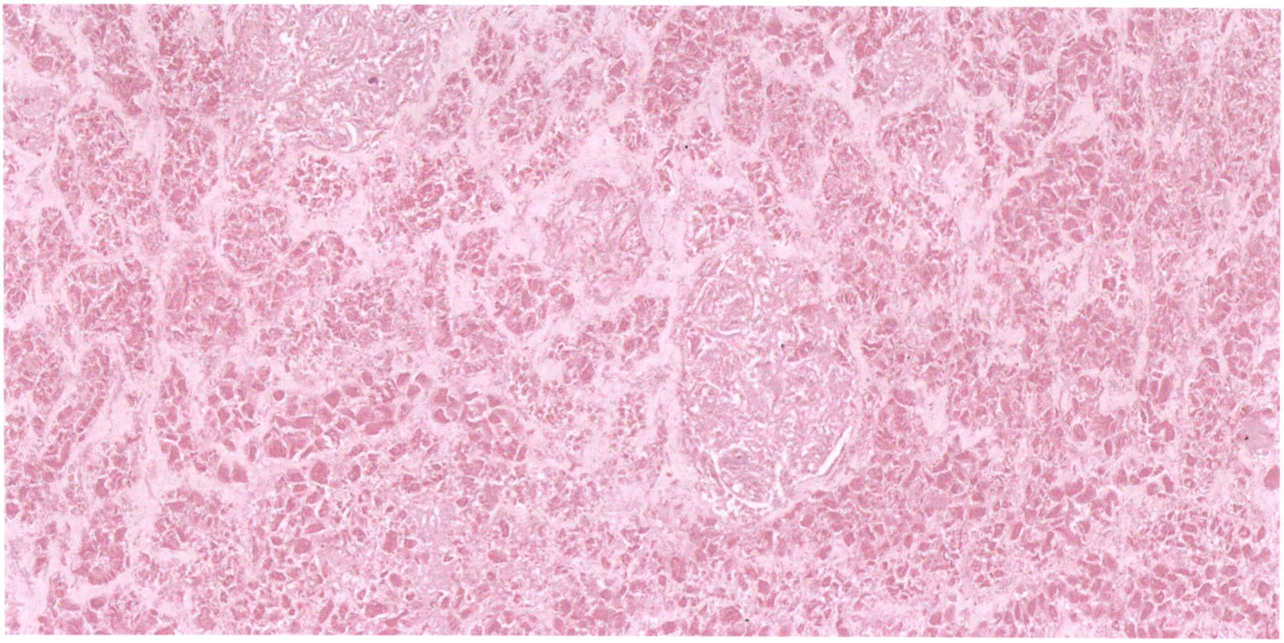

Fig. 14.1 Autolysis, as seen in this kidney section, can affect post mortem tissues to varying degrees. It may be possible to interpret some findings, whilst acknowledging the limitations of the autolysis. In some cases it may be very difficult to identify any pathology and this should be acknowledged

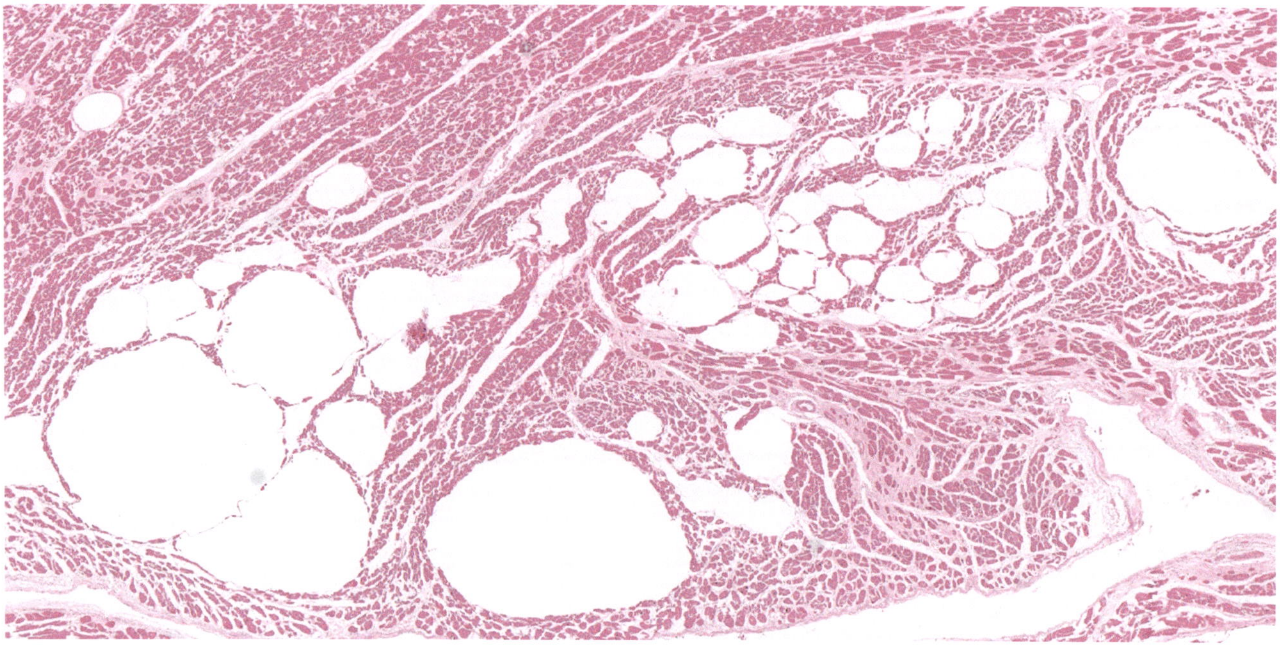

Fig. 14.2 In this heart tissue, gas forming artefact can be seen as a result of post mortem bacterial gas production. Even in autolysed heart it is possible to identify established fibrosis which may be relevant to the cause of death, therefore histology from a decomposed body can still be instructive

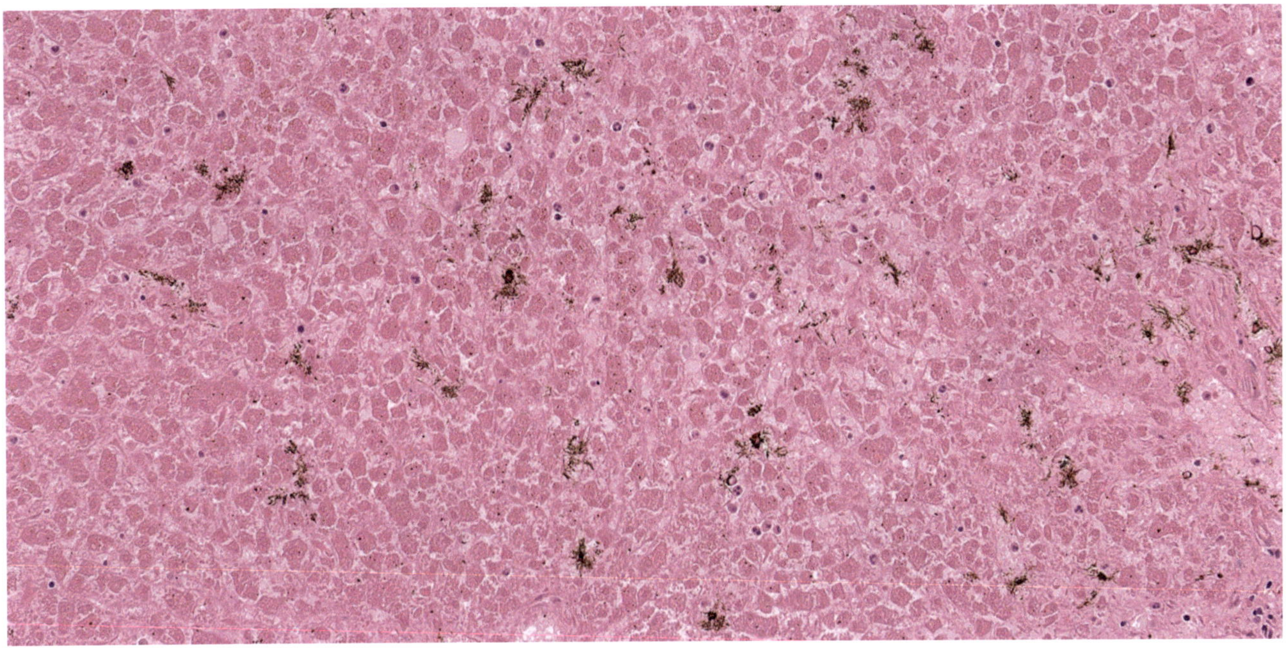

Fig. 14.3 It is common to see formalin pigment in post mortem tissues, such as in this section of liver. This should not be mistaken for other pathological pigments. Common pigments seen in the liver include lipofuscin (intracellular, fine, yellow/brown pigment) and bile (yellow or green pigment) which can be intracytoplasmic, intracanalicular or in Kupffer cells

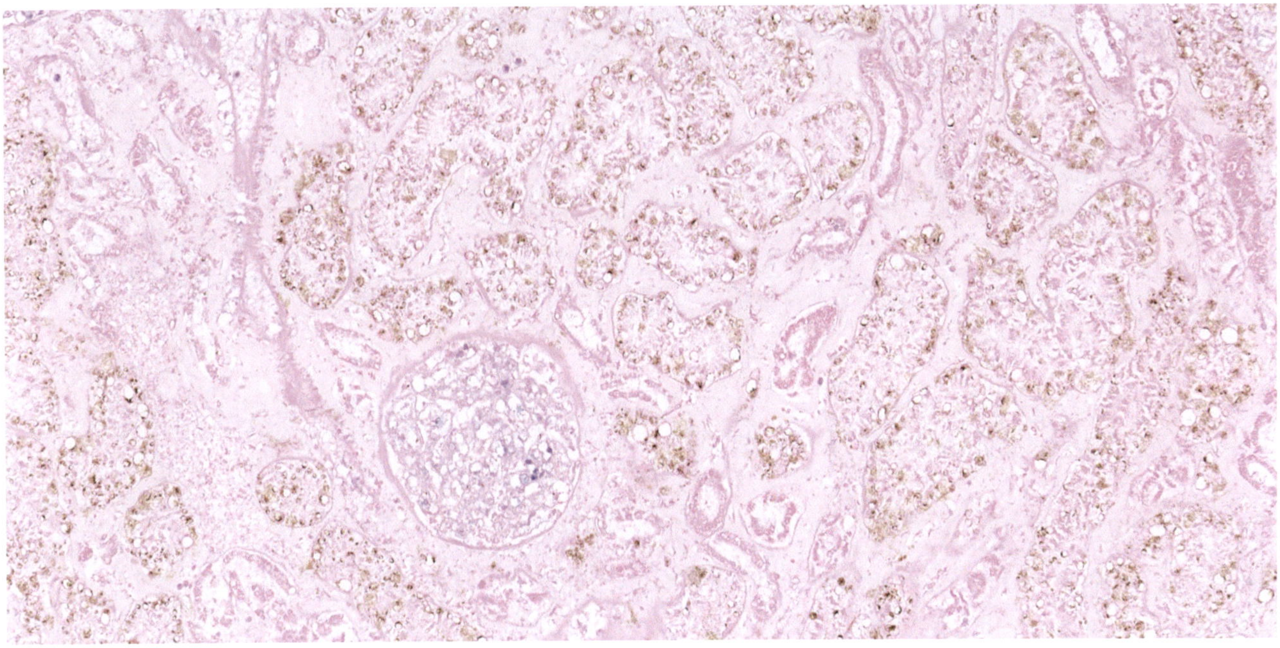

Fig. 14.4 This image shows another example of formalin pigment, this time involving the kidney

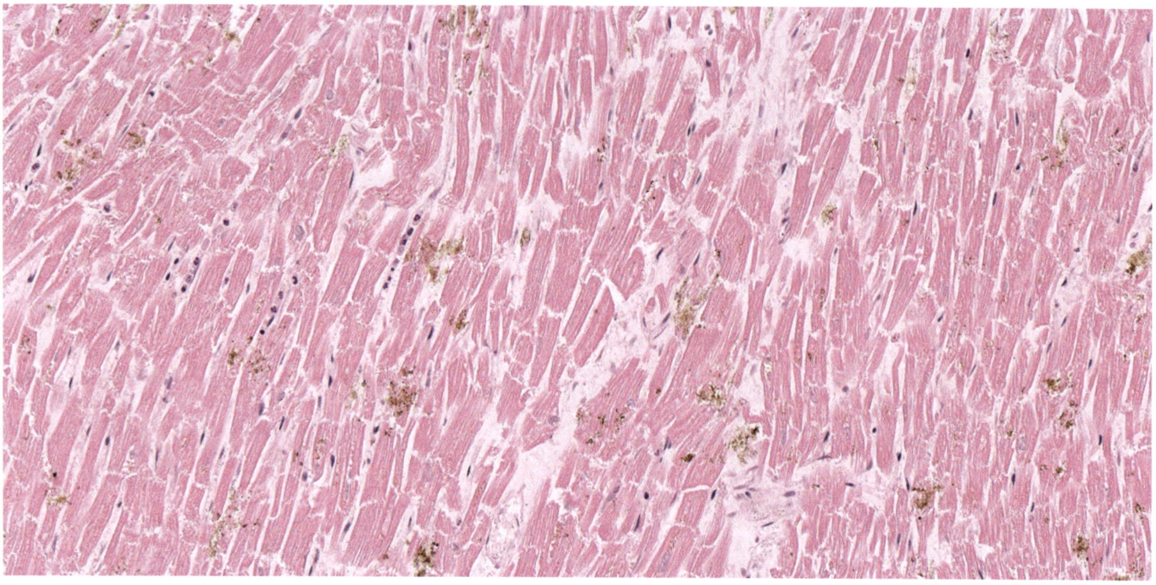

Fig. 14.5 Formalin pigment is seen here in the heart

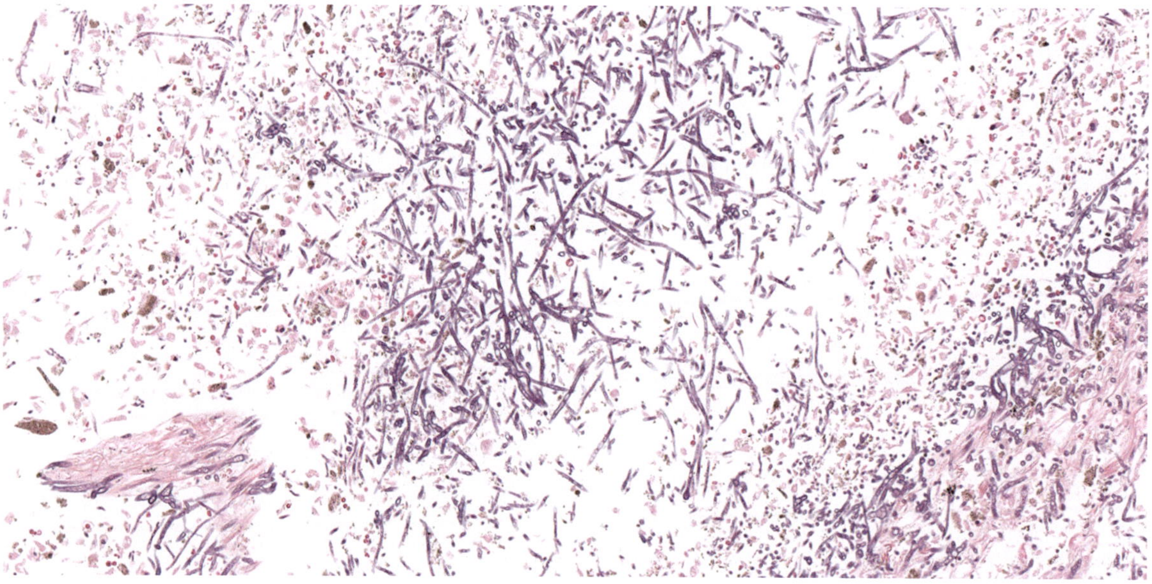

Fig. 14.6 It is not uncommon to see bacterial or fungal overgrowth in post mortem tissues. This should not be over-interpreted as evidence of infection in life. This section of lung shows the characteristic appearance of fungal overgrowth. It is important to note that there is no associated inflammatory reaction, making this clearly a post mortem phenomenon

Cardiovascular System

Pathology within the cardiovascular system is one of the most common findings in adult autopsy practice, particularly in the UK. Many findings can be assessed well macroscopically (see earlier chapters) but histological assessment can often add value in confirming or refining the diagnosis. Histology also provides positive feedback in learning about macroscopic interpretation.

In a medico-legal setting, histology of common pathologies, including ischaemic heart disease, may be important, for example in dating a myocardial infarction in a person who may have interacted with a healthcare system in the days prior to death.

Many cardiac pathology diagnoses can be made by the general pathologist. Histological assessment of more unusual cardiac disease, for example the inherited cardiomyopathies, may require the pathologist to consult with an expert cardiac pathologist to confirm a diagnosis. However, it is important for the general pathologist to make a good macroscopic assessment of the heart and sample the heart well for histology. Recommended sampling includes the anterior left ventricle (LV), lateral LV, posterior LV and interventricular septum, the anterior and posterior walls of the right ventricle, and any abnormal areas. Consideration should be given to sampling the coronary arteries, conduction system and the right and left ventricular outflow tracts.

The illustrations that follow cover normal appearances of the heart, autopsy artefacts, acquired disease including ischaemic heart disease, hypertension, valve disease and inflammatory conditions, the inheritable cardiomyopathies, and cardiac tumours (Figs. 14.7, 14.8, 14.9, 14.10, 14.11, 14.12, 14.13, 14.14, 14.15, 14.16, 14.17, 14.18, 14.19, 14.20, 14.21, 14.22, 14.23, 14.24, 14.25, 14.26, 14.27, 14.28, 14.29, 14.30, 14.31, 14.32, 14.33, 14.34, 14.35, 14.36, 14.37, 14.38, 14.39, 14.40, 14.41, 14.42, 14.43, 14.44, 14.45, 14.46, 14.47, 14.48, 14.49, 14.50, 14.51, 14.52, 14.53, 14.54, 14.55, 14.56, 14.57, 14.58, 14.59, 14.60, 14.61, 14.62, 14.63, 14.64, 14.65, 14.66, 14.67, 14.68, 14.69, 14.70, 14.71, 14.72, and 14.73).

Normal aorta (Figs. 14.74, 14.75, and 14.76) and pathology of the aorta (Figs. 14.77, 14.78, 14.79, 14.80, 14.81, 14.82, 14.83, and 14.84) is also shown, including aortitis and inheritable connective tissue disorders which can be associated with aortic dissection.

Heart

Normal and Artefacts

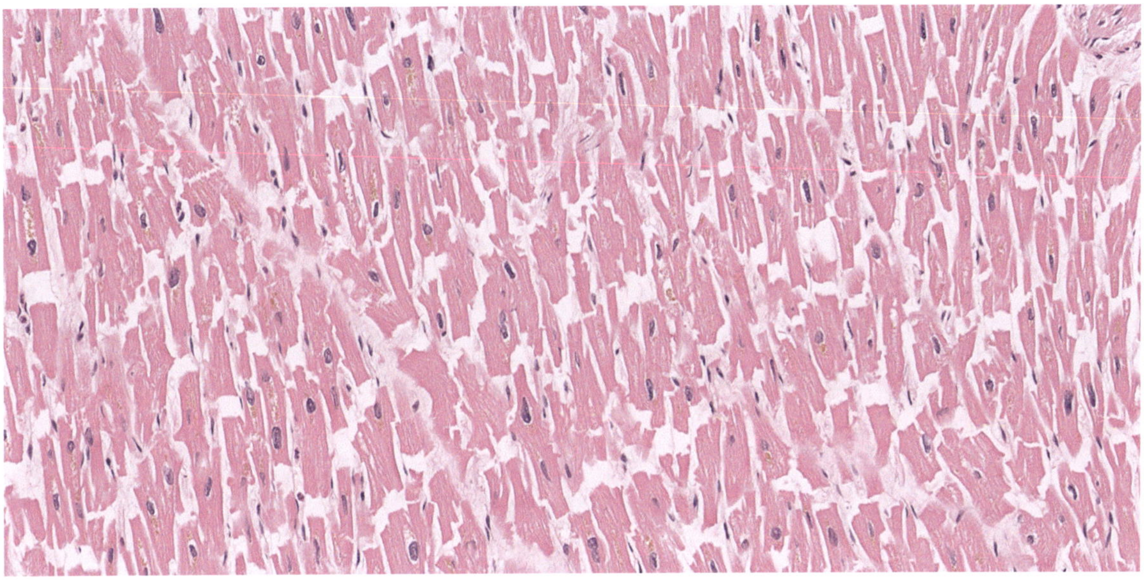

Fig. 14.7 This is normal heart in which lipofuscin pigment is seen. Lipofuscin is a degenerative finding of no pathological significance

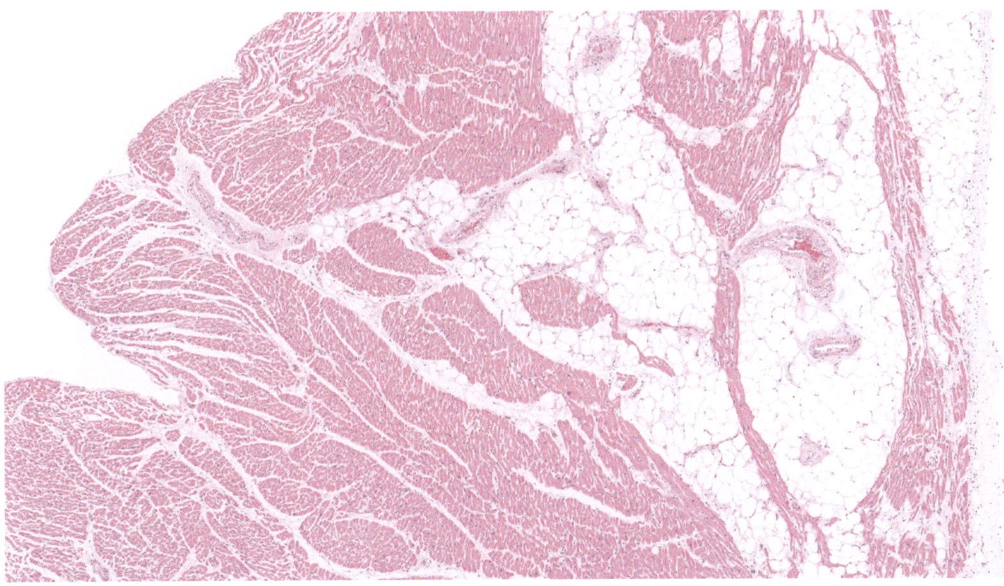

Fig. 14.8 The normal right ventricle may include a significant component of adipose tissue, particularly surrounding intra-cardiac vessels. Adipose tissue may also be seen with increasing frequency in older people and may be quite prominent, splaying apart bundles of myocytes rather than replacing them. Pathological adipose replacement occurs in arrhythmogenic right ventricular cardiomyopathy (see Fig. 14.47) but the pathologist should become familiar with the range of normal adipose tissue that can be seen within the right ventricle

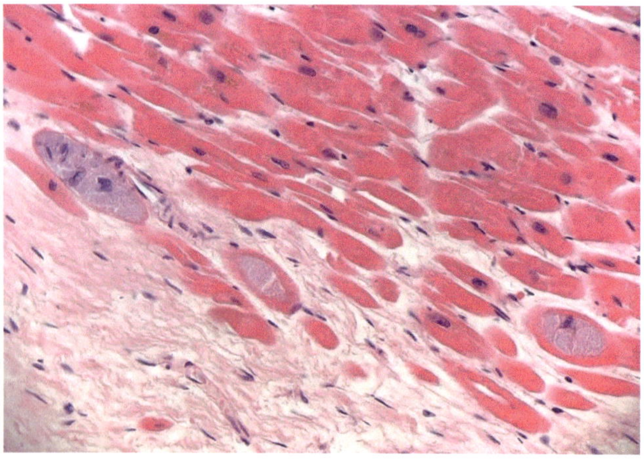

Fig. 14.9 With increasing age, basophilic degeneration of cardiac myocytes may be seen

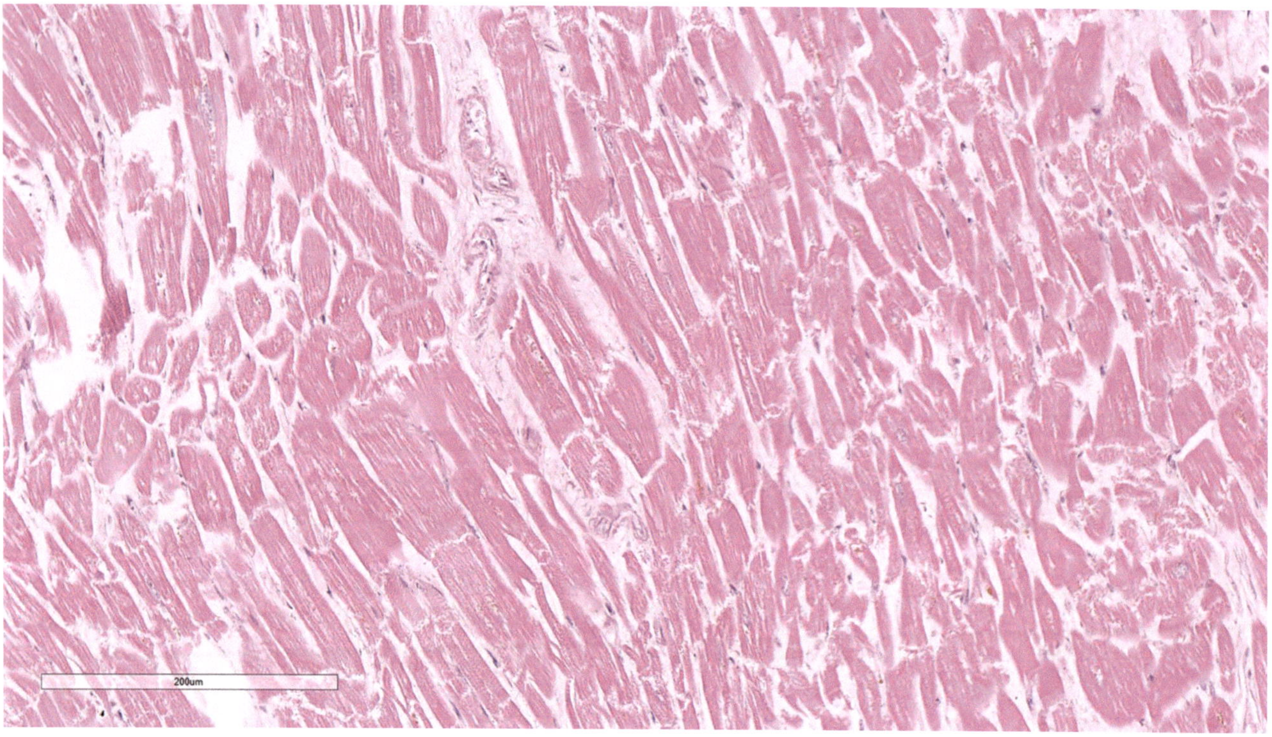

Fig. 14.10 In decomposition the myocardium becomes autolysed. The features seen include loss of the cardiac myocyte nuclei and breakdown of the cytoplasm

Ischaemic Heart Disease

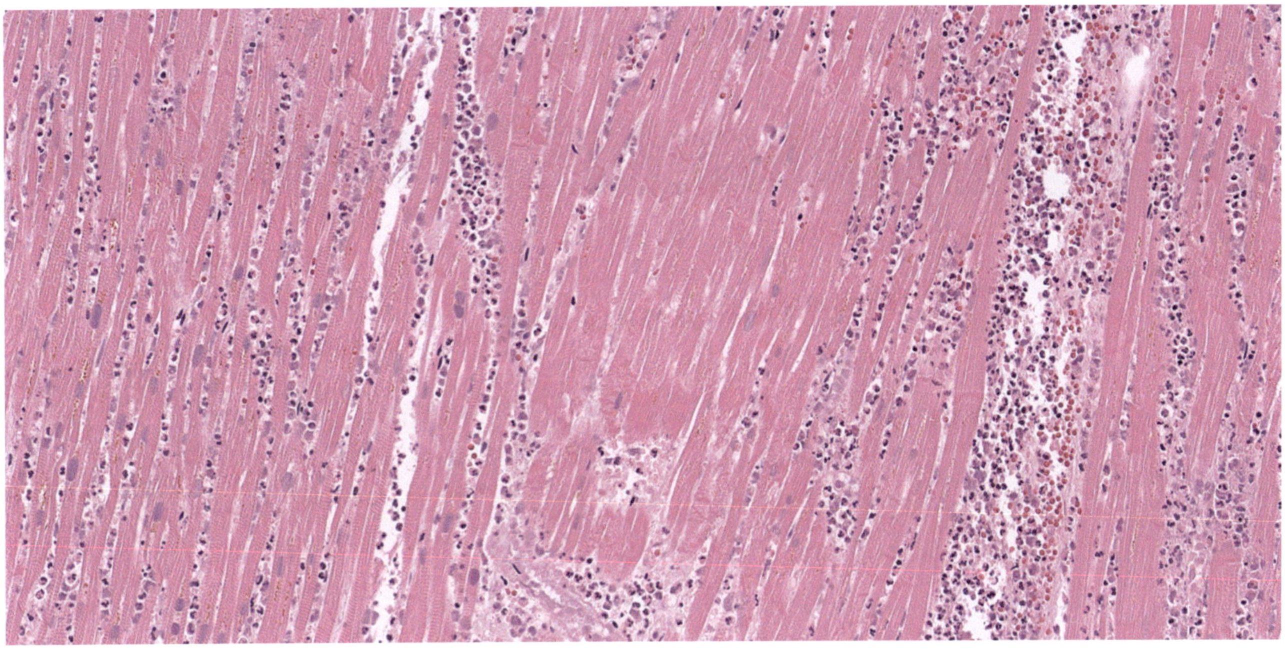

Fig. 14.11 In acute myocardial infarction there is loss of cardiac myocyte nuclei, formation of contraction bands and infiltration by neutrophils. Microscopic examination of acute myocardial infarction allows an estimation of the timing of the infarct. The autopsy pathologist may consult general pathology texts for tables of such timings

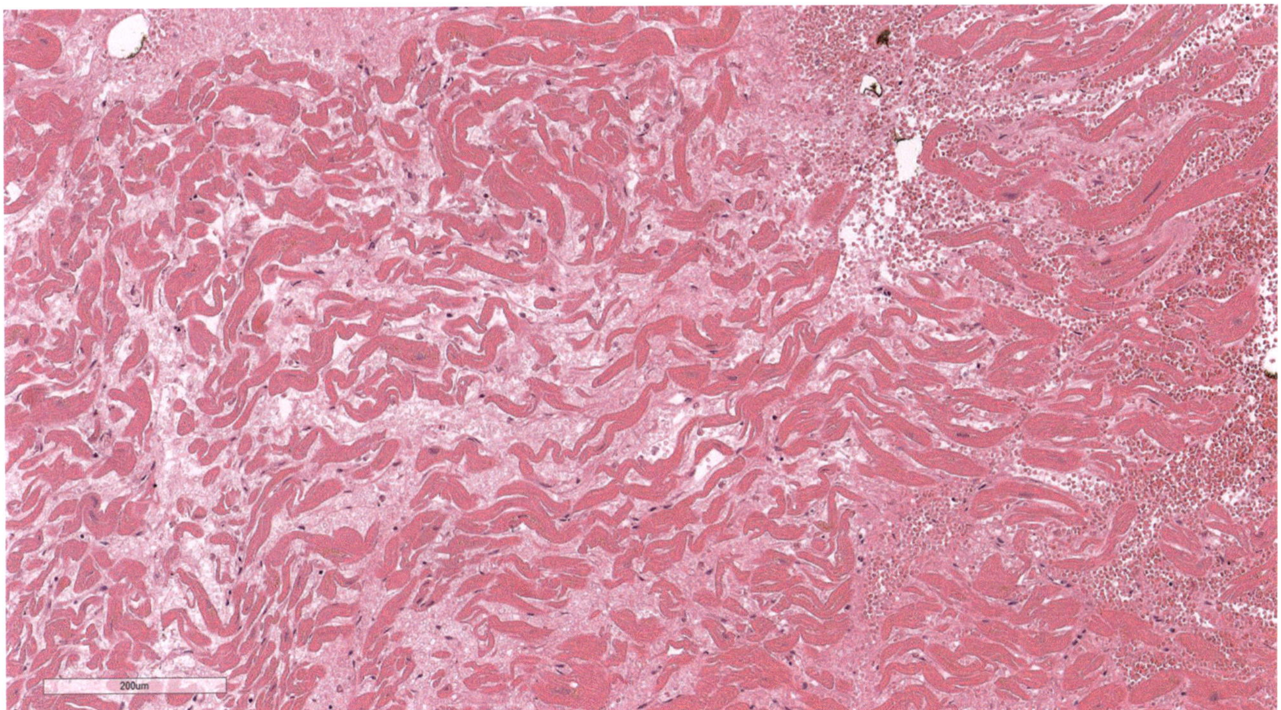

Fig. 14.12 This image shows an acute myocardial infarction, with dead myocytes and wavy fibres. There is haemorrhage between the fibres. Although wavy fibres are described as an early sign of acute myocardial infarct, they are most often seen associated with cardiac rupture, as in this case, as a rebound effect following stretching of the dead fibres and subsequent rupture

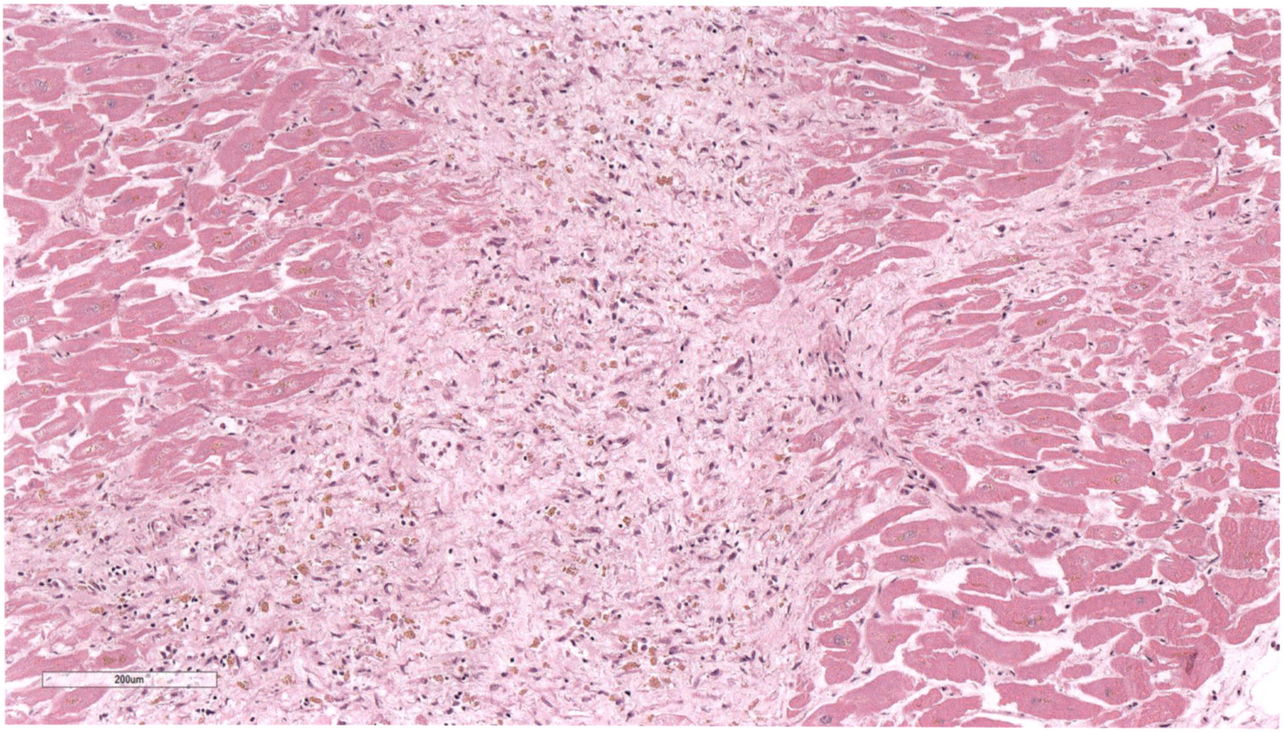

Fig. 14.13 Another image of acute myocardial infarction is shown here. This is an older, healing infarct. There are fibroblasts and haemosiderin pigment present

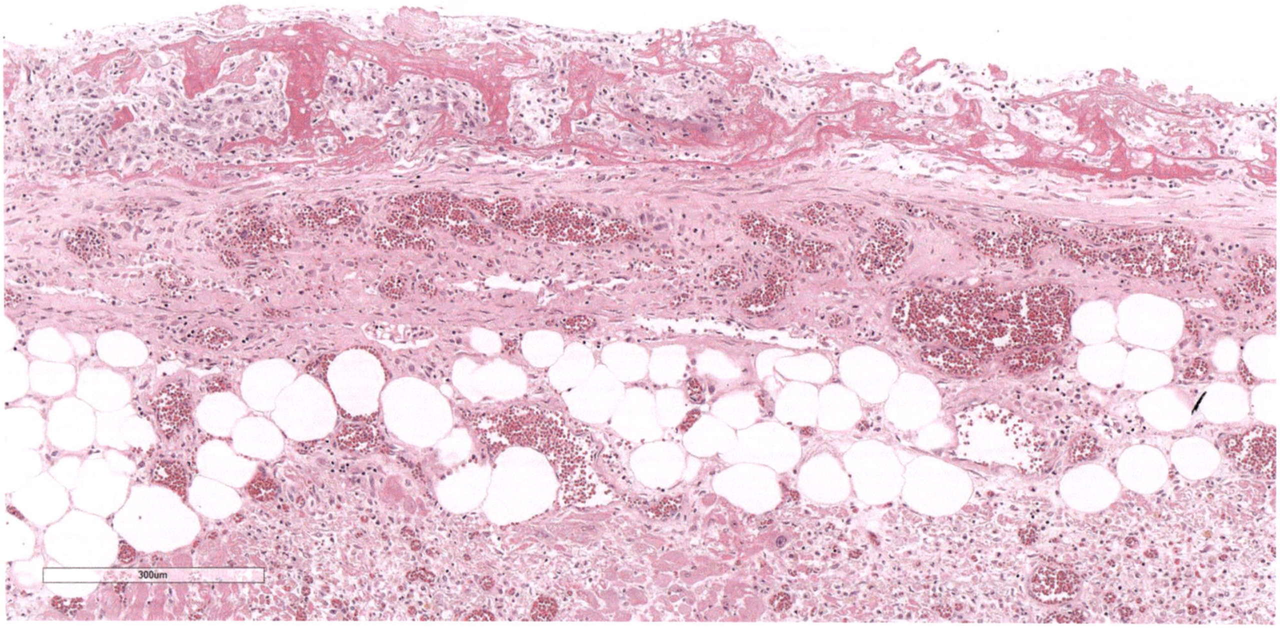

Fig. 14.14 Acute myocardial infarction may be complicated by fibrinous pericarditis. There is inflammation and fibrin deposition on the epicardial surface of the heart

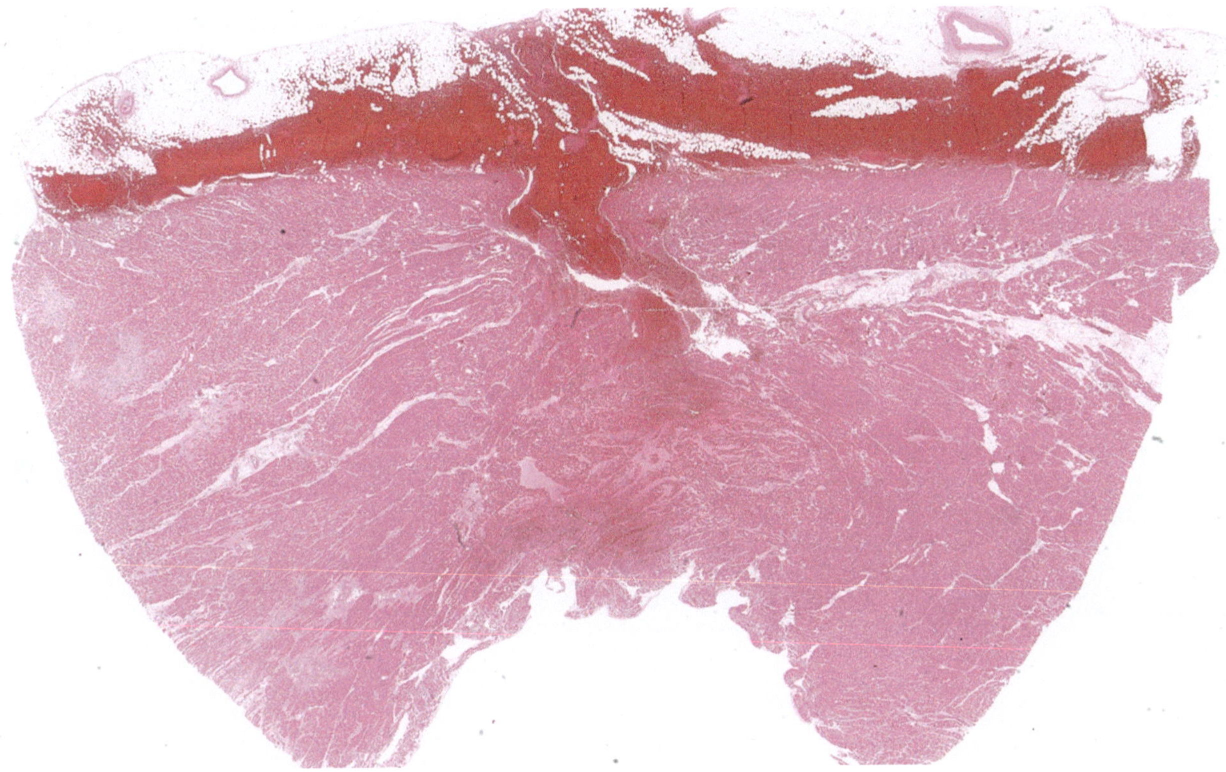

Fig. 14.15 Acute myocardial infarction may also be complicated by rupture of the ventricular wall, with consequent haemopericardium causing cardiac tamponade and cardiac arrest. Rupture of the wall can occur from 1 to 10 days following an acute infarct

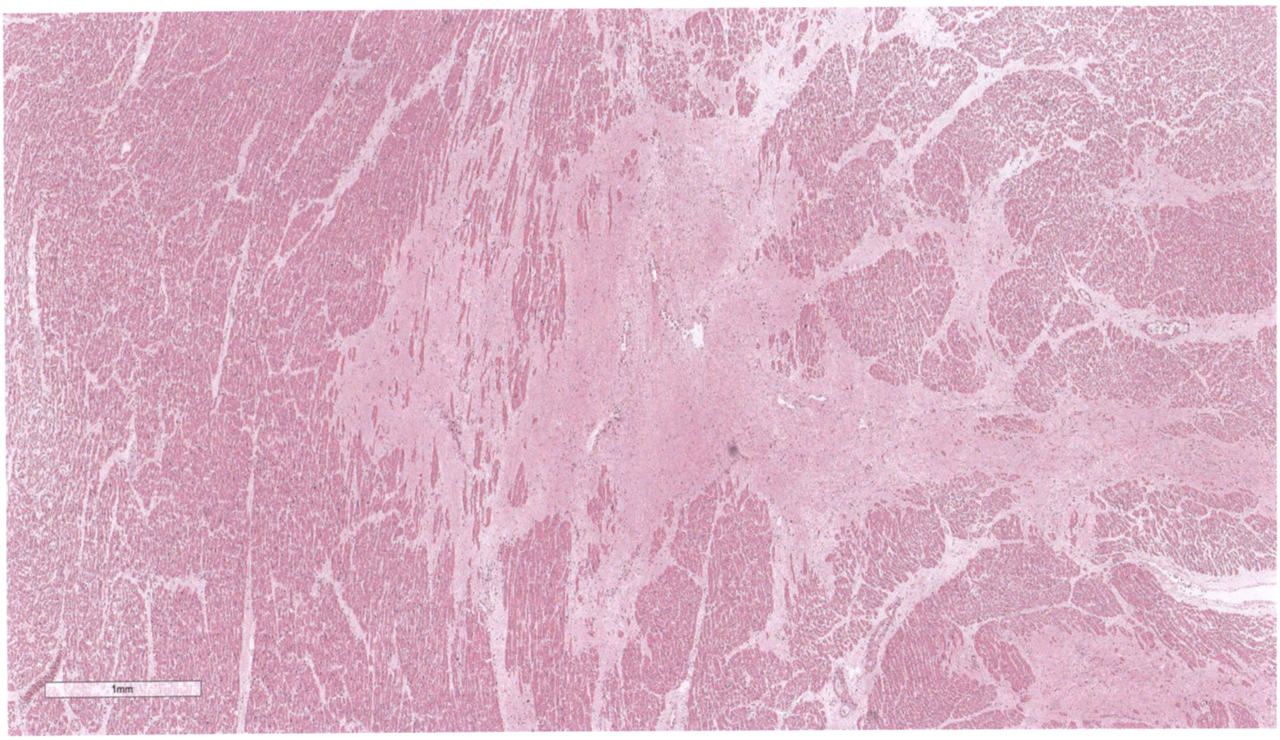

Fig. 14.16 Fibrosis in the heart can show different patterns which give a clue as to the aetiology. A large chunk of fibrosis which replaces a cluster of myocytes, as seen in this case following healing of an acute myocardial infarction, is termed "replacement type fibrosis" and is due to some form of damage to the myocytes, most commonly ischaemic damage. Healed myocarditis can also show a similar pattern but without a regional association with coronary artery disease

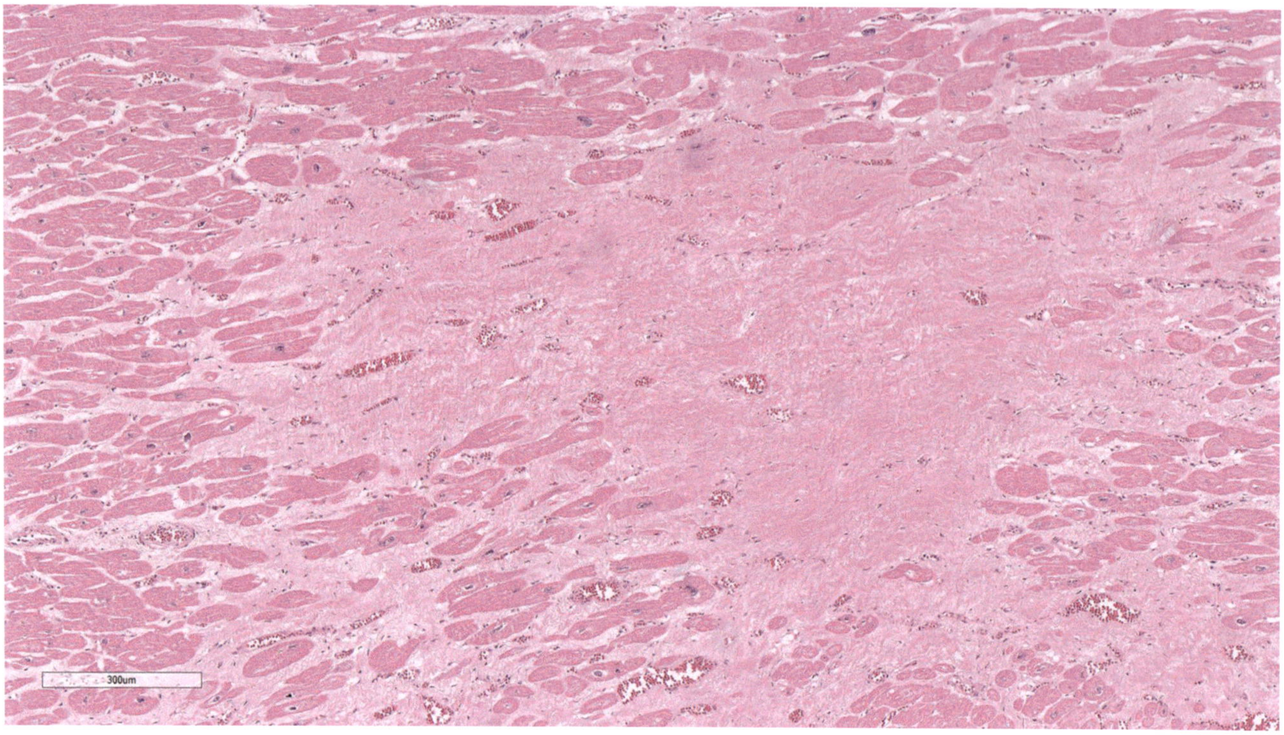

Fig. 14.17 This is another example of replacement type fibrosis in the heart, following healing of a myocardial infarct

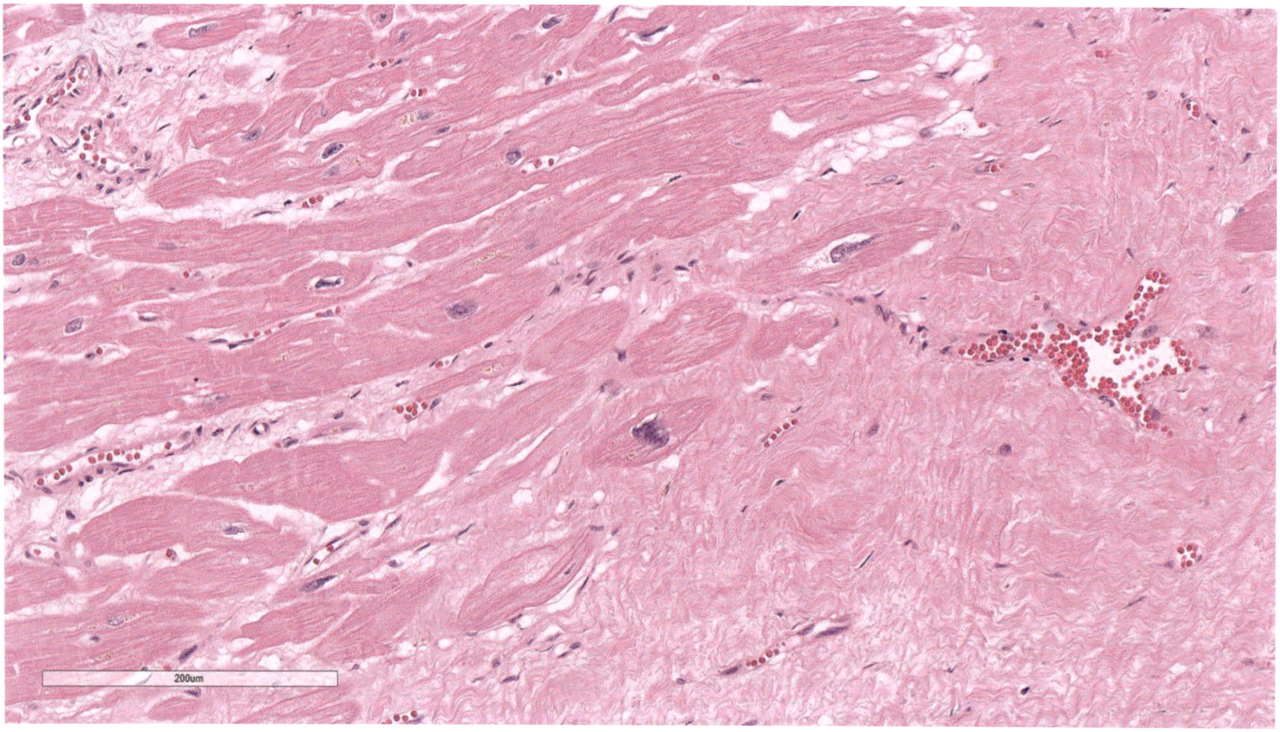

Fig. 14.18 Compensatory hypertrophy of surviving cardiac myocytes can be seen surrounding areas of replacement type fibrosis. This image shows enlargement of cardiac myocyte nuclei adjacent to an area of fibrosis

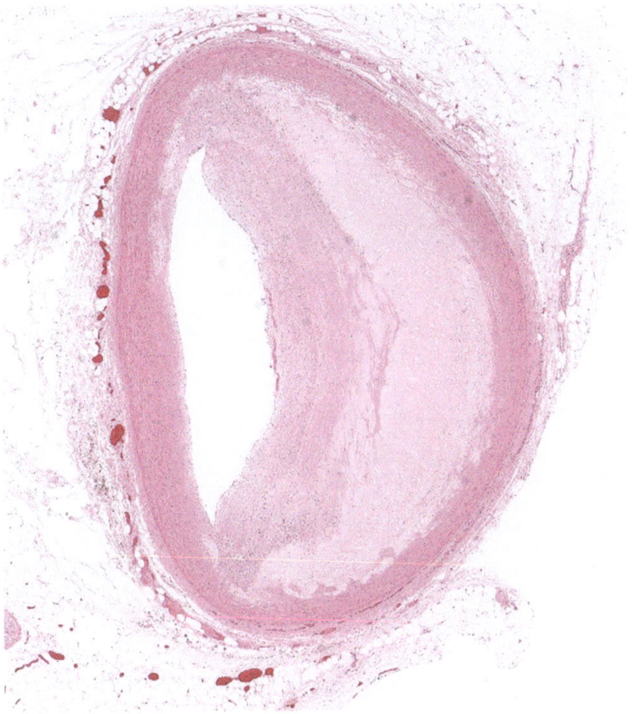

Fig. 14.19 Histology of coronary artery disease can help confirm macroscopic findings, estimate the degree of stenosis of the artery and identify high risk features such as a thin fibrous cap, erosion of the fibrous cap, rupture of a plaque and thrombus formation. This image shows atherosclerosis in the form of a lipid plaque with a thick fibrous cap. The atheroma is causing significant stenosis of the artery lumen

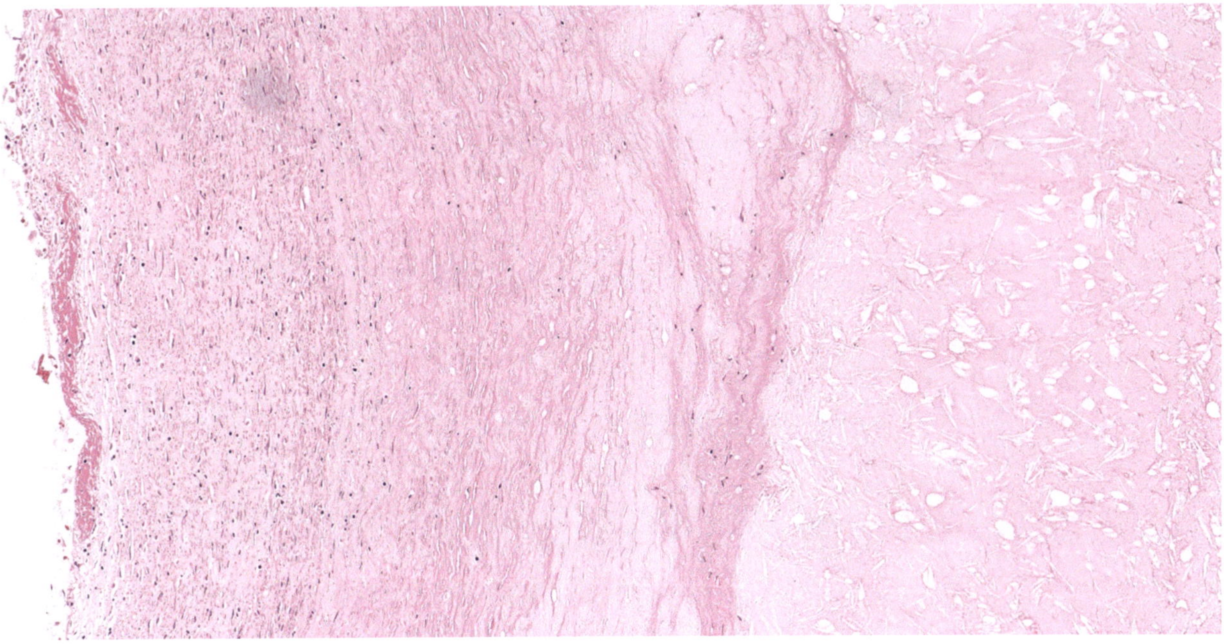

Fig. 14.20 This is a high power view of the same artery shown in Fig. 14.19, highlighting the lipid plaque on the right with cholesterol clefts, and the fibrous cap on the left, with some fibrin on the intimal surface

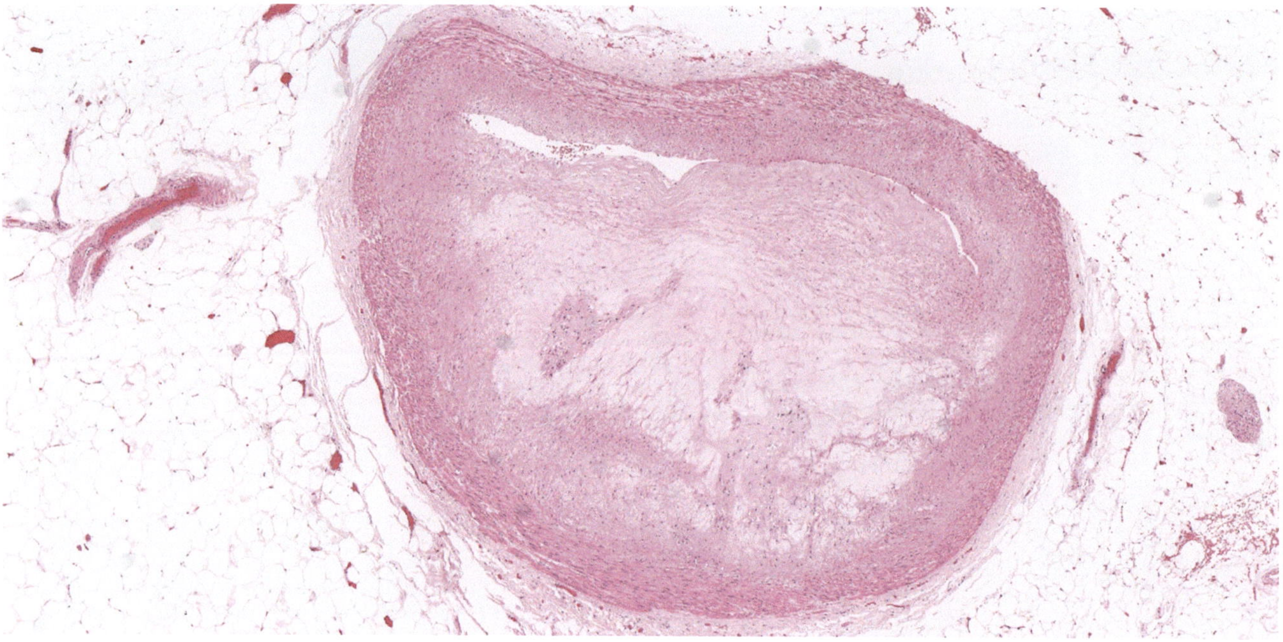

Fig. 14.21 This example of coronary artery atherosclerosis shows significant stenosis of the artery, leaving a slit-like lumen. Arteries can become distorted in processing and a single image may over- or under-estimate the true degree of stenosis

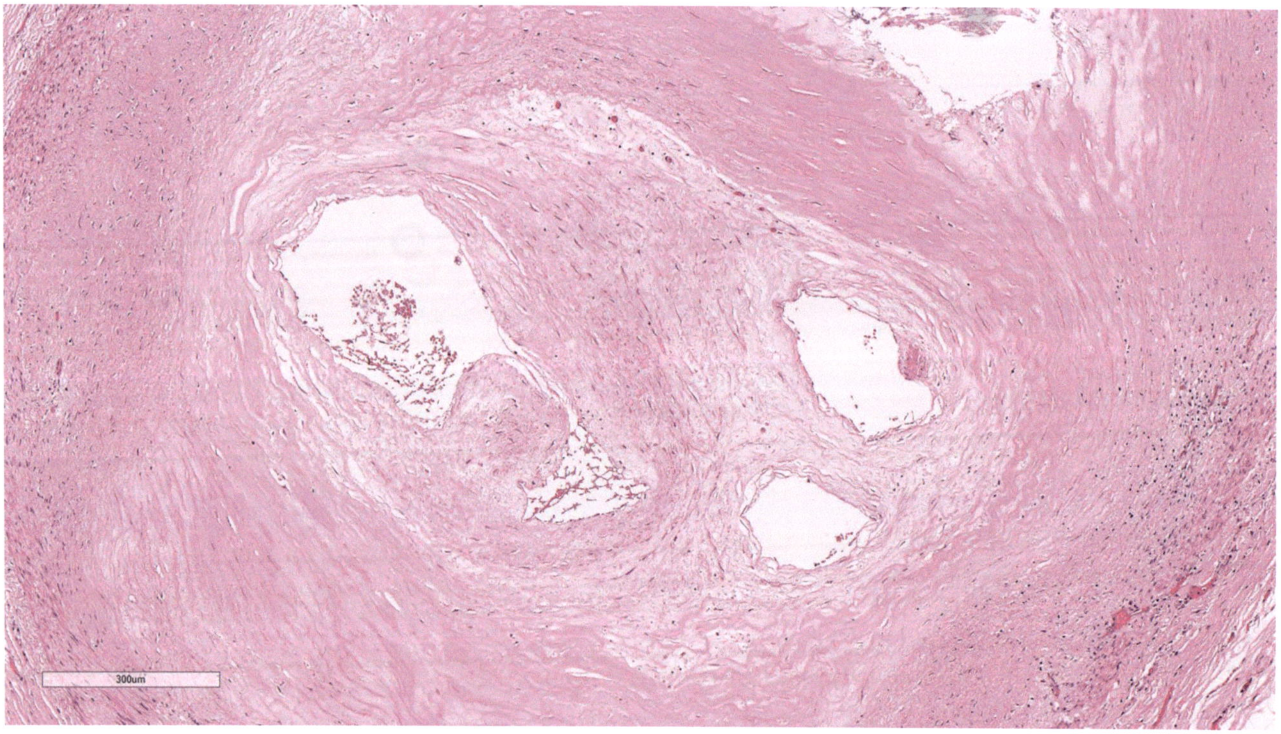

Fig. 14.22 Over time, an occluded artery can become recanalised. This image shows multiple small neo-lumina, re-opening the artery re-establishing some blood flow

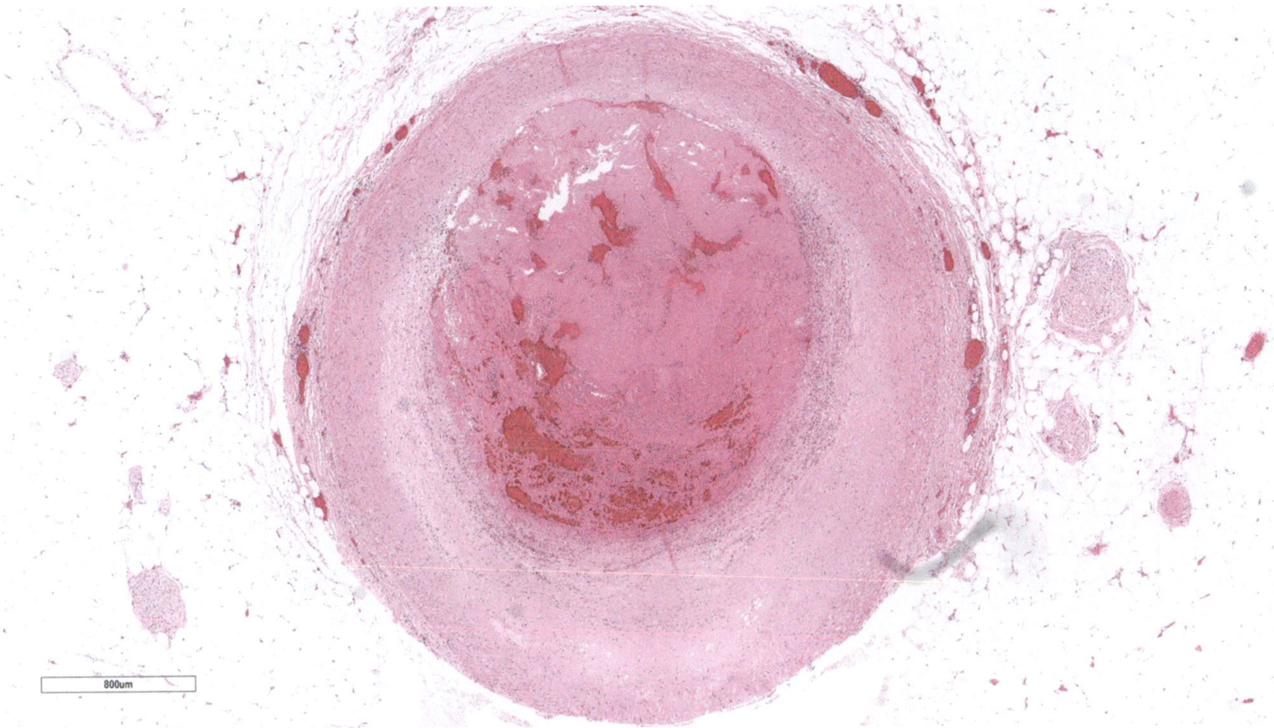

Fig. 14.23 Thrombosis of a coronary artery causes occlusion of the blood supply causing distant ischaemia and infarction of the heart. This section shows complete occlusion of the coronary artery by a thrombus. At times it can be difficult to judge the macroscopic appearance of a possible thrombus, as opposed to post mortem "clot", and histology can be valuable in confirming true thrombosis

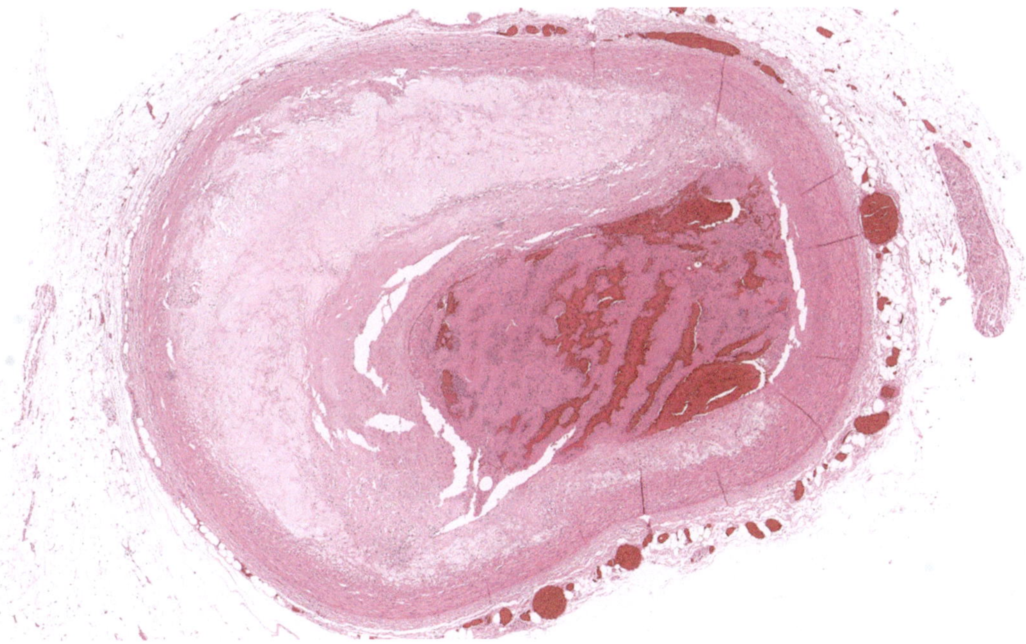

Fig. 14.24 This image shows another example of a coronary artery thrombus, occluding the artery, on a background of atherosclerosis

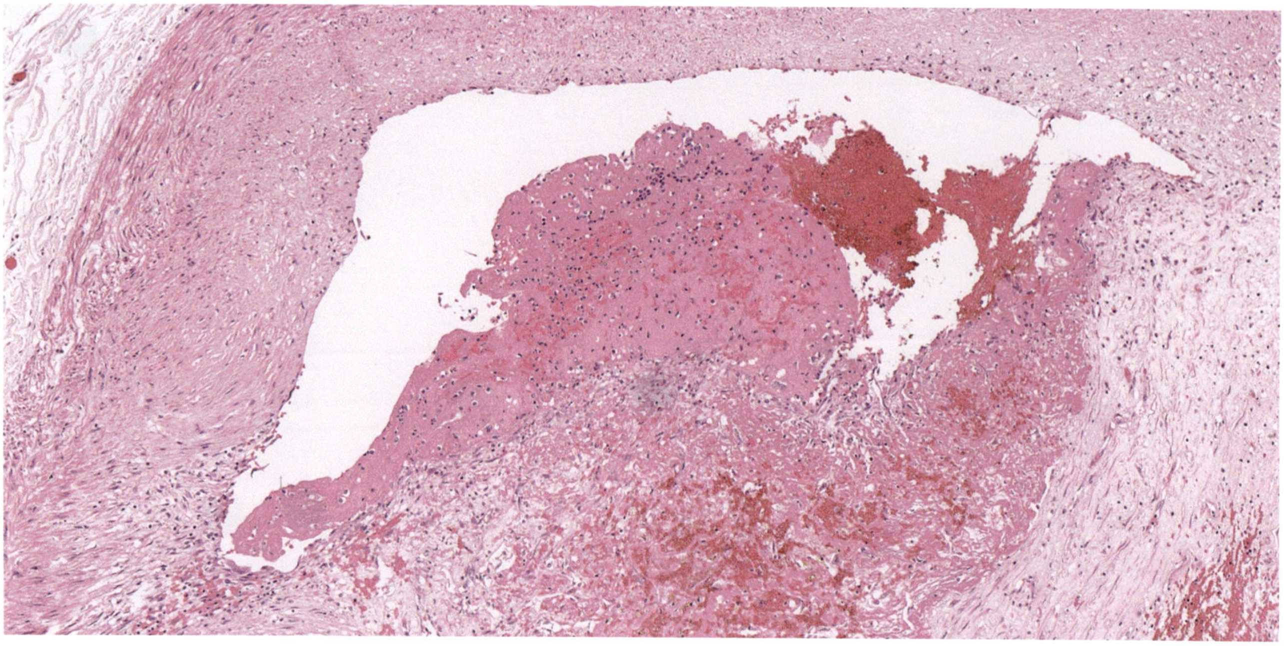

Fig. 14.25 In this high power view a fibrin thrombus is shown overlying a ruptured atherosclerotic plaque within a coronary artery

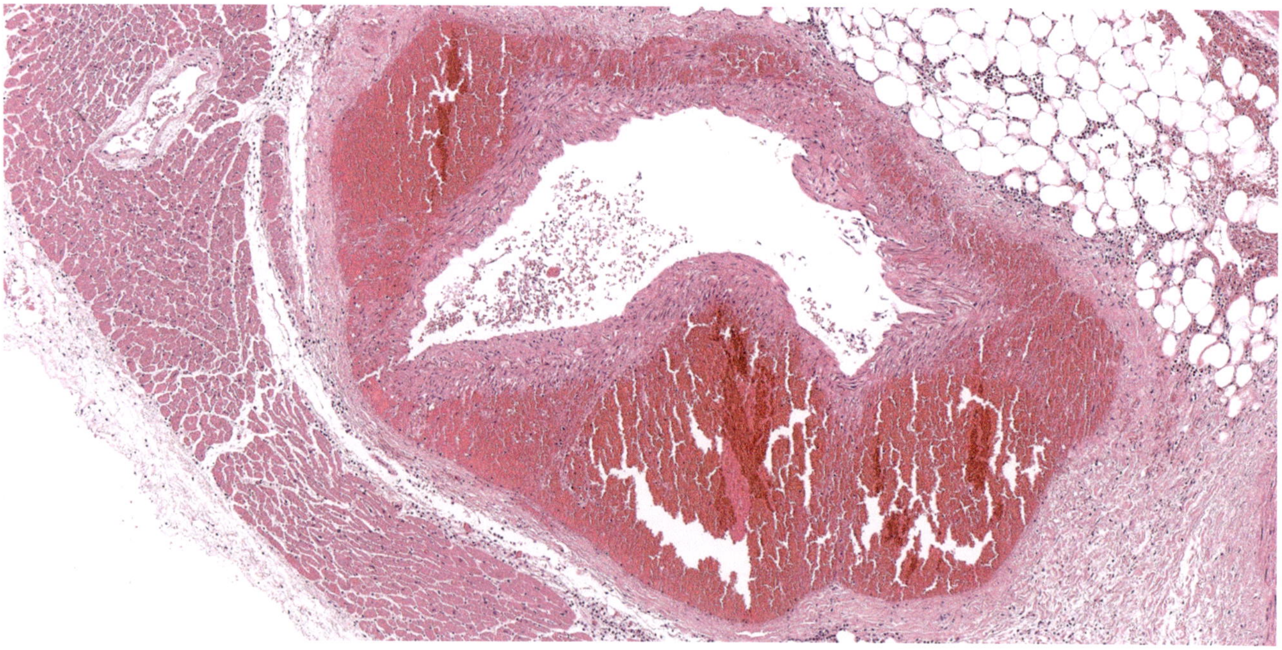

Fig. 14.26 Dissection of the coronary arteries is a rare cause of acute cardiac ischaemia and sudden death. It is associated with pregnancy but can also be seen in association with stimulant drug use or as a complication of instrumentation of the coronary arteries. This image shows blood tracking within the media and causing stenosis of the lumen. It can be difficult to distinguish coronary artery dissection from a coronary artery thrombus with the naked eye, but histology can aid the pathologist in making this distinction

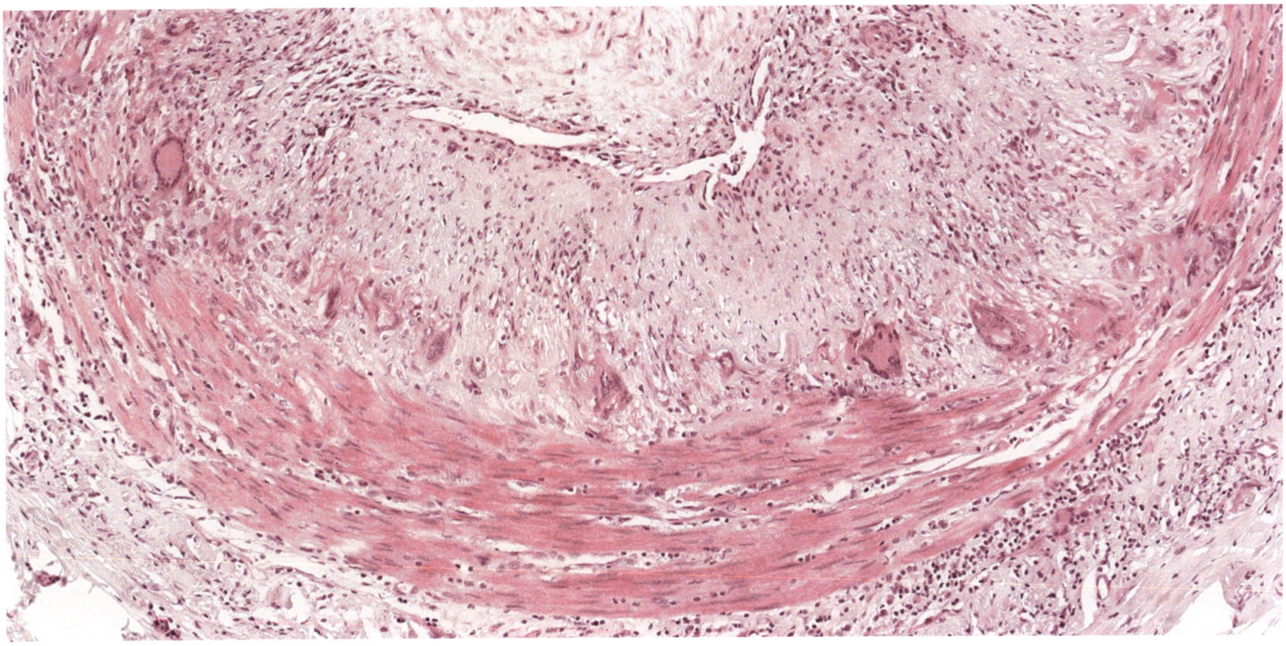

Fig. 14.27 Inflammatory conditions causing vasculitis, as in this case of giant cell arteritis, can lead to significant stenosis of the coronary arteries, with consequent ischaemia and sudden death

Hypertensive Heart Disease

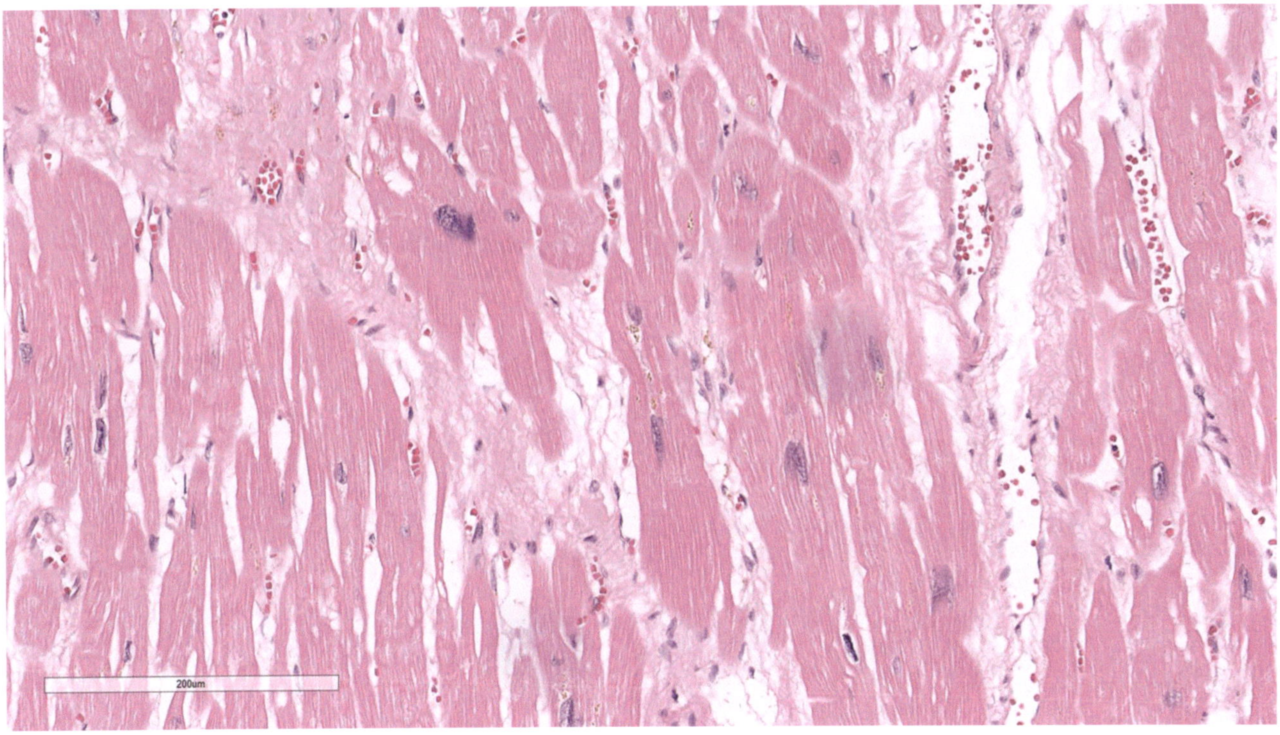

Fig. 14.28 Hypertension is one of the most common causes of left ventricular hypertrophy. Hypertensive heart disease is a common form of cardiac disease. This image shows cardiac myocyte nuclear hypertrophy as seen in hypertensive heart disease

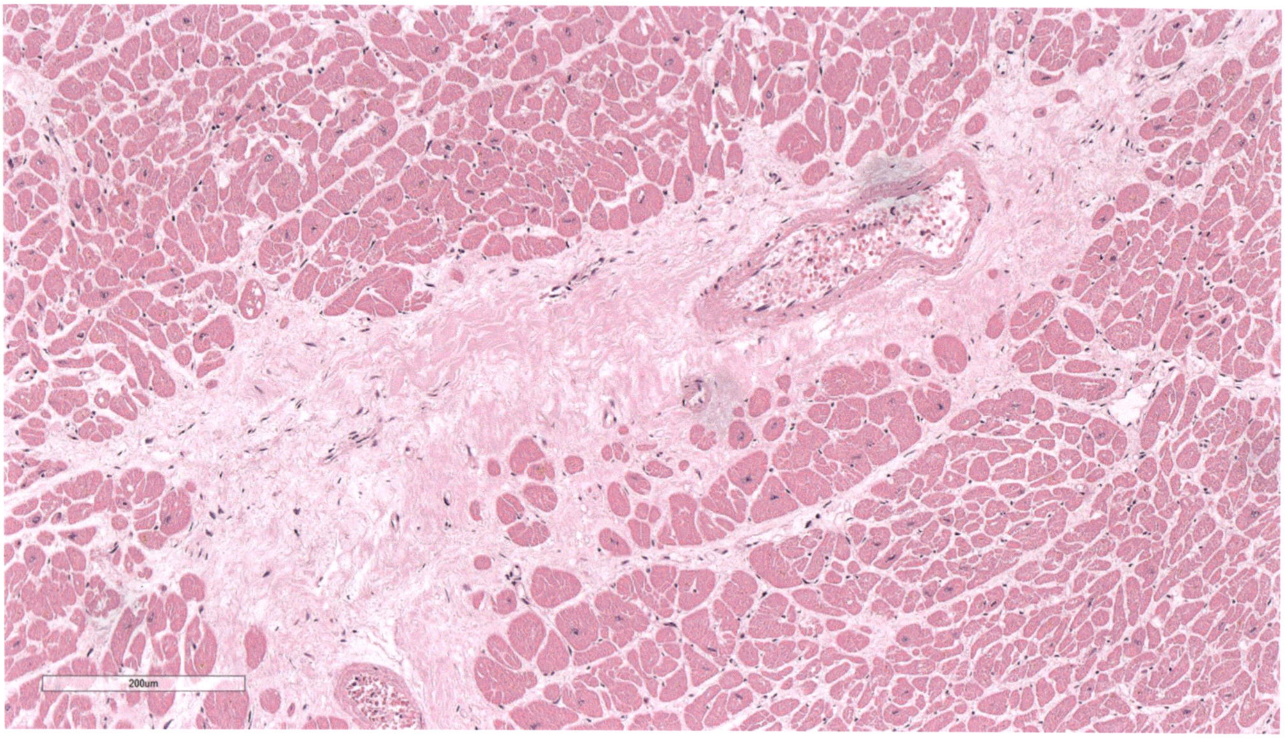

Fig. 14.29 Hypertensive heart disease is also associated with perivascular fibrosis. As the heart, particularly the left ventricle, enlarges, the inner half of the thickened ventricle wall becomes vulnerable to ischaemia which can lead to fatal arrhythmia

Valve Disease

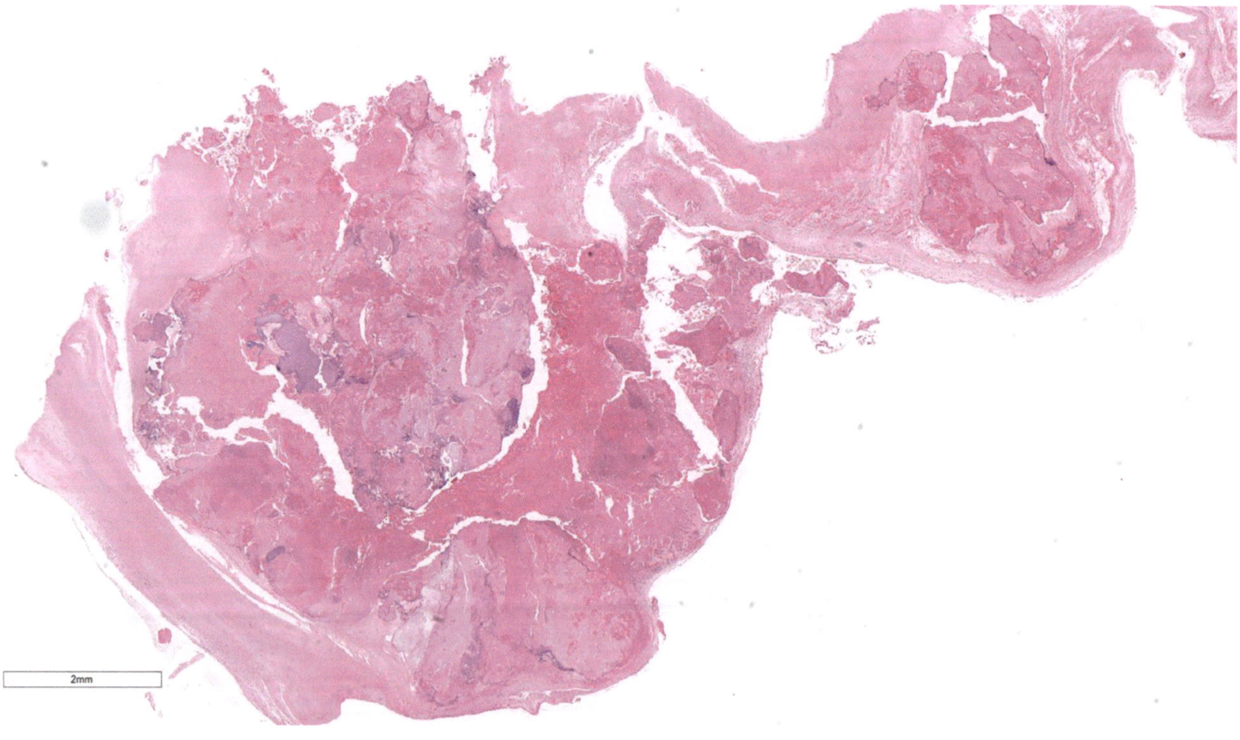

Fig. 14.30 Calcific aortic stenosis is another common cause of left ventricular hypertrophy and can be associated with sudden arrhythmic death. This image shows large, calcified masses thickening the aortic valve leaflet

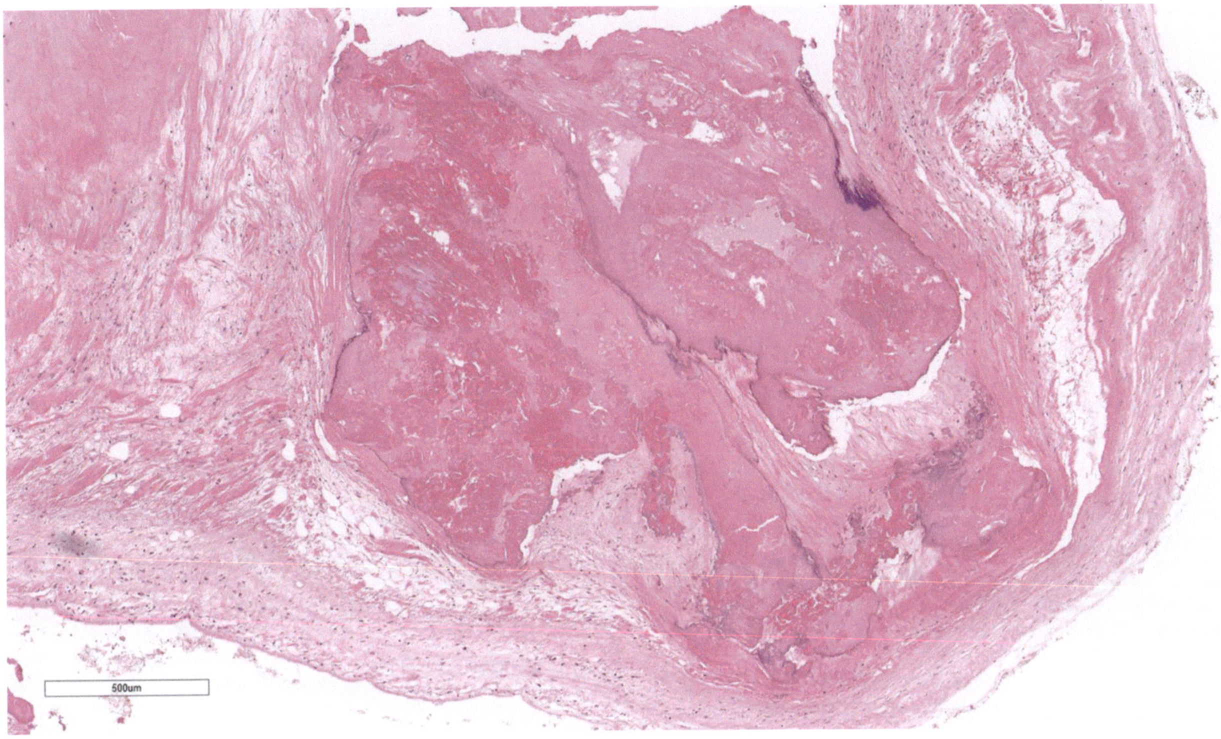

Fig. 14.31 This higher power view of the valve shown in Fig. 14.30 shows the deposits of calcium in calcific aortic stenosis

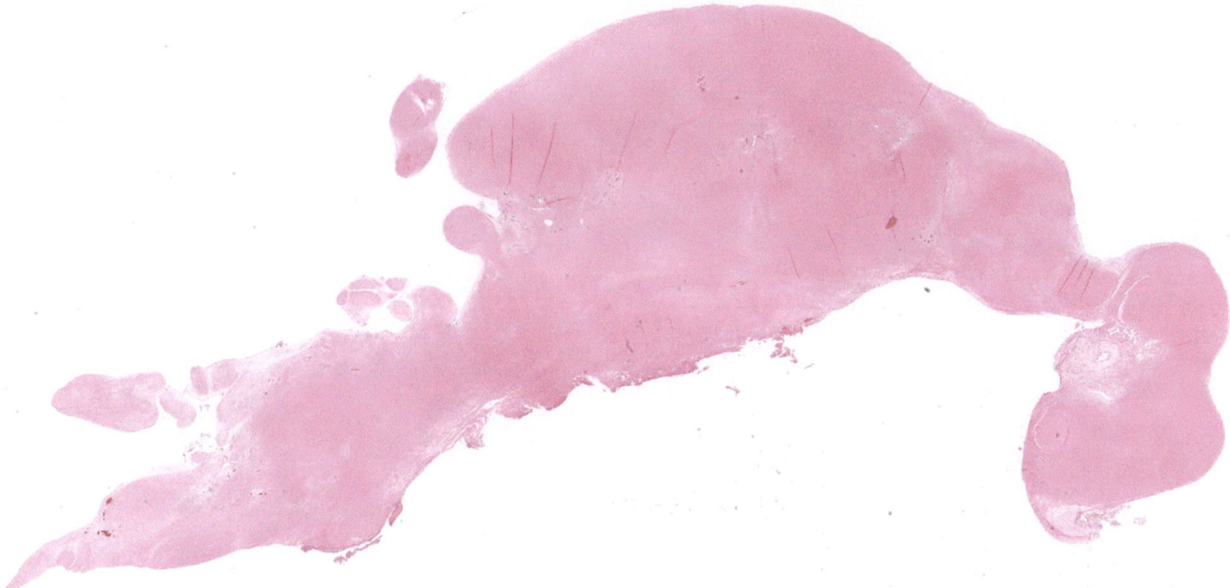

Fig. 14.32 The most common cause of mitral valve stenosis is rheumatic fever. This image shows the bland thickening of the mitral valve typically associated with rheumatic valve disease

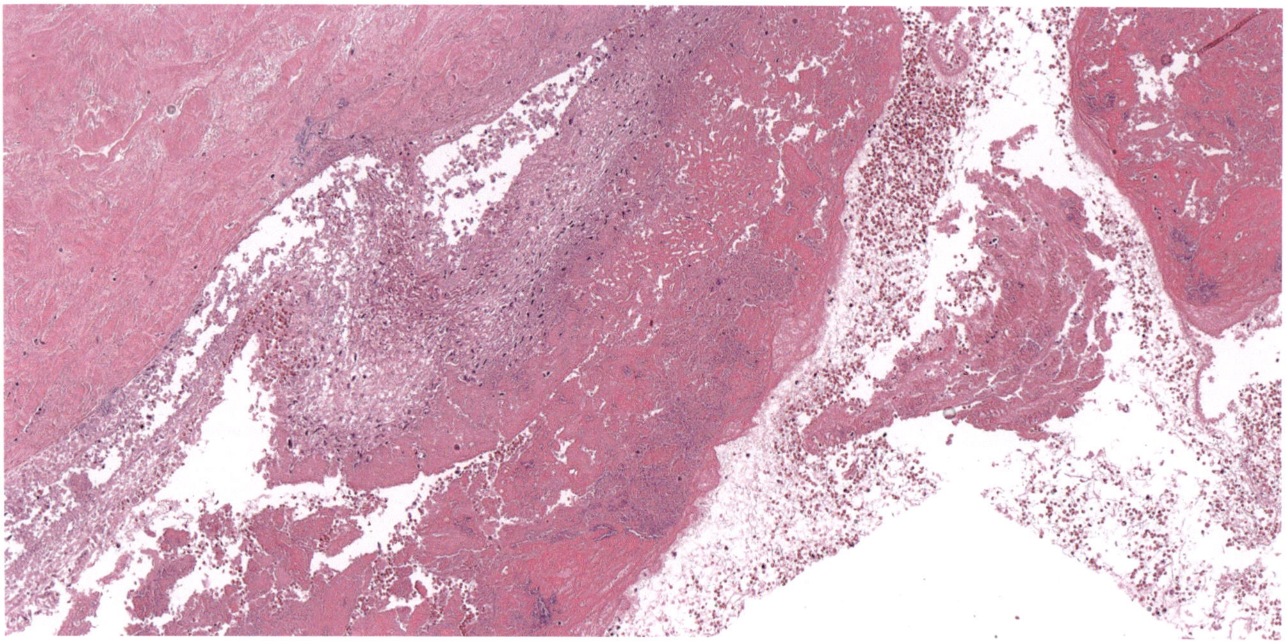

Fig. 14.33 Diseased heart valves are at risk of becoming colonised by bacterial vegetations. This image of bacterial endocarditis shows the valve leaflet with fibrin vegetations containing numerous bacterial colonies

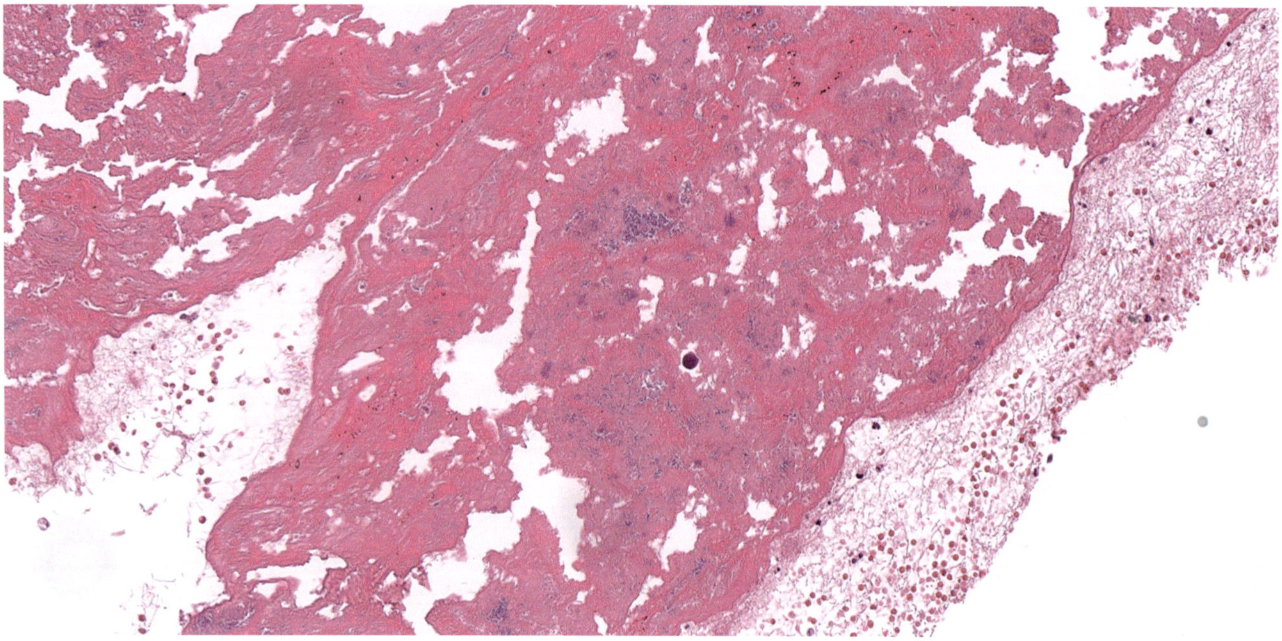

Fig. 14.34 A higher power view of the case of bacterial endocarditis from Fig. 14.33 showing a fibrinous vegetation containing bacteria

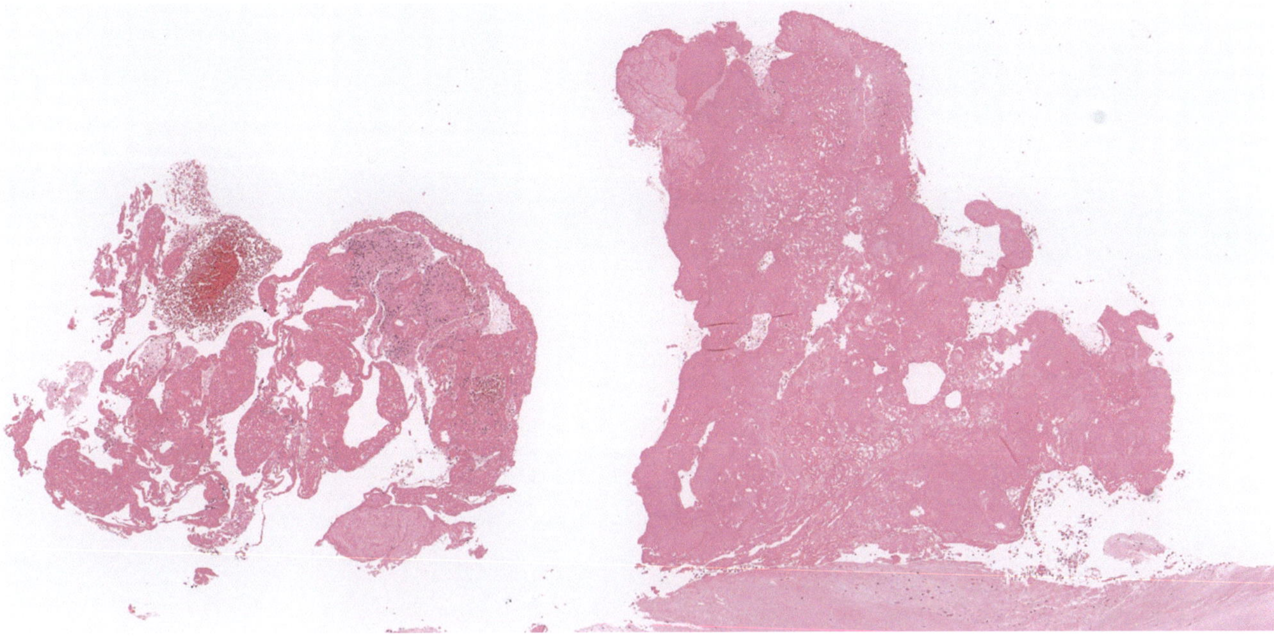

Fig. 14.35 Not all vegetations on heart valves are infective in origin. This case shows a non-infective endocarditis. The image shows the valve leaflet with fibrinous vegetations, with no bacterial colonies and a negative gram stain

Inflammatory and Degenerative Conditions

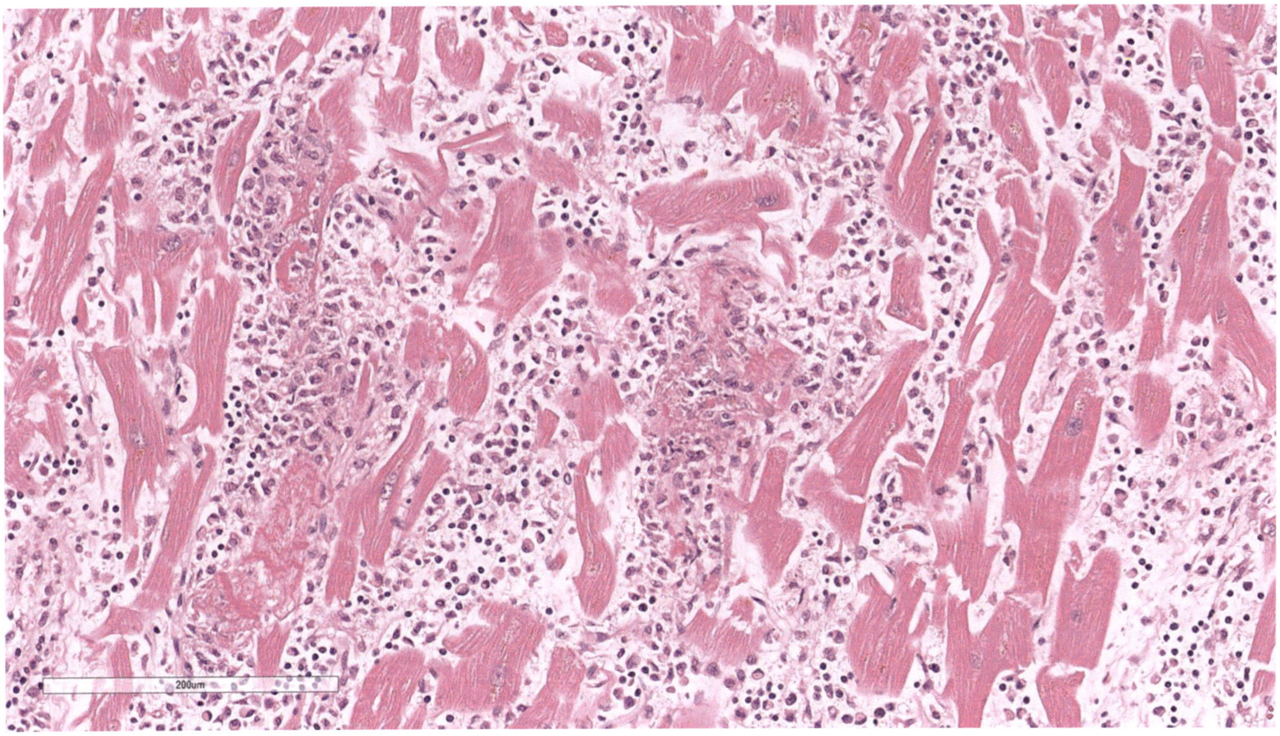

Fig. 14.36 Myocarditis, as seen here, can cause sudden death. It may be associated with symptoms of progressive cardiac failure. However, the symptoms may be non-specific and a diagnosis may be elusive in life. At autopsy the heart may appear macroscopically normal, or may appear mottled, and in many cases myocarditis is diagnosed only on histology. This image shows an infiltrate of lymphocytes, plasma cells and neutrophils infiltrating the myocardium, causing myocyte damage. There are many different causes of myocarditis, viral infections being most common, and several different histological patterns

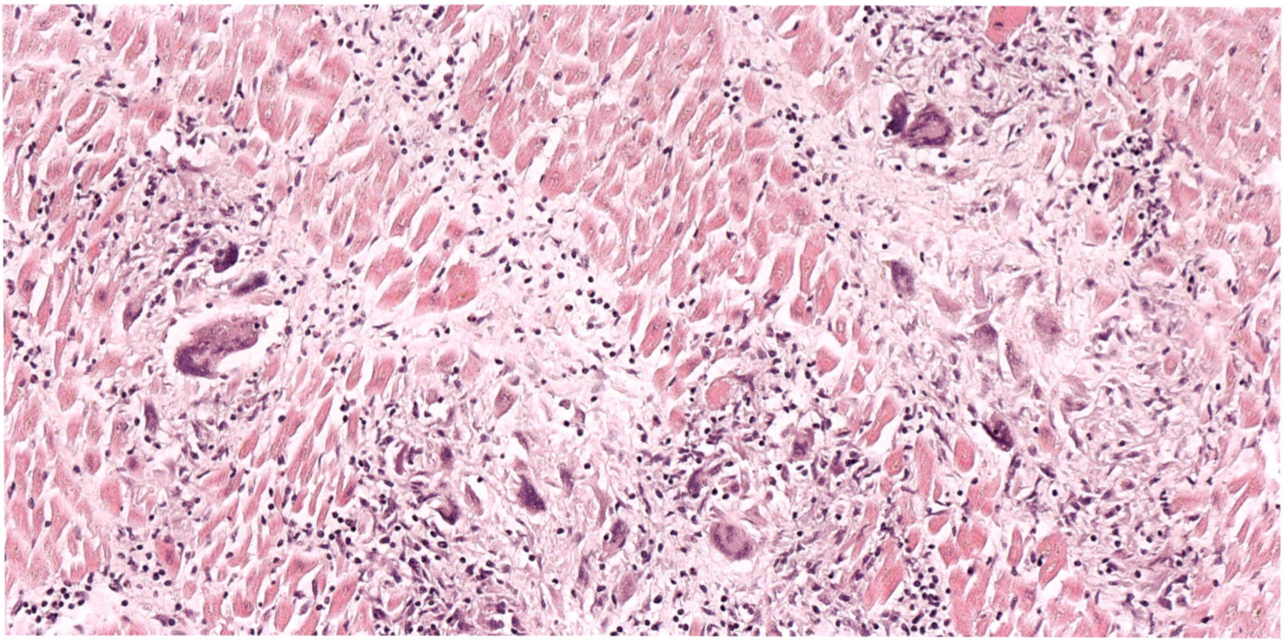

Fig. 14.37 Giant cell myocarditis usually presents with a rapidly progressive cardiac failure. It can be distinguished from sarcoidosis by the lack of granulomas and lack of fibrosis. This image shows multinucleate giant cells, lymphocytes and eosinophils infiltrating the myocardium with cardiac myocyte damage

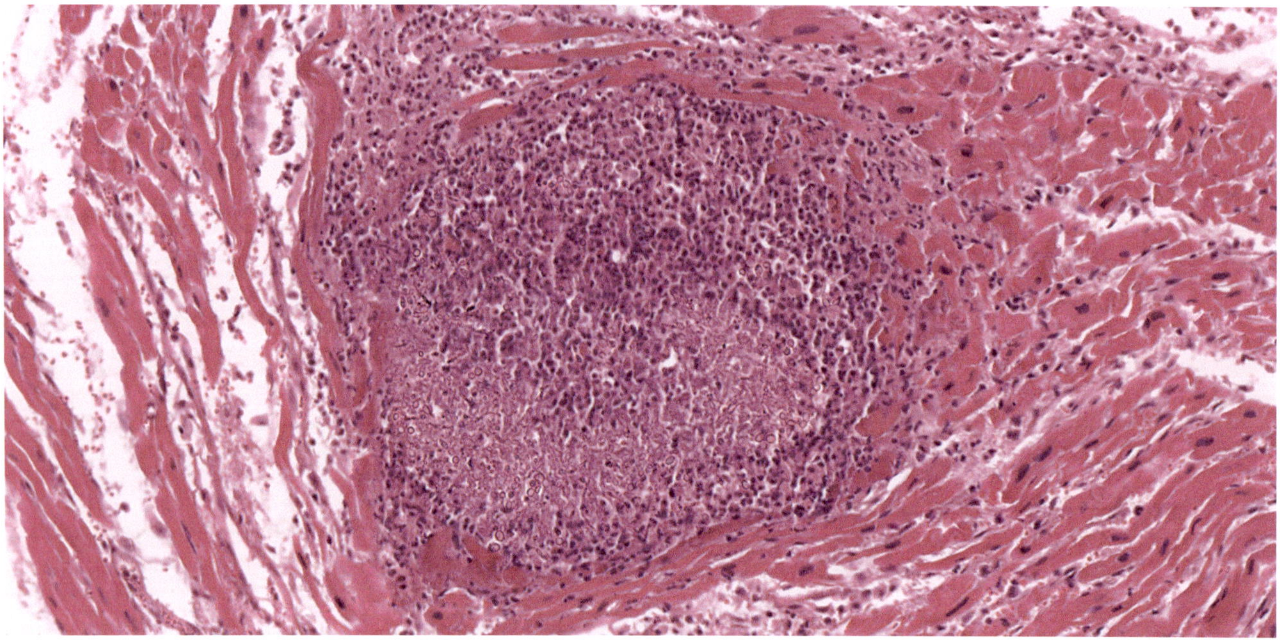

Fig. 14.38 This image shows a microabscess within the heart, containing fungal spores and hyphae within the abscess. Septic emboli from elsewhere in the body can cause microabscesses within the heart

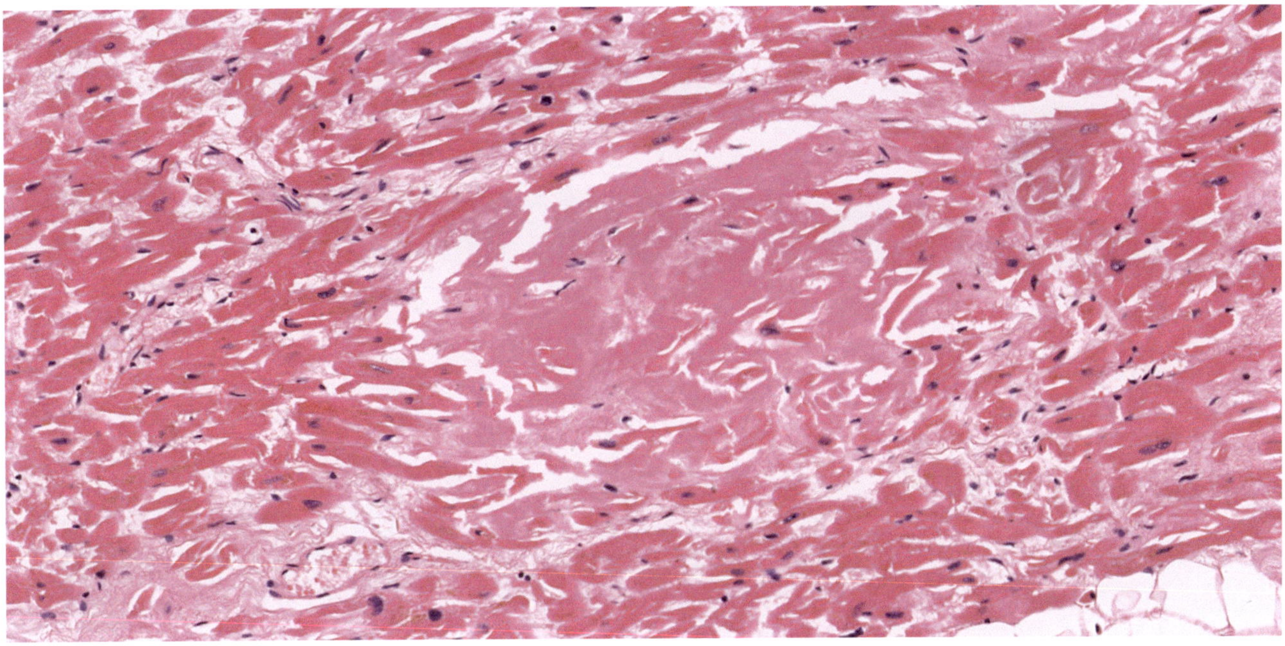

Fig. 14.39 This case of cardiac amyloidosis shows a dense deposit of eosinophilic material between the cardiac myocytes. On first glance, these deposits may look like areas of fibrosis, but the amyloid deposits tend to be scattered throughout the myocardium, rather than having a regional distribution as you would see with ischaemic damage. On closer inspection the bland eosinophilic appearance prompts the confirmatory staining with Congo red to confirm the material to be amyloid. Amyloidosis can affect the heart as part of a systemic amyloidosis, a plasma cell dyscrasia, or (most commonly in autopsy practice) as an isolated involvement of the heart in senile amyloidosis (transthyretin deposition). Amyloidosis can affect the atria and is a rare cause of atrial fibrillation

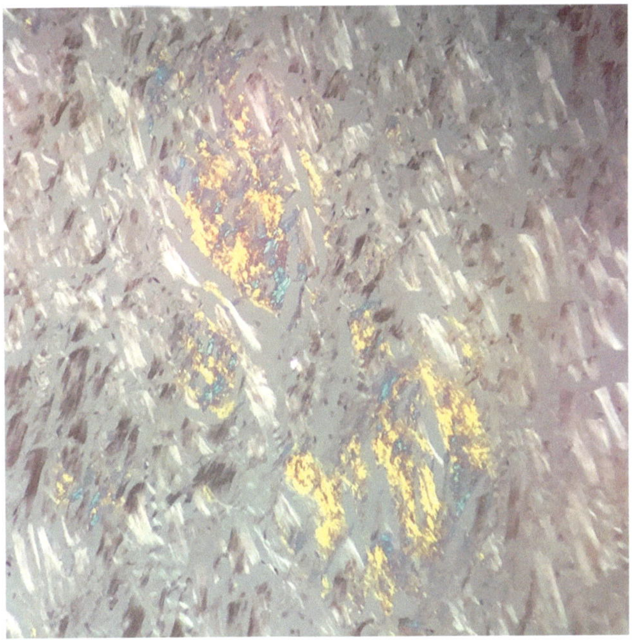

Fig. 14.40 Cardiac amyloidosis. Congo red staining confirms amyloid. Although traditionally described as showing apple-green birefringence, the colour may be yellow, green or blue-tinged

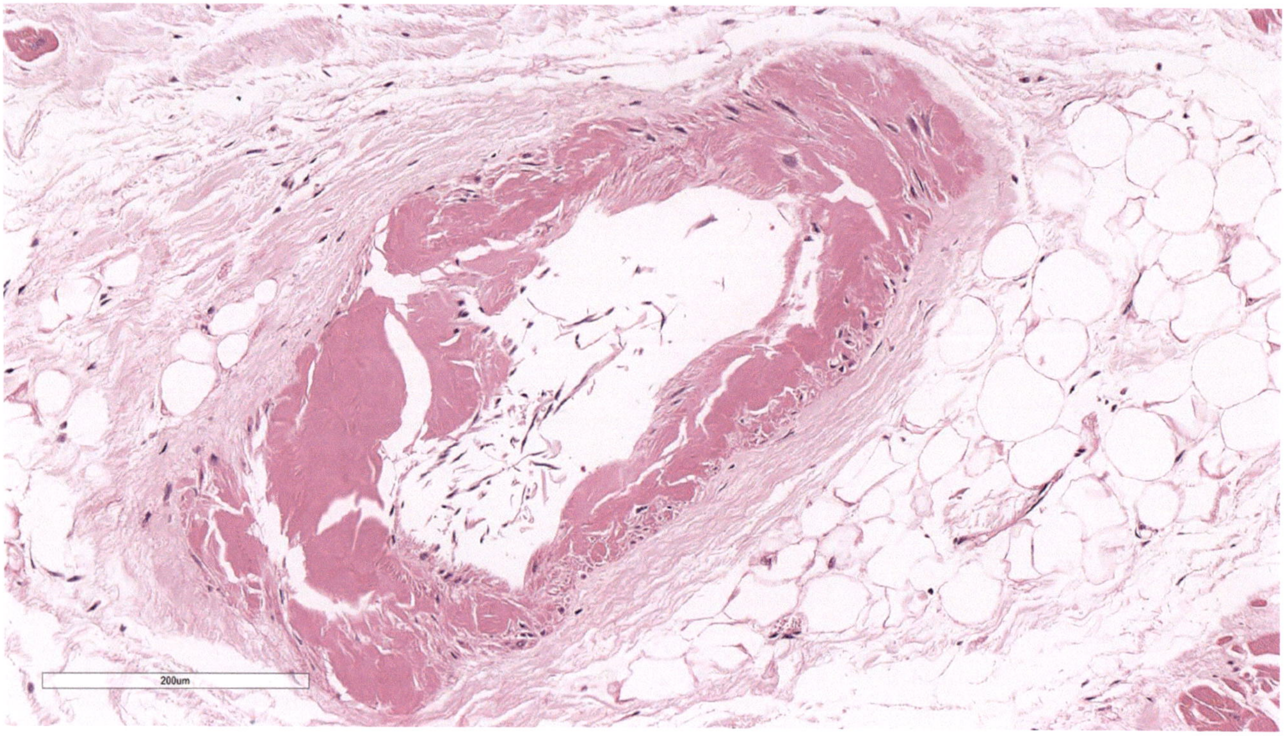

Fig. 14.41 Amyloidosis may also involve intra-cardiac arteries

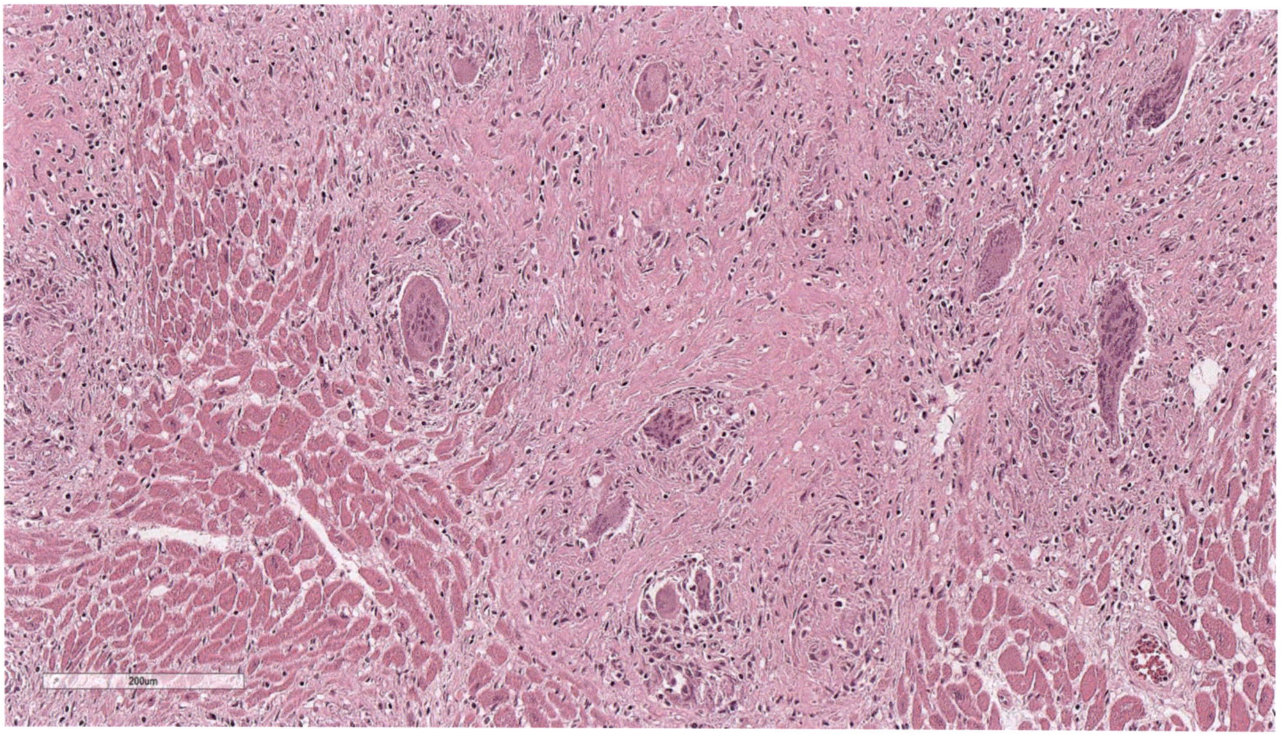

Fig. 14.42 Sarcoidosis is a systemic inflammatory condition which may show involvement of the heart. In this image there is granulomatous inflammation with multi-nucleated giant cells and fibrosis. Cardiac sarcoidosis can be a cause of sudden death. It typically causes a sudden cardiac arrhythmia due to the granulomatous inflammation and/or the associated fibrosis acting as an arrhythmogenic focus

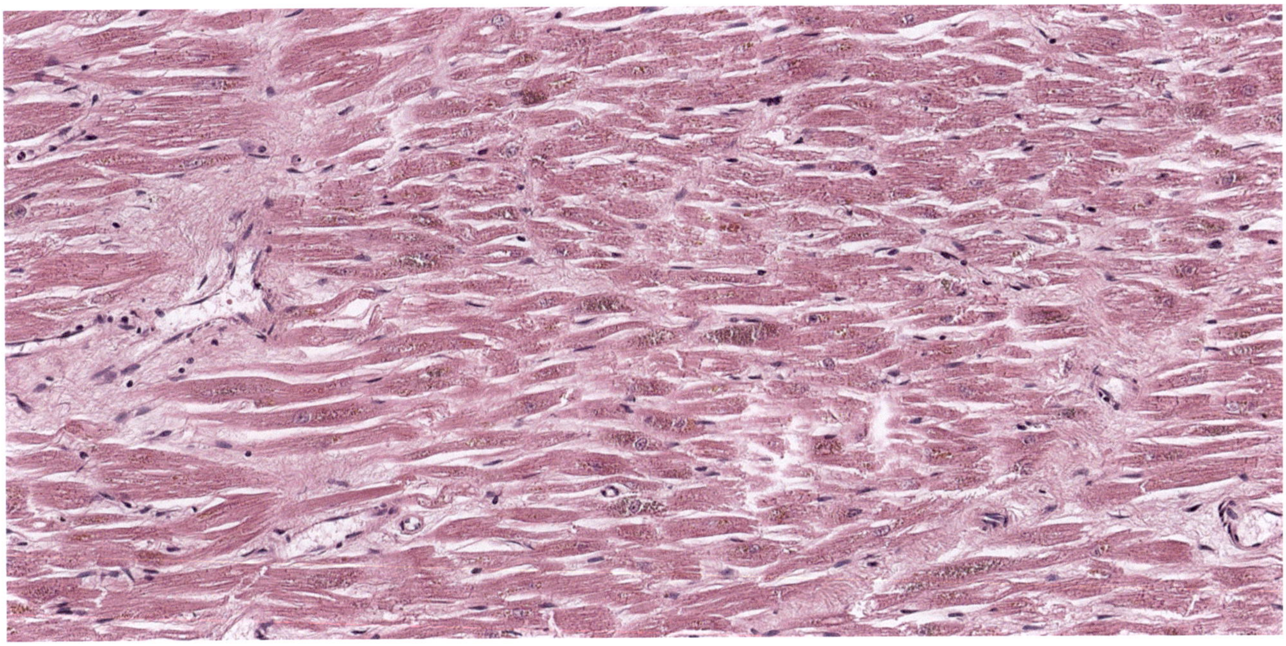

Fig. 14.43 Haemochromatosis, a disorder of iron storage, can affect the heart and other organs. Histology of the heart shows the brown pigment of iron deposition within myocytes. Perls' staining is confirmatory

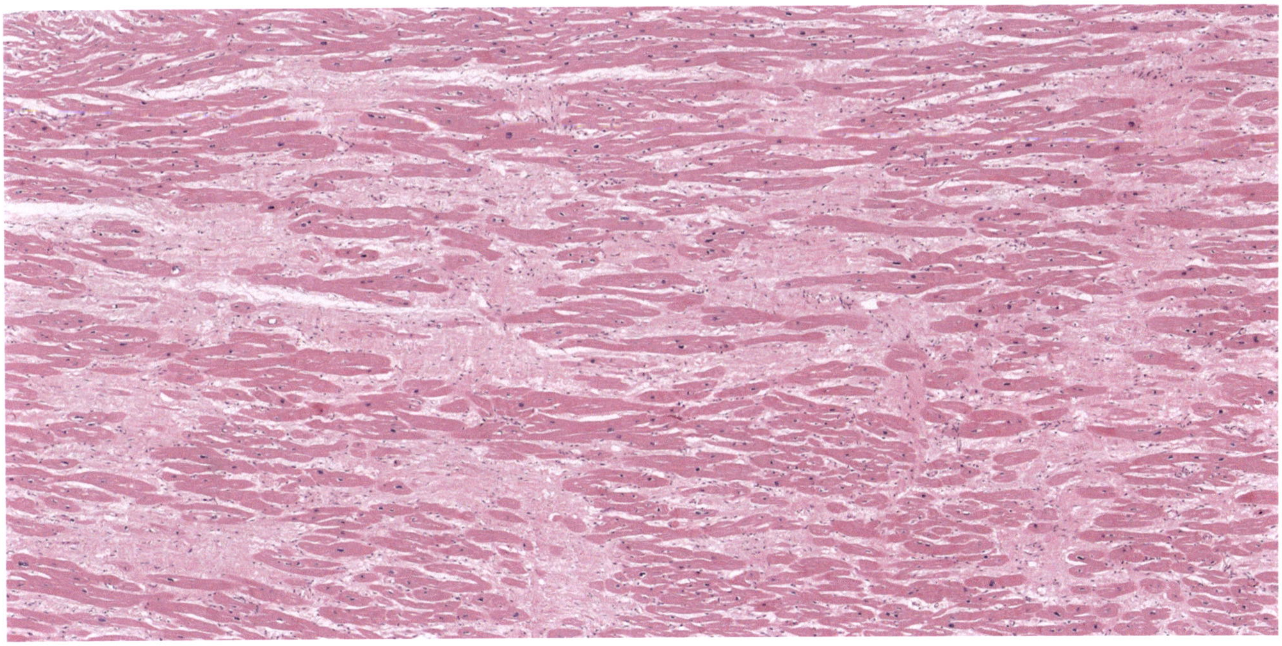

Fig. 14.44 Cobalt cardiomyopathy is rare. It is associated with excessive exposure to cobalt, in this case due to a prosthetic hip implant. It can cause myocardial hypertrophy and interstitial fibrosis

Inheritable Cardiomyopathies

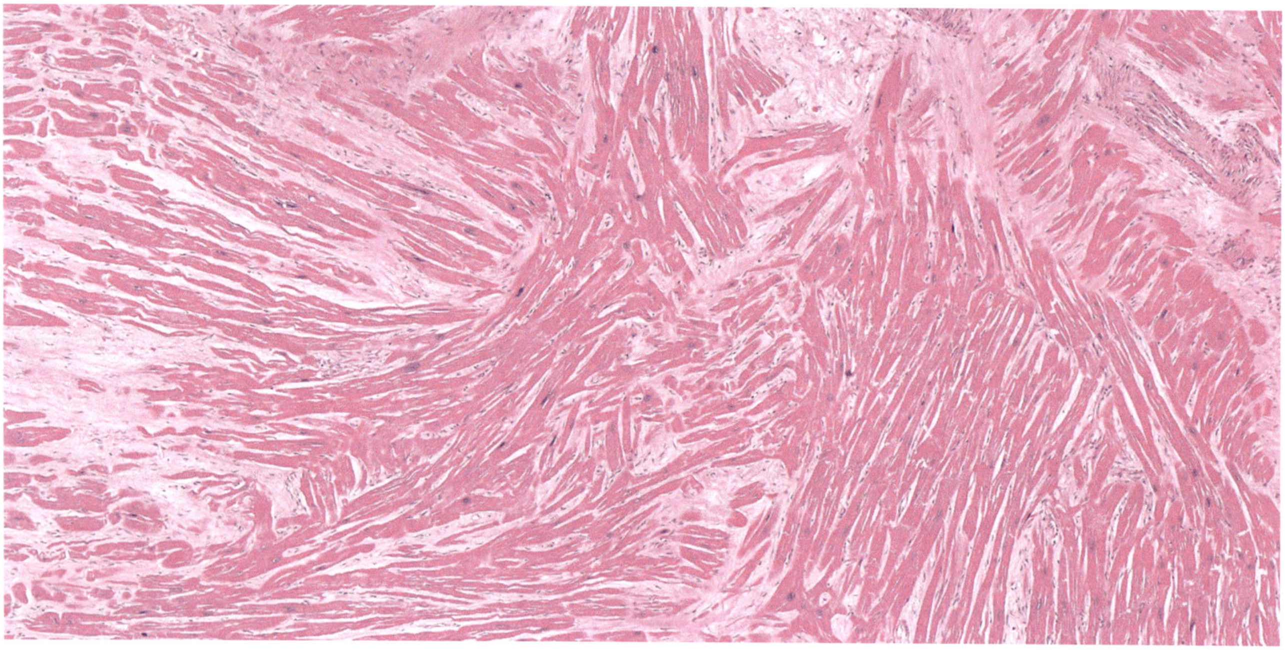

Fig. 14.45 Hypertrophic cardiomyopathy is the most common inheritable cardiomyopathy. It is associated with cardiac arrhythmia and an increased risk of sudden death. The hallmark histological feature is fibre disarray where individual myocytes and muscle fibres intersect at atypical angles. Other histological features include cardiac myocyte hypertrophy, fibrosis and vascular changes (medial thickening and stenosis) which contribute to hypoxia and fibrosis

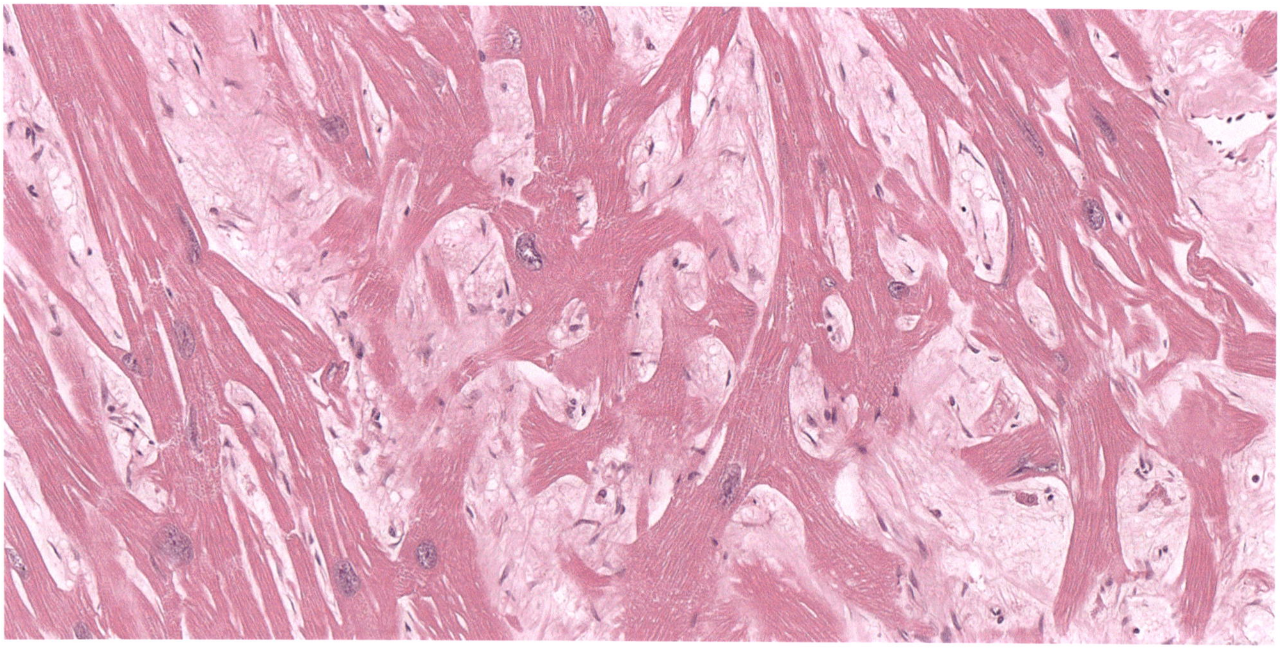

Fig. 14.46 A higher power view of the cardiac myocyte disarray and hypertrophy seen in hypertrophic cardiomyopathy is shown here

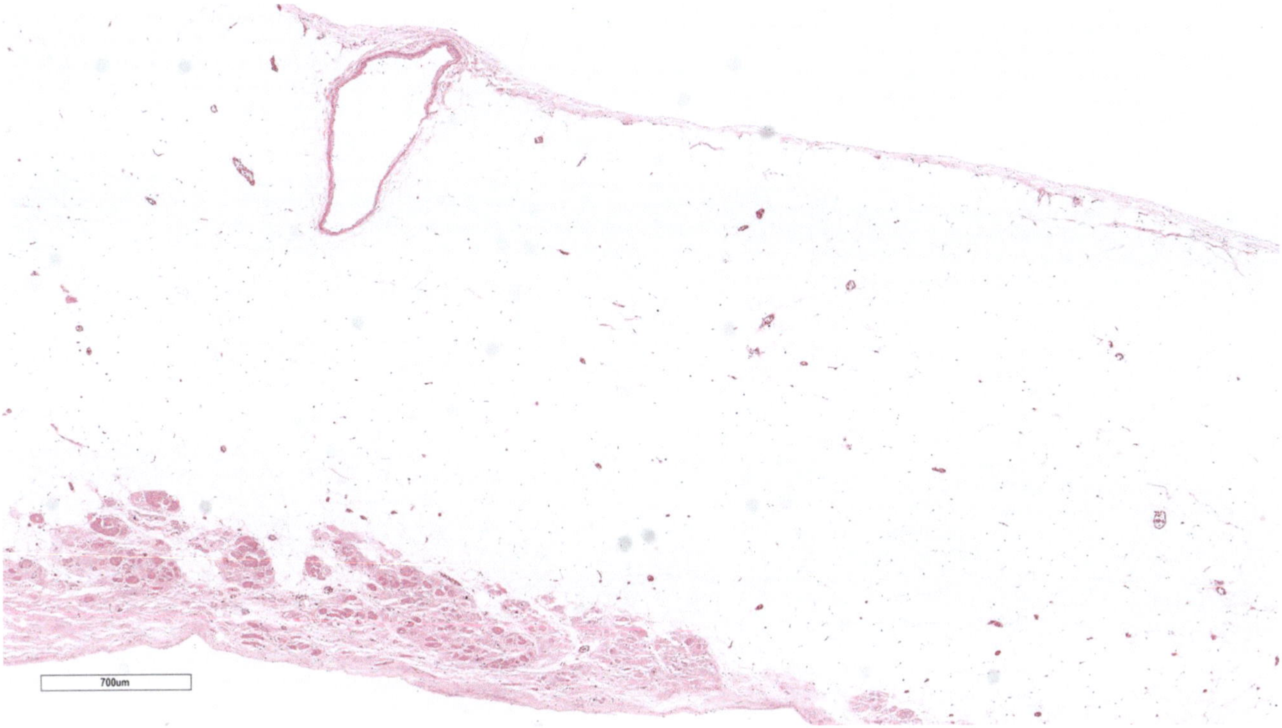

Fig. 14.47 Arrhythmogenic (right ventricular) cardiomyopathy is caused by mutations in desmosomal genes. These cause poor cell adhesion, and lead to apoptosis with replacement of the myocytes by adipose tissue or fibrosis. This image shows right ventricular myocardium replaced by adipose tissue and fibrosis. This case was associated with a PKP2 gene mutation

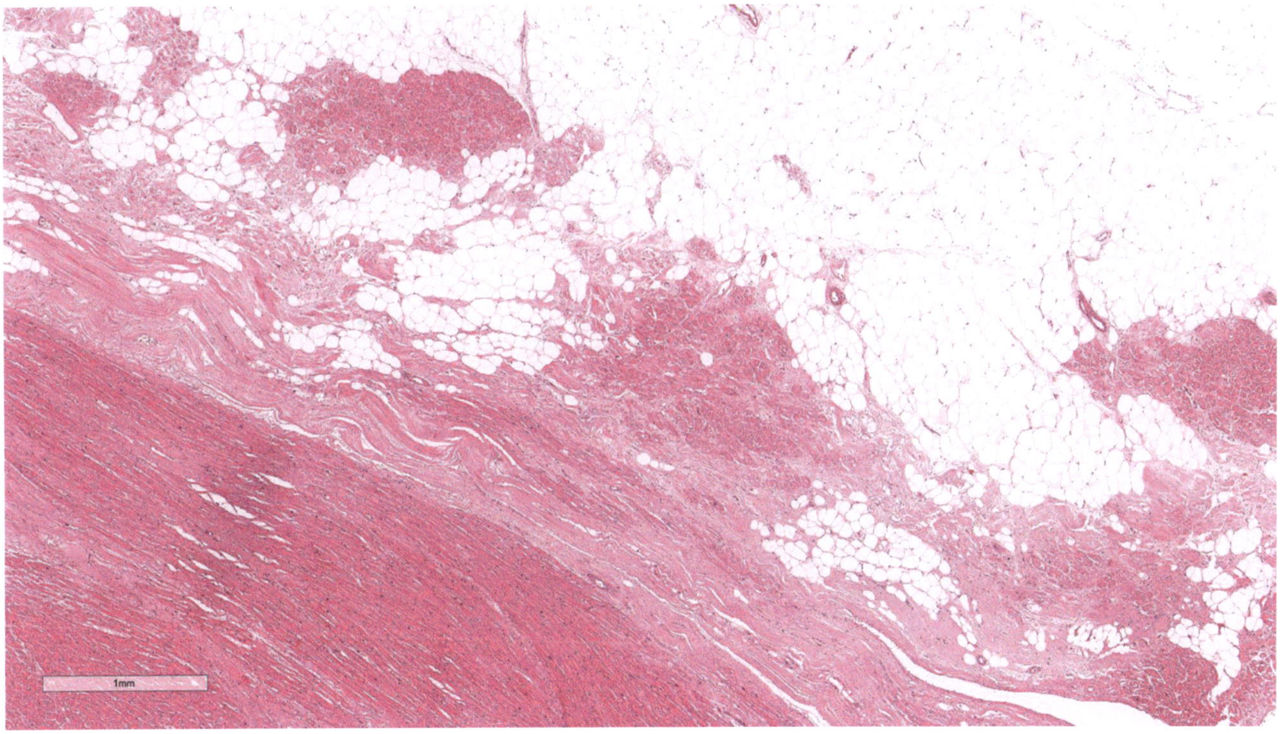

Fig. 14.48 This is an example of arrhythmogenic cardiomyopathy involving the left ventricle. Adipose tissue and fibrosis replaces the myocardium, extending from the outside in

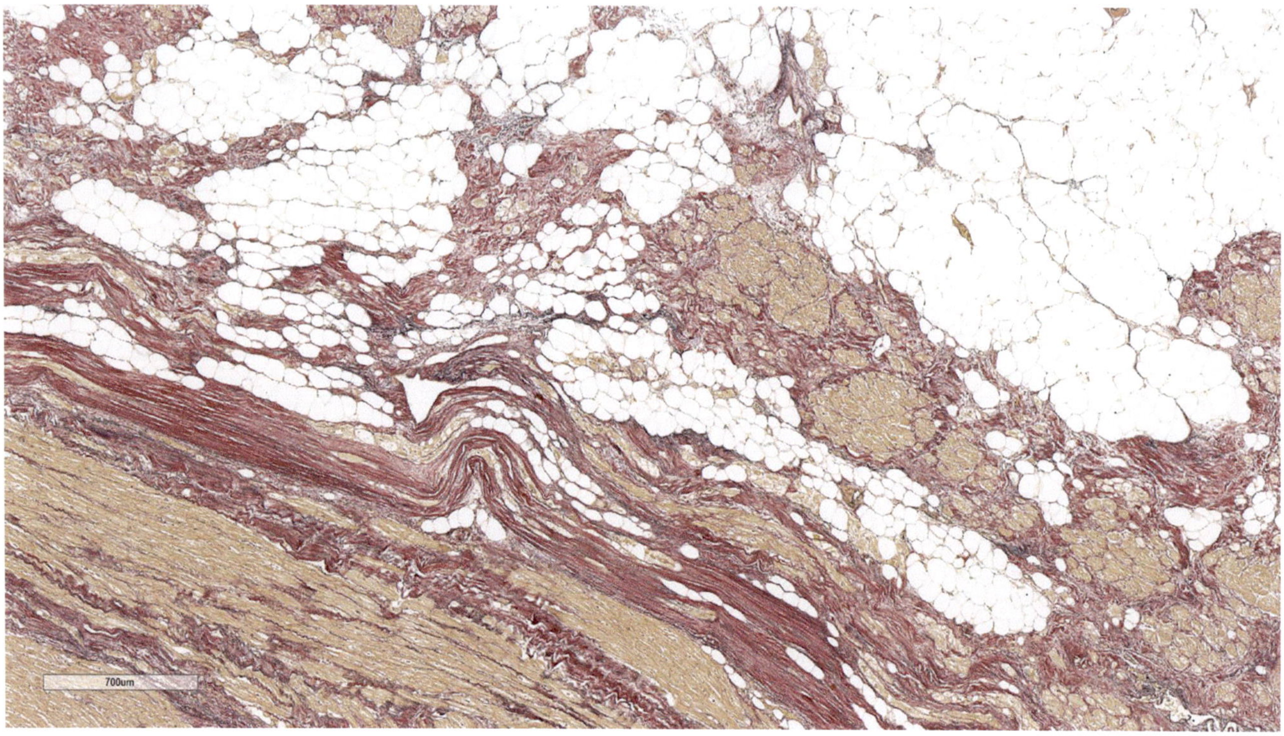

Fig. 14.49 Arrhythmogenic cardiomyopathy with left ventricular involvement. The elastic Van Gieson (EVG) stain shown here highlights the fibrosis

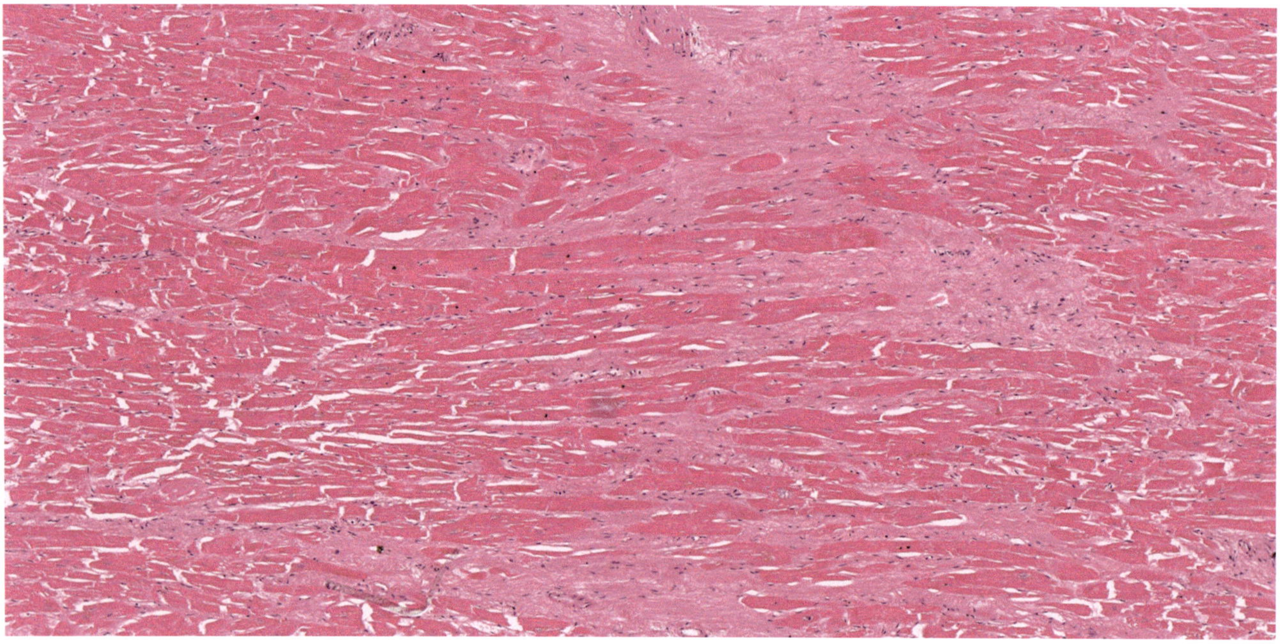

Fig. 14.50 Dilated cardiomyopathy (DCM) may be primary or acquired. Some cases may be familial. Histology tends to show an interstitial pattern of fibrosis as in this case. There are no specific histological features to distinguish the causes of DCM

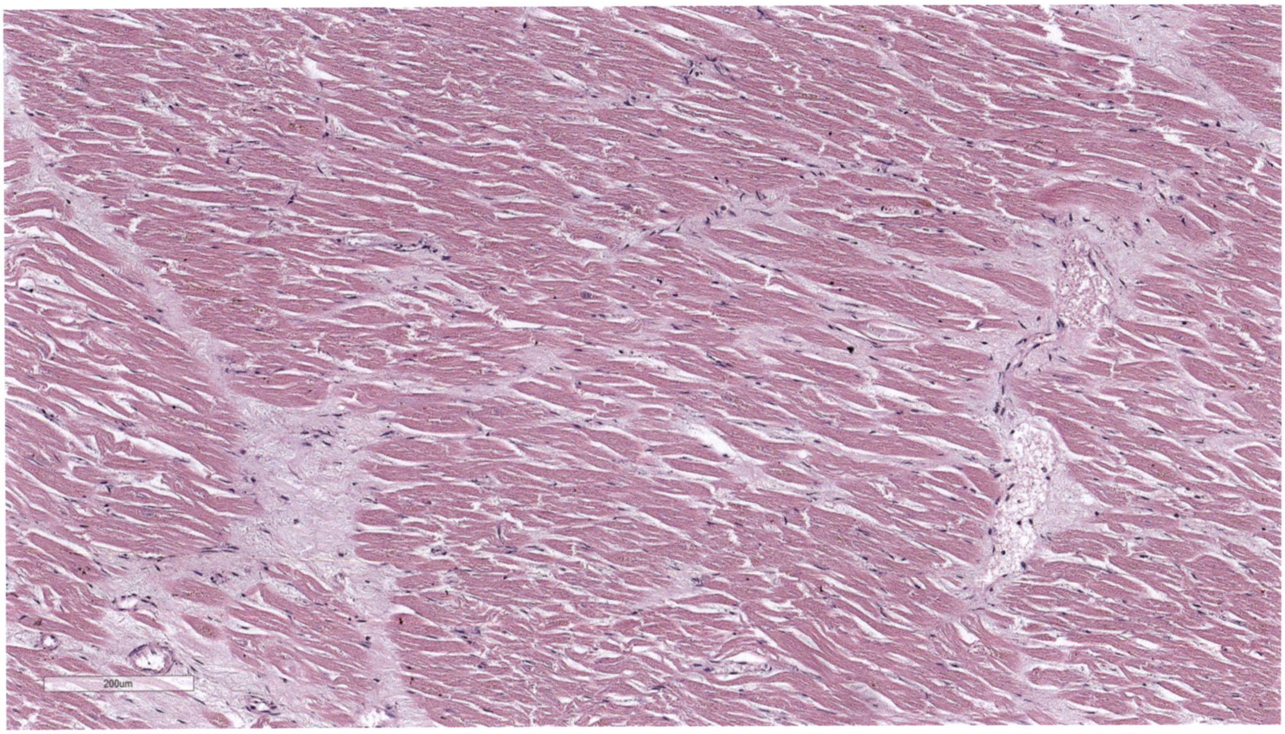

Fig. 14.51 In this example of dilated cardiomyopathy there is interstitial fibrosis with a peri-myocytic pattern

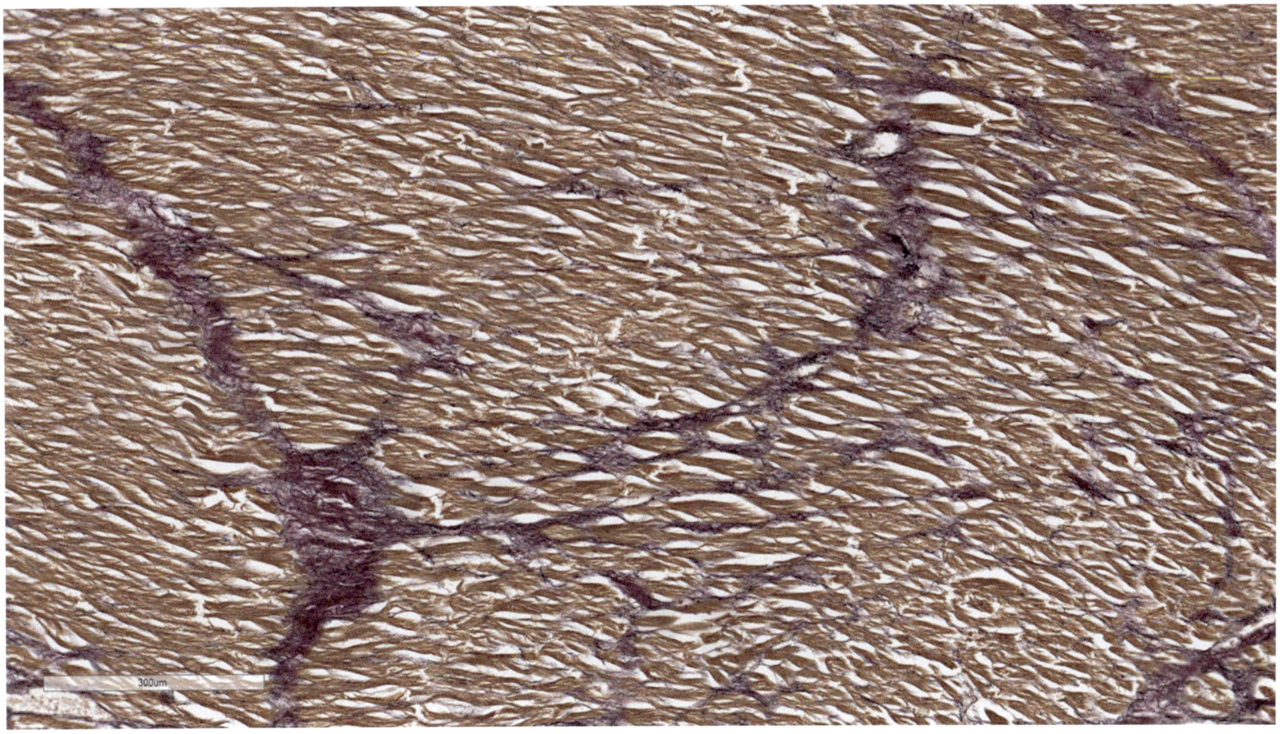

Fig. 14.52 Here is another example of dilated cardiomyopathy, this time showing interstitial fibrosis with a peri-myocytic pattern highlighted by EVG staining

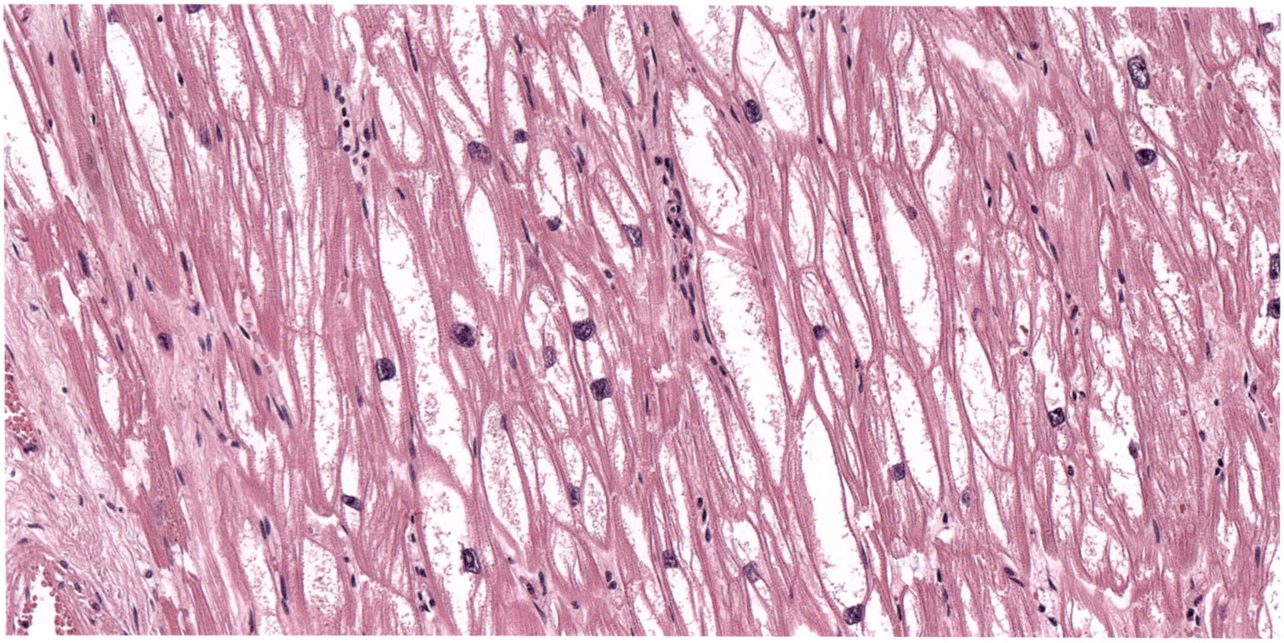

Fig. 14.53 Fabry disease is an X-linked disorder which can cause left ventricular hypertrophy. The histological hallmark is vacuolation of the cardiac myocytes

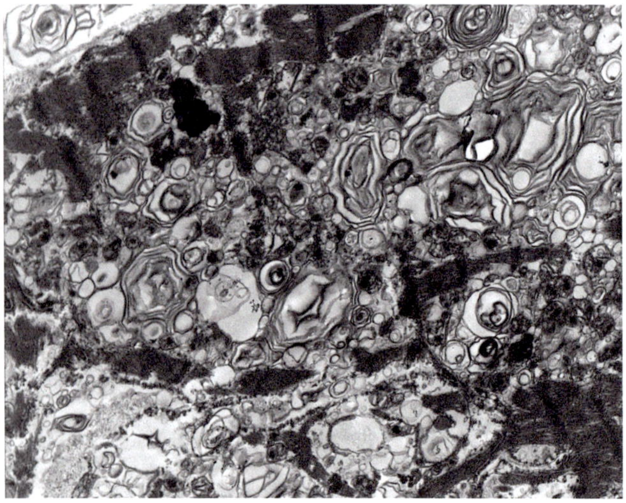

Fig. 14.54 In Fabry disease, intracellular round lamellated bodies are seen on electron microscopy which confirms the diagnosis

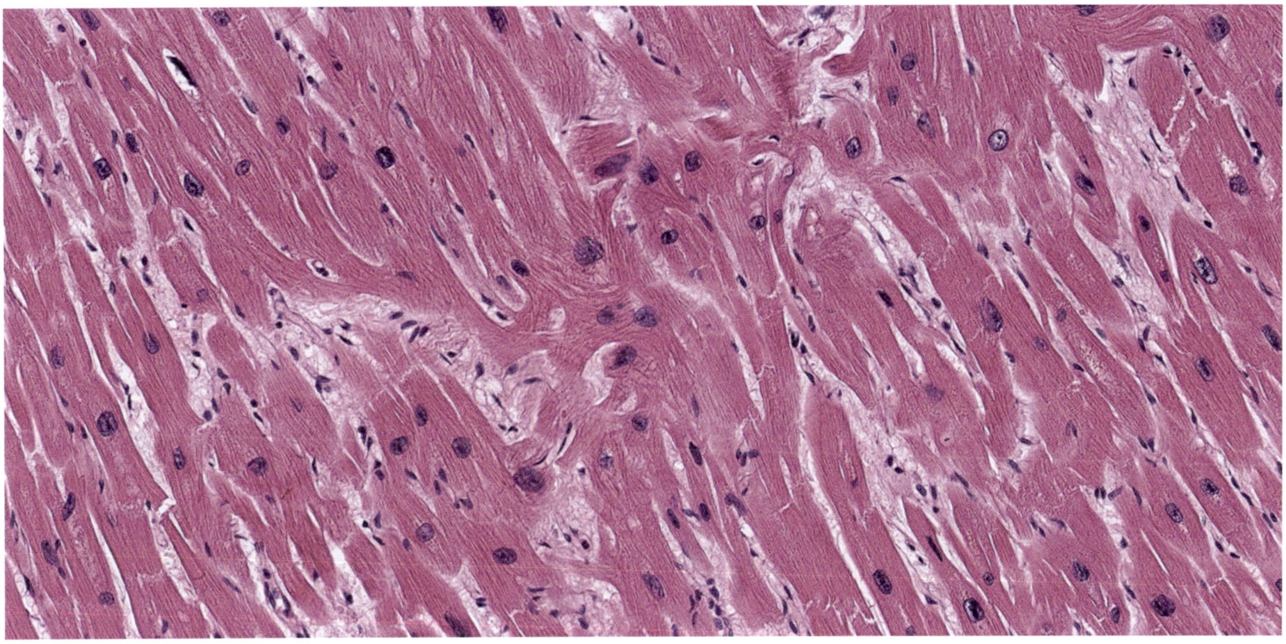

Fig. 14.55 There are several muscular disorders which can affect the heart. In Friedreich's ataxia there can be left ventricular hypertrophy and cardiac myocyte disarray which resembles hypertrophic cardiomyopathy microscopically

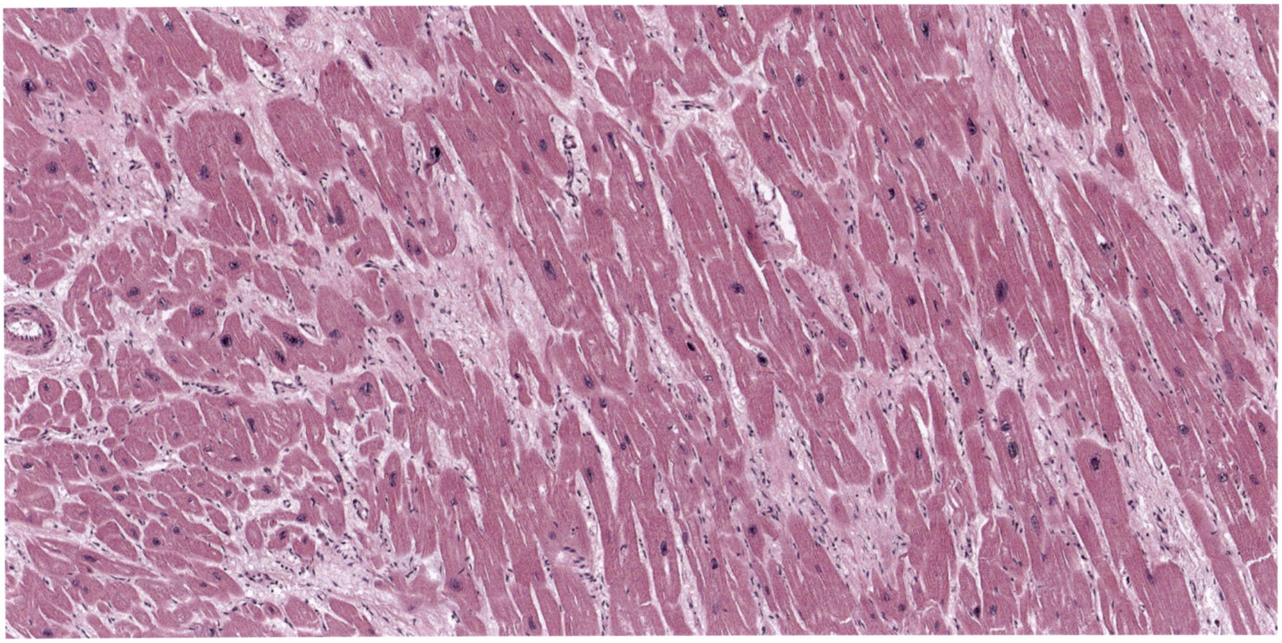

Fig. 14.56 Another example of Friedreich's ataxia involving the heart is seen here. There is cardiac myocyte nuclear hypertrophy and interstitial fibrosis

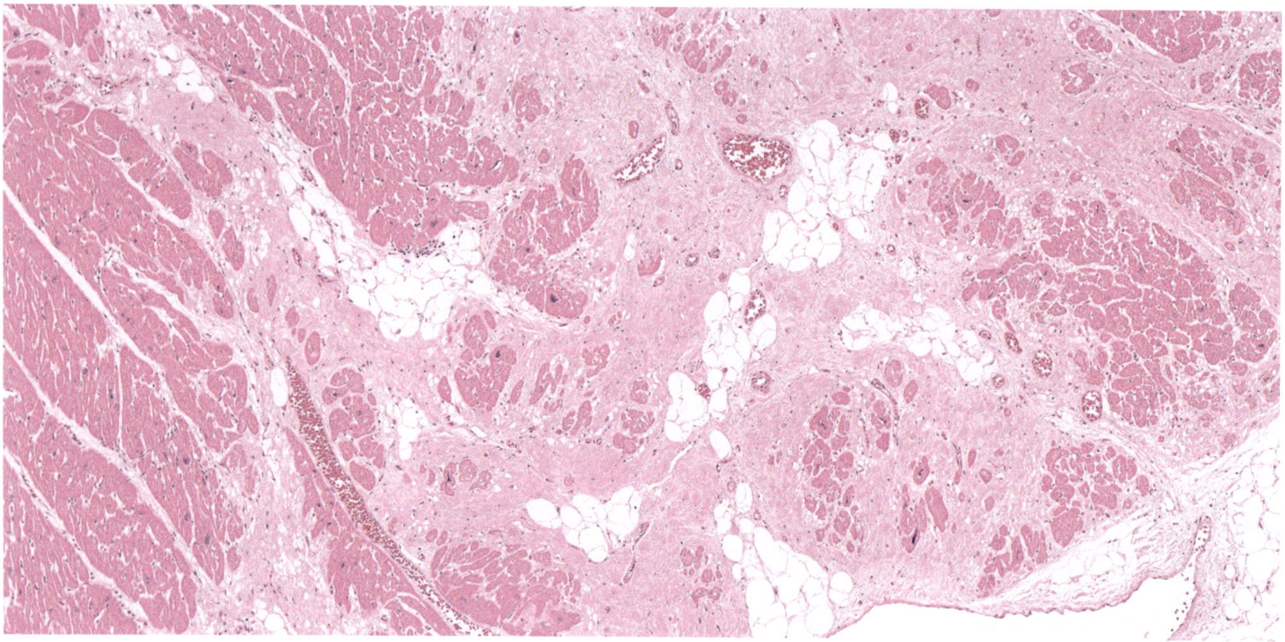

Fig. 14.57 In Duchenne muscular dystrophy, absence of dystrophin leads to successive myocyte micro-ruptures during contraction, resulting in cell death and replacement by fibrosis and adipose tissue

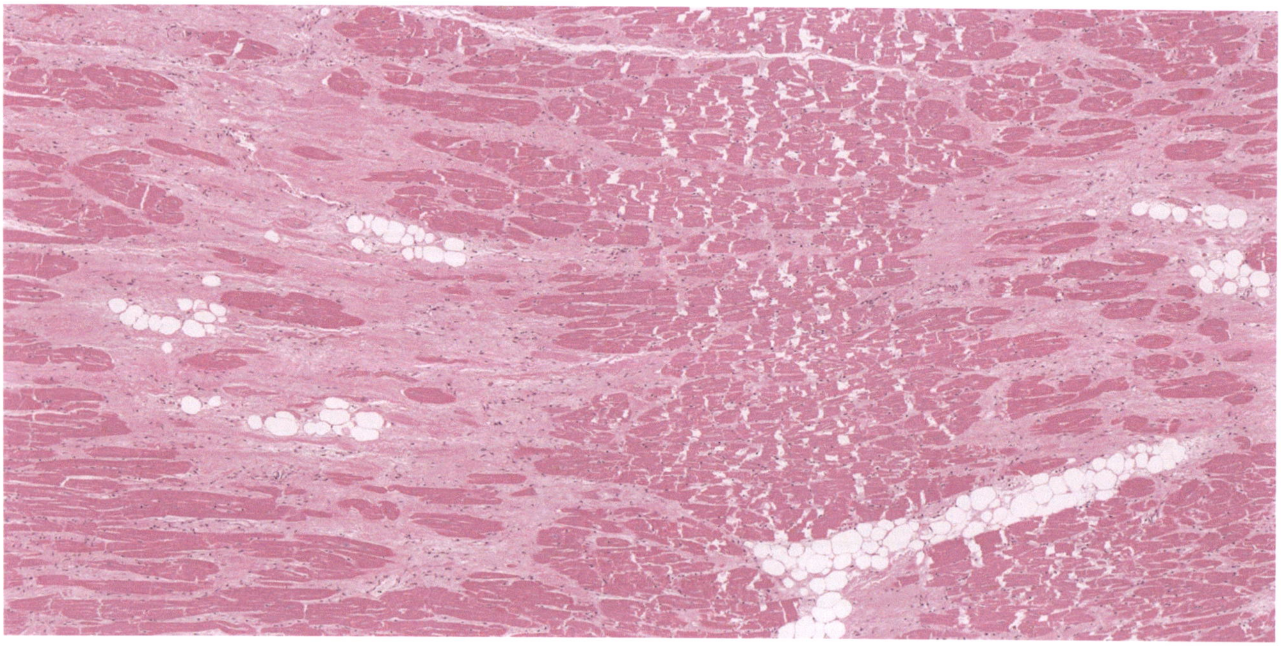

Fig. 14.58 In myotonic dystrophy involvement of the heart is common, although the mechanism is not well understood. Histological features can include fibrosis, myocyte hypertrophy and fatty replacement, which are shown here. These changes can affect the sino-atrial node and conduction system

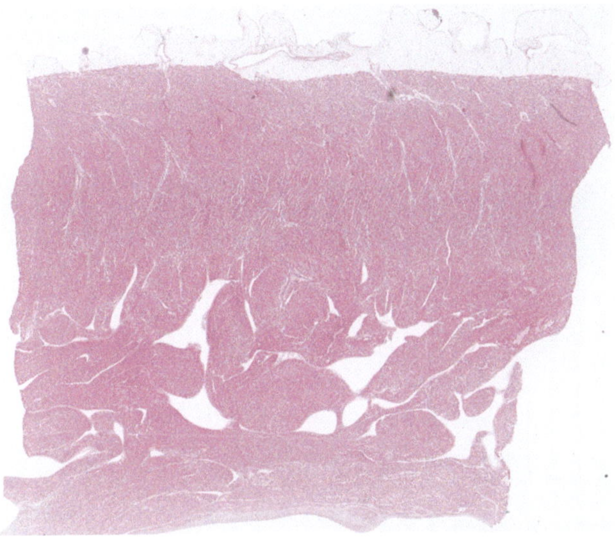

Fig. 14.59 Left ventricular non-compaction, a disorder of cardiac development, is a diagnosis made chiefly macroscopically or at low power microscopically. Finger-like trabeculae extend deep within the ventricle wall

Tumours of the Heart

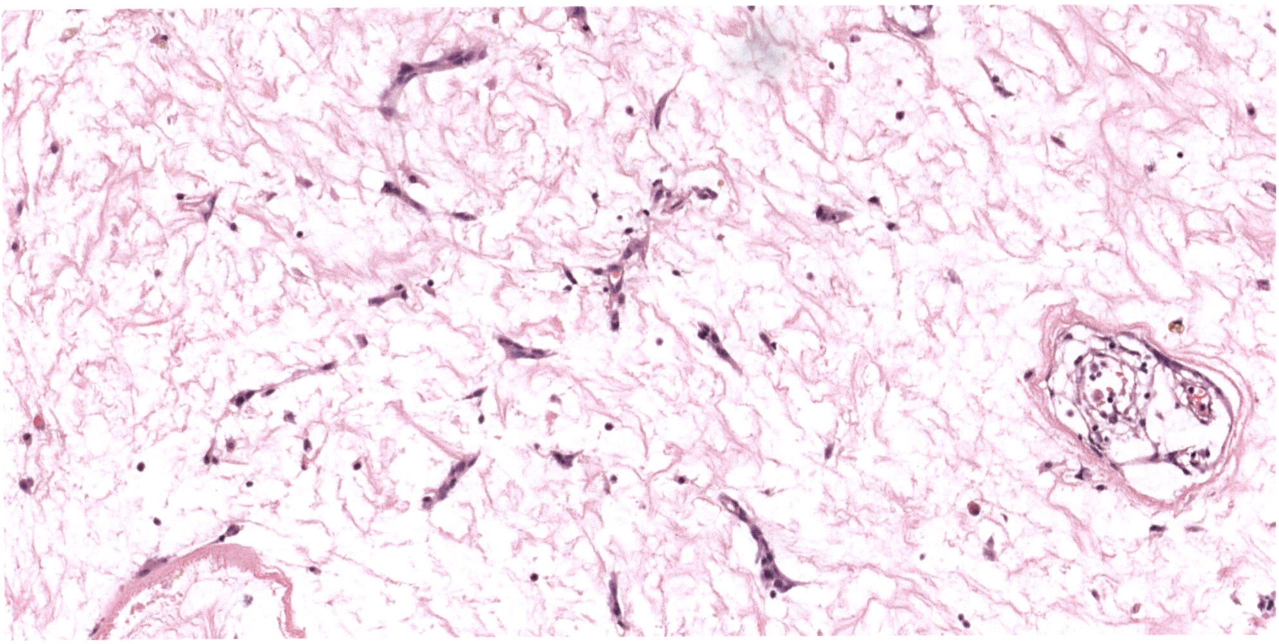

Fig. 14.60 Atrial myxoma is the most common primary tumour of the heart. Stellate myxoma cells are set in a myxoid background. Haemorrhage, haemosiderin and calcification are common

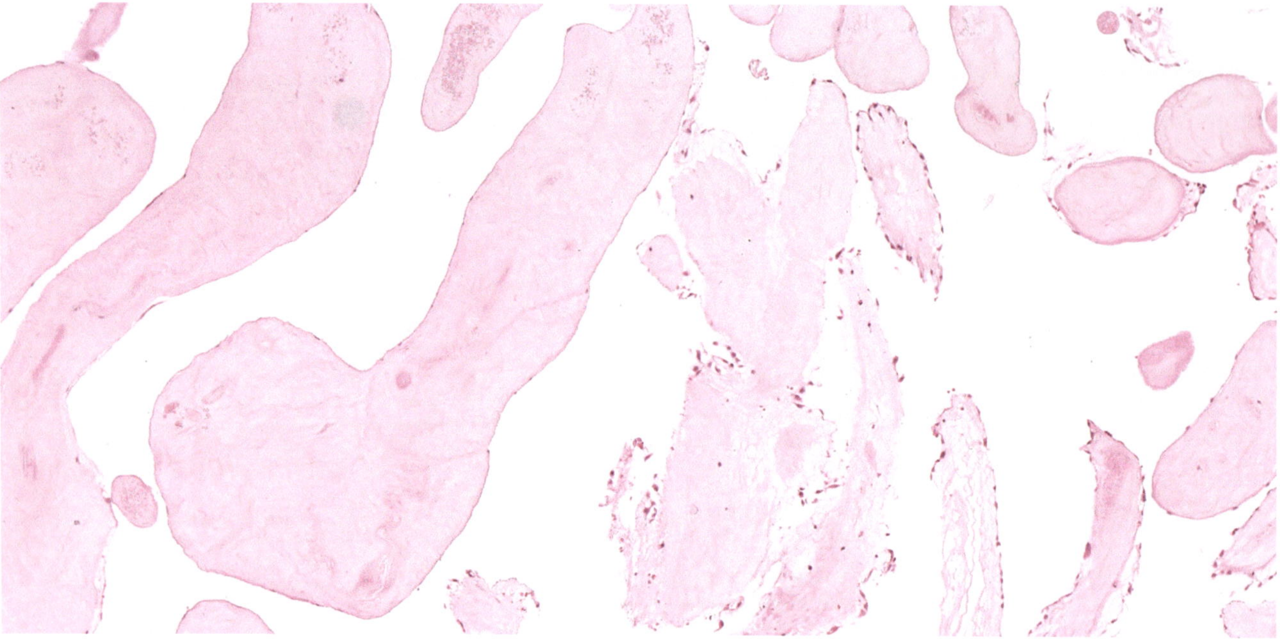

Fig. 14.61 Papillary fibroelastoma is a benign primary cardiac tumour. Microscopic features include bland, avascular, finger-like papillae lined by a thin endocardial layer

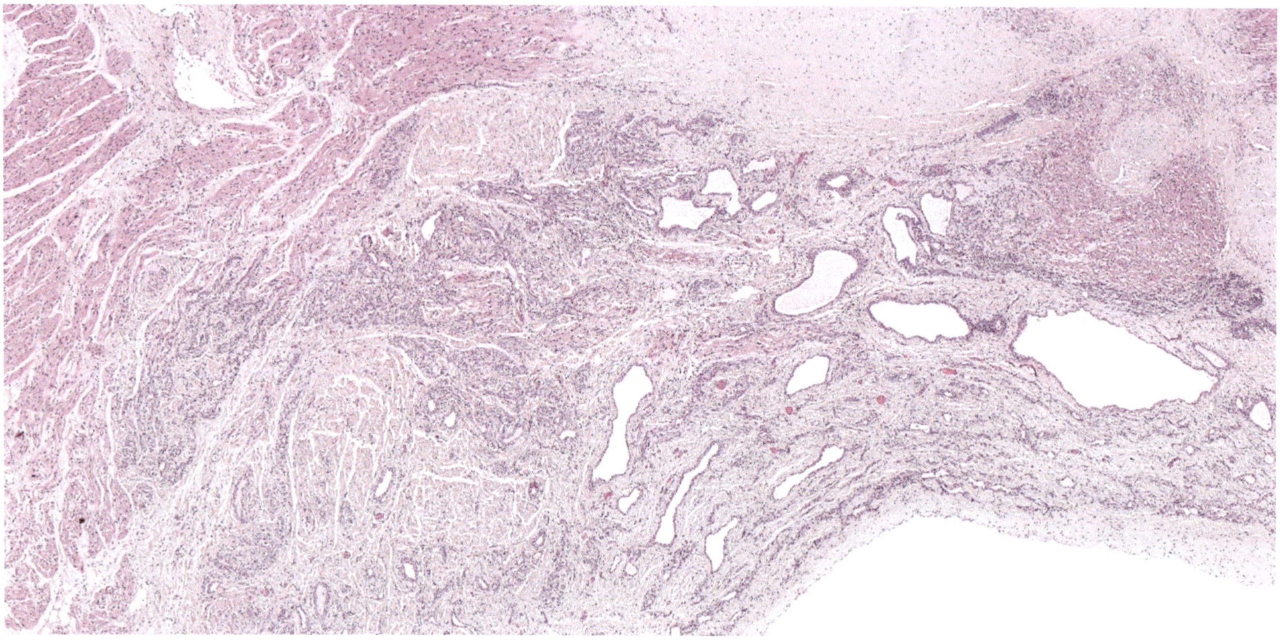

Fig. 14.62 Cystic tumour of the atrio-ventricular (AV) node is a rare tumour which can be a cause of sudden death, usually in children or young adults. Microscopically there are solid nests and cystic spaces lined by a bland cuboidal epithelium. These tumours may be very small and difficult to identify with the naked eye. However, their location near the AV node means even a small tumour can be fatal. Sampling of the conduction system will allow the pathologist to identify these tumours

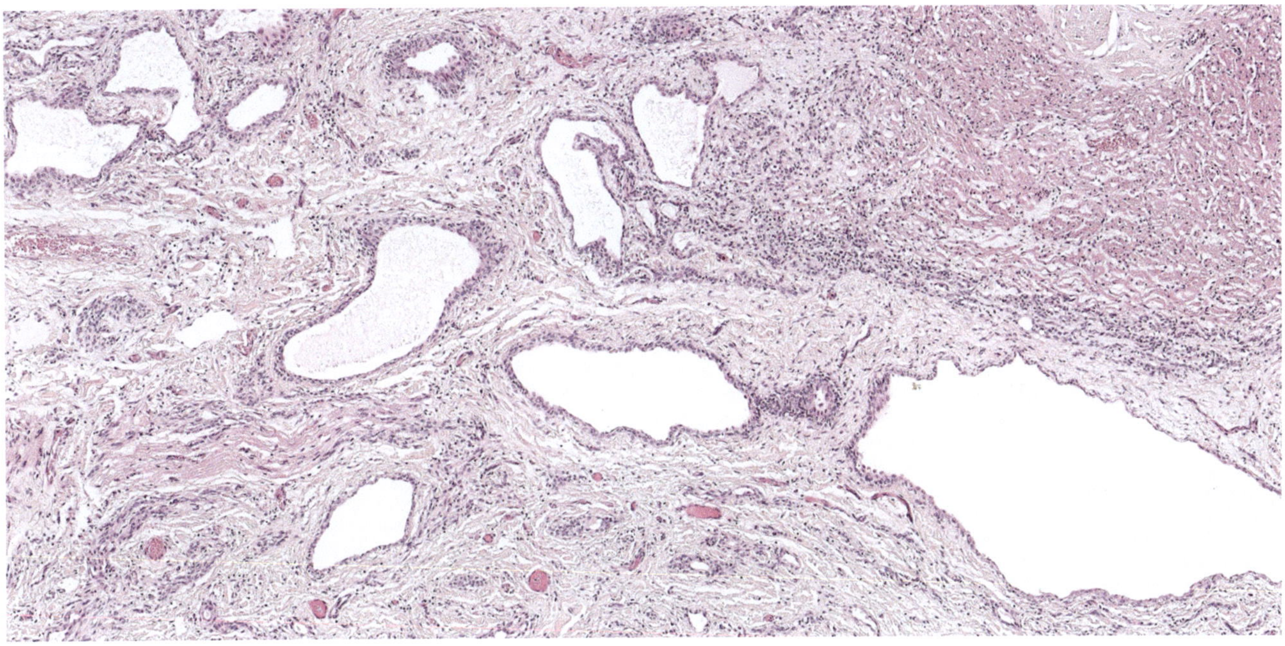

Fig. 14.63 A higher power view of the cystic tumour of the atrio-ventricular node shown in Fig. 14.62

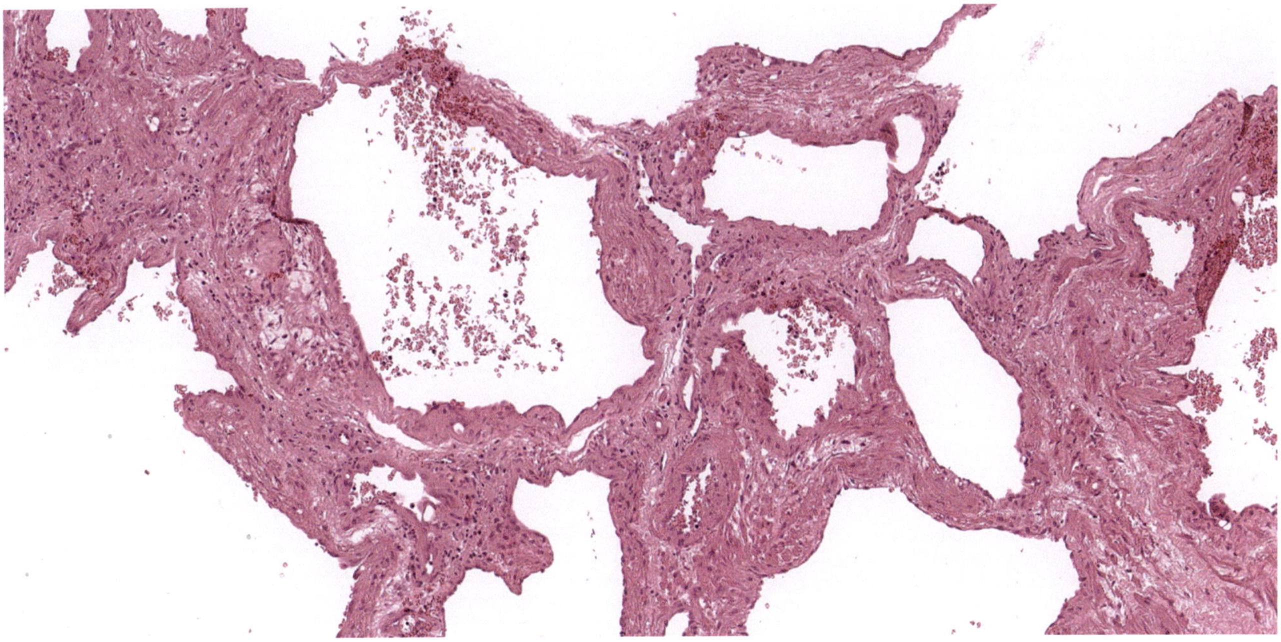

Fig. 14.64 Haemangiomas may be seen in the heart

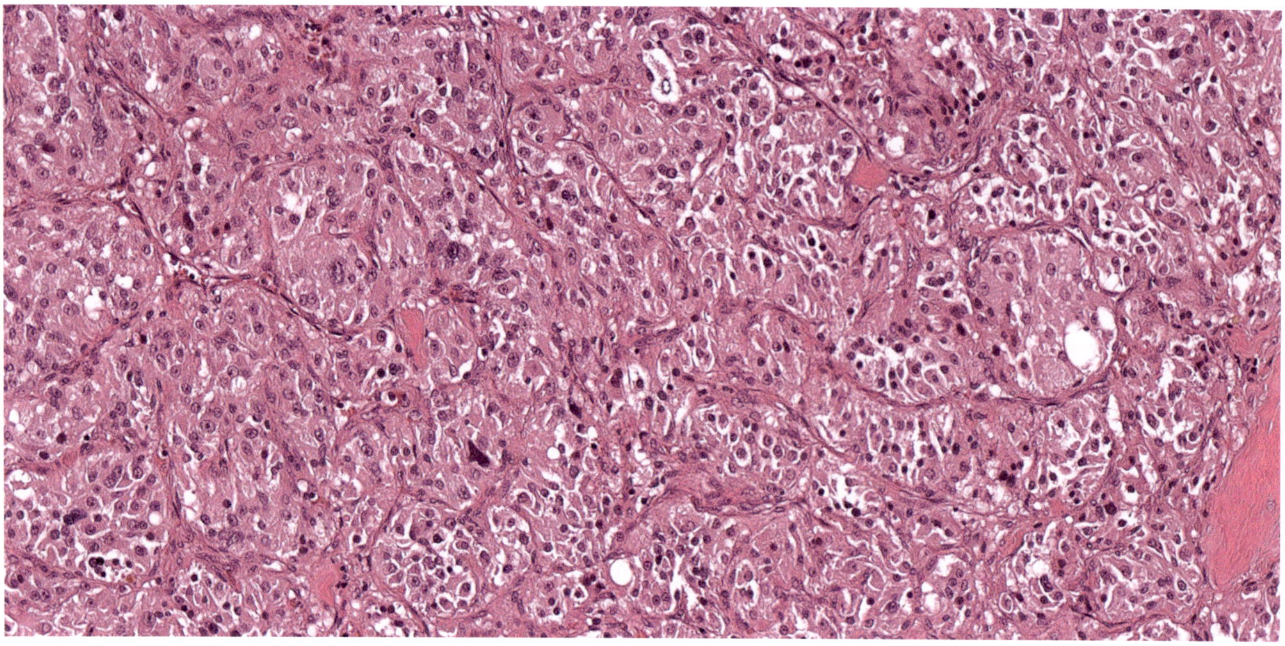

Fig. 14.65 The heart is one of the sites where paragangliomas can occur. Their microscopic features are similar to elsewhere in the body; a nested pattern separated by fibrous bands. Nuclear atypia is common

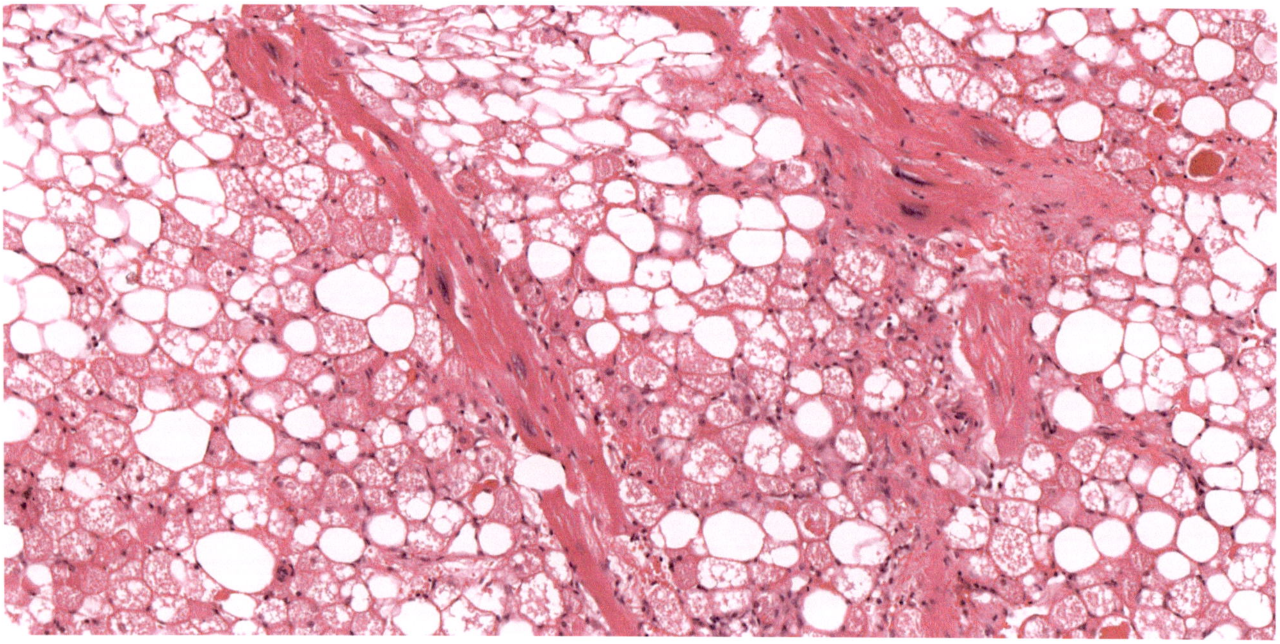

Fig. 14.66 The interatrial septum in the heart can become thickened with adipose tissue, known as lipomatous hypertrophy of the interatrial septum. Microscopically there is adipose tissue, including brown fat, admixed with cardiac myocytes

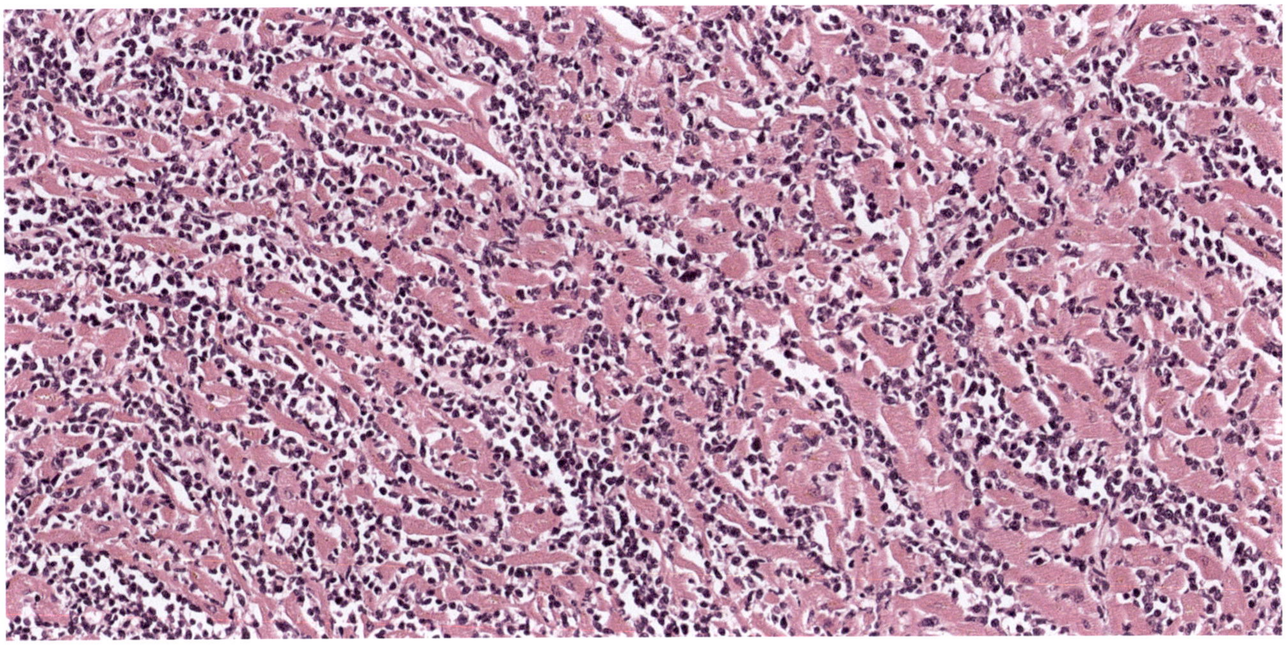

Fig. 14.67 Lymphomas may be primary to the heart as in this case which shows a primary B-cell lymphoma of the heart. There are lymphoma cells infiltrating between cardiac myocytes. Immunohistochemistry is required to confirm the lymphoid and neoplastic nature of these cells and to subtype the lymphoma

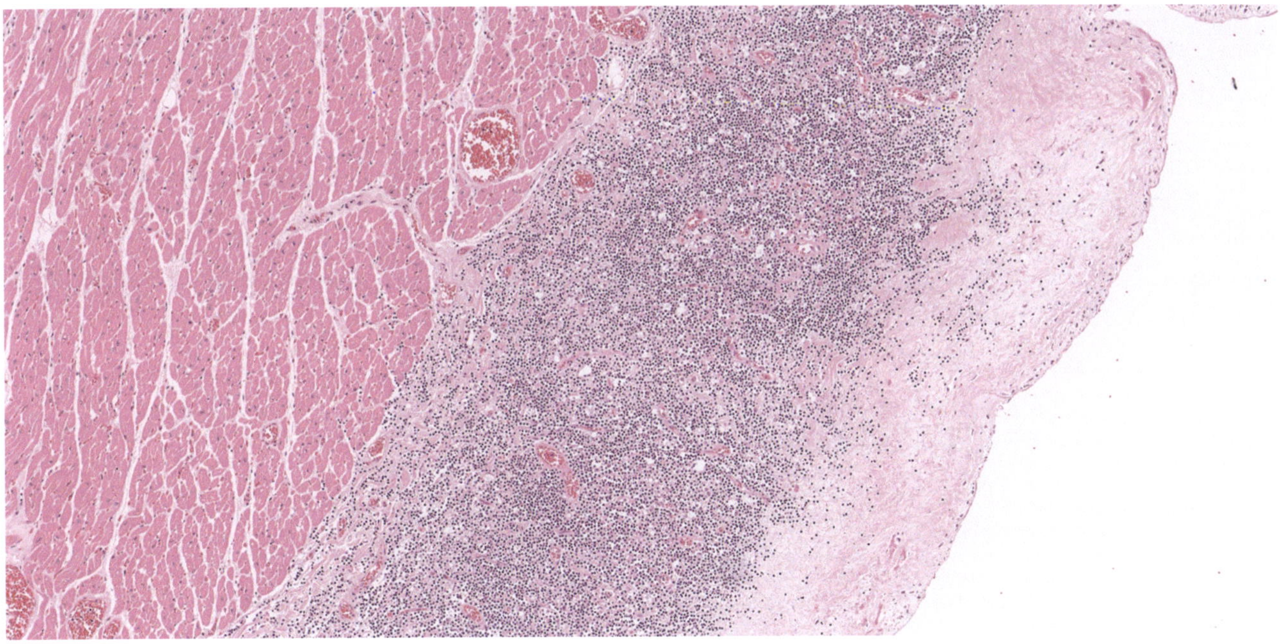

Fig. 14.68 This is an example of a systemic chronic lymphocytic leukaemia/small lymphocytic lymphoma involving the heart. There is an epicardial infiltrate of lymphoma cells. Precise typing of lymphoma would require immunohistochemistry. However, if there is a known diagnosis this may not be necessary

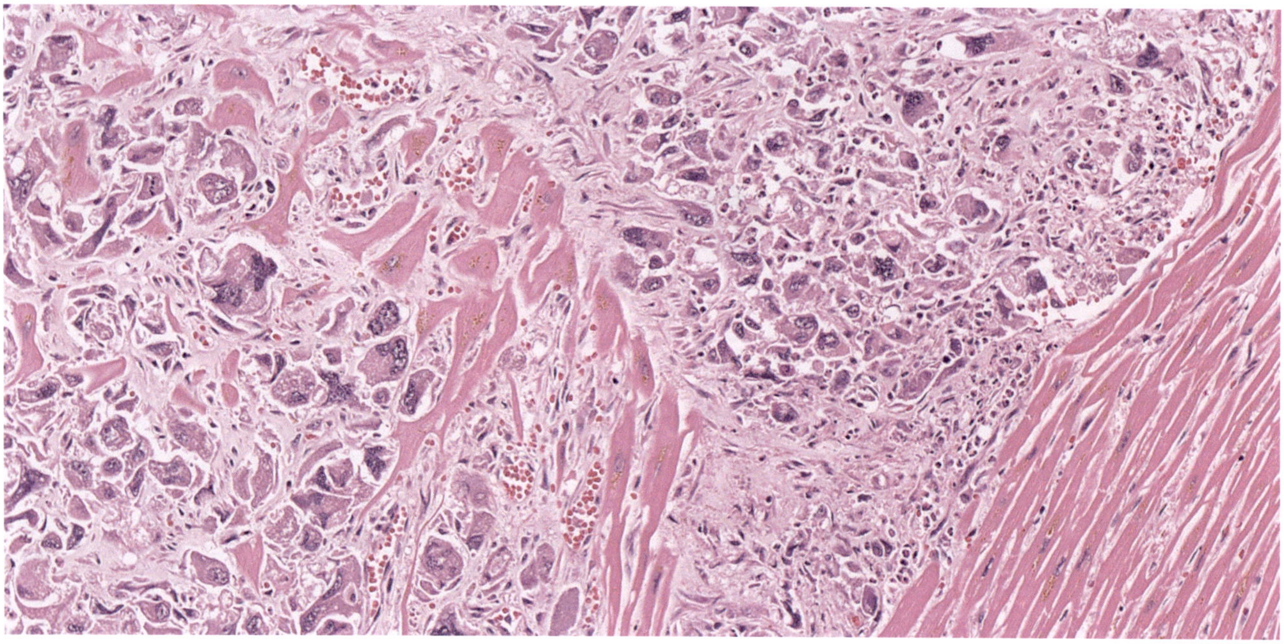

Fig. 14.69 Malignant tumours may metastasise to the heart. This image shows a metastatic pancreatic carcinoma. There are anaplastic carcinoma cells within the myocardium

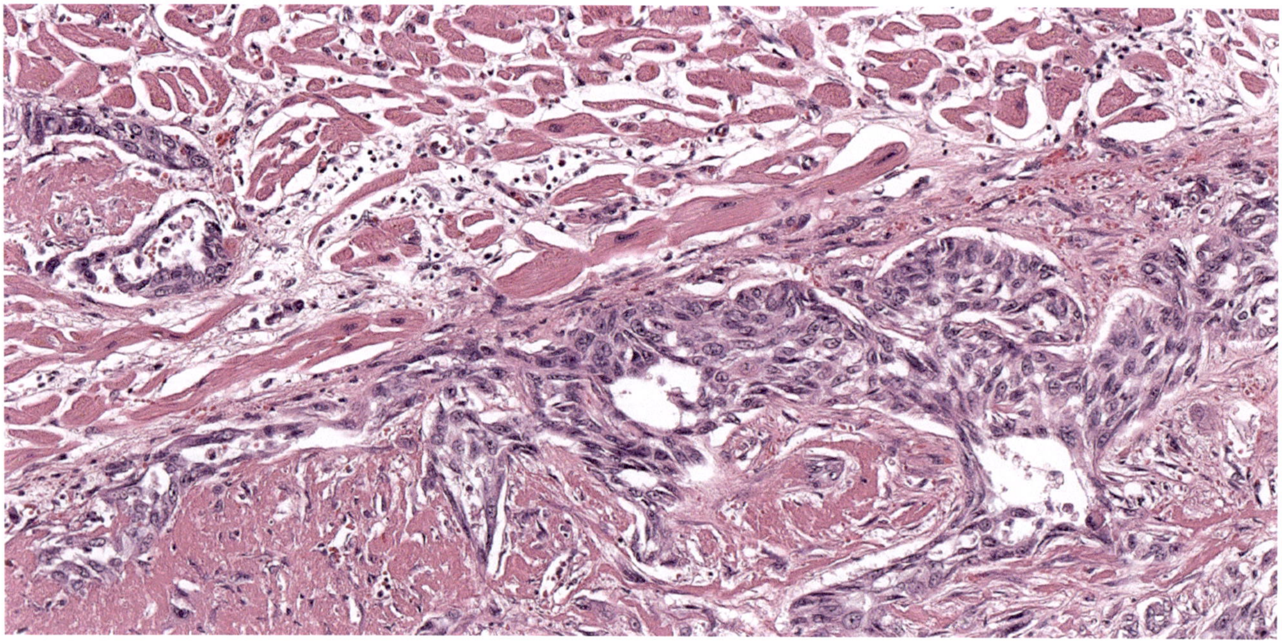

Fig. 14.70 This is an example of metastatic urothelial carcinoma in the heart

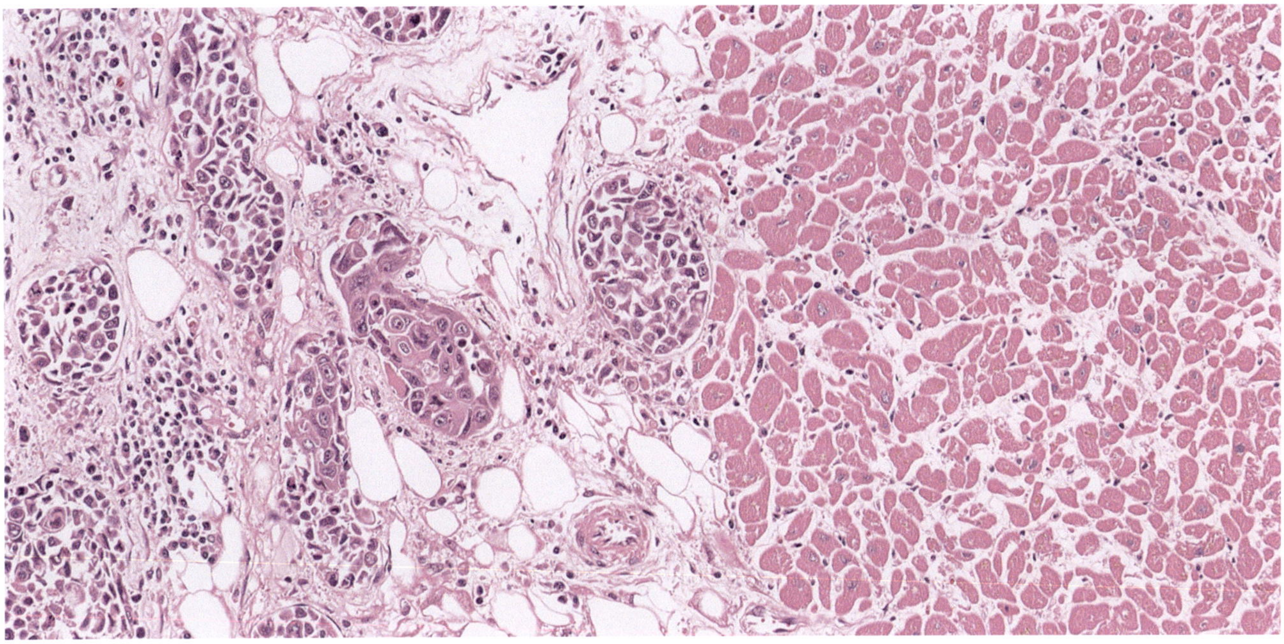

Fig. 14.71 Metastatic lung squamous cell carcinoma involving the heart is shown here

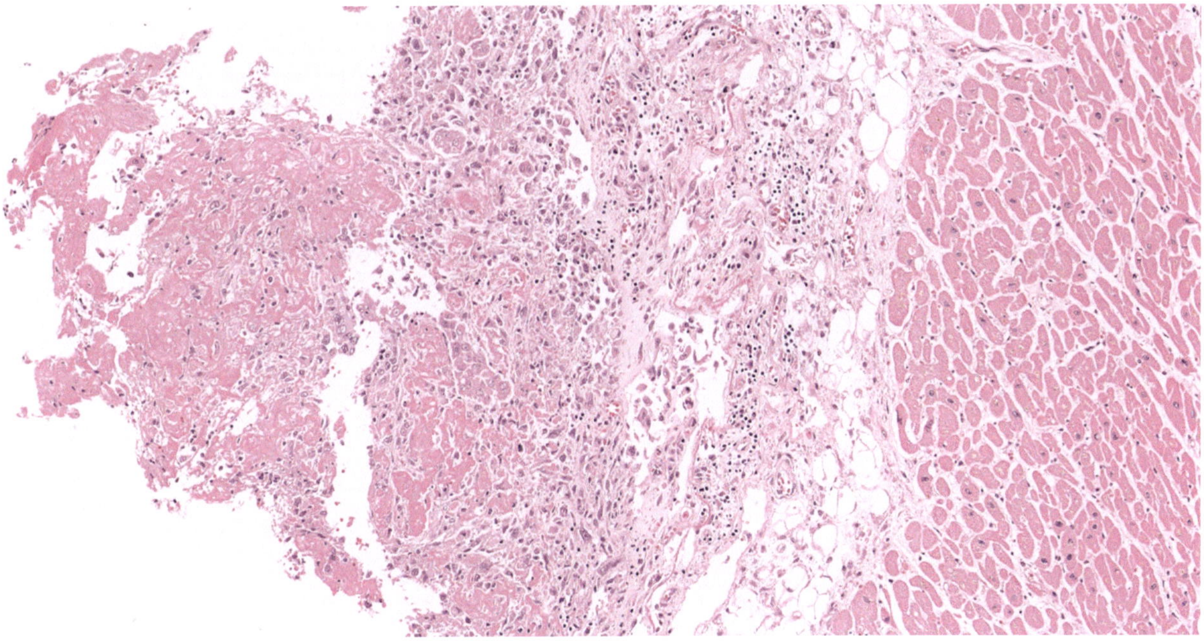

Fig. 14.72 In this case there are epicardial tumour deposits associated with fibrinous pericarditis

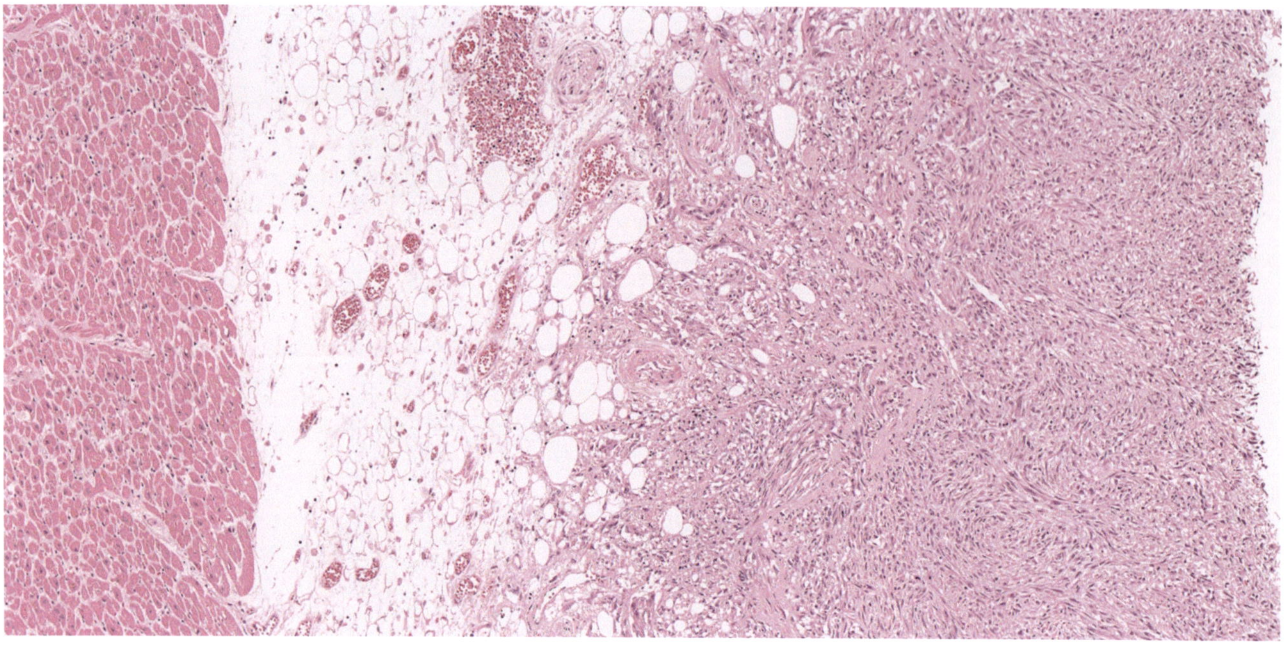

Fig. 14.73 Direct spread of pleural mesothelioma can commonly involve the pericardial sac and can involve the heart. In this image there is an epicardial deposit of a pleural mesothelioma

Aorta

Normal

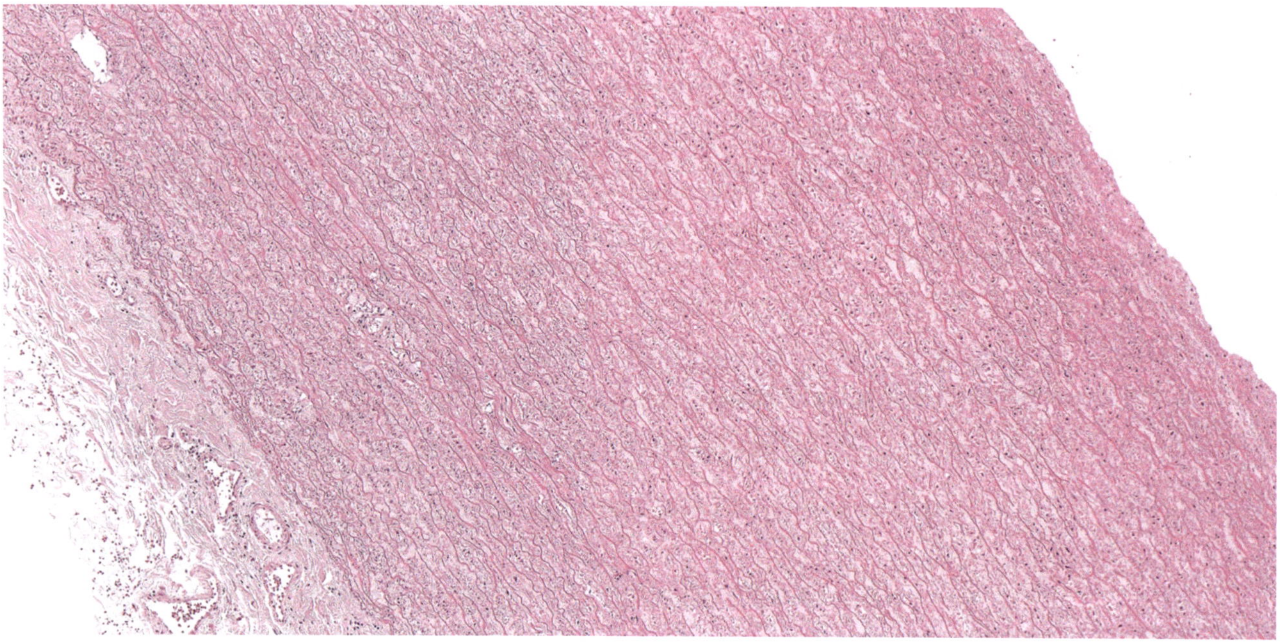

Fig. 14.74 This image shows the normal aorta. The aorta is an elastic artery. Note the densely packed elastic fibres in the media, visible on routine H&E staining

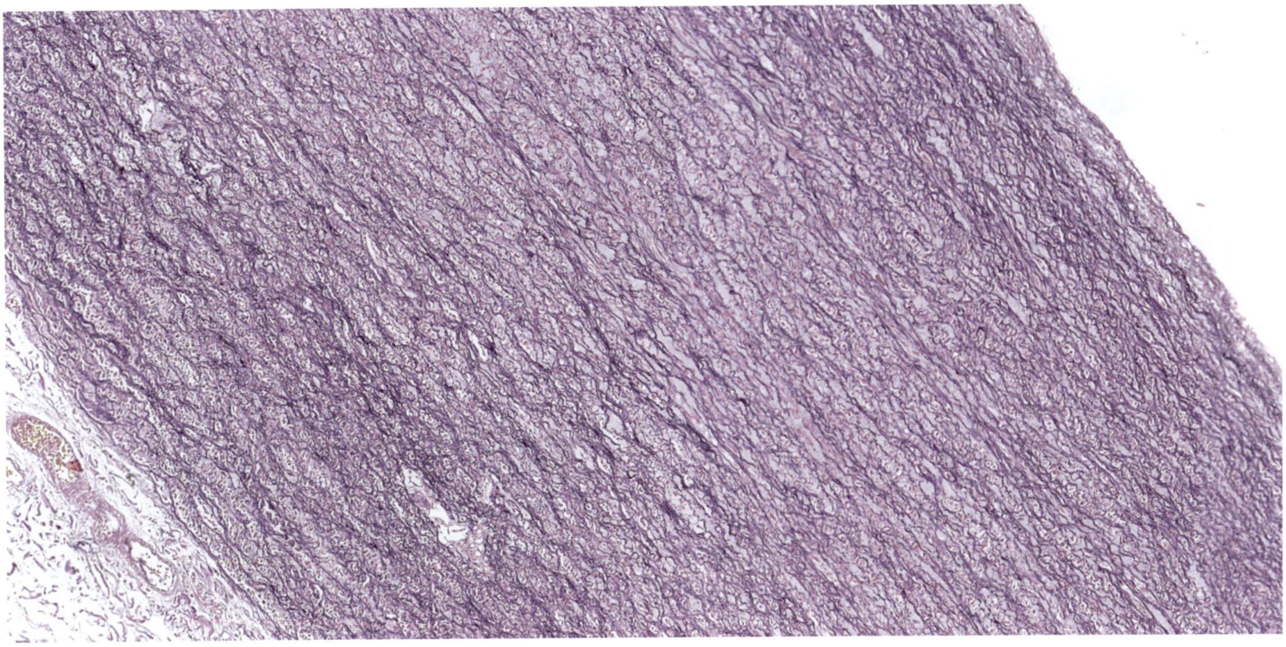

Fig. 14.75 In this image of normal aorta, EVG staining further highlights the densely packed elastic fibres in the media

Fig. 14.76 Alcian blue staining highlights the evenly distributed mucin in this normal section of aorta. EVG and alcian blue are standard special stains used to evaluate the aorta

Dissection

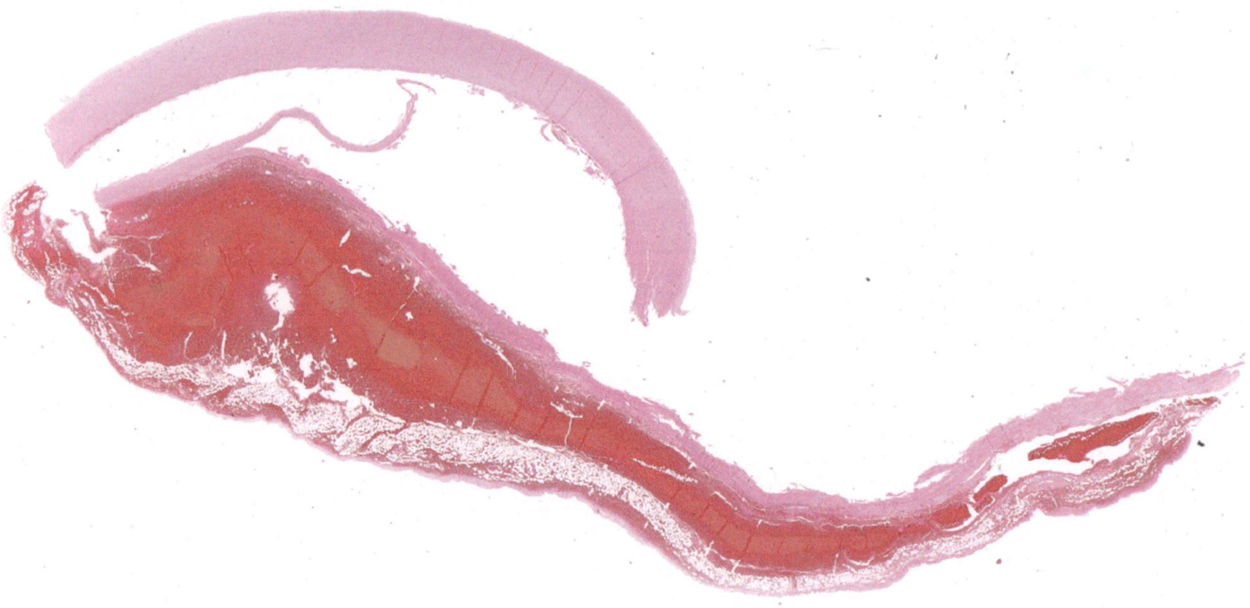

Fig. 14.77 This image shows dissection of the aorta. There is a splitting of the wall of the aorta with blood tracking outside of the media, into the adventitia. Dissection of the aorta may be associated with acquired disease such as hypertension or atherosclerosis, or inflammatory aortopathies, but may also be associated with inheritable connective tissue disorders. Histology evaluation of the aorta in the setting of dissection is important to delineate the underlying aetiology and consider the possibility of an inheritable disorder. Consensus terminology for the assessment of aortic disease is published by the Society for Cardiovascular Pathology and the Association for European Cardiovascular Pathology

Inflammatory Aortitis

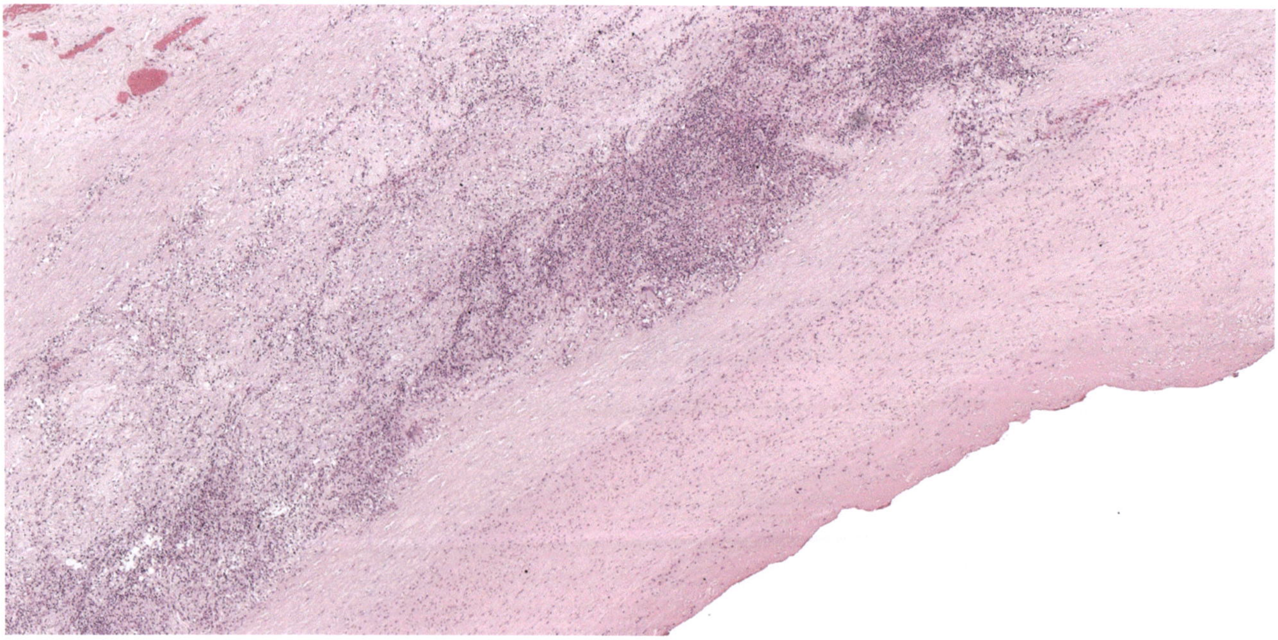

Fig. 14.78 In giant cell aortitis there is medial inflammation with multinucleated giant cells

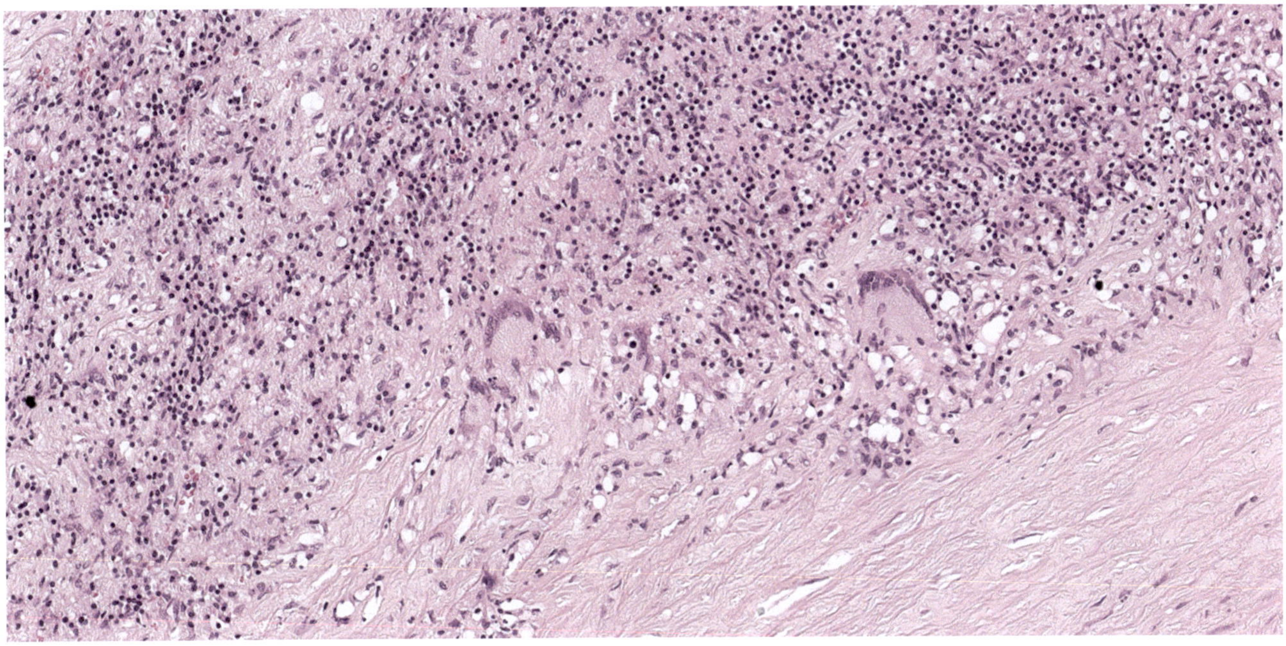

Fig. 14.79 This higher power view of Fig. 14.78 shows the multinucleated giant cells of giant cell aortitis

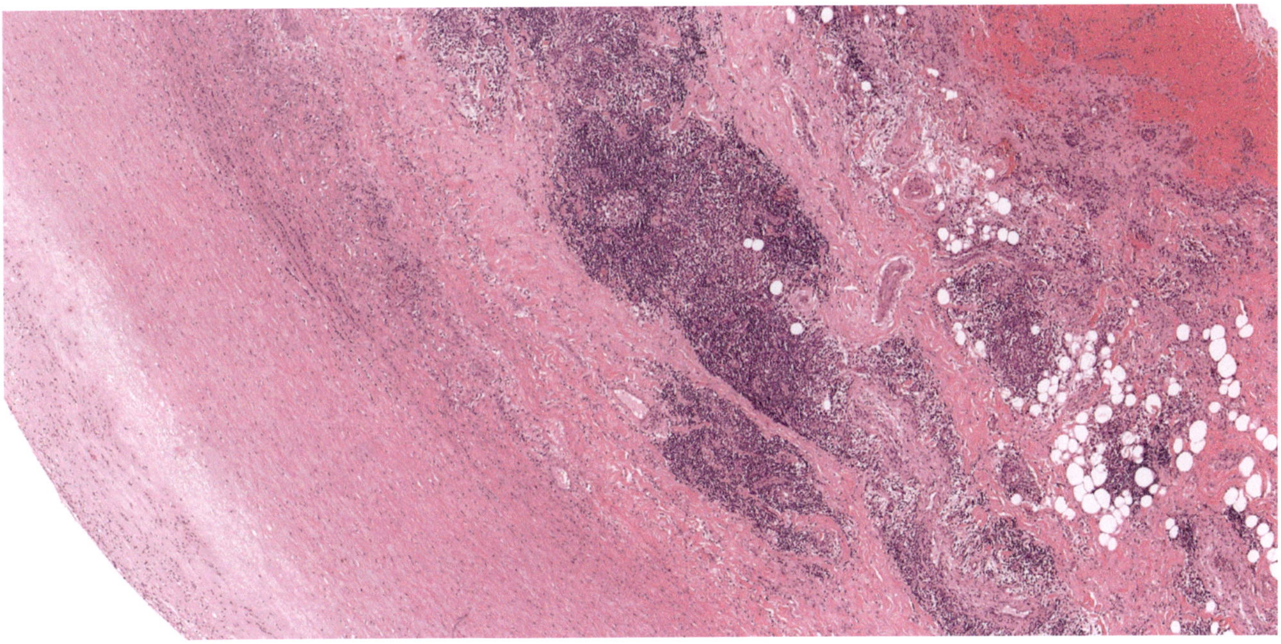

Fig. 14.80 Ankylosing spondylitis may involve the aorta, causing medial and adventitial inflammation, as seen here

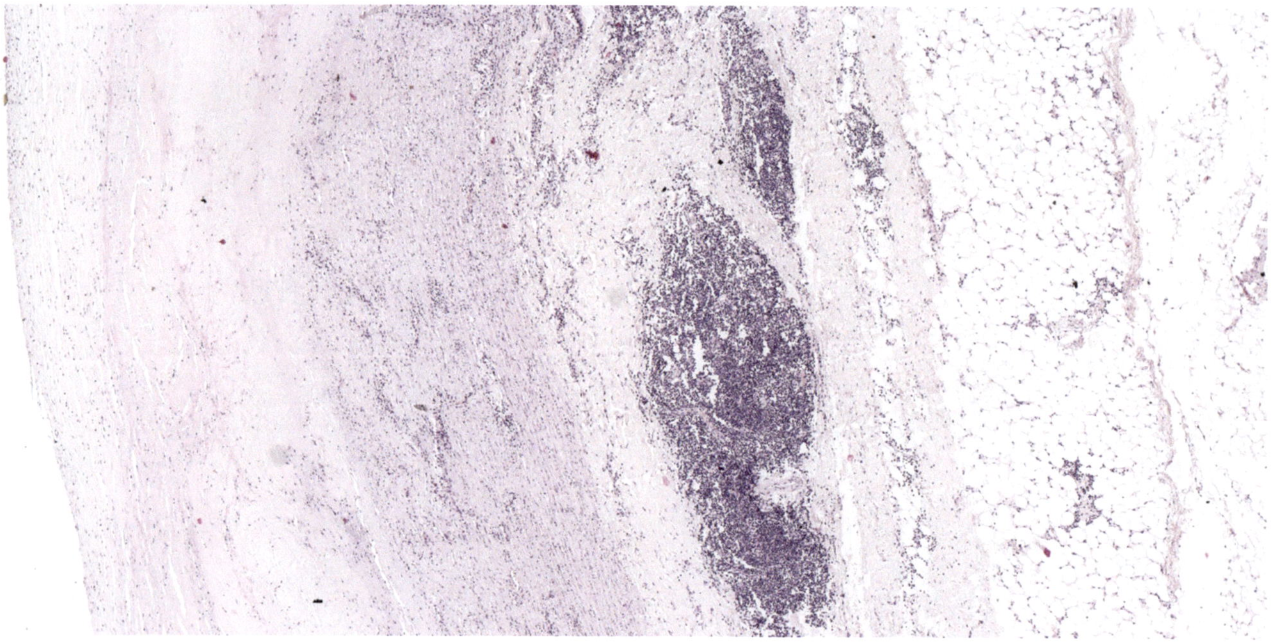

Fig. 14.81 Syphilis may involve large vessels such as the aorta. This image shows medial and adventitial inflammation. Obliterative endarteritis involving the vasa vasorum may also be seen

Non-inflammatory Aortopathy

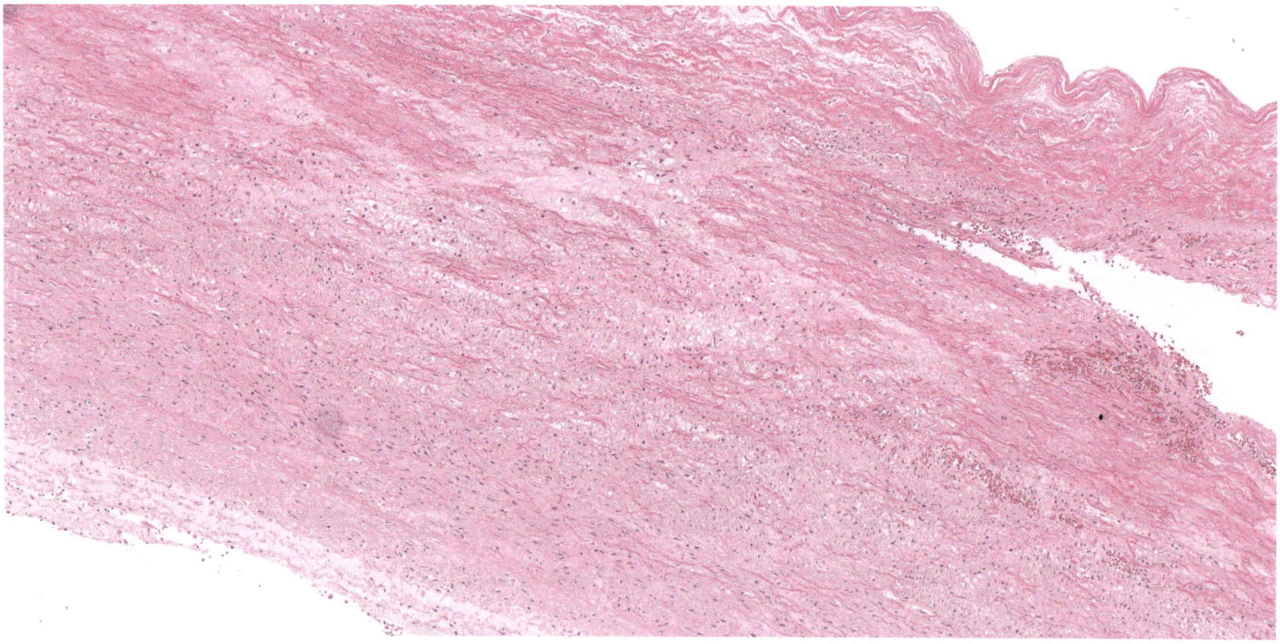

Fig. 14.82 Non-inflammatory aortopathies may be due to inheritable connective tissue disorders and can cause aortic dissection and death, particularly in young adults. This image of the aorta shows disruption of the lamellar units and loss of smooth muscle cells

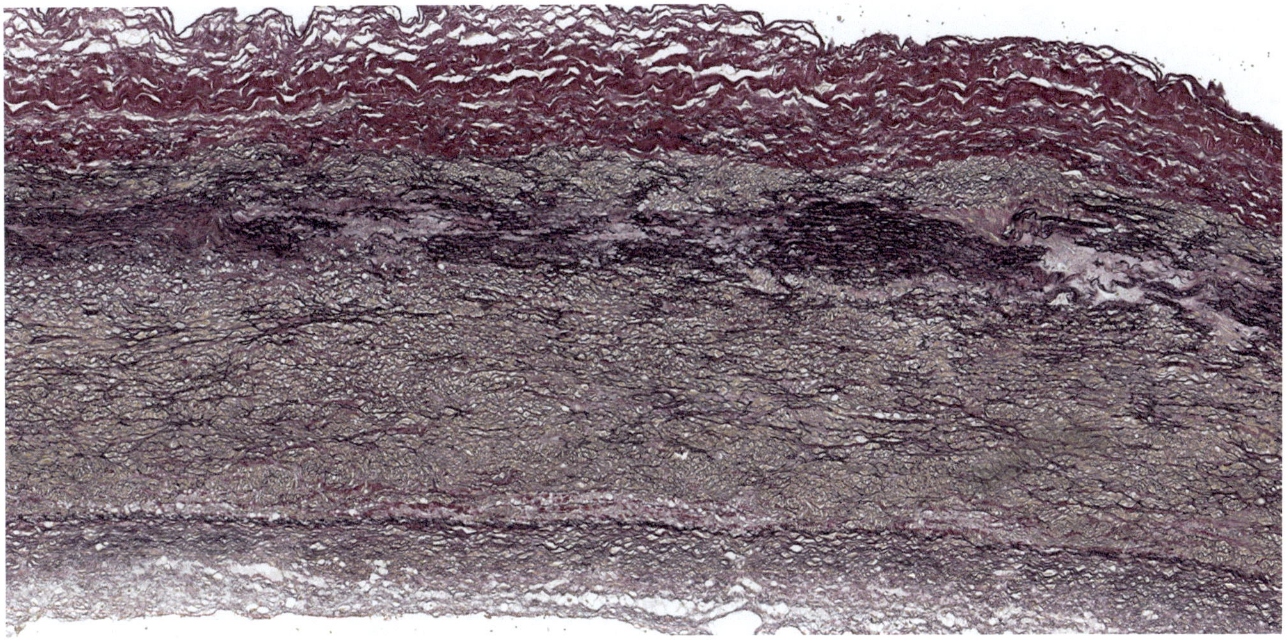

Fig. 14.83 Fragmentation of elastin is shown in this EVG stain of non-inflammatory aortopathy

Fig. 14.84 In this alcian blue stain of non-inflammatory aortopathy, there is clumpy accumulation of mucin

Lung

Pathology involving the lungs is commonly encountered at autopsy (Figs. 14.85, 14.86, 14.87, 14.88, 14.89, 14.90, 14.91, 14.92, 14.93, 14.94, 14.95, 14.96, 14.97, 14.98, 14.99, 14.100, 14.101, 14.102, 14.103, 14.104, 14.105, 14.106, 14.107, 14.108, 14.109, 14.110, 14.111, 14.112, 14.113, 14.114, 14.115, 14.116, 14.117, 14.118, 14.119, 14.120, 14.121, 14.122, 14.123, 14.124, 14.125, 14.126, 14.127, 14.128, 14.129, 14.130, 14.131, 14.132, 14.133, and 14.134). It may be the immediate cause of death, such as pneumonia, lung cancers or pulmonary thromboembolism, or may reflect other systemic pathology, such as pulmonary oedema as a consequence of cardiac failure or acute respiratory distress syndrome (ARDS) in sepsis.

Pulmonary pathology seen at autopsy in a medicolegal setting also incorporates a range of occupational diseases from exposure to asbestos, coal, silica and other inhaled particulates.

Unnatural lung and airways pathology such as aspiration and inhalation of smoke in fire deaths are also included in this section.

Lung

Normal and Artefacts

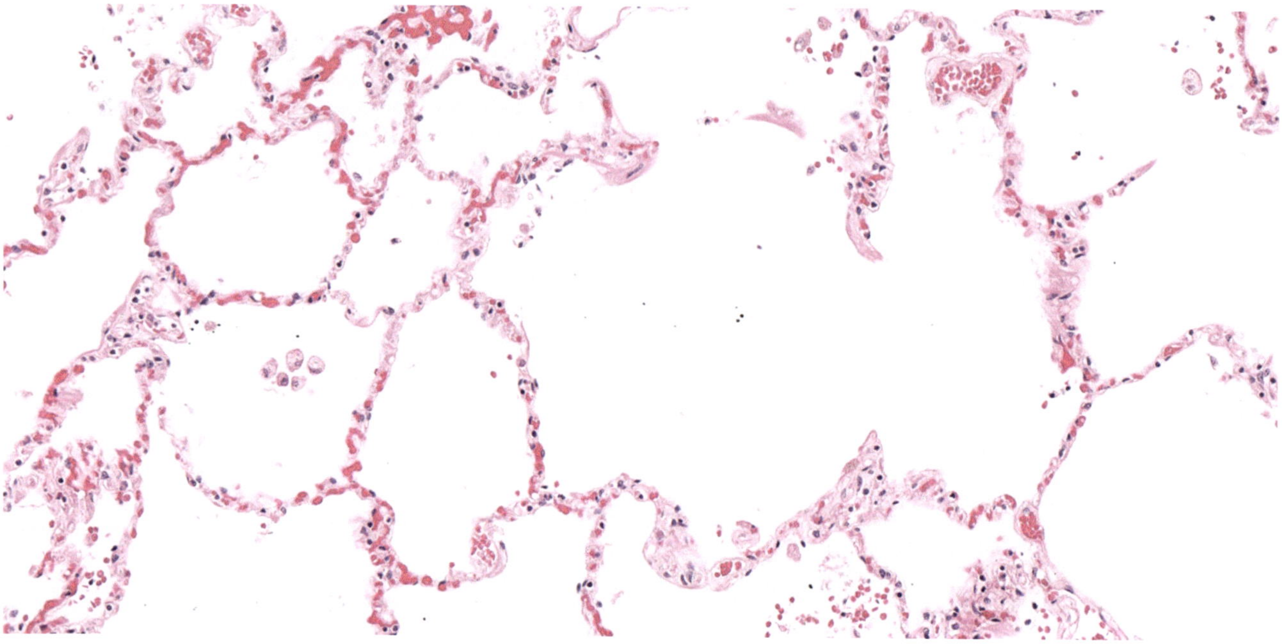

Fig. 14.85 The normal lung has thin alveolar walls with red blood cells visible in alveolar capillaries and inconspicuous pneumocytes lining the alveoli. Within the alveolar space there are resident macrophages

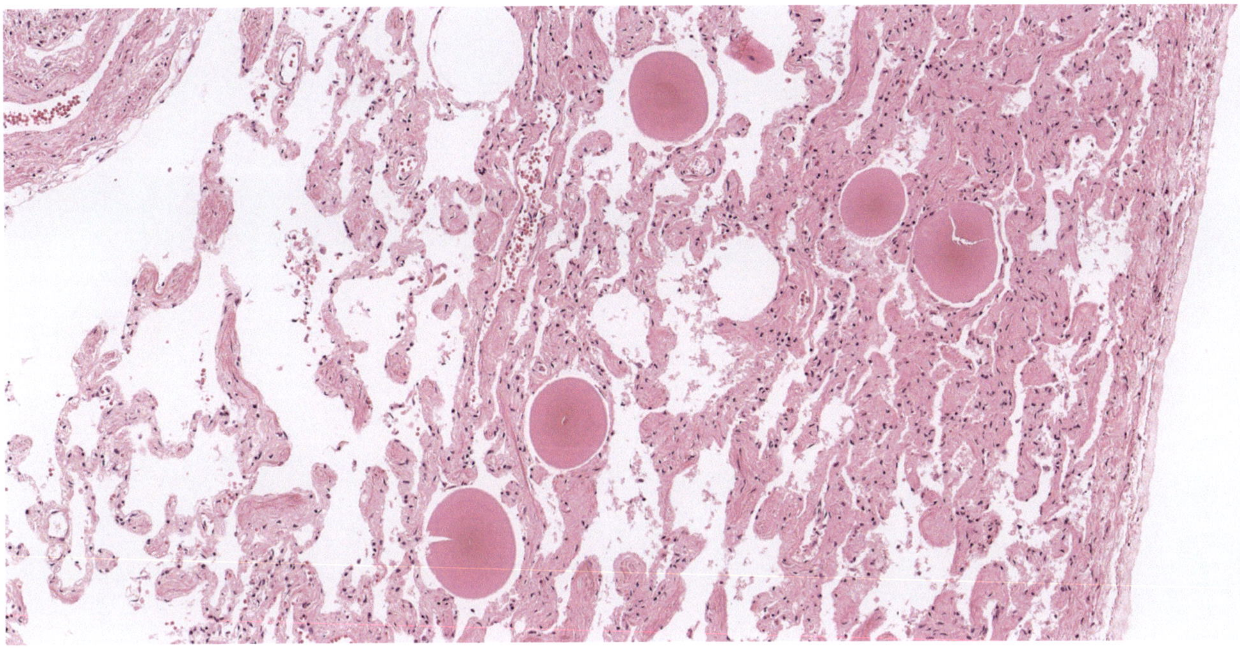

Fig. 14.86 Corpora amylacea may be seen in the lungs. These round eosinophilic concretions are similar in appearance to those seen in the prostate gland. They are a common finding of no pathological significance

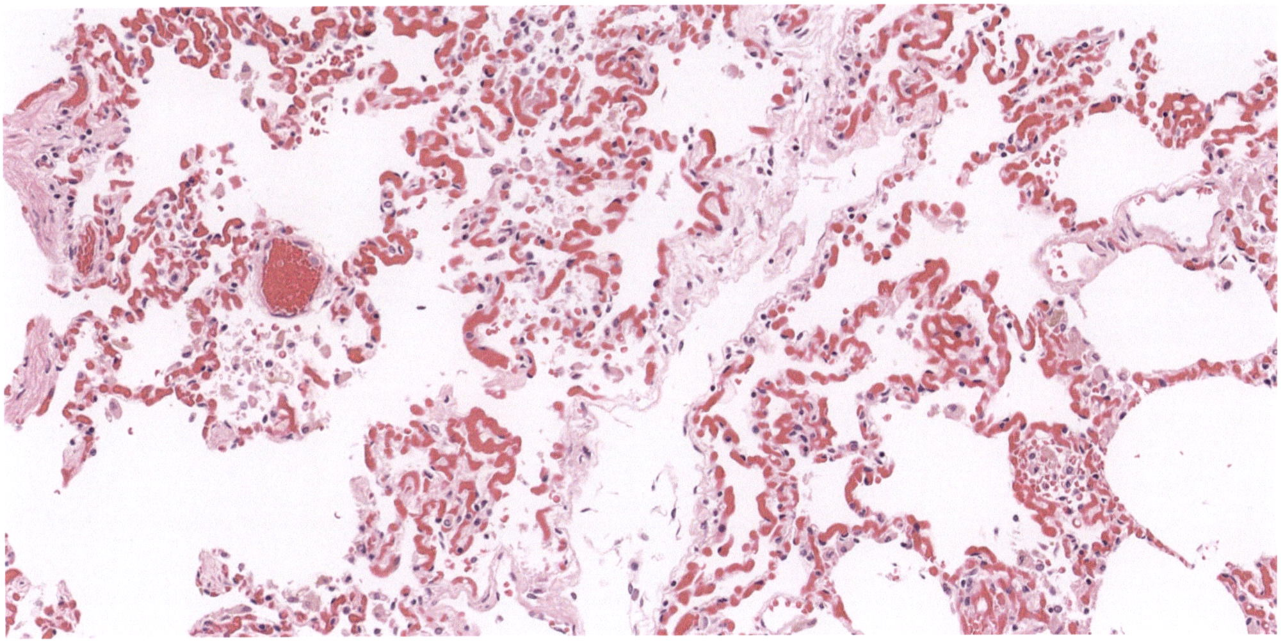

Fig. 14.87 This is also a normal lung section. Congestion of alveolar capillaries is common in the post mortem setting

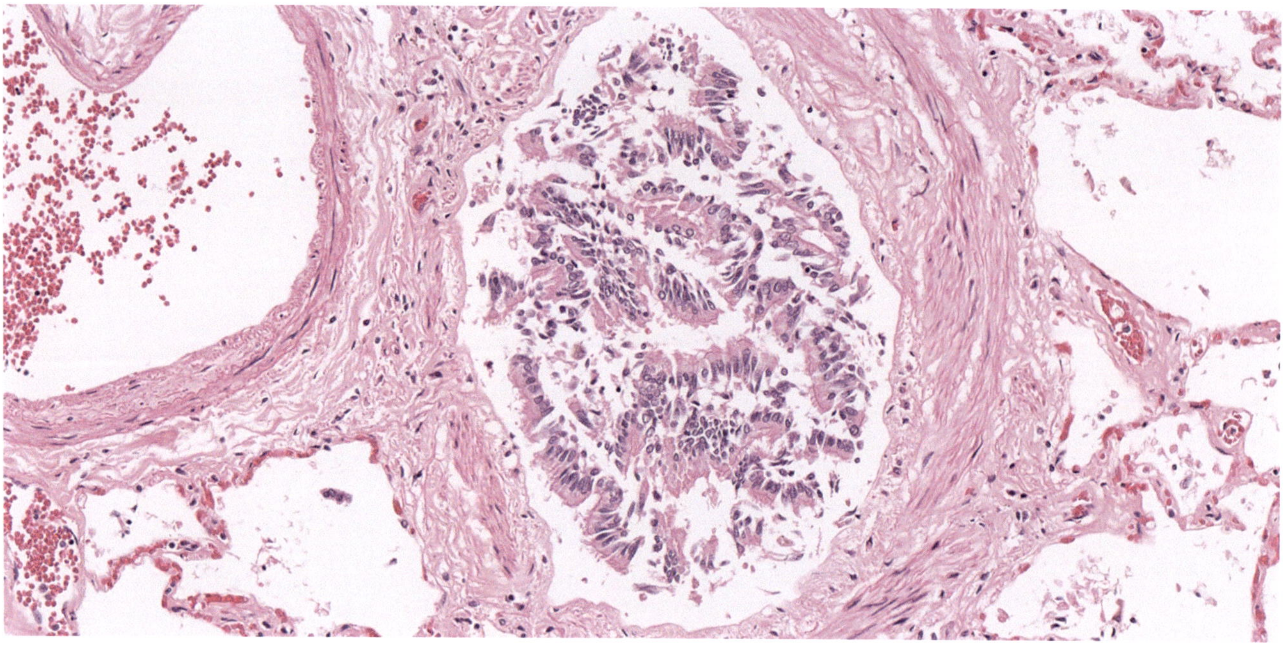

Fig. 14.88 This is a bronchus. Autolysis of the bronchial epithelium is common in the post mortem setting

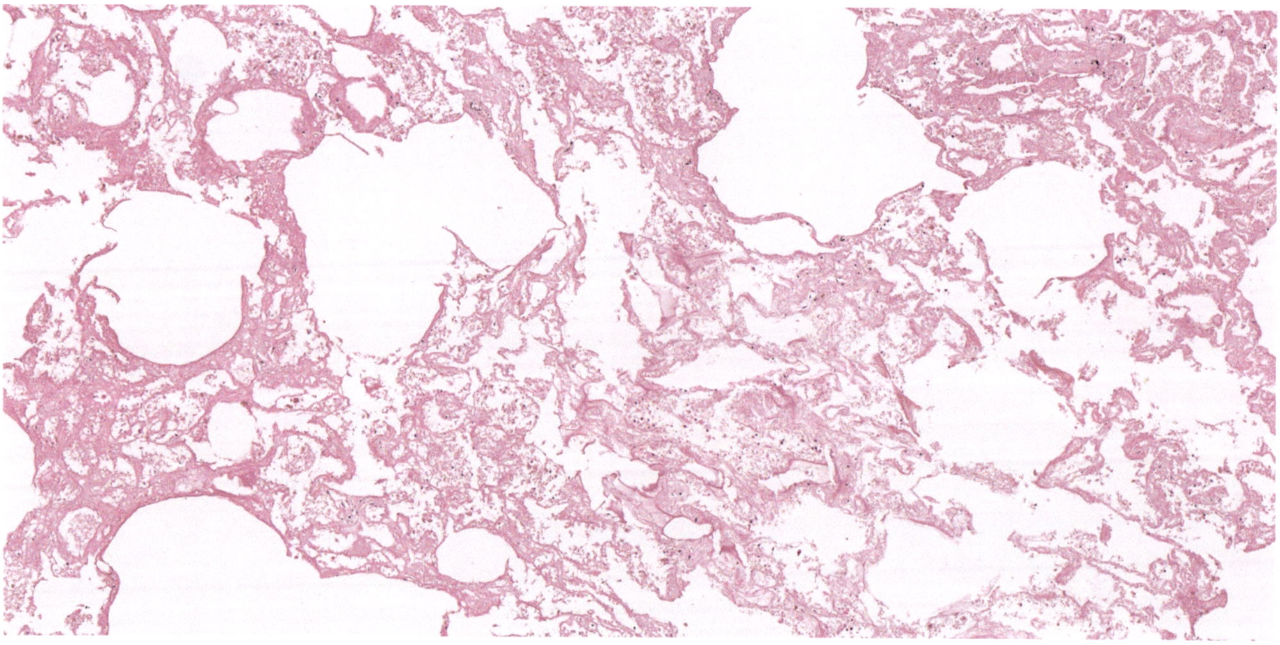

Fig. 14.89 This section of lung is autolysed. Autolysis may hamper interpretation and the pathologist should acknowledge the limits posed by decomposition changes

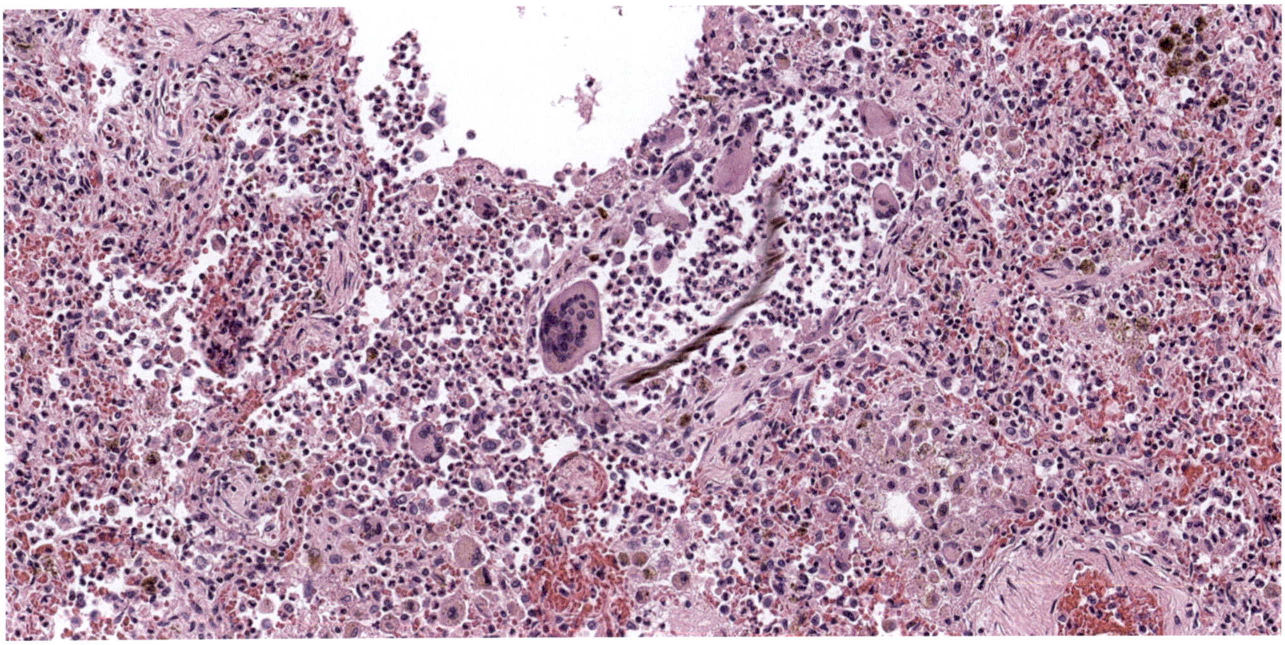

Fig. 14.90 This is a case of aspiration. There is foreign material within the lung, with a giant cell and neutrophil reaction

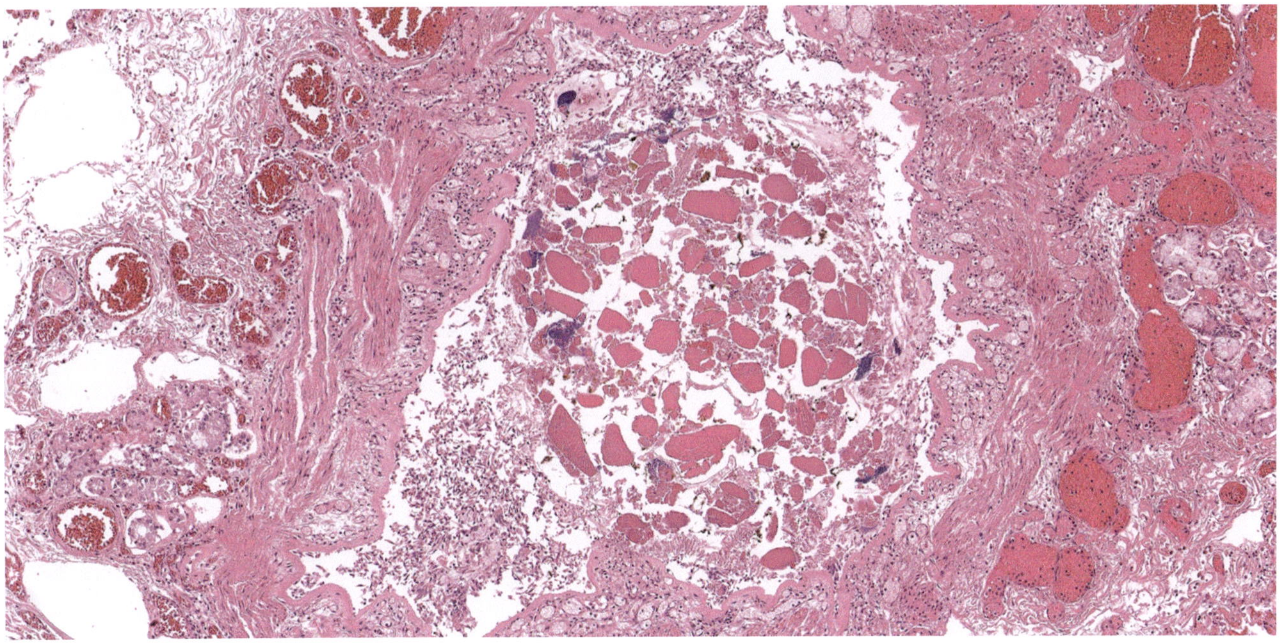

Fig. 14.91 This is another case of aspiration. In this image there are fragments of meat in the bronchus

Pulmonary Oedema

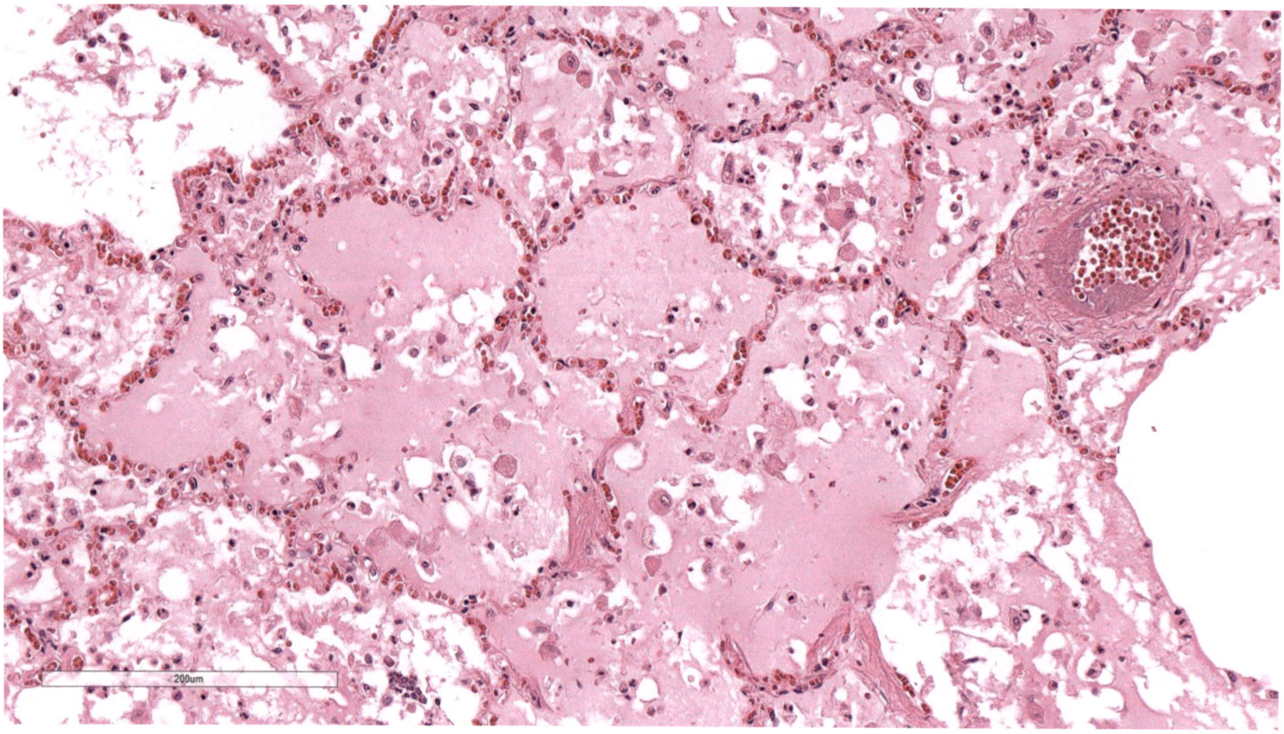

Fig. 14.92 Pulmonary oedema is commonly seen in many causes of sudden death. It is associated with sudden cardiac death or congestive cardiac failure, but also commonly seen in pulmonary infections, neurological deaths and drug and alcohol causes of death. Microscopically there is bland proteinaceous fluid within alveoli

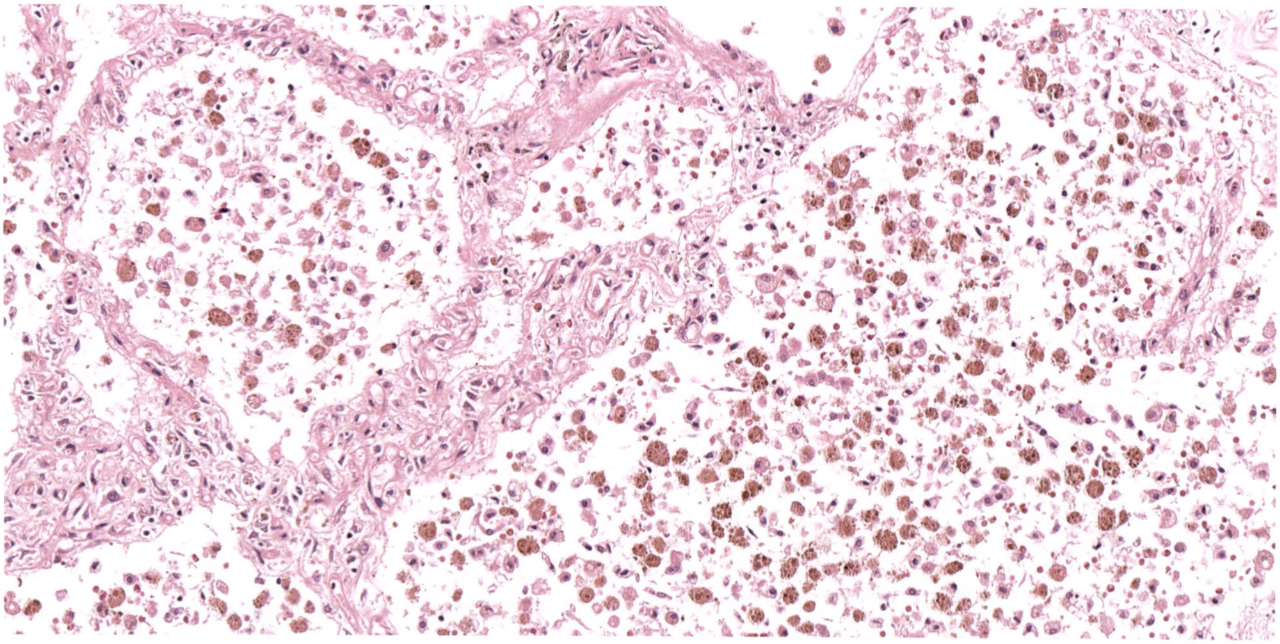

Fig. 14.93 This image shows so-called "heart failure cells". Pigmented alveolar macrophages may be seen within alveolar spaces in congestive cardiac failure. Contrast this appearance with the pigmentation of macrophages seen in cigarette smoking in Fig. 14.120

Infections

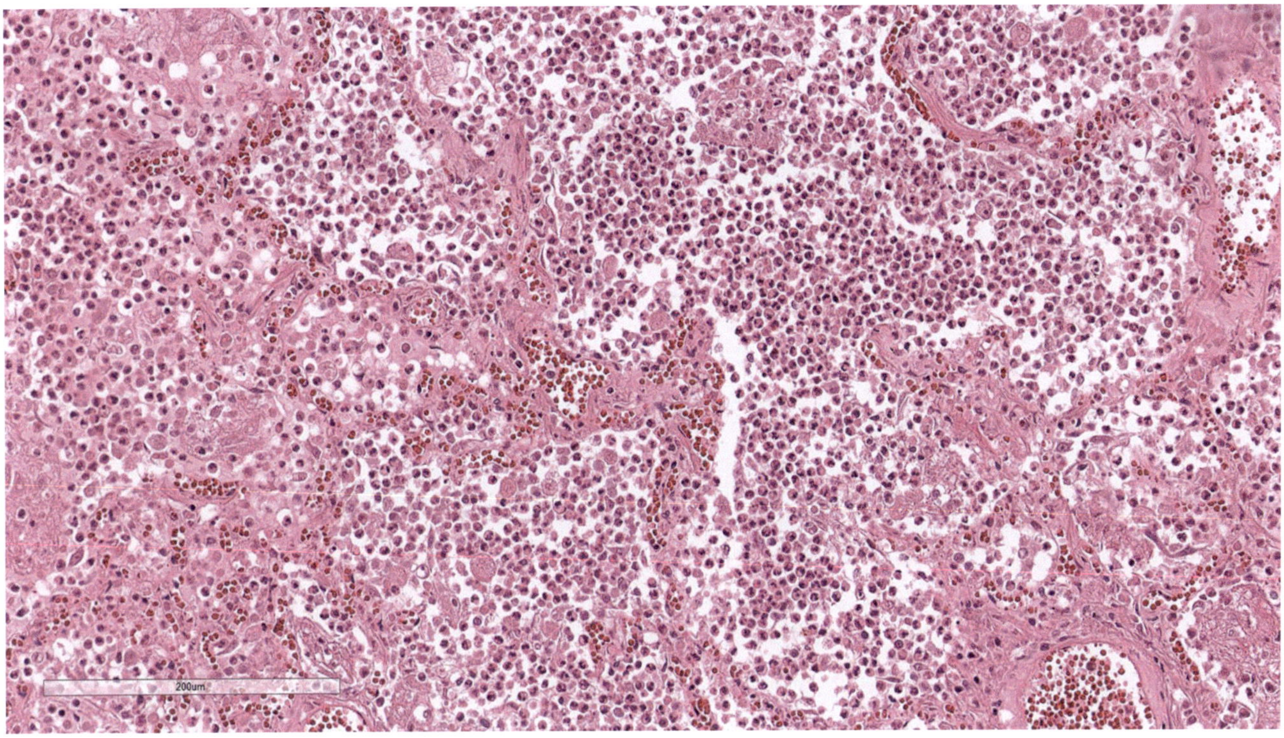

Fig. 14.94 Bronchopneumonia is a common cause of death. It may be evident with the naked eye. However it is well established that pneumonia is under-recognised macroscopically and may be identified on histology, where neutrophils are identified, filling alveoli, as shown in this image. Bronchopneumonia is a common end point of many different pathologies, including natural and unnatural pathology, for example chronic obstructive pulmonary disease, advanced cancers, trauma or respiratory depressant drugs. The underlying cause of the pneumonia should be considered when formulating the cause of death

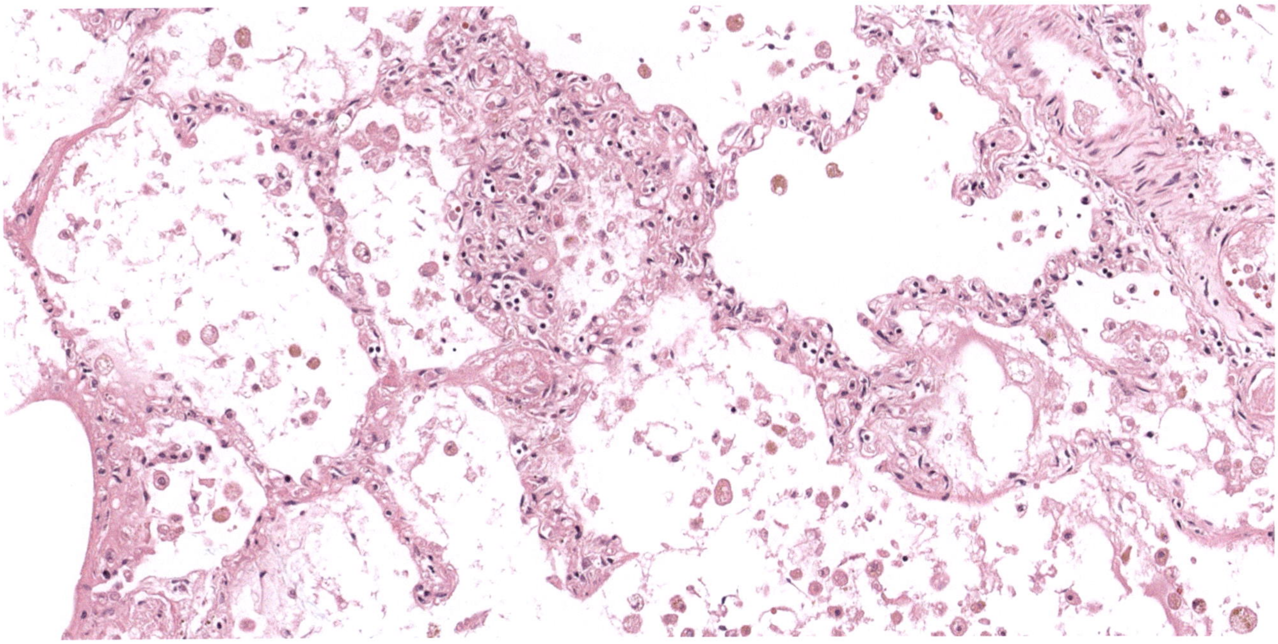

Fig. 14.95 Viral infections may involve the upper respiratory tract or the lower respiratory tract and can be a cause of death. In this case of influenza A infection, the lungs show thickened alveolar walls with lymphocytic infiltrate

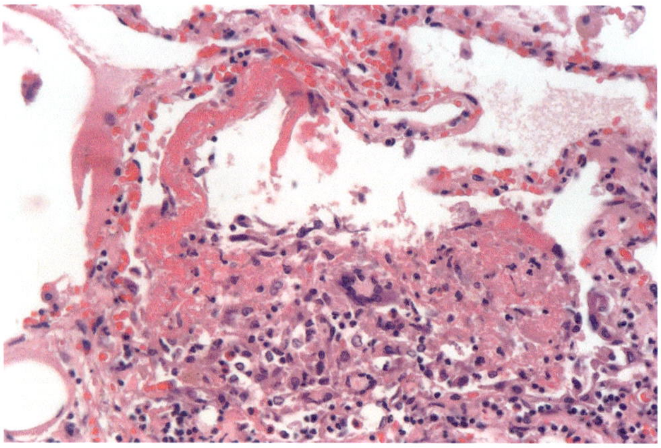

Fig. 14.96 This is a case of rhinovirus infection involving the lungs. There is thickening of the interstitium with lymphocytes and giant cells. Fibrin is seen within the alveoli

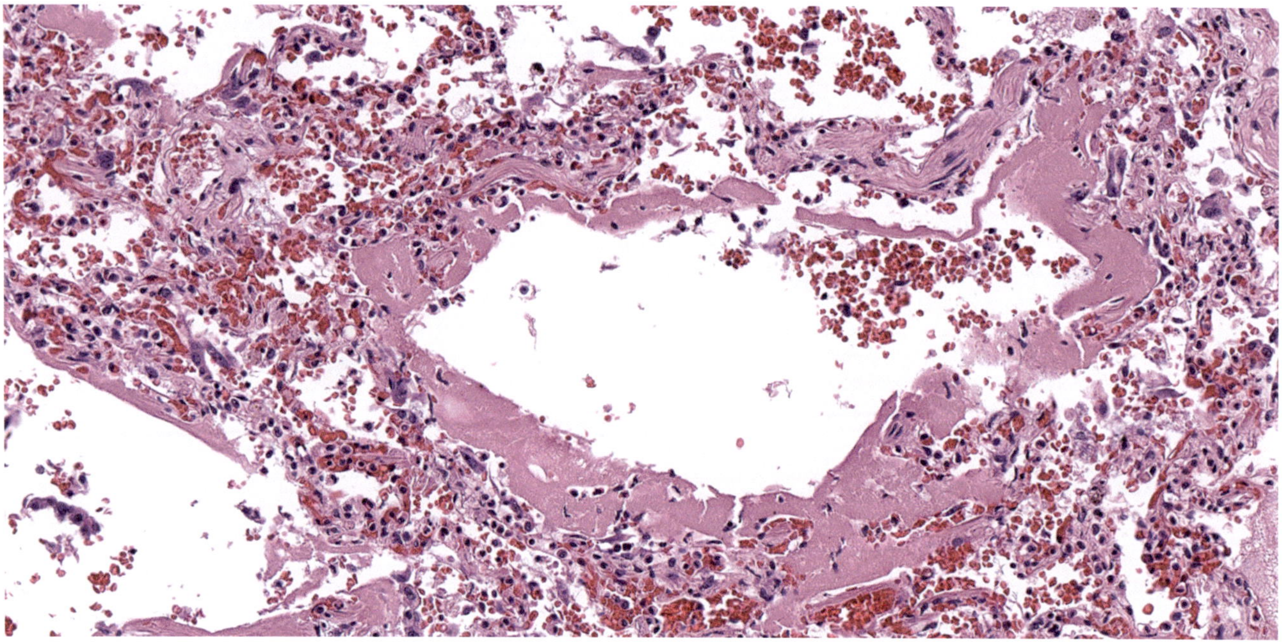

Fig. 14.97 This is a case of COVID-19 (SARS-CoV-2 infection). Histology of the lung shows thickening of the interstitium with lymphocyte infiltrate, exudative phase of diffuse alveolar damage with fibrin membranes, type 2 pneumocyte hyperplasia and shedding. It should be noted that the histological features of viral pneumonitis are not specific for the virus involved. The viral agent must be confirmed by PCR testing

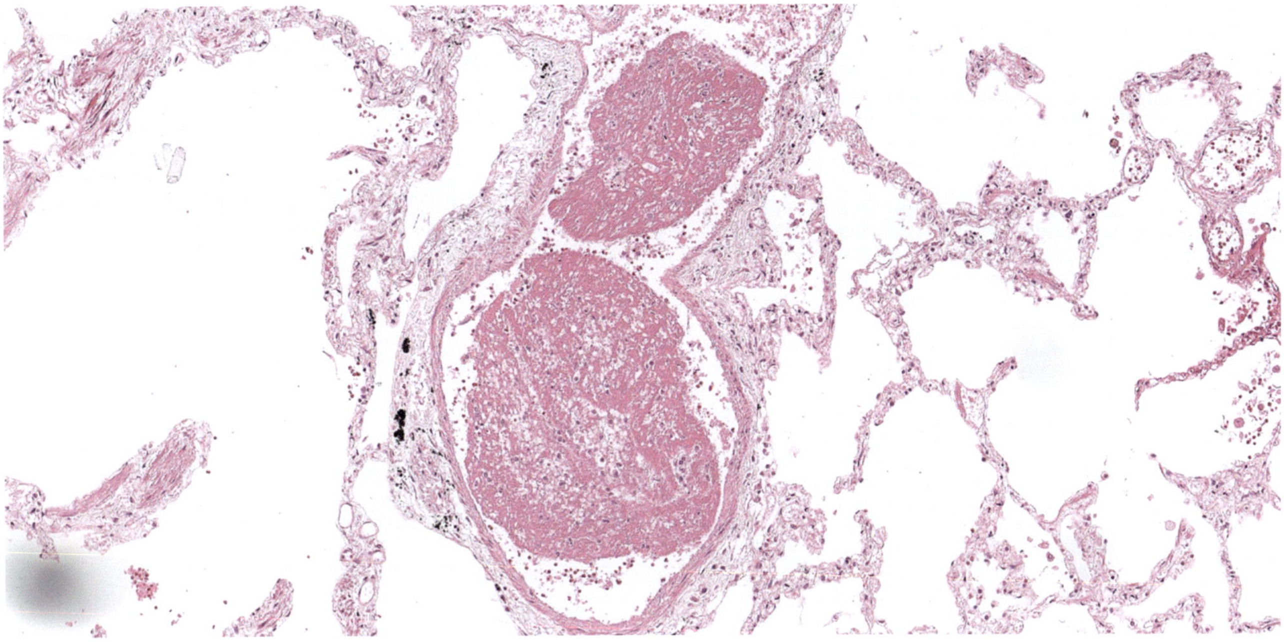

Fig. 14.98 COVID-19 can also be associated with thrombosis. In this case there are thrombi in a pulmonary artery. Thrombosis is also commonly seen associated with diffuse alveolar damage

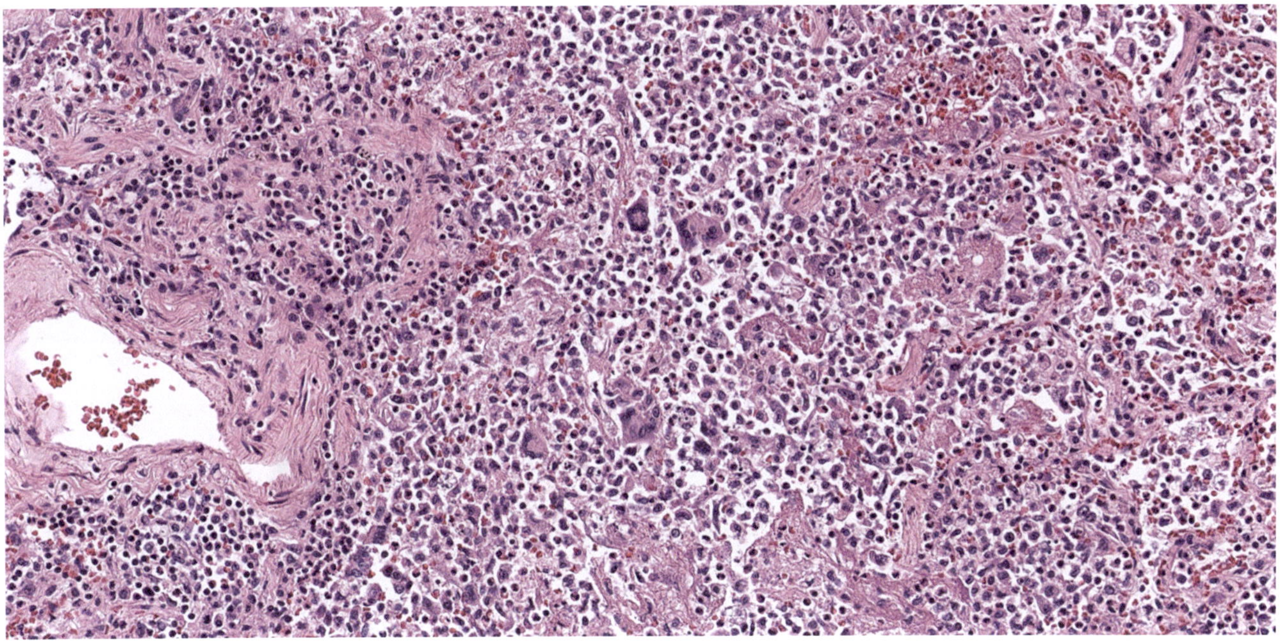

Fig. 14.99 This is a giant cell pneumonia caused by measles infection associated with a local measles outbreak

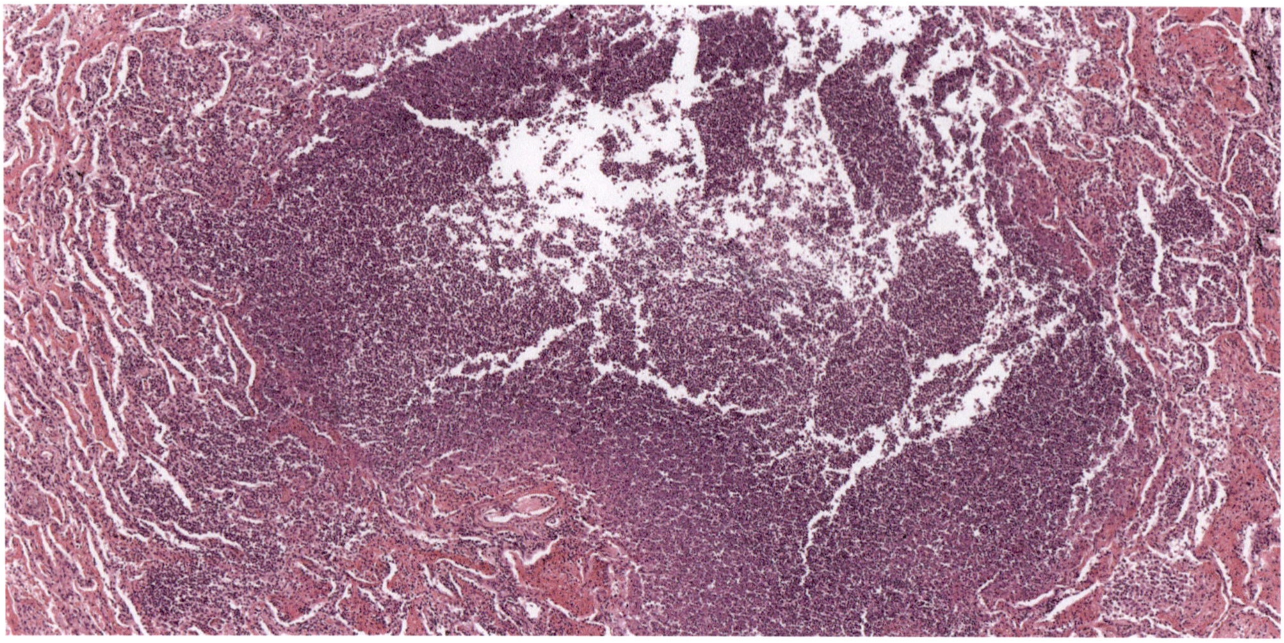

Fig. 14.100 This is a large abscess in the lung. There are several bacterial infections which are commonly associated with abscess formation

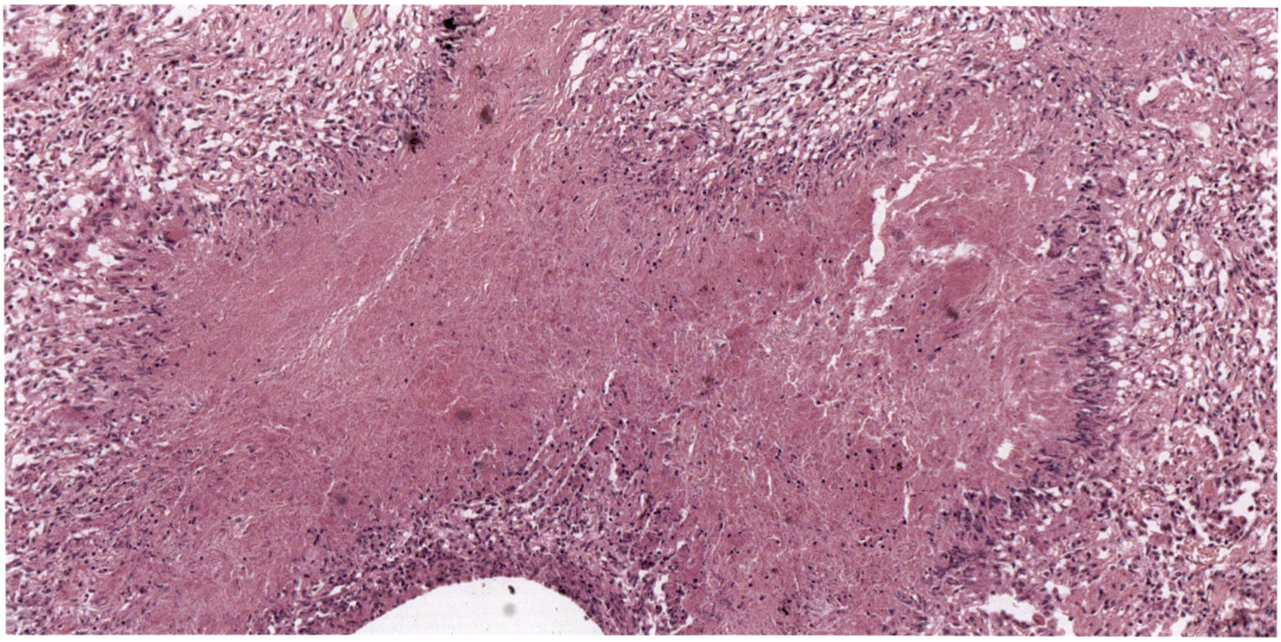

Fig. 14.101 In pulmonary tuberculosis, necrotising granulomatous inflammation is seen. Ziehl-Neelsen (ZN) staining can identify the causative organisms, although microbiological culture is much more sensitive. A sample of fresh lung tissue should be sent to microbiology for culture

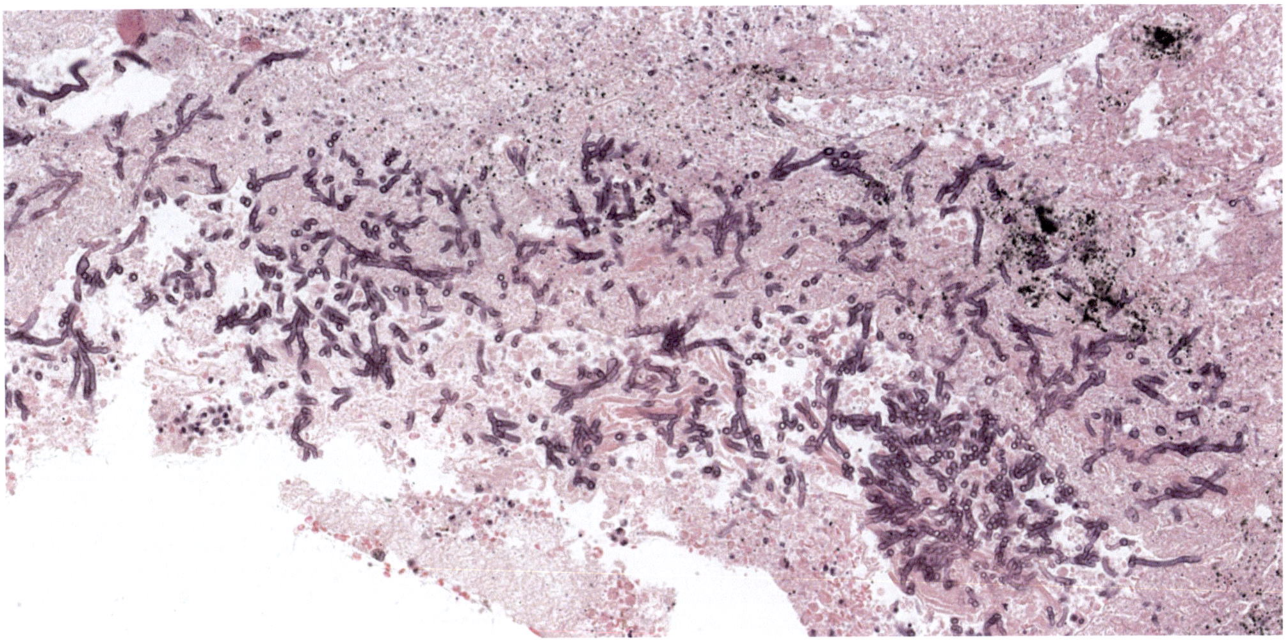

Fig. 14.102 Fungal infections can be established in the lungs or fungi can colonise pre-existing cavities in the lungs. Fungal overgrowth can also be seen as a post mortem artefact so it is important to look for a vital reaction to the organism. Bear in mind that in immunodeficiency the immune response may be limited and opportunistic fungal infections are common in this setting

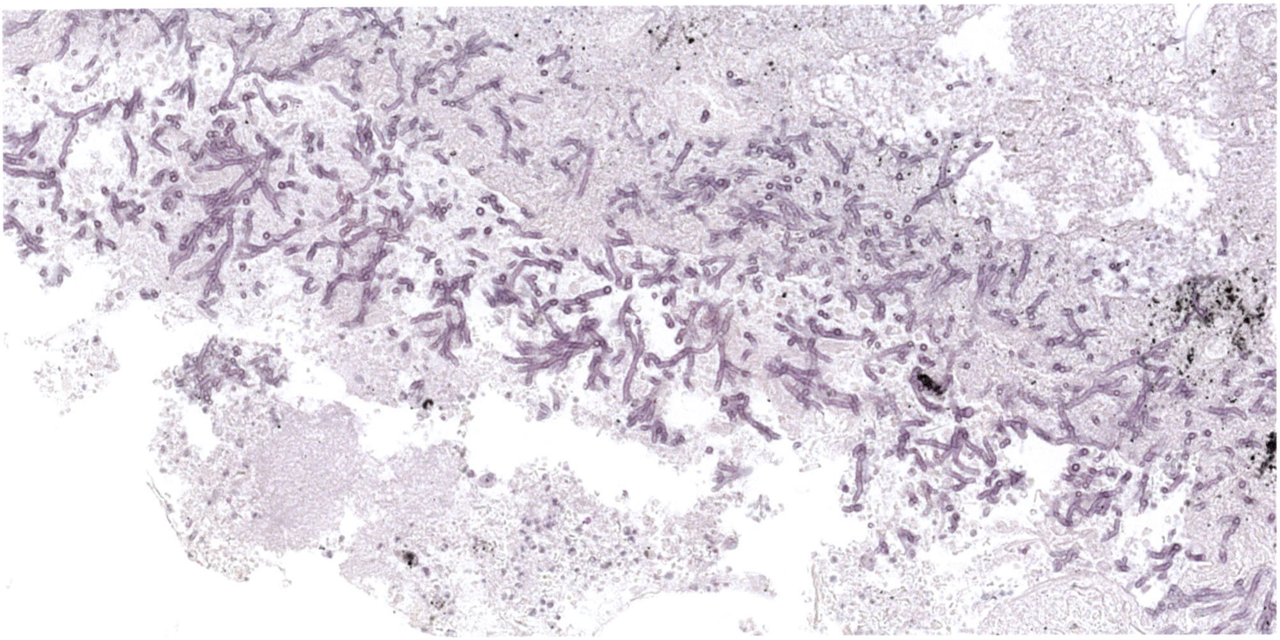

Fig. 14.103 Periodic acid-Schiff-diastase (DPAS) staining highlights the fungal organisms in this fungal pneumonia

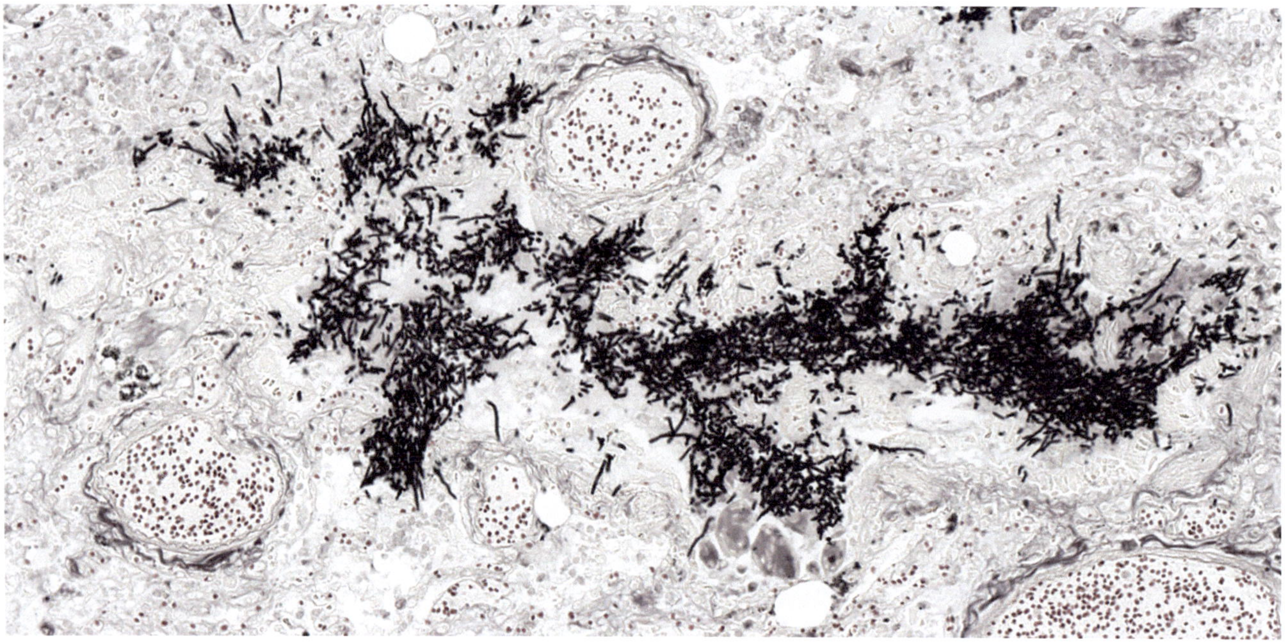

Fig. 14.104 Grocott staining highlights the fungal organisms in this further case of fungal pneumonia

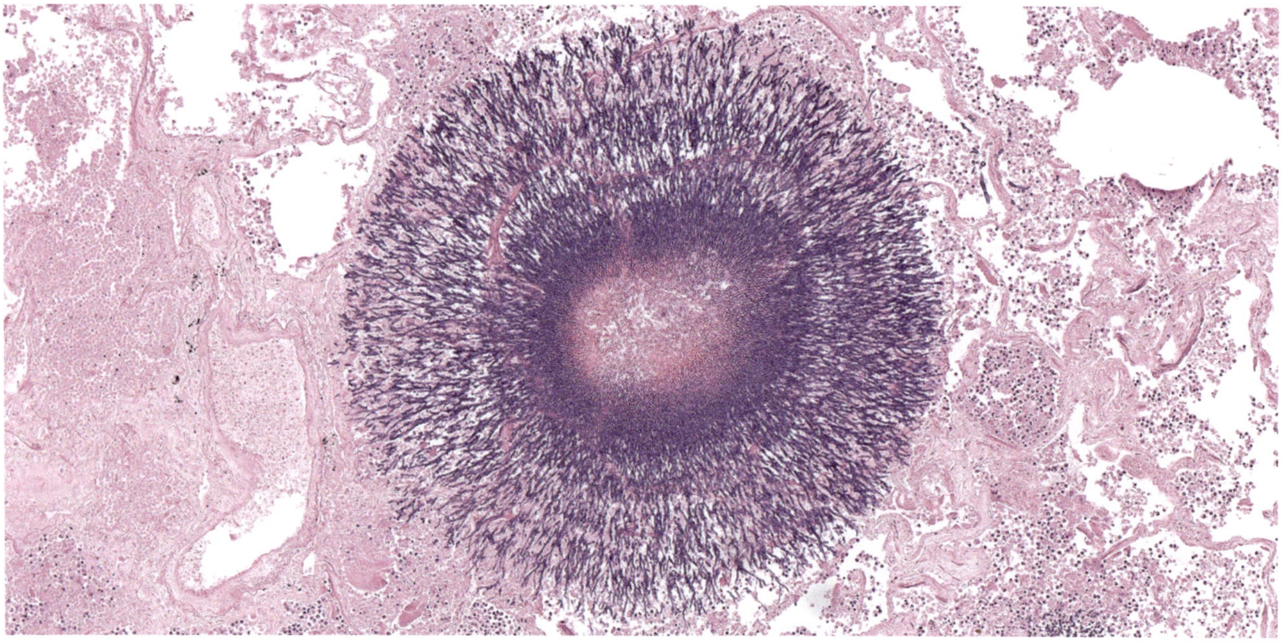

Fig. 14.105 This is pulmonary aspergillosis in a person with advanced pulmonary fibrosis. The fungal organisms are clearly evident on H&E staining. Morphological study and precise species identification should be confirmed by the microbiology department

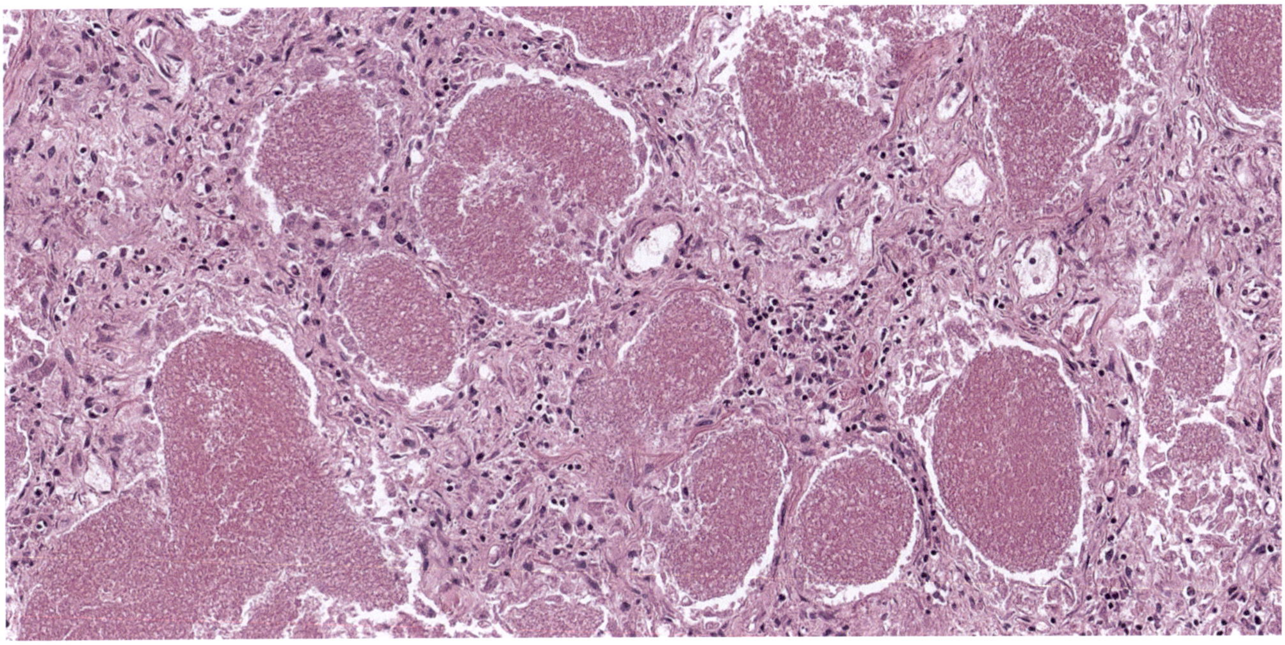

Fig. 14.106 This is an example of pneumocystis infection. Pneumocystis infection is typically associated with immunodeficiency, particularly HIV/AIDS. Clusters of organisms can be seen filling the alveoli

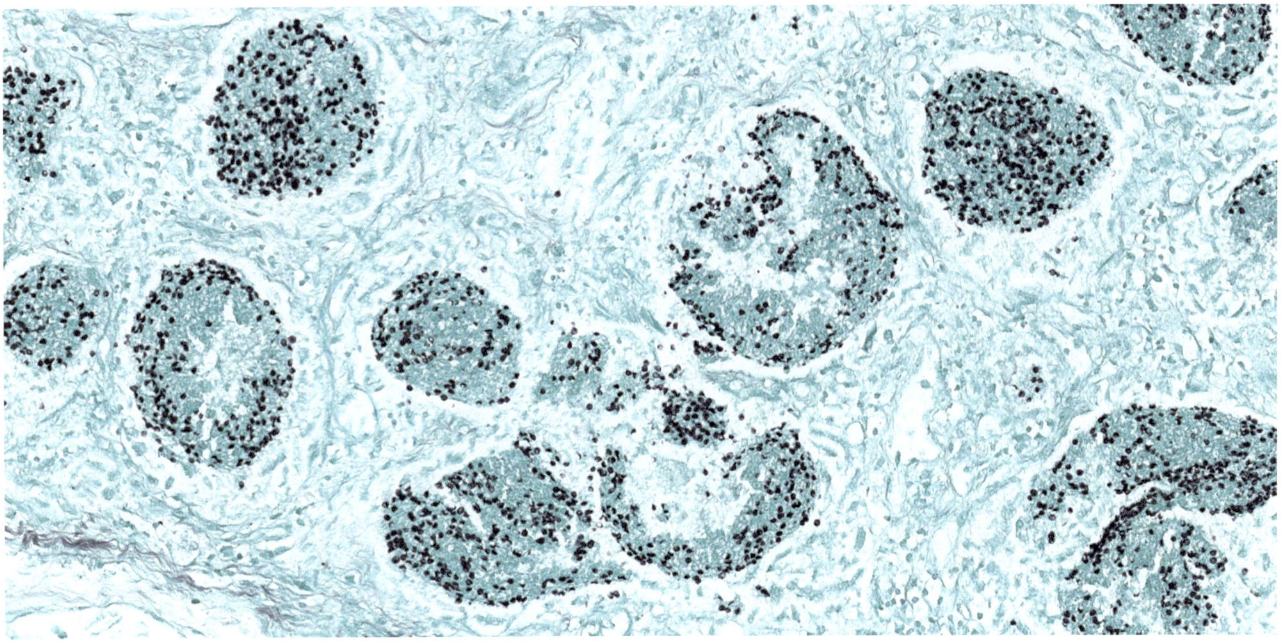

Fig. 14.107 This Grocott stain highlights the pneumocystis organisms from Fig. 14.106

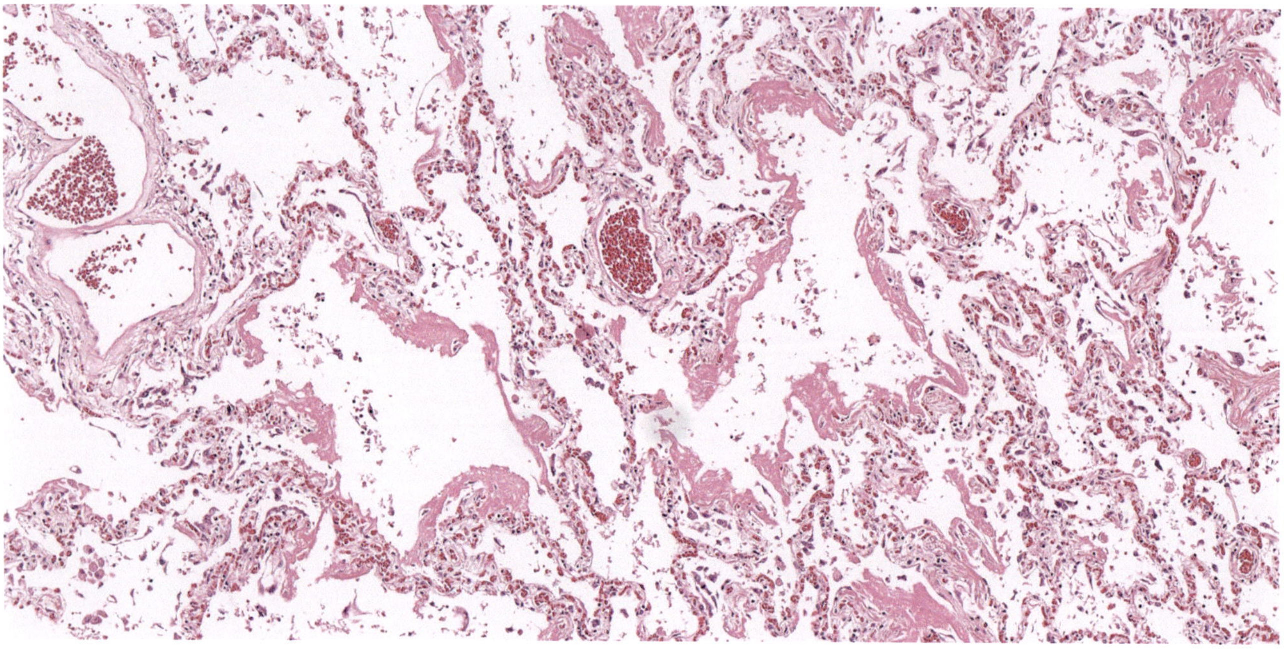

Fig. 14.108 There are many causes of diffuse alveolar damage (DAD). The most common cause is infections. There are several histological patterns which may be seen. An example of exudative phase of DAD is shown here. This image shows fibrin membrane formation lining alveolar walls, with type 2 pneumocyte hypertrophy and shedding

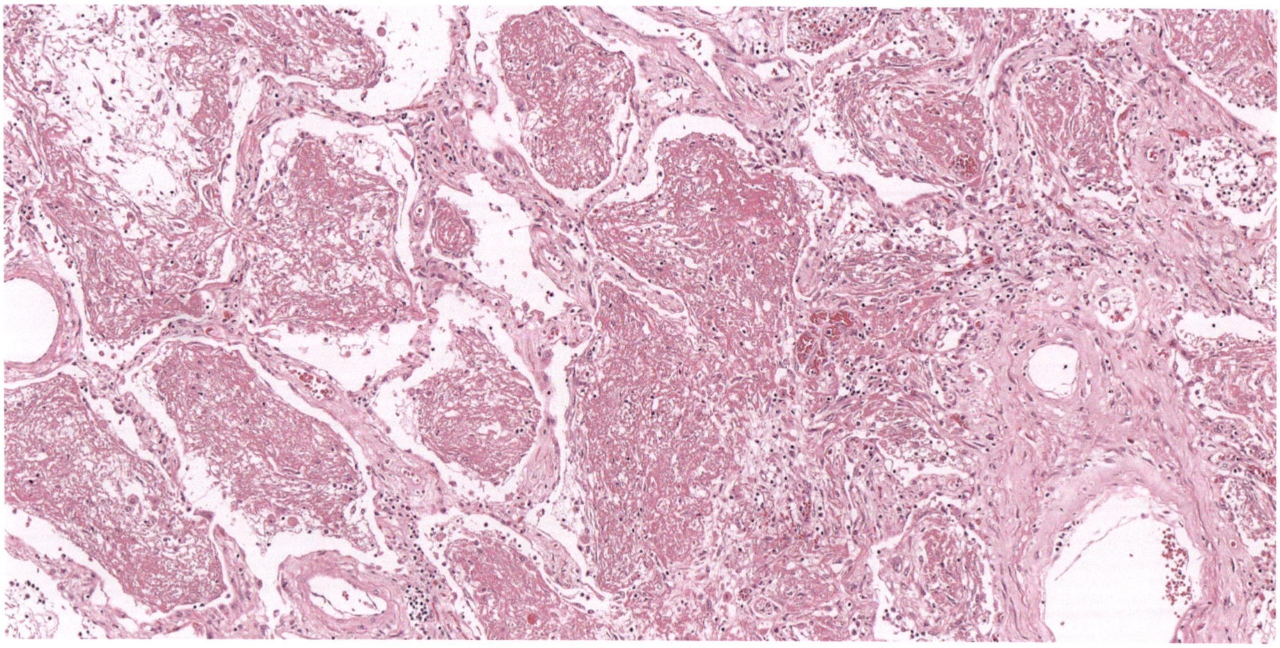

Fig. 14.109 This is another example of diffuse alveolar damage exudative phase with a different histological pattern. In this image there are balls of fibrin filling alveoli. This pattern has been termed acute fibrinous organising pneumonia (AFOP)

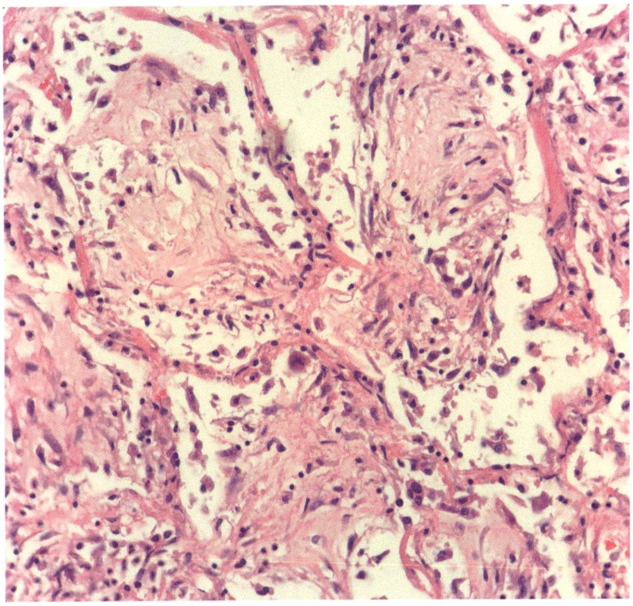

Fig. 14.110 Diffuse alveolar damage proliferative/fibrotic phase. This is the resolving phase of diffuse alveolar damage. In this image fibroblast clumps are seen filling the alveoli

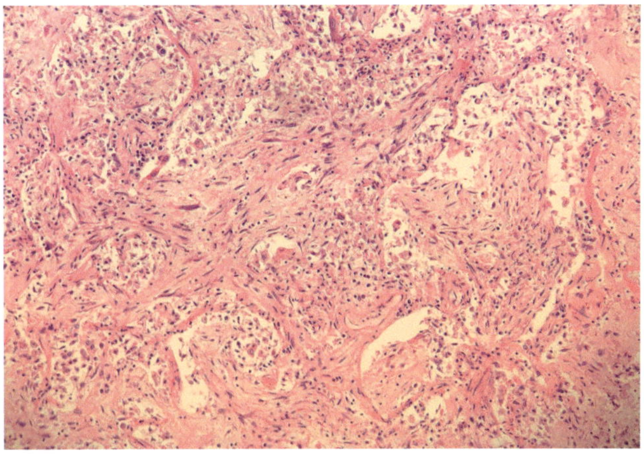

Fig. 14.111 This image shows another example of diffuse alveolar damage proliferative/fibrotic phase. There is fibroblast proliferation within alveoli and in the interstitium

Thromboembolism and Other Embolism

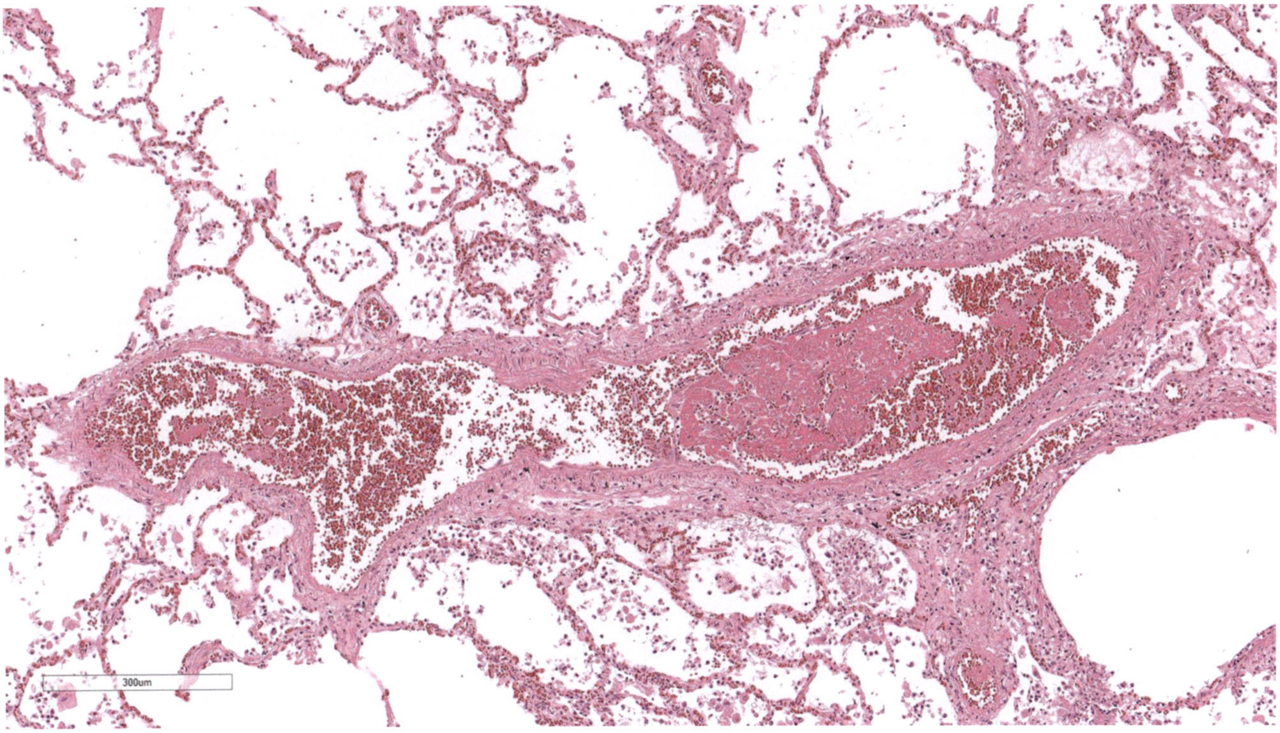

Fig. 14.112 There is a thromboembolus within a pulmonary artery. Pulmonary thromboembolism (PTE) is a common cause of sudden death. Histological evaluation of pulmonary thromboembolism may be important particularly in the medicolegal setting. However, dating of a PTE is not particularly precise. The earliest changes involve a cellular reaction where the thrombus becomes adherent to the vessel wall (the beginnings of organisation). Haemosiderin may be identified early. Equally it may be helpful to demonstrate a lack of organisation in a fresh thrombus

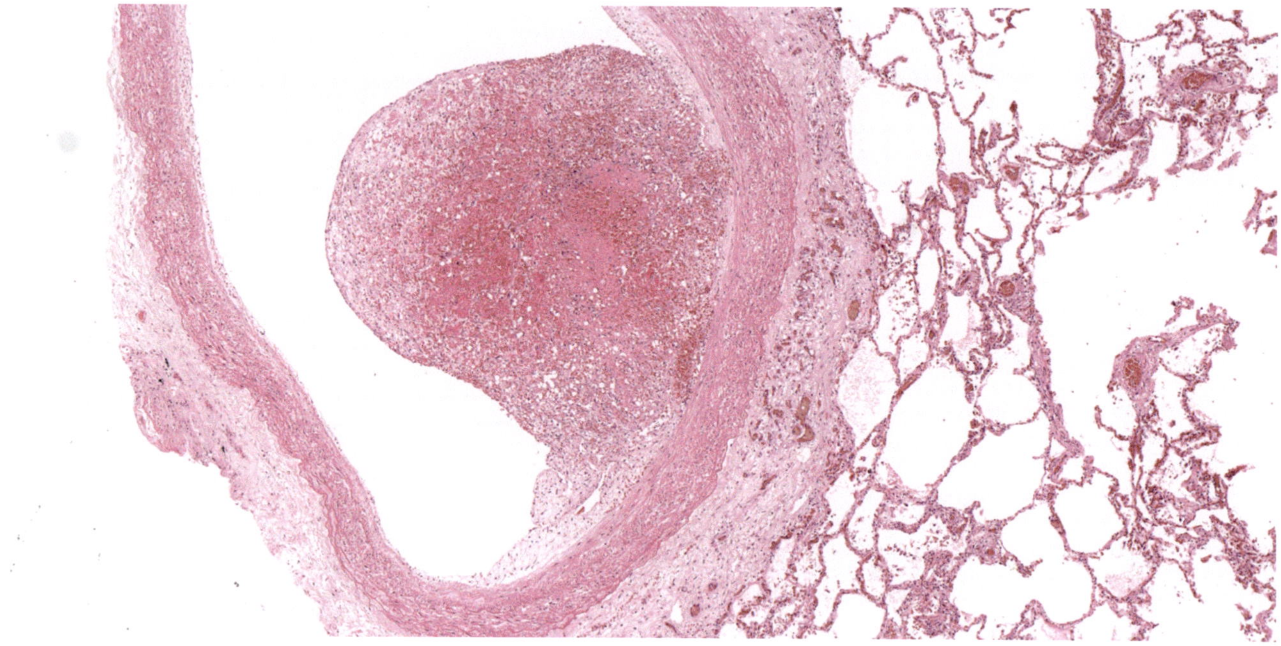

Fig. 14.113 This is an organising pulmonary thromboembolism. There is a cellular reaction at the vessel wall with adherence and early organisation of the thrombus

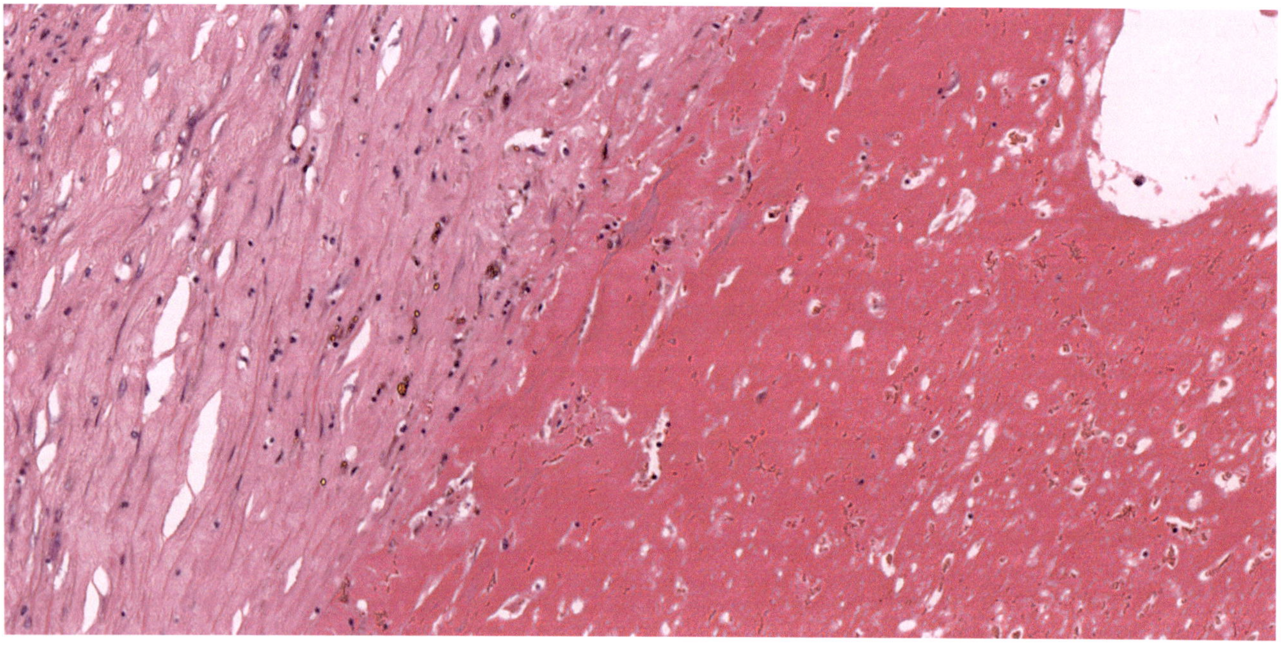

Fig. 14.114 In pulmonary thromboembolism haemosiderin may be seen in the artery wall within the first 24 h. This can be highlighted with Perls' staining for iron

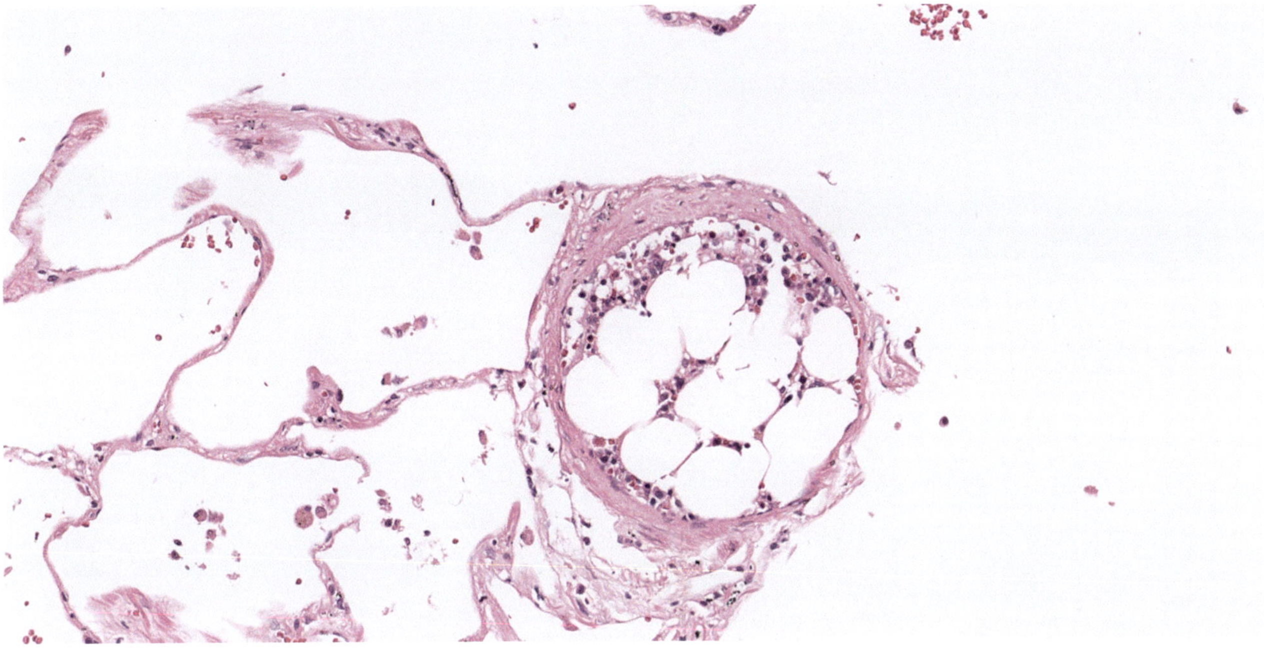

Fig. 14.115 Bone marrow embolism is a common autopsy finding in lung histology following attempts at resuscitation with chest compressions. Adipose tissue and haematopoietic cells are seen within a small artery

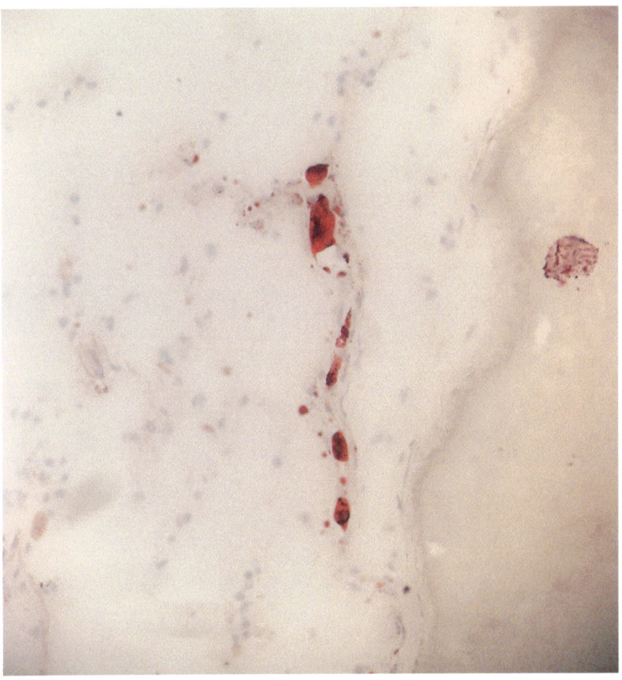

Fig. 14.116 This is an example of fat embolism. The fat stains red with this oil red O stain, which must be performed on fresh tissue by frozen section, not formalin fixed paraffin embedded tissue. There are fine fragments of fat which may occlude the alveolar capillaries and cause fat embolism syndrome. Fat embolism syndrome can follow traumatic injuries to the bones or soft tissue and presents with cardiovascular collapse or neurological symptoms of confusion, headache or seizures. Other autopsy findings can include a petechial skin rash and petechial haemorrhages in the brain

Asthma

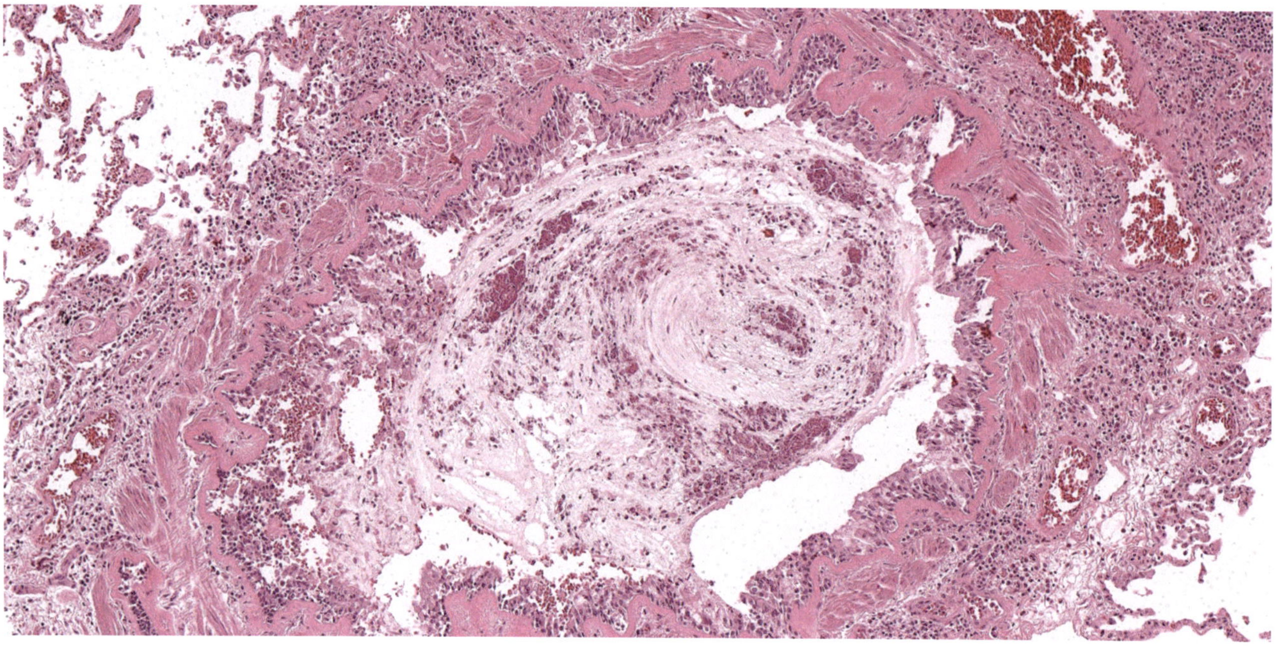

Fig. 14.117 Acute asthma may be a cause of sudden death. The histological features seen here include mucus plugging of the airway, marked thickening of the bronchial epithelial basement membrane, and eosinophil-rich inflammation around the bronchus

Emphysema

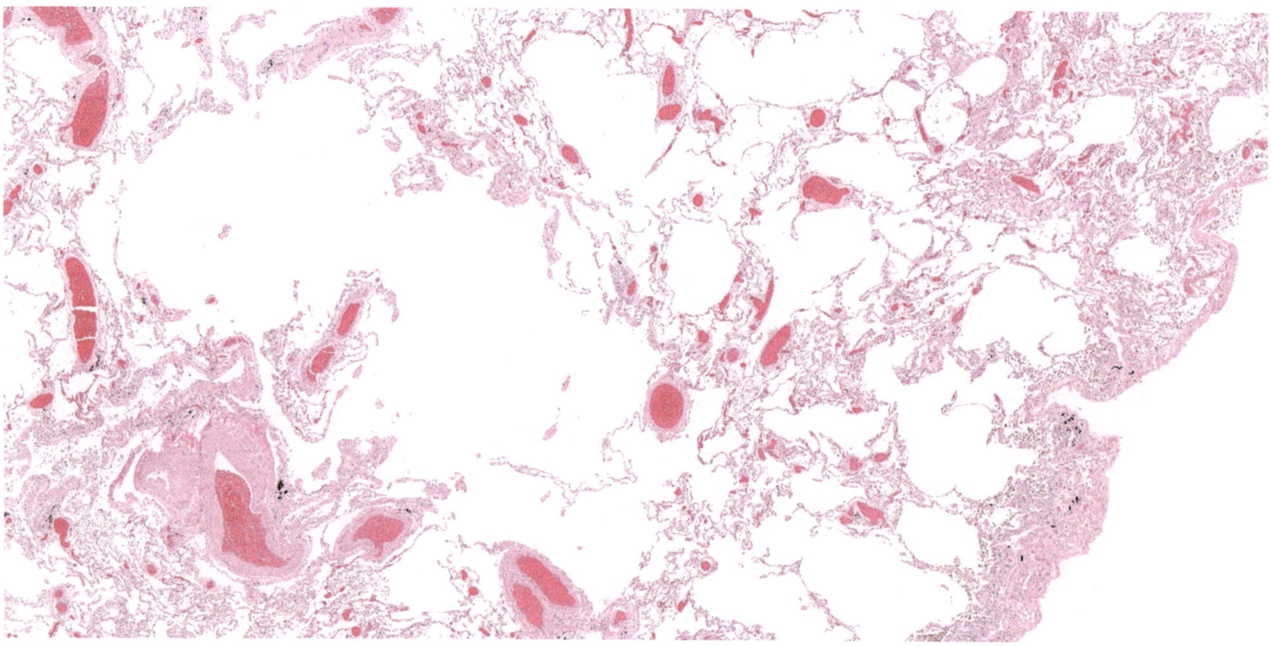

Fig. 14.118 Emphysema is best appreciated with the naked eye. Post mortem artefacts in the lung histology may cause difficulty in assessing true airspace widening due to emphysema

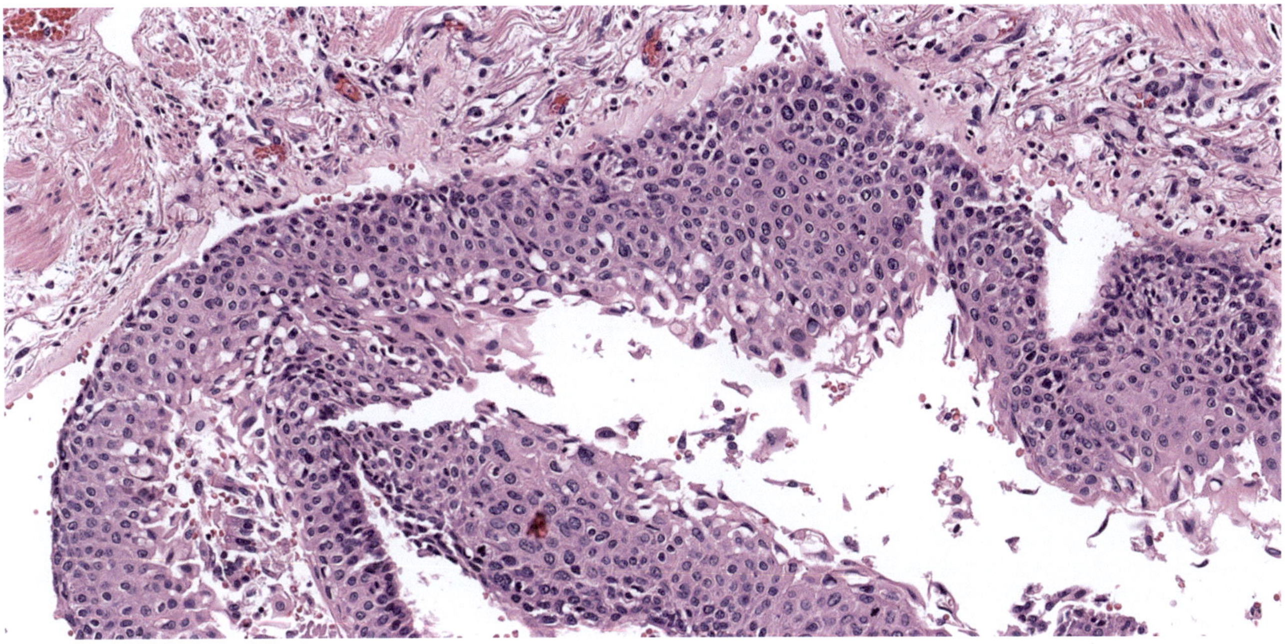

Fig. 14.119 Other histological changes in the lungs associated with cigarette smoking include squamous metaplasia in the trachea and bronchus as seen in this image

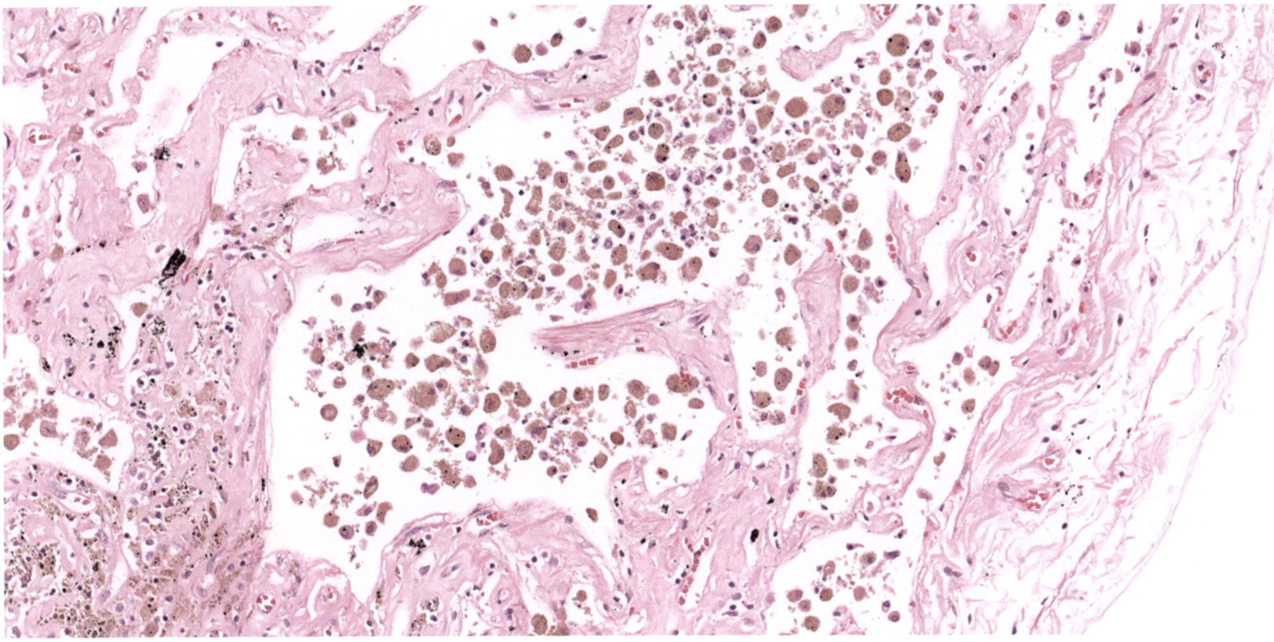

Fig. 14.120 In cigarette smoking it is common to see pigmented macrophages within the alveoli, with black and brown pigment

Sarcoidosis

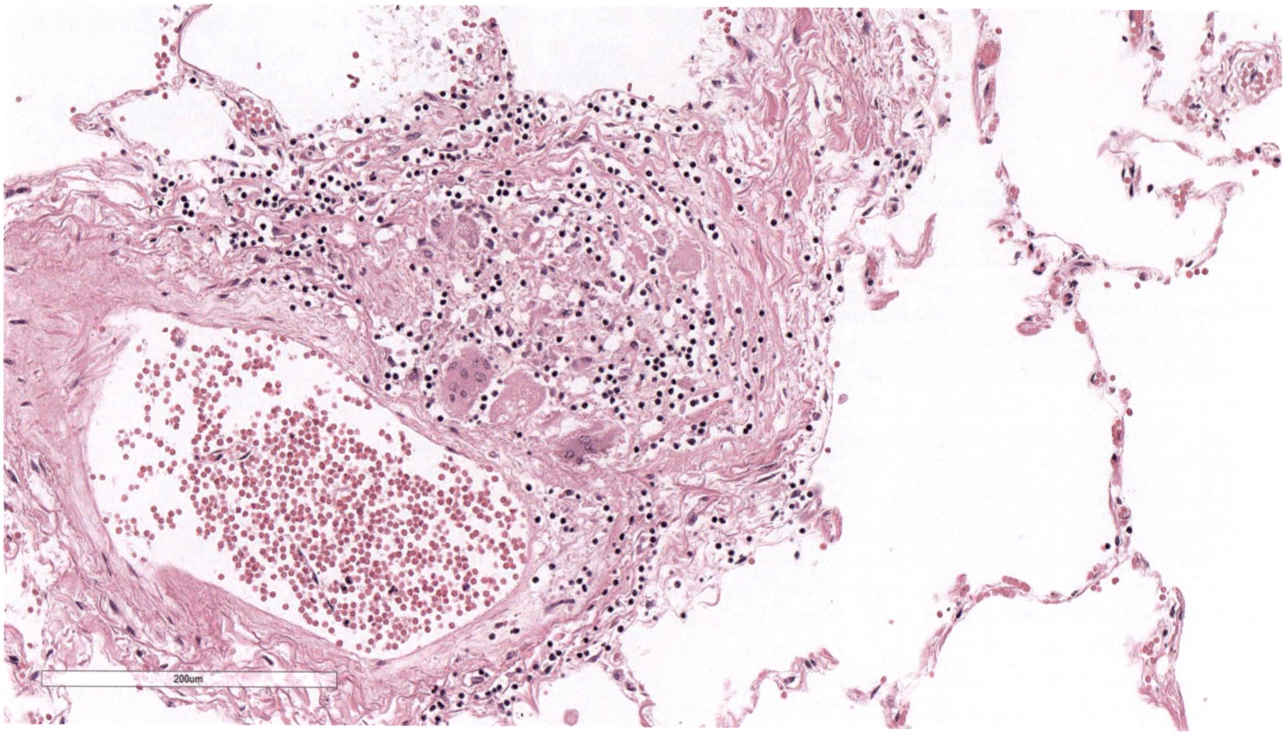

Fig. 14.121 In this example of pulmonary sarcoidosis there is non-necrotising granulomatous inflammation, in a bronchocentric arrangement. Sarcoidosis may be associated with lung infections, and cardiac involvement may be a cause of sudden cardiac death

Amyloid

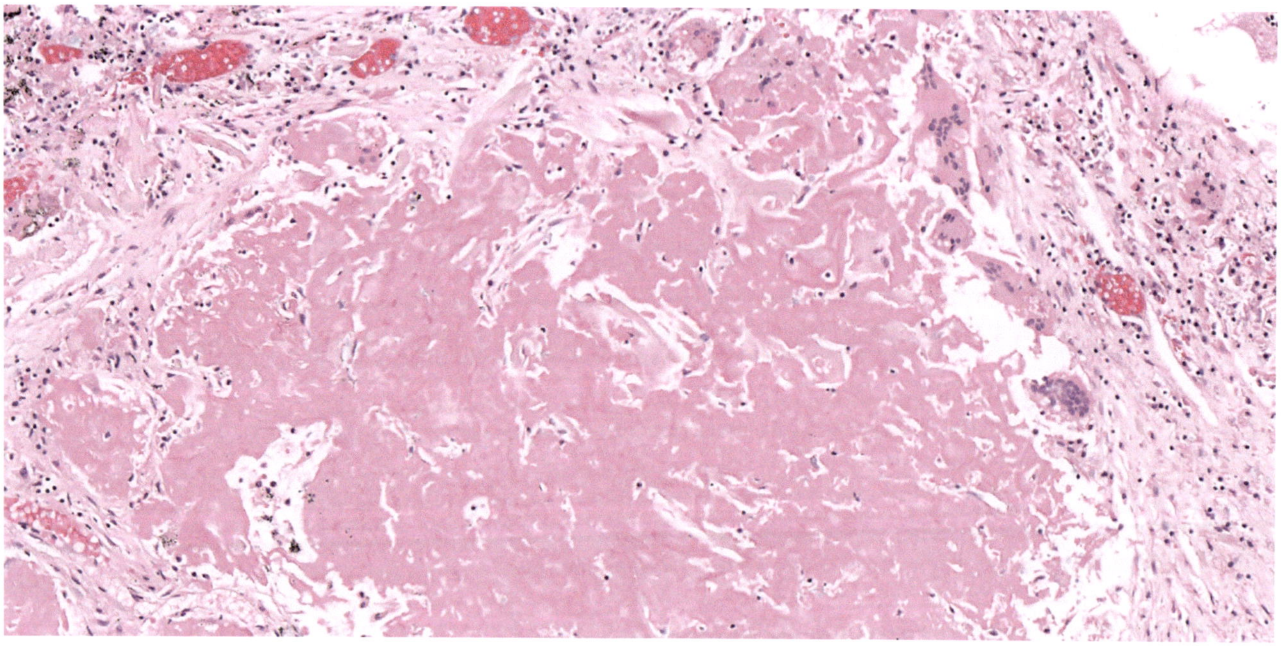

Fig. 14.122 Nodular pulmonary amyloid may cause lung masses but is not typically associated with systemic amyloidosis. Deposits of bland eosinophilic material are surrounded by multinucleated giant cells, which are a good diagnostic feature of this condition

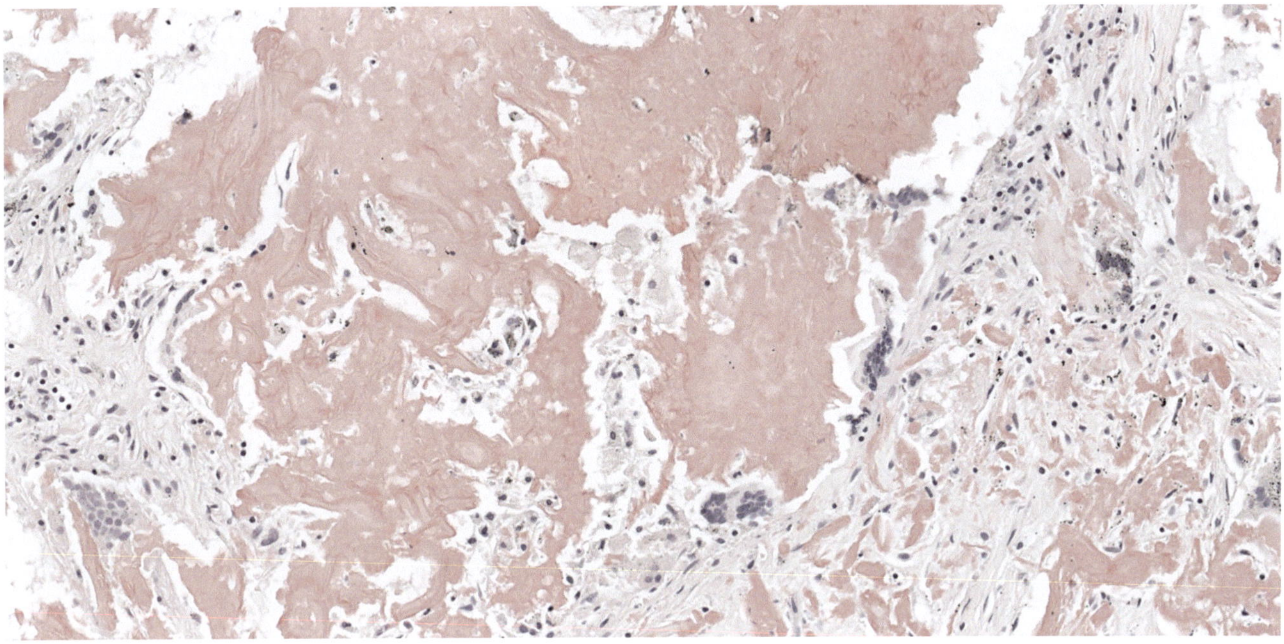

Fig. 14.123 This is Congo red staining of a case of nodular pulmonary amyloid

Pulmonary Fibrosis

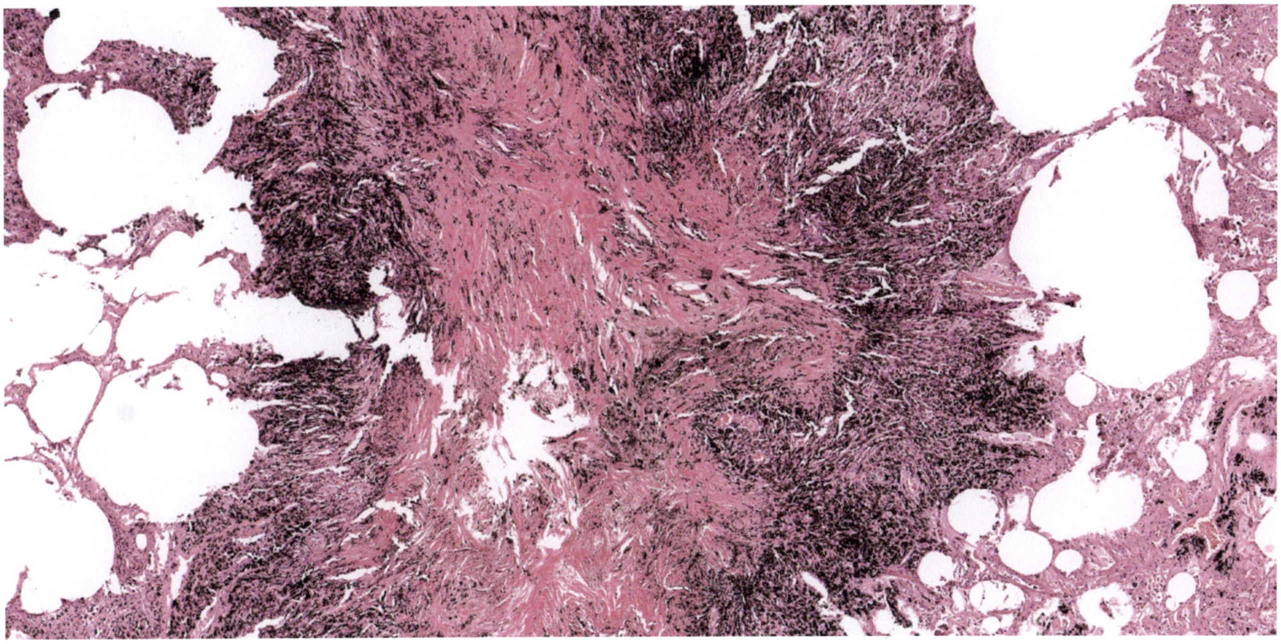

Fig. 14.124 Coal worker's pneumoconiosis (CWP) is mainly a macroscopic diagnosis. The advanced changes of progressive massive fibrosis, once common in mining areas, are rarely seen in the UK, but coal nodules and emphysema are still encountered in areas with high prevalence of coal mining. In this case there were multiple palpable coal nodules throughout the lungs. Histologically these are nodules of fibrosis surrounded by heavy coal dust deposition

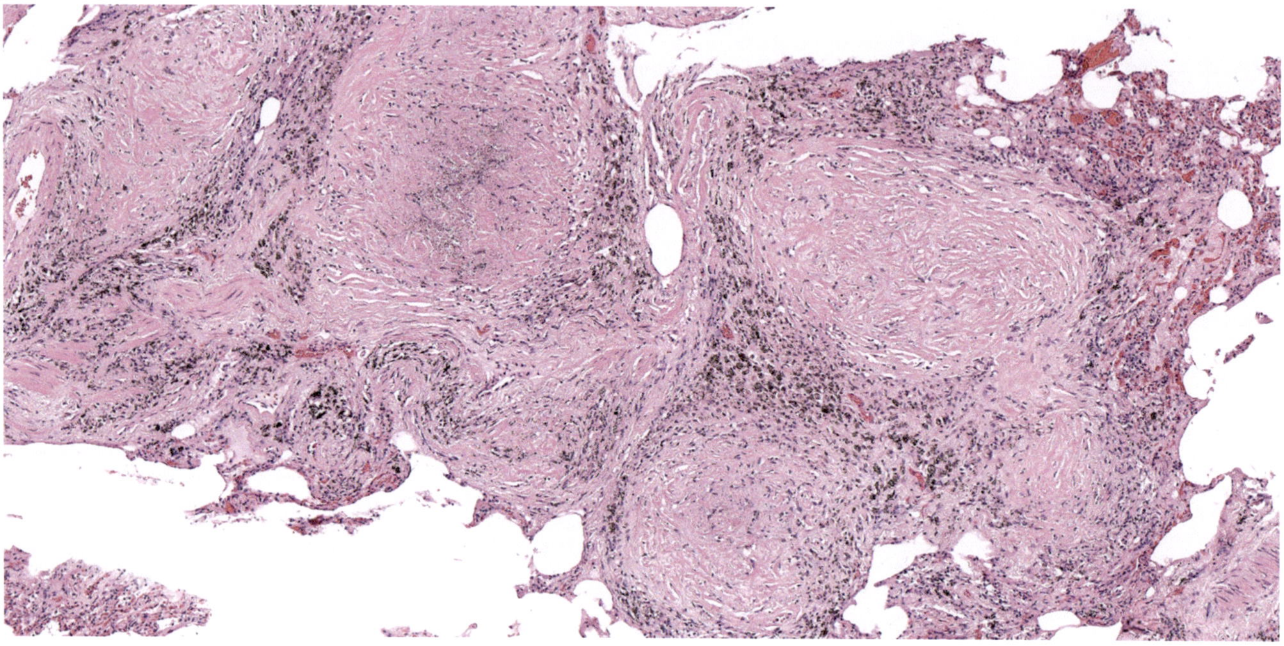

Fig. 14.125 Silicosis is a similar pneumoconiosis to coal worker's pneumoconiosis, with palpable nodules seen throughout the lungs and on the pleural surface. Histologically these are fibrotic nodules surrounded by silica dust particles, some of which are birefringent

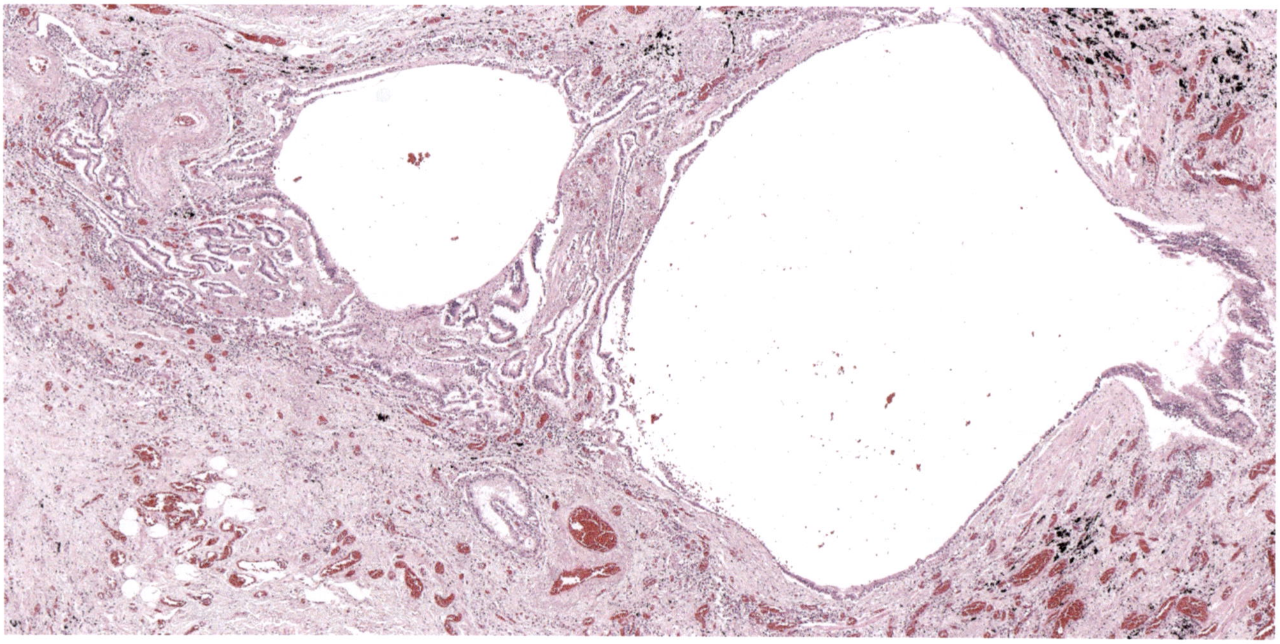

Fig. 14.126 Asbestosis is a cause of pulmonary fibrosis. It is associated with a high level of asbestos fibre exposure. The Helsinki criteria define the diagnostic criteria for asbestosis and other asbestos related diseases. This image shows honeycomb change with bronchial metaplasia in asbestosis

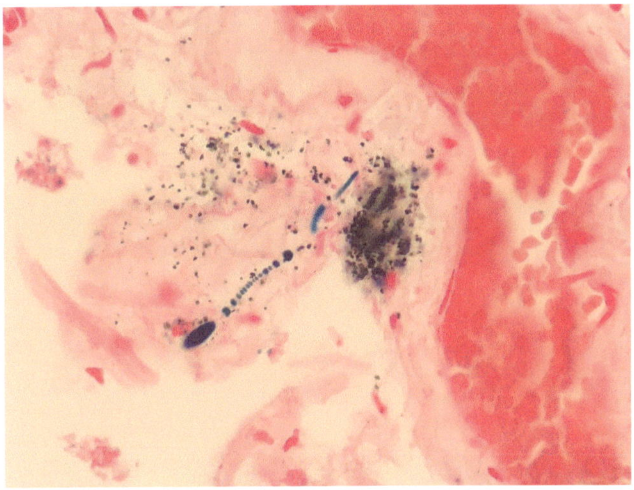

Fig. 14.127 Identification of asbestos bodies by light microscopy is part of the evaluation of pulmonary fibrosis in possible cases of asbestosis. In this image an asbestos body is seen. It has a colourless core with beaded iron deposition, highlighted by the Perls' stain. An alveolar macrophage containing black pigment is seen adjacent to the asbestos body

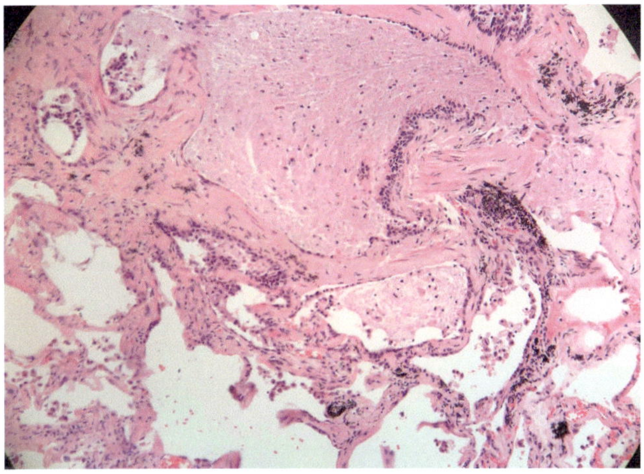

Fig. 14.128 Not all pulmonary fibrosis is related to occupational exposure. Idiopathic pulmonary fibrosis/usual interstitial pneumonitis (UIP) can cause a progressive respiratory failure. This image shows pulmonary fibrosis with honeycomb change. Superimposed lung infections are common in this context. Other important features of UIP include temporal heterogeneity and fibroblastic foci

Lung Tumours

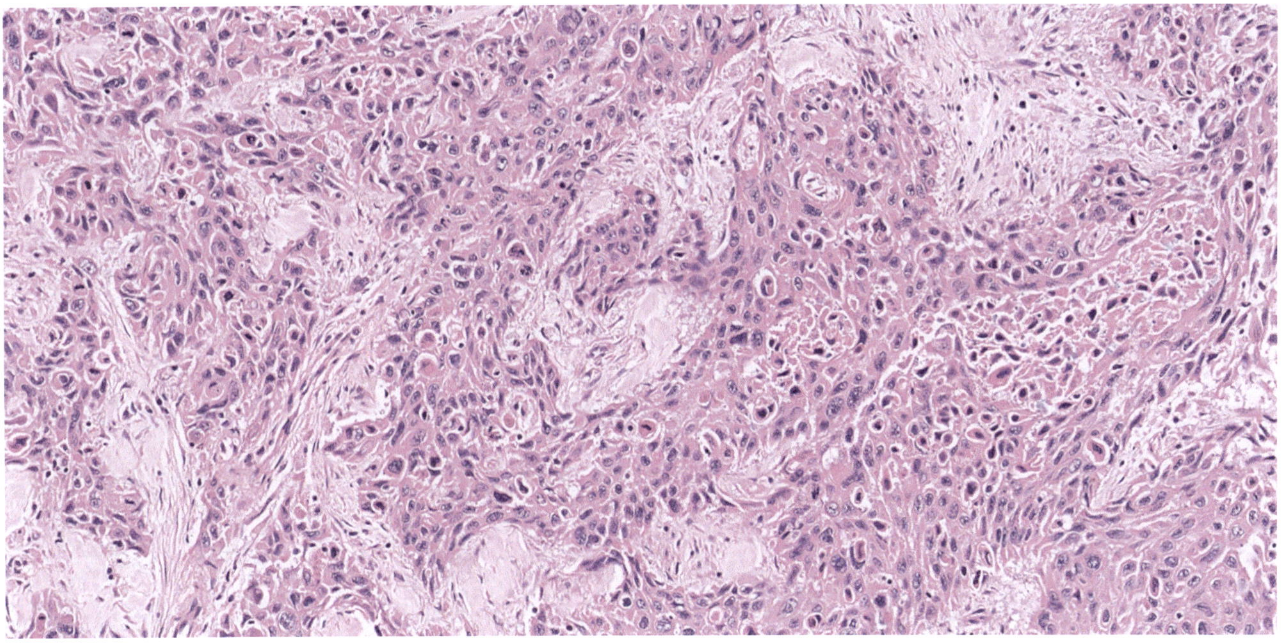

Fig. 14.129 Squamous cell carcinoma is one of the most common types of lung cancer. As seen here, it is characterised by keratinising or non-keratinising epithelium with prominent intercellular bridges and islands of cohesive tumour cells. The histological appearances are indistinguishable from squamous cell carcinomas of other sites such as the cervix or larynx

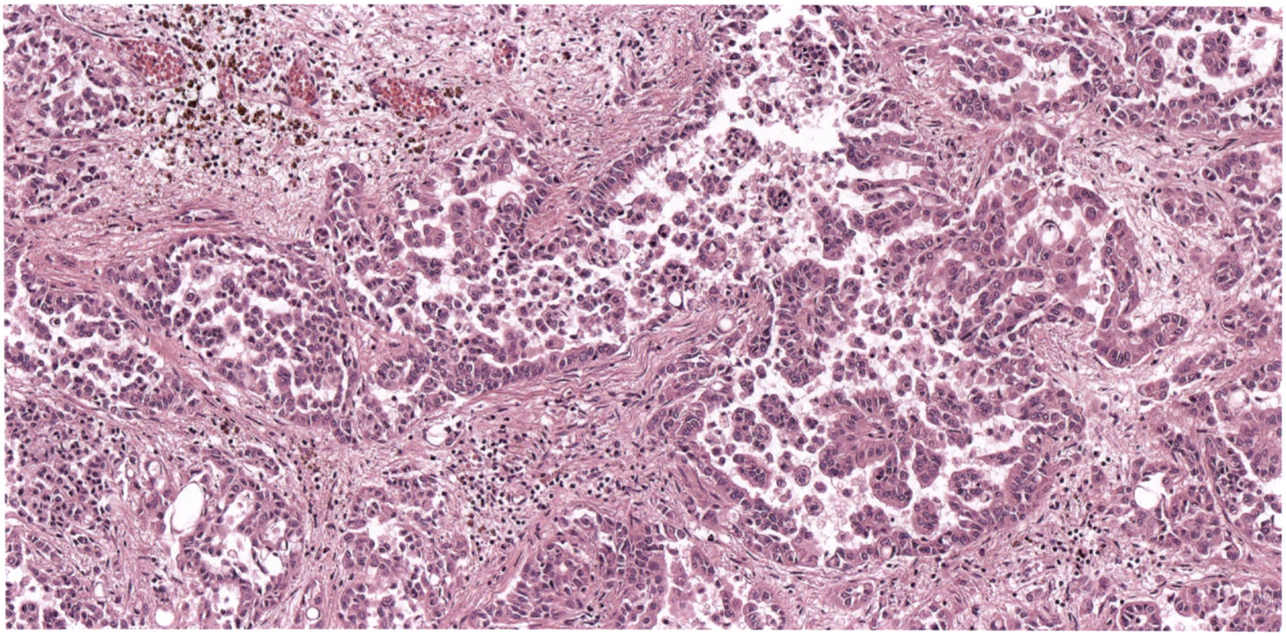

Fig. 14.130 Mesothelioma is a malignant tumour of the pleura (or rarely, the peritoneum) associated with asbestos exposure. There is usually a lag time of several decades between asbestos exposure and the development of mesothelioma. Mesotheliomas may have a variety of appearances, typically divided into those which show an epithelioid pattern and those which show a sarcomatoid pattern, and some tumours may show a mixture of patterns. In this image there is an epithelioid tumour with gland formation and micropapillary pattern

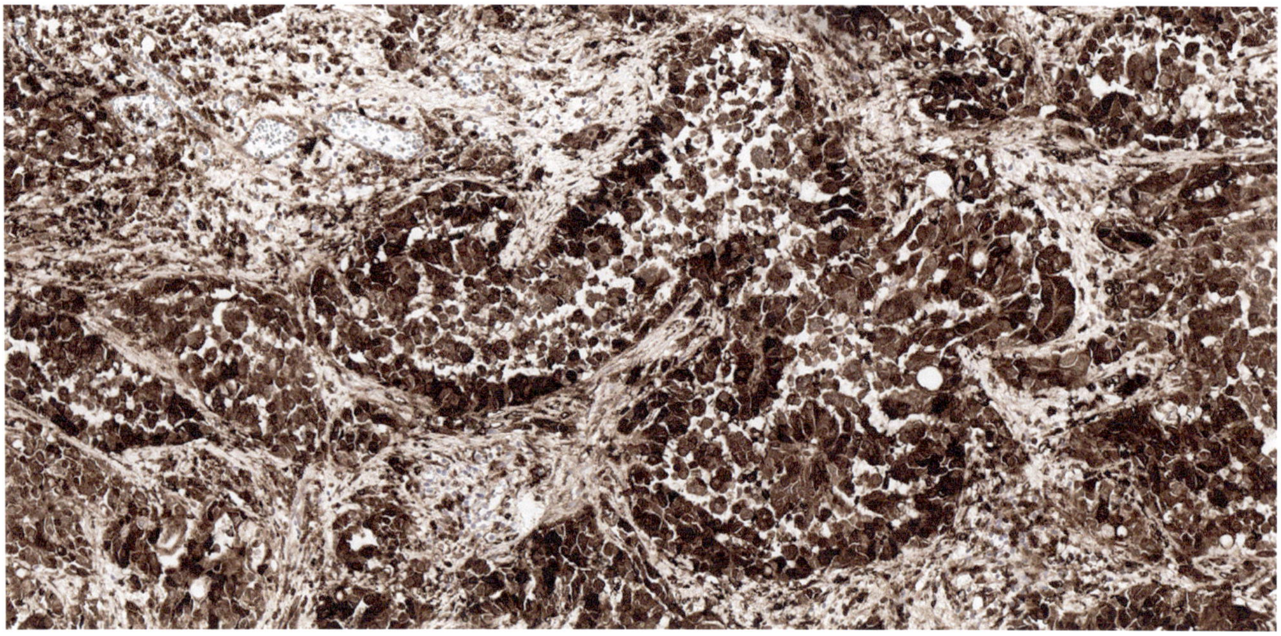

Fig. 14.131 Although the macroscopic features of mesothelioma may be characteristic (a pleural based tumour, encasing the lung) it may be necessary, and is often prudent, to confirm the diagnosis with immunohistochemical (IHC) staining. In this image IHC for calretinin shows positive nuclear and cytoplasmic staining, confirming the diagnosis of mesothelioma

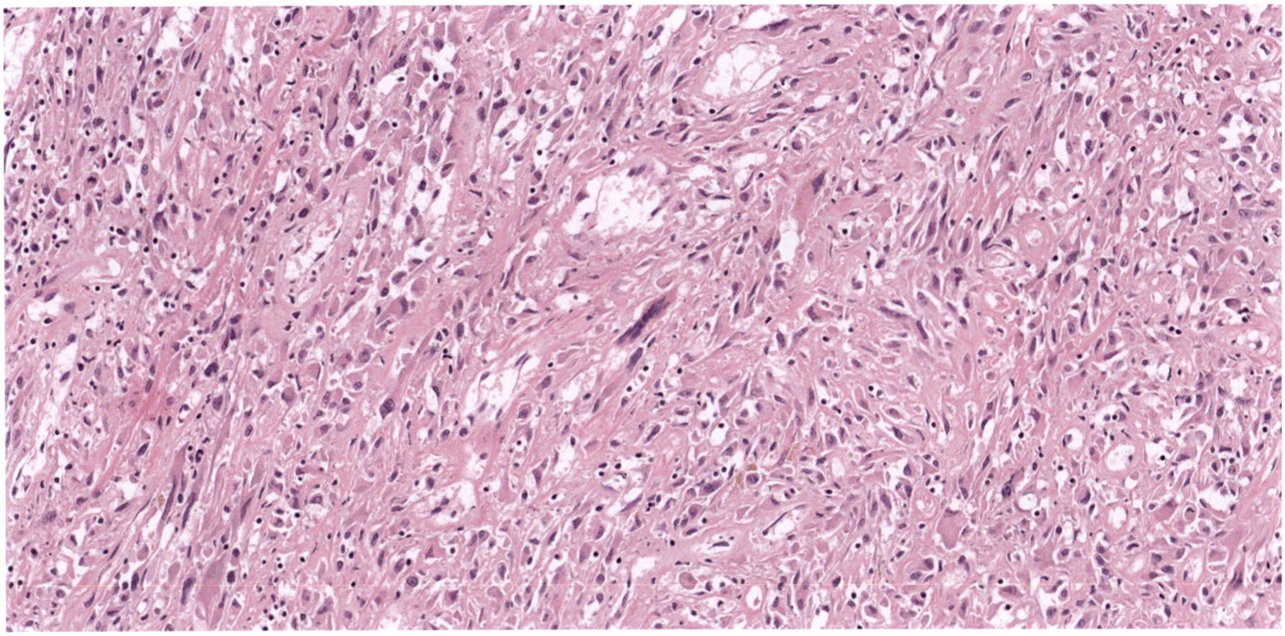

Fig. 14.132 This is an example of a sarcomatoid mesothelioma. This tumour has a spindle cell morphology with marked pleomorphism and no identifiable epithelial-type structures

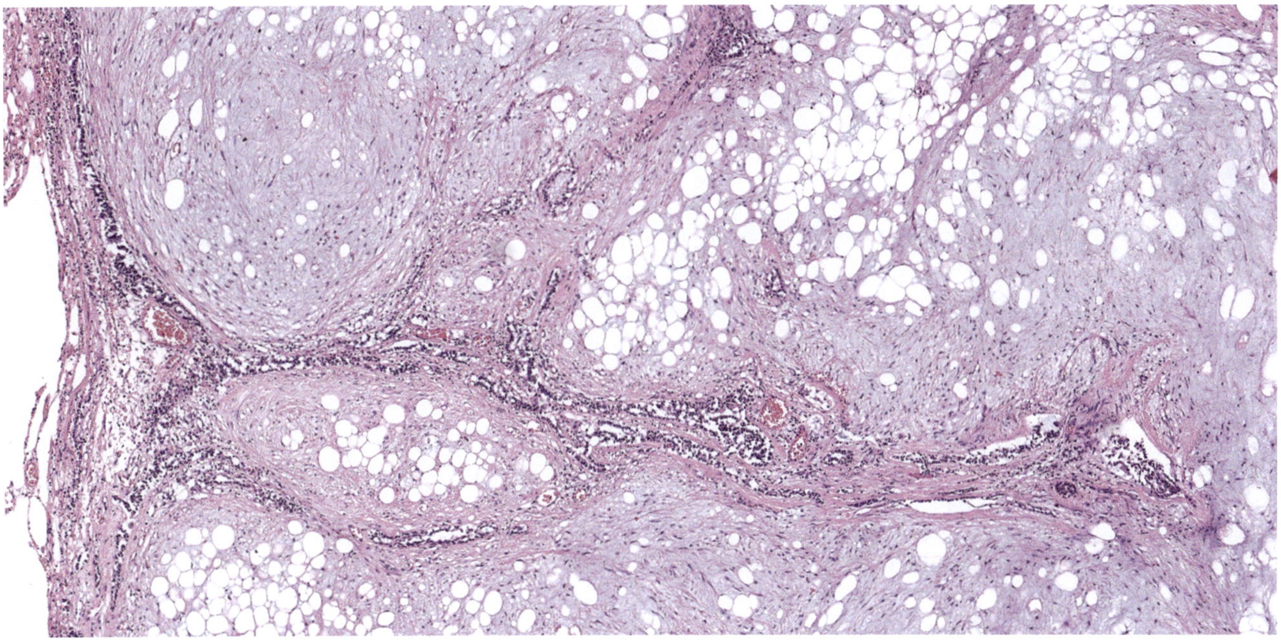

Fig. 14.133 A pulmonary hamartoma (chondroid hamartoma) is a benign tumour which may be encountered as an incidental finding at autopsy. There are nodules of chondroid type matrix with adipose tissue and bronchial epithelial elements

Fire Death

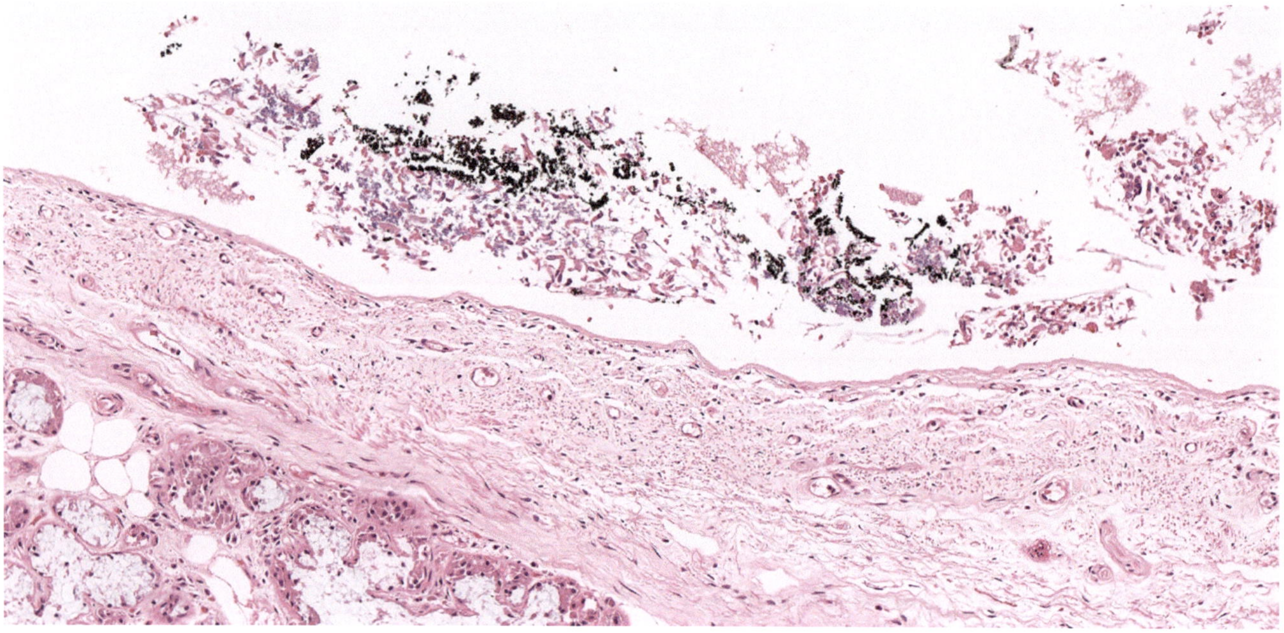

Fig. 14.134 Fire deaths often involve a combination of inhalation of smoke (including carbon monoxide) and other toxic fire gases such as cyanides. In such deaths, soot in the trachea is an indication that the deceased was alive and breathing during the smoky phase of the fire. This can be correlated with measurement of carboxyhaemoglobin in the blood

Gastrointestinal System

Of all the gastrointestinal organs, the liver is probably the most commonly examined microscopically at autopsy. It can show a range of pathologies considered either directly accountable for death or reflecting other disease processes.

Fatty change (steatosis) of the liver is commonly seen in association with alcohol excess, diabetes and obesity, with cirrhosis most commonly being associated with alcoholic liver disease and viral hepatitis.

The liver is a common site for metastatic spread of many cancers, including the lung and gastrointestinal tract.

Given the liver's metabolic and synthetic functions, liver disease can be associated with many pathological manifestations relevant to death, including a bleeding propensity, metabolic derangements and drug toxicity, with drugs directly toxic to the liver such as paracetamol and the effects of poor metabolism of drugs leading to poor clearance, accumulation and toxic effects.

The luminal organs (oesophagus, stomach, small and large bowel) suffer immensely from autolysis which hampers histological assessment of bowel pathology. However, meaningful interpretation is still possible. It can be helpful to sample any affected bowel together with an area of unaffected bowel to compare the effects of autolysis with the effects of true pathology.

Pancreatic pathology similarly suffers from the effects of autolysis. However, microscopic examination of the apparently macroscopically normal pancreas can identify pancreatitis as a cause of death.

Figures 14.135, 14.136, 14.137, 14.138, 14.139, 14.140, 14.141, 14.142, 14.143, 14.144, 14.145, 14.146, 14.147, 14.148, 14.149, 14.150, 14.151, 14.152, 14.153, 14.154, 14.155, 14.156, 14.157, 14.158, 14.159, 14.160, 14.161, 14.162, 14.163, 14.164, 14.165, 14.166, 14.167, and 14.168 illustrate the normal tissues of the gastrointestinal and hepatobiliary organs, with examples of associated pathologies.

Bowel

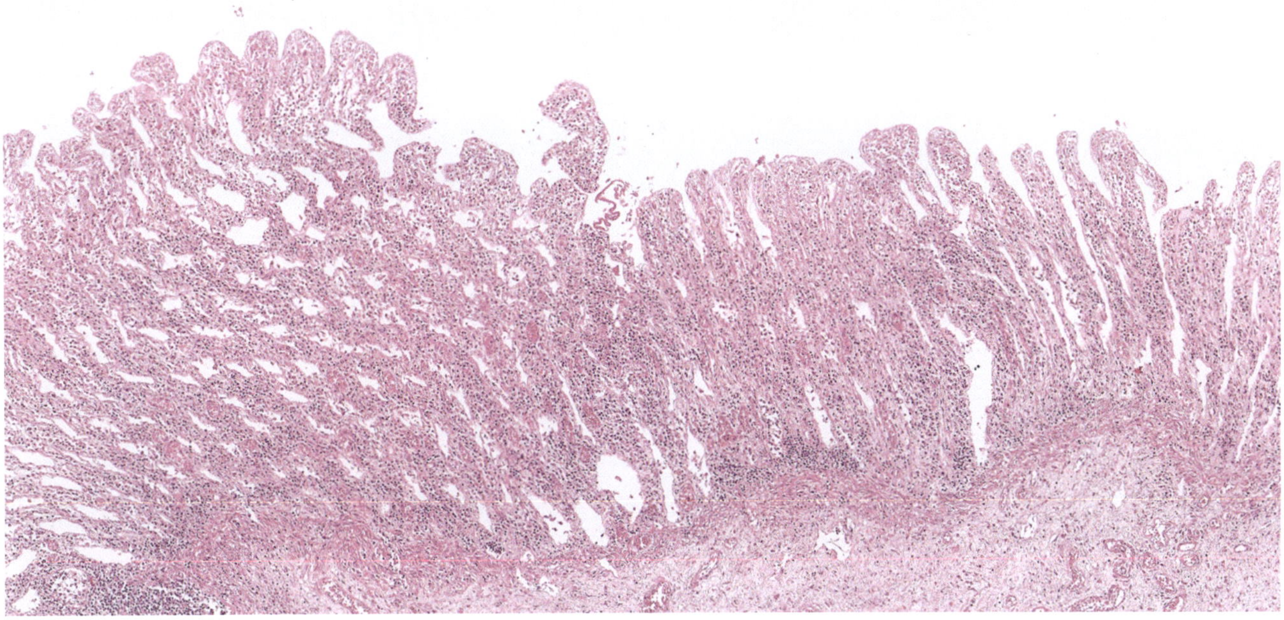

Fig. 14.135 Autolysis is very common in the post mortem setting in sections of the bowel, as seen in this image of the colon. It can be helpful to sample any affected bowel together with an area of unaffected bowel to compare the effects of autolysis with the effects of true pathology

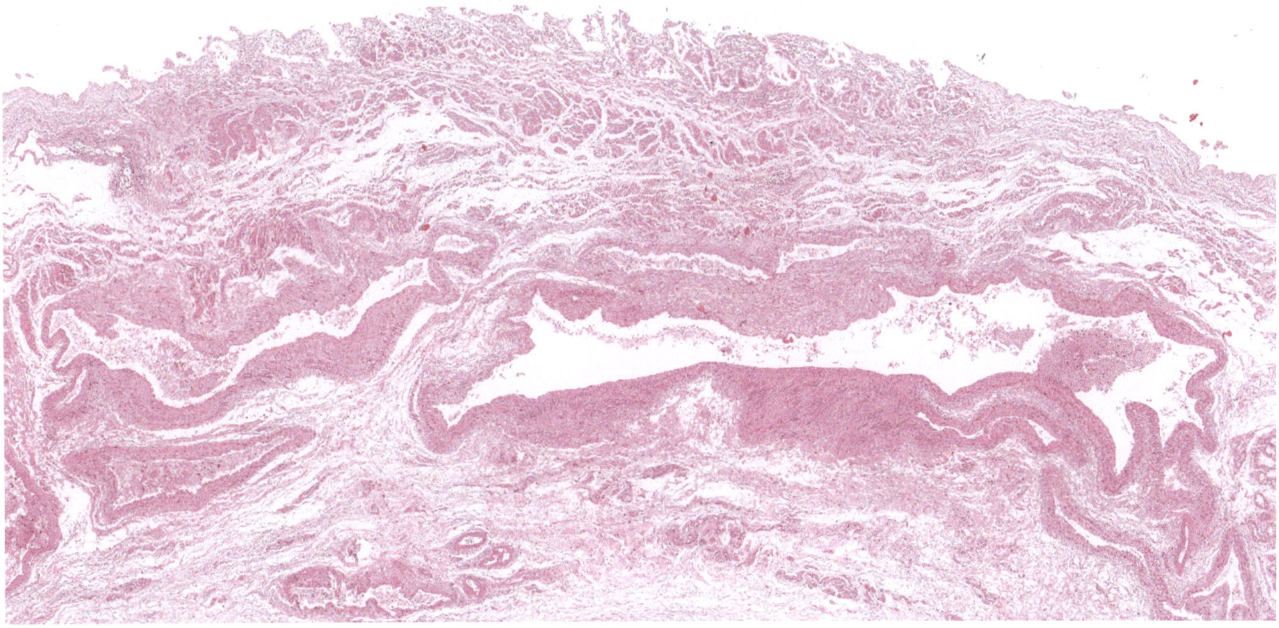

Fig. 14.136 Oesophageal varices are most commonly associated with cirrhosis of the liver and may be a source of fatal gastrointestinal haemorrhage. In this image there are dilated submucosal veins confirming the presence of varices

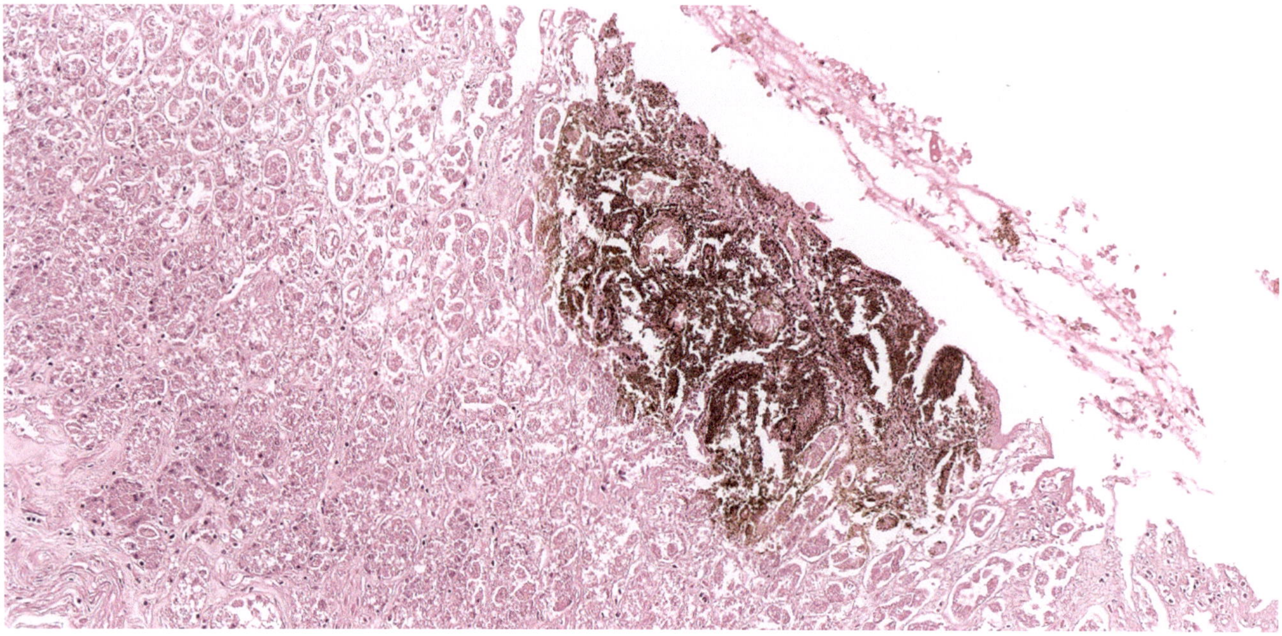

Fig. 14.137 Gastric erosions, as seen here, may be seen in many conditions, including hypothermia when they are known as Wischnewsky spots

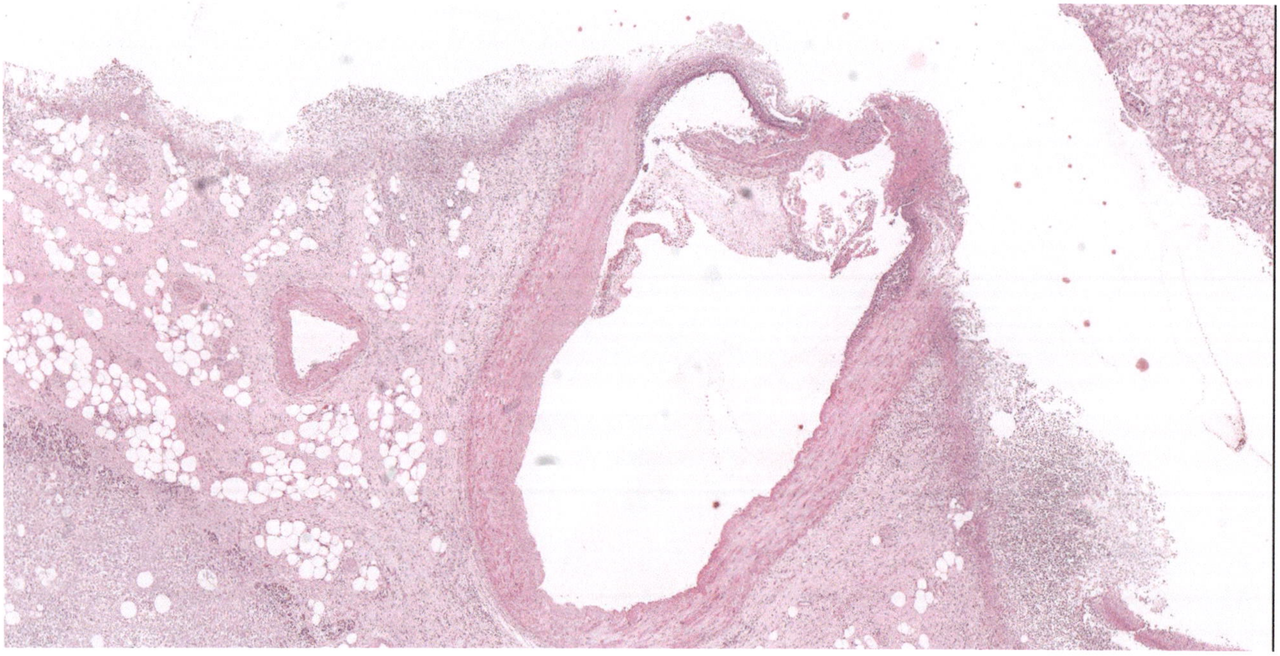

Fig. 14.138 Gastric and duodenal ulcers can cause bleeding or perforation and result in death. This image shows an eroded artery at the base of the ulcer

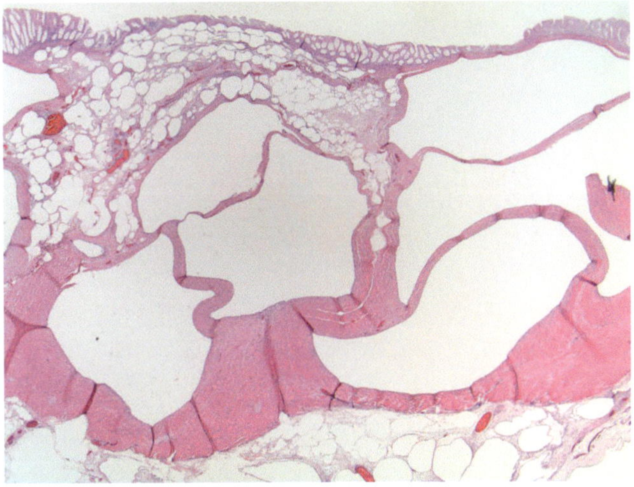

Fig. 14.139 This is an example of pneumatosis intestinalis, seen as large air spaces within the wall of the bowel. This condition may be idiopathic or iatrogenic and can cause perforation of the bowel

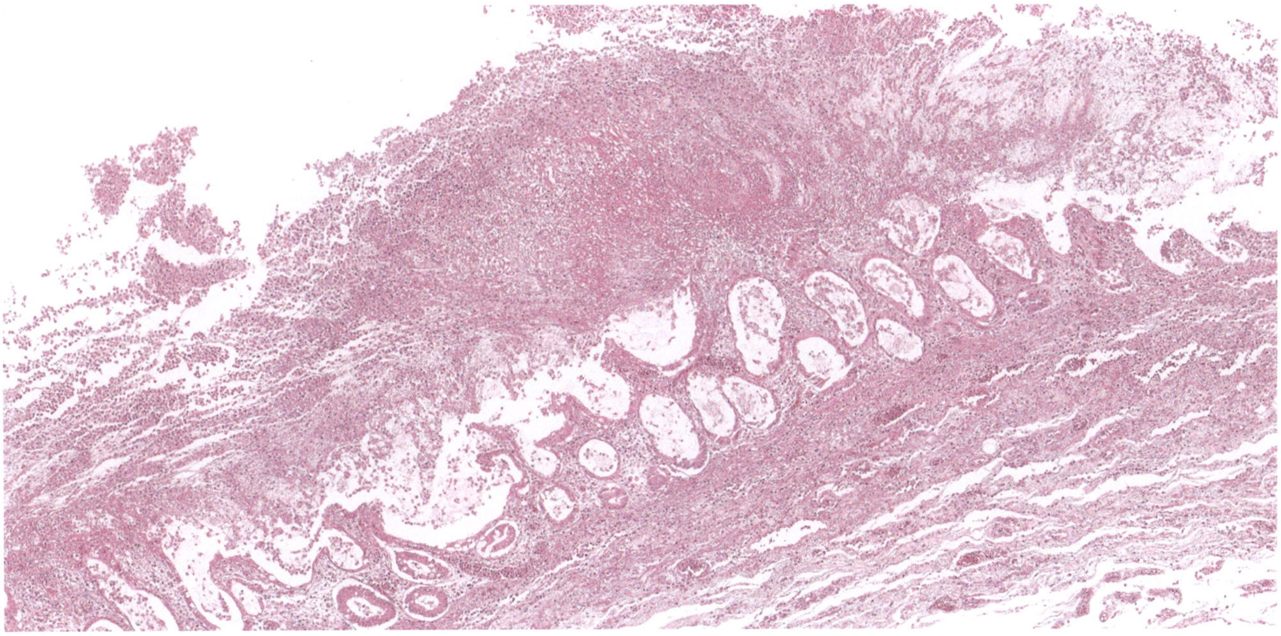

Fig. 14.140 Pseudomembranous colitis is caused by *Clostridium difficile* infection, typically associated with antibiotic therapy for another infection such as pneumonia. The antibiotic wipes out normal commensal bacteria in the large bowel allowing *C. difficile* to proliferate and cause colitis. In this image there are eruptive inflammatory lesions overlying the mucosa

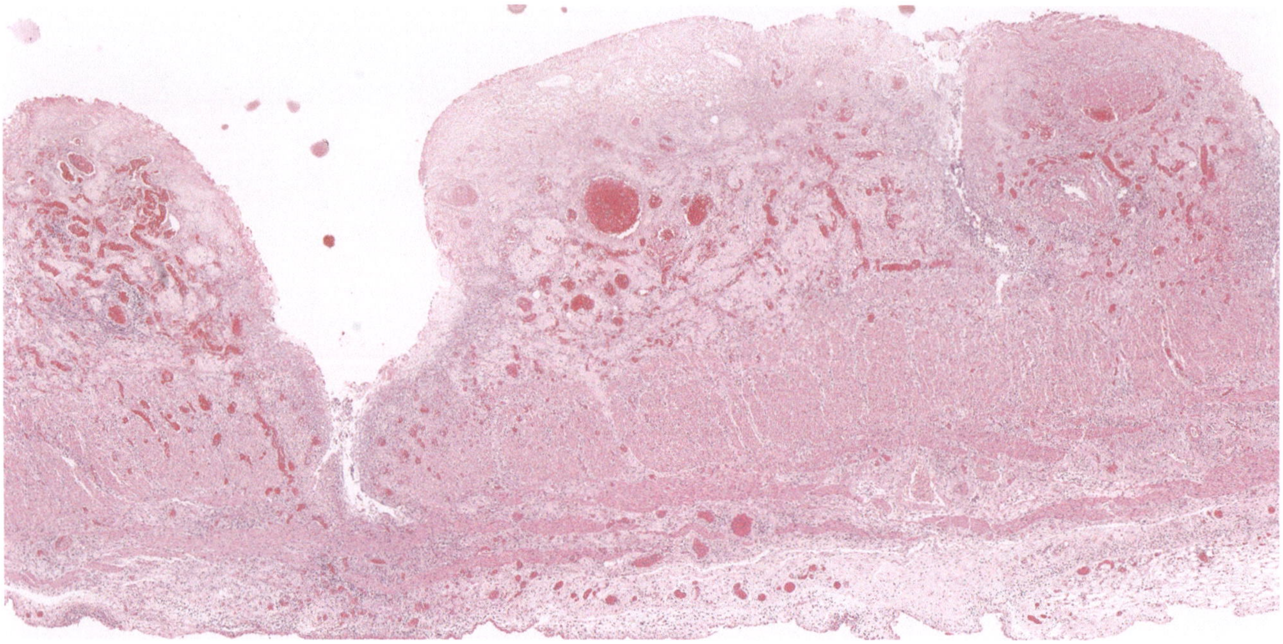

Fig. 14.141 Occasionally a fulminant colitis may present acutely and result in death without any established diagnosis of bowel disease. The precise typing of inflammatory bowel disease can be difficult at autopsy and is often hampered by autolysis of the mucosa. This image shows transmural inflammation and fissuring ulcers

Liver

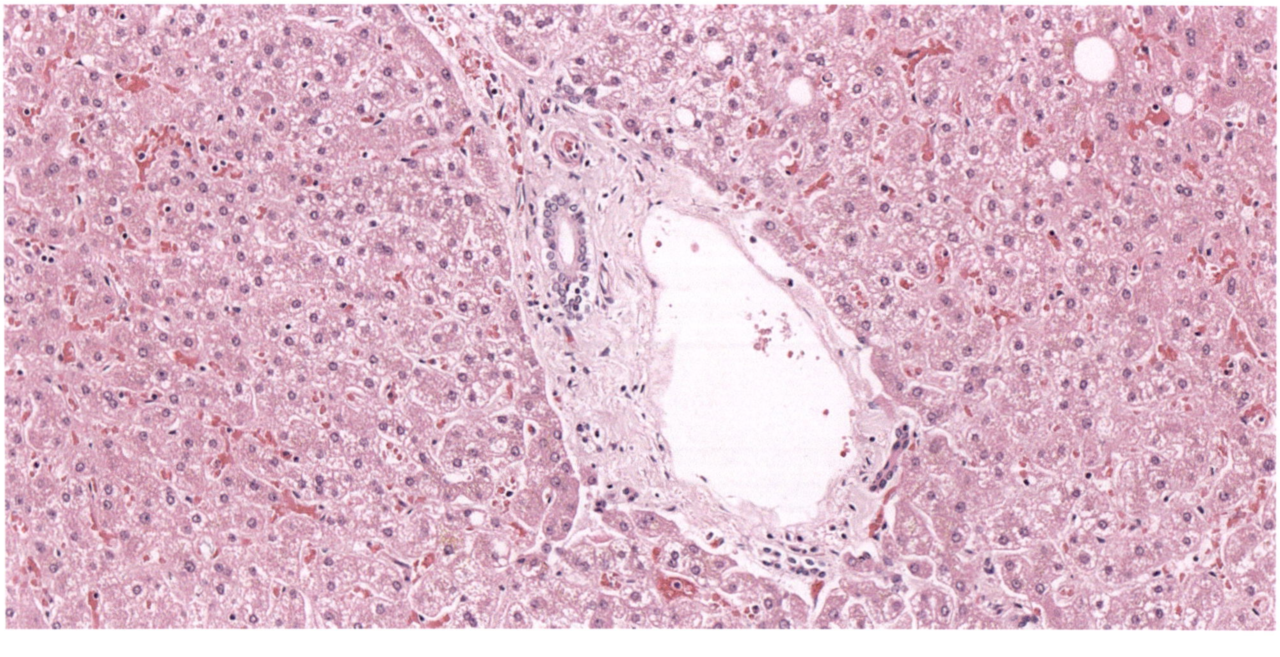

Fig. 14.142 This is an image of normal liver with a portal tract. The basic cell of the liver is the hepatocyte. These are large cells with a small nucleus and abundant cytoplasm. Clearing of the cytoplasm is commonly seen due to the glycogen content. The liver unit consists of a portal tract, within which a triad of bile ductule, vein and arteriole are seen, the lobule of hepatocytes with layers of 1–2 cells thick and intervening sinusoids, and a central vein

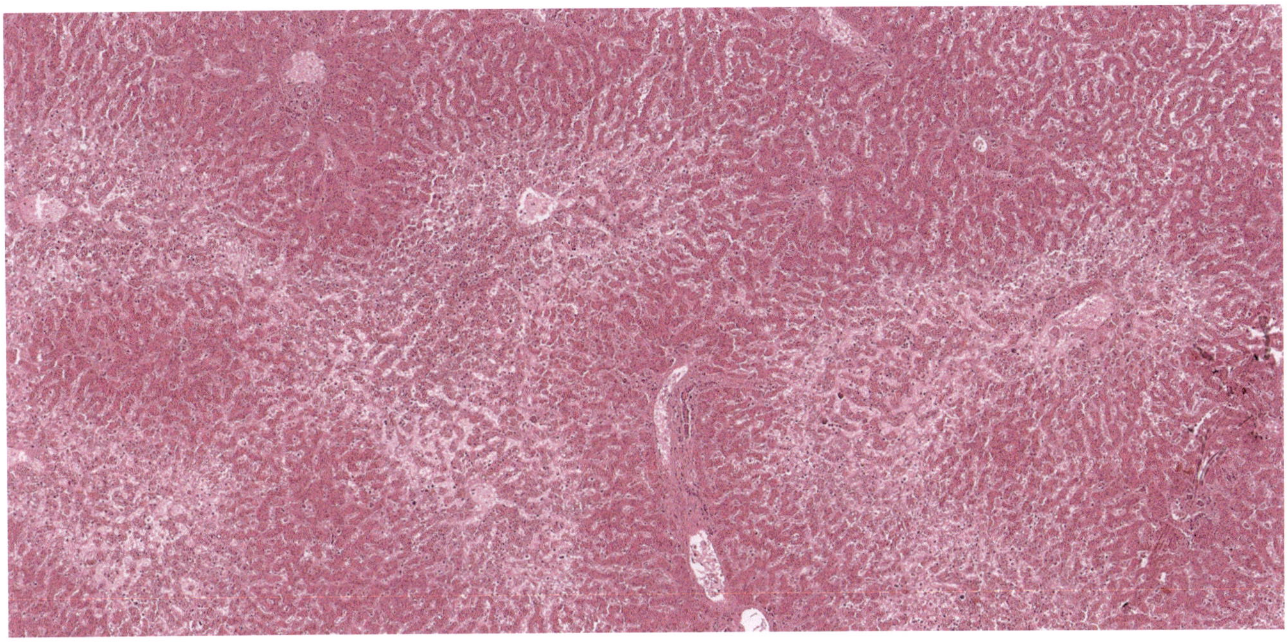

Fig. 14.143 In chronic venous congestion there is pallor and congestion of sinusoids around central veins. Classically associated with congestive cardiac failure, a similar pattern of sinusoidal congestion can be seen in any cause of right sided heart failure, including acutely in pulmonary thromboembolism

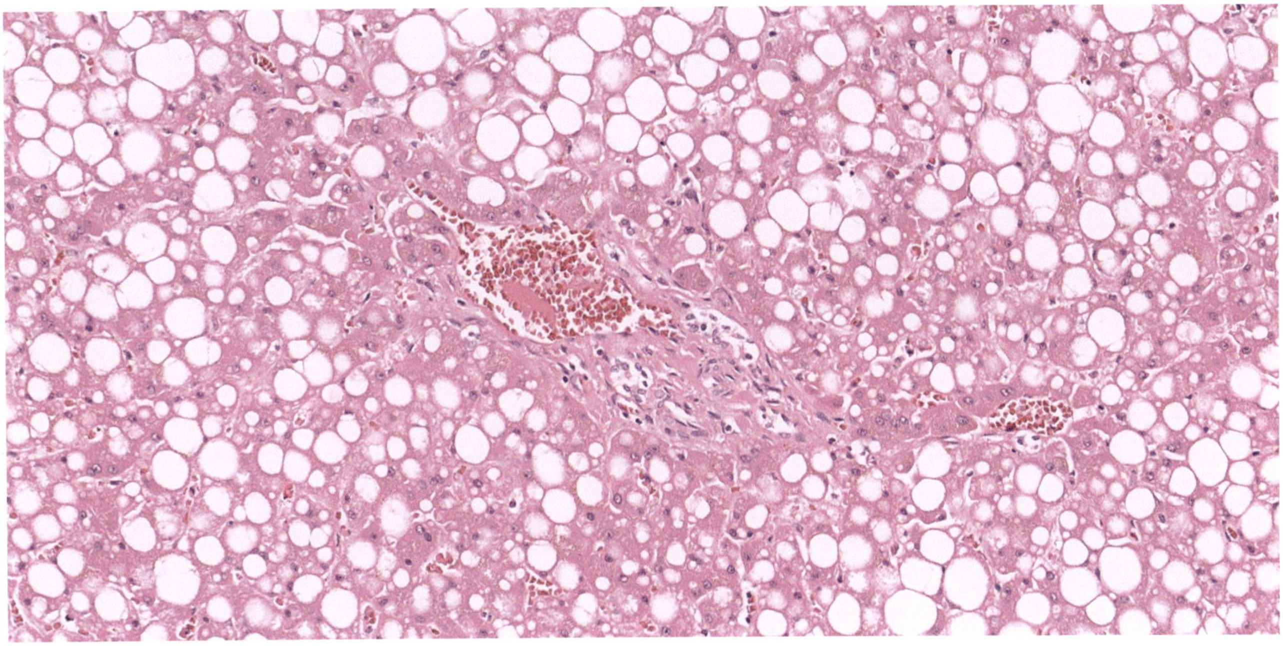

Fig. 14.144 This image shows liver with globules of fat within the cytoplasm of the hepatocytes, known as steatosis. In this case the steatosis involves more than two thirds of hepatocytes, in keeping with grade 3 steatosis. Fatty change of the liver is most commonly associated with alcohol excess. It can also be seen commonly in diabetes and obesity

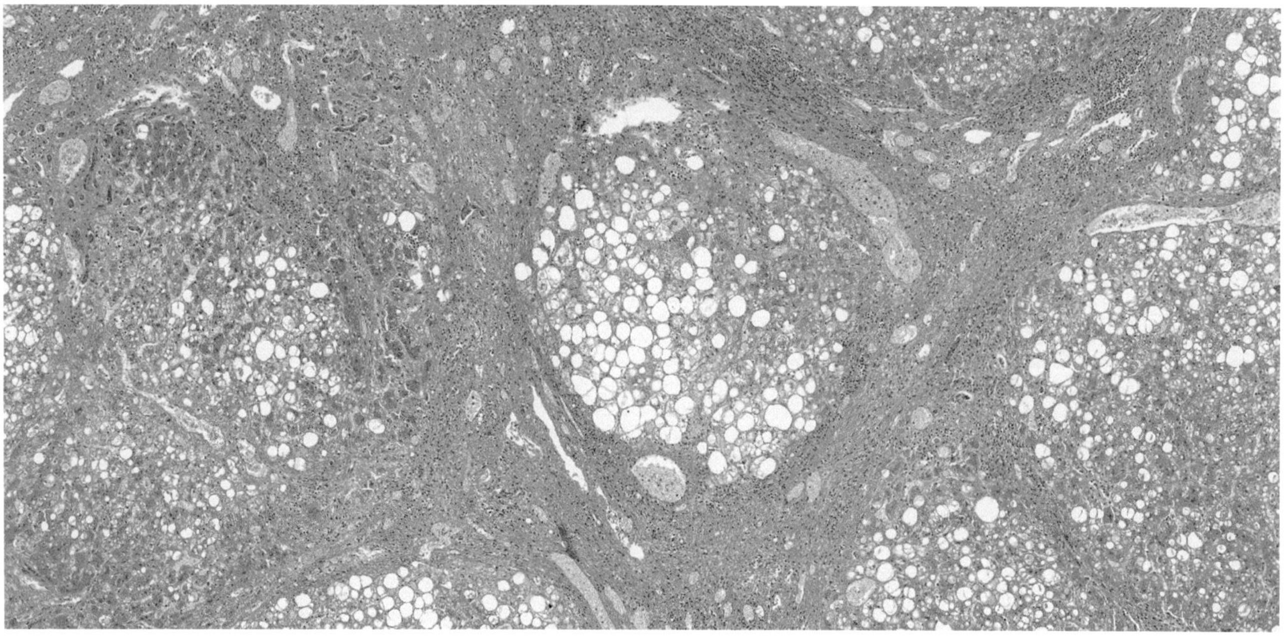

Fig. 14.145 The liver has a remarkable propensity to regenerate following injury. In alcoholic liver disease the liver regenerates but the nodules of new hepatocytes lack the normal liver lobule arrangement. This is an example of cirrhosis of the liver in alcoholic liver disease. Note also the steatosis and portal inflammation

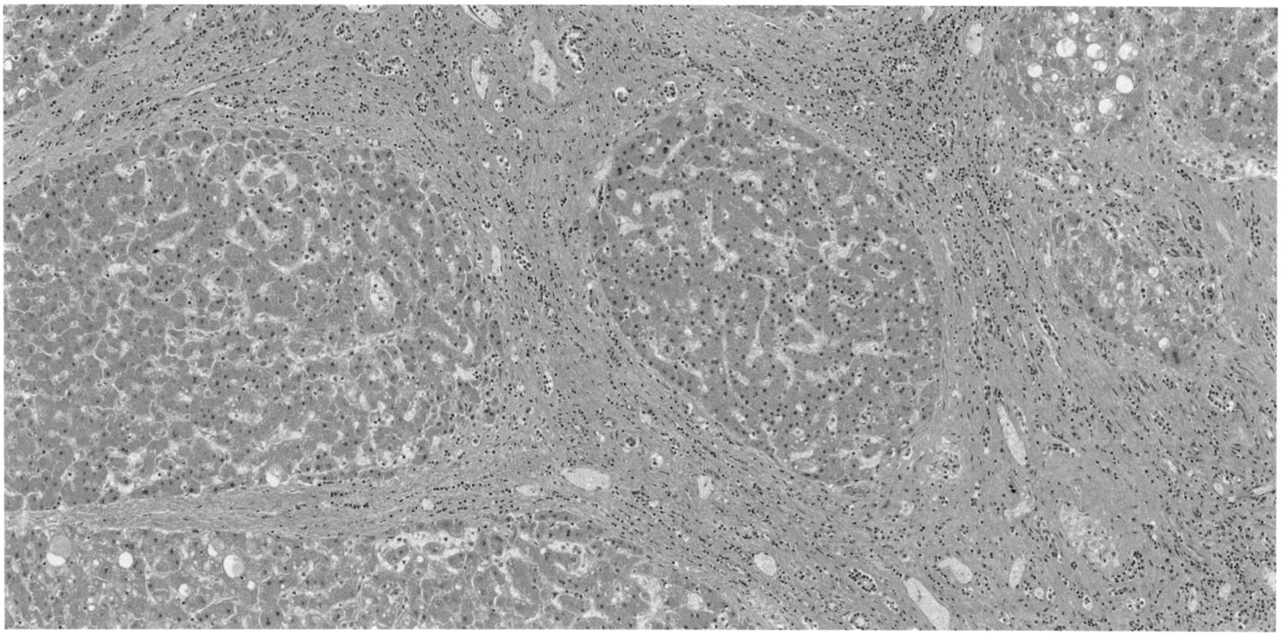

Fig. 14.146 This image shows cirrhosis of the liver in hepatitis C infection. Note the portal lymphocytic infiltrate and lack of steatosis

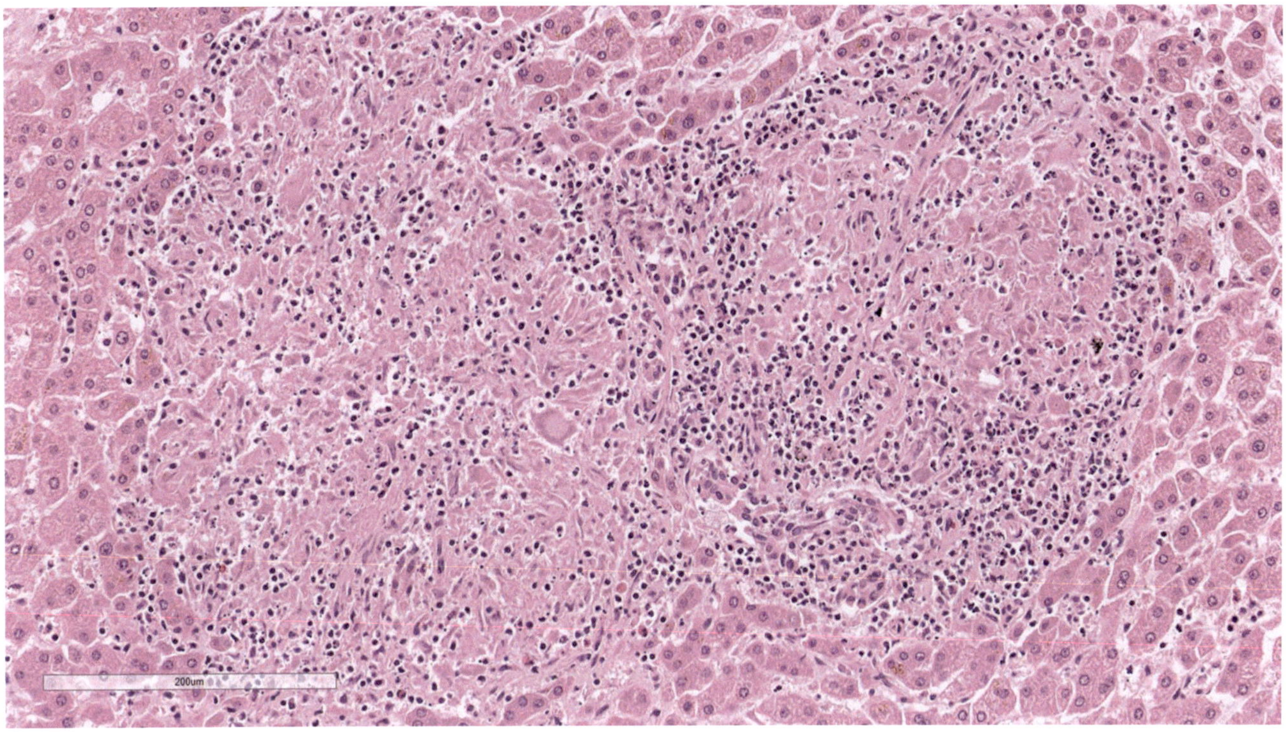

Fig. 14.147 Granulomatous inflammation in the liver has many causes. In this case it was secondary to intravenous drug use

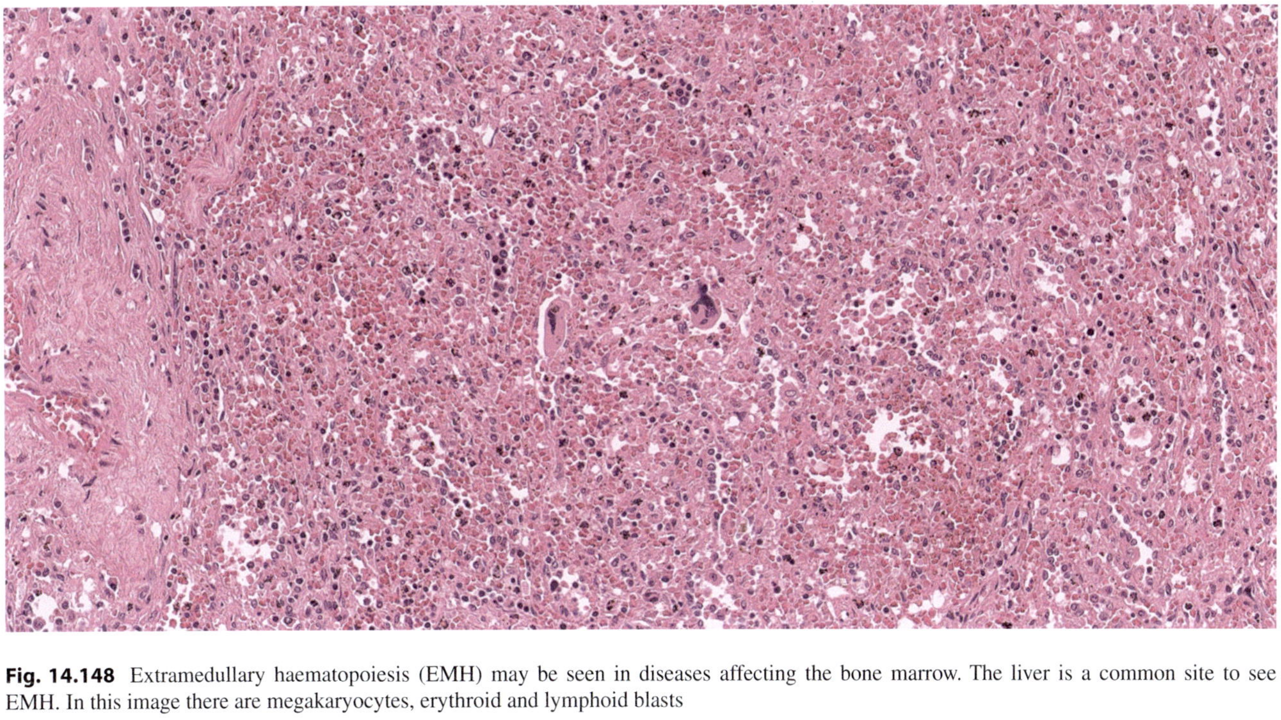

Fig. 14.148 Extramedullary haematopoiesis (EMH) may be seen in diseases affecting the bone marrow. The liver is a common site to see EMH. In this image there are megakaryocytes, erythroid and lymphoid blasts

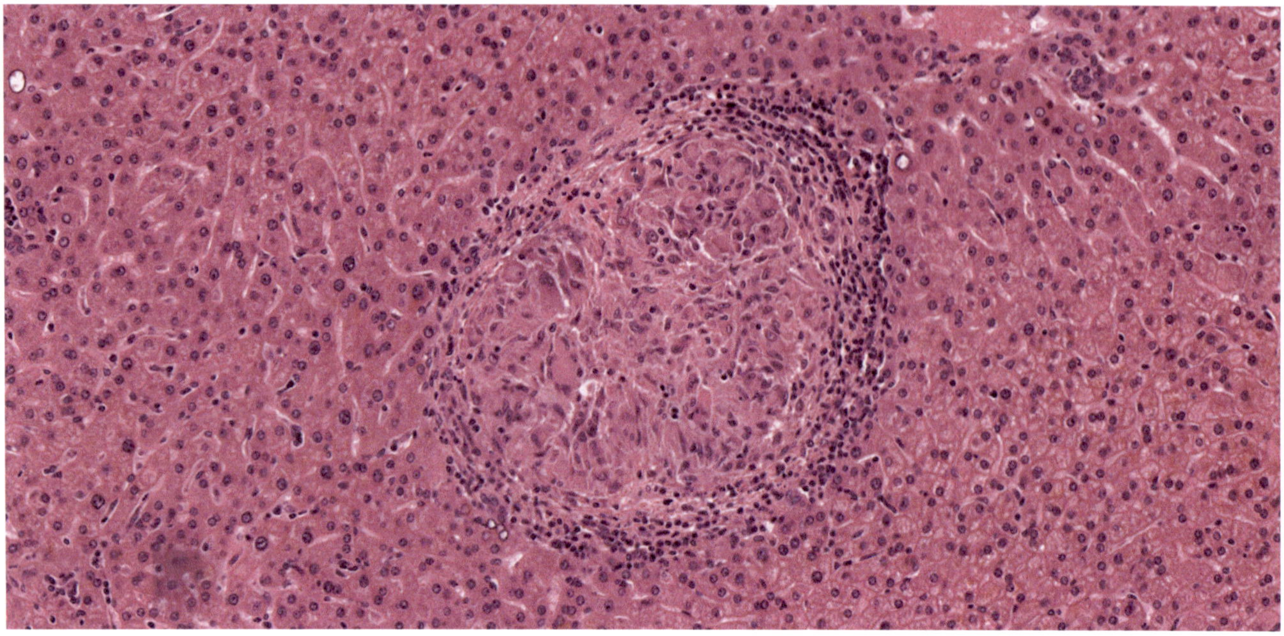

Fig. 14.149 Sarcoidosis is a multi-system inflammatory disease. Although primarily affecting the lungs, granulomas may be seen in other organs including the liver, and involvement of the heart can lead to sudden arrhythmic death. In this image there is non-necrotising granulomatous inflammation in the liver

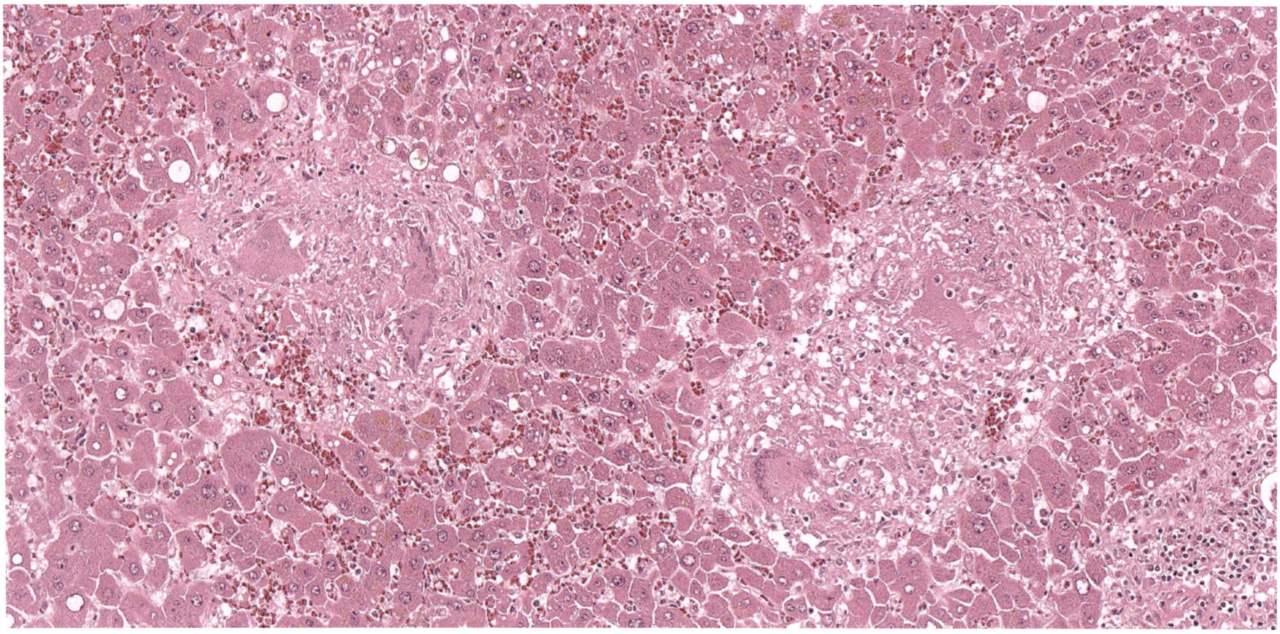

Fig. 14.150 Tuberculosis with miliary spread can involve many organs. In this image there is necrotising granulomatous inflammation in the liver

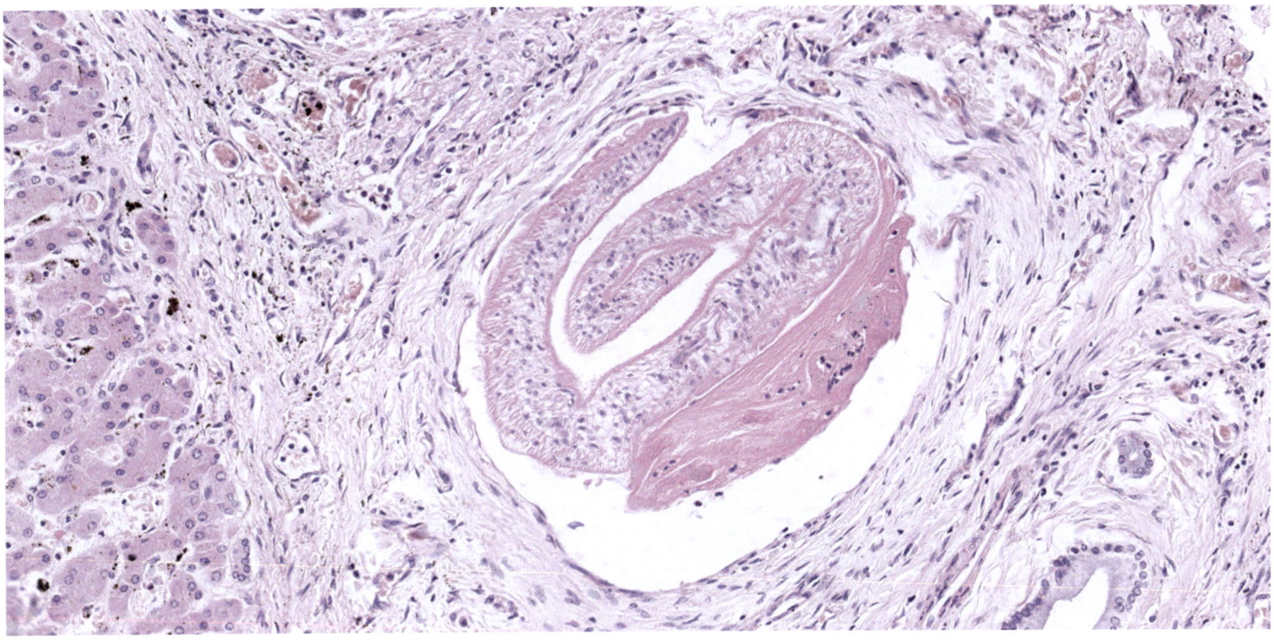

Fig. 14.151 This image shows a Schistosome worm in the liver. Schistosomiasis most commonly affects the bladder, kidneys and liver. Worms and eggs may be identified histologically. It can cause cirrhosis of the liver. More rare involvement of the lungs and heart may be seen

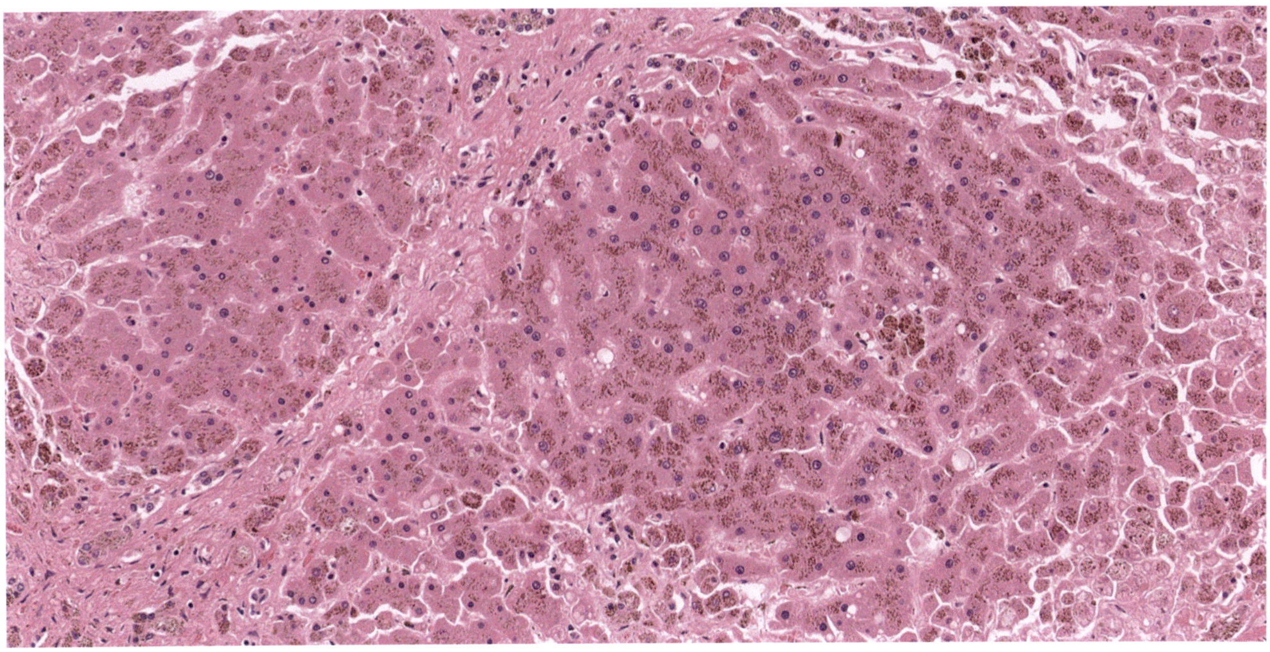

Fig. 14.152 Haemochromatosis, a disorder of iron storage, particularly affects the liver. This image shows an abundance of coarse brown haemosiderin pigment within hepatocytes

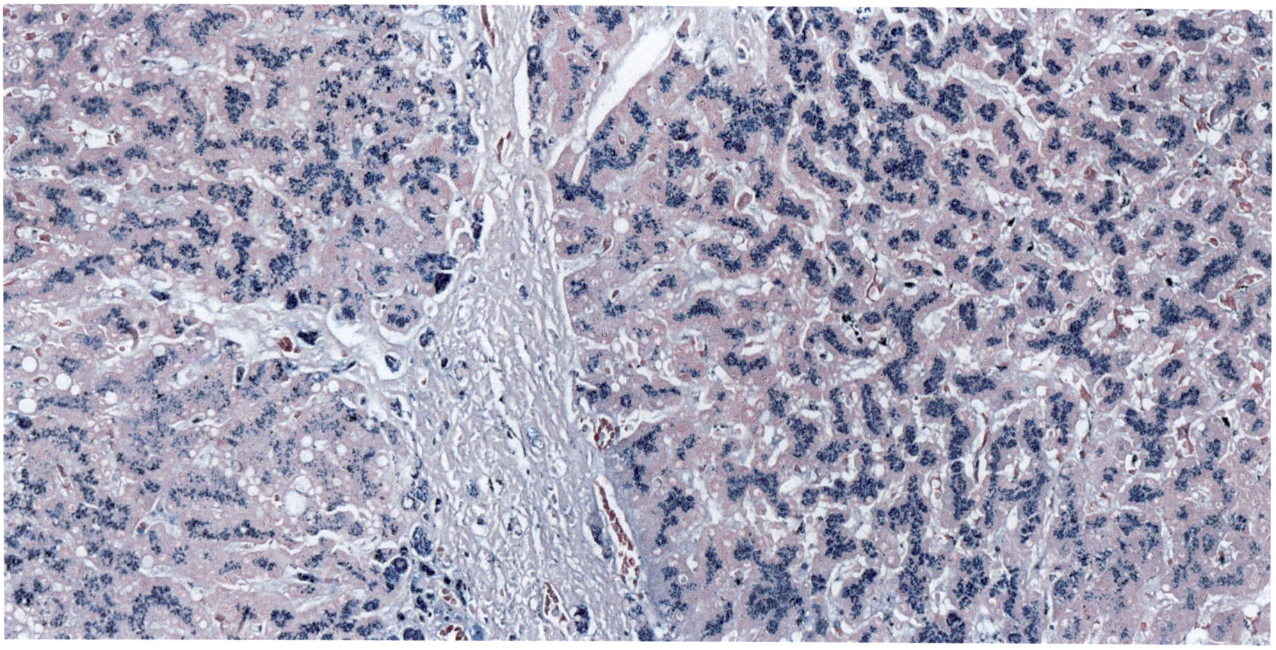

Fig. 14.153 Haemochromatosis in the liver, confirmed with Perls' stain

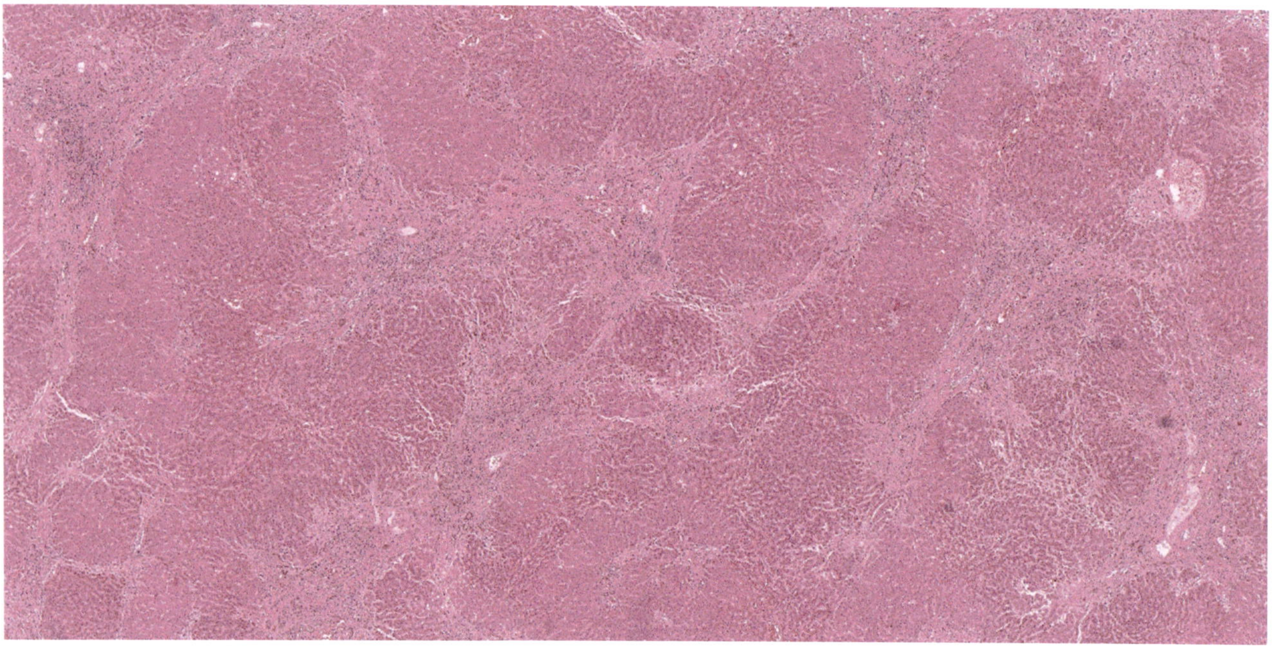

Fig. 14.154 Haemochromatosis can be a cause of cirrhosis of the liver and can be associated with hepatocellular carcinoma

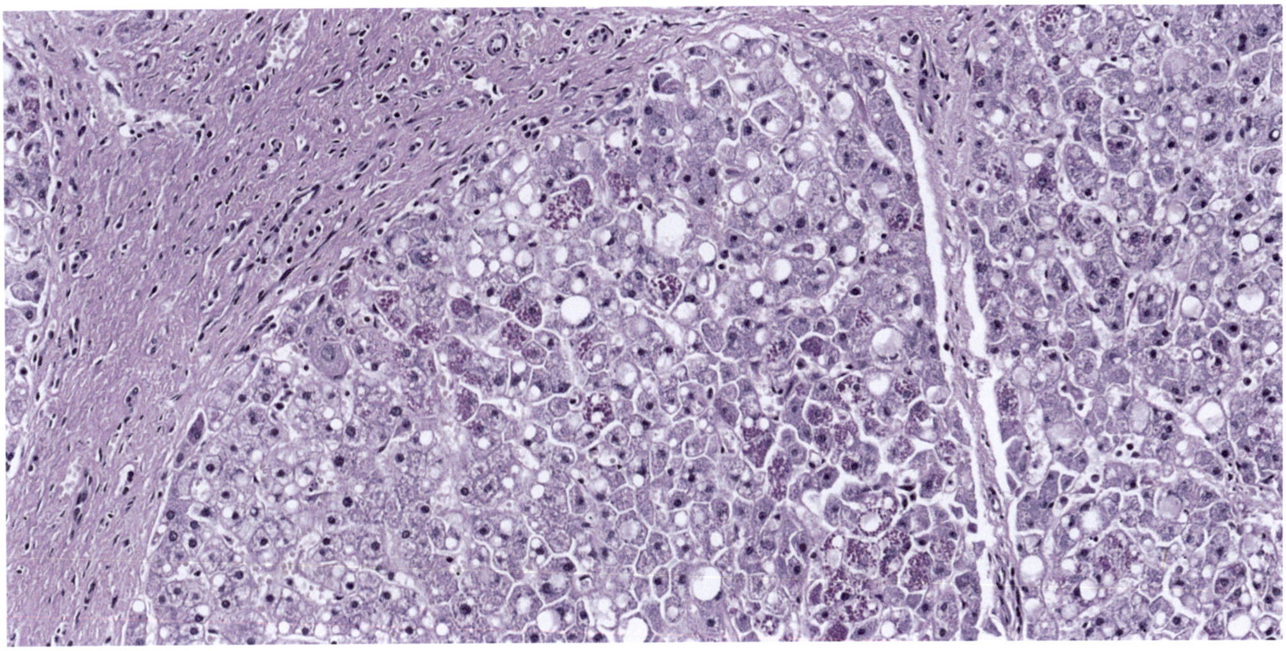

Fig. 14.155 Alpha-1 antitrypsin deficiency is another cause of cirrhosis of the liver and is a rare cause of emphysema of the lungs. In this image the DPAS stain highlights diastase-resistant alpha-1 antitrypsin globules within hepatocytes

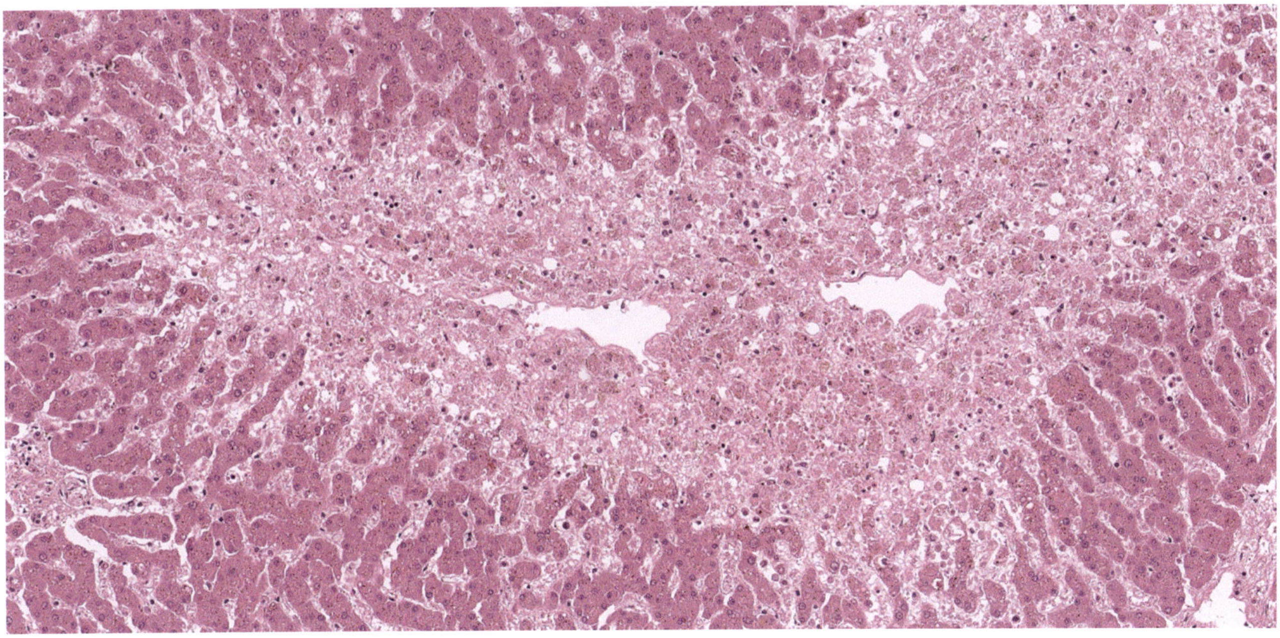

Fig. 14.156 The liver is often affected by drugs, given its function in the metabolism of many substances. In this image of liver in a case of paracetamol toxicity there is necrosis of hepatocytes in zone 3, around central veins. Whilst this distribution of hepatocyte necrosis is very typical of paracetamol toxicity, occurring several days or weeks after initial ingestion, this pattern of hepatocyte necrosis can also be seen in other causes such as under-perfusion due to hypovolaemia or hypotension

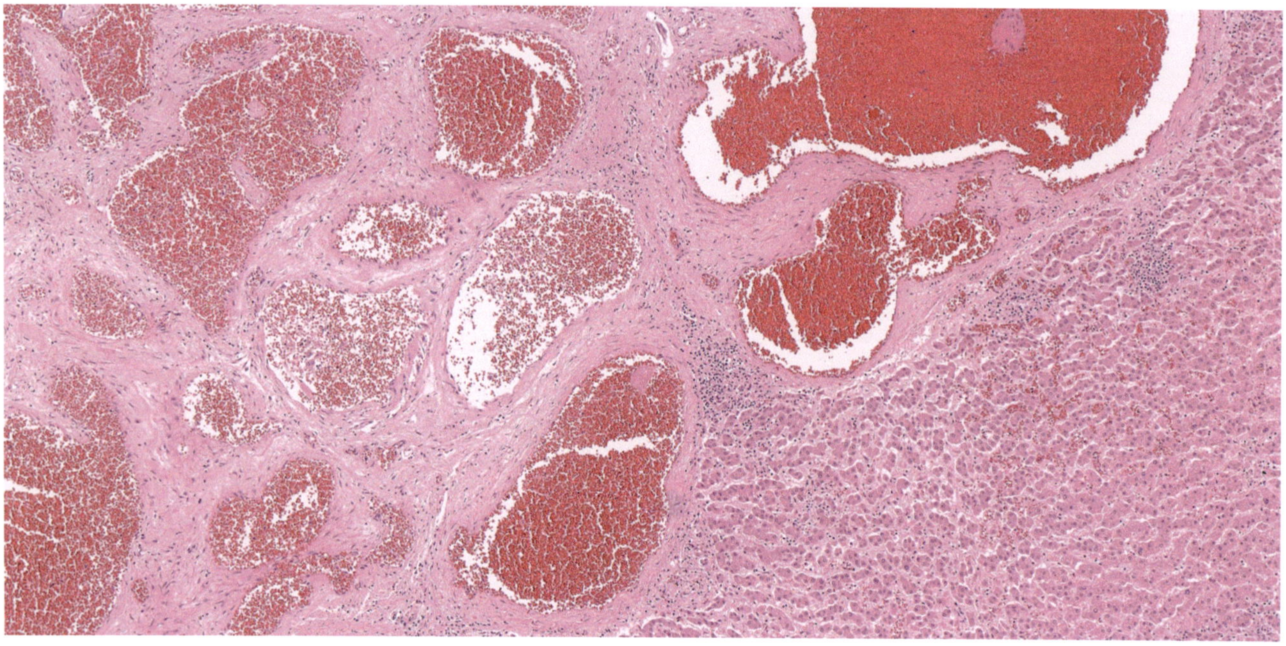

Fig. 14.157 This is a haemangioma in the liver. The image shows a proliferation of thin walled blood vessels. Haemangiomas are the most common primary liver tumour and are usually an incidental finding at autopsy

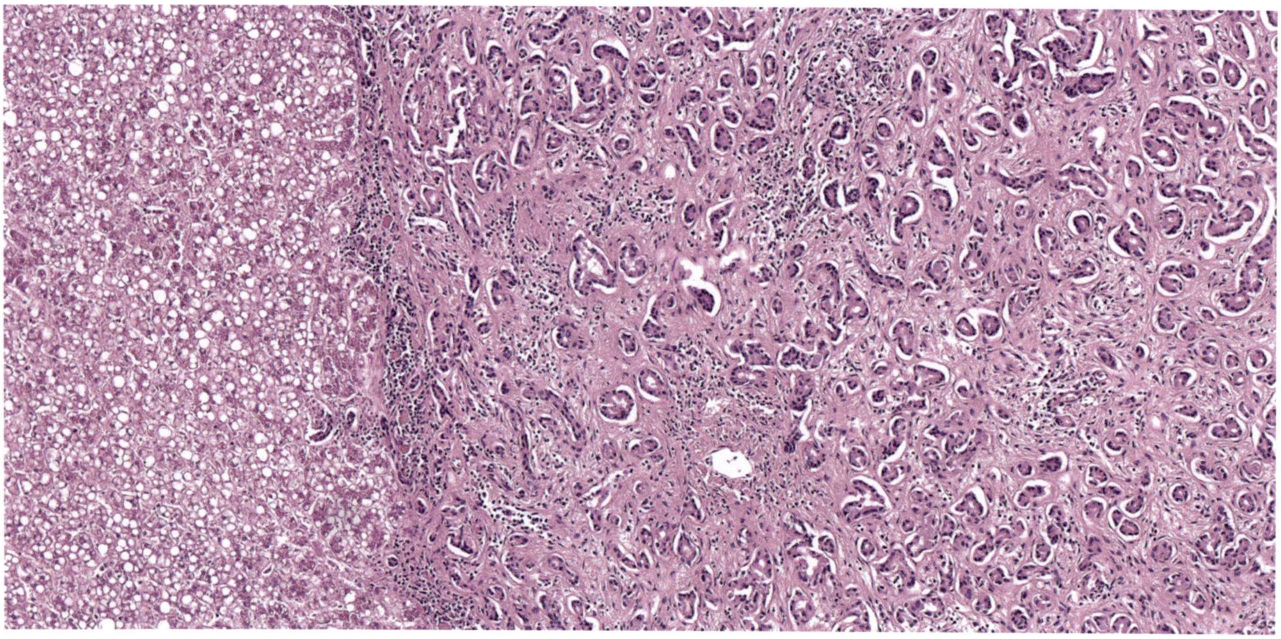

Fig. 14.158 This image shows a bile duct adenoma. There is a proliferation of small ducts resembling bile ductules. These are small tumours often measuring <1 cm, commonly seen just deep to the liver capsule. The background liver on the left side of the image shows grade 3 steatosis

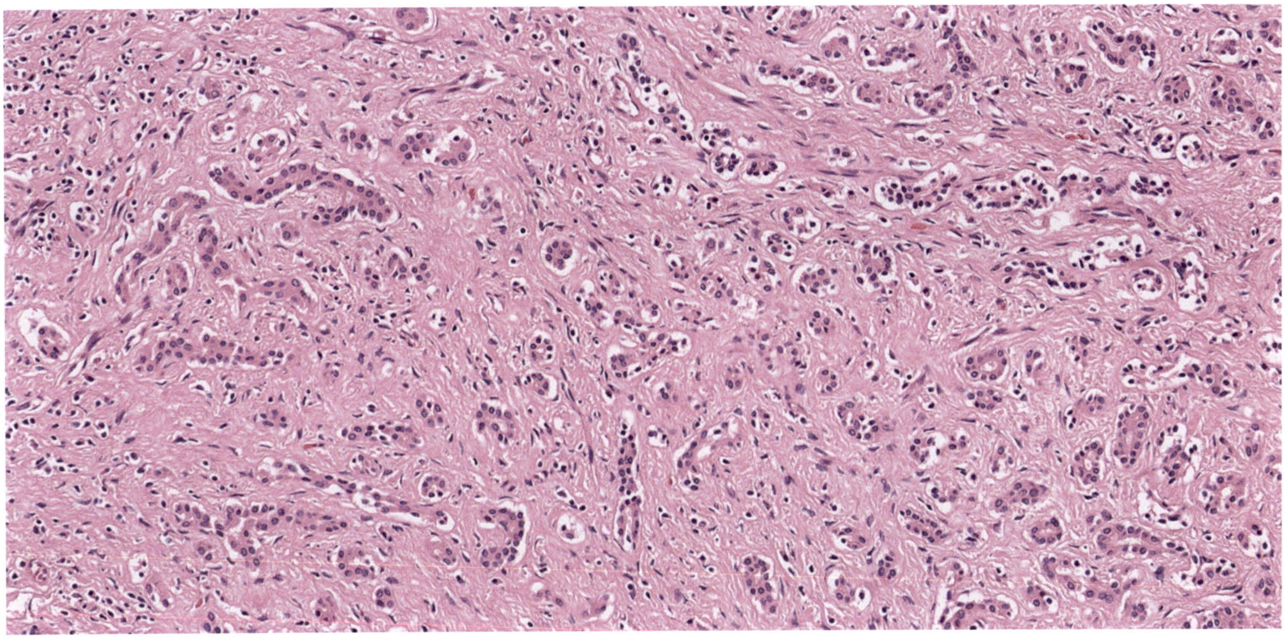

Fig. 14.159 Cholangiocarcinoma is one type of malignant tumour which is primary to the liver. In this image there are bland malignant ducts set in a fibrotic stroma. This was a large tumour involving most of the liver

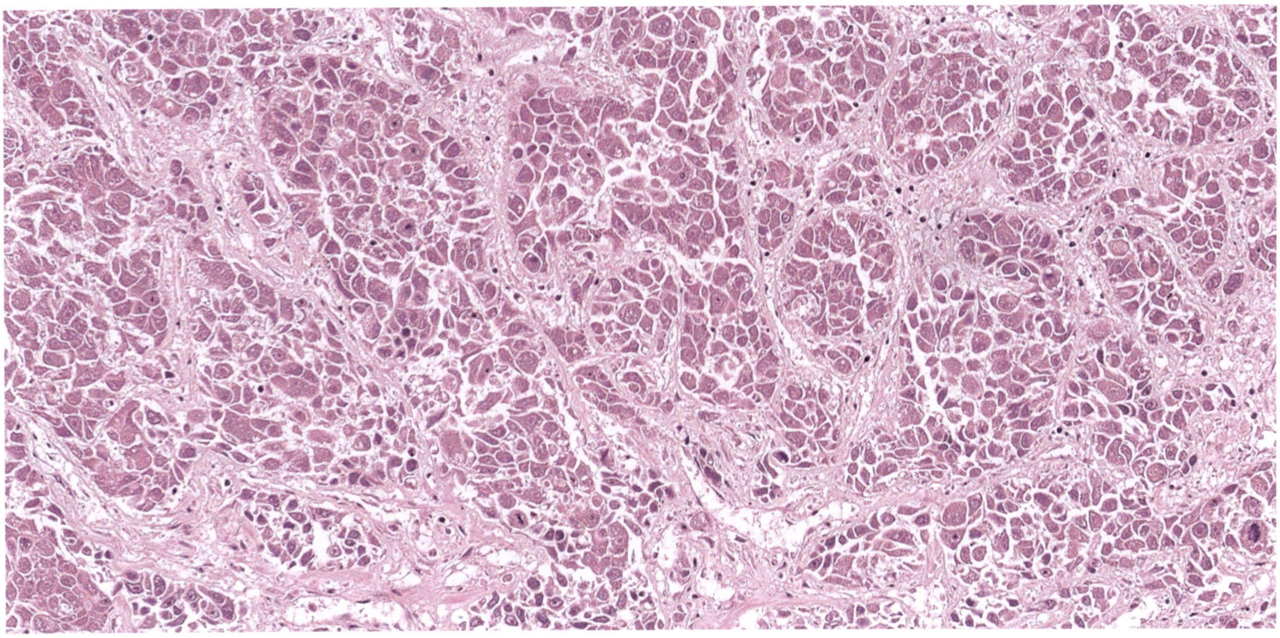

Fig. 14.160 Hepatocellular carcinoma often occurs in the setting of cirrhosis of the liver. The cells resemble normal hepatocytes and different architectural patterns can be seen including trabecular, solid and pseudo-glandular

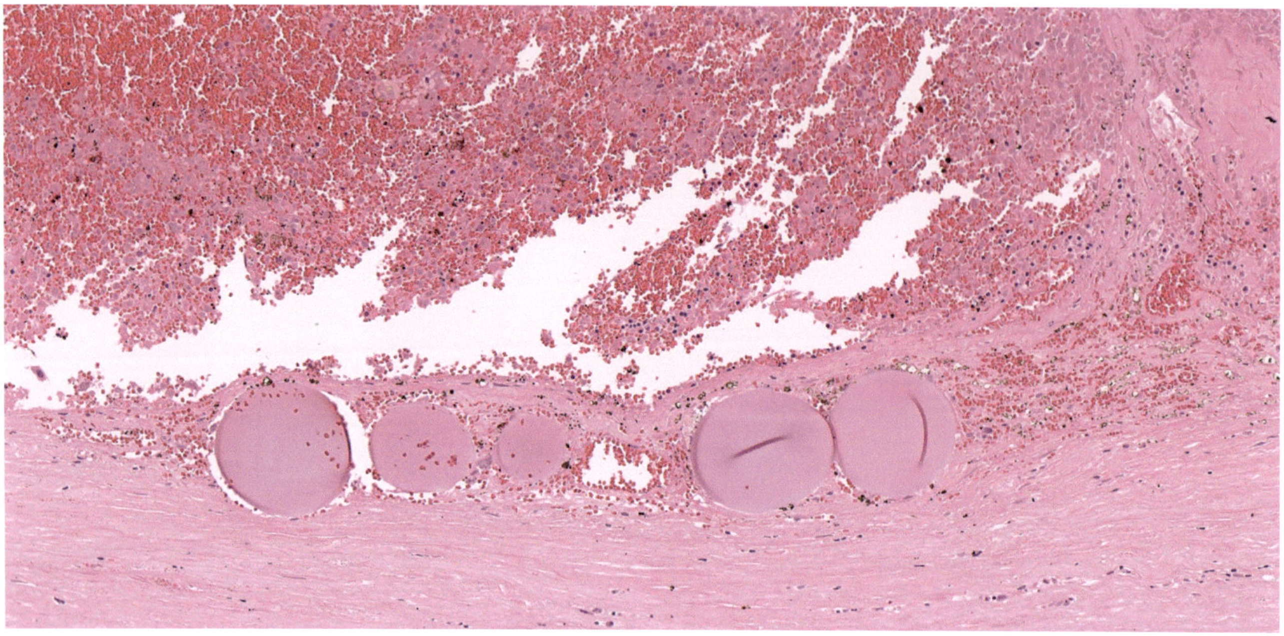

Fig. 14.161 The artefacts of medical treatment may be encountered in autopsy histology. In this case there was chemoembolisation of a hepatocellular carcinoma. In this image there are several round embolisation beads within a vein at the edge of the tumour. As a result of embolisation, the tumour now appears haemorrhagic and necrotic

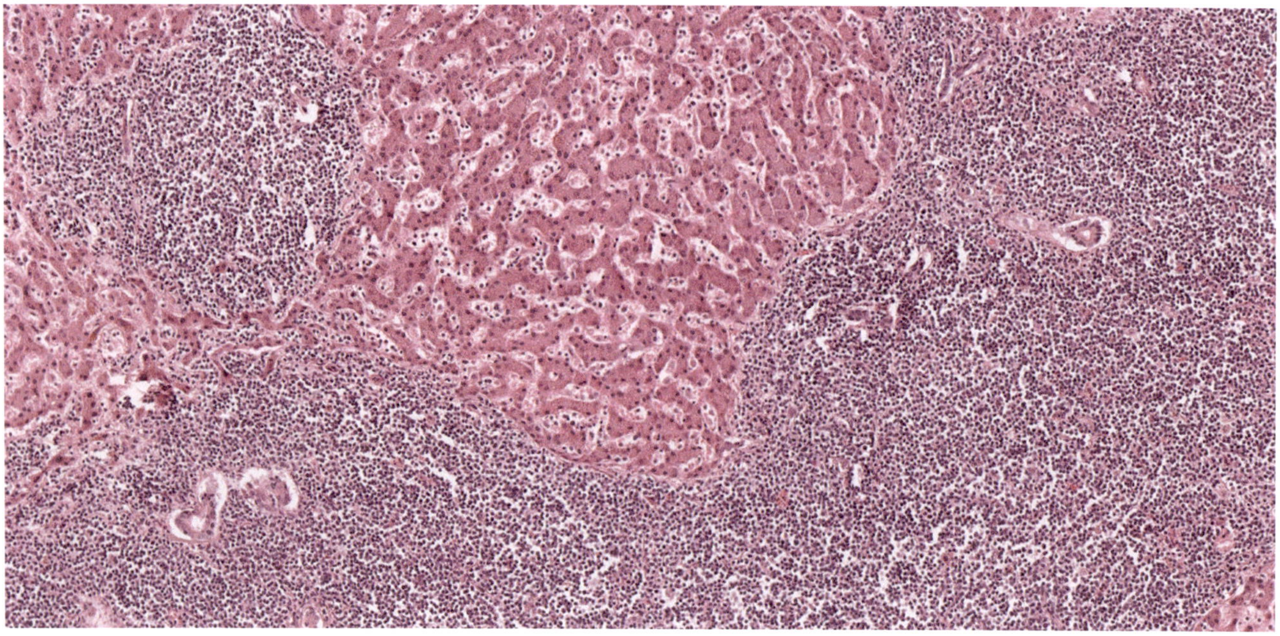

Fig. 14.162 Chronic lymphocytic leukaemia/small lymphocytic lymphoma can involve the liver. This image shows a dense infiltrate of small lymphoid cells in the liver. Precise typing of lymphoma would require immunohistochemistry. However, if there is a known diagnosis this may not be necessary

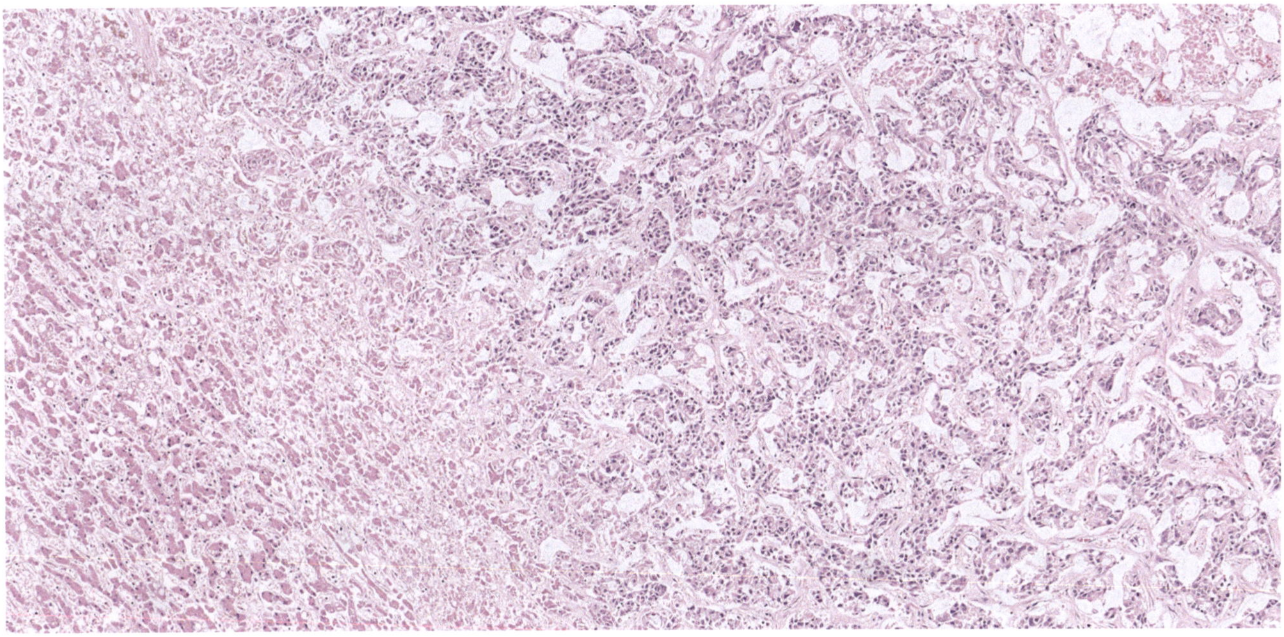

Fig. 14.163 The liver is a common site of metastasis of many tumours, in particular those from the gastrointestinal tract. In this image there is a deposit of tumour which has metastasised from a colorectal adenocarcinoma. Note the gland-forming tumour (adenocarcinoma) on the right side of the image

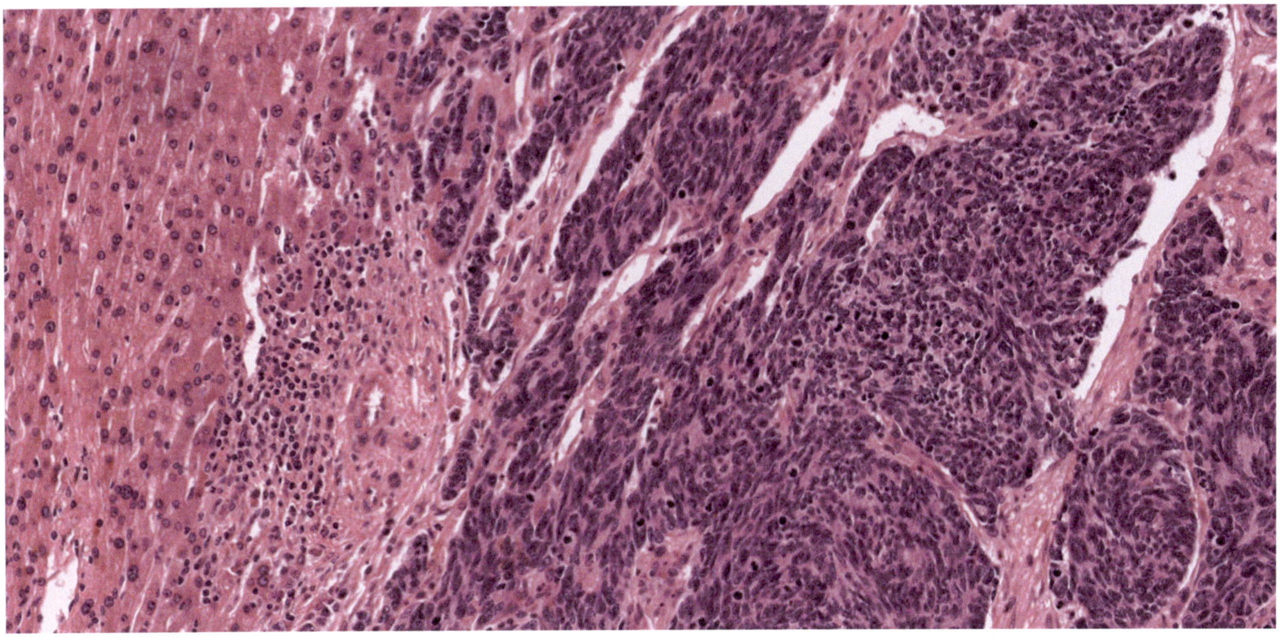

Fig. 14.164 This image shows a metastatic deposit of small cell lung carcinoma. The liver is a common site of metastasis from lung tumours. At autopsy it is often straightforward to identify the primary site of a metastatic tumour, but in some cases the primary site may not be obvious and microscopic evaluation can be helpful to determine the primary site of origin and the extent of tumour metastasis

Pancreas

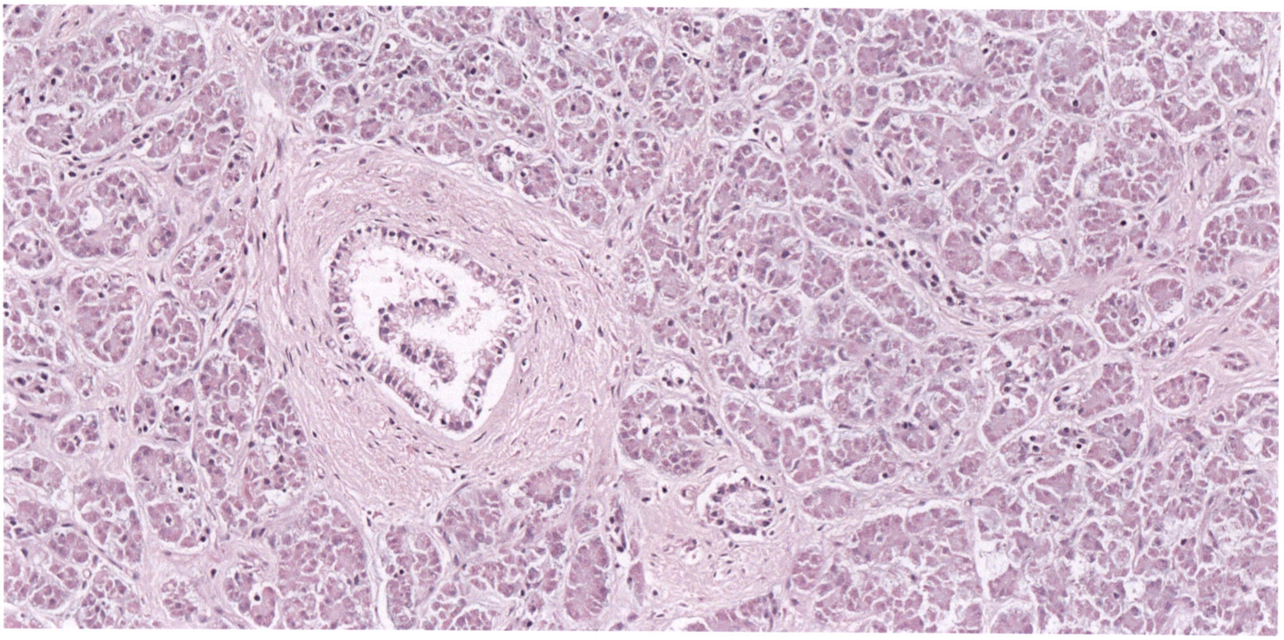

Fig. 14.165 This is normal pancreas. This organ is often affected by autolysis in post mortem histology which can hamper interpretation

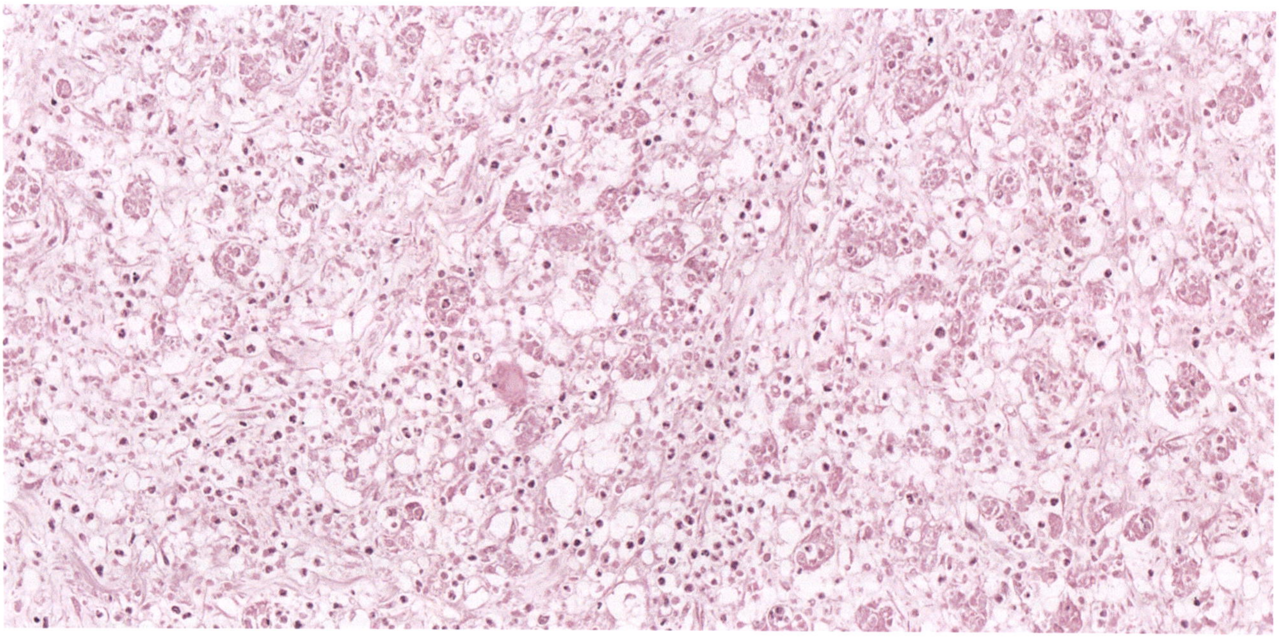

Fig. 14.166 Acute pancreatitis is usually evident to the naked eye, but microscopic confirmation can be helpful and occasionally acute pancreatitis may be identified microscopically when not so obvious macroscopically. In this image there is a neutrophilic infiltrate within the partially autolysed pancreas

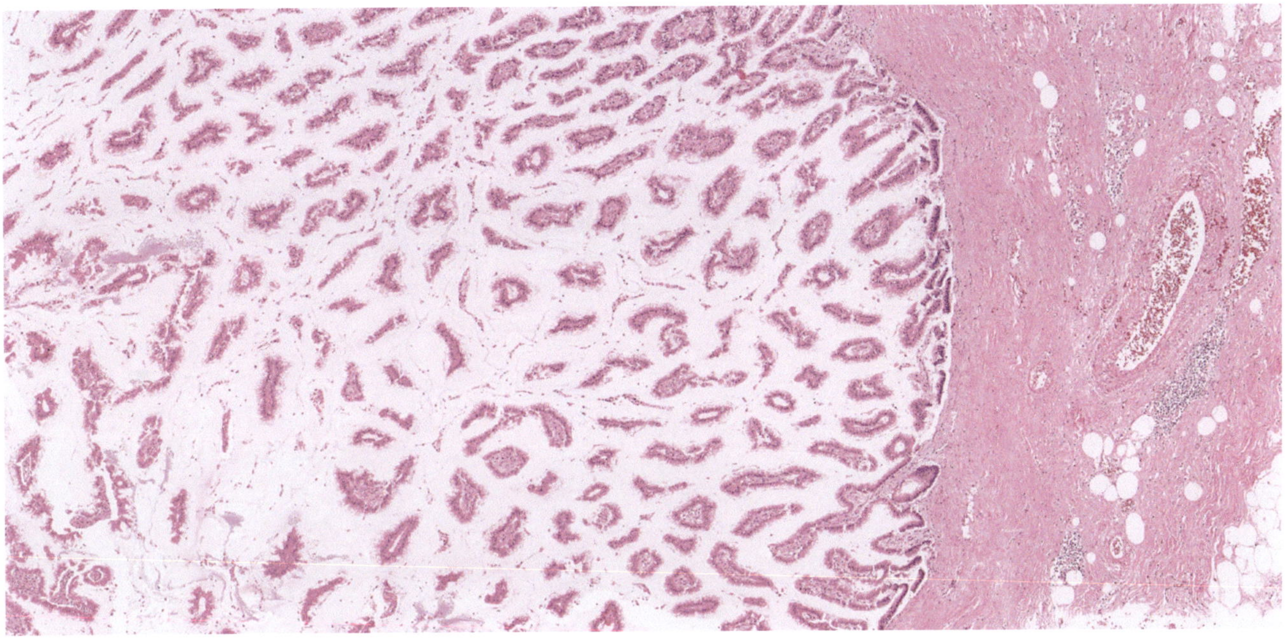

Fig. 14.167 Intraductal papillary mucinous neoplasms are less common than pancreatic adenocarcinomas. They may be confined to the pancreas, as in this case

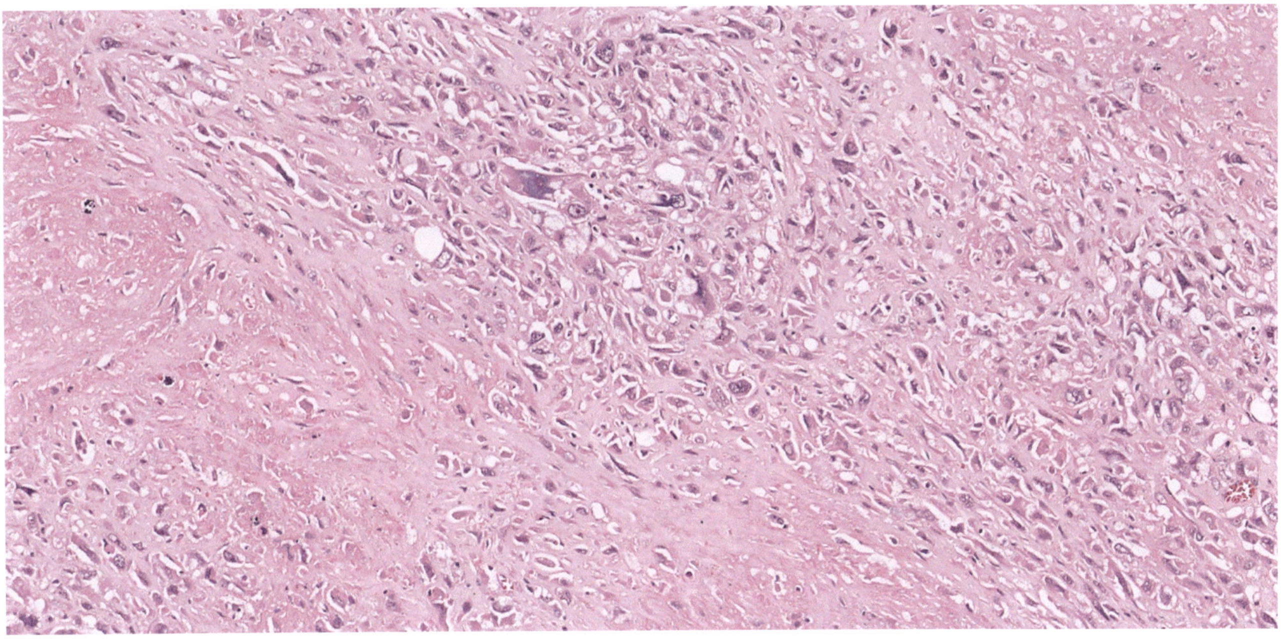

Fig. 14.168 This is an anaplastic carcinoma of the pancreas. Pancreatic tumours often present late and survival is often short. The first presentation may be at autopsy

Genitourinary System

In the autopsy setting, pathology of the kidneys most commonly reflects systemic disease, particularly hypertension, diabetes and vascular disease. A microscopic understanding of the features of these diseases in the kidney is a vital part of the autopsy pathologist's work. Primary conditions of the kidney are less commonly seen at autopsy. Other common pathologies encountered include ascending urinary tract infections, stones and infarcts (consider cholesterol embolism, septic embolism, endocarditis).

The excretory function of the kidney can illuminate systemic conditions such as rhabdomyolysis (excretion of myoglobin), ketoacidosis (typically associated with type 1 diabetes or alcoholism) and poisoning (ethylene glycol or renal papillary necrosis associated with non-steroidal anti-inflammatory drug use).

Tumours of the kidney, particularly renal cell carcinoma, can involve the renal vein with tumour embolism to the lungs being a rare cause of sudden death.

A range of kidney pathologies are shown in Figs. 14.169, 14.170, 14.171, 14.172, 14.173, 14.174, 14.175, 14.176, 14.177, 14.178, 14.179, 14.180, 14.181, 14.182, 14.183, 14.184, 14.185, 14.186, and 14.187.

Kidney

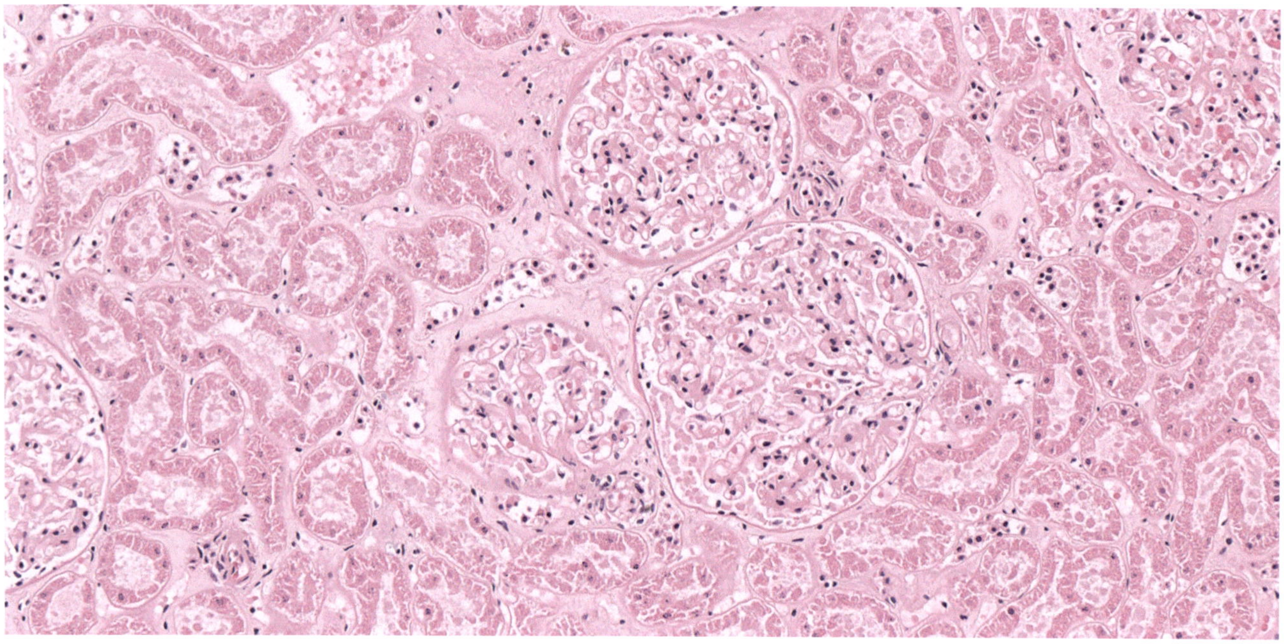

Fig. 14.169 This is normal kidney. In this image there is autolysis of the tubular epithelium. This occurs early in the post mortem period and is commonly seen in autopsy histology of the kidney to a variable degree

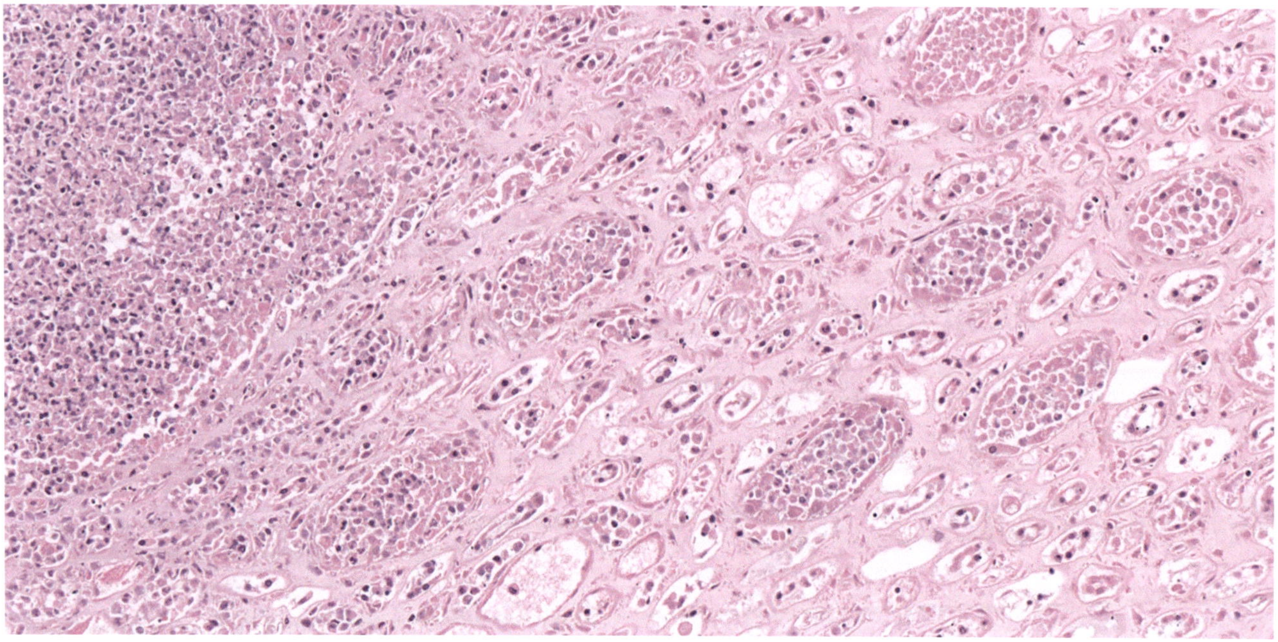

Fig. 14.170 Ascending urinary tract infection can result in pyelonephritis. This may be macroscopically evident but can be picked up as an unexpected finding on microscopic examination. This picture shows an acute inflammatory infiltrate and neutrophil tubule casts

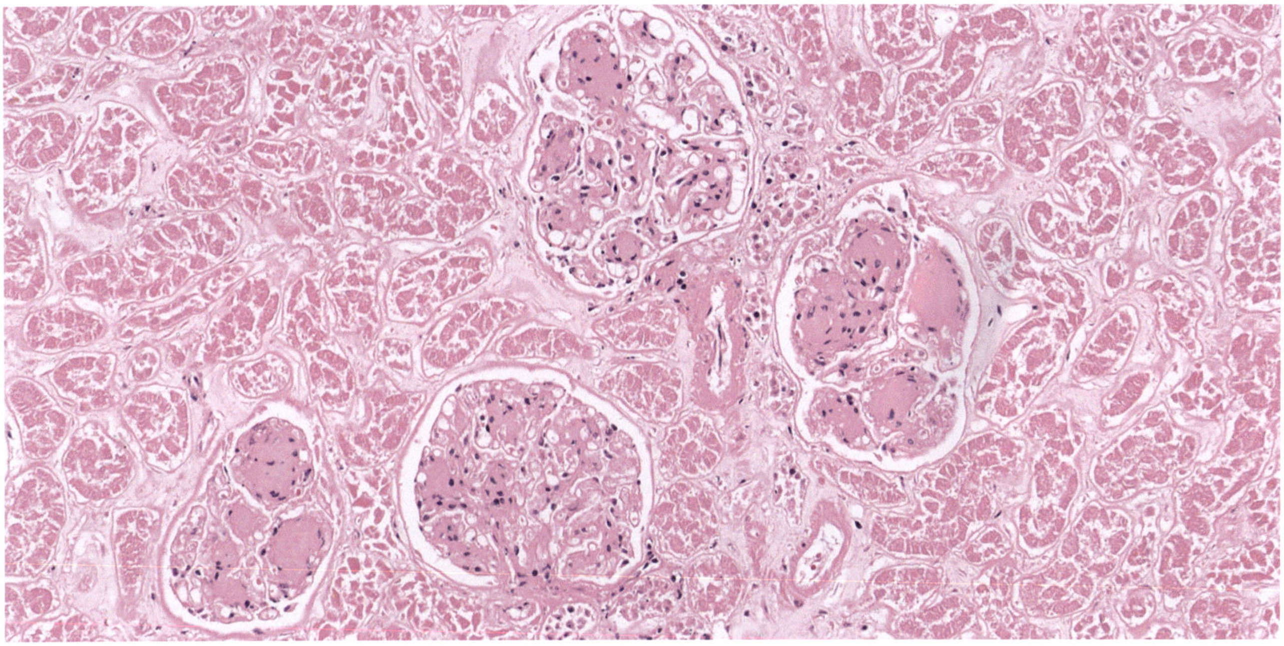

Fig. 14.171 Diabetic nephropathy is commonly seen at autopsy. In this image there is nodular segmental glomerulosclerosis (called Kimmelstiel-Wilson (K-W) nodules when associated with diabetic ketoacidosis) and hyaline arteriolosclerosis. K-W nodules are a classic lesion of diabetic nephropathy. However, several other microscopic features are seen involving vessels and tubules and K-W nodules are not always seen. It is therefore necessary to appreciate the range of histological features in order to recognise diabetic nephropathy (see Figs. 14.172 and 14.173)

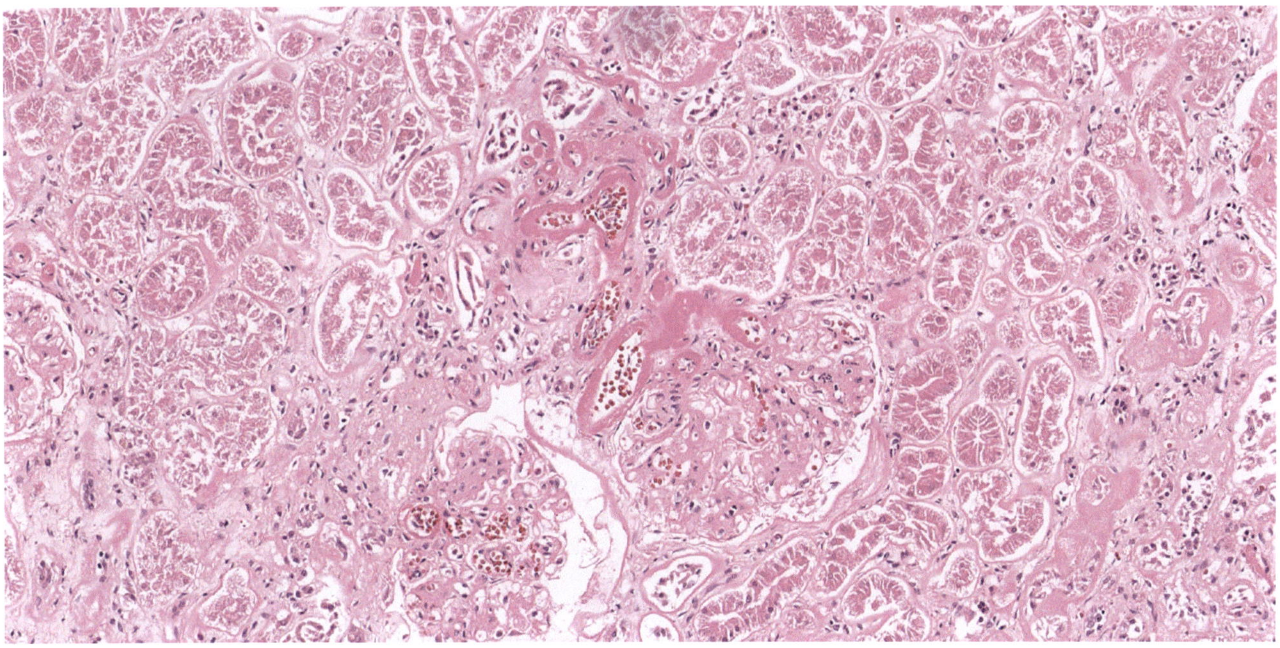

Fig. 14.172 Further features of diabetic nephropathy are shown in this image. There is hyaline arteriolosclerosis, which involves the glomerular capillaries, and afferent and efferent vessels

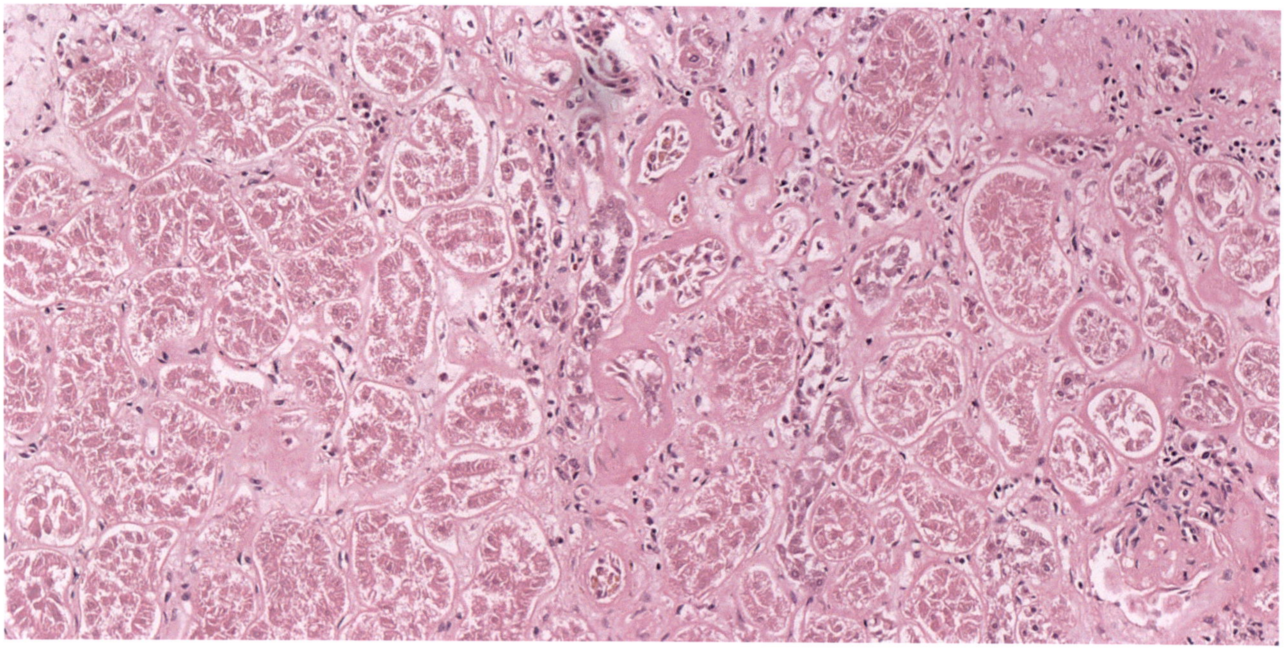

Fig. 14.173 In this image of diabetic nephropathy there is hyaline change of the tubular basement membrane

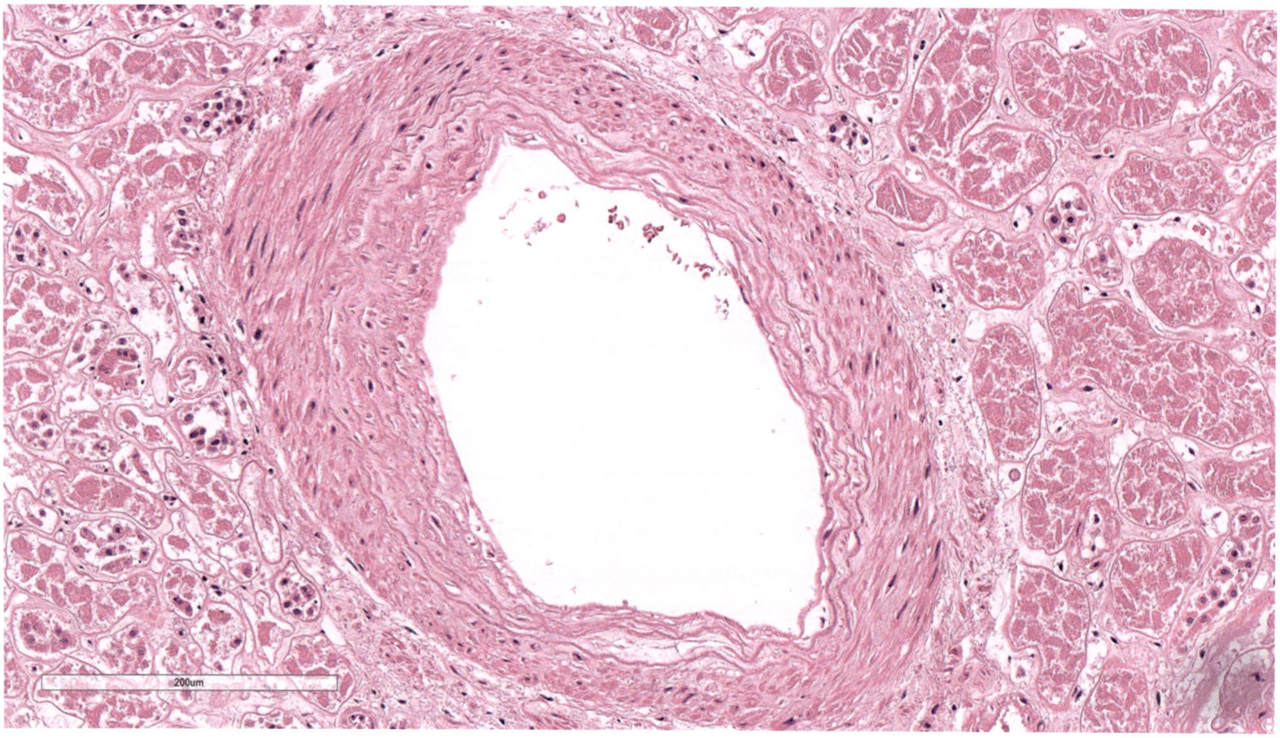

Fig. 14.174 Hypertension is common in countries with a Western diet, including the UK. The effects of hypertension are frequently seen at autopsy, including effects on the heart, kidneys and aorta. Shown here is elastic reduplication due to hypertension in a lobular artery in the kidney. The renal features of hypertension can involve small and large arteries, arterioles and glomeruli

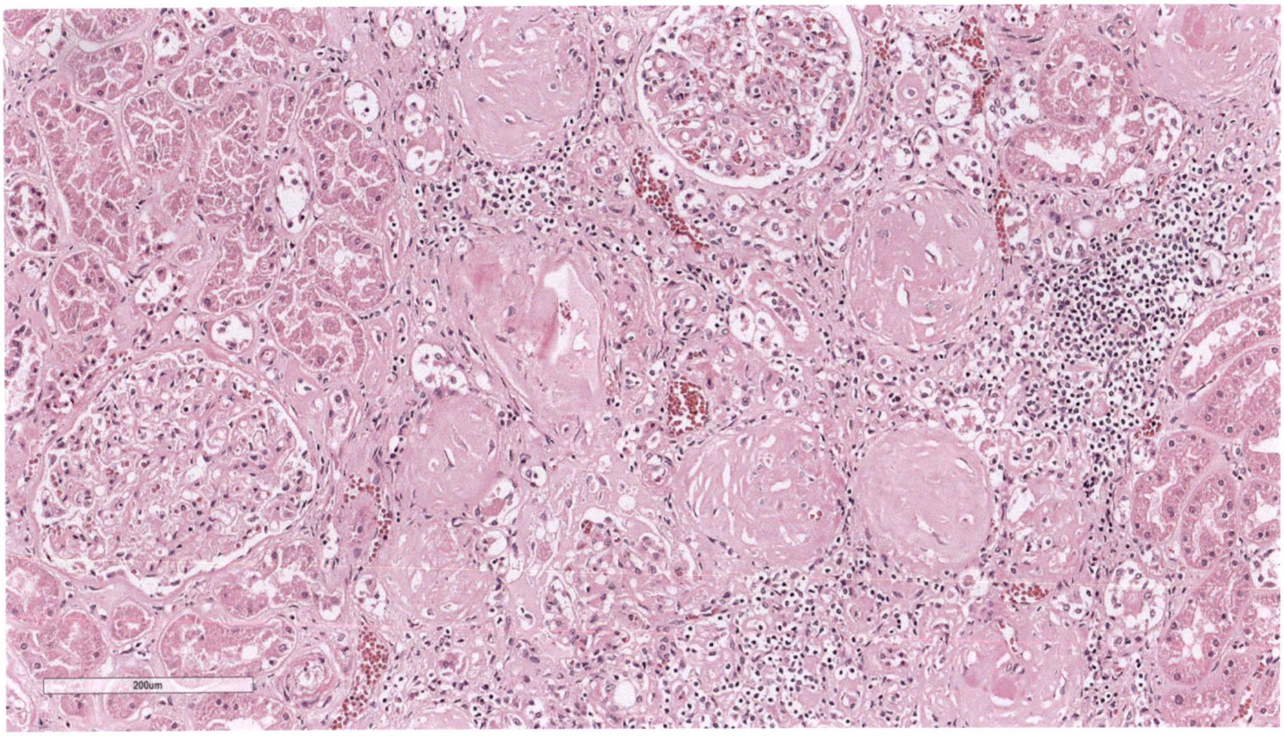

Fig. 14.175 Further features of hypertension are seen in this image in the form of sclerosed glomeruli and cortical chronic inflammation

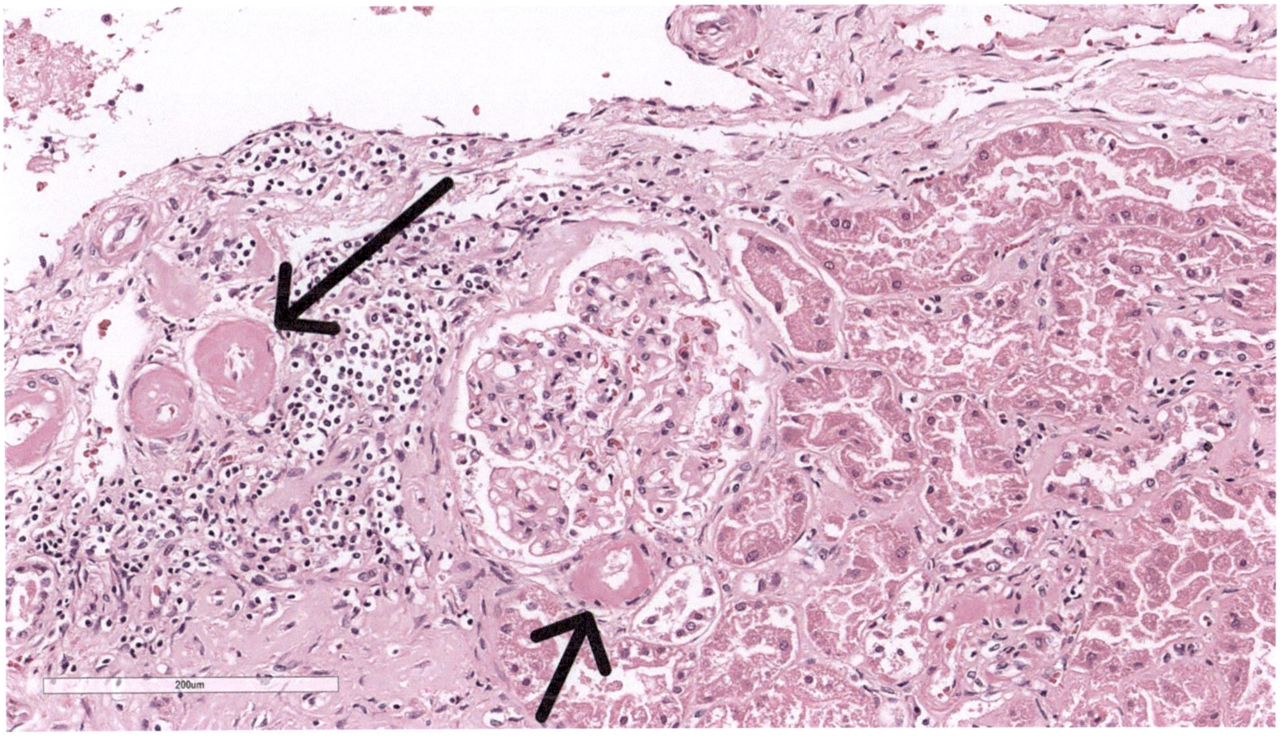

Fig. 14.176 In this image of the kidney in hypertension there is hyaline arteriolosclerosis (arrows)

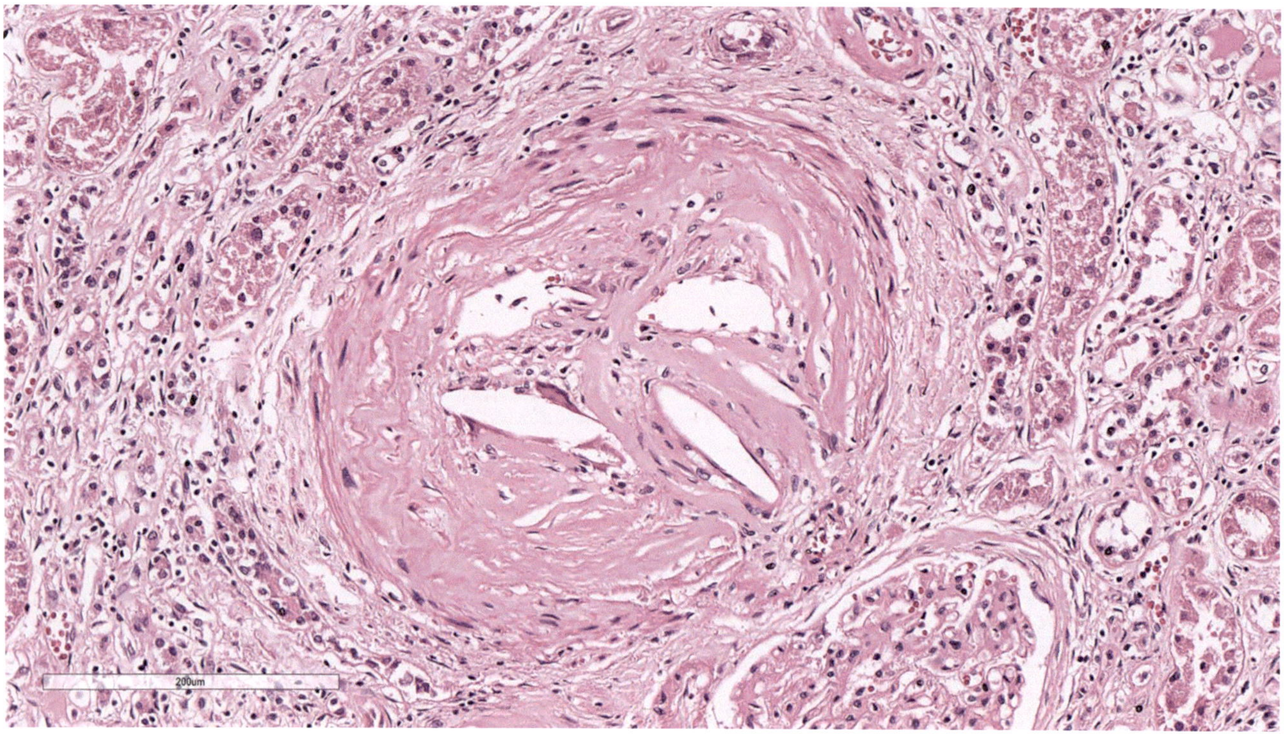

Fig. 14.177 Hypertension is a risk factor for atherosclerosis, and embolism of fragments of atheroma can lodge in end-organs such as the kidney, causing infarction. This image shows such pathology of a near-occluded artery containing a cholesterol embolus. The empty slit-like spaces within the artery lumen represent outlines of cholesterol emboli (dissolved out of the section in the tissue processing) and there is associated giant cell reaction

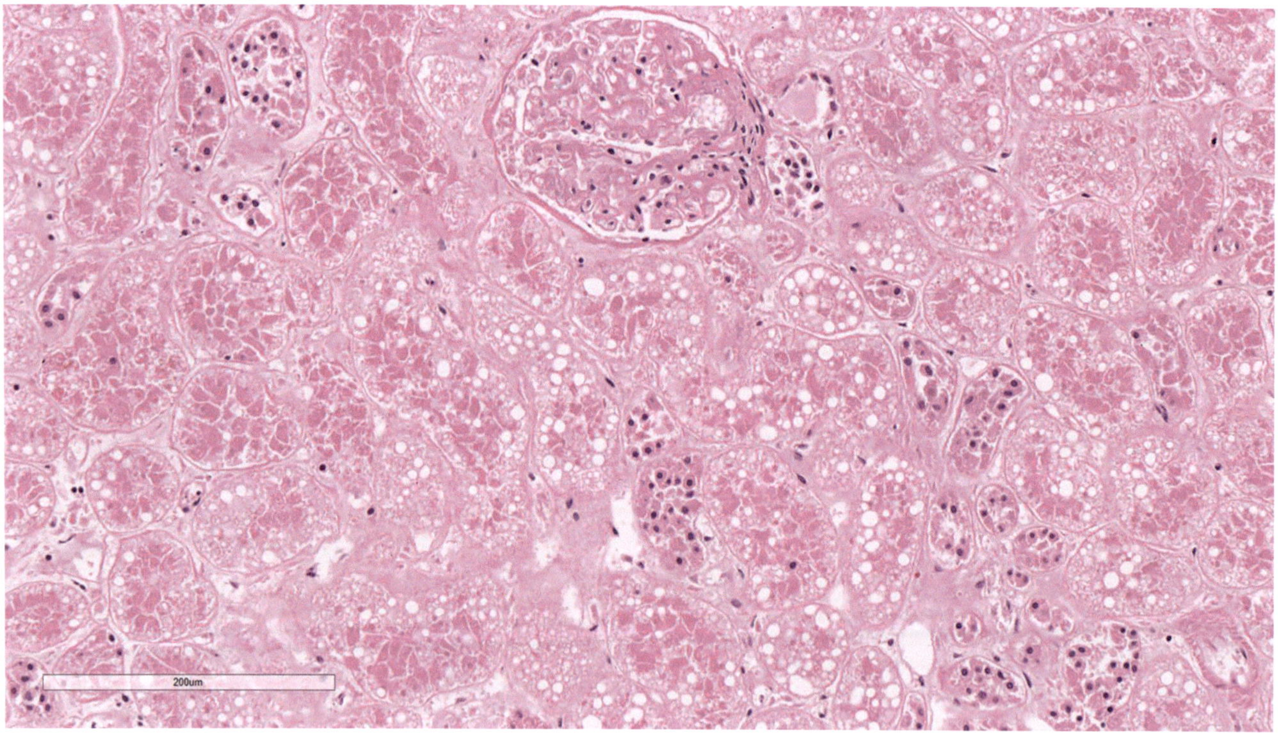

Fig. 14.178 Ketoacidosis is a severe, potentially fatal metabolic derangement, associated with type 1 diabetes, alcoholism and starvation. The typical histological feature of vacuolation of the tubular epithelium is seen here. These changes are called Armanni-Ebstein lesions. Ketoacidosis is confirmed by testing the blood for beta-hydroxybutyrate. A similar microscopic appearance, with vacuolation of the tubule epithelium, is also seen in other causes of acidosis

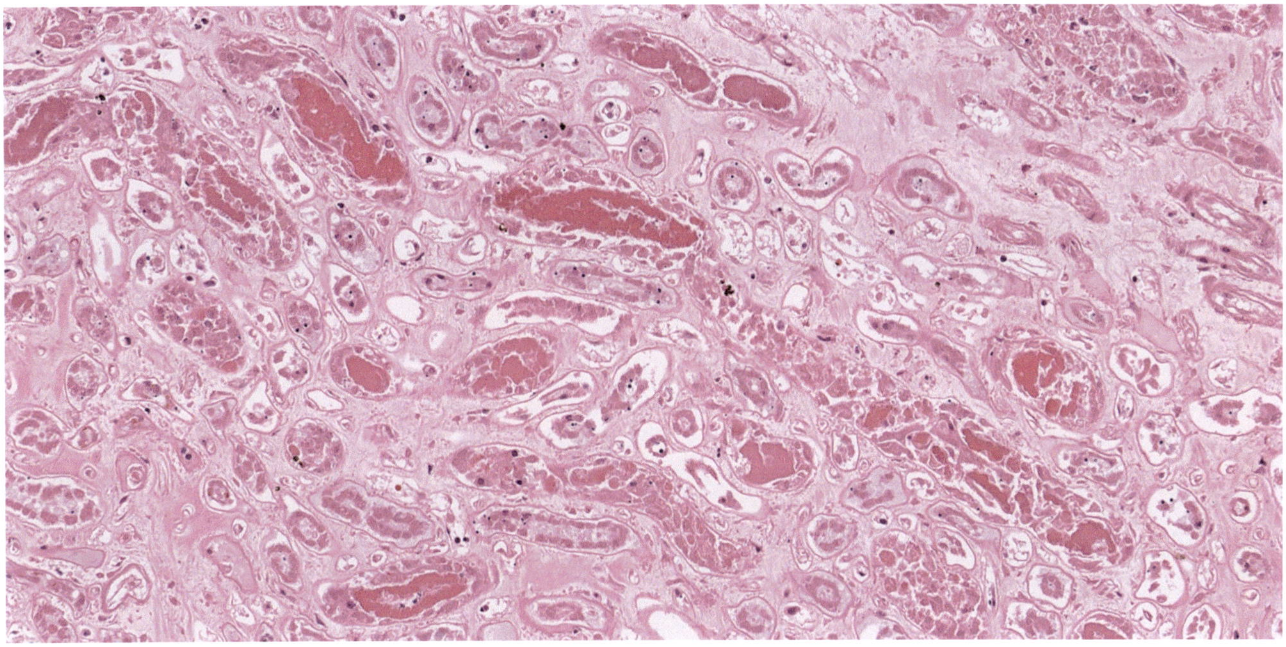

Fig. 14.179 Rhabdomyolysis may be seen in the setting of crush injury, trauma, or associated with some drugs such as statins, antidepressants, cocaine and many more. This image shows the dark red tubule casts of myoglobin

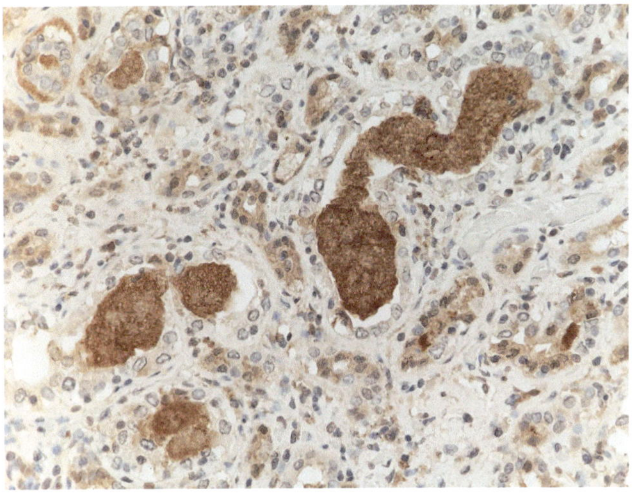

Fig. 14.180 Myoglobin immunohistochemistry confirms the nature of the tubule casts in this case of rhabdomyolysis

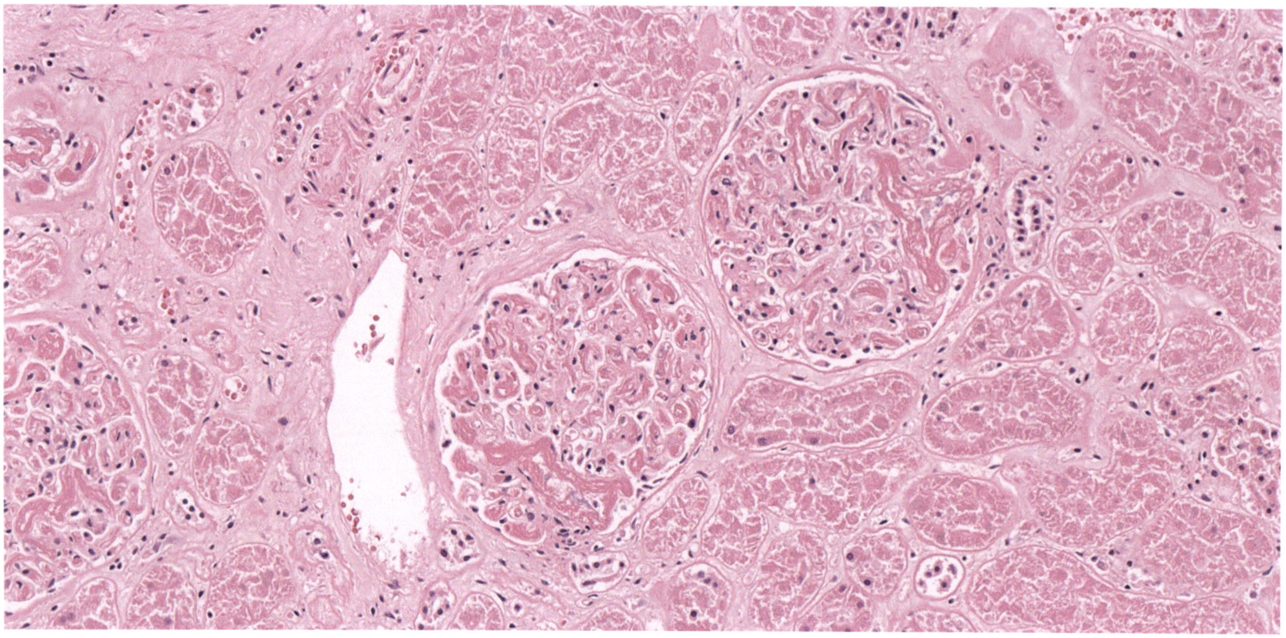

Fig. 14.181 Disseminated intravascular coagulation (DIC) is a systemic activation of the coagulation system which results in multiple microthrombi. These can be seen in multiple organs microscopically, particularly the kidneys, lungs and brain. This image shows these fibrin thrombi within glomerular capillary loops. DIC has many causes including sepsis, malignancy, trauma, liver disease and vascular anomalies

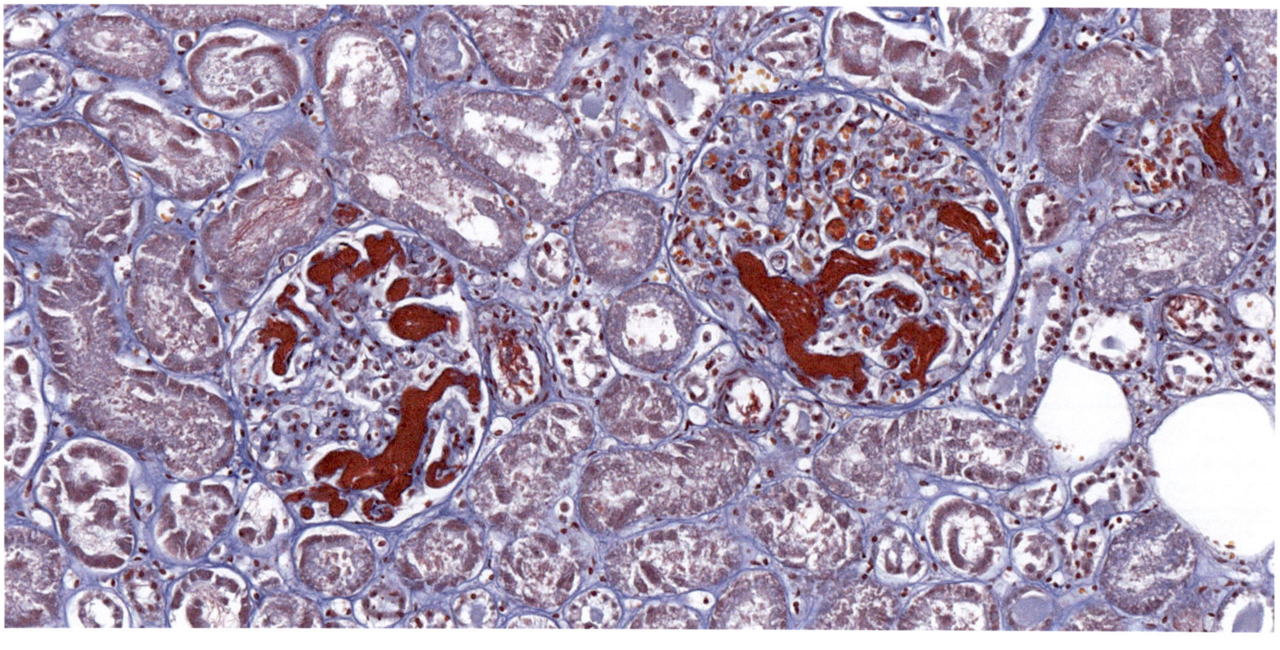

Fig. 14.182 Martius Scarlet Blue (MSB) stain highlights the fibrin thrombi (red) within the glomerulus in this case of disseminated intravascular coagulation

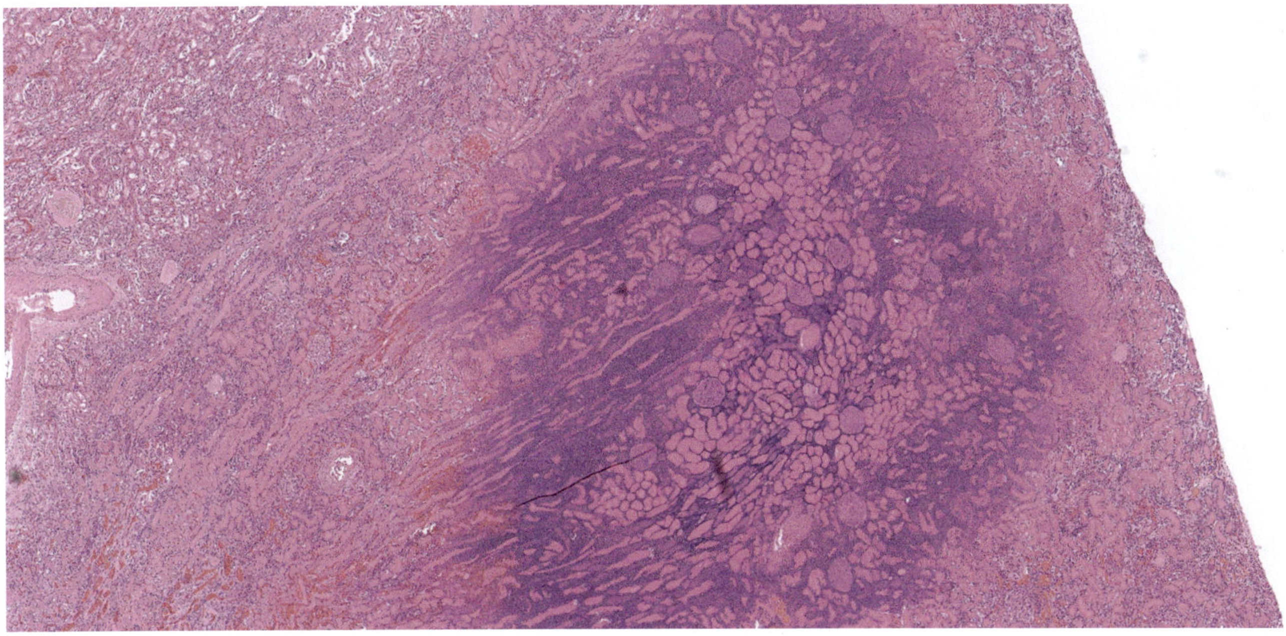

Fig. 14.183 This low power image of a recent renal infarct shows dead tissue with an intense inflammatory reaction and karyorrhectic debris. Renal infarcts can be associated with embolism of thrombi, cholesterol and other material, lodging in end organs such as the kidney, causing infarction

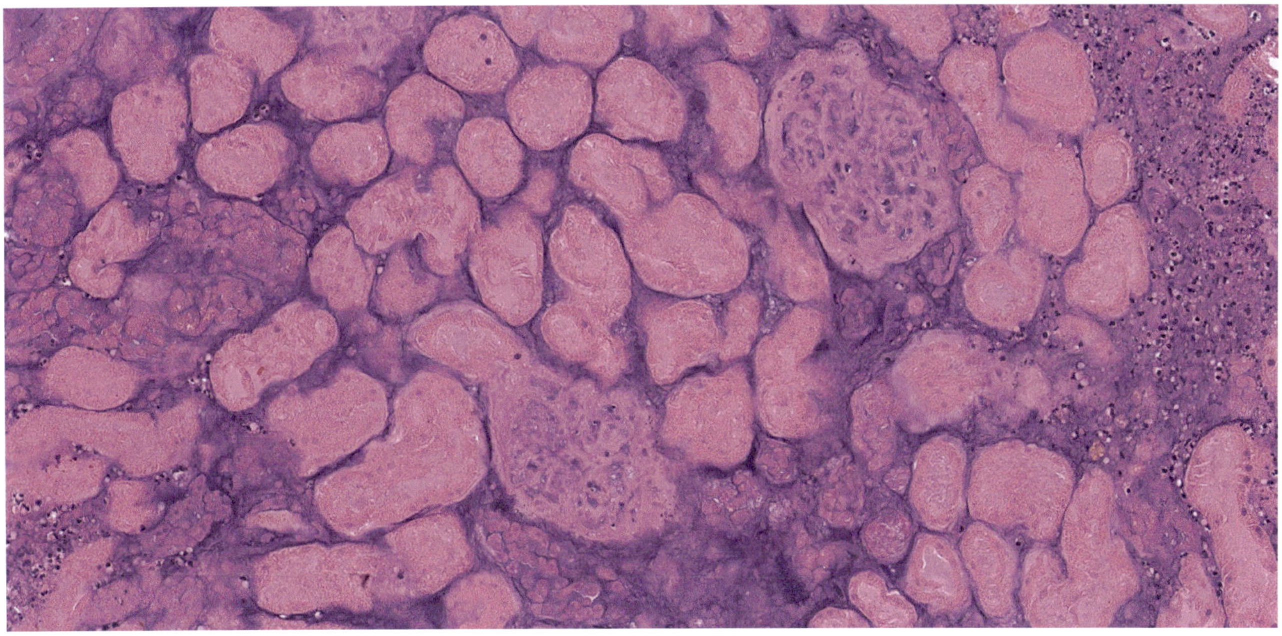

Fig. 14.184 This is a higher power of Fig. 14.183 showing dead tissue with an intense inflammatory reaction and karyorrhectic debris

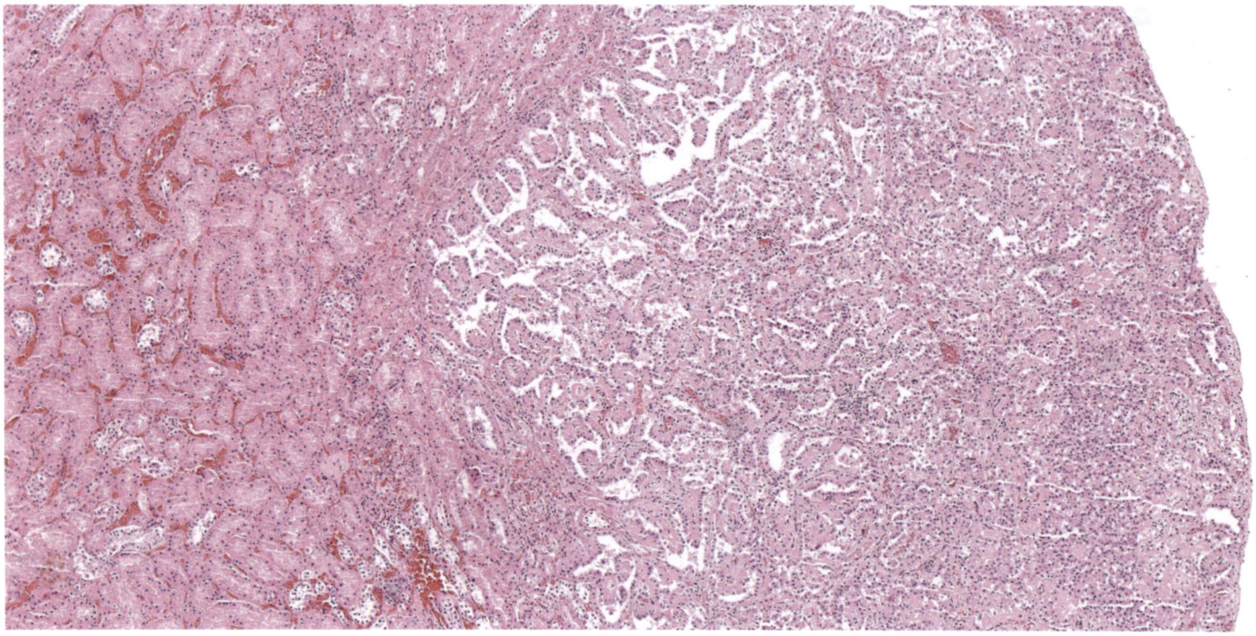

Fig. 14.185 The autopsy pathologist will often encounter lesions in the kidney, such as this papillary adenoma, a common incidental finding at autopsy

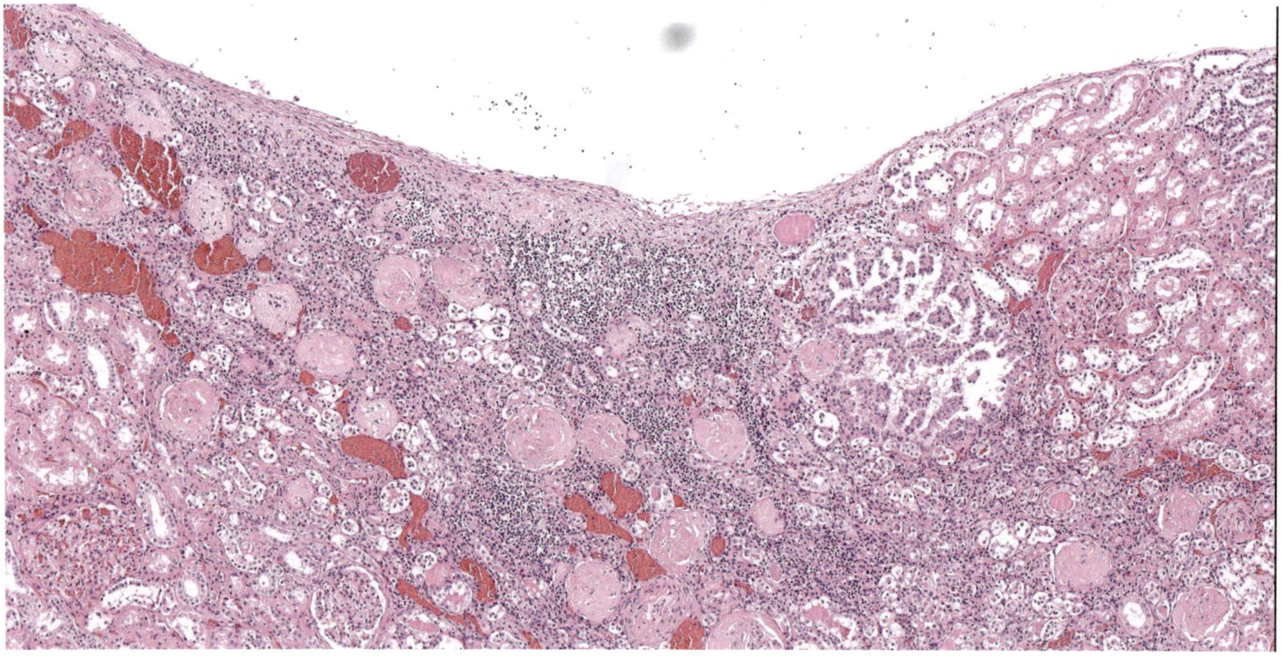

Fig. 14.186 This renal papillary adenoma is associated with a cortical pitted scar. Papillary adenomas are often seen in association with previous renal damage

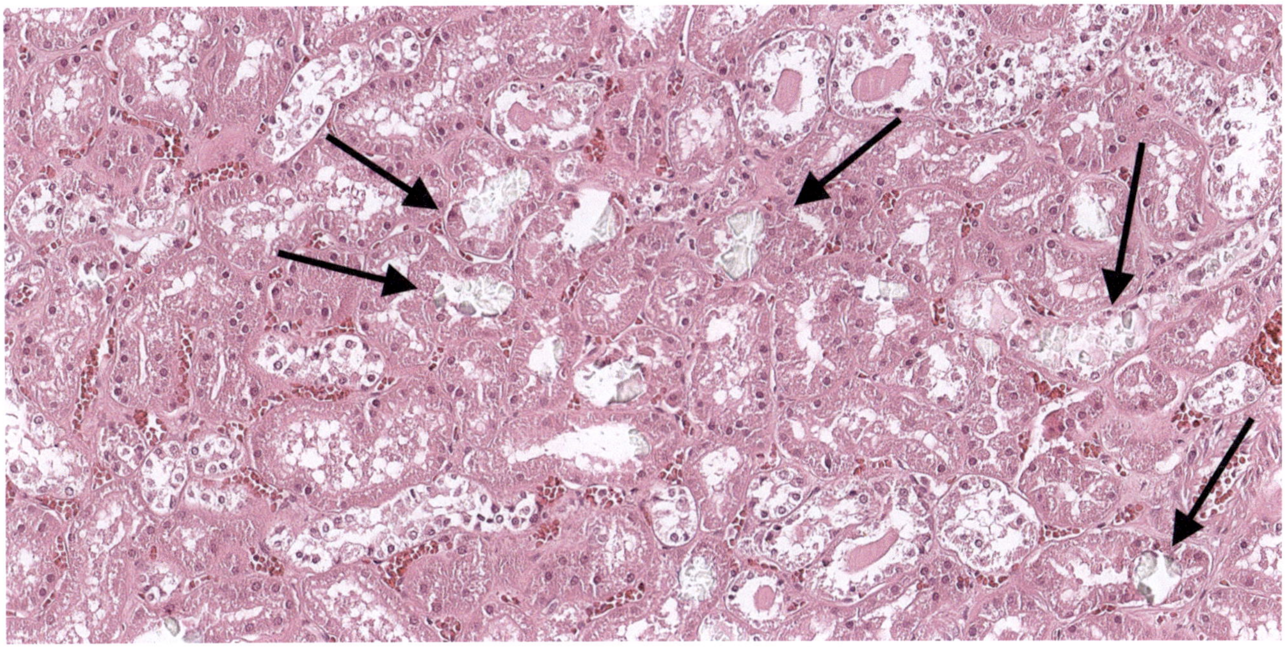

Fig. 14.187 This image of the kidney shows the consequence of ethylene glycol poisoning. There are oxalate crystals visible within renal tubules (arrows). These are birefringent under cross-polarised light

Maternal Death

Maternal death is an uncommon scenario for many autopsy pathologists, particularly in the UK which has a low maternal death rate. The most common causes of maternal death are infections, cardiac disease and thromboembolism. Other pregnancy-associated pathologies include pre-eclampsia, obstetric haemorrhage and amniotic fluid embolism. Histology is an important part of the assessment of the cause of maternal death and may involve sampling organs which are less familiar to the autopsy pathologist, including the uterus and placenta. Examples of pathology encountered in maternal deaths are illustrated in Figs. 14.188, 14.189, 14.190, 14.191, and 14.192.

Maternal Death

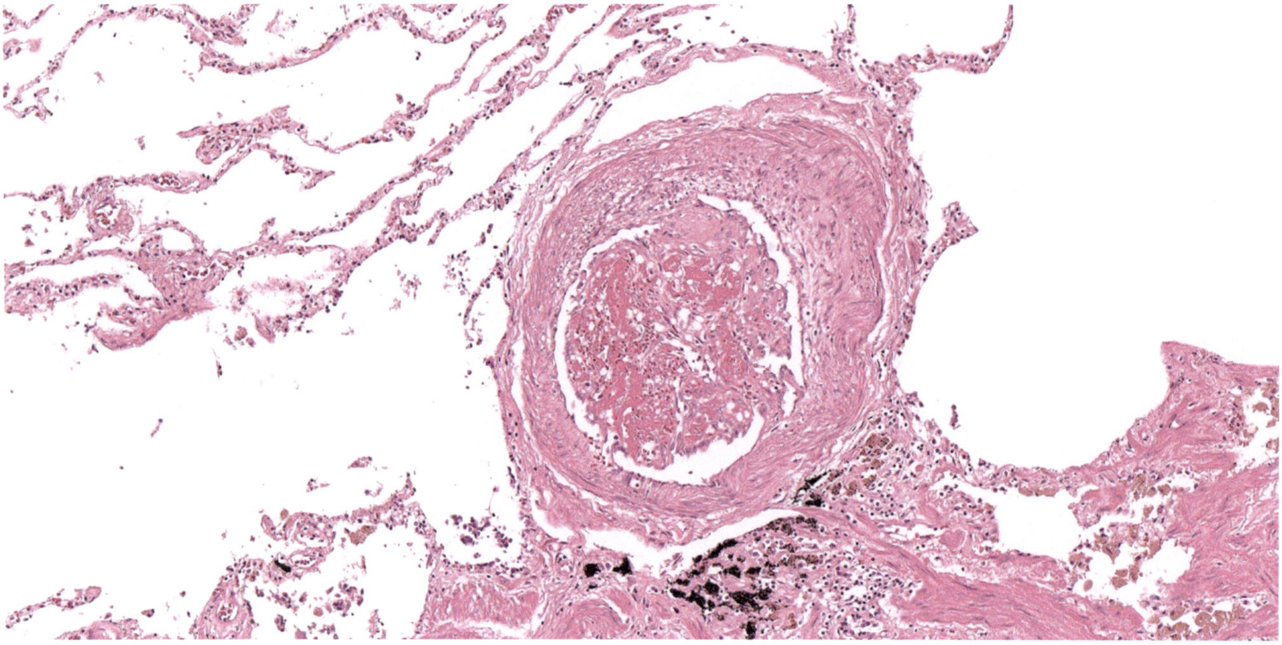

Fig. 14.188 Pulmonary thromboembolism remains a common cause of direct maternal death in the UK. This image shows early organisation of the thrombus to the vessel walls. Histology assessment of pulmonary thromboemboli can be important to assess chronology. See also Figs. 14.112, 14.113 and 14.114

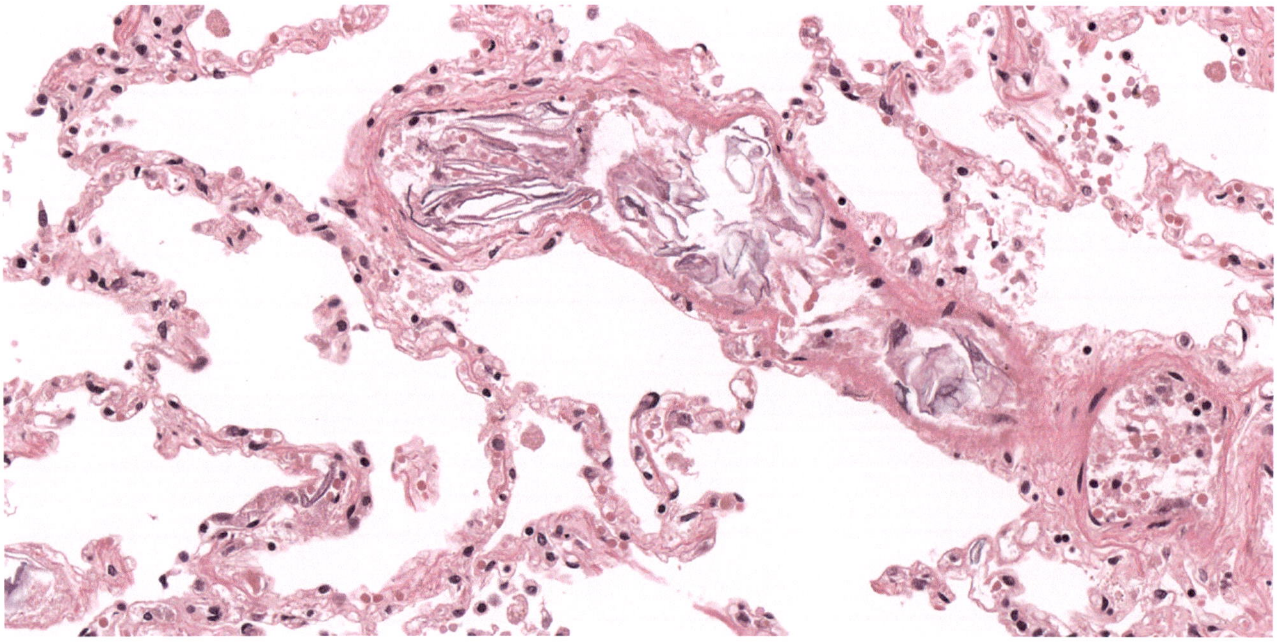

Fig. 14.189 Amniotic fluid embolism is a rare cause of maternal death. In this image fetal squames and mucins are filling the pulmonary arteriole and alveolar capillaries

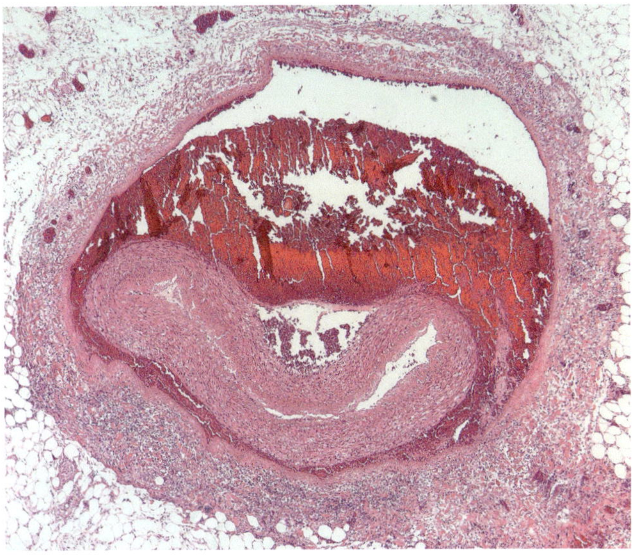

Fig. 14.190 Pregnancy can be associated with coronary artery dissection which causes myocardial ischaemia and infarction and can cause sudden death. The image shows blood tracking within a false lumen, compressing the true artery lumen, causing ischaemia and death

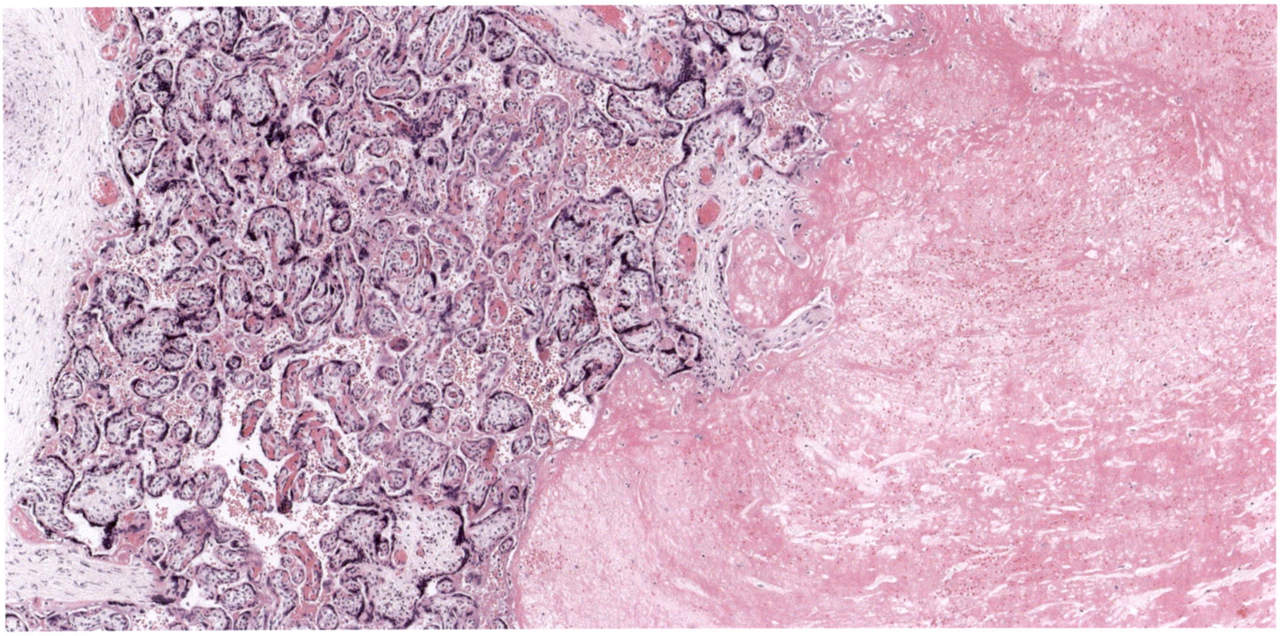

Fig. 14.191 Pre-eclampsia and hypertensive disorders of pregnancy are relatively common and can be an underlying cause of sudden death in late pregnancy. This image shows the effects of pre-eclampsia in the placenta. There is a placental infarct on the right side, a common pathological finding associated with pre-eclampsia. The other important organ to examine in pre-eclampsia/eclampsia is the kidney. Glomerular endotheliosis (mesangial and endothelial cell swelling and hypertrophy) causes narrowing and obstruction of the capillary loops and glomeruli appear bloodless

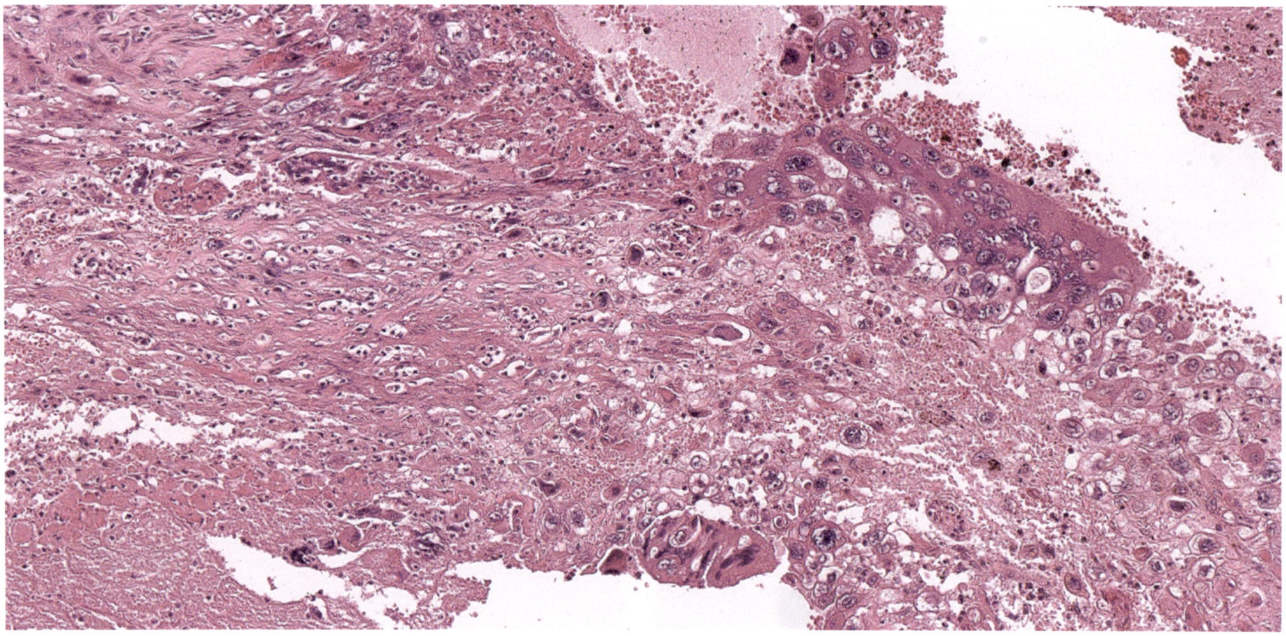

Fig. 14.192 Choriocarcinoma is a highly pleomorphic tumour composed of syncytiotrophoblast and cytotrophoblast cells, as shown here. Haemorrhage and necrosis are frequent. Metastases to the lungs can happen early

Reticuloendothelial System

Pathology of the spleen (Figs. 14.193, 14.194, 14.195, and 14.196) and lymph nodes (Figs. 14.197, 14.198, and 14.199) may be encountered as part of systemic conditions, such as infection-associated splenomegaly, portal hypertension, causing splenomegaly and fibrosis, end organ infarction in conditions such as endocarditis, or haematological conditions, particularly lymphomas involving the spleen.

Metastatic spread of malignant tumour via the lymphatics may be evident macroscopically and microscopic examination of the lymph nodes may confirm the extent of dissemination.

Spleen

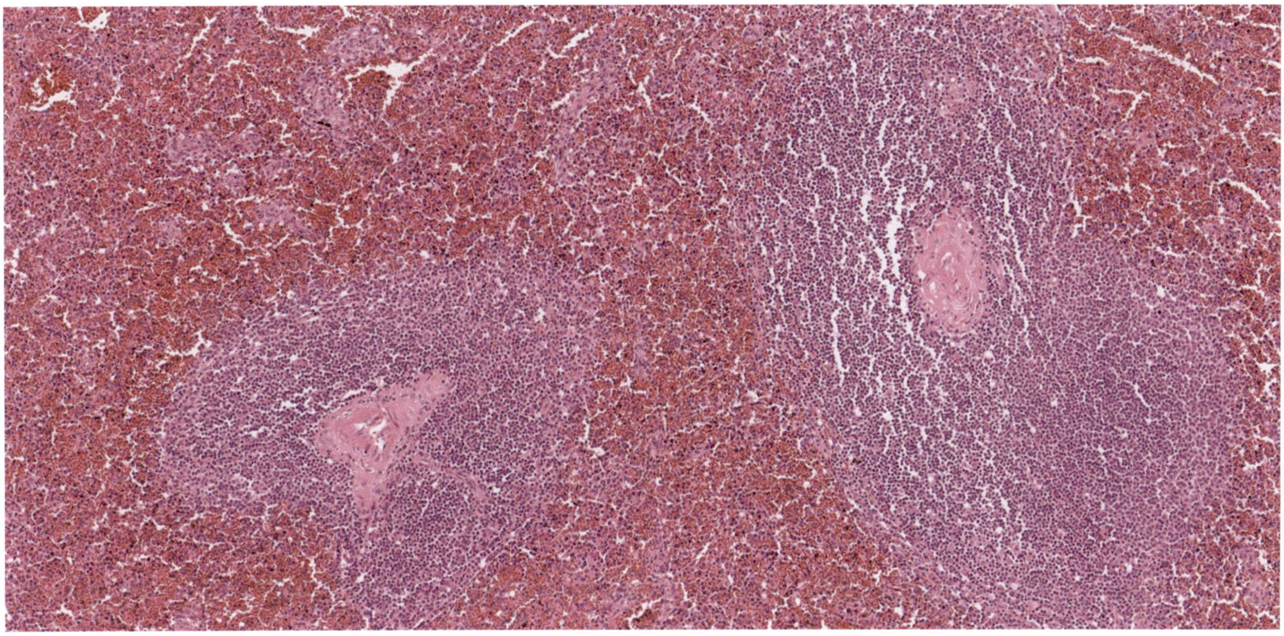

Fig. 14.193 This image shows normal spleen. Note the periarteriolar lymphoid sheath (white pulp) and red pulp

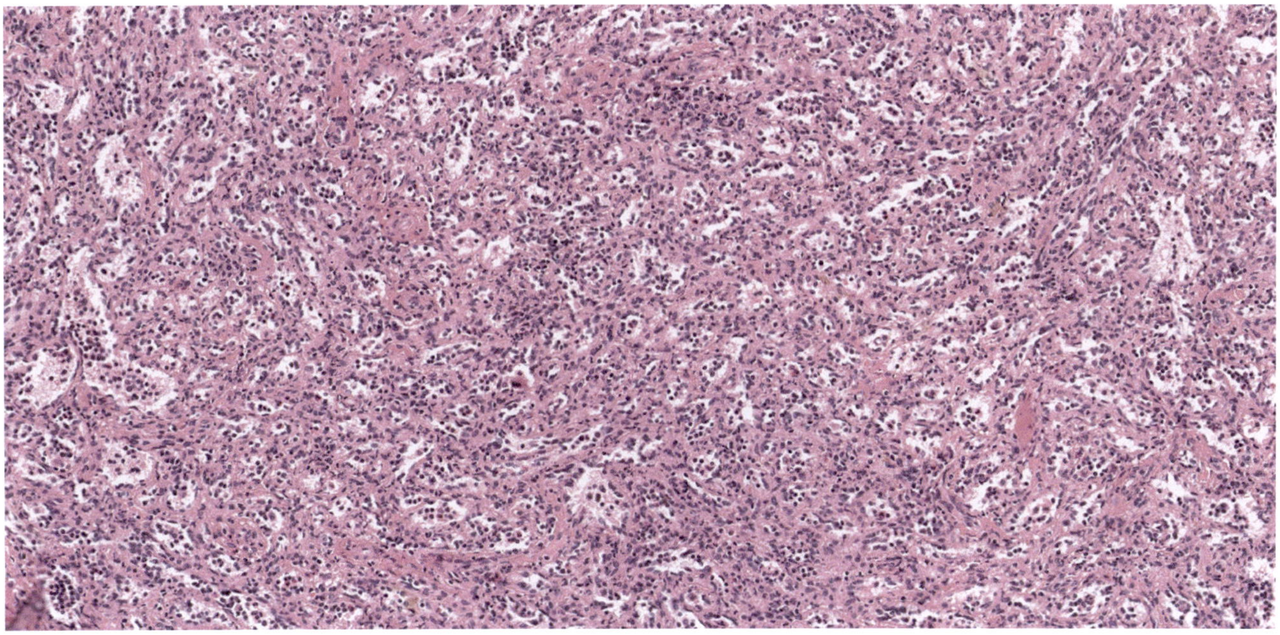

Fig. 14.194 In portal hypertension due to chronic liver disease it is common to see splenomegaly and fibrotic change of the red pulp. This image shows fibrotic change of the red pulp cords

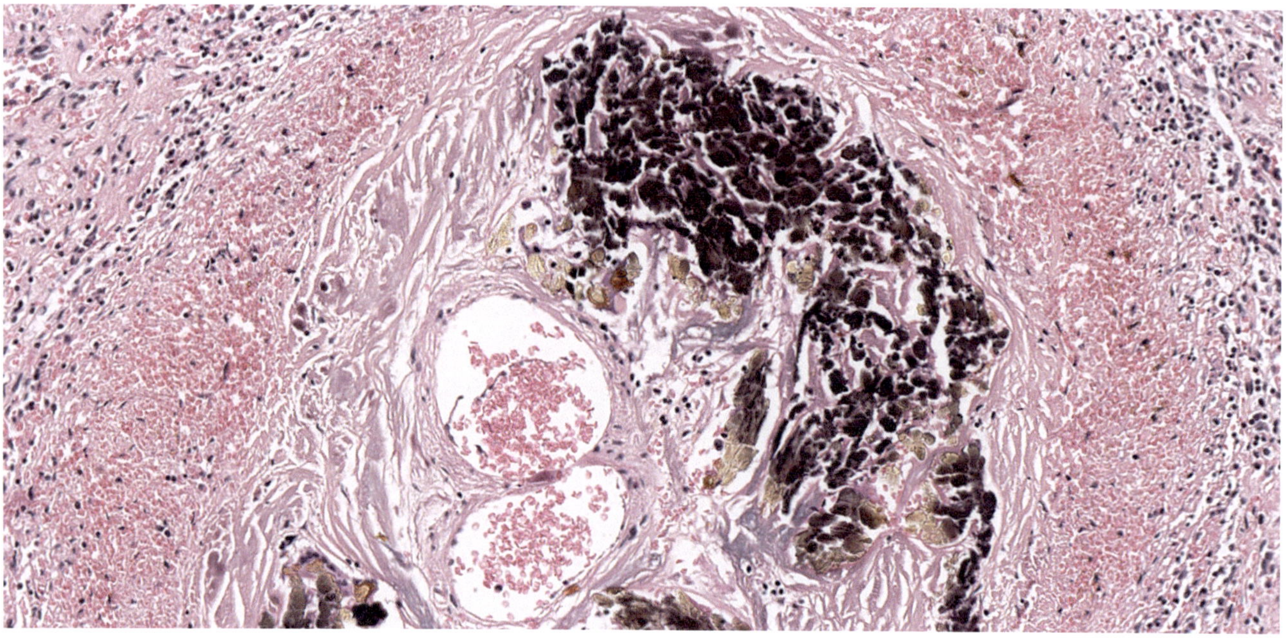

Fig. 14.195 This is a Gamna-Gandy body, a non-specific nodule of iron, calcium and other deposits seen in the spleen in association with portal hypertension, sickle cell disease and other diseases

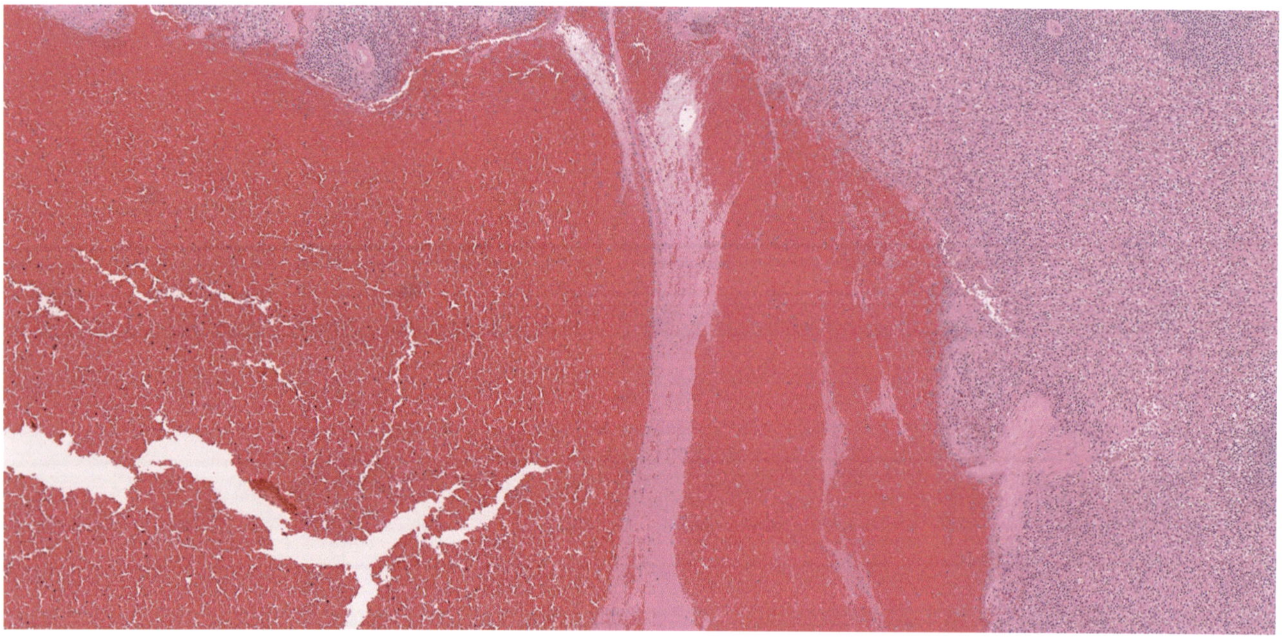

Fig. 14.196 The spleen is vulnerable to rupture in traumatic injury. Microscopic examination of the capsule may reveal a vital reaction if the rupture occurred some time before death

Lymph Node

The spleen is also a frequent casualty of trauma, although spontaneous or traumatic rupture of the spleen may be associated with underlying splenic pathology, and histology can be vital in establishing such a diagnosis.

Lymphomas may present for the first time at autopsy. Precise typing of a newly diagnosed lymphoma will require immunohistochemistry and referral to a lymphoma specialist would be prudent. Infections such as tuberculosis, EBV and HIV can cause dramatic lymphadenopathy and histological examination may point towards the causative agent.

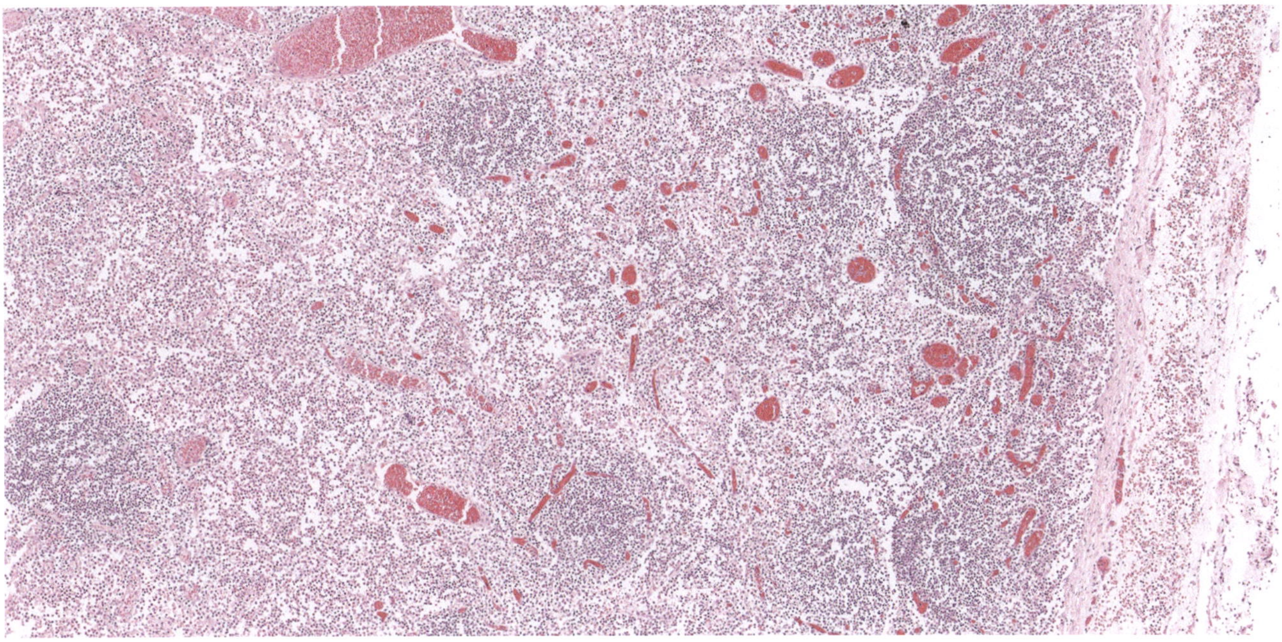

Fig. 14.197 This image shows normal lymph node. Autolysis often affects lymph node histology in the post mortem period

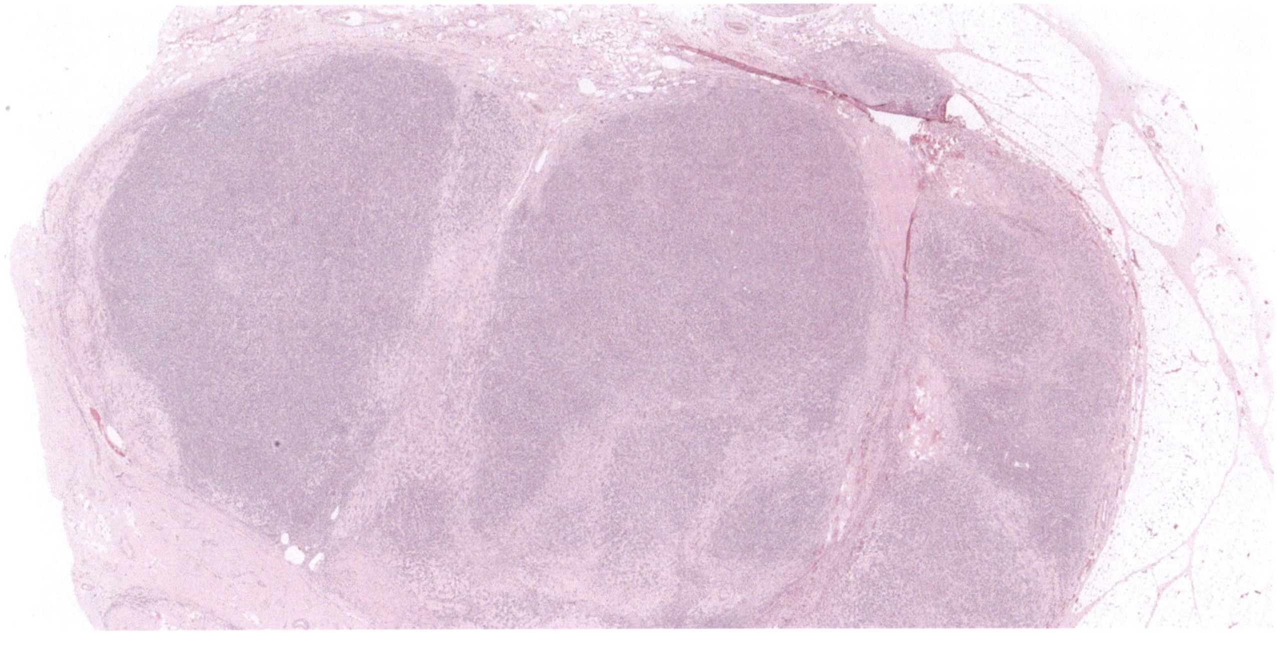

Fig. 14.198 Lymphadenopathy may be encountered at autopsy and microscopic examination is helpful to determine the pathological cause. In this image of nodular sclerosing Hodgkin lymphoma the lymph node is traversed by broad bands of fibrosis. Precise typing of lymphomas requires immunohistochemistry

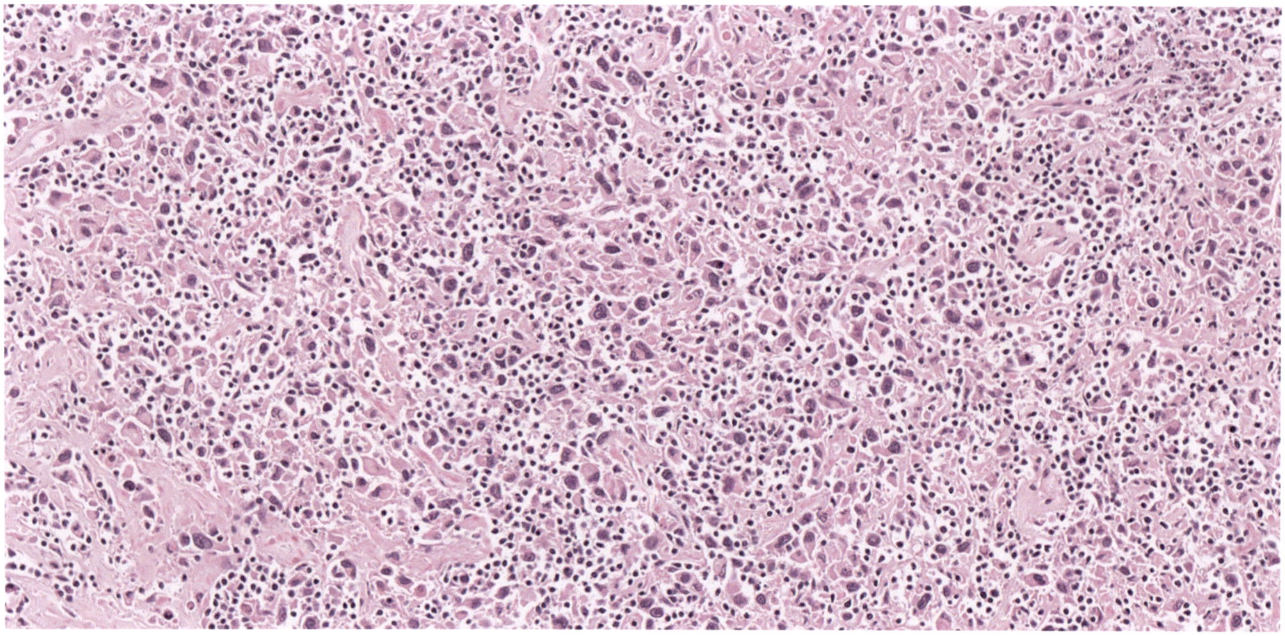

Fig. 14.199 In this higher power view of Fig. 14.198 there is effacement of the architecture and replacement by an infiltrate containing numerous Hodgkin cells and Reed-Sternberg cells

Endocrine System

Endocrine causes of death are quite rare. However, they are encountered frequently enough for the pathologist to require a good understanding of endocrine pathology and proficiency in microscopic diagnosis.

For example, Addisonian crisis can occur related to an underlying endocrine disorder or due to another pathological process overwhelming the adrenal gland, such as bilateral adrenal haemorrhage or tumour metastasis.

Tumours of the adrenal gland are most commonly an incidental finding. However, the association between phaeochromocytoma and high blood pressure may mean the tumour can be linked to cardiac, cerebral or vascular causes of death.

Thyroid gland pathology is common, particularly hypothyroidism. Histology of the thyroid can help distinguish between neoplastic and non-neoplastic disease when a mass is identified macroscopically. Anaplastic tumours can cause respiratory compromise and result in fairly rapid death requiring autopsy diagnosis via microscopy.

Figures 14.200, 14.201, 14.202, 14.203, 14.204, 14.205, 14.206, 14.207, and 14.208 illustrate some pathologies encountered in the adrenal glands and thyroid gland.

Adrenal Gland

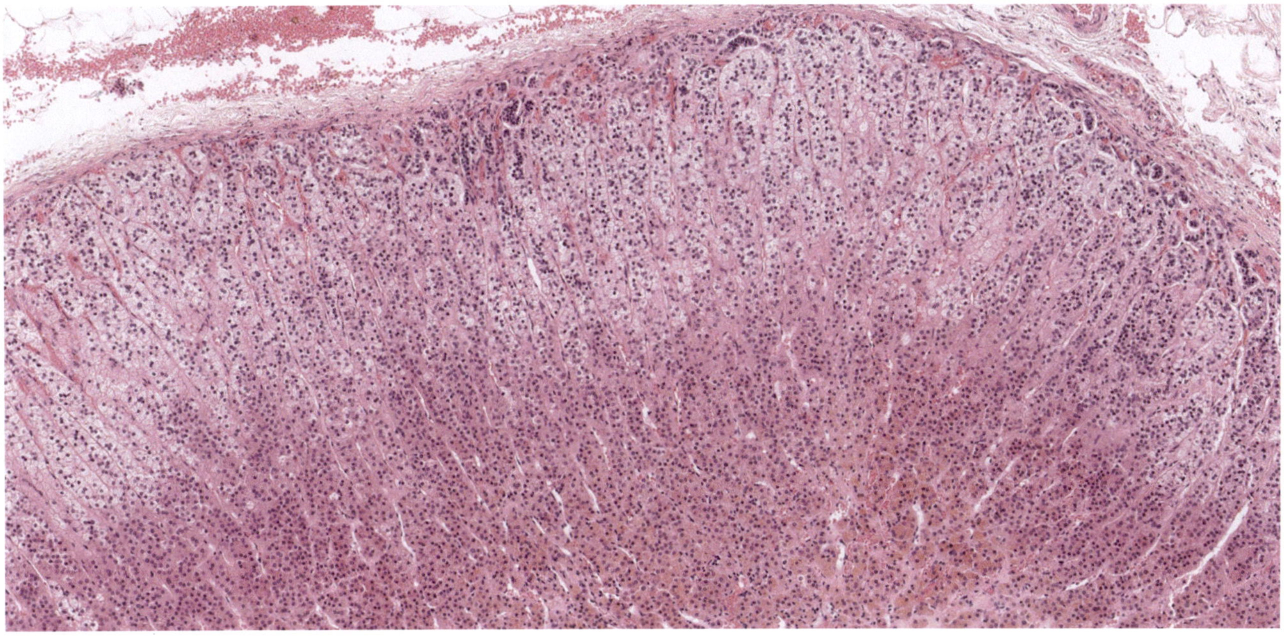

Fig. 14.200 This image shows normal adrenal gland. The normal layers of the gland are seen from the outermost zona glomerulosa, to the zona fasciculata and zona reticularis

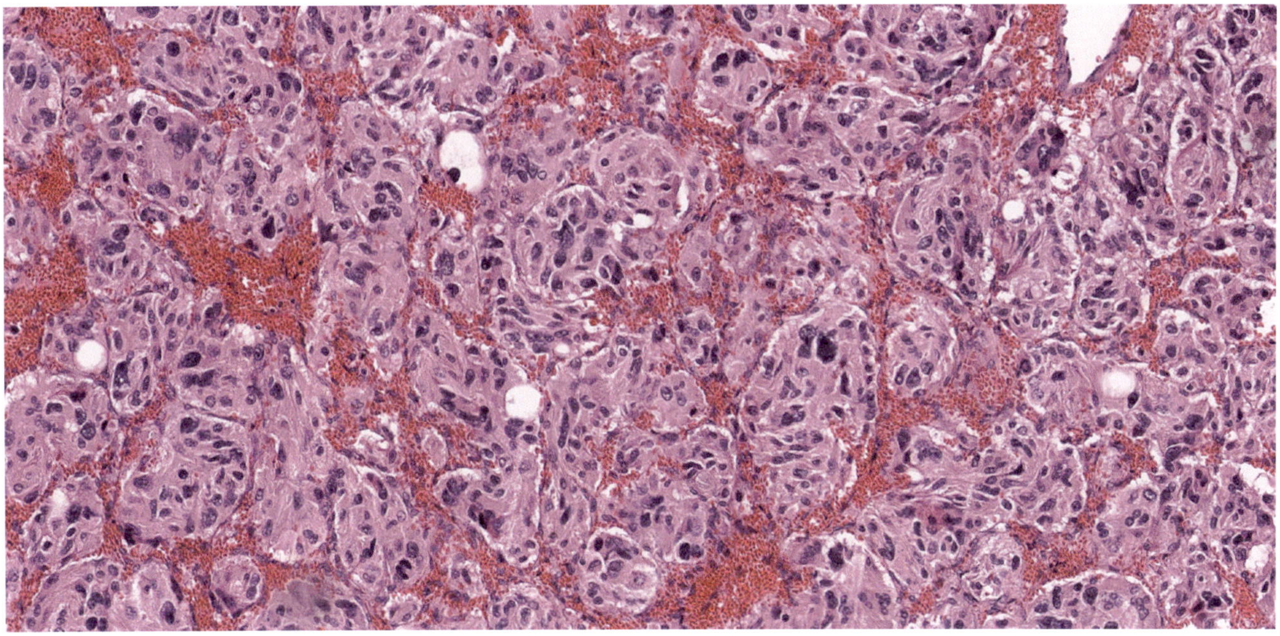

Fig. 14.201 Tumours in the adrenal gland may be primary or metastatic. This is a phaeochromocytoma, a primary adrenal tumour. There are nests of tumour cells with marked "endocrine atypia". Phaeochromocytomas may be linked to hypertension and may therefore be implicated in cardiac, cerebral or vascular causes of death

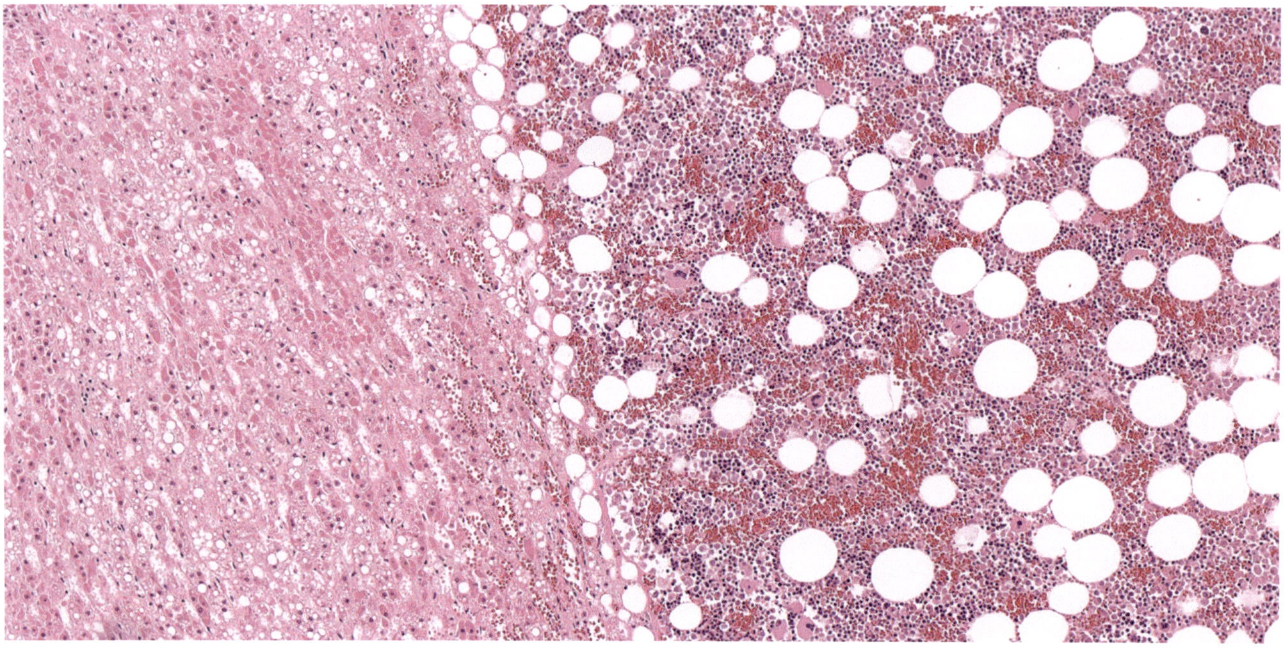

Fig. 14.203 Another benign adrenal tumour is shown on the right side of this image. This is a myelolipoma which is composed of adipose tissue and myeloid elements

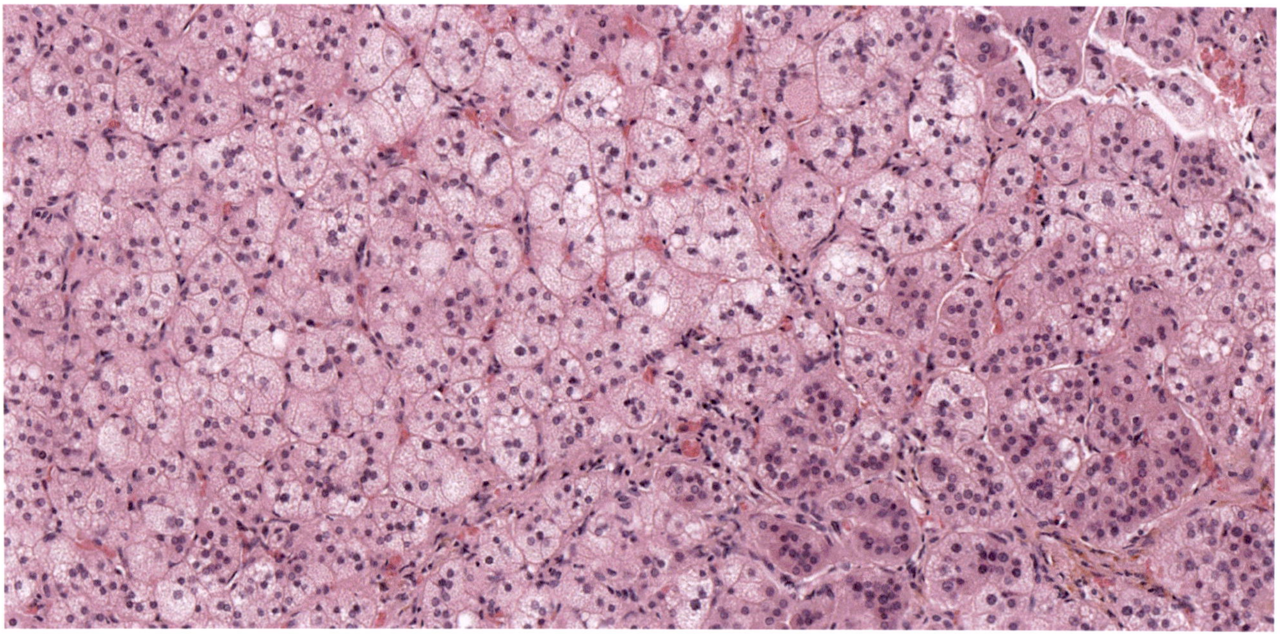

Fig. 14.202 This is an adrenal cortical adenoma, a benign adrenal tumour. The tumour cells resemble the cells of the zona fasciculata and zona reticularis

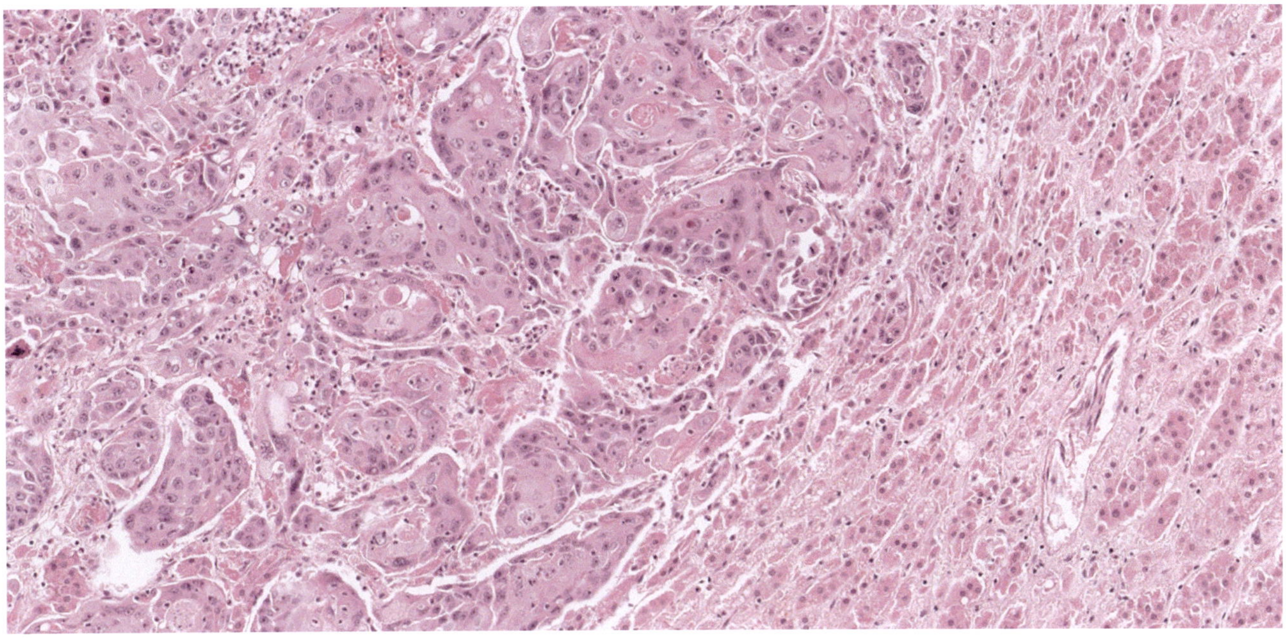

Fig. 14.204 The adrenal gland is a common site of metastasis of lung tumours. This image shows a metastatic deposit of lung squamous cell carcinoma

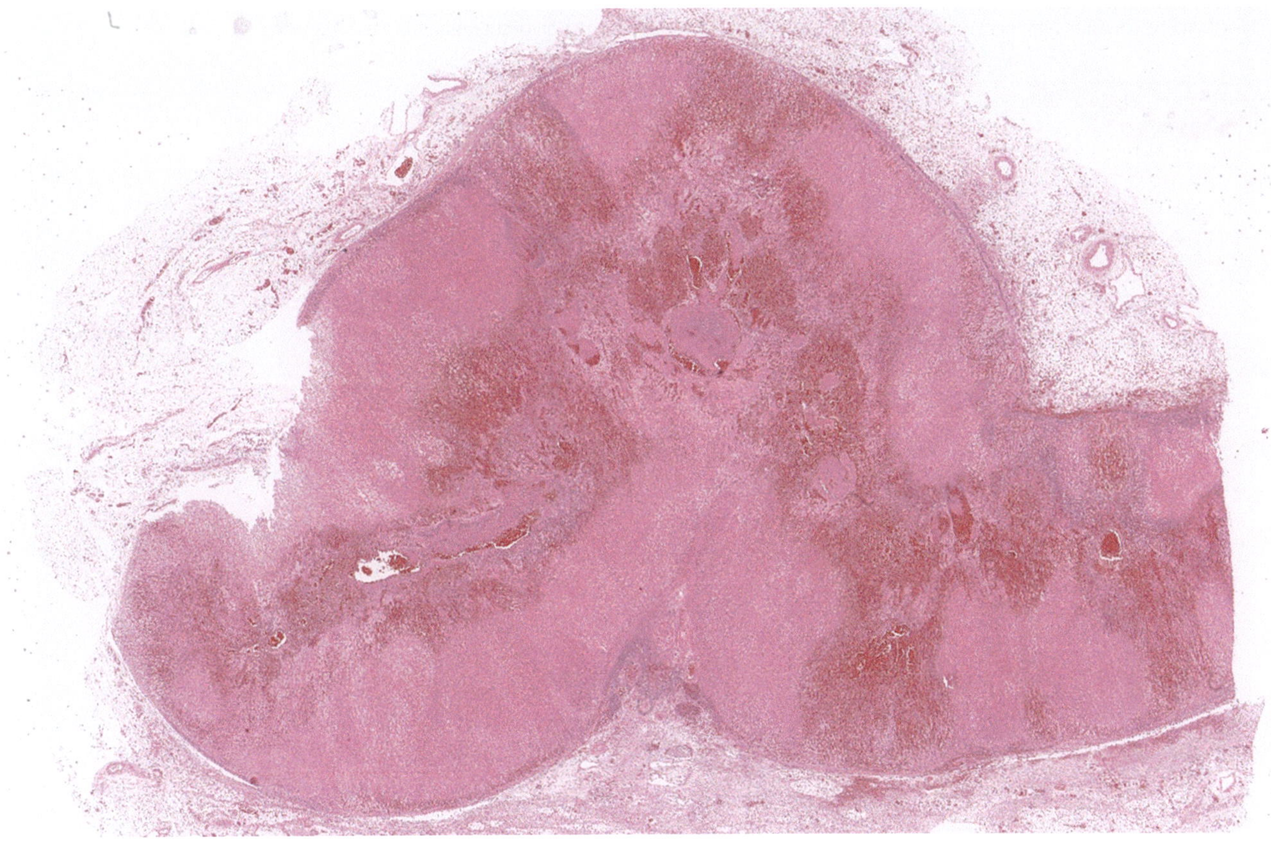

Fig. 14.205 When bilateral, adrenal haemorrhage (shown here) can cause acute adrenal insufficiency (Addisonian crisis) which can be fatal if not recognised and treated

Thyroid Gland

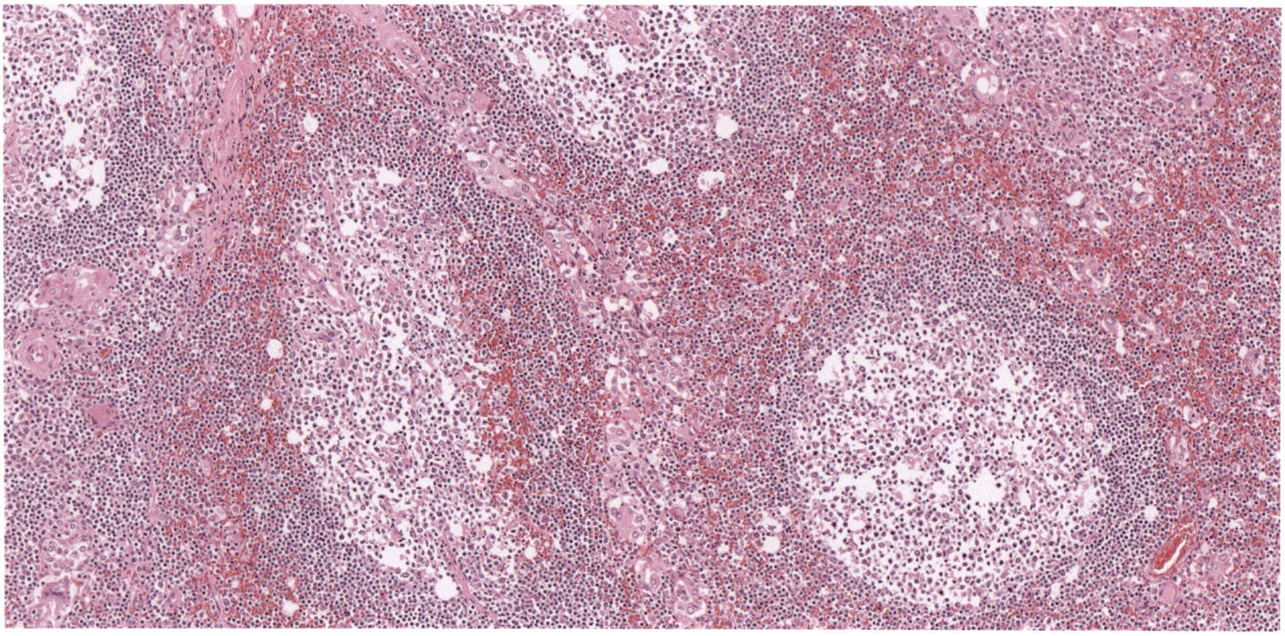

Fig. 14.206 Inflammatory conditions of the thyroid gland can have dramatic obliterative effects. This image shows a lymphocytic thyroiditis (Hashimoto's). There is lymphocytic inflammation with lymphoid follicle formation obliterating the thyroid gland

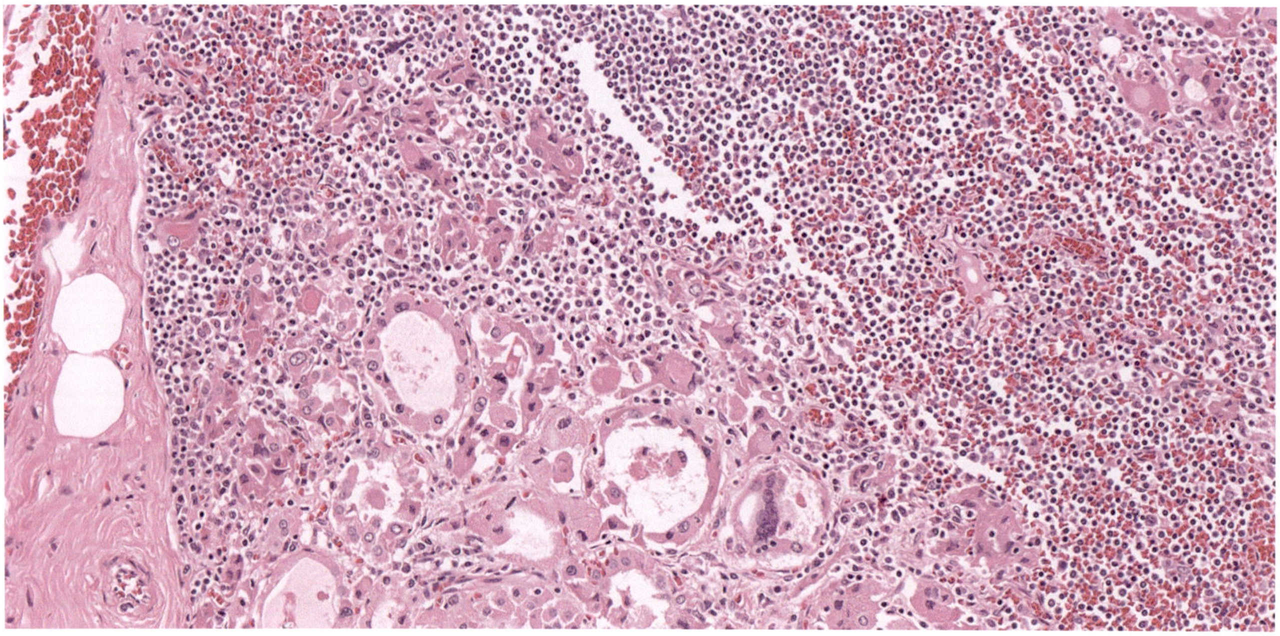

Fig. 14.207 In this image of lymphocytic thyroiditis (Hashimoto's) there is prominent Hurthle cell change

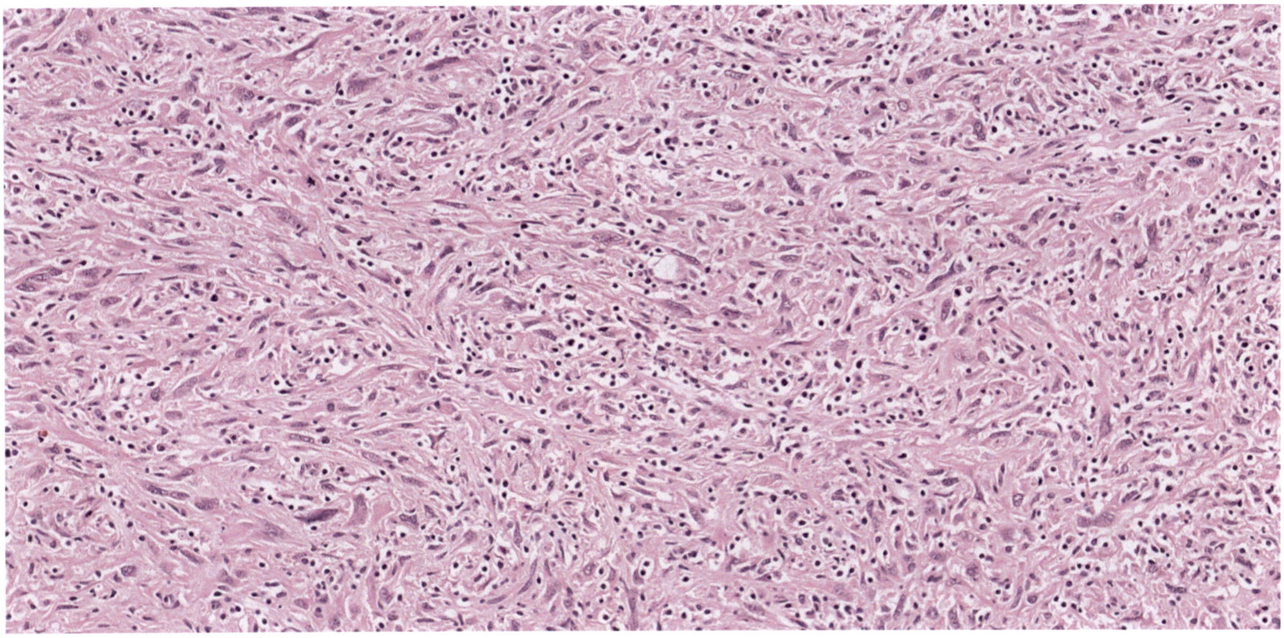

Fig. 14.208 Anaplastic carcinoma of the thyroid gland can cause acute respiratory compromise. Progression of such tumours can be rapid and the diagnosis may not be made until an autopsy and therefore microscopic examination of the tumour can facilitate a diagnosis, as in this case

Brain

Interpretation of the histology of the brain and spinal cord is, of course, the expertise of a neuropathologist. However, the general autopsy pathologist should have a basic understanding of the interpretation of histology of the brain (Figs. 14.209, 14.210, 14.211, 14.212, 14.213, 14.214, 14.215, 14.216, 14.217, 14.218, 14.219, 14.220, 14.221, 14.222, and 14.223). Commonly encountered pathology such as cerebral haemorrhage, infarction, hypoxic ischaemic injury and meningitis are perfectly within the realms of interpretation by an autopsy pathologist.

Specialist neuropathology should be consulted whenever the pathologist feels out of their depth, and particularly in cases of traumatic brain injury where there may be legal consequences, tumours and degenerative conditions. Sudden death in epilepsy should also prompt neuropathology referral.

Brain

Normal

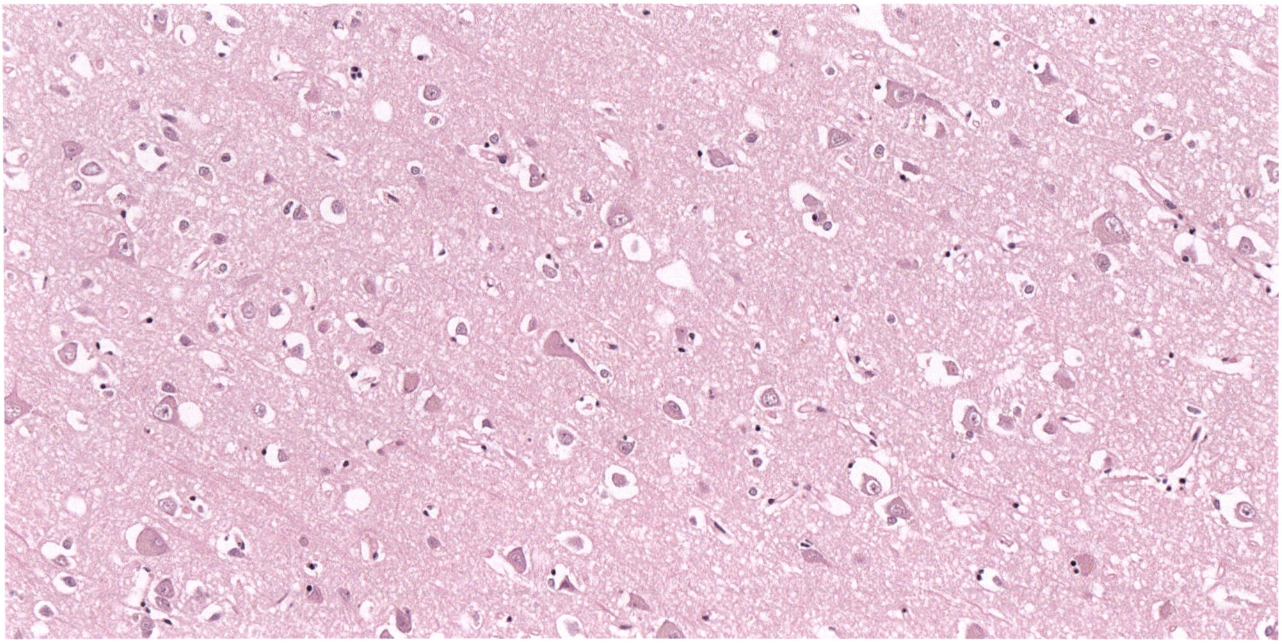

Fig. 14.209 This is an image from the brain, of normal grey matter. Note the large polygonal neuronal cell bodies. Familiarity with the appearance of normal brain tissue can help identify abnormalities. The expertise of a neuropathologist may be required when interpreting some brain pathology

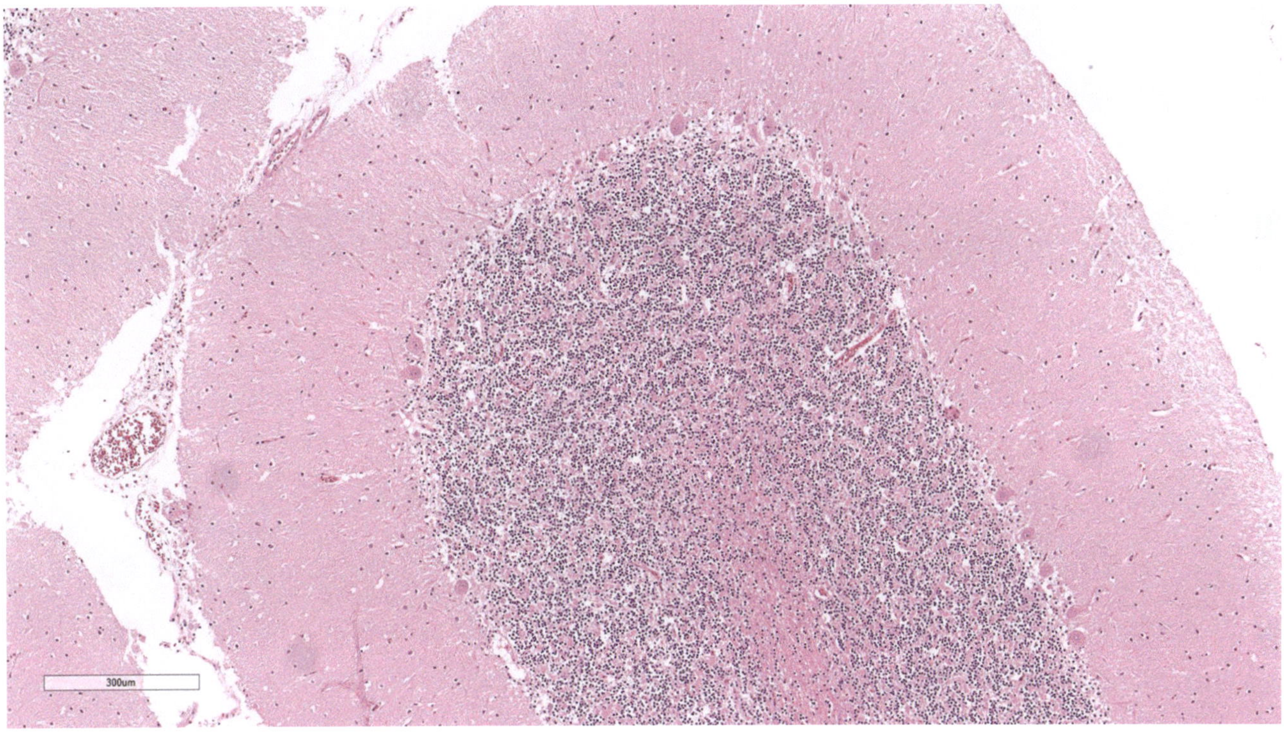

Fig. 14.210 This is normal cerebellum. Note the white matter, Purkinje cells, granular layer and molecular layer

Inflammatory

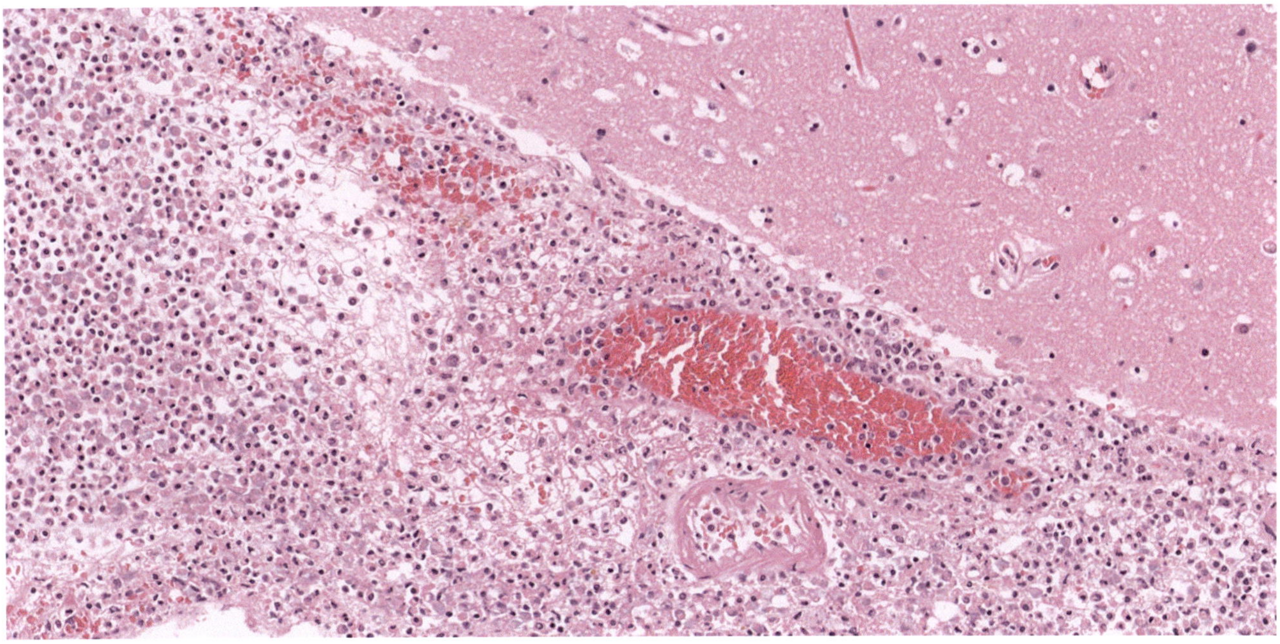

Fig. 14.211 In bacterial meningitis there may be obvious exudate over the surface of the brain, which is evident with the naked eye. However, meningitis can be identified as an unexpected finding on microscopic examination of apparently normal brain/meninges. In this image there are numerous neutrophils within the arachnoid layer, in keeping with meningitis

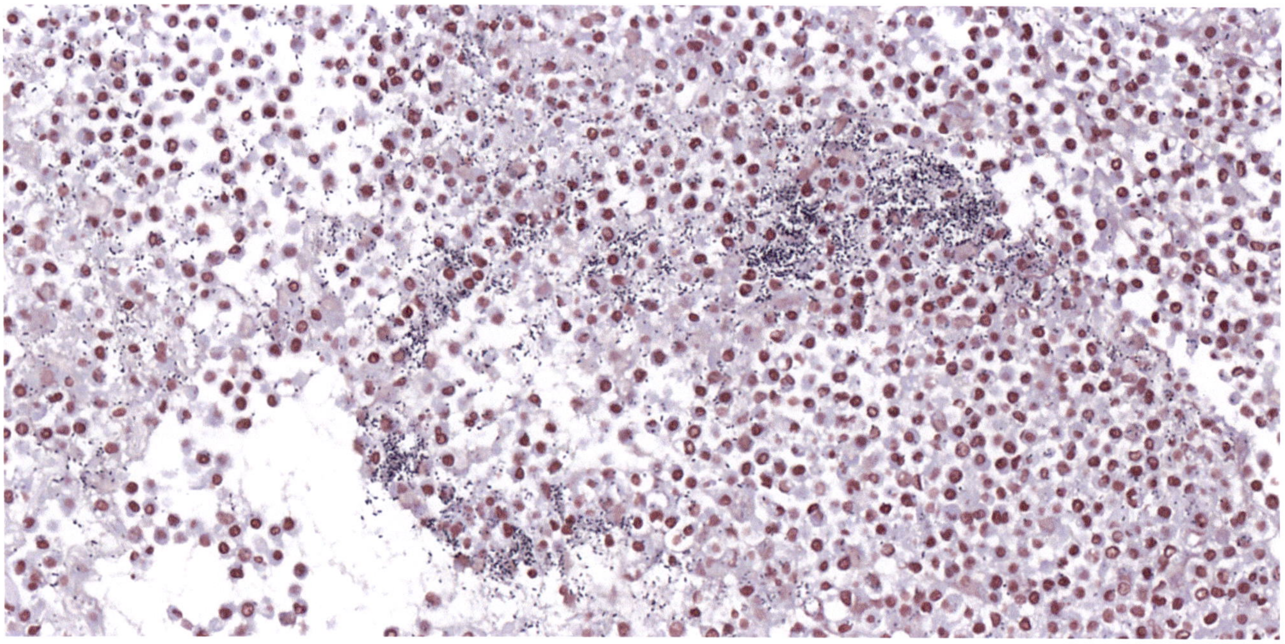

Fig. 14.212 Bacterial meningitis with numerous gram positive cocci

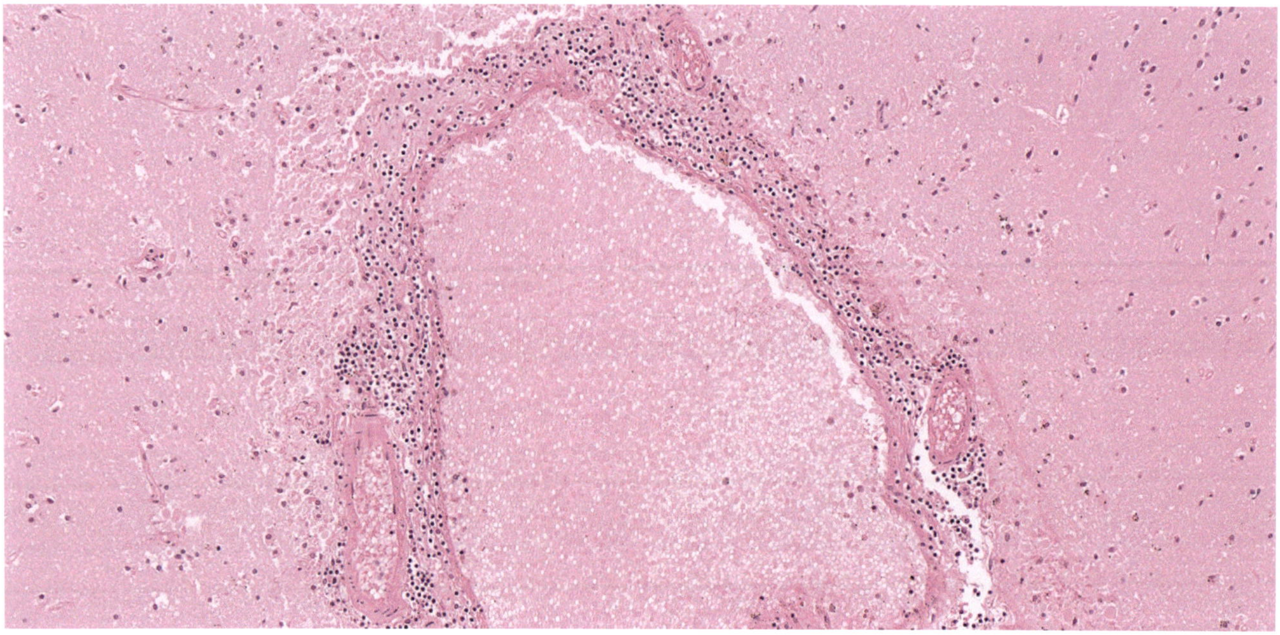

Fig. 14.213 Encephalitis can only be diagnosed microscopically. The brain may appear swollen and oedematous but there may be many causes of cerebral oedema. Microscopy can identify inflammation in the brain, as shown in this image. Note the peri-vascular cuffing by lymphocytes

Trauma

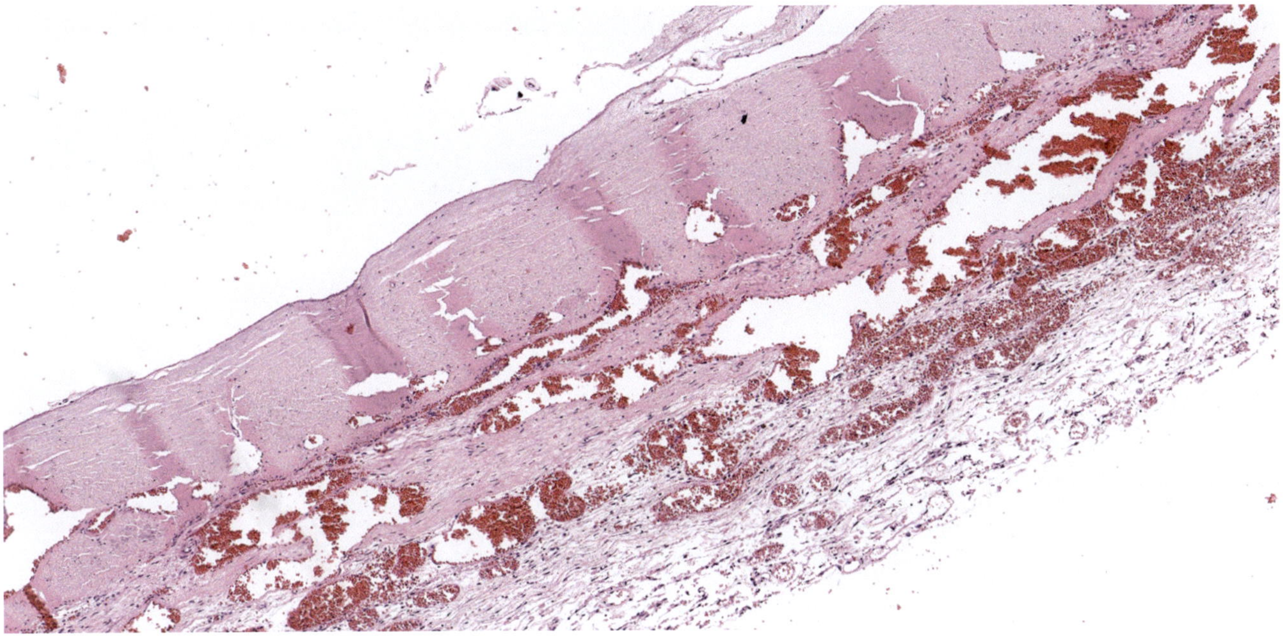

Fig. 14.214 Head injury, even minor injury in the elderly, can cause subdural haemorrhage (SDH). Given the association of SDH with traumatic injury it is often useful to take samples for histology and assess the likely age of the SDH. In this image the haemorrhage is organising, with large capillaries evident. A guide to dating subdural haemorrhage is available in neuropathology texts

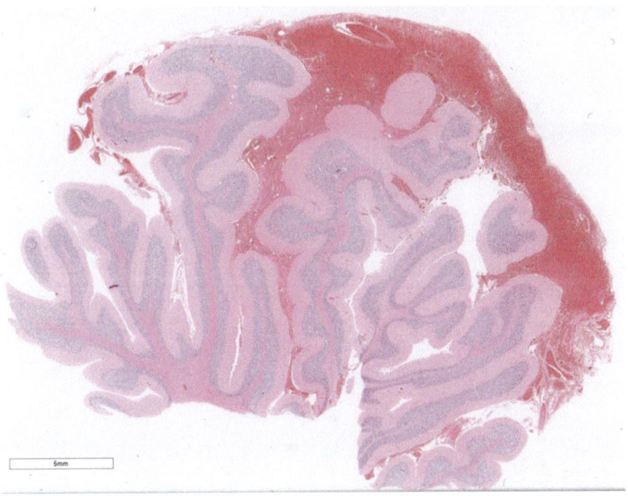

Fig. 14.215 Head injury may result in haemorrhage at different, or multiple, layers of the brain. In this image there is subarachnoid haemorrhage over the cerebellum

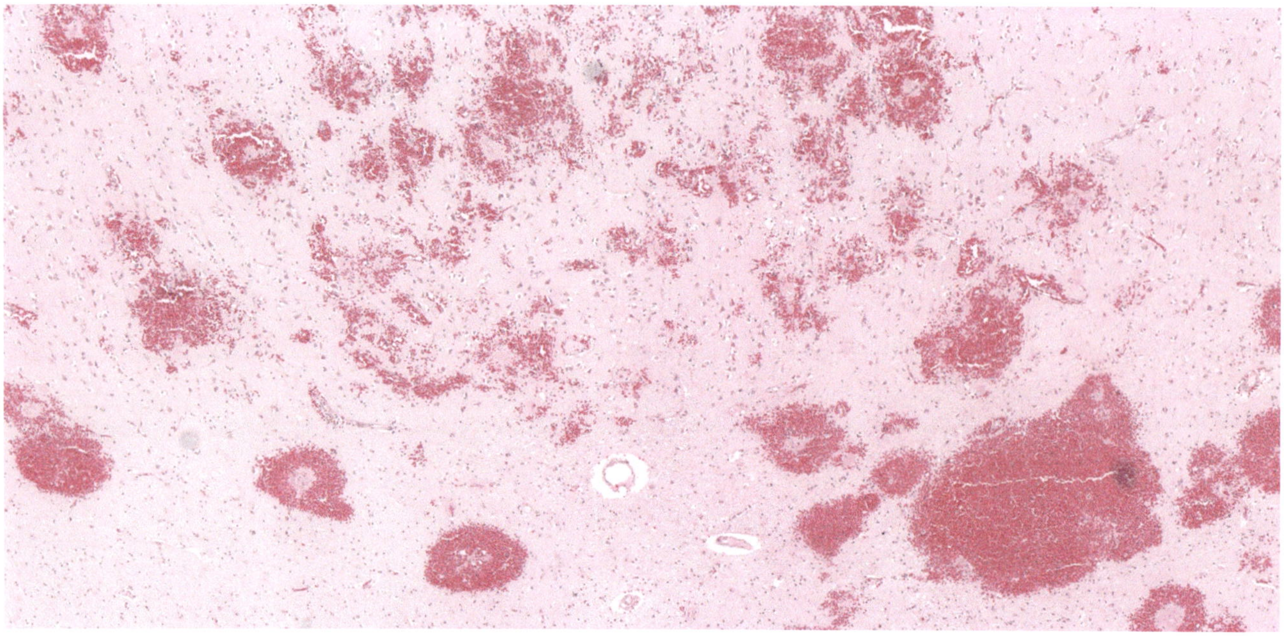

Fig. 14.216 Head injury may cause contusion of the brain. The microscopic appearances of contusion are shown in this image. There is spotty haemorrhage within the grey and white matter

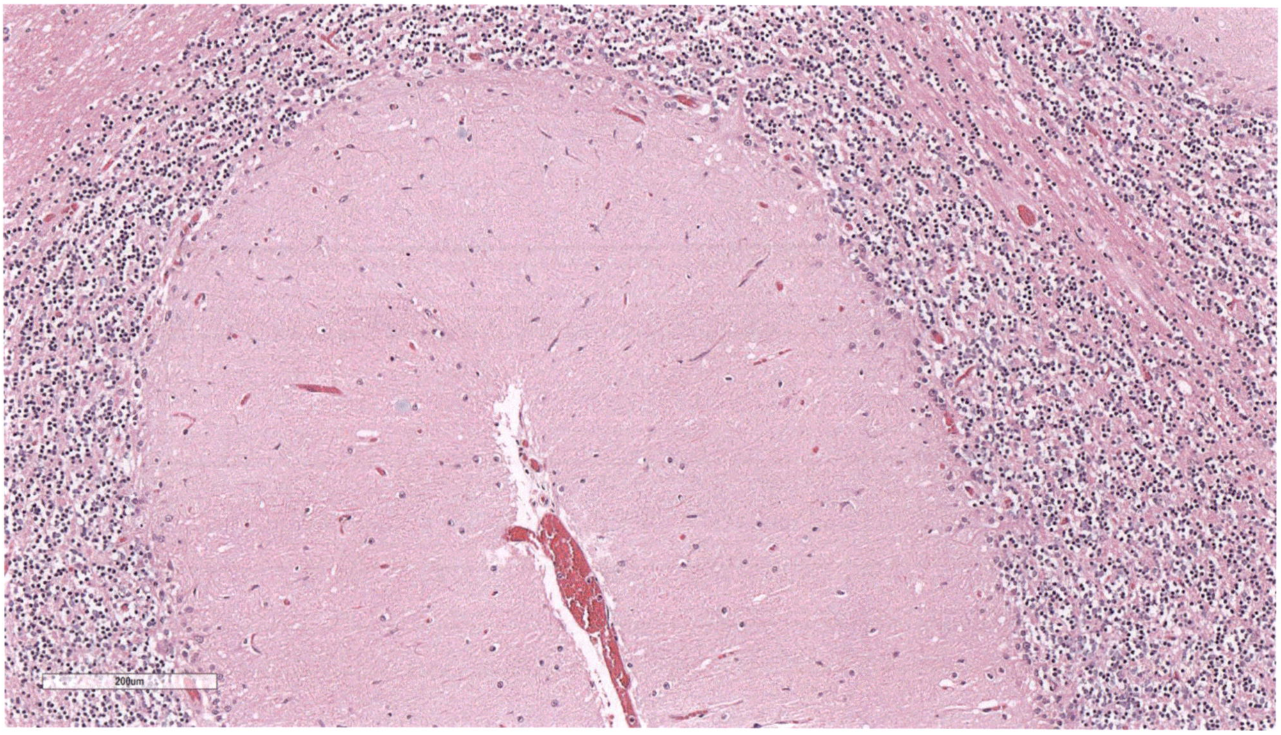

Fig. 14.217 In hypoxic brain injury different areas of the brain are affected at different stages. The Purkinje cells of the cerebellum are particularly vulnerable to hypoxia and are absent in this image

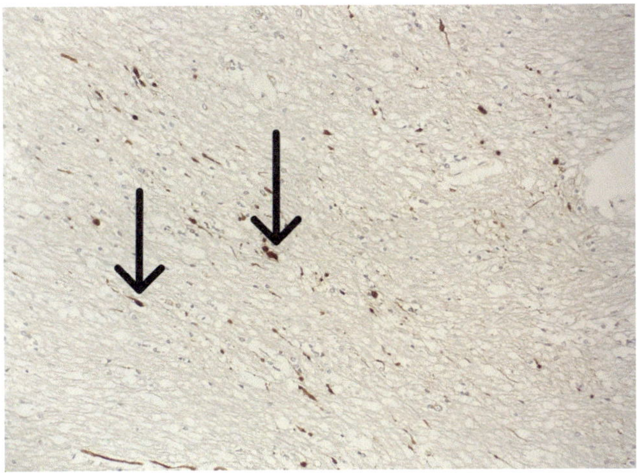

Fig. 14.218 This image shows diffuse traumatic axonal injury highlighted by β-APP immunohistochemistry. There are several immunoreactive axonal profiles indicating axonal injury, some of which show obvious axonal swelling and beading (arrows). Image courtesy of Dr. Kevin Kinch, University of Edinburgh

Brain Tumours

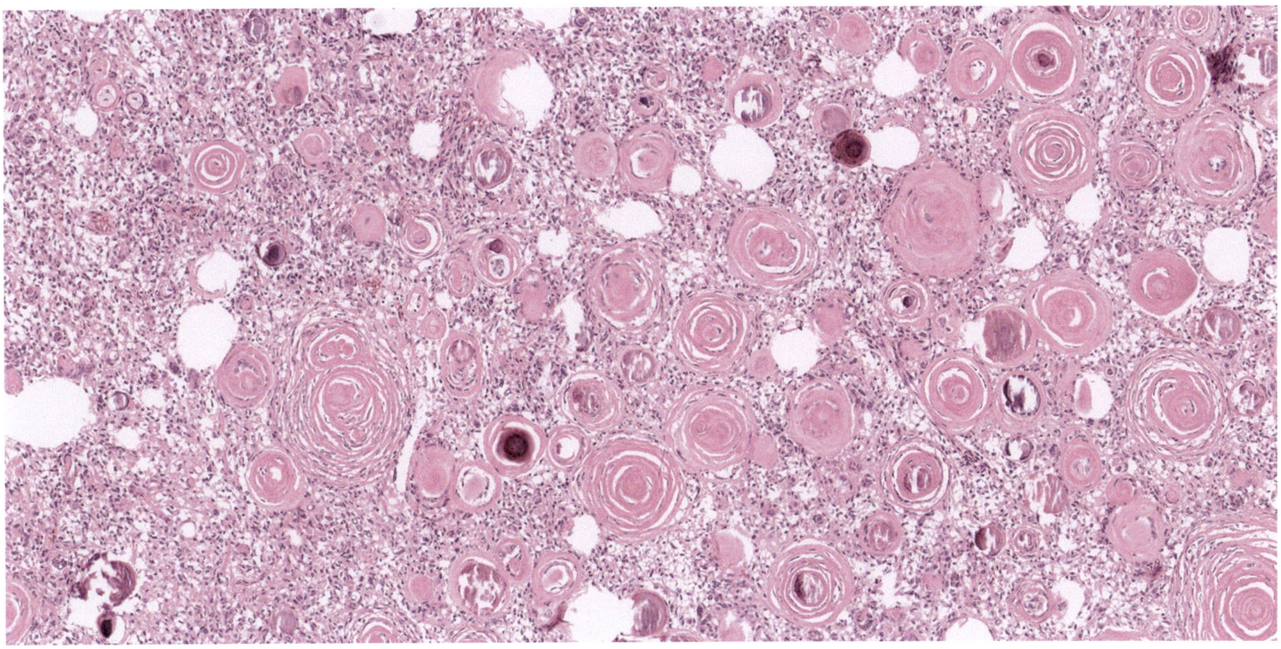

Fig. 14.219 Meningiomas are common benign tumours attached to the meninges. This image shows a meningioma with numerous psammoma bodies

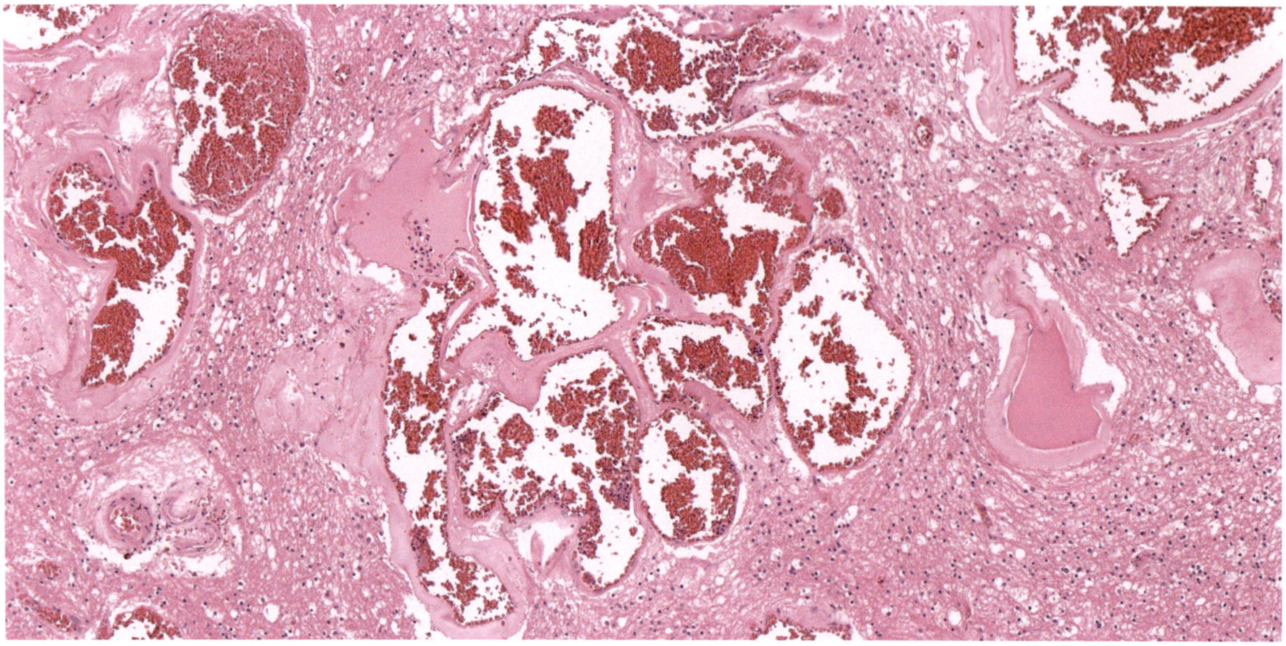

Fig. 14.220 This is a cerebral haemangioma. Even benign lesions like this can be a focus for an epileptic seizure and can be linked to sudden death

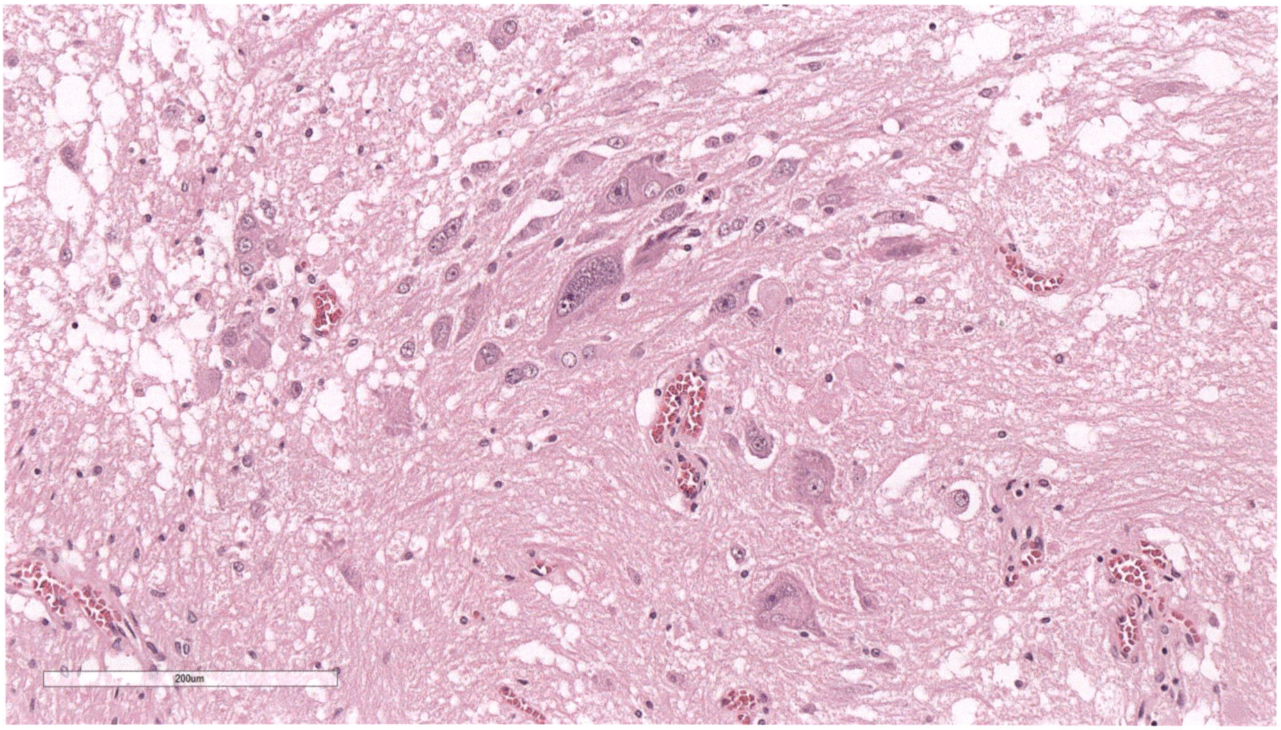

Fig. 14.221 This image shows a ganglioglioma. This rare primary brain tumour was associated with epileptic seizures and led to sudden unexpected death in epilepsy. Tumour typing of common or uncommon brain tumours is most appropriately done by a neuropathologist

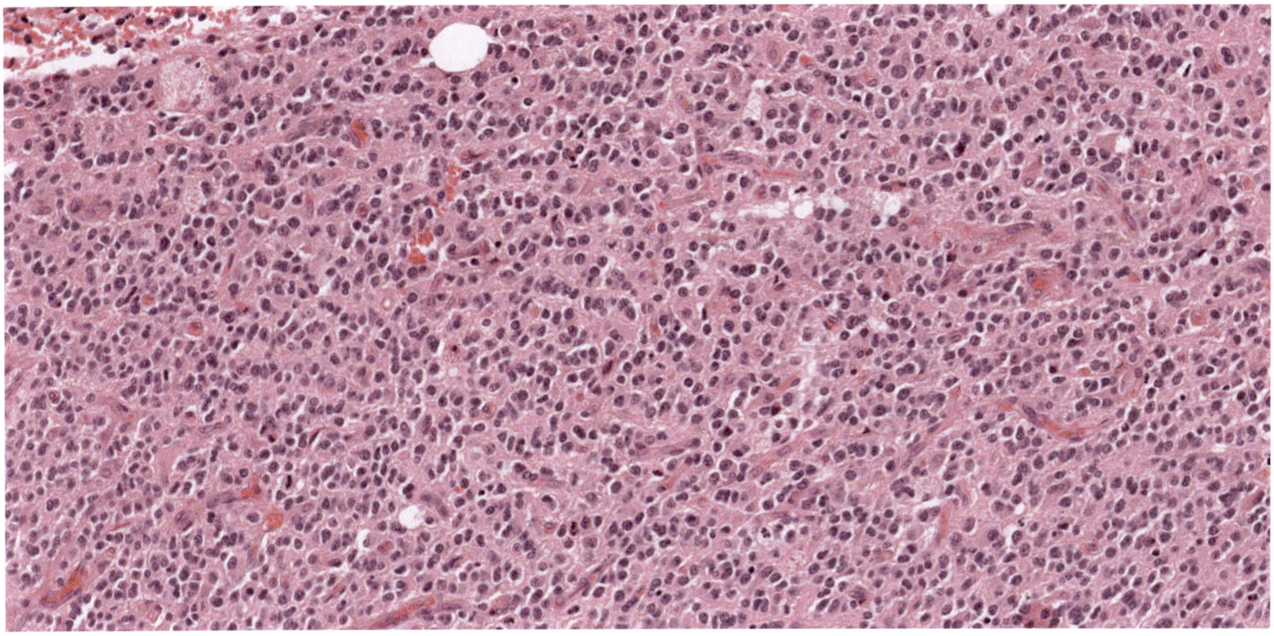

Fig. 14.222 This is an oligodendroglioma. The tumour cells have a fried egg appearance with round monotonous nuclei and peri-nuclear halos

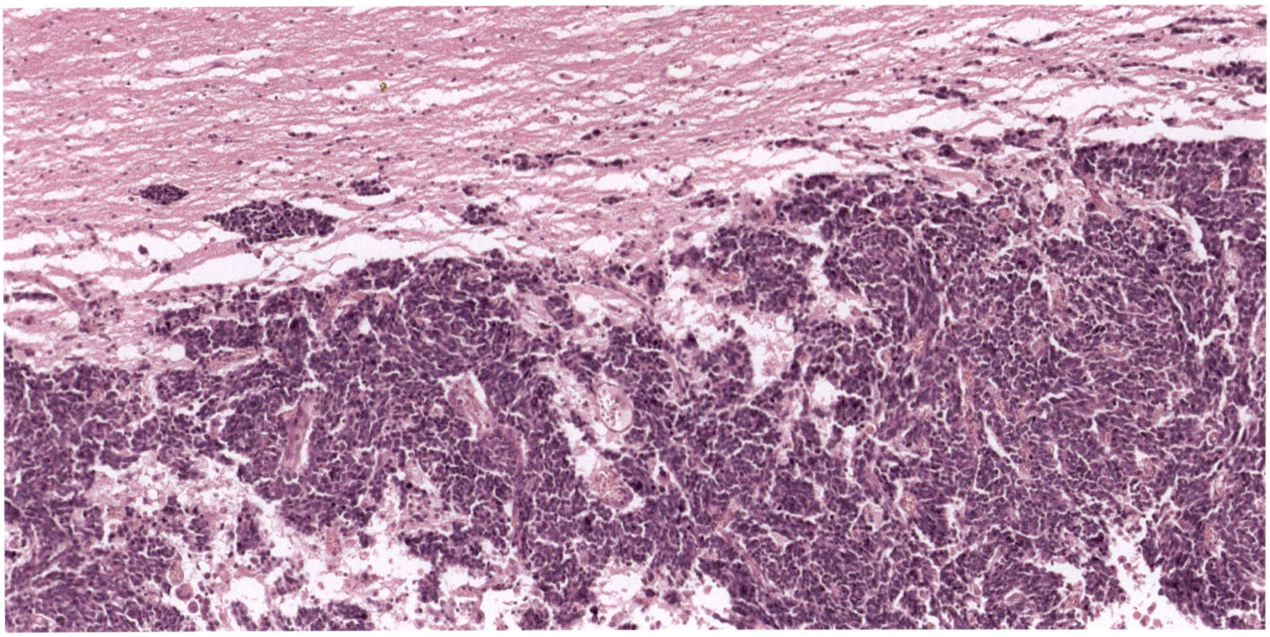

Fig. 14.223 This is a case of metastatic small cell lung carcinoma in the brain

Suggested Reading

Basso C, Calabrese F, Angelini A, Carturan E, Thiene G. Classification and histological, immunohistochemical, and molecular diagnosis of inflammatory myocardial disease. Heart Fail Rev. 2013;18(6):673–81.

Fogo A. Atlas of renal pathology. Pre-eclampsia/eclampsia. Am J Kidney Dis. 2001;38(2):E4–5.

Halushka MK, Angelini A, Bartoloni G, et al. Consensus statement on surgical pathology of the aorta from the Society for Cardiovascular Pathology and the Association For European Cardiovascular Pathology: II. Noninflammatory, degenerative diseases - nomenclature and diagnostic criteria. Cardiovasc Pathol. 2016;25(3):247–57. https://doi.org/10.1016/j.carpath.2016.03.002.

Kumar V, Abbas AK, Aster JC. Robbins & Cotran pathologic basis of disease. 10th ed. Elsevier; 2020.

Levi M, Toh CH, Thachil J, Watson HG. Guidelines for the diagnosis and management of disseminated intravascular coagulation. Br J Haematol. 2009;145:24–33.

Raghu G, Collard R, Egan JJ, et al. Idiopathic pulmonary fibrosis: evidence based guidelines for diagnosis and management. Am J Respir Crit Care Med. 2011;183:788–824.

Saukko P, Knight B. Knight's forensic pathology. 4th ed. CRC Press; 2015.

Stone JR, Bruneval P, Angelini A, et al. Consensus statement on surgical pathology of the aorta from the Society for Cardiovascular Pathology and the Association for European Cardiovascular Pathology: I. Inflammatory diseases. Cardiovasc Pathol. 2015;24(5):267–78. https://doi.org/10.1016/j.carpath.2015.05.001.

Suvarna SK. Cardiac pathology: a guide to current practice. Springer; 2013.

Thom A, Allinson K. Guidelines on autopsy practice: deaths in patients with epilepsy including sudden deaths. Royal College of Pathologists; 2019.

Whitwell HL. Forensic neuropathology. CRC Press; 2005.

Wolff H, Vehmas T, Oksa P, Rantanen J, Vainio H. Asbestos, asbestosis, and cancer, the Helsinki criteria for diagnosis and attribution 2014: recommendations. Scand J Work Environ Health. 2015;41(1):5–15.

Toxicology 15

Stephen R. Morley

Introduction

Post-mortem toxicological analysis should be considered in all deaths in which there is a possibility of an overdose or drug toxicity. It should also be used to consider the cognitive function of an individual prior to death in scenarios such as road traffic collisions and suicides.

Toxicology can be used to identify the presence of any substance which might be relevant to the death. Post-mortem biochemical analysis may also be of value in a proportion of sudden deaths, particularly those involving people with alcoholism, diabetes, or renal impairment—where the disease states may have contributed to an alteration in drug excretion and hence toxicity.

As with all such cases when looking at any positive results, one should have some understanding of the background disease of the individual, and ideally take advice from the toxicologist.

Volume of Distribution (Vd), Half-Life (T½) and Pharmacokinetics

The level of any drug or toxin may be different post-mortem compared with those encountered in life and in studies of healthy subjects. In life, drugs are absorbed into the bloodstream and tissues by active processes. The apparent volume into which drugs distribute is based primarily on protein binding, along with fat and water solubility. Drugs such as warfarin (primarily water soluble) have a volume of distribution of approximately 1 litre (L) per kilogram (kg), whereas many of the lipophilic compounds such as the antipsychotics (which have the primary effect in the brain, a tissue with high fat content) have volumes of distribution over 20 L/kg.

After death, the drugs will either decouple from protein binding or move out of the tissues in which they have been stored, to redistribute and re-equilibrate back into the blood. Therefore, drugs with a high volume of distribution (Vd), pragmatically defined as >3 L/kg) have a tendency to be higher in post-mortem blood than may be expected from ante-mortem blood.

The other factor that contributes to post-mortem redistribution is the proximity to the bowel, liver, or other organs in which drugs may be concentrated. It is considered that any drugs which remain in the bowel after death are no longer actively retained in the bowel. They may undergo variable passive diffusion into surrounding tissues.

It is therefore essential that when interpreting post-mortem blood concentrations, the site of sampling and the volume of distribution are known. Indeed, one should be mindful that it can be difficult to ascertain in some cases whether a high drug concentration is due to an overdose or redistribution.

If a drug is injected then it immediately enters the bloodstream. The same is essentially true for inhaled drugs as they pass easily into the pulmonary vasculature. Oral drugs will reach a peak concentration within approximately 30–45 min.

Drugs are recognised as foreign substances and so the body will metabolise them as rapidly as possible. This requires a functioning liver and, when the drugs have been made water soluble by metabolism in the liver, excretion by functioning kidneys. The time taken for the removal of the drug is defined by its half-life (T½). The half-life is the time taken for the drug concentration to halve.

S. R. Morley (✉)
Forensic Toxicology Unit, Leicester Royal Infirmary,
Leicester, UK
e-mail: stephen.morley1@nhs.net

S. K. Suvarna (represented by Grace Horne), A. K. Sharp (eds.), *Atlas of Adult Autopsy*,
https://doi.org/10.1007/978-3-031-72207-3_15

Drug Concentrations

There is no standard nomenclature for reporting post mortem drug concentrations. It is recommended that drugs are reported in mass units within either millilitres or litres.

$$1000 \text{ nanograms } (\text{ng}) = 1 \text{ microgram } (\mu g) = 0.001 \text{ milligram } (\text{mg})$$

$$1000 \text{ millilitres } (\text{mL}) = 1 \text{ litre } (\text{L})$$

There is a wide variation in the drug concentrations required for clinical effects. As an example, fentanyl has effects at 10 μg/L, whereas the antiepileptic drug valproate may require a blood concentration of up to 100 mg/L (100,000 μg/L) to be effective.

One other nuance is that in the UK, forensic blood alcohols are reported as mg/100 mL (mg/%) whereas clinical cases are reported as mg/L.

Metal concentrations (including lithium) are reported as millimoles per litre (mmol/L).

Samples Required for Toxicology Analysis

Most bodies are recovered soon after death and many different samples are possible. However, this is to be contrasted with the decomposed body and those after embalming has taken place. See also Chap. 10 regarding samples used for special tests.

Routine Cases

It is possible to screen and quantify on either preserved or unpreserved samples, but the sample type should be recorded as there may be differences in drug stability. As an example, cocaine is less stable in unpreserved blood, but is still detectable.

Although the toxicology laboratories are using more sensitive analysers, due to the consistency of post mortem blood, relatively large volumes are still used to reduce the effect of sample consistency.

In routine cases, the following samples are recommended:

Blood

- Unpreserved (plain) blood—ideally 20 mL or greater (drug screen and quantitation).
- Fluoride oxalate preserved blood—ideally 10 mL or greater (ideal for ethanol, cocaine, diazepam quantitation).

Urine

- Unpreserved (plain) urine—ideally 20 mL or greater (general screen).
- Fluoride oxalate preserved urine—ideally 10 mL or greater (ideal for ethanol analysis).

Vitreous Fluid

- Unpreserved vitreous fluid—as much as is available for biochemical analysis.
- Fluoride oxalate preserved vitreous fluid—1 mL for ethanol analysis.

Stomach Content

This is only worth sending if there is a suspicion of an overdose close to the time of death. Ideally all content should be sent, or an aliquot detailing the overall volume found.

Solid Tissues

Liver (deep within the right lobe) and muscle (e.g., psoas) may be sent. A 1 cm cube is often sufficient for screening purposes.

Rarely sampled sites are covered in Table 15.1.

Table 15.1 Sample requirements for toxicology analysis

Specimen	Common uses
Blood/plasma/serum	Preferred specimen (recent use with respect to death)
Urine	Preferred specimen after blood, although not useful for acute exposure
Vitreous	Ethanol, some biochemistry, glucose, electrolytes
Muscle (preferably psoas)	Most drugs—useful to screen in decomposition if no other fluids
Liver (deep in right lobe)	Most drugs—useful to screen in decomposition if no other fluids
Bile (rarely collected)	Most drugs—useful to screen in decomposition if no other fluids
Bone/bone marrow (rarely collected)	
Fat (rarely collected)	Volatiles after increased post-exposure period
Gastric contents	Orally administered drugs and poisons
Hair (not often collected for Coroner's cases)	All substances, especially basic/most metals
Pleural effusion (rarely collected)	
Lung	Volatiles/anaesthetic gases
Kidney (rarely collected)	Heavy metals
Faeces (rarely collected)	Porphyria
Brain (rarely collected)	Volatiles

Embalmed Bodies

Embalming chemicals consist of a variety of preservatives, sanitising and disinfectant agents and additives used to temporarily prevent decomposition. Typically, embalming fluid contains a mixture of formaldehyde, methanol, ethanol, and other solvents. The formaldehyde content generally ranges from 5% to 29% and the ethanol content may range from 9% to 56% (i.e., there is no international standard).

It is self-evident that any embalming action to the corpse may cause considerable changes of initial drug levels. These changes are due to alterations of the biological matrix as well as to dilution of a sample, release or degradation of the drug or poison. If one can identify a source of 'uncontaminated fluid' then some testing may be possible, but liaison with the toxicologist is often beneficial.

One area to consider is the cavernous sinus veins if the head has not been perfused with embalming fluid/opened.

If one is sending any sample in these cases, one should always send an aliquot of the embalming fluid to compare to post-mortem fluid volatiles.

Commonly Encountered Drugs and Toxins

The following section deals with the various drugs and toxins regularly encountered in toxicology analysis.

Ethanol

Ethanol (C_2H_5OH) is an alcohol. It is consumed as a social drug, but is also, along with other alcohols, produced as part of the post-mortem process of the body breaking down. One unit of ethanol (10 g) will lead to a peak blood alcohol of approximately 20 mg/100 mL blood. Ethanol is excreted and/or metabolised at a rate of approximately 20 mg/100 mL/h (range 10–35 mg/100 mL/h).

Toxicology laboratories are often well versed in measuring ethanol levels and confounding realities (e.g., post-mortem production). Most laboratories should also measure ethyl glucuronide (a non-enzymatic metabolite of ethanol) as a confirmatory marker for ethanol consumption.

However, post-mortem ethanol is highly variable and depends on the ambient circumstances of death [1]. There is an increased production if there is infection/bacterial contamination of blood (and less commonly urine). It is common to see concentrations of up to 20 mg/100 mL in most cases. However, it is not unusual to see concentrations up to 100 mg/100 mL and some cases up to 250 mg/100 mL have been reported.

T½: Ethanol shows zero order kinetics, falling by approximately 20 mg/100 mL/h (range, 10–35 mg/100 mL)
Vd: 0.6 L/kg
Samples: Preserved blood, urine and vitreous

The clinical effects of ethanol vary with the blood concentrations (Table 15.2).

There is a legal limit for driving a motor vehicle; 80 mg/100 mL blood in England and Wales, 50 mg/100 mL in Scotland. Therefore, it is often difficult at times to be definitive as to whether a post-mortem blood alcohol repre-

Table 15.2 Blood alcohol concentrations and general effects

10–50 mg/100 mL	Minimal outward effects, feelings of relaxation and well-being, increased sociability
50–100 mg/100 mL	Increased self-confidence and talkativeness, mild euphoria, reduced co-ordination, and slightly slowed reactions. Legal limit for driving in England and Wales is 80 mg/100 mL, in Scotland it is 50 mg/100 mL
100–150 mg/100 mL	Impaired balance, clumsiness, reduced alertness, lowered social reserve, increased excitability
150–200 mg/100 mL	Slurred speech, glazed eyes, flushed complexion, staggered gait, drowsiness, exaggerated emotional responses, impaired co-ordination, reduced inhibitions, dizziness, nausea, disorientation
200–250 mg/100 mL	Marked or heavy drunkenness, confusion, grossly impaired co-ordination, vomiting, reduced awareness, short-term memory is often impaired
250–300 mg/100 mL	Extreme drunkenness, stupor, impaired consciousness, reduced reflexes, depressed respiration, incontinence
300–400 mg/100 mL	Unconsciousness, absence of reflexes, coma. Possible death
Around 400 mg/100 mL and above	Possible death by respiratory depression or cardiac arrest

This table is for guidance only and may not apply to any specific individual. Although compartmentalised, the symptoms can overlap considerably and gradually increase in severity with increasing concentrations. The effects described apply to a social drinker but depend on the degree of habituation. A heavy drinker will show fewer effects, and a person unaccustomed to alcohol will have more pronounced symptoms. Therefore, the effects of any given blood alcohol level cannot be determined simply by reference to a table. Tolerance should be considered, together with other information such as evidence from witnesses and the findings of any medical examination. It is not possible to determine a particular level of alcohol that may cause memory loss in a specific individual or render an individual unable to form an intent or to give informed consent to, for example, sexual activity

sents a level above the legal limit. Different legal limits apply in Europe and elsewhere in the world.

As vitreous fluid is within a "contained" space this is often the ideal sample for ethanol analysis.

Ethylene Glycol

Ethylene glycol ($C_2H_2(OH)_2$) is a toxic alcohol used in engine antifreeze or as a radiator coolant. It is metabolised to the four toxic metabolites: glycolaldehyde, glycolate, glycolic acid and glyoxylate. It can be used as an adulterant for other alcohols or even deliberately as a poison.

T½: 3 h
Vd: 0.8 L/kg
Samples: Preserved blood

Toxic effects are usually associated with serum ethylene glycol concentrations >50 mg/100 mL (500 mg/L).

During the first few hours after ingestion of ethylene glycol the individual may experience transient inebriation, euphoria, nausea, and vomiting. The clinical course of ethylene glycol poisoning has been described in three stages. A neurological stage occurs within the first 12 h in which the accumulation of toxic ethylene glycol metabolites produces neurological symptoms including nystagmus, ataxia, myoclonic jerking, hypotonia, seizures and coma. An intermediate cardiopulmonary stage at 12–24 h may lead to tachycardia, hypertension, metabolic acidosis with a compensatory hyperventilation, and multiple organ failure. It has been reported that death most commonly occurs during this second stage. A renal stage occurring at 24–72 h onwards may lead to renal failure with oliguria, even with non-fatal level ingestion of ethylene glycol. The ethylene glycol metabolites may also cause kidney tissue destruction primarily from calcium oxalate crystal deposition.

Methanol

Methanol (CH_3OH) is a toxic alcohol that is found in various household and industrial agents. Products that contain methanol include windshield washer fluid, gas line antifreeze, carburettor cleaner, copy machine fluid, perfumes, food warming fuel, and is sometimes present in contraband alcoholic spirits.

T½: 2–24 h (zero-order)
Vd: 0.6 L/kg
Samples: Preserved blood

It can be highly toxic. The main toxicity is secondary to metabolism to formaldehyde and formic acid which cause metabolic acidosis and blindness. Ocular toxicity results from formic acid accumulation and is made worse by any acidosis.

Similar to ethylene glycol, the patient may initially appear intoxicated, and then suffer multi-organ failure. Antidotes are the same as ethylene glycol, namely alcohol or fomepizole.

Betahydroxybutyrate, Ketoacids and Ketoacidosis

The toxicologist should suspect ketoacidosis when there is excess acetone detected on volatiles (ethanol) analysis. This should prompt measurement of blood and/or vitreous beta-hydroxybutyrate (BHB) measurement. Acetone may also result from post-mortem autolysis, but BHB is unlikely to result from changes in the post-mortem period.

Ketonaemia is relevant in two main scenarios, namely chronic alcoholism, and diabetes mellitus (see Table 15.3). Excessive formation of ketone bodies (acetone and BHB) is also observed in conditions associated with decreased availability of carbohydrate (such as starvation or frequent vomiting) or decreased use of carbohydrates (such as diabetes mellitus and alkalosis).

T½: 3 h
Vd: 0.8 L/kg
Samples: Preserved blood (volatile screen), preserved urine (volatile screen), preserved and unpreserved vitreous (for BHB and vitreous glucose), plain blood if assessing HbA1c.

The confirmation of a toxic level of beta-hydroxybutyrate indicative of ketoacidosis is not well defined, with some papers quoting concentrations as low as 1 mmol/L as pathologically significant, but individuals may show no effects with concentrations up to 5 mmol/L. Hence 1–5 mmol/L is a grey area.

Table 15.3 Patterns of ketoacidosis

Diabetic	Alcoholic
History of type 1 diabetes mellitus	No history of type 1 diabetes mellitus
Vitreous glucose raised/detectable	Undetectable glucose
Raised HbA1c	Normal HbA1c
No alcohol history	History of chronic alcohol misuse

There is also ketosis with starvation, and beta-hydroxybutyrate may also be a marker for a chronic stress response such as hypothermia

Opiates and Opioids

Opiates are a wide family of drugs, which include morphine, heroin, codeine and pholcodine as examples. Opiates are drugs that are chemically related to the morphine molecule and so act on the morphine opiate receptors.

Opioids are not chemically related to morphine, but they act on some of the receptors that are reactive to opiates. In the early years of the 2020s, very potent synthetic opioids were being used to supplement heroin. These xylazines and nitazenes require specific screening. As with any post mortem toxicology investigation, the pathologist must be aware of the drugs that are screened for.

Heroin (Diacetyl Morphine) and Morphine

Diacetyl morphine (diamorphine) may be used therapeutically for pain relief in a hospital or palliative care setting. It is identical to illicit heroin (but the latter is likely to have contaminants and cutting agents added). Heroin is widely abused.

Heroin is metabolised almost instantaneously to 6-monoacetylmorphine (6-MAM), which is then further metabolised to morphine. Morphine is usually quantified in toxicology analyses. The presence of 6-MAM is consistent with the use of diamorphine/heroin within the previous 12–24 h. In the absence of 6-MAM, unless other contaminants such as papaverine, noscapine or meconin are detected, it is not possible analytically to distinguish morphine administration from the use of heroin/diamorphine. 6-MAM is detected better in vitreous and urine than blood, but detection in blood is likely to represent rapid death after use of illicit heroin or diamorphine.

Morphine is likewise used for pain relief. It is metabolised to morphine-3 and morphine-6 glucuronides in the liver. The morphine-3 glucuronide is pharmacologically inactive, whereas morphine-6 glucuronide is at least as potent with regard to sedation and respiratory depression as morphine.

Morphine in its nascent form is described as "free" morphine. The sum of the free, morphine-3 and morphine-6 glucuronide is described as "total" morphine. The ratio of total to free morphine has been found to range from 1:1 to 2:1 when death had occurred within 3 h of the administration of heroin in a naïve user. As the glucuronides are excreted by the kidney, renal impairment leads to accumulation of the morphine metabolites including the active morphine-6-glucuronide.

T½: 2–6 h
Vd: 3–5 L/kg
Specimens: Unpreserved blood and urine for screening, unpreserved blood for quantitation.

The fatal concentrations are highly dependent on tolerance and time from administration to death. In a naïve individual, concentrations as low as 100 ng/mL may be fatal. Deaths are more likely to occur at lower concentrations if there are other sedative drugs (e.g., alcohol, benzodiazepines, methadone) present concurrently. Tolerance may occur but is lost within a few days of abstinence.

Morphine toxicity is associated with progressive depression of the central nervous system, which may lead to coma, marked reduction of respiratory rate and respiratory arrest. Induction of vomiting increases the risk of aspiration pneumonia. Opiates may also cause a prolonged period of respiratory depression that then leads to pulmonary oedema. Morphine may be metabolised during this period, and this may account for what appears to be a low fatal opiate concentration.

Codeine

T½: 1.9–3.9 h
Vd: 3.5 L/kg
Specimens: Unpreserved blood and urine for screening, unpreserved blood for quantitation.

Codeine has analgesic properties, but the narcotic effects are substantially mediated by morphine. In the absence of other contributing factors there is strong evidence that free codeine concentrations of as low as 400 ng/mL may be sufficient to cause death [2].

Dihydrocodeine

T½: 3.5–4.5 h
Vd: 1–1.3 L/kg
Specimens: Unpreserved blood and urine for screening, unpreserved blood for quantitation.

In deaths attributed to dihydrocodeine alone, and poly-drug intoxication (including dihydrocodeine), the blood dihydrocodeine levels ranged between 900–19,900 ng/mL (median 3800 ng/mL) and 30–17,500 ng/mL (median 900 ng/mL) respectively [3].

Methadone

Methadone is a potent opioid narcotic analgesic. It is the commonest substitution drug in the treatment of heroin addiction. Methadone is metabolised to its major inactive metabolite EDDP (2-ethylidene-1,5-dimethyl-3,3-diphenylpyrrolidine). Peak methadone levels occur 2–4 h after ingestion.

The interpretation of the methadone result requires knowledge of the history of drug use and therefore the degree of tolerance that has been acquired.

T½: 10–35 h
Vd: 3–5 L/kg
Specimens: Unpreserved blood and urine for screening, unpreserved blood for quantitation.

In fatal cases in which methadone was the only drug found, the blood methadone concentrations vary greatly with a mean of about 500 ng/mL but with a range of 84–2700 ng/mL [4]. However, concentrations of up to approximately 1200 ng/mL are observed in "well" methadone users, so the interpretation is dependent on the details of death.

Methadone, in common with other opioids, causes respiratory depression even at therapeutic doses. It causes a prolonged period of unconsciousness that then leads to gradually worsening hypoventilation and respiratory failure. Methadone also causes arrhythmias, independent of its effects on respiration and hypoxia.

Fentanyl

Fentanyl is a potent synthetic narcotic analgesic usually administered in the form of a transdermal patch for the management of chronic pain, as a transmucosal lozenge or intravenously for enhancement of anaesthesia. Fentanyl is thought to be 75–100 times more potent than morphine.

T½: 3.7 h
Vd: 3–8 L/kg
Specimens: Unpreserved blood and urine for screening, unpreserved blood for quantitation.

Mean serum fentanyl concentrations have been reported to range from 0.3 to 2.5 ng/mL within 24 h after the administration of therapeutic use of 12.5–100 µg/h transdermal patches, respectively. There is a significant degree of tolerance in chronic users. In naïve individuals, death may be attributed to therapeutic range fentanyl levels, but it is not common for concentrations to be above 10 ng/mL [5].

Significant rises in blood fentanyl may occur if applied to damaged skin or if there is a rise in body temperature, such as occurs with infection. It is theoretically possible that there may be continued release of fentanyl from a patch in the post mortem period and so sampling should be distant from the patch application site.

As with other opioids the primary side effects are reduction of consciousness and respiratory depression. There is also an increased risk of potentially fatal tachyarrhythmias.

In addition to fentanyl, there has also been a rise in the use of even more potent opioids such as carfentanil. These are usually detected when spiked into heroin, as they are easier to produce and cheaper than heroin. Because of their potency, they are present at such low concentration that many standard toxicology screens may not be sensitive enough to detect them. The pathologist should confirm with their toxicology provider.

Tramadol

Tramadol is an analgesic. Its mode of action is complex and has both opioid and non-opioid analgesic effects as well as serotonin effects. Tramadol is metabolised to the active metabolite O-desmethyltramadol, which is thought to have a longer half-life.

T½: 6 h
Vd: 3 L/kg
Specimens: Unpreserved blood and urine for screening, unpreserved blood for quantitation.

The potentially lethal blood tramadol concentration has been reported as >2000 ng/mL. In some case reports where tramadol was the only drug thought to have caused intentional or unintentional death its concentration ranged between 6600 and 20,000 ng/mL. However, when tramadol was taken with other drugs its concentration in fatal cases ranged between 30 and 22,600 ng/mL [6].

Side effects include respiratory depression, lethargy, seizure, coma, cardiac arrest, and death. Concomitant use of tramadol with tricyclic antidepressants such as amitriptyline increases the risk of seizures and cardiac arrhythmias.

Oxycodone

Oxycodone is a semi-synthetic opioid analgesic used therapeutically in the management of moderate to severe pain. Oxycodone is metabolised to oxymorphone. Oxymorphone is prescribed in some countries, including the USA, but not in the UK.

T½: 3–6 h
Vd: 1.8–3.7 L/kg
Specimens: Unpreserved blood for screening and quantitation, unpreserved urine may be used to detect metabolite.

Numerous studies have been reported which show considerable overlap between oxycodone concentrations in oxycodone-related deaths (alone or in combination with a mixed drug ingestion) and deaths where the drug was determined to be an incidental finding. It is thought that the primary reason for the overlap between blood oxycodone concentrations in incidental findings at autopsy and cases where oxycodone played a role in the decedent's death may be the development of tolerance.

In various studies, the mean concentration of oxycodone in deaths attributed solely to oxycodone was around 700 ng/mL (with some levels as low as 200 ng/mL), whilst the mean oxycodone concentration in which death was associated with trauma (i.e., oxycodone was an incidental finding) was around 600 ng/mL (range 25–1990 ng/mL). Side effects include respiratory depression, lethargy, seizure, coma, cardiac arrest, and death.

Benzodiazepines

There are many benzodiazepines available for therapeutic use which are also abused. The chapter does not have space to cover all, and so uses the commonest (Diazepam) as the paradigm. Benzodiazepines are widely prescribed for the treatment of anxiety and insomnia. Diazepam (and other benzodiazepines) may be added to illicit heroin as a bulking agent.

Diazepam

Diazepam, like many benzodiazepines, is metabolised to other active benzodiazepines. In the case of diazepam, it is metabolised to nordiazepam, temazepam and oxazepam. This metabolism may occur in-vitro in blood samples. This can be reduced by sampling using fluoride oxalate preservative vials.

T½: Diazepam 20–40 h (nordiazepam 40–100 h)
Vd: Diazepam 0.6–2.4 L/kg
Specimens: Unpreserved blood and urine for screening, unpreserved blood for quantitation.

Acute toxicity of benzodiazepines is extremely low. Even large overdoses taken alone rarely cause death, although risks are increased in the presence of respiratory/cardiovascular disease. Post-mortem blood levels of diazepam above approximately 5000 ng/mL may be considered as causing death.

Over-sedation is thought to be a dose-related extension of the sedative-hypnotic effects of benzodiazepines. Symptoms include drowsiness, poor concentration and vigilance, ataxia, dysarthria, motor incoordination, diplopia, muscle weakness, vertigo, and mental confusion. In view of their prolonged half-lives the effects may persist for more than 24 h. In addition, the elderly appear to be particularly vulnerable to the amnesic/forgetfulness effects of benzodiazepines. However, tolerance to the sedative effects of benzodiazepines has been known to develop over 1 or 2 weeks of their use.

Chlordiazepoxide

Chlordiazepoxide is a benzodiazepine used for the treatment of anxiety and insomnia, and also as an adjunct in acute alcohol withdrawal. It is metabolised to nordiazepam, oxazepam and desmethylmedazepam, which are also active benzodiazepines.

T½: 5–30 h
Vd: 0.3–0.6 L/kg
Samples: Unpreserved blood and urine for screening, preserved blood sample for quantitation.

Post mortem blood levels above approximately 5000 ng/mL were associated with ataxia, hyperreflexia tachycardia and seizures. Blood levels above 20,000 ng/mL are reported as fatal when present as the only drug detected.

"Designer Benzodiazepines"

There has been a growing number of illicit benzodiazepines (etizolam, flualprazolam, clonazolam, flubromazolam, diclazepam etc) which appear and disappear in prevalence in post mortem cases. The primary issue is that individuals are now buying their prescribed medications online as they are cheaper. As some of these are sourced from non-accredited manufacturers, and illicit drugs are also not from accredited manufacturers, these tablets can contain any number of acute and toxic compounds. As well as being more potent than the standard benzodiazepines, there is also an increased risk of fatal arrhythmia, perhaps reflecting transient first degree and second-degree block and QT prolongation.

Cannabis (Tetrahydrocannabinol [THC])

There are over 100 different cannabinoids present in the cannabis plant. They are generally abused for their mind-altering properties, although a mild analgesic effect is recognised. Tetrahydrocannabinol (THC) is the main active ingredient of cannabis. The medicinal forms of cannabis contain only

THC. Metabolic degradation of THC produces 11-delta-9-THC-carboxylic acid (THC-COOH) as the main metabolite.

T½: 20–57 h (infrequent users) 3–13 days (frequent users)
Vd: 4–14 L/kg
Specimens: Unpreserved blood and urine for screening, unpreserved blood for quantitation.

A typical peak blood cannabis concentration of 100 ng/mL may be expected after use. THC is rapidly distributed from blood to tissues and blood levels drop quickly by >90% within 2 h of administration.

Blood THC levels >2 ng/mL are suggestive of recent use. 11-Delta-9-THC-carboxylic acid, the main metabolite of THC, is inactive. This product and other cannabinoid metabolites can be detected in the blood for up to 5 days and in the urine for up to about 30 days.

If cannabis is smoked, the effects are seen within 2–3 min, peaking at 10–20 min, and lasting for 90–120 min. At higher doses, the effects may last for up to 3–4 h. If taken orally, the onset of action is 30–60 min with symptoms typically persisting for 3–8 h.

The symptoms associated with low-to-moderate doses include relaxation, well-being, euphoria, drowsiness, distortions of perception of time, body image and distance, mild confusion, decreased concentration, decreased muscle strength and balance, impaired ability to perform complex motor tasks and panic or even mild paranoia. With high doses hallucinations may occur. Cannabis at high doses can induce acute psychotic symptoms, particularly in susceptible individuals, but there is debate as to whether regular (potent variety) cannabis usage causes chronic psychosis or schizophrenia. Cannabis can cause exercise-related tachyarrhythmias, although it is very rarely implicated as a cause of death.

Cannabis has a detrimental effect on complex tasks such as driving. In England and Wales there is a whole blood concentration limit of 2 ng/mL for driving in the UK [7].

Cocaine

Cocaine is a widely abused naturally occurring stimulant with mood altering (euphoric) actions. It also has anaesthetic properties, used in local anaesthetics. Cocaine is metabolised to the inactive metabolites benzoylecgonine and methylecgonine, both of which are inactive. In persons co-consuming ethanol, cocaine is also metabolised to cocaethylene, which has similar toxicity to cocaine.

Hydrolysis of cocaine to its metabolites is thought to start immediately after exposure and continue in the post mortem period. Sampling into fluoride oxalate preserved tubes reduces the rate of hydrolysis.

T½: Cocaine 0.7–1.5 h, benzoylecgonine 3.5–8 h, and methylecgonine 3.5–6 h, respectively.
Vd: Cocaine 1.6–2.7 L/kg
Samples: blood (preferably fluoride preserved) for screening and quantitation, urine for initial screening.

Cocaine levels <50 ng/mL are generally thought not to produce measurable physiologic effects, let alone toxicity. Thus, in the absence of any confirmatory histopathologic change, cocaine levels <50 ng/mL should not be deemed to be the cause of death. However, if appropriate histopathologic changes are present, cocaine may be the cause of death even when the blood cocaine levels are zero. Due to the dose, route of administration, period of survival, and storage of the sample "fatal" ranges are wide, but the associate appears stronger when concentrations are greater than approximately 500 ng/mL [8].

Cardiovascular damage is relatively common in young cocaine users. Ischaemic events have been reported regularly (due to both intravascular thrombus formation and vasoconstriction). There is a strong relationship between cocaine use, heart contraction bands, and sudden arrhythmic death. Associations have also been made with myocarditis, cardiomyopathy, accelerated coronary atheroma and valvular heart disease in those who abuse cocaine. Chronic use can lead to significant tolerance to the stimulant effects of cocaine.

Amphetamine

Amphetamine is a stimulant that is pharmacologically related to the catecholamines, adrenaline and noradrenaline. It is used for its euphoric effect and ability to augment physical and mental work speeds. Tolerance develops to both the stimulant and euphoric effects of amphetamine. There is considerable overlap between the non-toxic and toxic blood drug levels.

T½: 12 h
Vd: 3–4 L/kg
Specimens: Unpreserved blood and urine for screening, unpreserved blood for quantitation.

Amphetamine use may lead to reactions such as agitation, fever, and aggression, which can lead to very high body temperatures (malignant hyperpyrexia), and elevated heart rate and blood pressure. This may lead to rhabdomyolysis (muscle breakdown), intravascular coagulation, convulsions, haemorrhages from blood vessels and renal failure. Cardiotoxicity associated with the use or abuse of amphetamine, or its synthetic derivatives can manifest itself as acute myocardial infarction, cardiomyopathy, or arrhythmia. It may also be associated by poor cognition and decision making, putting one at risk of traumatic deaths.

Death from amphetamine toxicity will often not occur immediately, but rather after a few hours of agitation, fever, aggression, and hyperthermia and so post-mortem blood levels may not reflect peak concentrations. Arrhythmias can occur at blood concentrations of 20 ng/mL, but tolerant individuals may have minimal effects with concentrations of 600 ng/mL. Death from amphetamine toxicity is usually considered with post mortem concentrations above 500 ng/mL [9].

MDMA (Ecstasy) and MDA

3,4-Methylenedioxymethamphetamine (MDMA) is a synthetic psychostimulant, used widely in the club scene. MDMA displays stimulant effects such as euphoria, well-being, happiness, stimulation, increased energy, extroversion, feeling close to others, increased empathy, increased sociability, enhanced mood, mild perceptual disturbances and changed perception of colours and sounds. About 10% of MDMA is metabolised to methylenedioxyamphetamine (MDA), which is also active and possesses similar properties to MDMA.

T½: 6 7 h
Vd: 6 L/kg
Specimens: Unpreserved blood and urine for screening, unpreserved blood for quantitation.

After oral administration peak blood levels of MDMA are reached within 1–3 h. A 75 mg dose of MDMA leads to peak blood MDMA level of 130 ng/mL within 2 h with MDA peaking at around 7.8 ng/mL within 5 h.

MDMA also has a range of effects that can lead to acute toxic reactions, including hyperthermia (that may result in rhabdomyolysis, dehydration, and renal failure), raised blood pressure, raised heart rate, cardiac arrhythmias, increased coagulability state, hypertension that may in turn lead strokes, and the 'serotonin syndrome' (increased muscle rigidity, hyperreflexia, seizures, and hyperthermia).

These acute effects of MDMA are not dose related. It has also been reported that chronic use of amphetamines including MDMA may result in cardiotoxicity in relatively young individuals without pre-existing cardiac disease. This cardiotoxicity may manifest itself as acute myocardial infarction (due to vascular spasm), cardiomyopathy or cardiac arrhythmia.

Pregabalin and Gabapentin

Both gabapentin and pregabalin have become common adjunct drugs in those who are abusing heroin and benzodiazepines.

T½: Pregabalin 5–11 h, Gabapentin 5–9 h
Vd: Pregabalin 0.5 L/kg, Gabapentin 0.8–1.3 L/kg
Specimens: Unpreserved blood for screening and quantitation, unpreserved urine may be used to detect metabolite.

Both are considered relatively safe drugs although they have additional sedative effects to those of the opioids and may increase the risk of arrhythmia. Death from either as a single drug are very unusual, with toxic concentration being considered above approximately 50 mg/L.

Carbon Monoxide

Carbon monoxide (CO) is often produced by poor combustion of carbon-based fuels (e.g. wood, coal). When produced and inspired, the CO may adhere tightly to the normal blood oxygen binding site, as it readily complexes with haemoglobin (Hb), in the form of carboxyhaemoglobin (COHb). This has a characteristic pink colour, which if it persists may deprive the body of oxygen, causing end-organ hypoxic damage.

Deaths usually occur from either domestic fires or due to ongoing inhalation of low levels of poorly combusted fuels.

T½: 4 h on air, 60 min when administered 100% oxygen
Vd: Not relevant
Specimens: Unpreserved blood and urine for screening, unpreserved blood for quantitation.

The COHb "normal" range (i.e., general population) is <10% total haemoglobin. Toxicity occurs variably between 15–50% and death is expected in a healthy individual at >50%. Death may occur at lower percentage haemoglobin in those with pre-existing heart and/or lung disease.

Although symptoms due to carbon monoxide exposure vary from person to person, prolonged or high exposure may result in nausea, dizziness, headaches, vomiting, confusion, collapse, loss of consciousness, angina, and muscle weakness. Severe exposure can result in brain and heart damage or death. Medical problems, such as heart and lung conditions, vascular disease, anaemic conditions, and cigarette smoking may increase susceptibility to carbon monoxide poisoning.

Cyanide

Cyanide (CN^-) is a pure toxin not normally encountered in life. Smoke inhalation during the burning of common substances such as rubber, plastic, and silk can create cyanide fumes. The main uses of cyanide are in the photographic, chemical research, synthetic plastic, metal processing and electroplating industries. During cyanide toxicity mitochondrial energy production is inhibited. The brain and heart are most vulnerable to the toxic effects of cyanide. Rarely, it is used in suicide and homicide cases.

The lethal range for cyanide is 1 mg/L. The reported symptoms of cyanide toxicity include nausea, headache, dizziness, disorientation, seizure, tachycardia, arrhythmia, and in severe cases cardiopulmonary arrest.

Note: Suspected cases of autopsy poisoning should be approached with caution to avoid the autopsy team breathing in cyanide fumes from the body; particularly from stomach generated prussic acid gas (HCN).

Paracetamol

Paracetamol is a mild analgesic being also available in many proprietary preparations, which may contain mild opiate analgesics such as codeine, e.g., co-codamol. The paracetamol is not toxic (apart from when levels are above 500 mg/L, in which case a de-novo metabolic acidosis may occur). Rather, the paracetamol metabolite causes fatalities, generally as a result of liver necrosis/failure.

T½: 1–4 h
Vd: 0.8–1 L/kg
Specimens: Unpreserved blood and urine for screening, unpreserved blood for quantitation.

The interpretation of blood paracetamol levels should take into account the time period between ingestion and blood sampling. The peak blood paracetamol level is reached 1–3 h (mean 1.4 h) after a single dose. The half-life of paracetamol in adults after a therapeutic dose is thought to be 1–3 h, but when liver damage is present the half-life may be >4 h. Liver necrosis (damage) is maximal 3–4 days after ingestion of paracetamol overdose.

Non-specific symptoms similarly may include anorexia, nausea, vomiting, malaise, and features of hypoglycaemia, coagulopathy, and encephalopathy. There may also be right upper quadrant pain or tenderness, hepatomegaly, and oliguria. Usually within the next 3–5 days the symptoms worsen, and central nervous system depression, shock, hypothermia, and metabolic acidosis may develop. It has been reported that repeated administration of as little as 20 mg/kg/day of paracetamol over a protracted period of time may be associated with liver failure.

New Psychoactive Substances

There are increasing numbers of new drugs causing harm and deaths, currently driving public and media concern. These drugs, known as new psychoactive substances (NPS), and often misleadingly referred to as 'legal highs,' pose a challenge to government, local authorities, healthcare services and the criminal justice system.

They will often contain stimulant compounds similar to cocaine or cannabinoid-like compounds, but with significantly greater potency than cannabis and often with stimulant characteristics.

As with the newer potent opioid drugs, many of these new psychoactive substance compounds will not be detected by the first line screens performed even in the leading toxicology laboratories, and will require specific analysis, often prompted by the history.

Sampling

At present there is no standardised sampling so collection of both blood and urine is recommended, wherever possible.

T½: unknown
Vd: unknown
Specimens: Unpreserved blood and urine for screening, unpreserved blood for quantitation.

Nitrogen (N_2)/Helium (He)/Nitrous Oxide (N_2O)

The measurement of volatiles in post mortem blood is only offered by a few laboratories internationally, so their contribution to death is based on non-analytical evidence in most cases.

Asphyxiant gases act mainly by displacing oxygen from the atmosphere. This reduces the oxygen concentration in inspired air leading to hypoxaemia and brain death. Their presence stops the panic/distress of hypoxaemia.

Nitrous oxide is a relatively common drug of abuse in the UK. Fatalities have been reported after acute exposure, both as recreational abuse and self-harm. Deaths were most likely due to asphyxiation.

Helium is reported to cause respiratory depression, hypotension, cardiac dysrhythmias, pulmonary oedema and convulsions.

Insulin

Insulin is used therapeutically to control blood glucose in diabetes mellitus. There are both short acting (effective within approximately 1 h and lasting 3–4 h) and long acting (peaking within 2–3 h but providing a basal insulin over 24 h) insulins. The immunoassays used for measurement do not distinguish the natural or exogenous insulins. This requires mass spectrometry, which is only available in 1–2 places worldwide.

The primary toxic effect is hypoglycaemia with associated neuroglycopaenia, and changes in neural function. In life it is easy to measure blood glucose. In the post mortem period, the glucose will degrade to such an extent that even if normoglycaemic at death there may be none detected on post mortem testing. Glucose is best measured in vitreous at the post mortem.

Insulin will also cause a reduction in metabolism of fatty acids, so a further screening test is the measurement of beta hydroxybutyrate, which should be low.

Endogenous insulin is produced from proinsulin, with concurrent production of C peptide.

In an individual with a normally functioning pancreas, if there has been excess exogenous insulin use, in a post mortem case there would be a low glucose (with the caveat of the glucose degradation), a low beta hydroxybutyrate, a raised insulin, and low C peptide. In those with insulin dependent diabetes, they will have no endogenous C peptide, and so it is often impossible to be sure if there has been excess insulin use.

Other Drugs and Toxins

Many other drugs and toxins exist and for those not covered here, the reader is referred to specialist texts. Indeed, this chapter has by necessity been brief. Any specific questions should be directed to your toxicology supplier or use of the UK National Poisons Information Service is recommended.

References

1. Kugelberg FC, Jones AW. Interpreting results of ethanol analysis in post-mortem samples. A review of the literature. Forensic Sci Int. 2007;165:10–29.
2. Gerostamoulos J, Burke MP, Drummer OH. Involvement of codeine in drug-related deaths. Am J Forensic Med Pathol. 1996;17:327–35.
3. Skopp G, Klinder K, Pötsch L, et al. Postmortem distribution of dihydrocodeine and metabolites in a fatal case of dihydrocodeine intoxication. Forensic Sci Int. 1998;95(2):99–107.
4. Milroy CM, Forrest ARW. Methadone deaths: a toxicological analysis. J Clin Pathol. 2000;53:277–81.
5. Andresen H, Gullans A, Veselinovic M, et al. Fentanyl: toxic or therapeutic? Postmortem and antemortem blood concentrations after transdermal fentanyl application. J Anal Toxicol. 2012;36:182–94.
6. De Decker K, Cordonnier J, Jacobs W, Coucke V, Schepens P, Jorens PG. Postmortem distribution of dihydrocodeine and metabolites in a fatal case of dihydrocodeine intoxication. Forensic Sci Int. 1998;95:99–107.
7. Wolff K, Johnston A. Cannabis use: a perspective in relation to the proposed UK drug-driving legislation. Drug Test Anal. 2014;6(1–2):143–54.
8. Jenkins AJ, Levine B, Titus J, Smialek JE. The interpretation of cocaine and benzoylecgonine concentrations in postmortem cases. Forensic Sci Int. 1999;101:17–25.
9. De Letter EA, Piette MHA, Lambert WE, Cordonnier JACM. Amphetamines as potential inducers of fatalities: a review in the district of Ghent from 1976–2004. Med Sci Law. 2006;46:37–65.

Suggested Reading

Baselt RC. Disposition of toxic drugs and chemicals in man. 11th ed. Seal Beach: Biomedical Publications; 2017.

Moffat AC, Osselton MD, Widdop B, Watts J. Clarke's analysis of drugs and poisons. 4th ed. London: Pharmaceutical Press; 2011.

Appendix

Three items merit inclusion at the end of this book.

The first item is a single page document (used in the United Kingdom) to indicate the initial data after an autopsy has been performed. This details the name of the deceased along with basic information such as the date of death and that of the examination. There are choices regarding whether the case is concluded without histology or other tests, or that the case requires more work. The cause of death is given on this form, although on occasion "*awaiting further tests*" or "*pending*" is a reasonable response if the case has no clear/immediate solution. Clearly one should always indicate what samples have been taken. This can be generic or precise in terms of the volume/weight/number of samples. Of particular use is the box for comments. This allows initial thoughts to be given by the pathologist before the sign off at the base of the form.

This form is not meant to be proscriptive, or all encompassing. It is a guide for the reasonable end point of the case analysis.

The second item is a two-sided document. It is recommended that it is copied onto an A3 sheet, which is then folded in half. The first page is the generic data and external examination sheet, with the second page detailing the internal examination data, weights of the organs, and a summary of what samples were taken (if any). It is recommended to have both pages on the outer side of the folded A3 sheet (rather like the external cover of a book). This leaves two blank sides internally for additional notes, documents, correspondence and so on. In effect, it is its own file binder. The boxes for data entry are largely self-explanatory, but this simple document serves to provide a quick written summary sheet for those working in the mortuary.

Finally, Professor Suvarna developed a short form written guide for evisceration and organ dissection. It is informal and curt by necessity so that it can be printed, laminated and displayed in the mortuary as a memory aid for those training to refer to at the dissection bench. The order is prescriptive to teach a way of dissection which allows consideration of pathologies in each organ, in turn, without destroying findings of importance, in most cases. However, with experience, those training will likely adapt the order of dissection to suit the case data and personal preference. This document has purposefully been left in its informal format.

S. K. Suvarna (represented by Grace Horne), A. K. Sharp (eds.), *Atlas of Adult Autopsy*,
https://doi.org/10.1007/978-3-031-72207-3

Notification to coroner upon completion of post-mortem examination

Regs 14 &15 Coroners (Investigations) Regulations 2013

FORM 1

Name of deceased:		**Date of death:**	
☐	I have completed my examination of the body and consider the cause of death to be as shown below. I have not retained any material and do not consider that further examination of the body is required. **OR**		
☐	I have completed my examination of the body, which may be released, but in the circumstances of this particular case I believe it necessary to retain the material set out below in order to verify my macroscopic findings. At this stage I consider the cause of death to be as shown below. I believe that the retained material should be held for a period of _________ months *(Please justify retention for longer than six months in the comments section).* **OR**		
☐	I have completed my examination of the body and have retained the materials set out below under Regs 14 &15 Coroners (Investigations) Regulations 2013 and as exhibits under the Police and Criminal Evidence Act 1984.		
Cause of death:	**1a.** **1b.** **1c.** **2**		

The following investigations are to be made: Histology ☐ Toxicology ☐ Neuropathology ☐
Cardiac Pathology ☐ Bacteriology ☐ Virology ☐

Retained Materials

Whole Organs ☐ Brain ☐ Heart ☐ Kidney ☐ Other ___________

Histology tissues ☐ Brain ☐ Heart ☐ Lung ☐ Liver ☐ Kidney ☐ Pancreas
☐ Spleen ☐ Adrenal ☐ Thyroid No of blocks_____________

Toxicology ☐ Blood ☐ Urine ☐ Vitreous ☐ Stomach contents ☐ Muscle

Comments:

Pathologist:	**Signature:**	**Date:**

Autopsy number / consent / legal

Surname .... Admission date ....

Forename .... Date of death ....

DOB .... M F Time death ....

Hospital / mortuary number .... Date autopsy ....

Cons Ward ? observers

Clinical History

External

Identified OK ☐

height .... m. mass .... kg

- violence/trauma/neglect
- scars
- venepuncture
- rings or jewellery

- jaundice
- clubbing
- oedema
- lymphadenopathy
- tattoos

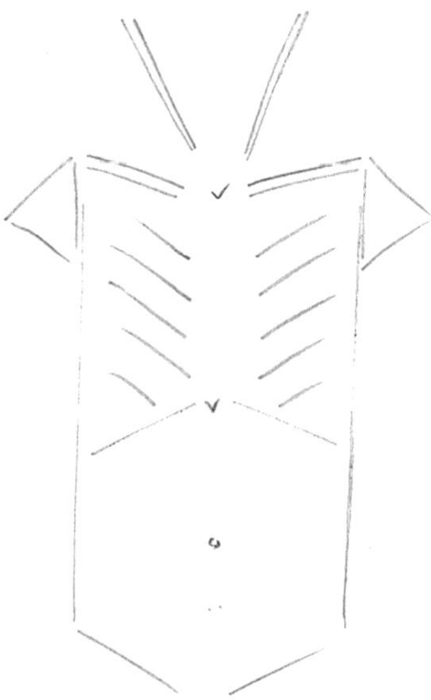

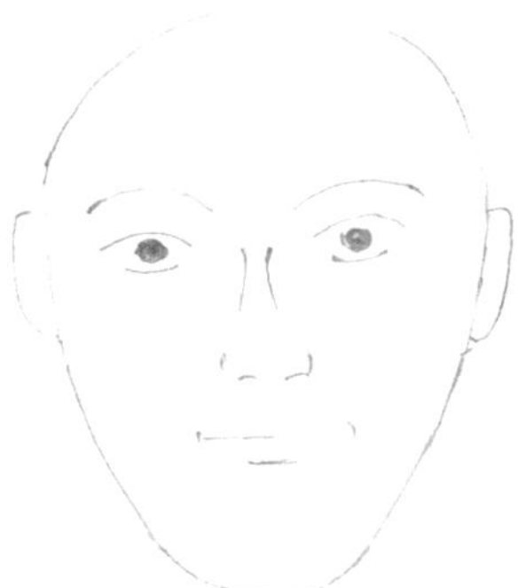

1a
1b
1c
1d
2

CVS
pericardium
heart ext
myocardium
chambers tvs diam R/L
valves / / /

LAD RCA CxA etc
aorta large artery
venae cavae RV LV/S

RS
larynx ETT ☐
trachea

bronchi pleural cavity R / L

lungs parenchyma

arteries emboli ☐

GIT mouth teeth tongue
oesophagus
stomach
small intestine
appendix
colon
mesenteries peritoneum

liver ext section
gallbladder bile ducts
pancreas

B
H
RL
LL
Liv
RK
LK
S

GU kidney surfaces
parenchyma

pelves ureters bladder

prostate testes/ext genitalia

ut/cx FT ov
breasts

Endocrine
thyroid ○
parathyroids ○
adrenals ○
pituitary ○

RES thymus
spleen ext cut section
LN thorax abdo
bone marrow

CNS skull venous sinuses
dura leptomeninges
cranial n arteries
brain
cerebrum
cerebellum
midbrain pons medulla

Tissue retained Y / N **Histology blocks n=** **Retained organs Y / N = which one/s**

Toxicology Y / N **Microbiology Y / N** **Additional data**

Dissection at post mortem examination – Prof S. Kim Suvarna's protocol

1. U or Y-shaped incision to open abdomen down to pubic symphysis – take blood and urine samples if required
2. Dissect neck flap back to mandible
3. Reflect soft tissue from chest wall
4. Check for pneumothoraces
5. Use rib shears to remove rib shield, cut soft tissue attachments close to ribs
6. Remove bowel, from jejunum to rectum – consider tying off if need to test stomach contents
7. Cut around mandible to free neck structures, try to keep above carotid bifurcation
8. Cut down both diaphragms, close to cavity wall
9. Pull thoracic contents over to each side and cut along vertebrae to free thoracic organs
10. Once thoracic block is free, put back in chest
11. Use blunt dissection down tissue plane behind pubic symphysis to free up pelvic organs and transect at pelvic floor
12. Pull thoracic contents down and continue cut bilaterally to free abdominal organs – follow line of psoas muscles
13. Pull up pelvic contents and cut remaining soft tissue attachments to pelvis
14. Remove organ block (Rokitansky)
15. Check cavities for collections, bruising, rib fractures, plaques etc
16. Approach the organ block posteriorly
17. Remove diaphragms
18. Find and remove adrenals, slice
19. Remove spleen, weigh and cut once, along long axis
20. Cut across proximal descending aorta and open along length, into both iliac arteries
21. Open and examine IVC and renal veins
22. Follow renal arteries to kidneys
23. Cut kidneys/ perinephric fat along long axis, peel back capsule
24. Follow ureters from renal pelvis to bladder
25. Open bladder +/- prostate
26. Consider extraction of testes at this point
27. Cut one slice into uterus/cervix/ovaries
28. Remove kidneys and weigh
29. Remove aorta
30. Open oesophagus and follow to GOJ
31. Dissect oesophagus from trachea, but leave attached to stomach
32. Find thyroid, remove in one piece – look out for parathyroids and save if found
33. Separate off thoracic and abdominal organs
34. Open gallbladder posteriorly and cut up to spiral valve
35. Open CBD and trace to duodenum
36. Remove ligaments / soft tissue from liver, remove and weigh
37. Serially slice liver at 1 cm intervals – ?save one slice to display
38. Continue cut in oesophagus along greater curve of stomach, continue and open duodenum
39. Lift up stomach to find pancreas, serially slice at 1 cm intervals
40. Approach thoracic block anteriorly
41. Inverted T cut to open pericardium, then remove pericardium

42. Find pulmonary valve externally and protect with fingers, cut horizontally into anterior of pulmonary trunk
43. Feel into pulmonary arteries for clots
44. Put fingers behind aorta and pulmonary artery and cut across with scissors
45. Cut above SAN at SVC and RA interface
46. Cut across rest of vessels to free heart - *NB. weigh heart after full dissection, not at this point*
47. Remove lungs from mediastinum, weigh
48. Cut into lungs between lobes to reveal vessels
49. Follow along vessels peripherally with scissors, in all lobes
50. Turn lungs over and follow bronchi and small airways peripherally, in all lobes
51. Follow neck vessels up from aortic arch, check for atherosclerosis, narrowing
52. Find coronary arteries in heart
53. Start looking for LAD mid way down septum and follow both ways, cut at 5mm intervals
54. Find and follow circumflex and RCA – ? atherosclerosis ? stenosis ? thrombosis ? normal architecture
55. Take 3 horizontal slices through left and right ventricles, from apex of heart
56. Cut into heart following flow of blood
57. Cut across posterior RA between venae cavae – look into auricle and at tricuspid valve from above
58. Cut down posterior aspect right atrium, though tricuspid valve, into right ventricle
59. Turn over, cut up anterior aspect right ventricle, though pulmonary outflow tract
60. Inspect pulmonary valve, note thickness of RVOT
61. Cut across pulmonary veins to open left atrium, look at auricle and mitral valve from above
62. Cut down back of left atrium, though mitral valve, into left ventricle
63. Turn over, cut up anterior aspect of left ventricle, keeping close to septum, through aortic valve, curve around left side, between left main stem and left auricle to open aorta
64. Inspect aortic valve
65. Look for coronary ostia – is it a 1-1-0 pattern? Weigh
66. Inspect brain surface, weigh, are vessels of CoW intact?
67. Cut off cerebellum and brainstem
68. Cut off lateral attachments of brain stem to look into 4th ventricle
69. Serially slice brain stem from behind
70. Cut cerebellum into two hemispheres and again at 45 degree angle
71. Serially slice cerebrum at approximately 1-1.5 cm intervals

Display examples of each organ for presentation... smile when applause starts !!

Index

S. K. Suvarna (represented by Grace Horne), A. K. Sharp (eds.), *Atlas of Adult Autopsy*,
https://doi.org/10.1007/978-3-031-72207-3

R

S

MIX
Papier aus verantwortungsvollen Quellen
Paper from responsible sources
FSC® C105338

If you have any concerns about our products,
you can contact us on
ProductSafety@springernature.com

In case Publisher is established outside the EU,
the EU authorized representative is:
Springer Nature Customer Service Center GmbH
Europaplatz 3, 69115 Heidelberg, Germany

Printed by Libri Plureos GmbH
in Hamburg, Germany